PHARMACOLOGY
and the NURSING PROCESS

PHARMACOLOGY
and the
NURSING PROCESS

LINDA LANE LILLEY, RN, MS
Associate Professor
School of Nursing
Old Dominion University
Norfolk, Virginia

ROBERT S. AUCKER, PHARMD
Clinical Pharmacist
St. Joseph's Hospital of Atlanta;
Adjunct Professor
Mercer Southern School of Pharmacy;
Adjunct Assistant Professor
Kennesaw State College
School of Nursing
Atlanta, Georgia

JOSEPH A. ALBANESE, RPH, PHD
Professor Emeritus
College of Staten Island
City University of New York
Staten Island, New York

with
contributions
by Richard E. Lake, BS, MS, MLA
DIRECTOR, CENTER FOR STUDENT SUCCESS;
PROFESSOR, READING DEPARTMENT
ST. LOUIS COMMUNITY COLLEGE AT
FLORISSANT VALLEY
ST. LOUIS, MISSOURI

Carol Ruscin, MSN, RN
CLINICAL NURSE SPECIALIST
HEALTH SOURCE ARKANSAS
LITTLE ROCK, ARKANSAS

with 188 illustrations

 Mosby

St. Louis Baltimore Boston Carlsbad Chicago Naples New York Philadelphia Portland
London Madrid Mexico City Singapore Sydney Tokyo Toronto Wiesbaden

Mosby
Dedicated to Publishing Excellence

A Times Mirror
Company

Publisher: Nancy Coon
Editor: Robin Carter
Developmental Editor: Gina Wright
Project Manager: Dana Peick
Senior Production Editor: Catherine Albright
Manufacturing Manager: Betty Richmond
Designer: Amy Buxton
Editorial Assistant: Kristin Geen

A NOTE TO THE READER:
The author and publisher have made every attempt to check dosages and nursing content for accuracy. Because the science of pharmacology is continually advancing, our knowledge base continues to expand. Therefore we recommend that the reader always check product information for changes in dosage or administration before administering any medication. This is particularly important with new or rarely used drugs.

Printed in the United States of America
Composition by University Graphics, Inc.
Printing and binding by Von Hoffmann Press, Inc.

Mosby–Year Book, Inc.
11830 Westline Industrial Drive
St. Louis, Missouri 63146

Library of Congress Cataloging in Publication Data

Lilley, Linda Lane.
    Pharmacology and the nursing process / Linda Lane Lilley, Robert
S. Aucker, Joseph A. Albanese ; with contributions by Richard E.
Lake, Carol Ruscin.
        p.   cm.
    Includes bibliographical references and index.
    ISBN 0-8016-7893-5
    1. Pharmacology. 2. Nursing. I. Aucker, Robert S.
II. Albanese, Joseph A. III. Title.
    [DNLM: 1. Pharmacology—nurses' instruction. 2. Drug Therapy—
nurses' instruction. 3. Drugs—administration & dosage. QV 4
L729p 1996]
RM301.L466   1996
615'.1—dc20
DNLM/DLC
for Library of Congress   95-46811
                               CIP

96 97 98 99 / 9 8 7 6 5 4 3 2

Preface

INTRODUCTION

Pharmacology and the Nursing Process provides the most up-to-date, clinically relevant information on pharmacology and nursing in an appealing, understandable, and practical format. This text's accessible size, readable writing style, and full-color design are ideal for today's busy nursing student. A unique approach to the study of pharmacology is taken by presenting study skills content that will help students understand and learn the particularly demanding subject of pharmacology. The text begins with Chapter 1: Study Skills. In addition, each part begins with a Study Skills Brief, which features a discussion of researched and proven study skills and applies that discussion to content in the part. Students are therefore encouraged to use research-based study skills to enhance their study of the subject of pharmacology.

MARKET RESEARCH

This text has incorporated many suggestions by focus group participants in the early 1990s. These focus groups, composed of nursing instructors from two-, three-, and four-year degree programs in Chicago, Philadelphia, and Los Angeles, assessed changes that have occurred in the teaching of pharmacology and determined what was needed to better teach pharmacology to nursing students. Based on faculty descriptions of their courses and students, these general recommendations were made:

- Accommodate the reading styles and abilities of the growing number of non-traditional nursing students.
- Increase the use of tables, illustrations, graphs, and other visually-oriented approaches.
- Utilize color to increase interest and highlight important drug interactions and processes.

We have taken a truly collaborative approach with this new text. The concerns raised by faculty in market research have been addressed, as have several additional improvements suggested by faculty who served as reviewers or consultants, either formally or informally, throughout the manuscript's development, and by the authors and editors of this text.

ORGANIZATION

The book includes 55 chapters presented in 11 parts organized by body system. The seven concepts chapters in Part 1 lay a solid foundation for the subsequent drug units and address the following topics:

- Study skills applied to learning pharmacology
- The nurse's role in pharmacotherapeutics
- Pharmacologic principles
- Neonatal, pediatric, and geriatric considerations related to pharmacology
- Legal, ethical, and cultural considerations
- Math calculations
- Photo atlas of medication administration techniques

Parts 2 through 11 present pharmacology and nursing management in a traditional *body systems/drug function framework*. This accepted approach facilitates learning by grouping functionally related drugs and drug groups. It provides an effective means to integrate the content into medical-surgical or adult health nursing courses or for teaching pharmacology in a separate course.

The 48 drug chapters in these parts constitute the main part of the book. Drugs are presented in a *consistent format*, with an emphasis on drug groups and key similarities and differences among the drugs in each group. Each chapter is subdivided into two discussions, beginning with a complete, clear discussion of pharmacology, followed by a comprehensive yet succinct discussion of the nursing process. *Pharmacology* is presented for each drug group in a consistent format:

- Mechanism of action
- Drug effects
- Therapeutic uses
- Side effects
- Contraindications (when appropriate)
- Toxicity/management of overdose (when appropriate)
- Interactions
- Dosages

Drug group discussions are followed by *Drug Profiles*, or brief narrative capsules of individual drugs in the class or group with pharmacokinetics tables for each drug. *Key drugs,* or prototypical drugs within a class, are identified with a ⚓ symbol for easy identification. These individual drug profiles are followed by *Nursing Process* discussions, which relate to the entire drug group and are also covered in a functional, six-step nursing process format of:

■ Assessment
■ Nursing diagnosis
■ Planning
■ Outcome criteria
■ Implementation
■ Evaluation

Each nursing process section provides a *Patient Teaching Tips* box that summarizes key points to cover in educating the patient about uses and effects of drugs within a given group. Because the role of the nurse as patient educator will continue to grow in importance, we have given an emphasis to this key content.

Each part begins with a *Study Skills Brief* that presents a study skills topic, such as time management, note taking, studying, and test taking, and relates it to the unit being discussed. This unique approach to teaching pharmacology is intended to aid those students who find pharmacology difficult and to provide a tool that may prove beneficial in their entire nursing school careers. Coverage of this study skills content is limited to Chapter 1 and the beginning of each part so that instructors who choose not to require their students to read this material can readily eliminate it. However, this arrangement of content may be very beneficial to those faculty teaching pharmacology through an integrated approach, as it helps the student identify key context and concepts. This arrangement also facilitates locating the content for either required or optional reading.

FEATURES

This book features numerous *pedagogic features* that prepare the student for important content to be covered in each chapter and encourage review and reinforcement of that content. Pedagogy that begins each chapter includes:

■ Learning objectives
■ Chapter outline
■ Glossaries of key terms with pronunciations, definitions, and page-number references

Each chapter concludes with *Take Home Points* that summarize key points subdivided by key topic, drug group, or nursing management, and *Critical Thinking Activities* that provide a variety of exercises to address different learning needs or styles. These exercises include critical thinking questions, multiple-choice questions, NCLEX-review questions, detailed case studies, and minicases.

Special topics have been highlighted for emphasis. *Special-emphasis boxes* include:

■ Cultural implications
■ Legal and ethical implications
■ Research issues
■ Home health, issues
■ Lifespan considerations, with separate boxes on neonatal, pediatric, and geriatric issues

COLOR

This is the first full-color pharmacology text for nursing students. Faculty suggested that color be used in both a functionally and visually appealing manner to more fully engage students in this typically demanding yet important content. We have used *full color throughout* to:

■ Highlight important content
■ Illustrate how drugs work in the body in over 95 newly developed anatomic and drug process color figures
■ Improve the visual appearance of the content to make it more engaging and appealing to today's more visually sophisticated reader

We believe the use of color in this approach will significantly improve students' involvement and understanding of pharmacology.

ANCILLARY PACKAGE

A carefully prepared ancillary package is available to instructors who adopt *Pharmacology and the Nursing Process*. These materials can significantly assist teaching and learning. The package and its features are:

INSTRUCTOR'S RESOURCE MANUAL AND TEST BANK INSTRUCTOR'S MANUAL SECTION

■ Chapter Overview
■ Key Terms
■ Chapter Outline
■ Teaching Strategies
■ Worksheet Answers
■ Answers to the Text's Critical Thinking Activities
■ How to Teach Pharmacology in an Integrated Curriculum
■ Disorders Index
   A duplication of the disorders index in the text, for your convenience

TEST BANK SECTION

- Over 300 NCLEX-type questions, coded for cognitive level

PHARMACOLOGY STUDY MANUAL

- Study skills chapter
  Reinforces study skills discussed in the text
  Allows practice in analyzing tests and applying test-taking strategies
- Worksheets from the *Instructor's Resource Manual*
- Perforated and three-hole punched for convenience

TRANSPARENCY ACETATE PACKAGE

- Contains 36 completely updated color illustrations
- Includes approximately 10 medication administration illustrations in full color

PHARMACOLOGY NEWSLETTER: *MOSBY'S PHARMACOLOGY UPDATE*

- A biannual publication of new drugs, drug news, feature articles, *and more!*

PHARMACOLOGY LECTURE VIDEO

- Discusses the *Five Rights of Drug Administration*
- Available to qualified adopters

We hope that we have provided the best teaching tools to help instructors' use their time most effectively both inside and outside the classroom. Our goal is to provide the resources needed to encourage student participation in the learning process and reinforce key content related to nursing pharmacology.

Acknowledgments

As mentioned earlier, this book has been truly a collaborative effort. We wish to thank the following instructors who provided input on an on-going basis throughout the development of this project: Donna Babao, RN, MSN; Pam Blake, RN, BSN, MSN; Sherry Currie, MSN; Janet Hicks Keen, RN, MS(N), CEN, CCRN; Lori A. Martell, PhD; Kathryn Moore, MEd; Mike Otto, PharmD, BCPS; Carolyn Smith Powell, ADN, BSN, MSN; Carol Ruscin, RN, BS, MSN; Sandra Mason Spengler, RN, BSN, MSN; Janice Traylor, MEd, MS, RN; Thomas Worms, MSN; and Bonnie Young, RN, MSN.

In addition, we would like to thank the following people: Ted Huff, Don O'Connor, Kristin Geen, Linda Wendling, Ken Turnbough, Greg McVicar, Anthony Saranita, and Susan Orf.

We also wish to thank Robin Carter and Gina Wright, our editors, who have worked with us side-by-side and whose help was invaluable in bringing this book about. Their support, encouragement, commitment to the project, empathy, and high level of professionalism have kept us motivated and excited about the end result. We are grateful to Dana Peick and Catherine Albright for very capably guiding the project through to publication and to Amy Buxton for her effective design. Richard Lake lent his study skills expertise and has created for us a unique and appropriate feature for students, and for his collaboration we are most grateful. And finally we thank Carol Ruscin for her willing and able assistance with galleys and page proofs.

Linda would like to thank her husband Les, for his constant support and words of encouragement, and her daughter Karen, for her understanding the time commitment and for her energy, smiles, and love, which has made this project easier to complete.

Bob would like to thank God, through whom all things are made possible. An endeavor of this magnitude requires divine intervention. The successful completion of this project required the support and guidance of many. To acknowledge the support of loved ones is not really adequately possible. They have had the patience and understanding of saints to put up with the demands placed on our personal lives by this project. Bob would also like to thank his wife Carol, whose love, support, and encouragement have no end.

Joe would like to thank the thousands of students he has had the privilege to teach. Your countless penetrating questions kept me current and truthful, and were my greatest teacher.

Finally, to those who teach, although your work may seem to go unnoticed or unappreciated, your impact will always be remembered in the accomplishments of your students. Your inspiration and motivation shapes the future.

We welcome comments from instructors and students who use this book so that we may continue to make improvements and be responsive to your needs in future editions. Please send any comments you may have in care of the publisher.

Linda Lane Lilley, RN, MS
Robert S. Aucker, PharmD
Joseph A. Albanese, RPh, PhD

Table of Contents

PART 1

Pharmacology Basics:
Study Skills Brief

1 Study Skills, 2

2 The Nursing Process and Medication Administration, 7

3 Pharmacologic Principles, 12

4 Neonatal, Pediatric, and Geriatric Considerations, 25

5 Legal, Ethical, and Cultural Considerations, 34

6 Mathematic Calculations, 44

7 Photo Atlas of Drug Administration, 49

PART 2

Central Nervous System:
Study Skills Brief

8 Narcotic Analgesic Agents, 88

9 General and Local Anesthetic Agents, 106

10 Hypnotic and Sedative Agents, 120

11 Antiepileptic Agents, 135

12 Antiparkinsonian Agents, 148

13 Psychotherapeutic Agents, 162

14 Central Nervous System Stimulant Agents, 194

PART 3

Autonomic Nervous System:
Study Skills Brief

15 Adrenergic Agents, 206

16 Adrenergic-Blocking Agents, 224

17 Cholinergic Agents, 238

18 Cholinergic-Blocking Agents, 246

19 Ganglionic-Blocking Agents, 255

PART 4

Cardiovascular System:
Study Skills Brief

20 Cardiac Glycosides, 264

21 Antidysrhythmic Agents, 276

22 Antianginal Agents, 300

23 Antihypertensive Agents, 319

24   *Coagulation Modifier Agents, 341*

25   *Antilipemic Agents, 367*

PART 5

Renal and Genitourinary System: *Study Skills Brief*

26   *Diuretic Agents, 384*

27   *Fluids and Electrolytes, 403*

28   *Female Reproductive Agents, 421*

29   *Male Reproductive Agents, 445*

PART 6

Endocrine System: *Study Skills Brief*

30   *Pituitary Agents, 454*

31   *Thyroid and Antithyroid Agents, 465*

32   *Antidiabetic and Hypoglycemic Agents, 475*

33   *Adrenal Agents, 489*

PART 7

Respiratory System: *Study Skills Brief*

34   *Antihistamines, Decongestants, Antitussives, and Expectorants, 502*

35   *Bronchodilators and Other Respiratory Agents, 519*

PART 8

Antiinfective and Antiinflammatory Agents: *Study Skills Brief*

36   *Antibiotics, 542*

37   *Antiviral Agents, 575*

38   *Antitubercular Agents, 587*

39   *Antifungal Agents, 597*

40   *Antimalarial, Antiprotozoal, and Antihelmintic Agents, 607*

41   *Antiseptic and Disinfectant Agents, 626*

42   *The NSAIDs (Nonsteroidal Antiinflammatory Drugs), 637*

PART 9

The Immune System and Biologic and Chemotherapeutic Modifiers: *Study Skills Brief*

43   *Immunosuppressant Agents, 656*

44   *Immunizing Agents, 663*

45   *Antineoplastic Agents, 676*

46   *Biologic Response Modifiers, 710*

PART 10

The Gastrointestinal System and Nutritional Agents: *Study Skills Brief*

47   *Antacids and Antiflatulents, 728*

48   *Antidiarrheals and Laxatives, 745*

Contents

49 *Antiemetic (Antinausea) Agents,* **764**

50 *Vitamins and Minerals,* **775**

51 *Nutritional Supplements,* **803**

PART *11*

**Miscellaneous Therapeutics:
Hematologic, Dermatologic,
Ophthalmic, and Otic Systems:**
Study Skills Brief

52 *Blood-Forming Agents,* **818**

53 *Dermatologic Agents,* **828**

54 *Ophthalmic Agents,* **842**

55 *Otic Agents,* **878**

Appendix

Canadian Trade Names, **885**

PART 1

PHARMACOLOGY BASICS: STUDY SKILLS BRIEF

This section will offer some specific examples for selected chapters in Part 1 to help you apply the study techniques and strategies from Chapter 1.

PURR, CHAPTER 1

Before beginning to apply the PURR text study model a quick overview of the steps might be useful. (For a more detailed explanation see Chapter 1.) The plan consists of four steps that will help to make you an active reader and an effective learner.

- **P** stands for Plan. This step is a prereading operation. Look at chapter objectives, chapter outline, and glossary, and read only the highlighted segments of the chapter body. As you do this you should be turning these elements into a series of questions. These questions will be essential in the next step.
- **U** stands for Understand. This is the second step, and the one in which concentrated learning and study take place. Read the chapter carefully and thoughtfully. Use the information gathered in the Plan step to activate your brain. The questions you generated in Plan are those that you are attempting to answer as you read.
- **R** The first R is for Rehearse. Practice what you have learned in the first two steps. Ask questions aloud. Attempt to answer those questions aloud. The idea is to practice what

you have learned soon after the reading. This reinforces learning and helps to identify what you will need to return to for mastery.

- **R** The second R (and final step) is Review. Within 24 to 48 hours after going through the P, U, and R steps, you must review material. Mastery, whether it is in a skill such as ice skating or an intellectual process such as learning nursing pharmacology, takes review and more review. In the PURR model, Review is the final step and should be repeated as often as needed. Review is done in the same way as rehearsal with the addition of some rereading. Ask questions, attempt to answer the questions, and when an answer is not forthcoming or is vague and unclear, then reread the needed portions of the text.

Plan

As you begin to work with individual chapters, consider how the first step in the PURR system can be used to help you set a purpose and become an active learner.

Chapter 2, Objectives

Consider Objective 1. *List the four phases of the nursing process.*

Now turn the objective into a question.

Objective 1 as a question: *What are the four phases of the nursing process?*

Now move to Objective 2 and make it a question. *What is/are the function and/or purposes of the nursing process?* Note that this question relates directly to Objective 1. By putting Objective 2 into a question format you will begin to expand and extend on the focus of the first objective and you will begin to focus on active learning with a clear purpose.

Move to the Chapter 2 outline. You should notice that the outline contains the answer to your first question. The four topic headings (Assessment, Nursing Diagnoses, Planning, and Implementation) are the four phases of the nursing process. In almost no time you have begun to learn from the chapter and to achieve the objectives set out for you. This is the value of using PURR as a technique for study. The questions focus your attention on the concepts, facts, and terms which are stressed by the author.

When you begin to read Chapter 2 you will discover that the four phases are repeated as topic headings and you have the Objective 2 question to focus your reading. Begin now to develop the habit of applying this strategy to the objectives in every chapter assigned before you begin to read. Remember to look at the chapter outline at this point as well. It is amazing how much can be learned by using the text structures provided.

VOCABULARY DEVELOPMENT

Objective 1 makes an important point. "Define common terms used in pharmacology." Success depends heavily on knowledge of the "language." The objective makes it clear that this chapter contains a number of terms that the author views as important to be mastered. This is only Chapter 3 and now is the time to begin to really apply yourself to mastering the language of this content. Look at the glossary. There are four terms that share the common element of "pharmaco-." While each of these four words will have different meanings, they will also have something in common. *Pharmaco-* is an example of a group word. No matter what prefixes, group words, and/or suffixes are added to it, a part of the meaning of any word containing pharmaco- will be drug or medicine. Look up pharmaco- in any dictionary and you will find drug or medicine to be the definition. (I used *The American Heritage Dictionary*.) Of course, you already knew that, but it is always ben-

eficial to start working on a new technique with something that is familiar. Look at the four words which begin pharmaco- and consider the rest of the word.

-dynamics   -genetics   -gnosy   -kinetics

What do each of these word parts mean? The meaning of pharmacodynamics is simply the combination of the meaning of pharmaco- and -dynamics. The definition, according to the glossary is, "The study of the biochemical and physiologic interactions of drug action." You could simply memorize this definition which would seem to accomplish Objective 1. But memorization does not always equal understanding. Let's try another approach. What does "dynamics" mean. Think about the word and relate it to your own experience and background. It appears to deal with movement or action. After looking it up in the dictionary, I find that all the meanings given seem to relate in some fashion to the idea of motion and/or action. A simplistic definition of pharmacodynamics would be drugs in action. Certainly this is not a technical or medical definition, but it contributes a great deal to an understanding of the definition provided in the glossary. This is the object of learning vocabulary. Do not memorize words without understanding. Apply a little thought and relate the term and definition in a way that makes the meaning personal for you. When you do that you will find that you understand the glossary definition better, and your ability to retain the meaning will be significantly improved. This means that the test item that asks you to select the definition for pharmacodynamics from a list of similar definitions will be much easier, because you will remember action and movement and look for the choice which best represents that concept.

Apply this same strategy to genetics. You already know what genetics means. Now you must determine how to connect that to the meaning in the text. After you have the definitions of gnosy and kinetics, you can apply the same procedure. When you have done this to all four words you will discover that you will not need to spend a great amount of time trying to memorize esoteric (look it up, it's a fun word to know) definitions. You will have personalized the meanings. Those meanings will stay with you much more readily than those learned by rote memorization. By the way, do you know what biochemical and physiologic mean? These terms are used in the glossary definition of pharmacodynamics. You need to know what they mean to fully understand pharmacodynamics.

Chapter 1

Study Skills

INTRODUCTION

What to study? When to study? How much to study? How to study? In the best of worlds every student would have all the skills necessary to be effective in all academic areas. Unfortunately, many students do not know how to study effectively or have developed techniques that work well in some circumstances but not in others. The purpose of this chapter is to introduce you to the steps to follow in learning text and maintain focus on the appropriate material. Extensive study skills covering time management, note-taking, mastering the text, preparing for and taking examinations, and developing vocabulary are presented in the *Study Skills Manual* that accompanies the text. These tools are important to any student, but in a challenging technical area such as nursing and pharmacology, they become even more valuable. The techniques described here and in the *Study Skills Manual* will not necessarily make learning easy, but they will help you to achieve your goals as a student.

PURR

PURR is a handy mnemonic device representing a four-step process that will lead to mastery of material, and these steps are to:

Prepare
Understand
Rehearse
Review

There is some good news and some bad news about PURR. The bad news is that it requires your going through every chapter four times. I can hear the screams at this point, but hang on because the good news is that you are not going to actually *read* the chapter four times. You are only going to *go through* it four times. Only one of those times is a slow, careful, intensive reading. The other trips through the chapter are much quicker. In fact, the first time you go through the chapter should only take 5 or 10 minutes. Each time you go through the chapter, you are processing the information in distinctly different ways. The PURR approach will really enhance your learning, and if you use it from the first assignment on, I know you will find in the end that it takes you less time to learn what you must than you were spending before you adopted the PURR approach.

Prepare

Reading the text, like any complex process, is not something to leap into without thought and planning. *Pharmacology and the Nursing Process* is organized to really help you learn the material, but you have to take advantage of what the authors have done for you to facilitate this. Preparing to read means setting goals and objectives for your own learning, but the tools you need to do this are already in place. Look at the opening pages of any chapter in the text and you will see a standard structure.

Every chapter begins with a **title.** Learn to use the title as the first step in preparing to learn. Chapter 4 is entitled "Neonatal, Pediatric, and Geriatric Considerations." This instantly identifies what the chapter is about. Don't immediately start reading; instead think about the title for a few seconds. Are there any unfamiliar terms? If your answer is "no," great!! If it is "yes," then you already have some focus for your reading because you know you will need to learn this unfamiliar term, or terms, and its meaning.

The next feature of every chapter are the **objectives.** You need objectives for learning, and the authors have anticipated this. Read the objectives, *actively.* Don't just look at the words, think about the objectives. Ask yourself the following questions: What do I already know about this material? How do these objectives relate to earlier assignments? How do they relate to objectives the instructor has given? The chapter objectives identify things you should be able to do after you have read the material. Don't wait until you have read the chapter to start trying to respond. *Prepare* means getting the brain engaged from the very beginning. Studying the chapter objectives establishes a direction and purpose for your reading. This will enable you to maintain your concentration and focus while you read.

The **chapter outline** shows the major points to be covered. Study it and notice the major headings (topics) and the indented headings (subtopics). This is essentially a picture of the chapter, and using the picture is an essential step in preparing to read. As you read the chapter outline, turn the topic and subtopics into a series of questions that you want to be able to answer when you finish reading. Think about the objectives and how these headings relate to them. Finally, in the outline of chapters devoted to specific classes of agents, notice there are elements that are common to every one. The last two headings are always "Implementation" and "Evaluation." This tells you that these are two common elements you will be expected to know at the end of every chapter. The minutes you spend *preparing* will pay off in a big way when you start to read.

The last feature in the opening pages of each chapter is the **glossary.** This is one of the most valuable tools the authors have provided. They know there are many terms to learn and are giving you a head start on learning them. Spend a few minutes with the glossary. Notice the terms that are also used in the chapter objectives and outline. Go back and look at the objectives and outline and think about what you have learned just from the glossary. As you study the glossary, look for shared root words, prefixes, or suffixes. If words share such common word elements, this means that these words also have a shared meaning. Learning the meaning of common word elements can really simplify the whole process of learning vocabulary. Perhaps you remember in grade school being told to "look for the little words in the big word." This is essentially the same technique—one that worked then and one that will work now.

Now make a quick pass through the chapter or the assigned pages from the chapter. Focus on the text conventions, which are described later in this chapter. Look for anything that stands out in the chapter, such as boldfaced text, boxed material, and tables. This provides a quick overview of the chapter, which will make the next steps in the PURR process much more effective and efficient.

Preparing makes the whole approach to learning an active one. It may not make the chapters the most exciting reading you will ever do, but it will help you to accomplish your personal learning objectives as well as those set by the authors.

On-the-Run Action. Preparing is great to do during "found" time. It should not take more than 5 or 10 minutes. Time between classes, time spent waiting for the coffee water to boil, or any other small block of time that usually just slips away can be used to accomplish this step.

Understand

The time has now come to read the assignment. Go to your desk, the library, or wherever it is you have chosen for serious study. Reading the assignment is where all your preparation pays off. If you did the "Prepare" step earlier in the day, it is not a bad idea to spend a minute or two going through the chapter features again to get your focus. As you read the assignment, remember the chapter objectives and notice the chapter outline headings repeated in the body of the chapter. As you read, rephrase the headings as questions to help keep you focused on the task at hand. Because this is the first time you are really homing in on the concepts and the details, this is not the time to do any of the text notations. Read and, as you read, think. Terms from the glossary are repeated and their meanings often expanded and clarified in the body of the text. Pay attention to these terms as you read. Think about what they mean and how you would define them to someone else. Read for meaning. Read to *understand.* Don't read just to get to the end of the assignment. That is a passive action. Ask yourself questions. Analyze, respond, and react as you read.

Often reading assignments are too long to be read with complete understanding in one session. If you find your concentration is flagging or you don't remember anything you read on the previous page, it is time to take a break. All too often students have only one objective—to finish the assignment. You might be able to force yourself to keep on reading, but you won't learn much. Mark your place and take a 5- or 10-minute break. Take a walk, read the daily comic strips, get a soda or a cup of coffee, and then go back to reading. When you come back to the assignment, spend the first 3 or 4 minutes reviewing. Look back at the previous chapter heading and think about what you were reading before the break. The chapter can be broken down into many small reading sessions, but it is critical that you don't lose sight of the chapter as a whole. Spending these minutes in review may seem like time that could be better spent continuing with the reading, but this quick review will save time in the long run.

There is no quick way to read a chapter. You won't find an "on-the-run action" for this step because it can't be done in this way. But, if you do the "Prepare" step first, you will be surprised at how much more easily you get the reading done and how much more learning you have achieved in the process.

Rehearse

Rehearsing is the third step in the process. It starts the process of consolidating your learning and establishing a basis for long-term memory. Rehearsal accomplishes two things. First, it helps you find out what you understand from the reading. Knowing what you know is really important. Second, it identifies what you don't understand, and this may be an even more important benefit. Knowing what you don't know before it comes to light during an exam is critical.

How to Rehearse. Everything you do in the "Prepare" and "Understand" steps comes into play in the "Rehearse" step. Rehearsal should begin with the features at the beginning of the chapter. Open the text to the beginning of the chapter. Start with the chapter title and begin to quiz yourself on what you have read. Compose three or four questions pertaining to the chapter title, and then try to answer them to your satisfaction. The questions you ask yourself should be

both literal, asking for specific information presented in the chapter, and interpretive, testing your comprehension of concepts and relationships. An example of a literal question using the Chapter 4 title might be: "What are the definitions of 'neonatal,' 'pediatric,' and 'geriatric'?" This question would help you determine whether you can satisfactorily define these terms in your own words. Asking and answering such questions as this always serves to move learning from short-term to long-term memory. Literal questions are very important to help you grasp the factual information and terminology contained in the reading assignment. However, it is also necessary to ask questions that stimulate thought about the concepts and the relationships between the facts and concepts presented in the chapter. An example of an interpretive question regarding the Chapter 4 title might be: "What is the most important concept pertaining to the use of drugs in neonatal, pediatric, and geriatric patients?" Sometimes you will find that, even though the question is interpretive, the authors have anticipated the question and the text does contain the direct answer to your question. Other times you will need to formulate your own response by pulling together bits and pieces of information from the entire reading assignment.

Once you have exhausted the question potential for the chapter title, move on to the chapter objectives. Use the same process here. Rephrase the objectives as questions and try to answer them. Remember the object of rehearsal is to reinforce what you have learned and to identify areas where you need to spend additional time (review).

Skip the chapter outline and go to the glossary. Cover the definitions and try to define each term in your own words. Or cover the term and on the basis of the definition name the term. Don't just memorize the definition, because you may find the information presented differently on an exam and you will then be unable to respond.

Now proceed to the chapter or assigned pages. The chapter headings, the same headings as in the chapter outline, are the main tools for rehearsal. Apply the same question-and-answer technique used for the title and objectives to test what you may already know about the chapter content. Turn the headings into questions and answer them. Look at the text for bold-faced and italicized items, lists, and other text conventions. These too can become the basis for questions. The tables and diagrams should also be used for this purpose. Keep in mind the importance of asking both literal and interpretive questions. Some of the questions you ask yourself should also tie different topic headings together. Ask yourself how topic A relates to topic B.

As you proceed through the chapter, don't worry if you can't answer the questions you ask. As stated earlier, one of the goals of the rehearsal process is to identify what you need to spend more time on. If you can give no response to a particular question, put a mark in the margin of the pertinent place in the text to remind yourself to come back and spend more time on this material, but move on at this point. Rehearsal should be a relatively quick procedure. Once you become accustomed to the PURR method, it should take no more than 15 or 20 minutes to rehearse 15 pages after doing the "Prepare" and "Understand" steps.

As you reach the end of the chapter, skim the "Implementation" and "Evaluation" sections. Make sure that the relationship between these sections and the information in the rest of the chapter is clear. If you have questions or concerns, note them in the margins and ask your instructor to clarify these points. Although the objective is to master the chapter content as an independent learner, sometimes it is essential to ask questions of the instructor to facilitate the process.

When to Rehearse. Ideally rehearsal should take place almost immediately after you finish reading the material. Take a 10- to 15-minute break, and then start the process. The longer the gap between reading and rehearsal, the more you will forget and the longer it will take to rehearse. If you are breaking a reading assignment down into smaller segments, do the rehearsal for each segment before you begin reading the new material. This helps to maintain the sense of continuity in the chapter. I know this seems like a lot of work to do in a study session, but with practice it will go quickly and you will be pleasantly surprised at the quality and quantity of your learning.

Review

The review aspect is the fourth and final step in the PURR process, and it is an essential step. No matter how well you have learned material in the preceding steps, forgetting will always occur. Reviewing is the only way to really store what you have learned in long-term memory. The good news is that, using the PURR model, the review can be done for small segments of material and can be done relatively quickly.

How to Review. The basic review process is essentially the same as the rehearsal process, with some limited rereading the one difference. When you cannot

immediately answer a question, read the pertinent material again. *This does not mean you should read the entire chapter again.* Often the answer to the question will pop into your mind after you've read only a few lines. When this happens, stop reading and go back to responding to your question. The idea is to reread only as much material as is necessary to make the answer clear. One or two words or one or two sentences may trigger personal recall, but it may also take two or three paragraphs for this to happen.

Frequency of Review. How many times should you review material in this way? This actually depends on many factors, such as the difficulty of the material, the length of the assignment, and your personal background. Only you can determine how often you need to review, but there are some guidelines that will help you decide this for yourself.

First, consider the difficulty of the material. If it is very complex, contains many new terms and difficult concepts, and seems difficult to grasp, then you should review very frequently. On the other hand, if the material is straightforward and you are able to relate it well to what you've already learned, then less frequent reviews will serve to keep the material in your memory.

Second, consider how well the review went. If you had difficulty answering many questions to your satisfaction or had to do a lot of rereading, you should schedule another review soon (a day or two later at most).

The success of each review session should be used to help you determine when to schedule another session. The review step is a means of monitoring the success of the learning process. If reviews go well, limited rereading is necessary, and you are able to give clear answers to your questions, this tells you that you can wait several days (four or five) before reviewing this material again. A so-so review, more extensive rereading, and poor answers indicate you should only let 2 or 3 days go by before reviewing the material again. If the review goes very poorly, you should plan to review the material again the next day. It is up to you to judge the success of each review and to decide how often you need to review. The nice thing about PURR is that it enables you to monitor your own success and to easily regulate the learning process.

Technique for Rehearsal and Review. Both rehearsal and review foster active learning, which helps you maintain interest in the material and strengthens your memory. For these benefits to occur, it is essential that the review and rehearsal processes be done orally. Simply talk aloud as you go through the material. Ask questions and give your answers out loud. This forces you to really think about the material. It helps you to organize it and to translate it into your own words. The object is not to memorize everything you have read but really to understand and be able to explain it. Eventually you will need to answer questions on an exam. Framing questions as a part of the learning process is a way to anticipate exam questions. The more questions you ask yourself during study time, the more likely some of the questions on the exam will be ones you've asked yourself. Further, by doing the rehearsal and review orally, you will find it easier to recall the answers during the exam because this oral model requires more than just remembering seeing the material; you will actually be able to hear the rehearsed answers in your mind. Another advantage of doing the rehearsal and review processes orally is, as stated earlier, that it helps to identify what needs further study. When your oral answer is fragmentary, contains many ''uhs,'' and is really disorganized, then you know you need to devote more time to learning this term, fact, or concept.

The PURR system may seem like a lot of work at first. The idea of going through a chapter four times understandably seems daunting. Add to this the need for several review sessions and the first reaction is likely to be: ''This won't work'' or ''I don't have the time to do this.'' Don't take that attitude. This system does work. It cultivates interest, aids concentration, fosters mastery of the material, and ensures long-term memory of the material, which, after all, is important not just for doing well on exams but also for doing well as a nurse with the safe care of patients at stake. The PURR system will work if you will use it. It may take 3 or 4 weeks to get comfortable with the system, but if you keep at it, pretty soon it will become a habit, and a good one. After awhile you won't be able to imagine studying in any other way.

One final note about the PURR method. Like all study systems it is a model. As you use it, you may discover ways of changing it that work better for you. That's okay. Don't hesitate to make adjustments that better suit your learning style and strategies. Just remember as you start out that *Preparation, Understanding, Rehearsal,* and *Review* are solid learning principles and cannot be ignored.

Study skills tips are included on the two pages at the beginning of each part. These hints are directly applied to the content found within the chapters of the following unit. Detailed information on specialized study skills, such as time management, note-taking, exam preparation, and vocabulary building are present in the *Sudy Skills Manual* that accompanies this text.

2

The Nursing Process
and Medication Administration

Objectives

When you reach the end of this chapter, you will be able to:

1 List the four phases of the nursing process.
2 Discuss the function and purposes of the nursing process.
3 Describe how the nursing process would be utilized in medication administration.
4 Identify the components of the assessment process in patients receiving medications, including both the subjective and objective data.
5 Discuss how nursing diagnoses are formulated for patients receiving medications.
6 Identify possible goals and outcome criteria for patients receiving medications.
7 List specific nursing interventions that would be appropriate for patients receiving medications.
8 Discuss the evaluation process as it relates to the administration of medications.

CHAPTER OUTLINE

Overview
Assessment
Nursing Diagnoses
Planning
  Goals and outcome criteria
Implementation
  Right drug
  Right dose
  Right time
  Right route
  Right patient
Evaluation

Glossary

Goals Objective, measurable, and realistic changes of behavior in the patient, achieved through nursing care, with an established time period for achieving the outcome. (p. 7)

Nursing process An organizational framework for the practice of nursing. It encompasses all steps taken by the nurse in caring for a patient: assessment, nursing di-agnosis, planning (with outcome criteria), implementa-tion of the plan (with patient teaching), and evaluation. The rationale for each step is founded on nursing the-ory. (p. 7)

Outcome criteria Descriptions of patient goals that are succinct, well thought-out. They include behavioral expectations to be met by specific deadlines and always bear in mind the ultimate goal of patient safety. (p. 7)

OVERVIEW

The **nursing process** is an orderly and systematic method of identifying the following components of a patient's health status and care: the specific health sta-tus; specific problems, defined as alterations in human needs; the plans to solve the problems through the es-tablishment of **goals** and **outcome criteria**; implemen-tation of the plans; and the evaluation of how effective, or ineffective, your plans were in promoting optimal wellness and health and solving the identified prob-lems.

The nursing process is central to all nursing ac-tions. It is flexible, adaptable, and adjustable to nu-merous situations, including the administration of medications. There are specific phases within the nurs-ing process; these include assessment, planning, im-

Nursing Process: Patient Care and Medication Administration

ASSESSMENT

Objective data
43 y/o black male
Family history of DM
VS normal
FBS 239
Diminished pedal pulses

Subjective data
c/o frequent urination, increase in thirst, weight loss, headache, lethargy, confusion.

Nursing diagnosis
Alteration in urinary elimination, frequency, due to possible pathophysiologic changes from ? DM as evidenced by frequent trips to bathroom at night.

PLANNING/OUTCOME CRITERIA

Goal:
Patient will return to normal urinary patterns.
Outcome Criteria:
Patient will awaken to void no more than once per night and void per usual routine during the day.

Patient Care Situation and the Nursing Process

EVALUATION

Sleeping most of the night; only gets up once during the night to void.
Normal urinary patterns during the day.

IMPLEMENTATION

Monitor FBS as ordered.
Monitor fluid intake and output daily for excessive output or any other imbalance.
Assess skin turgor daily.
Assess pre-illness elimination patterns.
Educate patient about the disease process and management of symptoms once therapy initiated.

ASSESSMENT

Objective data
43 y/o male
Recent Dx of IDDM
New insulin regimen of regular and NPH
No history of previous illnesses
No other health problems

Subjective data
States "uneasy with treatment plan"
States "knows very little about DM, its treatment and complications"
States "fearful of giving self injections"

Nursing diagnosis
Knowledge deficit related to newly diagnosed DM and new treatment regimen with insulin as evidenced by voicing fears and anxieties and asking many questions.

PLANNING/OUTCOME CRITERIA

Goal:
Patient adheres to new insulin treatment regimen without complications.
Outcome Criteria:
Patient will state reasons for taking insulin therapy to help regulate blood sugars.
Patient will state side effects of insulin therapy, such as hypoglycemia.
Patient will state importance of daily glucometer testing to maintain consistent blood sugar levels.
Patient will state the S&S of hypoglycemia and means of treatment.
Patient understands importance of follow-up with physician for close monitoring.
Patient demonstrates safe "drawing-up" of insulin and injection technique with rotation of sites of injection.

Medication Administration and the Nursing Process

EVALUATION

Has normal FBS and monitors blood sugar levels daily with glucometer.
Able to continue insulin therapy at home.
Has minimal to no complications related to insulin therapy.
Able to treat S&S of hypoglycemia, should they occur.

IMPLEMENTATION

Educate patient and family re: DM, its treatment with insulin, and side effects of therapy.
Use AV aids, films, pamphlets for education about insulin therapy, injection sites, etc.
Monitor FBS as ordered.
Assess patient's response to Dx of DM and to its treatment.
5 "Rs": right dose, right drug, right time, right patient, right route.

AV, audiovisual; *c/o,* complains of; *DM,* diabetes mellitus; *Dx,* diagnosis; *FBS,* fasting blood sugar; *IDDM,* insulin-dependent diabetes mellitus; *NPH,* insulin; *S&S,* signs and symptoms; *VS,* vital signs; *y/o,* years old.

plementation, and evaluation. See the box on p. 8 for an example of the application of this nursing process to a particular patient care situation and its very specific use in the administration of medications.

ASSESSMENT

During the assessment phase of the nursing process, both subjective and objective data on the patient are collected. Subjective data, supplied by the patient or family, may include some of the following: the chief complaint, a detailed history of the present illness and any past medical problems, the family medical history, the sociocultural profile and socioeconomic status, and the cognitive and motor ability. The objective data may be obtained through physical assessment and include the vital signs, weight, height, laboratory results, and results of diagnostic tests.

A thorough medication history is very important to ensure the safe use of medications in patients. It may involve both subjective and objective data collection. The following information is all part of a complete medication history: over-the-counter medications (aspirin, vitamins, Tylenol [acetaminophen] products, laxatives, cold preparations, sinus medications, and antacids), any prescription medications (including birth control pills), street drugs (marijuana, cocaine, angel dust, LSD, etc.), problems with drug therapy in the past (allergies, adverse effects, side effects, diseases that may contraindicate or limit the use of some medications), and growth and development issues as related to the patient's age. A thorough health assessment and head-to-toe physical assessment are also part of the assessment phase.

NURSING DIAGNOSES

Once the complete assessment data have been obtained, the next step is to analyze the information before formulating the nursing diagnoses. A nursing diagnosis as it relates to drug therapy should be a judgment or conclusion about the potential or actual need or problem of a particular patient. Remember, the two major tasks in the assessment phase are the collection of subjective and objective data and the formulation of nursing diagnoses. Most nursing diagnoses will probably have as their basis the patient's knowledge deficit and the possibility of side effects and other complications of therapy.

PLANNING

After the data are collected, the planning phase can start. Planning includes the identification of goals and outcome criteria.

The major aims of the planning phase are to prioritize all the nursing diagnoses and to specify the

goals and outcome criteria and the time when these should be achieved. After this the specific nursing care plan can be developed. The planning phase gives you time to get any special equipment, to review the possible procedures or techniques to be rendered, and to gather information either for yourself or on the patient. This step leads to the provision of safe care if you combine professional judgment-making with the acquisition of knowledge about the patient and the medication to be given.

Goals and Outcome Criteria

Goals are objective, measurable, and realistic, with an established time period for achievement of the outcome, which is more specifically stated in the outcome criteria. Patient goals are reflected in expected changes through nursing care. The outcome criteria, or description of goals, should be succinct, well thought out, and patient and nursing focused, and should include behavioral expectations to be met by certain deadlines, bearing in mind that the ultimate aim of these criteria is the safe and effective administration of medications. These criteria should relate to each nursing diagnosis and direct the implementation of the nursing care plan. The formulation of these criteria begins with the analysis of the judgments made about all the patient data and subsequent nursing diagnoses and ends with the development of a nursing care plan. Outcome criteria provide a standard of measure that can be used to move toward the goal. They may address special storage and handling techniques, administration procedures, equipment needed, drug interactions, side effects, and contraindications. In this text, specific timeframes will usually not be included in the goals and outcome criteria, as this process must be individualized for *each* patient situation and reflect such individual and specific planning and nursing judgment.

The patient-oriented outcome criteria must apply to any medications the patient will receive. For example, in the sample situation described in the box on p. 8 the outcome criteria of the 43-year-old man with diabetes mellitus were focused on the administration and general aspects of insulin therapy. In this patient the nurse-oriented outcome criteria include specific patient education about insulin, its side effects, contraindications to its use, and injection techniques, as well as what you the nurse should know about the physician's order, patient, and medication before the medication is administered. If you have any questions about the order, its appropriateness, or safety in a given patient, you should get answers to your questions and then use your professional judgment in the implementation of the order. During the planning phase, if you find your patient's condition is changing and could be worsened by the medication or that the physician's order is unclear or incorrect, you should withhold the medication, contact the physician for clarification or further instructions, and document this. If you are unable to contact the physician, notify your nurse manager or nursing supervisor immediately about the problem and check your nursing policy guidelines to find out who else to contact. Never do nothing!

IMPLEMENTATION

Implementation consists of the initiation and completion of the nursing care plan, as defined by the nursing diagnoses and the outcome criteria. When it comes to medication administration, you need to know and understand all the information about each medication prescribed and especially about your patient. Some of the questions to ask yourself include: What is the patient's medical diagnosis? What are the laboratory and diagnostic test findings? What have been the patient's past experiences with medicines and with hospital and health care facilities? What are the patient's vital signs? What are the medications ordered and the medications the patient is already taking? What does the particular drug do? and What are the drug's adverse effects, the contraindications to its use, the appropriate dosages, and the routes of administration? In addition, it is important to always go by the five "rights" of medication administration: right drug, right dose, right patient, right time, and right route.

Right Drug

To ensure that the right drug is administered, attention must be paid to both the drug orders and the medication labels when preparing medications for administration. In addition, you should consider whether the drug is appropriate for the patient. For you to be sure that the right drug is being administered and is appropriate, you must obtain information about the patient, such as his or her past and present medical history and a thorough and updated medication history, including any over-the-counter medications used. Information about the drug is also important. Sources of information include drug reference books, drug inserts (manufacturer's information), and a pharmacist. Be careful *not* to rely on information from your peers and co-workers because *you* are the one responsible for administering the right drug.

Right Dose

Before administering any drug by any route, you must know the particulars about each drug given. No matter how busy you may be, you must check the order and the label on the medication and check for all the five rights at least *three* times before giving the medication to the patient. If you have any questions, contact the physician to clarify the order and never assume anything when it comes to the dose of a drug. Always ask yourself, is the dose appropriate to the patient's age and size? Always recheck your mathematical calculations.

Patient information to obtain before you administer a dose of a medication includes the patient's weight, height, vital signs, and age. Remember that neonates, pediatric patients, and elderly patients are more sensitive to medications.

Right Time

When it comes to the right time of medication administration, often you will be confronted with a conflict between the pharmacokinetic and pharmacodynamic properties of the drugs prescribed and the patient's life-style and likelihood of compliance. For example, the right time for the administration of antihypertensive agents may be four times a day, but for the active, working, 42-year-old newlywed man, taking a medication with side effects of impotency on time four times a day may lead to decreased compliance. This emphasis on and teaching about the right time for the administration of medications to your patients must be reflected in your own practice, so that no matter how busy you are with patients, you must concentrate on the patient and assess every patient individually to identify any special time considerations.

In addition, medications must be given either one-half hour before or after the actual time specified in the physician's orders (that is, if a medication is ordered to be given at 9:00 every morning, you may give the drug any time between 8:30 and 9:30 AM), except for stat. medications, which must be given within one-half hour of the order. Always check the hospital or facility policy and procedure for any other specific information concerning the "half hour before/after" rule.

If medications are ordered every day on a bid, tid, or even qid basis, the times may be changed if this is not harmful to the patient, if the medication and the patient's condition do not require adherence to an exact schedule, and with physician approval or notification. For example, if an antacid is ordered to be given tid at 9:00 AM, 1:00 PM, and 5:00 PM but the nurse has misread the order and gives it at 11:00 AM, depending on the hospital or facility policy, the medication, and the patient's condition, this may not be considered an error and the dosing times simply changed to 11:00 AM, 3:00 PM, and 7:00 PM without harm to the patient and without incident to the nurse.

There are other factors to consider when it comes to the right time. These include multiple-drug therapy, drug-drug or drug-food compatibility, diagnostic studies, the bioavailability of the drug (such as the need for consistent timing of doses around the clock to maintain blood levels), drug actions, and any biorhythm effects, as occur with steroids.

Right Route

As already stated, you must know the particulars about each medication before administering it to ensure the right drug, dose, and routes are being used. Never assume what the route for administration is—always check with the physician if in any doubt.

Right Patient

It is critical to the patient's safety that you check his or her identity each time before you give a medication. Ask for his or her name and always check for an identification band or bracelet for clarification and confirmation of the patient's name, ID number, age, and allergies.

EVALUATION

Evaluation occurs after the plan has been implemented but is actually an ongoing part of the nursing process and the drug therapy. Evaluation in the context of drug therapy is the monitoring of the patient's response to the drug—the expected and unexpected responses, the therapeutic effects (produced intended effects), the side effects, and the toxic effects.

The nursing process is an ongoing and essentially circular process (see the box on p. 8), and the evaluation of the patient's response to previous therapy and other components of his or her medical or surgical reg-

imen is an important facet of the safe and effective delivery of drug therapy. The documentation of any findings and cautions regarding medication use and the continuous assessment of patients are critical aspects of safe and effective nursing care.

In summary, the nursing process as it relates to drug therapy is the way you organize and provide drug therapy in the context of prudent nursing care. Astute assessments, the establishment of outcome criteria, a correct administration technique and procedure related to the drug, and continual evaluation will become easier and more comprehensible with additional experience and knowledge.

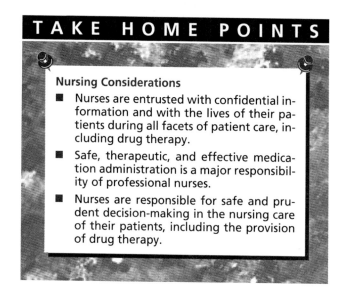

TAKE HOME POINTS

Nursing Considerations
- Nurses are entrusted with confidential information and with the lives of their patients during all facets of patient care, including drug therapy.
- Safe, therapeutic, and effective medication administration is a major responsibility of professional nurses.
- Nurses are responsible for safe and prudent decision-making in the nursing care of their patients, including the provision of drug therapy.

Critical Thinking ACTIVITY

1. Because of the changes in the ordering, distribution, and administration of drugs, the advances in technology, and the increased potency of medications, what is the *crucial* responsibility of the nurse when implementing drug therapy?

BIBLIOGRAPHY

Cohen M: Medication errors . . . misprinted doses; FDA precautions, *Nursing 94* 24(10):15, 1994.

Davis NM: Med errors: a well-informed patient is a valuable asset, *AJN* 94(3):14, 1994.

Lilley LL, Guanci R: Med errors, *AJN* 95(5): 1995.

United States Pharmacopeial Convention: *USP DI drug information for the health care professional*, ed 14, Rockville, Md, 1994, The US Pharmacopeial Convention.

Chapter 3

Pharmacologic Principles

Objectives

When you reach the end of this chapter, you will be able to:

1 Define common terms used in pharmacology.
2 Understand the role of pharmacokinetics and pharmacodynamics in medication administration.
3 List and understand the application of the four principles of pharmacotherapeutics.
4 Discuss the utilization of natural drug sources in the development of new drugs.

CHAPTER OUTLINE

Overview
Pharmacokinetics
  Absorption
    Process
    Route
      Parenteral
        Subcutaneous and intramuscular injections
      Enteral
      Sublingual
      Oral
      Topical
        Transdermal
      Inhalation
  Distribution
  Metabolism
  Excretion
  Half-life
  Onset, peak, and duration
Pharmacodynamics
  Mechanism of action
    Receptor interaction
    Enzyme interaction
    Nonspecific interactions
Pharmacotherapeutics
  Assessment
  Implementation
    Acute therapy
    Maintenance therapy
    Supplemental therapy
    Palliative therapy
    Supportive therapy
    Prophylactic therapy

Monitoring
  Therapeutic index
  Drug concentration
  Patient's condition
  Tolerance and dependence
  Interactions
    Adverse reactions
  Other drug effects
    Teratogenic
    Mutagenic
    Carcinogenic
  Reassessment
Pharmacognosy

Glossary

Drug-induced teratogenesis (ter ah tō jen' ĕ sis) The study of drug-induced congenital anomalies. It deals with the toxic effects that drugs can have on the developing fetus. (p. 23)

Pharmacodynamics (fahr mah kō dī na' miks) The study of the biochemical and physiologic interactions of drugs. It examines the physicochemical properties of drugs and their pharmacologic interactions with suitable body receptors. (p. 13)

Pharmacogenetics (fahr mah kō ge ne' tiks) The study of genetic factors and their influence on drug response. It investigates the nature of genetic aberrations that result in the absence, overabundance, or insufficiency of drug metabolizing enzymes. Vogel has defined the term as meaning "genetically determined variations that are revealed solely by the effects of drugs." (p. 22)

Pharmacognosy (fahr mah kog no sē) The study of drugs that are obtained from natural plant and animal sources. This science was formerly called *materia medica* (materials of medicines) and is concerned with the botanical or zoological origin, biochemical composition, and therapeutic effects of natural drugs, their derivatives, and constituents. (p. 13)

Pharmacokinetics (fahr mah kō ki ne' tiks) The study of drug distribution rates between various body compartments during a drug's biophase. It deals with the absorption, distribution, metabolism, and excretion of drugs. (p. 13)

Pharmacotherapeutics (fahr mah kō ther ah pu' tiks) The treatment of pathologic conditions through the use of drugs. There are two forms of therapeutics: empirical and rational. In empirical therapeutics there is no suitable explanation for effectiveness of the drugs involved. In rational therapeutics the drugs have known mechanisms of action. Pharmacotherapeutics has also been called *therapeutics*. (p. 13)

Toxicology (tok si kol' ah jē) The study of poisons. It deals with the effects of drugs and chemicals in living systems, their detection, and the treatment to counteract their poisonous effects. (p. 13)

OVERVIEW

The collective scientific study of the origin, nature, chemistry, effects, and uses of drugs is called *pharmacology*. It may also be defined as the study of all the interactions that can occur between drugs and living organisms. Defining pharmacology and its scope is essential to an understanding of medicine and how you practice your profession. Without a sound understanding of basic pharmacologic principles, you cannot appreciate the therapeutic benefits and potential toxicity of drugs. Pharmacology is an extensive science that incorporates five interrelated sciences: pharmacokinetics, pharmacodynamics, pharmacotherapeutics, toxicology, and pharmacognosy. The various pharmacologic agents discussed within each chapter are described from the standpoint of these five interrelated sciences. Other commonly used terms such as *therapeutic index, tolerance, dependence,* and *dose-response curves* are also discussed within this chapter.

Pharmacokinetics examines four characteristics of drugs in the body: drug absorption, distribution, metabolism, and excretion. These four characteristics and their relationship to drug and drug metabolite concentrations are then determined for various body sites over specified periods. The onset of action, the peak effect of a drug, and the duration of a drug's effect are also properties studied by pharmacokinetics. **Pharmacodynamics** investigates the biochemical and physical effects of drugs in the body. More specifically, it determines a drug's mechanism of action. The use of drugs and the clinical indications for drugs to prevent and treat diseases constitute the focus of **pharmacotherapeutics**. Pharmacotherapeutics incorporates the principles of drug actions. An understanding of phar-

macotherapeutics is essential for nurses in their role as the persons implementing drug therapy. The study of the adverse effects of drugs on living systems is termed **toxicology**. Such toxicologic effects are often an extension of a drug's therapeutic action. Therefore toxicology often involves overlapping principles of both pharmacotherapy and toxicology. Plants are the source for many drugs, and the study of these natural drug sources (plants, animals) is called **pharmacognosy**.

Pharmacology is a very dynamic discipline that incorporates several different disciplines. Traditionally chemistry is seen as the primary basis of pharmacology, but pharmacology also relies heavily on the physical, biologic, and social sciences.

PHARMACOKINETICS

A particular drug's onset of action, time to peak effect, and duration of action are all characteristics defined by pharmacokinetics. Pharmacokinetics is the study of what actually happens to a drug from the time it is put into the body until the time all of it and its metabolites have left the body. Therefore drug absorption into, distribution to, metabolism within, and excretion from a living organism represent the combined focus of pharmacokinetics.

Absorption
Process

Drug absorption is the process of incorporating a drug into the body and its various tissues, organs, and other biologic sites. Unless a drug is administered directly into the circulation by intravenous injection, it must first be transformed from a dosage form to a biologically available substance for it to gain entry into the systemic circulation. Bioavailability is the amount of a drug in a particular dosage form that is absorbed into the circulation. If two medications have the same bioavailability, they are said to be bioequivalent. There are various factors affecting the rate of drug absorption. These include the administration route of the drug, food, or fluids administered with the drug; the dosage formulation; the status of the absorptive surface; the rate of blood flow to the small intestine; the acidity of the stomach; and the status of gastrointestinal motility.

Route

How a drug is administered, or its route of administration, affects the rate and extent of absorption of that drug. Although there are several different dosage formulations available for delivering medications to the body, they can all be broken down into three basic categories, or routes of administration: oral (enteral), parenteral, and topical. Absorption characteristics vary depending on the particular dosage form and the particular category.

Parenteral. The parenteral route is the fastest route by which a drug can be absorbed, followed by the enteral and the topical routes. Intravenous injections deliver the drug directly into the circulation, where it is distributed with the blood throughout the body. An intravenous drug formulation is absorbed the fastest. At the other end of the spectrum are transdermal patches, intramuscular injections, and subcutaneous injections. These drug formulations may take several hours to days before they are totally absorbed by the body.

Parenterally administered drugs can be given intradermally, subcutaneously, intramuscularly, intrathecally, intraarticularly, and intravenously. The medications that are commonly given by the parenteral route offer the advantage of bypassing the first-pass effect and are in general quickly absorbed. The parenteral route of administration offers an alternative route of delivery for those medications that cannot be given orally. The problems posed by acid changes within the stomach, absorption changes in the intestines, and the presence or absence of food and fluid are not then a concern. There are fewer obstacles to absorption in the parenteral administration than in the enteral administration of drugs. However, drugs that are administered by the parenteral route must still be absorbed into cells and tissues before they can exert their pharmacologic effect.

SUBCUTANEOUS AND INTRAMUSCULAR INJECTIONS. Parenteral injections under the skin are referred to as subcutaneous injections, and parenteral injections into the muscle are called intramuscular injections. Muscles have a greater blood supply than the skin does, therefore drugs injected intramuscularly (IM) are typically absorbed faster than ones injected subcutaneously (SC). Absorption from either of these sites may be increased by applying heat to the injection site or by massaging the site. This increases the blood flow to the area and therefore enhances absorption.

Absorption can be decreased by administering cold packs to the site of injection. This is typically done to localize an injection. This would be done, for example, if an intravenously administered vasopressor, like epinephrine, has extravasated or leaked out of the vein and into the surrounding tissue and has begun to cause ischemia and tissue damage. Cool compresses produce vasoconstriction, which reduces cellular activity and in turn may limit tissue injury. Sometimes injections may be given with a vasoconstrictor-like epinephrine to confine an injected drug to the site of injection, thereby limiting its pharmacologic action to that particular area.

Some intramuscular drugs are suspensions and are poorly absorbed. This is by design. The slow absorption of the intramuscular suspension allows for delivery over a longer period. Such injections are commonly called depot injections.

Enteral. In enteral drug administration the drug is absorbed into the systemic circulation through the oral or gastric mucosa, the small intestine, or the rectum. The rate of absorption of these drugs can be altered by many factors. When drugs are taken orally, they are absorbed from the gastrointestinal tract into the portal circulation (liver). Depending on the particular drug, it may be extensively metabolized in the liver before it reaches the systemic circulation. Normally, orally administered drugs are absorbed from the intestinal lumen into the mesenteric blood system and conveyed by the portal vein and to the liver. Once the drug is in the liver, the enzyme system metabolizes it and it is passed into the general circulation. The metabolism of a drug and its passage from the liver into the circulation is called the first-pass effect (Fig. 3-1).

When drugs with a high first-pass effect are administered orally, a large amount of drug may be metabolized before it reaches the systemic circulation. The same drug given intravenously will bypass the liver. This prevents the first-pass effect from taking place, and therefore more drug reaches the circulation. Parenteral doses of drugs with a high first-pass effect are much smaller than enterally administered oral doses, yet they produce the same pharmacologic response.

Sublingual. Drugs administered by the sublingual route are absorbed into the highly vascularized tissue under the tongue—the oral mucosa. Sublingual nitroglycerin is an example. These drugs are absorbed rapidly because this area has a large blood supply, and such drugs bypass the liver. Drugs administered by the buccal or sublingual, vaginal, and intravenous routes bypass the liver. By doing so, drugs like sublingual nitroglycerin are absorbed rapidly into the bloodstream and delivered to their site of action, in this case coronary arteries. These same characteristics are true for rectally administered medications. Enemas and suppositories (rectal and vaginal) are absorbed directly into the bloodstream, thus bypassing the liver and the first-pass effect. A listing of the various drug routes according to whether they are affected by first-pass effects in the liver is given in the box on p. 15.

Oral. There are many factors that can alter the absorption of orally (enterally) administered drugs. Acid changes within the stomach, absorption changes in the intestines, and the presence or absence of food and fluid can alter the rate and extent of absorption of drugs administered enterally. Various factors that affect the acidity of the stomach are the time of day, the

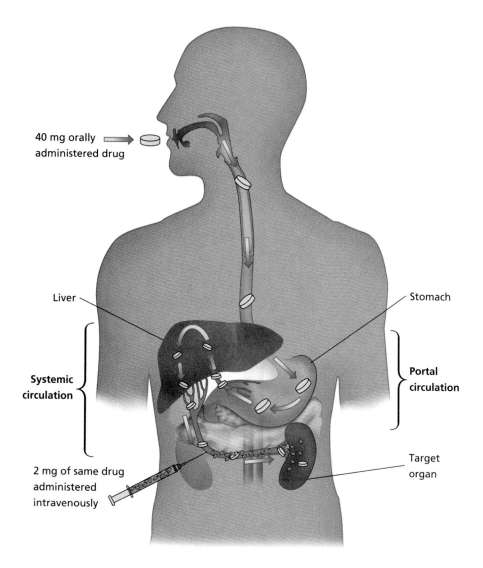

40 mg orally
administered drug

Liver

Stomach

**Systemic
circulation**

**Portal
circulation**

2 mg of same drug
administered
intravenously

Target
organ

▼ FIG. 3-1 First-pass effect is the metabolism of a drug and its passage from the liver into the circulation.

Drug Routes and First-Pass Effects

First-Pass Routes
Oral
Rectal
Hepatic artery
Portal vein

Non–First-Pass Routes

Intravenous	Intraocular
Subcutaneous	Transdermal
Inhalation	Intramuscular
Intranasal	Buccal
Intraarterial	Intravaginal
Sublingual	

age of the patient, the presence of food, and the type of food. If there is food in the stomach during the dissolution of an orally administered medication, this may interfere with its dissolution and absorption and delay its transit from the stomach to the small intestine, where most drugs are absorbed. On the other hand, food may enhance the absorption of some fat-soluble drugs or drugs that are easily broken down in an acidic environment.

Most orally administered drugs are absorbed in the small intestine, which has an enormous surface area. Drug absorption may be altered in patients who have had portions of their small intestine removed because of disease. Anticholinergic drugs may slow down the gastrointestinal transit time, or the time it takes substances in the stomach to be dissolved and passed into the intestines. This may allow more time for an acid-susceptible drug to be in contact with the acid in the stomach and subsequently broken down.

The stomach and small intestine are highly vascularized. When blood flow to that area is decreased, absorption may also be decreased. Sepsis and exercise are examples of conditions in which blood flow is decreased. In both cases, blood is shunted away from the gastrointestinal tract to other areas.

Topical. Topical routes of drug administration involve the application of medications to body surfaces. Several different drug delivery systems exist for doing this. Topically administered drugs can be applied to the skin, eyes, ears, nose, and lungs, to name just a few. As with the other routes (enteral and parenteral), there are both benefits and drawbacks to using the topical route of administration. Topically applied drugs typically deliver a constant amount of drug over long periods, but the drug's effects are usually very slow in their onset and very prolonged in their offset. This can be a problem if the patient begins to experience side effects from the drug and there is already a considerable amount of drug in the subcutaneous tissues.

Topical ointments, gels, and creams are examples of topically administered drugs. They are commonly used for their local effects, and they include sunscreens, antibiotics, and nitroglycerin paste and ointment. The drawback to their use is that their systemic absorption is very unreliable. Therefore topically applied ointments, gels, and creams are seldom used for the treatment of any systemic illnesses.

Topically applied drugs can also be utilized in the treatment of various illnesses of the eye, ear, and sinuses. In such conditions most frequently the required drug is delivered topically to the actual site of illness and bypasses the first-pass effect in the liver.

TRANSDERMAL. Transdermal drug delivery is a topical route of drug administration that has been utilized commonly. Some examples of drugs administered by this route are fentanyl, nitroglycerin, nicotine, and clonidine. This route offers the advantage of bypassing the liver and its first-pass effects; it is suitable for patients who cannot tolerate orally administered medications, and the effect of such drugs can last for as long as 3 days.

Inhalation. Inhaled drugs are delivered to the lungs as micron-sized drug particles. This small drug size is necessary to get the drug to the small airways within the lungs—the alveoli. Once the small particle of drug is in the alveolus, drug absorption is fairly easy. At this site the thin-walled pulmonary alveolus is in contact with the capillaries, where the drug can be absorbed quickly. Many pulmonary-related diseases can be treated with such topically applied (inhaled) drugs. Examples of inhaled drugs include pentamidine, which is used to treat *Pneumocystis carinii* infections in the lung; albuterol, which is used for the treatment of bronchial constriction in asthmatics; and vasopressin, which is used to treat diabetes insipidus.

Distribution

Once a drug enters the bloodstream (circulation), it is distributed throughout the body. At this point it is also beginning to be eliminated by the organs that metabolize and excrete drugs—the liver and the kidney. A drug can be freely distributed to extravascular tissue only if it is not bound to protein. If a drug is bound to protein, it is generally too large to pass into tissues. The transport of a drug in the body by the bloodstream to its site of action is referred to as distribution. There are three primary proteins that bind to and carry drugs throughout the body. They are albumin, alpha-1-acid glycoprotein, and corticosteroid-binding globulin. By far the most important of these is albumin. When a patient has a low albumin level, for instance when he or she is malnourished or burned, there is more free, unbound drug as a result. Unbound drug is free to be distributed to and to diffuse into tissues and cells where it can cause a pharmacologic action. The areas where the drug is distributed first are those that are most extensively supplied with blood.

Rapid distribution: heart, liver, kidney, and brain
Slow distribution: muscle, skin, and fat

A theoretical volume, called the *volume of distribution*, is sometimes used to describe the various areas where drugs may be distributed. These areas, or compartments, can be the blood, total body water, or fat. Typically a drug that is highly water soluble will have a small volume of distribution and high blood concentrations. The opposite is true for drugs that are highly fat soluble. Fat-soluble drugs have a large volume of distribution and low blood concentrations. Drugs that are water soluble and highly protein bound are more strongly bound to proteins in the blood and less likely to be absorbed into tissues. Because of this their distribution and onset of action can be slow. Drugs that are highly lipid soluble and poorly bound to protein are easily taken up into tissues and distributed throughout the body. They may even be resorbed back into the circulation from fatty tissue.

There are some sites in the body where it may be very difficult to distribute drug. These sites typically either have a poor blood supply, like the bone, or have barriers that make it difficult for drugs to pass through, like the blood-brain barrier.

Metabolism

Metabolism is also referred to as *biotransformation* because it involves the biologic transformation of a drug into an inactive metabolite, a more soluble compound, or a more potent metabolite. Biotransformation is the next step after absorption and distribution. The organ most responsible for the biotransformation or metabolism of drugs is the liver. Other tissues and organs that aid in the metabolism of drugs are the kidneys, lungs, plasma, and intestinal mucosa.

Hepatic biotransformation involves the use of an enormous variety of microsomal enzymes that control a variety of chemical reactions and aid in transforming medications. These microsomal enzymes are targeted against lipid-soluble, nonpolar drugs, which are typically very difficult to eliminate. Some of the ways in which the liver can metabolize drugs are listed in Table 3-1.

The biotransformation capabilities of the liver can vary considerably from patient to patient. Various factors, diseases, conditions, and medications that can alter biotransformation are listed in Table 3-2.

Delayed drug metabolism results in the accumulation of drugs and a prolonged action of the effects or responses to drugs. Stimulating drug metabolism can thus cause diminishing pharmacologic effects. This is often the case with the repeated administration of some drugs that may stimulate the formation of new microsomal enzymes.

Excretion

The elimination of drugs from the body is referred to as excretion. Whether they are active, metabolized, or changed, all drugs must eventually be removed from the body. The primary organ responsible for this is the kidney. Two other organs that also play an important role in the excretion of drugs are the liver and the bowel. Most drugs are metabolized or biotransformed in the liver by various glucuronidases and by hydroxylation and acetylation. Therefore, by the time most drugs reach the kidneys, they have been extensively metabolized and only a small fraction of the original drug is excreted as the original compound. Other drugs may circumvent metabolism and reach the kidneys in their original form. Drugs that have been metabolized by the liver become very polar and water soluble. This makes their elimination by the kidney much easier. The kidney itself is capable of forming glucuronides and sulfates from various drugs and their metabolites.

The actual act of excretion is accomplished through glomerular filtration, resorption, and tubular secretion. Free, unbound water-soluble drugs and metabolites go through passive glomerular filtration, and

Table 3-1	Mechanisms of Biotransformation		
Type of Biotransformation	**Mechanism**	**Result**	
Oxidation Reduction Hydrolysis	Chemical reactions	Increase polarity of chemical, making it more water soluble and more easily excretable. Often this results in a loss of pharmacologic activity.	
Conjugation	Combination with another substance, e.g., glucuronide, glycine, methyl, or alkyl groups		

Table 3-2	Conditions and Drug-Induced Changes in Biotransformation		
		Biotransformation	
Condition or Drug-Induced	**Actual Disease or Drug**	**Increased**	**Decreased**
Diseases	Cardiovascular dysfunction		X
	Renal insufficiency		X
Condition	Starvation		X
	Obstructive jaundice		X
	Genetics		
	Fast acetylator	X	
	Slow acetylator		X
Drugs	Central nervous system depressants	X	
	Xanthines	X	
	Barbiturates	X	

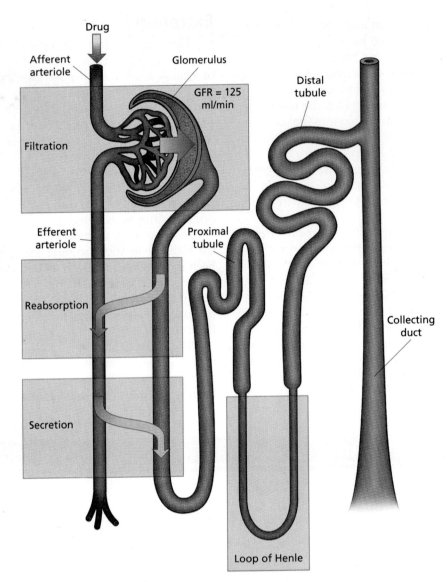

▼ **FIG. 3-2** Drug excretion. The primary processes involved in drug excretion and the approximate location that these processes take place in the kidney are illustrated.

this takes place between the blood vessels of the afferent arterioles and the glomeruli. Many substances present in the nephrons go through active tubular resorption. Resorption occurs at the level of the tubules, where substances are taken back up into the circulation and transported away from the kidney. This is done in an attempt by the body to retain needed substances. These substances are actively resorbed back into the systemic circulation. Some substances may also be secreted into the nephron from the vasculature surrounding it. The processes of filtration, resorption, and secretion are shown in Fig. 3-2.

The excretion of drugs by the intestines is another common route of elimination. This is also referred to as *biliary excretion*. Drugs that are eliminated by this route are taken up by the liver, released into the bile,

and eliminated in the feces. Once certain drugs, like fat-soluble drugs, are in the bile, they may be resorbed into the bloodstream, returned to the liver, and again secreted into the bile. This process is called enterohepatic circulation. Enterohepatic-recycled drugs persist in the body for much longer periods.

Other less common routes of elimination are the lungs and sweat, salivary, and mammary glands. Depending on the particular drug, these organs can be highly effective eliminators of drugs.

Half-life

Another pharmacokinetic variable is the half-life. It is the time it takes for one half of the original amount of a drug in the body to be removed and is a measure

Table 3-3	The Concept of Drug Half-Life					
DIFFERENT PERSPECTIVES				**CHANGING VALUES**		
Drug concentration (mg/L)	100	50	25	12.5	6.25	3.125
Hours after peak concentration	0	8	16	24	32	40
Number of half-lives	0	1	2	3	4	5
Percentage of drug removed	0	50	75	88	94	97

of the rate at which drugs are removed from the body. For instance, if the maximum level that a particular dosage could achieve in the body is 100 mg/L and in 8 hours the measured drug level is 50 mg/L, the estimated half-life for that drug is 8 hours. The concept of drug half-life from several different perspectives is illustrated in Table 3-3.

After about five half-lives most drugs are considered removed from the body. At that time approximately 97% of the drug has been removed and what little is remaining is too small to have any beneficial or toxic effects.

Onset, Peak, and Duration

The pharmacokinetic terms *absorption, distribution, metabolism,* and *excretion* are all used to describe a drug's action. Drug actions are the cellular processes involved in the drug and cell interaction, and an example of this would be a drug's action on a receptor. This is in contrast to a *drug effect,* which is the physiologic reaction of the body to the drug. It is similar to a drug's therapeutic effect in that it constitutes how the function of the body is affected as a whole by the drug. The terms *onset, peak,* and *duration* are used to describe drug effects.

A drug's onset of action is the time it takes for the drug to elicit a therapeutic response. The time it takes for a drug to reach its maximum therapeutic response is its peak effect. Physiologically this corresponds to increasing drug concentrations at the site of action. The duration of action of a drug is the time that drug concentration is sufficient to elicit a therapeutic response. The processes of drug absorption, distribution, and elimination directly determine the duration of action of a particular drug.

PHARMACODYNAMICS

The study of the mechanism of drug actions in living tissues is called *pharmacodynamics.* Anatomy and physiology study how and why the body functions the way it does. Drug-induced alterations in these normal physiologic functions are explained by the concept of pharmacodynamics. A positive change in a faulty physiologic system is called the therapeutic effect of a drug, and this is the goal of drug therapy. Understanding the pharmacodynamic characteristics of a drug can aid in assessing a drug's therapeutic effect.

Mechanism of Action

There are several ways by which drugs can produce therapeutic effects. The mechanism by which a drug does this is called its *mechanism of action.* The effects that a particular drug has depend on the cells or tissue targeted by the drug. Once the drug is at the site of action, it can modify the rate (increase or decrease) at which that cell or tissue functions or it can modify the function of that cell or tissue. A drug cannot, however, make a cell or tissue perform a function that it was not intended to do.

Receptor Interaction

There are three basic ways by which drugs can exert their mechanism of action: receptors, enzymes, and nonspecific interactions. If a drug's mechanism of action is the result of a receptor interaction, then the drug's structure is essential. This drug-receptor interaction involves the selective joining of the drug molecule with a reactive site on the surface of a cell or tissue. This in turn elicits a biologic effect. Therefore a receptor is a reactive site on the surface of a cell or tissue. Once a substance (drug or chemical) binds to and interacts with the receptor, a pharmacologic response is produced. The degree to which a drug attacks and binds with a receptor is called its affinity. The drug with the best "fit" and strongest affinity for the receptor will elicit the greatest response from the cell or tissue. A drug becomes bound to the receptor through the formation of chemical bonds between receptors on the cell and the active site of the drug. Drugs that bind to receptors interact with receptors in several different

Drug-Receptor Interactions: Definitions

INTERACTION TERM	DEFINITION
Agonist	Drug binds to receptor, and there is a response.
Partial agonist	Drug binds to receptor, and there is a diminished response compared with that elicited by the agonist.
Antagonist	Drug binds to receptor, but there is no response. Drug prevents binding of agonists.
Competitive antagonist	Drug competes with the agonist for binding to receptor. If it binds, there is no response.
Noncompetitive antagonist	Drug combines with different parts of receptor and inactivates it, so agonist has no effect.

ways to either elicit or block a physiologic response. The box above lists the different types of drug-receptor interactions and their definitions.

Enzyme Interaction

Enzymes are substances that catalyze nearly every biochemical reaction in a cell. The second way drugs can produce effects is by interacting with these enzyme systems. For a drug to alter a physiologic response this way, it must inhibit the action of a specific enzyme. To do this the drug "fools" the enzyme into binding to it instead of its normal target cell. This protects these target cells from the actions of the enzymes. For example, angiotensin-converting enzyme (ACE) causes an enzymatic reaction that results in the production of a substance called *angiotensin II*, which is a potent vasoconstrictor and mediator of several other processes. The group of drugs called *ACE inhibitors* fools the ACE into binding to it rather than the angiotensin I and thereby prevents the formation of angiotensin II. This in turn causes vasodilation and helps to reduce blood pressure.

Nonspecific Interactions

Nonspecific mechanisms of drug action do *not* involve a receptor or an enzyme in the alteration of a physiologic or biologic function of the body. Instead cell membranes and various cellular processes such as metabolic processes are their main site of action. Such drugs can either physically interfere with or chemically alter these cellular processes. Some cancer drugs and antibiotics have this mechanism of action. By incorporating themselves into the normal metabolic process, they alter the final product, causing the formation of a defective final product. This final product could be a cell wall that, if not properly formed, results in cell death caused by cell lysis, or it could be the lack of a needed energy substrate that leads to cell starvation and death.

PHARMACOTHERAPEUTICS

The use of a medication to treat a pathologic condition is called pharmacotherapeutics. Pharmacotherapy is a dynamic process that should be occurring continuously throughout a patient's therapy, and it involves assessment, implementation of a treatment plan, monitoring of that plan, and reassessment. Besides being an ongoing process, it should be an ever-changing one that accommodates the varying therapeutic needs of the patient.

Assessment

Assessment involves obtaining an accurate history and performing a careful clinical examination. This may include having appropriate laboratory tests or necessary diagnostic procedures performed. The knowledge gained from this first step is invaluable. This information combined with information on the patient's socioeconomic status and the risks and benefits of therapy provide the basis for the implementation of an appropriate drug therapy, the pharmacotherapy. The type of therapy initiated is dictated by the severity and urgency of the patient's condition and the prognosis.

Implementation

The implementation of a treatment plan can involve several types and combinations of therapies. Therapy can be acute, maintenance, supplemental (or replacement), palliative, supportive, or prophylactic.

Acute Therapy

Acute therapy involves intensive drug therapy and is typically implemented in the critically ill patient. It is generally needed to sustain life. Examples are the administration of vasopressors to maintain blood pressure and cardiac output after open heart surgery or the use of volume expanders in a patient who is in shock.

Maintenance Therapy

Maintenance therapy typically does not eradicate the problems the patient may have but does prevent progression of the disease. It is used for the treatment of chronic illnesses such as hypertension. The drug therapy maintains the patient's blood pressure within certain limits, which prevents certain end-organ damage.

Supplemental Therapy

Supplemental or replacement therapy supplies the body with a substance needed to maintain normal function. This substance may be needed either because it cannot be made or because it is deficient in quantity. Examples are the administration of insulin to diabetic patients or iron to patients with iron-deficiency anemia.

Palliative Therapy

The goal of palliative therapy is to make the patient as comfortable as possible. It is typically used in the end stages of an illness when all possible therapy has failed. The use of high-dose narcotic analgesics to relieve pain in the final stages of cancer is an example. The use of oxygen in end-stage pulmonary disease is another.

Supportive Therapy

Supportive therapy maintains the integrity of body functions while the patient is recovering. Providing fluids and electrolytes to prevent dehydration in a patient with the flu who is vomiting and has diarrhea is an example. Giving fluids, volume expanders, or blood products to a patient who has lost blood during surgery is another.

Prophylactic Therapy

Prophylactic therapy is drug therapy provided on the basis of prior practical experience. It is based on scientific knowledge often acquired during years of observation of a disease and its causes. For example, based on practical experience a surgeon knows that when he or she makes an incision through the skin there is the possibility that skin bacteria are present that can later infect that incision. Based on this knowledge, the surgeon administers an antibiotic before making the incision. The antibiotic is also chosen on the basis of prior experience. Empiric therapy, on the other hand, is not founded on a scientific or rational basis. It is the administration of a drug when a certain pathologic process is suspected on the basis of the patient's symptoms. For example, we give acetaminophen to a patient who has a fever. The cause of the fever may not be known, but empirically we give the patient acetaminophen because we believe it will lower the temperature.

Monitoring

Once the appropriate therapy has been implemented, the effectiveness of that therapy must be evaluated. This constitutes the clinical response of the patient to the therapy. Evaluating this clinical response requires that the evaluator be familiar with both the drug's intended therapeutic action and its unintended but potential side effects.

All drugs are potentially toxic and can have cumulative effects. Recognizing them and knowing their effect on the patient are integral components of this monitoring process. *A drug accumulates when it is being absorbed quicker than it can be eliminated, or when it is administered before the previous dose has been metabolized or cleared from the body.* Knowledge of the function of the organs responsible for metabolizing and eliminating a drug combined with knowledge of how a particular drug is metabolized and excreted will enable the nurse to anticipate problems or treat them appropriately if they occur.

Therapeutic Index

The ratio between a drug's therapeutic benefits and its toxic effects is referred to as its *therapeutic index*. The safety of a particular drug therapy is determined by this index. If a drug has a low therapeutic index, there is a narrow range between a therapeutically active dose of the drug and a toxic dose. Such a drug has a greater likelihood of causing an adverse reaction and therefore requires closer monitoring.

Drug Concentration

Drug concentrations in patients can also be an important tool for evaluating the clinical response to drug therapy. Certain drug levels correspond to therapeutic responses while others correspond to toxic effects. Toxic drug levels are typically seen when the body's normal mechanisms for metabolizing and excreting drugs are impaired. This commonly occurs when liver and kidney functions are impaired or in persons such as neonates who have an immature liver or kidneys. Dosage adjustments should be made in these patients to appropriately accommodate their impaired metabolism and excretion.

Patient's Condition

Another patient-specific factor to be considered when monitoring drug therapy is a patient's concurrent diseases or other medical conditions. A patient's response to a drug may vary greatly depending on his or her physiologic and psychologic demands.

Disease, infection, cardiovascular function, and gastrointestinal function are just a few such physiologic factors. Stress, depression, and anxiety are some psychologic factors that can alter a patient's therapeutic response.

Tolerance and Dependence

The monitoring of drug therapy requires a knowledge of tolerance and dependence and an understanding of the difference. Tolerance is the phenomenon of a decreasing response to repetitive drug doses, whereas dependence is a physiologic or psychologic need for a drug. Physical dependence is the physiologic need for a drug, for example, a narcotic in a patient with cancer-related pain. Psychologic dependence is the desire for the euphoric effects of drugs and typically involves the recreational use of various drugs such as benzodiazepines, narcotics, and amphetamines.

Interactions

Drugs may interact with other drugs, foods, or agents administered as part of laboratory tests. Knowledge of drug interactions is vital to the appropriate monitoring of drug therapy. The more drugs a patient receives, the more likely a drug interaction will occur. This is especially true in the elderly, who typically have an increased sensitivity to drug effects and are receiving several medications.

Adverse Reactions. Knowledge of adverse drug reactions is an essential component of pharmacotherapy. An adverse drug reaction is an undesirable response to drug therapy. The study of poisons and unwanted responses to therapeutic agents is commonly referred to as toxicology. An adverse drug reaction can be either a side effect or a harmful effect. Many are extensions of the drug's normal pharmacologic actions. Adverse drug reactions can be broken down into four basic categories: pharmacologic, idiosyncratic, drug interaction, and hypersensitivity reactions.

Pharmacologic adverse drug reactions are extensions of the drug's effects in the body. For example, a drug that is used to lower blood pressure in a patient with hypertension causes a pharmacologic adverse drug reaction when it lowers the blood pressure to the point where the patient becomes unconscious.

Idiosyncratic reactions are not the result of a known pharmacologic property of a drug or patient allergy but are peculiar to that patient. Such a reaction is a genetically determined abnormal response to ordinary doses of a drug. Genetically inherited traits that result in the abnormal metabolism of drugs are universally distributed throughout the population. The study of such traits that are solely revealed by drug administration is called **pharmacogenetics**. Idiosyncratic drug reactions are usually caused by abnormal levels of drug-metabolizing enzymes: a complete absence, a deficiency, or an overabundance of the enzyme.

There are many pharmacogenetic diseases. A common one is glucose-6-phosphate dehydrogenase (G6PD) deficiency. This pharmacogenetic disease is transmitted as a sex-linked trait and affects approximately 100 million people. Persons who lack proper levels of G6PD have idiosyncratic reactions to a wide range of drugs. There are more than 80 variations of the disease, and all produce varying degrees of drug-induced hemolysis. Drugs capable of inducing hemolysis in such patients are listed in the box below.

Hypersensitivity reactions involve the patient's immune system. The patient's immune system recognizes the drug, a drug metabolite, or an ingredient in a drug formulation as a dangerous foreign substance. This foreign substance is then attacked, neutralized, or destroyed by the immune system, causing a hypersensitivity reaction.

The final type of adverse drug reaction is a *drug interaction* and results when two drugs interact and produce an unwanted effect. This unwanted effect can be the result of one drug either making the other more potent and accentuating its effects or diminishing the effectiveness of another.

Other Drug Effects

Other drug-related effects that need to be monitored during therapy are teratogenic, mutagenic, and carcinogenic effects. These can result in devastating patient outcomes and can be prevented in many instances by appropriate monitoring.

Teratogenic. The teratogenic effects of drugs result in structural defects in the unborn fetus. Such agents are called teratogens. There are three major categories of exogenous human teratogens: viral diseases, radiation, and drugs or chemicals. Fetal development

---

Drugs to Avoid in Patients with Glucose-6-Phosphate Dehydrogenase Deficiency

- Para-aminosalicylic acid
- Furazolidone
- Sulfonamides
- Antimalarials
- Nitrofurantoin
- Sulfones
- Aspirin
- Phenacetin
- All oxidants
- Chloramphenicol
- Probenecid

involves a delicate programmed sequence of interrelated embryologic events. Any significant disruption in embryogenesis can result in a teratogenic effect. Drugs that are capable of crossing the placenta can act as teratogens and cause **drug-induced teratogenesis**. Drugs administered during pregnancy can produce different types of congenital anomalies. The period when the fetus is most vulnerable to teratogenic effects begins with the third week of fetal development and usually ends after the third month.

Mutagenic. Mutagenic effects are changes in the genetic composition of living organisms (permanent changes) and consist of alterations in the chromosome structure, the number of chromosomes, and the genetic code of the deoxyribonucleic acid (DNA) molecule. Agents capable of inducing mutations are called mutagens. Radiation, chemicals, and drugs can act as mutagenic agents in human beings. The largest genetic unit that can be involved in a mutation is a chromosome. The smallest is a base pair in a DNA molecule. Agents that affect genetic processes are active only during cell reproduction.

Carcinogenic. The carcinogenic effects of drugs cause cancer, and such chemicals and drugs are called carcinogens. There are several exogenous factors that contribute to the development of cancer besides drugs, and the list grows daily. Some of the more notable ones are listed in the box below.

Chemically induced carcinogenesis usually requires lengthy exposure to carcinogens. Even brief exposures to potent carcinogens will involve a long latent period before cancer develops.

Reassessment

The processes of assessment, implementation, and monitoring should be reassessed regularly. In this reassessment the nurse should appraise a patient's clinical symptoms in the context of the efficacy of drug therapy. This should be done regularly throughout the course of therapy. It is also a dynamic process that should change to reflect the changes in a patient's status. As the patient's condition improves or worsens the

treatment plan (pharmacotherapy) should be changed to accommodate the new therapeutic needs of the patient. Neglecting the reassessment component of pharmacotherapy heightens the risk of inappropriate and ineffective therapy being rendered.

Exogenous Carcinogens

- Dietary customs
- Environmental pollution
- Food-production procedures
- Oncogenic viruses
- Food-processing procedures
- Smoking
- Drug abuse

TAKE HOME POINTS

Pharmacology
- Study of all interactions between drugs and living things.
- Drug origin, nature, chemistry, effects, and uses.
- Essential to understanding medicines and how they work.

Pharmacokinetics
- Involves drug absorption, distribution, metabolism, and excretion.
- Used to explain a drug's actions in the body, such as its onset, peak, and duration.

Pharmacodynamics
- Effects of drugs in the body (both biochemical and physical).
- Example = receptor stimulation by a drug and the resulting biologic response.
- The way the drug works = mechanism of action.

Pharmacotherapy
- Use of a drug to treat a disease.
- Includes assessment, implementation, monitoring, and reassessment.

Prophylactic Therapy
- Starting drug therapy based on prior knowledge and experience.
- Based on scientific knowledge and years of observation.

Drug Actions
- Its pharmaceutical, pharmacokinetic, and pharmacodynamic properties—each having a specific effect on the overall way a drug works within a patient.

Adverse Reactions
- Predictable and unpredictable.
- Iatrogenic, carcinogenic, and teratogenic.

Nurse's Role
- More than just the memorization of the names of pharmacologic agents, their use, and associated interventions.
- Requires a sound comprehension and application of this knowledge to a variety of clinical situations.

PHARMACOGNOSY

The source of all our early drugs was nature, and the study of these natural drug sources (plants and animals) is called pharmacognosy. Although many of our current drugs are synthetically derived, most were first isolated in nature. By studying the composition of the natural substance and its physiologic effects in living systems, researchers can identify the exact chemical features of a substance that produce the desired response. Armed with this knowledge they can then go to the laboratory and produce that exact substance, but devoid of the unwanted effects that many naturally occurring substances may have. So, although most new drug products are synthetic, the underlying principle of pharmacognosy is that an understanding of the actions and effects of natural drug sources is essential to new drug development. The principles of pharmacognosy have enabled us to isolate the naturally occurring hormone insulin, determine its exact genetic sequence, and synthesize that exact sequence over and over again. This has enabled us to make human insulin synthetically.

The four main sources for drugs, then, are plants, animals, minerals, and laboratory synthesis. An example of a plant from which a drug is derived is foxglove. It is the source of cardiac glycosides, and has yielded the present-day drug digoxin. The plant family (belladonna, poppy plant, etc.) also provides alkaloids, which are very useful and potent drugs. Examples include atropine (belladonna), caffeine (coffee), and nicotine (tobacco). Animals are the source of many of our hormone therapies. Premarin (conjugated estrogen) is derived from pregnant female horses, *pregnant mares*. Insulin is isolated from pigs and cows because the amino acid sequence of their insulin is very similar to that of ours. Heparin is another commonly used drug that is derived from cows and pigs (bovine and porcine heparin). Some common mineral sources of currently used drugs are salicylic acid, aluminum hydroxide, and sodium chloride. Recombinant DNA techniques provide many laboratory-derived drug products, such as erythropoietin (Epogen and Procrit), granulocyte-macrophage–colony stimulating factor (Sargramostim), granulocyte-colony stimulating factor (Filgrastim), and human insulin (Humulin and Novolin).

The interrelated pharmacologic principles of pharmacokinetics, pharmacodynamics, pharmacotherapeutics, toxicology, and pharmacognosy are essential to a sound understanding of pharmacology and the nursing practice. Medications are very powerful and effective. Without a thorough knowledge and appreciation of these principles, a potentially very useful treatment modality could become a very harmful and dangerous one in your hands. Therefore an understanding of pharmacologic principles ensures the provision of safe and effective drug therapy.

Critical Thinking A C T I V I T Y

1. To produce a desired effect, a drug must:
   a. Be completely metabolized by the GI tract and stomach.
   b. Undergo the first-pass effect in the liver.
   c. Be identifiable as a plasma protein or receptor.
   d. Have an appropriate concentration at its site of action.

BIBLIOGRAPHY

Chernow B: *The pharmacologic approach to the critically ill patient*, ed 3, Baltimore, 1994, Williams & Wilkins.

DiPiro JT et al: *Pharmacotherapy: a pathophysiologic approach*, ed 2, New York, 1992, Elsevier Science Publishing.

Fitzgerald M: Pharmacologic highlights. Principles of pharmacokinetics, *J Am Acad Nurse Pract* 6(12):581, 1994.

Johnson KB: *The Harriet Lane handbook*, ed 13, St Louis, 1993, Mosby.

Keen JH: *Critical care and emergency drug reference*, St Louis, 1994, Mosby.

Knoben JE, Anderson PO: *Handbook of clinical drug data*, ed 6, Hamilton, Ill, 1988, Drug Intelligence Publications.

McEvoy GK: *AHFS drug information*, Bethesda, Md, 1994, American Society of Hospital Pharmacists.

McKenry LM, Salerno E: *Mosby's pharmacology in nursing*, ed 19, St Louis, 1995, Mosby.

Skidmore-Roth L: *Mosby's 1995 nursing drug reference*, St Louis, 1995, Mosby.

Chapter 4

Neonatal, Pediatric, and Geriatric Considerations

Objectives

When you reach the end of this chapter, you will be able to:

1 Discuss how age can have an impact on the effects of medications in a patient, especially the pediatric or geriatric patient.

2 Identify specific age-related considerations to be borne in mind when administering medications to the pediatric or geriatric patient.

3 Develop a nursing care plan in the framework of the nursing process for the administration of medications to the pediatric or geriatric patient.

CHAPTER OUTLINE

Neonatal and Pediatric Considerations
  Physiology and pharmacokinetics
  Pharmacodynamics
  Dose calculations
Geriatric Considerations
  Polypharmacy and drug use
  Physiologic changes
  Pharmacokinetics
    Absorption
    Distribution
    Metabolism
    Excretion
  Problematic geriatric medications

Nursing Process
Assessment
Nursing Diagnoses
Planning
  Pediatric or geriatric goals
  Pediatric or geriatric outcome criteria
Implementation
Evaluation

Glossary

Geriatric (jer ē a′ trik) Pertaining to a person who is 65 years of age or older. (p. 28)

Polypharmacy (pol ē fahr′ mah sē) The use of many different drugs in treating a patient who may have one or several health problems. (p. 28)

Most of our experience with drugs and pharmacology has been gained from the adult population, and by far the greater majority of drug studies and articles on drugs have focused on the population between the ages of 13 and 65 years. To further compound the problem, it has been estimated that 75% of our currently approved drugs lack Food and Drug Administration approval for pediatric use and therefore lack specific dosage guidelines for use in neonates and children. Drug usage, however, extends far beyond just patients between 13 and 65 years of age. Most drugs are also effective in younger and older patients, but drugs oftentimes behave very differently in these patients at the opposite ends of the age spectrum. It is therefore vitally important from the standpoint of the safe and effective administration of drugs to understand what these differences are and how to adjust for them.

During the time from the beginning to the end of life, our bodies change in many ways. These changes have a dramatic effect on the pharmacokinetics (absorption, distribution, metabolism, and excretion) of drugs. The newborn, pediatric, and geriatric patient each has special needs, and these are discussed in this chapter. Drug therapy at the two ends of the spectrum of life is much more likely to result in adverse effects and toxicity. This is especially true if certain basic principles are not understood and followed.

NEONATAL AND PEDIATRIC CONSIDERATIONS

The definition of a *child* in terms of age is vastly different from that of a neonate or infant and therefore *child* (i.e., the age ranges) should not be mistakenly used to refer to a patient less than 2 years of age. Definitions of the terms used to refer to the patient are given in Table 4-1. This is the classification that applies throughout this chapter.

Physiology and Pharmacokinetics

The physiology unique to neonates accounts for most of the differences in the pharmacokinetic and pharmacodynamic behavior of drugs between neonates and adults. The immaturity of organs is the physiologic factor most responsible for these differences. The various physiologic characteristics of the neonatal population also apply to the pediatric population, but to a lesser extent. In both groups anatomic structures and physiologic systems and functions are still in the process of developing. The box on the next page lists those physiologic factors responsible for altering the pharmacokinetic properties of drugs.

Table 4-1	Classification of Young Patients	
AGE RANGE	**CLASSIFICATION**	
<38 wk gestation	Premature or preterm infant	
<1 mo old	Neonate or newborn infant	
1 mo to <2 yr old	Infant	
2 to <12 yr old	Child	

Pharmacodynamics

As just mentioned, drug actions, or pharmacodynamics, are altered in young patients and the maturity of various organs plays a role in how drugs act in the body. Certain drugs may be more toxic while others may be less toxic in young patients. Drugs that are more toxic in children are phenobarbital, morphine, and aspirin. Drugs that children tolerate the same as or better than adults are atropine, codeine, digoxin, and phenylephrine. The sensitivity of receptor sites may also vary with age, thus higher or lower doses are required depending on the drug. In addition, rapidly developing tissues may be more sensitive to certain drugs, and therefore smaller doses are required. Drugs may also be contraindicated during the growth years. For instance, tetracycline may discolor teeth, and corticosteroids may suppress growth.

Dose Calculations

Many drugs commonly used in adults have not been sufficiently investigated to ensure their safety and effectiveness in children. Most drugs administered in children are given on an empirical basis, with little in the way of formal studies supporting their use. Because newborns are small and immature in many respects, this makes them very susceptible to many insults. They lack many of the protective mechanisms that allow adults to resist these same stressors in the environment. The skin of young patients is thin and permeable, their stomachs lack acid to kill bacteria and other invaders, their lungs lack mucous barriers, their body temperatures are poorly regulated and they can easily become dehydrated, and their liver and kidneys are immature and cannot manage foreign substances as well as older patients. Because of such factors, the doses used in young patients must differ from those used in adults. Several formulas for calculating drug doses in young patients have been devised, as noted in the following:

PEDIATRIC CONSIDERATIONS
Pharmacokinetic Changes in the Neonate and Pediatric Patient

Absorption
- Gastric pH is less acidic because acid-producing cells in the stomach are immature until approximately 3 years of age.
- Gastric emptying is slowed because of slow or irregular peristalsis.
- First-pass elimination by liver is reduced due to immaturity of liver and reduced levels of microsomal enzymes.
- Topical absorption is faster because of a proportionally greater body surface area and thin skin.
- Intramuscular absorption is faster and irregular

Distribution
- Total body water (TBW) content is much greater: 65% to 75% more in infants and 85% more in premature infants than in adults.
- Fat content is less in young patients because of the greater TBW content.
- Protein binding is decreased because of decreased production of protein by immature liver.
- More drugs enter the brain because of an immature blood-brain barrier.

Metabolism
- The levels of microsomal enzymes are decreased because the immature liver has not yet started producing enough.
- Older children may have increased metabolism and require higher doses once hepatic enzymes are produced.
- There are many variables that affect metabolism in premature infants, infants, and children, including the status of liver enzyme production, genetic differences, and what the mother has been exposed to during pregnancy.

Kidney
- Glomerular filtration rate as well as tubular secretion and resorption are all decreased in young patients because of the immaturity of the kidney.
- Perfusion to the kidneys is often low, resulting in immature glomeruli and renal tubules and a shorter loop of Henle. This causes reduced renal function and concentrating ability.

Clark's rule
Based on Weight—for Children >2 years old

$$\frac{\text{Weight (in pounds)}}{150} \times \text{Adult dose} = \text{Child's dose}$$

Young's rule
Based on Age*—for Children >2 years old

$$\frac{\text{Age (in years)}}{\text{Age (in years)} + 12} \times \text{Adult dose} = \text{Child's dose}$$

Fried's rule
Based on Age—for Children <1 year old

$$\frac{\text{Age (in months)}}{150} \times \text{Adult dose} = \text{Child's dose}$$

Height and weight
Based on Body surface area†—for any Child

$$\frac{\text{Body surface area (m}^2)}{1.73 \text{ (m}^2)} \times \text{Adult dose} = \text{Child's dose}$$

These four methods are used to calculate a starting dose from which to work. Dose calculations based on the body surface area are the most accurate because this method takes into consideration the relationship between the child's height and weight and more precisely gauges the maturity of a child's organs and metabolic rate. Dose calculations based on weight alone make the assumption that a child is a miniature adult, which is incorrect.

The child's response to the dose calculated is ultimately the most important dosing tool, and titrating to the desired response should be the goal. The potential problems in younger patients are many, so dose calculations and the drug preparation should always be double-checked. Small mistakes can translate into far greater consequences in these fragile human systems.

To accurately administer medications to pediatric patients, their weight, height, or age, and the maturity of their organs (kidney and liver), along with their response to the medication, must all be taken into account. If this is done, the safe and effective administration of medications is assured.

GERIATRIC CONSIDERATIONS

Between the beginning and end of life, our bodies change in many ways. These changes have a dramatic effect on the pharmacokinetics of drugs. The geriatric

---

*Age is considered less desirable than the weight or body surface area as a basis to calculate a child's dose.
†Body surface area is considered more accurate than age or weight as the basis for dose calculations in pediatric patients.

GERIATRIC CONSIDERATIONS
Percentage of Population
Over the Age of 65

Year	Percentage >65 years
1900	4%
1990	12%
2000	20%

Risk of Polypharmacy-Induced Drug Interactions

No. of Drugs	Risk
2	6%
5	50%
8	100%

patient has special needs, and drug therapy at this end of the spectrum of life is much more likely to result in adverse effects and toxicity. This is especially true if certain basic principles are not understood and adhered to.

For the sake of the discussion here, a **geriatric** patient is defined as one 65 years of age or older. This segment of the population is growing at a dramatic pace (see box above). At the beginning of this century, geriatric persons constituted a mere 4% of the total population. At that time more people died of infections than of degenerative, chronic illnesses such as heart disease, cancer, and diabetes. As medical technology has advanced, so has our ability to prolong life, oftentimes by treating and curing illnesses that at one time people commonly died of. This has resulted in a growing population of older adults. Today patients over the age of 65 constitute 12% of the population. By the year 2000 it is estimated that this figure will increase to 20%. The elderly represent the fastest-growing segment of the population, increasing by about 2% a year. This is only expected to continue as new disease prevention and treatment methods are developed.

Polypharmacy and Drug Use

The growing aged population also consumes a larger proportion of all medications. It is estimated that the geriatric patient population consumes more than 25% of all the medications produced. For this and many physiologic reasons, the elderly are at a greater risk (three to seven times greater) for suffering adverse drug reactions and drug interactions. Over-the-counter (OTC) medications are primarily used by those over the age of 65. It has been estimated that 70% of all OTC medications are used by the geriatric population while only 10% of the adult population younger than 65 uses OTC medications. Not only does the geriatric population consume a greater proportion of prescription and OTC medications, they frequently take

multiple medications on a daily basis. One third of all persons in the geriatric age group take more than eight different drugs a day, and many take as much as 15. More than 80% of these patients have one or more chronic illnesses. In this age of medical specialization, patients may see several different physicians for their many illnesses. These different specialists may all prescribe medications for the illness they are treating, which often explains why a patient is taking 8 to 15 medications plus OTC drugs. This practice is called **polypharmacy**. The risk of drug interactions, adverse reactions, and potentially a hospitalization or prolonged hospitalization is far greater in this setting. As the number of medications a person takes increases so does the risk of a drug interaction (see box above). For example, a patient receiving two medications has approximately a 6% chance of suffering a drug interaction. This risk drastically increases as the number of drugs the patient is taking increases. A patient taking five medications has a 50% chance of a drug interaction. This chance rises to 100% if he or she is taking eight medications.

Along with the risk of drug interactions come multiple other risks—more hospitalizations for the treatment of adverse drug effects, greater likelihood of drug-induced falls that lead to hip fractures, and heightened risk of addiction are just a few. All of these are preventable. Recognizing polypharmacy in a patient and taking steps to reduce it by seeing to it that drugs are eliminated or changed or the dosages altered can dramatically lower the incidence of these undesirable drug effects.

Physiologic Changes

The physiologic changes that geriatric persons undergo also affect how many drugs act. An understanding of these physiologic changes and how they affect pharmacokinetics and pharmacodynamics (drug action) will help ensure the provision of safe and effective drug therapy.

As we progress in years, the body ages and the function of several organ systems slowly deteriorates

Table 4-2	Physiologic Changes in the Geriatric Patient
SYSTEM	**PHYSIOLOGIC CHANGE**
Cardiovascular	↓ Cardiac output = ↓ absorption and distribution ↓ Blood flow = ↓ absorption and distribution
Gastrointestinal	↑ pH (alkaline gastric secretions) ↓ Peristalsis = delayed gastric emptying
Hepatic	↓ Enzyme production = ↓ metabolism ↓ Blood flow = ↓ metabolism
Renal	↓ Blood flow = ↓ excretion ↓ Function = ↓ excretion ↓ Glomerular filtration rate = ↓ excretion

after many years of wear and tear. The collective physiologic changes associated with the aging process have a major effect on the disposition of drugs. Table 4-2 lists four of the most important body systems affected by the aging process.

These and other physiologic changes that take place in the elderly directly affect drug action. The sensitivity of the elderly patient to many drugs is altered as a result of these physiologic changes, and therefore drug usage should be adjusted to accommodate these changes. For instance, there is a general decrease in body weight, sometimes resulting in the elderly patient weighing the same as a child. However, the drug doses administered in the elderly are often the same as those administered to healthy adults. The criteria for drug doses in the elderly should therefore be based more on weight and less on age (i.e., adult versus pediatric doses).

Laboratory values are important to monitor in the elderly. They can serve as a gauge of organ function. The two most important organs from the standpoint of how drugs are broken down and eliminated are the liver and the kidneys.

Assessing kidney function—
  urine output: Blood urea nitrogen (BUN), and serum creatinine

Assessing liver function—liver
  enzymes: Aspartate aminotransferase (SGOT) and alanine aminotransferase (SGPT)

These laboratory values can help in the assessment of an elderly patient's ability to metabolize and eliminate medications.

GERIATRIC CONSIDERATIONS
Pharmacokinetic Changes in the Geriatric Patient

Absorption
- Gastric pH is less acidic because of a gradual reduction in the production of hydrochloric acid in the stomach.
- Gastric emptying is slowed because of a decline in muscle tone and motor activity.
- Movement throughout the gastrointestinal (GI) tract is slower because of decreased muscle tone and motor activity.
- Blood flow to GI tract is reduced by 40% to 50% because of decreased cardiac output and decreased blood flow.
- The absorptive surface area is decreased because the aging process blunts and flattens villi.

Distribution
- Total body water (TBW) content is decreased as body composition changes (ratio of fat to water increases).
- Fat content is increased because of decreased lean body mass and increased TBW content.
- Protein (albumin) binding sites are reduced because of decreased production of proteins by aging liver and reduced intake.

Metabolism
- The levels of microsomal enzymes are decreased because the capacity of the aging liver to produce them is reduced.
- Liver blood flow is reduced by approximately 1.5% per year after age of 25, decreasing hepatic metabolism.

Kidney
- Glomerular filtration rate is decreased by 40% to 50% primarily because of decreased blood flow.
- Number of intact nephrons is decreased.

Pharmacokinetics

The pharmacokinetic properties of absorption, distribution, metabolism, and excretion may be quite different in the elderly than in the younger adult. An awareness of these helps in the appropriate administration of drugs and monitoring of the geriatric patient taking medications. The box above lists the four pharmacokinetic phases and summarizes how they are altered by the aging process.

Absorption

Absorption in the elderly can be altered by many mechanisms. Advancing age not only results in a reduction in the absorption of nutrients from the elderly patient's diet but also in the absorption of drugs. There are several physiologic changes that account for this. There is a gradual reduction in the stomach's ability to produce hydrochloric acid, which results in a decrease in gastric acidity. This may alter the absorption of weakly acidic drugs like barbiturates and aspirin. The combination of decreased cardiac output and advancing atherosclerosis results in a general reduction in the flow of blood to major organs such as the stomach. By 65 years of age there is an approximate 50% reduction in blood flow to the gastrointestinal (GI) tract. Absorption, whether nutrient or drug, is dependent on good blood supply to the stomach and intestine. Once the drug is absorbed it must be carried by the bloodstream to its eventual site of action.

GI motility is important not only for moving substances out of the stomach but also for moving them throughout the GI tract. Muscle tone and motor activity in the GI tract are reduced, and this often results in constipation in geriatric patients, for which they frequently take laxatives. This use of laxatives may accelerate GI motility and reduce the absorption of drugs. One particular category of laxatives, the bulk-forming laxatives, has been shown to reduce the absorption of certain medications such as cardiac glycosides (digoxin). Bran and high-fiber foods may have the same effect. Another consequence of aging is an overall reduction in the absorptive surface area of the GI tract. The aging process also causes the villi to become flattened and blunted, reducing their overall absorptive capabilities.

Distribution

The distribution of medications throughout the body is vastly different in the elderly than it is in younger adults. There seems to be a gradual reduction in the total body water content with aging. Therefore the concentrations of highly water soluble drugs may be higher in geriatric patients because they have less water for them to be diluted in. The composition of the body also changes with aging. The lean muscle mass decreases, resulting in increased body fat. In both men and women there is an approximate 20% reduction in muscle mass between the ages of 25 to 65 years and a corresponding 20% increase in the fat content. Drugs such as hypnotics and sedatives that are primarily distributed to the fat will therefore have a prolonged effect.

Many drugs distributed by means of the blood are carried by proteins. By far the most important of these is albumin. Reduced protein concentrations, including that of albumin, result from aging. This may be due in part to reduced liver function, which produces many of these proteins, or to decreased intake or poor absorption despite adequate intake, or, to a combination of these factors. Whatever the cause, a reduced number of protein-binding sites for highly protein bound drugs results in higher levels of unbound drug. Drugs that are not bound to proteins are active. Therefore the effects of highly protein bound drugs may be enhanced if their doses are not adjusted in keeping with the albumin concentrations.

Metabolism

Metabolism declines with advancing age. The transformation of active drugs into inactive metabolites is primarily performed by the liver, but the liver slowly loses its ability to metabolize drugs effectively because the production of microsomal enzymes is reduced. There is also a reduction in blood flow to the liver because of reduced cardiac output and atherosclerosis. A reduction in the hepatic blood flow of approximately 1.5% per year occurs after the age of 25. All these factors contribute to prolonging the half-life of many drugs, which can potentially result in drug accumulation if drug intervals are not adjusted accordingly.

Excretion

The excretion of drugs is reduced in the geriatric population. A reduction in the glomerular filtration of 40% to 50% in the elderly combined with a reduction in blood flow, for the same reasons that apply to the liver, can result in extremely delayed drug excretion, and hence drug accumulation. Renal function should be monitored frequently in the elderly to prevent drug accumulation. Appropriate dose and interval adjustments can be made easily based on a patient's renal function, and the potentially dangerous complications that can result from inappropriate dosing can thereby be prevented.

Problematic Geriatric Medications

Drugs in certain classes are more likely to cause problems in the elderly because of many of the physiologic alterations and pharmacokinetic changes already discussed. Table 4-3 lists the most common problematic geriatric medications.

Knowledge of the physiologic changes in the elderly combined with an understanding of the various pharmacokinetic changes that occur is extremely useful in the management of the geriatric patient and can lead to improvements in drug therapy and thereby the prevention of unwanted consequences of inappropriate dosing.

Table 4-3	Problematic Geriatric Medications
MEDICATION	**COMMON GERIATRIC COMPLICATIONS**
Analgesics	
Opioids	Confusion, constipation, urinary retention, nausea, vomiting, and respiratory depression
NSAIDs	Edema, nausea, abdominal distress, gastric ulceration, and bleeding
Anticoagulants (heparin and coumadin)	Major and minor bleeding episodes, many drug interactions, and dietary interactions
Anticholinergics	Blurred vision, dry mouth, constipation, confusion, urinary retention, and tachycardia
Antihypertensives	Nausea, hypotension, diarrhea, bradycardia, and heart failure
Cardiac glycosides (digoxin)	Visual disorders, nausea, diarrhea, arrhythmias, hallucinations, decreased appetite, and weight loss
Sedatives and hypnotics	Confusion, daytime sedation, ataxia, lethargy, and increased forgetfulness
Thiazide diuretics	Electrolyte imbalance, rashes, fatigue, leg cramps, and dehydration

NSAIDs, nonsteroidal antiinflammatory drugs.

NURSING PROCESS

ASSESSMENT

Before administering any medication to a pediatric patient, a thorough health and medication history must be obtained that includes the patient's age, information on allergies to drugs and food, the medical and medication history (including adverse drug reactions), head-to-toe assessment findings, baseline vital signs, weight (important because many doses are calculated per kilogram of body weight), height, and level of growth and development. The prescriber's orders should be triple-checked because there is no room for error when working with pediatric patients.

General assessment data to be gathered in the elderly patient include age, allergies to drug and food, present and past medical and medication history (especially prescription and OTC medications being taken), results of renal and liver function studies, visual acuity, and cognitive or skill abilities. Just because patients appear to be alert does not mean they understand what you are saying or can self-administer medications without difficulty or without causing themselves harm.

You should assess the family support systems and the patient's ability to take medications safely. Whenever possible, always opt, unless ordered otherwise,

to use a nonpharmacologic approach to treatment in geriatric patients. The patient's financial status is also important to assess because this may affect compliance.

Other general questions that should be posed to both the pediatric patient (most likely to their caregiver or parent) and the geriatric patient include: Are there any chronic illnesses, nutritional problems, or GI tract disorders?, Are there certain attitudes toward medical treatment?, and What is ability of the patient or family to understand information about the medication, instructions concerning its use, and the importance of medication compliance?

NURSING DIAGNOSES

Nursing diagnoses related to the administration of medications to pediatric and geriatric patients include:

- Risk for injury to self related to side effects of medications;
- Risk for altered nutritional status related to either age (especially the elderly) or medication therapy.
- Risk for injury related to idiosyncratic reactions due to age.
- Knowledge deficit related to information about medications and their side effects or about when to contact the physician.

PLANNING
Pediatric or Geriatric Goals

Goals related to the pediatric or geriatric patient include:

- Patient will be free of complications associated with the adverse effects of medications.
- Patient will remain compliant (or take medication as prescribed with assistance) until medication is discontinued by physician.
- Patient (or caregiver/parent/legal guardian) will contact physician when appropriate as related to medication therapy.

Pediatric or Geriatric Outcome Criteria

Outcome criteria related to the administration of medications to the pediatric or geriatric patient include:
- Patient (or parent/legal guardian/caregiver) will state the importance of taking medication as prescribed (e.g., improved condition, decreased symptoms).
- Patient (or parent/legal guardian/caregiver) can follow instructions specific to the administration of the medication ordered (e.g., the special application of an ointment).
- Patient (or parent/legal guardian/caregiver) will state therapeutic and side effects of specific medication therapy.
- Patient will show improvement in condition related to compliance and successful medication therapy.
- Patient will take or receive medications safely and without injury.
- Patient (or parent/legal guardian/caregiver) can state specific situations when the physician must be contacted (e.g., occurrence of fever, pain, vomiting, rash or diarrhea, worsening of condition, bronchospasms, dyspnea).

IMPLEMENTATION

Always practice the five "rights" concerning the administration of medications and follow the label and medication instructions. Patients should be encouraged to take medications as directed and not to discontinue them, "double-up" on doses, or take any OTC medications unless they clear this with the prescriber *first*! In general, when it comes to pediatric or geriatric patients, be sure the patient, parents, or caregiver understands instructions specific to the medication and that all medications should be kept out of the reach of small children. Provide written and oral instructions concerning the drug name, action, purpose, dose, time of administration, route, side effects, safety of administration, storage, and interactions, and any cautions about or contraindications to its use. Specific guidelines for administration are given in Chapter 7

TAKE HOME POINTS

Age-Related Pharmacokinetic Effect
- Dramatic differences in drug absorption, distribution, metabolism, and excretion at the beginning and end of life.
- At one end neonates and pediatrics; at the other end geriatric patients.

Preterm, Newborn, Infant, and Child
- Preterm = <38 weeks.
- Newborn = <1 month.
- Infant = 1 month to <2 years.
- Child = 2 to <12 years.

Dose Calculations in Children
- Based on *weight* = *CLARK's rule*.
- Based on *age* = *YOUNG's rule and FRIED's rule*.
- Based on *height and weight* = *body surface area*.

Geriatric Patients
- >65 years of age.
- In 1990, 12% of total population; in 2000, 20% of total population.
- Fastest-growing segment of the population.
- Consume >25% of all medications and >70% of OTC medications.

Polypharmacy
- One patient may have several illnesses and be taking many drugs.
- Drastically increases the risk of drug interactions, adverse reactions, and hospitalization.
- One patient on five medications has 50% chance of a drug interaction, a 100% chance if on eight.

Nurse's Role
- Nurse must be well informed and knowledgeable about growth and development principles and the effects of various agents during each life phase and in various phases of illness.
- Always follow the five "rights" of medication administration to prevent drug errors and harm to patients of all ages.
- Thorough patient education for all involved in the patient's care should include written and oral instructions.

and are discussed throughout the book where appropriate.

EVALUATION

In general, when dealing with pediatric or geriatric patients, the nurse should be constantly observing for the expected effects of the medication. Side effects should also be watched for, and the nurse should know when the effects represent toxicity or overdosage and inform the prescriber immediately. The patient, parent, legal guardian, or caregiver should also be aware of these.

Critical Thinking **A C T I V I T Y**

1. Select one of the following drugs, phenytoin or tetracycline, and discuss its potential risks to the fetus or breast-feeding newborn in relation to the needed benefits to the mother.

BIBLIOGRAPHY

Chernow B: *The pharmacologic approach to the critically ill patient*, ed 3, Baltimore, 1994, Williams & Wilkins.

Cohen M: Medication errors, *Nursing, 94* 24(2):17, 1994.

DiPiro JT et al: *Pharmacotherapy: a pathophysiologic approach*, ed 2, New York, 1992, Elsevier Science Publishing.

Johnson KB: *The Harriet Lane handbook*, ed 13, St Louis, 1993, Mosby.

Keen JH: *Critical care and emergency drug reference*, St Louis, 1994, Mosby.

Lilley LL, Guanci R: Med errors, *AJN* 95(5): 1995.

McEvoy GK: *AHFS drug information*, Bethesda, Md, 1994, American Society of Hospital Pharmacists.

McKenry LM, Salerno E: *Mosby's pharmacology in nursing*, ed 19, 1995, Mosby.

Raju T et al: Medication errors in neonatal and pediatric intensive care units: a quality assurance, *Lancet* 2:4, 1989.

Skidmore-Roth L: *Mosby's 1995 nursing drug reference*, St Louis, 1995, Mosby.

Chapter 5

Legal, Ethical, and Cultural Considerations

Objectives

When you reach the end of this chapter, you will be able to:

1 Identify various drug legislation passed at the state and federal levels.
2 Discuss the impact of drug legislation on drug therapy and nursing.
3 Provide examples of the scheduled categories for controlled substances.
4 Identify the process involved in the development of new drugs, including investigational new drug application, phases of investigational drug studies, and informed consent.
5 Discuss the nurse's role in the development of new and investigational drugs.
6 Discuss the ethical aspects of drug administration and the nurse's role.
7 Explain the effect of culture on a patient's response to and compliance with drug therapy.

CHAPTER OUTLINE

U.S. Drug Legislation
  The Pure Food and Drug Act of 1906
  The Food, Drug, and Cosmetic Act of 1938
  1952: The Durham-Humphrey Amendment of the 1938 Act
  1962: The Kefauver-Harris Amendment of the 1938 Act
  1970: The Comprehensive Drug Abuse Prevention and Control Act
New Drug Development
  Investigational new drug application
  Informed consent
  Phases of investigational drug studies
    Phase I
    Phase II
    Phase III
    Phase IV
  New drug application
  Expedited drug approval
Canadian Legislation
  Canadian Food and Drugs Act
  Canadian Narcotic Control Act
Nursing Implications
  Legal issues
  Ethical practice
  Cultural aspects

Glossary

Blinded investigational drug study A research method in which the subject taking the drug under study is purposely unaware of a key element or elements in the study (e.g., which administered substance is the drug under study versus a *placebo*). This method eliminates bias on the part of the subject. (p. 38)

Canadian Food and Drugs Act Amended many times since its inception in 1953, this act is the main piece of drug legislation in Canada. It protects consumers from contaminated, adulterated, or unsafe drugs and unsafe labeling practices; and addresses appropriate advertising and selling of drugs, food, cosmetics, or devices. (p. 38)

Canadian Narcotic Control Act of 1961 Addresses the possession, sale, manufacture, production, and distribution of narcotics. It was enacted in response to increasing misuse and abuse of drugs in the mid-to-late 1960s. (p. 39)

Controlled Substance Act of 1970 Also known as the Comprehensive Drug Abuse Prevention and Control Act, it promotes research on drug abuse; the prevention of drug abuse through education, treatment, and rehabilitation for drug-addicted persons; and enhancement of law enforcement. It also created the classification system for *controlled substances* that is used to regulate the manufacture, distribution, and dispensing of drugs. (p. 36)

Double-blind, placebo-controlled study A research method in which both the investigator and subject are purposely unaware of key elements in the study (e.g., which administered substance is the drug under study versus a *placebo*). This method eliminates bias on the part of both the investigator and the subject. (p. 38)

Durham-Humphrey Amendment of 1952 A modification of the Food, Drug, and Cosmetic Act of 1938 that differentiated between prescription (i.e., *legend*) drugs and *over-the-counter* medications and medications that could and could not be refilled without another prescription, as well as identified which original prescriptions and refills could be authorized over the telephone. (p. 36)

Expedited drug approval A hastening of the usual investigational new drug approval process by the Food and Drug Administration and pharmaceutical companies in response to a public health threat (e.g., AIDS). Drugs showing promise in phase I and II clinical trials are given to qualified patients, and the drug approval process is shortened if the drug continues to show promise. (p. 38)

Food, Drug, and Cosmetic Act of 1938 This act required drug manufacturers to apply for an investigational new drug exemption for a safety review before marketing new drugs. (p. 36)

Informed consent Permission obtained from a patient consenting to the performance of a specific test or procedure. Informed consent is required before most invasive procedures can be performed and before a patient can be admitted into a research study. The document must be written in a language understood by the patient and be dated and signed by the patient and at least one witness. Included in the document are clear, rational descriptions of the procedure or test. Also required is a statement that care will not be withheld if the patient does not consent to this; informed consent is voluntary. By law, informed consent must be obtained more than a given number of days or hours before certain procedures are performed and must always be obtained when the patient is fully mentally competent. (p. 37)

Investigational new drug A drug approved for marketing by the Food and Drug Administration and available only for use in experiments to determine its safety and efficacy. (p. 37)

Kefauver-Harris Amendment of 1962 This act required drugs to be proved both safe and effective before being granted an approved status. Because of this act many drugs found to be ineffective have been removed from the market. (p. 36)

Legend drugs Another name for prescription drugs. The Durham-Humphrey Amendment required that prescription drug labels include the legend stating, ''Caution—Federal law prohibits dispensing without prescription.'' (p. 36)

New drug application Once a drug successfully completes the first three phases of an investigational new drug study, the drug manufacturer may submit a new drug application to the Food and Drug Administration. If this application is approved, the company may sell the drug exclusively. (p. 38)

Over-the-counter drugs Drugs that are available to consumers without a prescription. Also called *nonprescription drugs*. (p. 36)

Placebo (plĕ sē′ bō) An inactive substance (e.g., saline, distilled water, or sugar) or a less-than-effective dose of a harmless substance (e.g., a water-soluble vitamin). Placebos are used in experimental drug studies to compare the ''effects'' of the inactive substance with the bona fide effects of the experimental drug. They are also prescribed to satisfy the requests of patients who cannot be given the medication they request or who, in the judgment of the health care provider, do not need this medication. (p. 38)

Pure Food and Drug Act of 1906 The first federal law that attempted to protect the public from dangerous, adulterated, and mislabeled products. It established the *United States Pharmacopeia* and *The National Formulary* and gave the federal government authority to enforce the standards these contained. The act applied only to drugs sold in interstate commerce. (p. 35)

U.S. DRUG LEGISLATION

Up until the beginning of the 20th century there were no federal rules and regulations to protect consumers from the dangers of medications. Not until numerous devastating drug-induced catastrophes occurred did the government intervene. The first act passed by the federal government in response to these catastrophes was the **Pure Food and Drug Act**, passed in 1906. Since 1906, several acts have been passed to further ensure the safe and effective use of drugs. This federal legislation protects the public from drugs that are impure, toxic, or ineffective, or that have not been tested before public sale. The primary purpose of this federal legislation is to ensure safety. A brief understanding of the most important acts provides both an overview of the past and a view into the possible future of drug development and usage.

The Pure Food and Drug Act of 1906

In 1906 the federal government passed the Pure Food and Drug Act to protect the public from adulterated or mislabeled drugs. It required drug companies to declare on the package label the presence of identified dangerous and possibly addicting drugs. This act designated *The United States Pharmacopeia* and *The National Formulary* as official standards for therapeutic use, patient safety, quality, purity, strength, packaging safety, and dosage form. ''USP'' can be put after the names of drugs that meet these standards. This act also empowered the federal government to enforce these standards and to take legal action against those companies that do not comply with the provisions of the act.

The Food, Drug, and Cosmetic Act of 1938

There were several shortcomings to the 1906 act that resulted in new legislation. The Food and Drug Act only specified that drug labeling not contain false or misleading claims about the therapeutic benefits of a particular drug. It did not address the issue of proper testing for safety before a drug could be marketed. In 1937 more than 100 deaths occurred as a result of the

Table 5-1	Controlled Substances: Schedule Categories		
SCHEDULE	**ABUSE POTENTIAL**	**MEDICAL USE**	**DEPENDENCY**
C-I	High	None	Severe
C-II	High	Accepted	Severe physical and/or psychologic
C-III	<C-II	Accepted	Moderate/low physical or high psychologic
C-IV	<C-III	Accepted	Limited physical or psychologic
C-V	<C-IV	Accepted	Limited physical or psychologic

ingestion of a diethyleneglycol solution of sulfanilamide. This product had been marketed as an "elixir of sulfanilamide" without its toxicity being investigated. This stimulated the government to enact The **Food, Drug, and Cosmetic Act of 1938**, which prohibited the marketing of new drugs before proper testing of their safety had been done. Now pharmaceutical companies had to submit an investigational new drug exemption to the government for review of a drug's safety before it could sell the product.

1952: The Durham-Humphrey Amendment of the 1938 Act

To provide further safety to the consumers of drugs, The **Durham-Humphrey Amendment** was passed. This amendment distinguished between drugs that could be sold with or without a prescription and identified those that should not be refilled without a new prescription. Drugs for which a prescription is needed before they can be sold are called **legend drugs** because the labels have to carry the legend: "Caution—Federal law prohibits dispensing without a prescription." These drugs are also called *prescription drugs*. Drugs for which a prescription is not needed are referred to as *nonprescription* or **over-the-counter** (OTC) **drugs**. This act also specified that certain drugs such as narcotics, hypnotics, and tranquilizers could not be refilled without a new prescription from a physician.

1962: The Kefauver-Harris Amendment of the 1938 Act

The **Kefauver-Harris Amendment** came into being partly because of concern on the part of a senator from Tennessee and also in response to the thalidomide tragedy. In 1958 Senator Estes Kefauver began a Senate investigation into the drug industry. Drug companies were making huge profits through the use of false or misleading promotions. Not much attention was paid to Senator Kefauver's concerns until the thalidomide tragedy occurred in Europe. Thalidomide

was a widely used sedative-hypnotic marketed in Europe at this time that was found to cause severe deformities in the babies of mothers who took the drug during pregnancy. The European thalidomide experience prompted the United States to enact the Kefauver-Harris Amendment of 1962. Before 1962 the safety but not the efficacy of a new drug had be proved prior to its approval and marketing. After this amendment was passed, both safety and efficacy had to be proved before a new drug could be approved for use.

1970: The Comprehensive Drug Abuse Prevention and Control Act

Much like the previous acts, The Comprehensive Drug Abuse Prevention and Control Act was enacted by Congress in response to the growing misuse and abuse of drugs in the middle and late 1960s. This act is also known as The **Controlled Substance Act** and was designed to address the problem of drug abuse at this time. It promoted drug education and research into the prevention and treatment of drug dependence, strengthened enforcement authority, established treatment and rehabilitation facilities, and designed schedules or categories for controlled substances. These categories of drugs were defined according to their abuse potential and are listed in Table 5-1. Each controlled substance category has specific dispensing restrictions, which are listed in Table 5-2. Examples of drugs that fall into the various controlled substance categories are given in Table 5-3.

NEW DRUG DEVELOPMENT

The research into and development of new drugs is an ongoing process in the pharmaceutical industry, a multibillion-dollar industry that must continuously develop new and better drugs to maintain their competitive edge. The research required for the development of new and better drugs may take several years. Hundreds of substances are isolated that never make

Table 5-2	Controlled Substances: Dispensing Restrictions
SCHEDULE	**DISPENSING RESTRICTIONS**
C-I	■ Only with approved protocol
C-II	■ Written prescription only (if telephoned in, need written prescription within 24 hours) ■ No prescription refills ■ Container must have warning label
C-III	■ Written or oral prescription that expires in 6 months ■ No more than 5 refills in 6-month period ■ Container must have warning label
C-IV	■ Written or oral prescription that expires in 6 months ■ No more than 5 refills in 6-month period ■ Container must have warning label
C-V	■ Written prescription or over-the-counter varies with each state law

Table 5-3	Controlled Substances: Categories and Examples
SCHEDULE	**EXAMPLES**
C-I	Heroin, LSD, marijuana, mescaline, peyote, psilocybin, and methaqualone
C-II	Codeine, cocaine, hydromorphone, meperidine, morphine, oxycodone, methadone, secobarbital, pentobarbital, amphetamine, methylphenidate, and others
C-III	Codeine, hydrocodone, oxycodone, morphine, and dihydrocodeine combination products; paregoric and nonnarcotic preparations of pentazocine and propoxyphene
C-IV	Barbital, phenobarbital, chloral hydrate, meprobamate, fenfluramine, the benzodiazepines (e.g., diazepam, temazepam, lorazepam), dextropropoxyphene, pentazocine, and others
C-V	Medications generally for relief of coughs or diarrhea containing limited quantities of certain opioid controlled substances

it to market. Once a potentially beneficial drug has been isolated, there is a very regulated and systematic process that the pharmaceutical company must go through before the drug can be used in the open market). This highly sophisticated and systematic process is regulated and carefully monitored by the United States Food and Drug Administration (FDA), whose primary purpose is to ensure patient safety. Drug efficacy is also a top concern.

This system of drug research and development is one of the most stringent in the world. There are many benefits and drawbacks to it. It was developed out of concern for patient safety and drug efficacy. To ensure that these two very important objectives are met with some degree of certainty requires much time and paperwork. This is the downside to the system. Many drugs are marketed and used in foreign countries long before they get approval for use in the United States. However, many drug-related tragedies are averted by this strict system, as the thalidomide tragedy that occurred in Europe but not in the United States proves. There must be a balance between making new lifesaving therapies available and protecting consumers from potential drug-induced adverse effects.

Investigational New Drug Application

A pharmaceutical company must prove both the safety and efficacy of a newly isolated drug before it

can be used in the general population. Testing begins in animal models. The new medication must be tested for its pharmacologic use, dosage ranges, and possible toxic effects. After extensive animal testing that proves the safety and efficacy of the new drug, the pharmaceutical company can then submit an application for an **investigational new drug** (IND). Only after the FDA reviews and approves this application can the pharmaceutical company proceed with investigational studies of the IND in human subjects. There are four phases to this clinical evaluation process in human subjects. The collective goal of these phases is to provide information on the safety, toxicity, efficacy, potency, bioavailability, and purity of the IND. Informed consent must be obtained of all patients before they can be enrolled in an IND study.

Informed Consent

Informed consent involves the careful explanation of the purpose of the study, procedures to be used, and risks involved. Participants in experimental drug studies should be informed volunteers and not uninformed, coerced subjects. Some patients may have unrealistic expectations of the IND's usefulness. Often they have the misconception that because an investigational drug is ''new,'' it must automatically be better than existing forms of therapy. To prevent any bias introduced by such thinking, many studies are designed to incorporate a **placebo**. A placebo is an inert substance that is not a drug. An example of one is normal saline. A study incorporating a placebo is called a *placebo-controlled study*. It attempts to eliminate any bias that an IND study volunteer may have toward the new drug. Other volunteers may be reluctant to enter the study because they think they will be treated like "guinea pigs." Whatever the circumstances of the study, the study volunteers must be informed of all the potential hazards as well as the possible benefits of the new therapy. It should be stressed to the study volunteer that involvement in IND studies is truly voluntary and that the subject can quit the study at any time.

Phases of Investigational Drug Studies

Phase I

Phase I studies involve small numbers of healthy volunteers as opposed to volunteers afflicted with the disease or ailment that the new drug is meant to treat. The purpose of these studies is to determine the optimal dosage range and the pharmacokinetics of the drug (absorption, distribution, metabolism, and excretion). Also performed are blood tests, urinalyses, assessments of vital signs, and specific monitoring tests.

Phase II

Phase II studies involve small numbers of volunteers that have the disease or ailment the drug is supposed to diagnose or treat. Study participants are closely monitored for the drug's effectiveness and any side effects. If no serious side effects occur, the study can progress to phase III.

Phase III

Phase III studies involve large numbers of patients at medical research centers. The purpose of this larger sample size is to provide information about infrequent or rare adverse effects that may have been selected out in the studies consisting of small numbers of patients. Information obtained during this clinical phase helps to identify any risks associated with the new drug. Placebo-controlled studies are employed during this phase to eliminate any patient bias. To eliminate any bias on the part of the investigator, he or she is also **blinded** to the identity of the investigational substance. Neither the investigator nor the study subject knows whether the drug being administered is a placebo or the IND. This type of study is called a **double-blind, placebo-controlled study**. The three objectives of this phase are to establish the drug's clinical effectiveness, safety, and dosage range.

Phase IV

Phase IV studies are postmarketing studies voluntarily conducted by the pharmaceutical companies to obtain further proof of the therapeutic effects of the new drug. Often these studies compare the safety and efficacy of the new drug with that of another drug in the same therapeutic category. An example would be a comparison of a new NSAID (nonsteroidal anti-inflammatory drug) with ibuprofen in the treatment of osteoarthritis. Some medications make it through all phases of clinical trials without any problems, but not until they are used in the general population do severe adverse effects show up.

New Drug Application

After the first three phases are completed, the FDA reviews all the results. If these are favorable, the pharmaceutical company may submit a **new drug application** (NDA). Once the FDA has reviewed and approved the NDA, the pharmaceutical company is free to market the new drug exclusively.

Expedited Drug Approval

The FDA has attempted to make lifesaving investigational drug therapies available to the population sooner by offering an **expedited drug approval** process. The public health threat posed by the acquired immunodeficiency syndrome (AIDS) has motivated the FDA and pharmaceutical companies to shorten the IND approval process, allowing physicians to give qualified AIDS patients medications that have shown promise during early phase I and II clinical trials. If the drug then continues to show favorable results, the overall process of drug approval is hastened as much as possible.

CANADIAN LEGISLATION

In Canada concerns over the sale and use of foods, drugs, cosmetics, and medical devices began long before these concerns did in the United States. Canadian drug legislation began in 1875 when the Parliament of Canada passed an act to prevent the sale of adulterated food, drink, and drugs. Since that time foods and drugs have been controlled on a national basis.

Canadian Food and Drugs Act

The **Canadian Food and Drugs Act** is the main piece of legislation concerning drugs in Canada. The act has been amended several times since its beginning in 1953 and has two main purposes. The first purpose is to protect the consumer from drugs that are contaminated, adulterated, or unsafe for use. It also addresses drugs that are labeled falsely, may be misleading, or are deceptive. To determine if drugs comply with this act, one of six recognized pharmacopeias and formularies can be used as a reference. These are listed in one of the many "schedules" contained in this act, Schedule B. The references contained in Schedule B are listed below:

- Pharmacopoeia Internationalis
- The United States Pharmacopeia/National Formulary
- British Pharmaceutical Codex
- The British Pharmacopoeia
- Pharmacopée Française
- The Canadian Formulary

The second purpose of the Canadian Food and Drugs Act is to address appropriate advertising and selling of drugs, food, cosmetics, and devices. The Act stipulates that no food, drug, cosmetic, or device is to be advertised or sold to the general public as a treatment, preventive, or cure for certain diseases listed in Schedule A of the Act. Some examples of these diseases are alcoholism, arteriosclerosis, and cancer. When a drug meets these standards it is labeled with the legend *Canadian Standard Drug*, or CSD, on its inner and outer labels.

This particular Act has many more amendments or schedules that have been added over the years.

Table 5-4	Additional Schedules to the Canadian Food and Drug Act
SCHEDULE	**DESCRIPTION**
Schedules C and D	Drugs in these schedules must list where the drug was manufactured and the process and conditions of manufacturing.
Schedule F	List of drugs that can be sold and refilled only on prescription; refills cannot exceed 6 mo; labels on these drugs are marked *Pr*, or prescription required. *Examples:* Antibiotics, hormones, and tranquilizers
Schedule G	These drugs, also known as controlled drugs, affect the CNS; identified by *C* on the label. *Examples:* Amphetamines, barbiturates, and phenmetrazine
Schedule H	These are restricted drugs; only available to institutions for research; have dangerous physiologic and psychologic side effects; have no recognized medical use.

Some of the more important ones are listed in Table 5-4.

Canadian Narcotic Control Act

The regulations that address the possession, sale, manufacture, production, and distribution of narcotics are covered in the **Canadian Narcotic Control Act**. This act was passed in 1961 and replaced the previous act, the Canadian Opium and Narcotic Act of 1952. The Canadian Narcotic Control Act is similar in its purpose to the Comprehensive Drug Abuse Prevention and Control Act of 1970 in the United States, which was enacted in response to the growing misuse and abuse of drugs in the middle and late 1960s.

The administrative responsibility for this Act belongs to the Department of National Health and Welfare. The enforcement of this Act belongs to the members of the Royal Canadian Mounted Police.

NURSING IMPLICATIONS
Legal Issues

It is within the framework of the standards of nursing care and nurse practice acts that the nurse's role and responsibility are defined. Besides these standards, there are specific institutional policies and procedures with which nurses must be familiar to fulfill their legal obligation and responsibility to their patients. Some of the legal issues and concepts are listed and defined in the box on p. 40. The five "rights" of medication and the law provide necessary standards for safe patient care and should never be ignored. The law should be viewed as helpful and as a framework for practice, not as an impediment to care.

Ethical Practice

Ethical nursing practice is based on the basic ethical principles of beneficence, nonmalfeasance, autonomy, veracity, integrity, and justice. These basic principles are defined in the box on p. 40. The American Nurses Association Code of Ethics for nurses (see box on p. 40) should be a familiar framework of practice to all nurses and serve as an ethical guideline for nursing care. These ethical principles and code of ethics ensure that the nurse is acting on behalf of the patient and with his or her best interest at heart.

As a professional, the nurse has the responsibility to provide safe nursing care to patients regardless of the setting, person, group, community, or family involved. Although it is not within the nurse's realm of ethical and professional responsibility to impose his or her own values or standards on the patient, it is within his or her realm to provide information and assist the patient in facing decisions regarding health care.

(Text continued on p. 42.)

LEGAL/ETHICAL PRINCIPLES
Legal Issues and Concepts

1. Standards of care: Definitions of the specific standards of care that professional nurses must provide.
2. Nurse practice acts: Acts that establish educational requirements for professional nurses and distinguish between nursing and medical practice; they vary from state to state.
3. Licensure: All registered nurses must be licensed by the state board of nursing before they can practice nursing. The licensure process requires a registered nurse to pass the National Council Licensure Examinations.
4. Tort: A civil wrong committed against a person or property. An example of an unintentional tort is malpractice; an example of intentional tort is invasion of privacy.
5. Negligence: Conduct that falls below the established standard of care.
6. Malpractice: Professional misconduct and lack of skill in the performance of professional duties or tasks that is established if the following can be proved: The nurse owed a duty to the client; the nurse did not carry out the specific duty; the client was injured, and the injury was the result of the nurse's failure to carry out the specific duty.

LEGAL/ETHICAL PRINCIPLES
Ethical Principles and Nursing Implications

1. Beneficence: The doing or active promotion of good; implications include "how the patient is best served."
2. Nonmalfeasance: The duty to do no harm to a client; implications include avoiding doing any deliberate harm while rendering nursing care.
3. Autonomy: Self-determination and ability to act on one's own; implications include promoting a patient's decision-making process, supporting informed consent, and assisting in decisions or making a decision when a patient is posing harm to himself or herself.
4. Justice: Being fair or equal in one's actions; implications include the fair distribution of resources for the care of the patient and determination of when to treat.
5. Veracity: Duty to tell the truth; implications include telling the truth with regard to investigational new drugs and informed consent.
6. Confidentiality: The duty to respect privileged information about a patient; implications include not talking about a patient in public or outside the context of the health care setting.

American Nurses Association Code of Ethics

■ The nurse provides services with respect for human dignity and the uniqueness of the patient unrestricted by considerations of social or economic status, personal attributes, or the nature of health problems.

■ The nurse safeguards the patient's right to privacy by judiciously protecting information of a confidential nature.

■ The nurse acts to safeguard the patient and the public when health care and safety are affected by the incompetent, unethical, or illegal practice of any person.

■ The nurse assumes responsibility and accountability for individual nursing judgments and actions.

■ The nurse maintains competence in nursing.

■ The nurse exercises informed judgment and uses individual competence and qualifications as criteria in seeking consultation, accepting responsibilities, and delegating nursing activities to others.

■ The nurse participates in activities that contribute to the ongoing development of the profession's body of knowledge.

■ The nurse participates in the profession's efforts to implement and improve standards of nursing.

■ The nurse participates in the profession's efforts to establish and maintain conditions of employment conducive to high-quality nursing care.

■ The nurse participates in the profession's effort to protect the public from misinformation and misrepresentaiton and to maintain the integrity of nursing.

■ The nurse collaborates with members of the health professions and other citizens in promoting community and national efforts to meet the health needs of the public.

From American Nurses Association: *Code for nurses with interpretive statements*, Kansas City, Mo, 1985, The Association.

Canadian Nurses Association Code of Ethics

The body of the code is divided into the following sources of nursing obligations:

Patients

- A nurse is obliged to treat patients with respect for their individual needs and values.
- Based on respect for patients and regard for their rights to control their own care, nursing care should reflect respect for the clients' right of choice.
- The nurse is obliged to hold confidential all information about a patient learned in the health care setting.
- The nurse has an obligation to be guided by consideration for the dignity of patients.
- The nurse is obliged to represent the ethics of nursing before colleagues and others.
- The nurse is obliged to advocate all patients' interests.
- In all professional settings, including education, research, and administration, the nurse retains a commitment to the welfare of patients. The nurse has an obligation to act in a fashion that will maintain trust in nurses and nursing.

Health Team

- Patient care should represent a cooperative effort, drawing on the expertise of nursing and other health professions. By acknowledging personal or professional limitations, the nurse recognizes the perspective and expertise of colleagues from other disciplines.
- The nurse, as a member of the patient's health care team, is obliged to take steps to ensure that the patient receives competent and ethical medical and nursing care.

Social Context of Nursing

- Conditions of employment should contribute to patient care and to the professional satisfaction of nurses. Nurses are obliged to work toward securing and maintaining conditions of employment that satisfy these goals.

Responsibilities of the Profession

- Professional nurses' organizations recognize a responsibility to clarify, secure, and sustain ethical nursing conduct. The fulfillment of these tasks requires professional organizations to remain responsive to the rights, needs, and interests of patients and nurses.

From Canadian Nurses Association: *Code of ethics for nursing*, Ottawa, 1985, The Association.

LEGAL-ETHICAL PRINCIPLES

It is crucial to remember that a nurse cannot legally administer any medication without a prescriber's order, even in the case of placebo therapy. Even though a placebo may work effectively, its administration should never be taken "lightly." Placebos are often ordered for unusual situations and often when there are limited options available. Most prescribers who honor an open and honest relationship with their patients will write a placebo order only when it is necessary and when they have explained the rationale behind the decision. This is often an ethical dilemma for the nurse, but nurses usually agree and choose to administer the placebo after all other viable alternatives have been used.

McKenry L, Salerno E: *Pharmacology in nursing*, ed 19, St Louis, 1995, Mosby.

CULTURAL IMPLICATIONS
Cultural Practices

CULTURE	PRACTICE
Western	Increased participation in health care; demand more explanation about diseases and treatment, as well as the prevention of diseases.
Asian	Believe in traditional medicine and use physicians and herbalists in their health care.
African	Persons of African ancestry in the West Indies, Haiti, Jamaica, and Dominican Republic as well as natives of the continent of Africa practice folk medicine and also employ "root workers" as healers.
European	Traditional health beliefs are held, and there are some persons who still practice folk medicine.

The nurse also has the right to refuse to participate in any treatment or aspect of a patient's care that violates personal ethical principles. However, this should be done without deserting the patient. Should this situation arise, it is the nurse's responsibility to inform the appropriate persons about the conflict and to transfer the patient to the safe care of another professional nurse before the start of treatment.

It is a nurse's responsibility to always provide the highest-quality nursing care and practice within the standards of care. The American Nurses Association Code of Ethics and the previously mentioned ethical principles should constitute the framework for the professional practice of nursing.

Cultural Aspects

A patient's cultural background is another important variable to be considered in a patient's nursing care and in the administration of medications. Cultural factors are important to holistic nursing care because they affect the patient's health, health beliefs, and health care practices, including drug therapy. Some examples of cultural influences are presented in the box on p. 41. The nurse needs to acknowledge and accept the influences of a patient's cultural beliefs, values, and customs to prevent a conflict from arising between the goals of nursing and health care and the dictates of a patient's cultural background.

TAKE HOME POINTS

The Food and Drug Act of 1906
- Enacted to protect public from adulterated or mislabeled drugs.
- Designated the *United States Pharmacopeia* and the *National Formulary* as official standards for therapeutic use, patient safety, quality, purity, strength, packaging safety, and dosage form.

The Durham-Humphrey Amendment
- Specified which drugs need a prescription to be sold and which do not.
- Do need a prescription = legend drugs; do not need a prescription = over-the-counter drugs.

The Controlled Substance Act
- Passed in 1971 in response to growing misuse and abuse of drugs in the middle and late 1960s.
- Provides for increased research into, and prevention of, drug abuse and "drug dependence."
- Provides for treatment and rehabilitation of drug abusers and drug-dependent persons.
- Strengthens law enforcement authority.
- Controlled substances schedule (C-I through C-V).
- C-I = high abuse potential and no medical use.
- C-V = low abuse potential and accepted medical use.

Informed Consent
- Careful explanation of the purpose of a study.
- Describes procedures used and risk involved.
- Informed volunteers are not uninformed, coerced subjects.

FDA Drug Approval Process
- IND = investigation new drug; NDA = new drug application.
- Clinical phases I, II, and III (to determine safety, dose, and efficacy).
- Experimental phases = IND phases I, II, and III; put on market if NDA approved by FDA.
- Takes several years.

Canadian Food and Drugs Act
- Main piece of drug legislation in Canada.
- Enacted to protect consumer from adulterated or mislabeled drugs.
- Regulates advertising and selling of drugs, food, cosmetics, or devices.

Nurse's Role
- The five "rights" of medication administration include the right drug, patient, route, time, and dose.
- Nurses involved in drug research need to be knowledgeable about the research process, patient's rights, and informed consent.
- Legal guidelines, ethical principles, and the ANA Code of Ethics ensure that the nurse is acting on sound foundations of nursing care.

Critical Thinking **A C T I V I T Y**

1. Discuss the impact of advanced practice as it relates to safe and effective drug therapy.

▲▲

BIBLIOGRAPHY

American Nurses Association: *Code for nurses with interpretive statements*, Kansas City, Mo, 1985, The Association.

Canadian Nurses Association: *Code of ethics for nursing*, Ottawa, 1995, the Association.

DiPiro JT et al: *Pharmacotherapy: a pathophysiologic approach*, ed 2, New York, 1992, Elsevier Science Publishing.

Lilley L et al: Getting back to basics—"5 rights" of medication administration, *AJN* 94(9):15, 1994.

McEvoy GK: *AHFS drug information*, Bethesda, Md, 1994, American Society of Hospital Pharmacists.

McKenry LM, Salerno E: *Mosby's pharmacology in nursing*, ed 19, St Louis, 1995, Mosby.

Medication orders: looking for approval, *Nursing 94* (Advice PRN) 2:14, 1994.

Pharmaceutical Research Manufacturers Association, annual report, 1994.

Chapter 6

Mathematic Calculations

Objectives

When you reach the end of this chapter, you will be able to:

1 Discuss the significance of accurate math calculations in the administration of medications.
2 Describe the various parts of a drug order.
3 Identify the different abbreviations used in drug orders.
4 Identify the various metric measurements.
5 Utilize the abbreviations and metric measurements safely and accurately.
6 Convert among the apothecary and metric measurement systems.
7 Safely calculate drug medication orders.

CHAPTER OUTLINE

Responsibility and Common Sense
Reading Drug Orders
Drug Weights and Measures
  Metric system
  Apothecary system
  Household system
  Avoirdupois system
  Other systems of drug measurement
    Units
    International units and milliequivalents
Calculating Drug Doses
  Fraction method
  Dimensional analysis

Glossary

Apothecary system (ah pa′ thə ker ē) *Apothecary* is an obsolete term for a pharmacist. The apothecary system of measurement consists of graduated liquid volumes, called *apothecary measures*. The apothecary measure was originally based on a unit called a *minim*, which was equivalent to one drop of water. The minim has now been standardized to equal 0.06 ml; 60 minims equal 1 fluid dram, and 8 fluid drams equal 1 fluid ounce. *Apothecary weight* refers to a system of graduated heaviness based on the grain, which originally equaled the weight of a plump grain of wheat. The grain has been standardized to equal 65 mg; 20 grains

equal 1 scruple, 3 scruples equal 1 dram, and 8 drams equal 1 ounce. (p. 46)

Avoirdupois system (a ver dŭ poiz) The English system of weights in which there are 7000 grains, 256 drams, or 16 ounces to 1 pound. One ounce in this system equals 28.35 g, and 1 pound equals 453.59 g. (p. 46)

Household system A system of measurement popular in the United States, commonly used in cookery, in which the teaspoon is the basic unit of measurement. Three teaspoons equal 1 tablespoon, and 2 tablespoons equal 1 fluid ounce. (p. 46)

International units A unit of measurement in the Système International System de Unités (SI), an internationally accepted scientific system of expressing length, mass, and time in basic units (IU) of centimeters, grams, and seconds, replacing the former centimeter-gram-second system. The SI system also includes as standard measurements the ampere, kelvin, candela, and mole. (p. 47)

Metric system A decimal system of measurement in which the meter (39.37 inches) is the basic unit of length, the gram (15.432 grains) is the basic unit of weight or mass, and as a derived unit, the liter (0.908 U.S. dry quart or 1.0567 U.S. liquid quart) is the basic unit of volume. (p. 46)

Milliequivalent (mil ĭ ē kwiv′ ah lent) The number of grams of solute dissolved in 1 ml of a normal solution, or one thousandth of a gram equivalent. A milliequivalent per liter (mEq/L) is one thousandth of 1 gram of a specific substance dissolved in 1 L of plasma. The milliequivalent is used to measure electrolytes. (p. 47)

Units The amount of a particular drug in typically 1 ml of solution. This is unique for each drug. (p. 47)

RESPONSIBILITY AND COMMON SENSE

There are almost as many ways of doing mathematical calculations as there are persons doing them. This chapter will look at some of the most common ones and point out the strengths and weaknesses of each. There are many important aspects to consider when doing calculations, but probably the most important one is common sense! If a drug dose calculation does not seem right, then most likely it is not. The administration of drugs to patients is a shared responsibility among the patient, the physician, the pharmacist, and the nurse. All those involved have a moral and legal responsibility to ensure that this takes place in a safe and effective way. The nurse has a legal and a professional responsibility to ensure that his or her patients receive the right dose of the right medication at the right time in the right manner. There are many checks and balances in the system to guarantee that this happens. The necessary calculations involved in the safe and accurate administration of medications to patients are described in this chapter.

Calculating drug doses is one small part of the overall process of medically treating a patient. Before you actually calculate the drug dose, you must follow many steps. As described in Chapter 2, the nurse should evaluate the patient and the prescribed medication for the five ''rights'': the right patient, the right drug, the right dose, the right time, and right route. Other principles to follow to decrease the likelihood of mistakes are to calculate doses systematically and to do your calculations consistently time after time so that the process becomes easier with each calculation. It also helps to have a peer check your calculations, especially if the dose seems unusual or if the math is very difficult. Remember common sense should prevail! If a calculation shows you should give 25 mg of digoxin and the strongest strength is 0.25 mg, common sense should tell you that the patient should not be given 100 tablets, especially since drug dosage forms are usually manufactured with the most commonly prescribed dosages in mind.

READING DRUG ORDERS

Medication orders often employ Latin phrases and many abbreviations. To read the order these must be understood. The correct interpretation of these Latin terms and abbreviations is essential to the appropriate administration of calculated drug dosages. These abbreviations save time in the communication among medical personnel. The most commonly used Latin terms and abbreviations are listed in Table 6-1.

If the written order is confusing or unclear, then the pharmacist or physician should be consulted for clarification. It is also a good practice to administer medications that you are familiar with. If a nurse does not know what he or she is giving to a patient, he or she cannot determine the therapeutic or toxic effects of the administered drug. This is a very important aspect of drug therapy.

DRUG WEIGHTS AND MEASURES

There are at least four different systems of measurement: the metric system, the apothecary system, the avoirdupois system, and the household system. The metric and apothecary are by far the most commonly used for the ordering of medications.

Table 6-1	Pharmaceutical Abbreviations
ABBREVIATION	**TRANSLATION**
Drug Dosage	
cc	Cubic centimeter
g	Gram
gr	Grain
gtt	Drop
lb	Pound
m	Minim
ml	Milliliter
no	Number
qs	Quantity sufficient
ss	One half
oz	Ounce
tbsp	Tablespoon
tsp	Teaspoon
Drug Route	
ID	Intradermal
IM	Intramuscular
IV	Intravenous
OD	Right eye
OS	Left eye
OU	Both eyes
PO	By mouth
SC	Subcutaneous
SL	Sublingual
Drug Administration	
aa	Of each
ac	Before meals
ad lib	As desired
bid	Twice a day
h	Hour
hs	Hour of sleep/at bedtime
noct	Night
pc	After meals
prn	When needed
qd	Every day
qh	Every hour
qid	Four times a day
qod	Every other day
℞	Prescribe/take
sos	If necessary
stat	Immediately
tid	Three times a day

Metric System

The **metric system** is the most widely used and international system of measurement and utilizes numbers that are commonly used by health care professionals around the world. The *United States Pharmacopeia* uses this system. The metric system has many advantages, especially when converting up or down in increments. It can be used to measure either liquids or solids. Unfortunately, because the general public in the United States has not yet caught on to its use, this has meant that two systems of measurement, it and the household system, are both in use.

Apothecary System

The **apothecary system** is older than the metric system and is the only system of measurement that utilizes symbols to represent units of measure.

Household System

The **household system** is the system of measurement most people in the United States are familiar with. This system is used for home remedies, over-the-counter (OTC) medications, recipes, and food products. Although commonly used by the general population, it is seldom used by health care professionals.

Avoirdupois System

The final system of drug measurement is the **avoirdupois system**. It was popular many years ago when the compounding of prescriptions was common. Now the pharmaceutical industry handles the greater responsibility for drug compounding and measurements are standardized. The boxes at left list the various units of measurement for solids and liquids used in the four systems. These tables also show how a measurement in one system is converted into that in another.

Sometimes it is necessary to convert within a system of measurement. When doing this, it is necessary to know equivalents within a system. Table 6-2 lists these equivalents.

Liquid Systems of Measurement

METRIC	APOTHECARY	HOUSEHOLD
5 milliliter (ml)	1 fluid dram	1 teaspoon
15 ml	½ fluid ounce	1 tablespoon
30 ml	1 fluid ounce	2 tablespoons
240 ml	8 ounces	1 cupful
473 ml	16 ounces	1 pint
946 ml (1 liter)	32 ounces	1 quart
3785 ml	12 ounces	1 gallon

Solid Systems of Measurement

METRIC	APOTHECARY	AVOIRDUPOIS
1 gram (g)	15 grains (gr)	15.4 grains (gr)
28.35 g	480 gr	1 oz
31 g	1 ounce (oz)	437.5 gr
454 g	1.33 pounds (lbs)	1 pound (lb)
373 g	1 lb	0.75 lb
1 kg	2.7 lb	2.2 lb

Table 6-2 Conversions within Systems

LIQUIDS			SOLIDS		
Apothecary System					
60 minims	=	1 fluid dram	20 grains	=	1 scruple
8 fluid drams	=	1 fluid ounce	3 scruples	=	1 dram
16 fluid ounces	=	1 pint	8 drams	=	1 ounce
2 pints	=	1 quart	12 ounces	=	1 pound
4 quarts	=	1 gallon			
Household System					
3 teaspoons	=	1 tablespoon	16 ounces	=	1 pound
2 tablespoons	=	1 ounce			
16 ounces	=	1 pint			
2 pints	=	1 quart			
4 quarts	=	1 gallon			
Metric System					
1000 ml	=	1 liter	1000 μg	=	1 mg
			1000 mg	=	1 g
			1000 g	=	1 kg

Other Systems of Drug Measurement

Some medications are measured by specific manufacturer measurements. These measurements may be based on the biologic or chemical activity of the drug. Whichever the case, they differ from the traditional systems just described and are worth mentioning here.

Units

Units (U) is a term of measurement used to describe the amount of a particular drug in typically 1 ml of solution. Units express the biologic activity observed for the drug in animal tests, for example, the amount of drug required to produce a particular response. This is unique for each drug. A unit of insulin is not equivalent to a unit of heparin. The international standard of U-100 insulin means that 1 ml of insulin solution contains 100 units of insulin regardless of the type. Nystatin, an oral liquid preparation, contains 100,000 units of nystatin per milliliter of nystatin solution. Heparin is another medication that is typically measured in units.

International Units and Milliequivalents

International units (IU) are typically used to measure biologicals such as hormones, enzymes, and vitamins. **Milliequivalents** (mEq) are used to measure electrolytes and express the ionic activity of a drug. The total number of milliequivalents per a certain concentration of fluid is determined by the pharmaceutical manufacturer. The dose of these products should be based on their milliequivalent amount rather than on their actual volume (milliliter) amount.

CALCULATING DRUG DOSES

To arrive at the correct dose of a medication, it is essential to be able to perform drug dose calculations. The common units of measurement, the equivalents between the systems, and the methods of manipulating these data have already been discussed, and this will aid in the determination of a drug dose. In addition to this knowledge, you must have basic arithmetic skills, especially in the use of fractions and decimals. Several methods for drug dose calculation are presented. Selecting one of these methods and consistently using that one system is best.

Many drugs require individualized dosing. Such drug dose calculations must take into consideration the body weight or body surface area of the patient, especially those whose body weight is low (e.g., children and infants), who are obese, or who are elderly.

Before calculating a drug dose for a particular patient, you must first convert all units of measure to a single system, if this has not already been done. The boxes on p. 46 can be used to make these calculations. The best approach to this is to convert to the system used on the drug label. For example, if the drug is ordered in milligrams but the drug label shows the drug is prepared in 5-gr tablets, convert the ordered number of milligrams per dose to the equivalent number of grains to determine the total number of tablets that need to be given to the patient to make up one dose.

TAKE HOME POINTS

Five "Rights"
- Evaluate the patient's condition and the prescribed medication before administration.
- Right patient, right dose, right time, right route, and right drug.

Common Sense
- Most important concept in calculating appropriate dose.
- Drug dosage forms manufactured with the most commonly prescribed dosages in mind.

Weights and Measures
- Four different systems: metric, apothecary, avoirdupois, and household.
- Metric is the most widely used and the international system of measurement.

Fraction Method
- Uses ratios and proportions to arrive at answer.
- Takes many steps to get answer and no way to double-check it.

Dimensional Analysis
- Takes what information you know and works to get the lacking information.
- If final units are what you desired, your answer is correct = a double check.

Math Calculations
- Everyday presents a challenge to the mathematical skills of a professional nurse, calling for the nurse to always follow a logical sequence in performing drug dose calculations.
- If unsure of your mathematical skills or calculations, never hesitate to ask a colleague to check your calculations. The most minute error can be life-threatening!

Fraction Method

A patient has been given the following order: "Aspirin 650 mg PO qd." However, the aspirin product in stock is: "Aspirin 5 gr." Using the fraction method to calculate the number of tablets this patient must receive to make up a dose:

1. Convert the ordered 650 mg to grains.
2. By using Table 6-2 we know that there are 65 mg in 1 gr. What we want to know is how many grains constitute 650 mg.
3. Use ratios and proportions and set the ratio as follows:

$$\frac{65\ mg}{1\ gr} = \frac{650\ mg}{X\ gr}$$

4. Cross multiply to get: $X \cdot 65\ mg = 650\ mg \cdot 1\ gr$
5. Solve for X: $X = \dfrac{650\ mg \cdot 1\ gr}{65\ mg}$
6. X = 10 gr.

7. The aspirin comes in 5-gr tablets, so the patient should receive **two 5-gr** aspirin tablets.

Dimensional Analysis

To calculate the same dose using dimensional analysis:

1. Write down the desired units, in this case the number of tablets.
2. Take what information about the patient and the drug you have and manipulate it so that you can cancel out the unwanted units and leave behind the desired units, as follows:

Information known about the patient			Desired Unit
$\dfrac{1\ tablet}{5\ gr}$	$\dfrac{1\ gr}{65\ mg}$	$650\ mg$ =	→ ? tablets

Manipulation of information			Desired Unit
$\dfrac{1\ tablet}{5\ \cancel{gr}}$	$\dfrac{1\ \cancel{gr}}{65\ \cancel{mg}}$	$650\ \cancel{mg}$ =	→ 2 tablets

Critical Thinking A C T I V I T I E S

1. Amoxicillin has been ordered as "gr XV," but the tablets you have in the storage cart are labeled "gr V." How many tablets should you give to the patient?

2. Your 30 kg pediatric patient is prescribed amoxicillin for otitis media. The following prescription is written for his inner ear infection. Calculate how many days this 480 cc bottle will last if you give the medication as directed.
   Amoxil Suspension 125 mg/5 ml
   480 cc
   Take one tablespoon three times a day until gone
   a. What mg dose is your patient receiving every 8 hours?
   b. The recommended child's dose for amoxicillin is 20-50 mg/kg/24 hours in three divided doses (q8h). Has your patient been prescribed a correct dose for his weight?

3. An order is written for your patient to receive 33 mcg/min of nitroglycerin; the concentration of the bag of nitroglycerin handed to you is 100 mcg/ml. At what rate (in ml/hr) should you set your infusion pump to administer this nitroglycerin infusion at 33 μg/min?

BIBLIOGRAPHY

Blais K, Bath J: Drug calculation errors of baccalaureate nursing students, *Nurs Educ* 17:12, 1992.

Chernow B: *The pharmacologic approach to the critically ill patient*, ed 3, Baltimore, 1994, Williams & Wilkins.

Cohen M: Medication errors, *Nursing, 94,* 24(10):15, 1994.

DiPiro JT et al: *Pharmacotherapy: a pathophysiologic approach*, ed 2, New York, 1992, Elsevier Science Publishing.

Johnson KB: *The Harriet Lane handbook*, ed 13, St Louis, 1993, Mosby.

Keen JH: *Critical care and emergency drug reference*, St Louis, 1994, Mosby.

McEvoy GK: *AHFS drug information*, Bethesda, Md, 1994, American Society of Hospital Pharmacists.

McKenry LM, Salerno E: *Mosby's pharmacology in nursing*, ed 19, St Louis, 1995, Mosby.

Murphy M, Graveley E: The use of hand-held calculators for solving pharmacology problems, *Nurs Educ* 15:35; 41:43, 1990.

Chapter 7

Photo Atlas of Drug Administration

CHAPTER OUTLINE

Medication Orders and Documentation, p. 50

Syringes, p. 52

Preparing Injections from Ampules and Vials, p. 55

Assessment
Planning and Implementation
  Prepare injection from ampule
  Prepare injection from vial
  Prepare injection in one syringe by mixing two
    vials
Evaluation

Injection Sites, p. 59

Administering Injections, p. 62

Assessment
Planning and Implementation
Evaluation

Administering IV Medications by Piggyback or Volume Administration Sets, p. 65

Assessment
Planning and Implementation
Evaluation

Administering Medications by IV Bolus (Push), p. 67

Assessment
Planning and Implementation
Evaluation

Adding Medications to IV Fluid Containers, p. 69

Assessment
Planning and Implementation
Evaluation

Initiation of Patient-Controlled Analgesia, p. 71

Assessment
Planning and Implementation
Evaluation

Administering Oral Medications, p. 78

Assessment
Planning and Implementation
Evaluation

Instilling Ophthalmic Medications, p. 80

Assessment
Planning and Implementation
  To administer ointment
  To instill eyedrops
Evaluation

Administering Eardrops, p. 81

Assessment
Planning and Implementation
Evaluation

Administering Nasal Drops, p. 82

Assessment
Planning and Implementation
Evaluation

Administering Medications via a Nasogastric Tube, p. 83

Assessment
Planning and Implementation
Evaluation

Medication Orders and Documentation

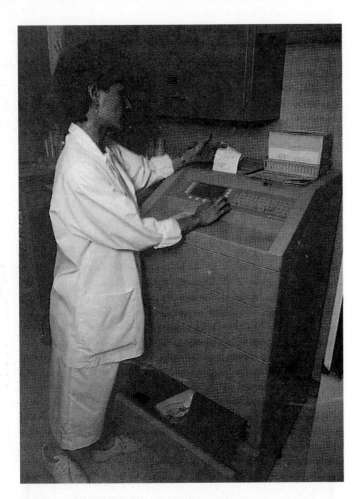

▼ **Fig. 7-1** Computer-controlled dispensing system. (From Potter P, Perry A: *Fundamentals of nursing: concepts, process, and practice,* ed 3, 1995, St Louis, Mosby.)

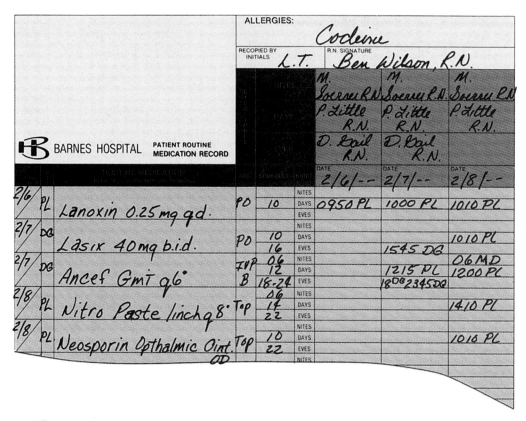

▼ **Fig. 7-2** Example of medication record. (From Potter P, Perry A: *Fundamentals of nursing: concepts, process, and practice,* ed 3, 1995, St Louis, Mosby.)

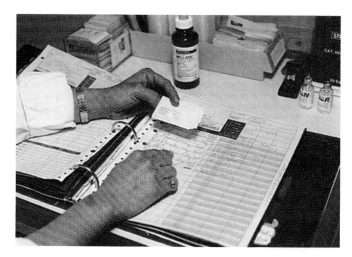

▼ **Fig. 7-3** The nurse is responsible for checking the label of the medication with the transcribed medication order. (From Potter P, Perry A: *Fundamentals of nursing: concepts, process, and practice,* ed 3, 1995, St Louis, Mosby.)

▼ **Fig. 7-4** Before administering any medication, the nurse should check the patient's identification and allergy bracelet. (From Potter P, Perry A: *Fundamentals of nursing: concepts, process, and practice,* ed 3, 1995, St Louis, Mosby.)

Syringes

▼ **Fig. 7-5** Parts of a syringe and hypodermic needle. (From Potter P, Perry A: *Fundamentals of nursing: concepts, process, and practice,* ed 3, 1995, St Louis, Mosby.)

▼ **Fig. 7-6** Types of syringes. *From top to bottom:* disposable 3-ml hypodermic syringe (intramuscular), 3-ml hypodermic syringe (subcutaneous), tuberculin syringe, and insulin syringe. (From Potter P, Perry A: *Fundamentals of nursing: concepts, process, and practice,* ed 3, 1995, St Louis, Mosby.)

▼ **Fig. 7-7** Hypodermic needles arranged in order of gauge. *Top to bottom:* 19-, 20-, 21-, 23-, and 25-gauge. (From Potter P, Perry A: *Fundamentals of nursing: concepts, process, and practice,* ed 3, 1995, St Louis, Mosby.)

▼ **Fig. 7-8 A,** Carpuject syringe and prefilled sterile cartridge with needle. **B,** Assembling the carpuject. **C,** The cartridge slides into the syringe barrel, turns, and locks at the needle end. The plunger then screws into the cartridge end. (From Potter P, Perry A: *Fundamentals of nursing: concepts, process, and practice,* ed 3, 1995, St Louis, Mosby.)

A

B

▼ **Fig. 7-9** Needle with plastic guard to prevent needle-sticks. **A,** Position of guard before injection. **B,** After injection, the guard locks in place, covering the needle. (From Potter P, Perry A: *Fundamentals of nursing: concepts, process, and practice,* ed 3, 1995, St Louis, Mosby.)

▼ **Fig. 7-10** Special containers are available in nursing units for the disposal of contaminated syringes. (From Potter P, Perry A: *Fundamentals of nursing: concepts, process, and practice,* ed 3, 1995, St Louis, Mosby.)

Preparing Injections from Ampules and Vials

ASSESSMENT

Wash hands. Check order.

PLANNING AND IMPLEMENTATION

1. Prepare needed equipment and supplies:
   - Ampules: see Fig. 7-11A.
     (1) Ampule containing medication
     (2) Syringe and needle
     (3) Small gauze pad or alcohol swab
     (4) Container for disposing of glass
   - Vials: see Fig. 7-11B.
     (1) Vial with medication
     (2) Syringe and needle
     (3) Alcohol swab
     (4) Solvent (e.g., normal saline or sterile water)
   - Medication cards, forms, or printouts
2. Assemble supplies at work area in medicine room.
3. Check each medication card, form, or computer printout against label on each ampule or vial.

A

▼ **Fig. 7-11** (From Potter P, Perry A: *Fundamentals of nursing: concepts, process, and practice,* ed 3, 1995, St Louis, Mosby.)

B

▼ **Fig. 7-13** (From Potter P, Perry A: *Fundamentals of nursing: concepts, process, and practice*, ed 3, 1995, St Louis, Mosby.)

▼ **Fig. 7-12** (From Potter P, Perry A: *Fundamentals of nursing: concepts, process, and practice*, ed 3, 1995, St Louis, Mosby.)

Prepare Injection from Ampule

- Tap top of ampule lightly and quickly with finger until fluid leaves neck (see Fig. 7-12A).
- Place small gauze pad or dry alcohol swab around neck of ampule.
- Snap neck quickly and firmly away from hands (see Fig. 7-12B).
- Draw up medication quickly. Hold ampule upside down or set it on flat surface. Insert syringe needle into center of ampule opening (see Fig. 7-13A). Do not allow needle tip or shaft to touch rim of ampule.

- Aspirate medication into syringe by gently pulling back on plunger (see Fig. 7-13B).
- Keep needle tip below surface of liquid. Tip ampule to bring all fluid within reach of needle.
- If air bubbles are aspirated, do not expel air into ampule.
- To expel excess air bubbles, remove needle. Hold syringe with needle pointing up. Tap side of syringe to cause bubbles to rise toward needle. Draw back slightly on plunger, and push plunger upward to eject air. *Do not eject fluid.*
- If syringe contains excess fluid, use sink for disposal. Hold syringe vertically with needle tip up and slanted slightly toward sink. Slowly eject excess fluid into sink. Recheck fluid level in syringe by holding it vertically.
- Cover needle with sheath or cap. Change needle on syringe.
- Dispose of soiled supplies. Place broken ampule in special container for glass.

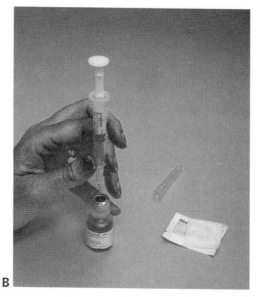

▼ **Fig. 7-14** (From Potter P, Perry A: *Fundamentals of nursing: concepts, process, and practice,* ed 3, 1995, St Louis, Mosby.)

▼ **Fig. 7-15** (From Potter P, Perry A: *Fundamentals of nursing: concepts, process, and practice,* ed 3, 1995, St Louis, Mosby.)

Prepare Injection from Vial

- Remove metal cap covering top of unused vial. Expose rubber seal.
- Wipe off surface of rubber seal with alcohol swab, if vial had been previously opened.
- Take syringe and remove needle cap. Pull back on plunger to draw amount of air into syringe equivalent to volume of medication to be aspirated from vial (see Fig. 7-14A).
- Insert tip of needle, with bevel pointing up, through center of rubber seal (see Fig. 7-14B). Apply pressure to tip of needle during insertion.
- Inject air into vial, holding on to plunger.
- Invert vial while keeping firm hold on syringe and plunger (see Fig. 7-15A). Hold vial between thumb and middle fingers of nondominant hand. Grasp end of syringe barrel and plunger with thumb and forefinger of dominant hand.
- Clean work area. Wash hands.
- Once again, check fluid level in syringe and compare with desired dose (see Fig. 7-15B).

▼ **Fig. 7-16** (From Potter P, Perry A: *Fundamentals of nursing: concepts, process, and practice,* ed 3, 1995, St Louis, Mosby.)

Prepare Injection in One Syringe by Mixing Two Vials

- Do not contaminate one medication with another.
- Ensure that the final dosage is accurate.
- Maintain aseptic technique.
- See Fig. 7-16. Take a syringe and aspirate the volume of air equivalent to the first drug's dosage (vial A).
- Inject air into vial A, making sure that the needle does not touch the solution.
- Withdraw the needle, aspirate air equivalent to the second drug's dose (vial B), then inject the volume of air into vial B.
- Immediately withdraw the required medication from vial B into the syringe. At this point the drug from vial A has not contaminated vial B. When preparing insulin injections, always withdraw the unmodified (Regular) insulin first.
- Apply a new, sterile needle to the syringe and insert it into vial A, being careful not to push the plunger and expel the drug within the syringe into the vial.

- Withdraw the desired amount of drug from vial A into the syringe. (*Note:* If a vial has excess positive pressure, the plunger may begin to move, causing an accidental withdrawal of too much of the drug.)
- Withdraw the needle, apply a new needle, and sheath the syringe.

EVALUATION

1. Return to patient in 10 to 30 minutes, depending on route, to monitor the therapeutic effectiveness of the medication administered.
2. Monitor for any side effects of medication.
3. Document and report any unusual responses.

Injection Sites

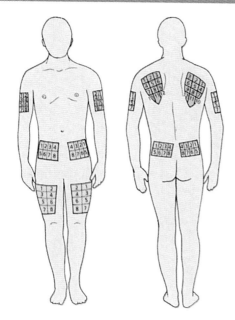

▼ **Fig. 7-17** Common sites for SC injections. Note how sites might be rotated. (From Potter P, Perry A: *Fundamentals of nursing: concepts, process, and practice*, ed 3, 1995, St Louis, Mosby.)

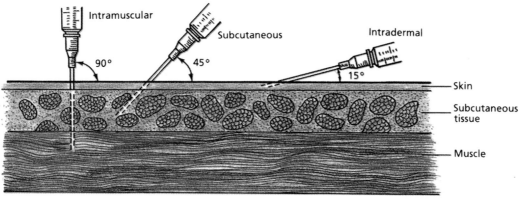

▼ **Fig. 7-18** A comparison of the angles of insertion for IM (90 degrees), SC (45 degrees), and ID (15 degrees) injections. (From Potter P, Perry A: *Fundamentals of nursing: concepts, process, and practice*, ed 3, 1995, St Louis, Mosby.)

▼ **Fig. 7-19 A,** Injection site into the vastus lateralis muscle. **B,** Anatomic view of the site for IM injection into the vastus lateralis muscle. (From Potter P, Perry A: *Fundamentals of nursing: concepts, process, and practice*, ed 3, 1995, St Louis, Mosby.)

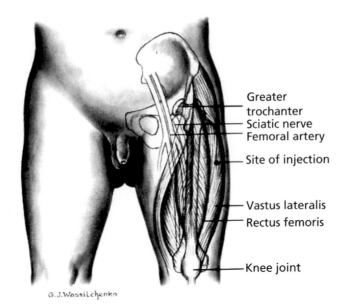

G.J.Wassilchenko

▼ **Fig. 7-20** Acceptable IM site for children, the vastus lateralis muscle. (From Potter P, Perry A: *Fundamentals of nursing: concepts, process, and practice*, ed 3, 1995, St Louis, Mosby.)

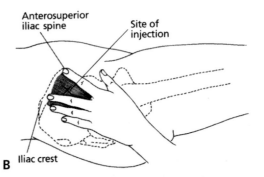

▼ **Fig. 7-21 A**, Injection site into ventrogluteal muscle avoids major nerves and blood vessels. **B**, Anatomical view of ventrogluteal muscle injection site. (From Potter P, Perry A: *Fundamentals of nursing: concepts, process, and practice*, ed 3, 1995, St Louis, Mosby.)

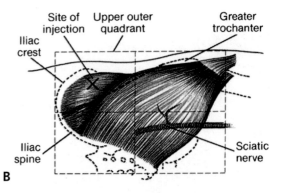

▼ **Fig. 7-22 A**, Site of injection into the left dorsogluteal muscle. **B**, Imaginary diagonal line extending from the posterior superior iliac spine to the greater trochanter is the landmark for selecting the dorsogluteal injection site. (From Potter P, Perry A: *Fundamentals of nursing: concepts, process, and practice*, ed 3, 1995, St Louis, Mosby.)

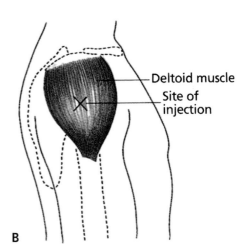

▼ **Fig. 7-23** **A**, Site of IM injection into the deltoid muscle. **B**, Site of deltoid muscle injection below acromion process. (From Potter P, Perry A: *Fundamentals of nursing: concepts, process, and practice,* ed 3, 1995, St Louis, Mosby.)

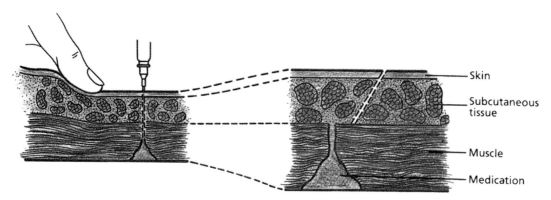

▼ **Fig. 7-24** The Z-track method of injection prevents the deposit of medication through sensitive tissues. (From Potter P, Perry A: *Fundamentals of nursing: concepts, process, and practice,* ed 3, 1995, St Louis, Mosby.)

▼ **Fig. 7-25** Administering IM injection by the air-lock technique prevents tracking of medication through SC tissues. (From Potter P, Perry A: *Fundamentals of nursing: concepts, process, and practice,* ed 3, 1995, St Louis, Mosby.)

Administering Injections

ASSESSMENT

1. Assess indications for proper route for medication.
2. Check medication order.
3. Assess medical history and history of allergies.
4. Observe verbal and nonverbal responses toward receiving injection.
5. Wash hands.

PLANNING AND IMPLEMENTATION

1. Prepare needed equipment and supplies:
   - Proper-size syringe:
     (1) SC: 1 to 2 ml
     (2) IM: 2 to 3 ml for adult, 1 to 2 ml for child
     (3) ID: 1-ml tuberculin
   - Proper-size needle:
     (1) SC: 25- to 27-gauge and ⅜ to ⅝ inches in length
     (2) IM: 18- to 23-gauge and 1 to 1½ inches in length for adults, 25- to 27-gauge and ½ to 1 inch in length for child and ⅝ for newborn
     (3) ID: preattached 26- to 27-gauge
   - Antiseptic swab (Betadine or alcohol)
   - Disposable gloves
   - Medication ampule or vial
   - Medication card, forms, or printouts

2. Check medication order again. (Three checks promotes safety!)
3. Prepare correct medication dose from ampule or vial. Check carefully. Be sure all air is expelled. (For IM medications that are particularly irritating to tissues, draw 0.2 cc of air into syringe, being careful not to expel drug dose. See Z-track method.)
4. For IM injection, change needle if medication is irritating to SC tissue.
5. Apply disposable gloves. (*Note:* Always adhere to Universal Precautions with patient contact.)
6. Identify patient by checking identification armband and asking name.
7. Explain procedure to patient and proceed in calm, confident manner.
8. Close room curtains or door.
9. Keep sheet or gown draped over body parts not requiring exposure.
10. Select appropriate injection site. Inspect skin surface over sites for bruises, inflammation, or edema:
    - SC: palpate sites for masses of tenderness.
    - IM: note integrity and size of muscle and palpate for tenderness.
    - ID: note lesions or discolorations of forearm.
11. If injections are given frequently, rotate sites.

▼ **Fig. 7-26** (From Potter P, Perry A: *Fundamentals of nursing: concepts, process, and practice,* ed 3, 1995, St Louis, Mosby.)

12. Assist patient to comfortable position:
    - ■ SC: have patient relax arm, leg, or abdomen, depending on site chosen.
    - ■ IM: have patient lie flat, on side, or prone or have client sit, depending on site chosen.
    - ■ ID: have patient extend elbow and support it and forearm on flat surface.
13. Relocate site using anatomical landmarks.
14. Cleanse site with antiseptic swab. Apply swab at center of site and rotate outward in circular direction for about 5 cm (2 inches) (see Fig. 7-26A).
15. Hold swab between third and fourth fingers of nondominant hand.
16. Remove cap from needle by pulling it straight off.
17. Hold syringe correctly between thumb and forefinger of dominant hand:
    - ■ SC: hold as dart (see Fig. 7-26B) at 45- or 90-degree angle.
    - ■ IM: hold as dart.
    - ■ ID: hold bevel of needle pointing up.
18. Administer injection:
    - ■ SC:
      - (1) For average-size patient, spread skin tightly across injection site or pinch skin with nondominant hand.
      - (2) Inject needle quickly and firmly at 45- to 90-degree angle (see Fig. 7-27A). (Then release skin, if pinched.)
      - (3) For obese patient, pinch skin at site and inject needle below tissue fold.

- ■ IM:
  - (1) Position nondominant hand at proper anatomic landmarks and spread skin tightly. Inject needle quickly at 90-degree angle into muscle.
  - (2) If client's muscle mass is small, grasp body of muscle between thumb and other fingers.
  - (3) If medication is irritating, use Z-track method (see section on Z-track methods).
- ■ ID:
  - (1) With nondominant hand, stretch skin over site with forefinger or thumb.
  - (2) With needle almost against client's skin, insert it slowly at 5- to 15-degree angle until resistance is felt. Then advance needle through epidermis to approximately 3 mm (⅛ inch) below surface. Needle tip can be seen through skin.
19. After needle enters site of SC or IM injections *only*, grasp lower end of syringe barrel with nondominant hand. Move dominant hand to end of plunger. Avoid moving syringe while slowly pulling back on plunger to aspirate drug (see Fig. 7-27B). If blood appears in syringe, remove needle, discard medication and syringe, and repeat procedure. (It is unnecessary to aspirate ID injection.)
20. Inject medication slowly. (For ID injections, it is normal to feel resistance; if not, needle is too deep.)

A   B

▼ **Fig. 7-27** (From Potter P, Perry A: *Fundamentals of nursing: concepts, process, and practice*, ed 3, 1995, St Louis, Mosby.)

▼ **Fig. 7-28** (From Potter P, Perry A: *Fundamentals of nursing: concepts, process, and practice,* ed 3, 1995, St Louis, Mosby.)

21. During ID injection, note formation of small bleb on skin's surface (see Fig. 7-28).
22. Withdraw needle while applying alcohol swab gently above or over injection site.
23. For SC or IM injections, massage skin lightly. OPTIONAL: apply bandage for ID injections, *do not massage site.*
24. Assist patient to comfortable position.
25. Discard unsheathed needle and attached syringe into appropriately labeled receptacles.
26. Remove disposable gloves. Wash hands.
27. For ID injection, draw circle around perimeter of injection site with skin pencil.
28. For SC and IM injections, chart medication dose, route, and site and time and date given in medication record. Correctly sign according to institutional policy.
29. For ID injections, record area of injection, amount and type of testing substance, and date and time on medication record.

EVALUATION

1. Return to room and ask if patient feels acute pain, burning, numbness, or tingling at injection site. Observe for allergic reaction after injection.
2. Return to evaluate therapeutic or adverse response to medication in 10 to 30 minutes.
3. Document and report any unusual responses.

LEGAL PRINCIPLES
Infiltrating IV

Nurses often encounter an infiltrating IV in the routine care of many of their patients and every action taken is very important to the standard of care of that patient and in ensuring that the nurse has acted as any prudent nurse would. The assessment and action taken by the nurse can be important for the patient as in the case of **Macon-Bibb Hosp. Authority vs. Ross (335 S.E. 2d 633-GA)**.

Situation
Ms. Ross was brought to the ER of the hospital with dyspnea, bradycardia, and a blood pressure of 250/150. She went into respiratory arrest at 2:55 PM; she was intubated with an endotracheal tube, and nitroprusside was administered IV to decrease her blood pressure. Because of the rapid drop in blood pressure, an IV administration of dopamine was started at 3:28 PM in her right wrist to increase her blood pressure. When her BP was stable, she was transferred to the cardiac care unit at 4:30 PM. At midnight, a nurse noted that the IV site had a "bruise bluish in color." The next notation was at 11:00 AM the following day, in which it was recorded that the patient's right arm was swollen and painful with a large blistered area around the IV site. The same notation was made at 4:00 PM. It was not until 6:50 PM that a note indicated that a physician was informed of the infiltration. As a result of the extravasation of dopamine, the patient's lower right arm was permanently scarred. On a jury verdict, the court entered judgement for the patient. The hospital appealed.

The court of appeals affirmed the judgment of the lower court. It was noted that, although an infiltration may result from an improper technique, it may also be due to the size of the needle, the status of the patient's veins, or specific intolerance to an IV. However, according to the expert nurse's testimony, supported by suitable references, dopamine should be infused into a "large vein," such as in the antecubital fossa, to minimize the risk of extravasation. In addition, dopamine should be monitored continuously for free flow. If extravasation of dopamine occurs, the recommended treatment of the site is infiltration with a saline solution of phentolamine (Regitine) within 12 hours.

The nurses were criticized for not being sufficiently knowledgeable regarding dopamine, which resulted in their failure to notify a physician of the patient's impaired tissue integrity.

From McKenry L, Salerno E: *Mosby's pharmacology in nursing,* ed 19, St Louis, 1995, Mosby.

Administering IV Medications by Piggyback or Volume Administration Sets

ASSESSMENT

1. Check physician's order to determine type of medication and dosage.
2. Assess patency of existing IV infusion line by noting infusion rate of main IV line.
3. Assess insertion site for signs of infiltration or phlebitis.

PLANNING AND IMPLEMENTATION

1. Prepare following equipment and supplies:
   - Piggyback set:
     (1) Medication prepared in a 50 to 100 ml labeled infusion bag with IV line, microdrip, or macrodrip infusion tubing set
     (2) Needle (21- or 23-gauge)
     (3) Adhesive tape (optional)
     (4) Antiseptic swab
     (5) Metal hook (optional)
     (6) Disposable gloves
   - Volume-control administration set:
     (1) Volutrol, Pediatrol, or Burette
     (2) Infusion tubing
     (3) Syringe (5 to 20 ml)
     (4) Needle (1 to 1½ inches 21- or 23-gauge)
     (5) Vial or ampule of ordered medication
     (6) Medication label
2. Wash hands and apply gloves.
3. Administer medications by piggyback set:
   - Assemble supplies at bedside.
   - Connect infusion tubing to medication bag. Allow solution to fill tubing by opening regulator flow clamp.
   - Hang medication bag at or above level of main fluid bag. Hook may be used to lower main bag (see Fig. 7-29A).
   - Connect covered sterile needle to end of infusion tubing.
   - Check patient's identification by looking at armband and asking name.
   - Clean injection Y-port of main line with antiseptic swab.
   - Remove cover and insert needle of secondary piggyback line through injection port of main line. Secure with strip of adhesive tape if necessary. If available, use needle-lock devices to secure needle of secondary piggyback line through injection port of main line (see Figs. 7-29B and C, and Fig. 7-30A).

▼ **Fig. 7-29** (From Potter P, Perry A: *Fundamentals of nursing: concepts, process, and practice,* ed 3, 1995, St Louis, Mosby.)

4. Administer medication by volume-control administration set (e.g., Volutrol:)
   - Assemble supplies in medication room.
   - Prepare medication from vial or ampule.
   - Check patient's identification by looking at armband and asking name.
   - Fill Volutrol with desired amount of fluid (50 to 100 ml) by opening clamp between Volutrol and main IV bag (see Fig. 7-30B).
   - Close clamp and check to be sure clamp in air vent of Volutrol chamber is open.
   - Clean injection port on top of Volutrol with antiseptic swab.

   - Remove needle cap and insert syringe needle through port and then inject medication (see Fig. 7-30C). Gently rotate Volutrol between hands.
   - Regulate IV infusion rate appropriate for medication. Follow physician, pharmacist, or manufacturer recommendations for infusion rates.
   - Label Volutrol with name of drug, dose, total volume including diluent, and time of administration.
   - Dispose of uncapped needle and syringe in proper container.
5. Remove and dispose of gloves. Wash hands. Document.
6. Record drug, dose, route, and time administered on medication form. Record volume of fluid in medication bag or Volutrol on intake and output form.

EVALUATION

1. Observe client for signs of adverse reactions.
2. During infusion, periodically check infusion rate and condition of IV site.
3. Monitor for therapeutic effects.

A

B

C

▼ **Fig. 7-30** (From Potter P, Perry A: *Fundamentals of nursing: concepts, process, and practice,* ed 3, 1995, St Louis, Mosby.)

Administering Medications by IV Bolus (Push)

ASSESSMENT

1. Check physician's order for type of medication to be administered, dosage, and route.
2. Assess IV or heparin (saline) lock insertion site for signs of infiltration or phlebitis.
3. If medication is to be pushed into IV line, assess patency of line by noting infusion rate.
4. Assess for allergic reactions (applies to *all* medications).
5. Read package insert or procedure for proper IV dilution of medication and time to infuse.

PLANNING AND IMPLEMENTATION

1. Prepare equipment and supplies:
   - IV push (existing line)
     (1) Medication in vial or ampule
     (2) Syringe (3 to 5 ml)
     (3) Sterile needles (21- and 25-gauge)
     (4) Antiseptic swab
     (5) Watch with second hand or digital readout
   - IV push (IV lock):
     (1) Medication in vial or ampule
     (2) Syringe (3 to 5 ml)
     (3) Syringe (3 ml)
     (4) Vial of heparin flush solution (1 ml = 100 units or 1 ml = 10 units) or vial of normal saline (depending on agency policy)
     (5) Sterile needles (21- and 25-gauge)
     (6) Antiseptic swab
     (7) Watch with second hand or digital readout
     (8) Disposable gloves
2. Wash hands. Apply gloves.
3. After preparing medication, apply small-gauge needle to syringe.
4. Administer medication by IV push (existing line):
   - Check patient's identification by looking at armband and asking name.
   - Select injection port of IV tubing closest to patient. (Circle on port may indicate site for needle insertion.)
   - Clean off injection port with antiseptic swab.
   - Insert small-gauge needle of syringe containing prepared drug through center of port.
   - Occlude IV line by pinching tubing just above injection port. Pull back gently on syringe's plunger to aspirate for blood return (see Fig. 7-31A). (*Note:* The IV tubing above the injection site is clamped off.)
   - After noting blood return, inject medication slowly over several minutes. (Read directions on drug package.) Use watch to time administrations (see Fig. 7-31B).
   - After injecting medication, release tubing, withdraw syringe, and recheck fluid infusion rate.

A **B**

▼ **Fig. 7-31** (From Potter P, Perry A: *Fundamentals of nursing: concepts, process, and practice,* ed 3, 1995, St Louis, Mosby.)

5. Administer medications by IV push (IV lock):
   - ■ Check patient's identification by looking at armband and asking full name.
   - ■ Heparin flush:
     (1) Prepare syringe with 1 ml of heparin flush solution.
     (2) Prepare syringe with 3 ml of normal saline. Attach 25-gauge needle to syringe.
   - ■ Saline only:
     (1) Prepare 2 syringes with 2 ml of normal saline each. Attach 25-gauge needle to each syringe.
   - ■ Heparin and saline:
     (1) Clean lock's rubber diaphragm with antiseptic swab.
     (2) Insert needle of syringe containing normal saline through center of diaphragm. Pull back gently on syringe plunger and look for blood return.
     (3) Flush reservoir with 1 ml saline by pushing slowly on plunger.
     (4) Remove needle and saline-filled syringe.
     (5) Clean lock's diaphragm with antiseptic swab.
     (6) Insert needle of syringe containing prepared drug through center of diaphragm.
     (7) Inject medication bolus slowly over several minutes. (Each medication has recommended rate for bolus administration. Check package directions.) Use watch to time administration (see Fig. 7-32).
     (8) After administering bolus, withdraw syringe.
     (9) Clean lock's diaphragm with antiseptic swab.
     (10) Repeat injection of 1 ml of normal saline.
     (11) *Heparin flush:* Insert needle of syringe containing heparin through diaphragm. Inject heparin slowly, and remove syringe.
      Saline flush: If using only saline to flush reservoir, use 2 ml of saline before and after each use of IV lock.

6. Dispose of uncapped needles and syringes in proper receptacle.
7. Remove and dispose of gloves and sharps. Wash hands. Document.
8. Record drug, dose, route, and time administered on medication form. Also note adverse reactions.

EVALUATION

1. Observe patient closely for therapeutic versus adverse reactions as the drug is administered and for several minutes thereafter.
2. Document and report any unusual findings.

▼ **Fig. 7-32** (From Potter P, Perry A: *Fundamentals of nursing: concepts, process, and practice,* ed 3, 1995, St Louis, Mosby.)

Adding Medications to IV Fluid Containers

ASSESSMENT

1. Check physician's order for type of IV solution, medication, and dose.
2. When more than one medication is to be added to solution, assess for drug compatibility.

PLANNING AND IMPLEMENTATION

1. Prepare equipment and supplies:
    - Vial or ampule of prescribed medication
    - Syringe of appropriate size (5 to 20 ml)
    - Sterile needle (1 to 1½ in, 19- to 21-gauge) with special filters (optional)
    - Correct solvent (e.g., sterile water or normal saline)
    - Sterile IV fluid container (bag or bottle, 500 to 1000 ml in volume)
    - Alcohol or antiseptic swab
    - Label to attach to IV bag or bottle
2. Wash hands thoroughly.
3. Assemble supplies in medication room.
4. Prepare prescribed medication from vial or ampule. (If filter needle is used, replace it with regular needle before injecting medication into IV fluid container.)
5. Identify patient by reading identification band and asking name.
6. Prepare patient by explaining that medication is to be given through existing IV line or one to be started. Explain that no discomfort should be felt during infusion. Encourage patient to report symptoms of discomfort.
7. Add medication to new container:
    - Locate medication injection port on IV solution bag:
        (1) Remove plastic cover over port. Port has small rubber stopper at end. Do not select port for IV tubing insertion or air vent.
    - Locate injection site on IV solution bottle:
        (1) Remove metal or plastic cap and rubber disk. Place cap upside down on counter top.
        (2) Locate medication injection site on bottle's rubber stopper. Site is usually marked by X, circle, or triangle.
    - Wipe off port or injection site with alcohol or antiseptic swab (see Fig. 7-33A).
    - Remove needle cap from syringe and insert needle of syringe through center of injection port or site and inject medication (see Fig. 7-33B).

▼ **Fig. 7-33** (From Potter P, Perry A: *Fundamentals of nursing: concepts, process, and practice*, ed 3, 1995, St Louis, Mosby.)

■ Withdraw syringe from bag or bottle. Cover glass bottle top with antiseptic swab and sterile bottle cap.

■ Mix medication and IV solution by holding bag or bottle and turning it gently end to end.

■ Complete medication label with name and dose of medication, date, time, and your initials. Stick it upside down on bottle or bag (see Fig. 7-34A).

■ Spike bag or bottle with IV tubing and hang (see Chapter 39). Regulate infusion at ordered rate.

8. Add medication to existing container:
    ■ Prepare vented IV bottle or plastic bag:
        (1) Check volume of solution remaining in bottle.
        (2) Verify dilution of medication desired (amount of medication per milliliter).
        (3) Close off IV infusion clamp.
        (4) Wipe medication port with alcohol or antiseptic swab.
        (5) Lower bag or bottle from IV pole. Insert syringe needle through injection port and inject medication.
        (6) Gently mix bottle or bag.
        (7) Rehang bag and regulate infusion to desired rate.
    ■ Complete medication label and stick it to bag or bottle.

9. Properly dispose of equipment and supplies and chart appropriate places in patient's chart.

10. Record solution and medication added to parenteral fluid on appropriate form (see Fig. 7-34B).

EVALUATION

1. Monitor and report side effects (e.g., change in pulse rate, noisy respirations, or change in blood pressure).

2. Evaluate for therapeutic effects.

3. Document.

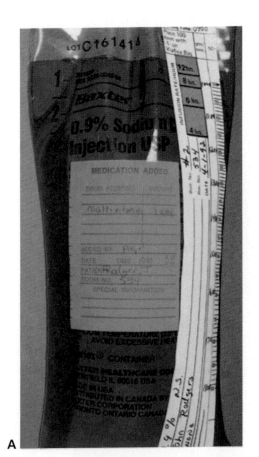

A

B

▼ **Fig. 7-34** (From Potter P, Perry A: *Fundamentals of nursing: concepts, process, and practice*, ed 3, 1995, St Louis, Mosby.)

Initiation of Patient-Controlled Analgesia

ASSESSMENT

With the advent and wide-spread use of patient-controlled analgesia (PCA) pumps in the management of pain, there are many issues and guidelines associated with their use, such as checking the physician's orders, assessment of pain, initiating and maintaining an IV line, using a specialized programmed syringe pump, and constant monitoring of the patient, pump, IV site, and response of the patient. PCA pumps are contraindicated in patients with chronic obstructive pulmonary disease, history of allergy to morphine or meperidine, and history of addiction or drug abuse and patients with major psychiatric disturbances. Always remember that patient education is a very critical part of the control of pain with PCA pumps.

PLANNING AND IMPLEMENTATION

1. Once you have verified the physician's order, check to see what is available on the unit and be sure to have all tubing, medication needed (checking calculations), filters, syringes, patent IV, and pump (with appropriate and functioning parts and equipment) at the bedside (see Fig. 7-35).

2. Always identify the patient prior to administering any medication or procedure and recheck for the 5 "Rs" of medication administration. In addition, explain to the patient everything that will take place and its purpose and how this will help in the management of pain.

▼ **Fig. 7-35**

3. Make sure you snap off the caps of the plunger or the injector piece and the prefilled vial. Connect the injector to the prefilled vial. This can be done with most pumps by screwing them together (see Fig. 7-36).

4. You must prime and remove all air from the pump and all of the corresponding equipment by pushing down on the injector (see Fig. 7-37).

▼ **Fig. 7-36**

▼ **Fig. 7-37**

5. Attach the female connector found on the long end of the PCA tubing to the male end of the injector located in the vial (see Fig. 7-38).

6. It is then recommended to flush the tubing up to the **Y-branch** or **Y-injection** site at the backcheck valve port. It is important to remember that flush-ing ALL the tubing would cause an excess dose of IV narcotic to be administered when first attached to the patient. Once this is completed, close off the slide clamp located on the PCA tubing (see Fig. 7-39).

▼ **Fig. 7-38**

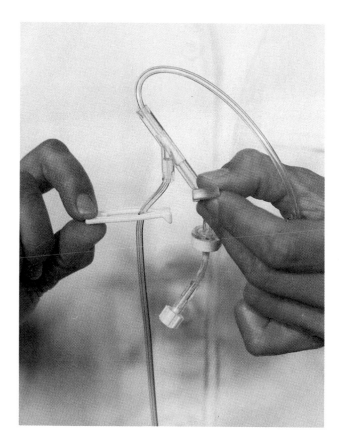

▼ **Fig. 7-39**

7. You may now activate the drive release mechanism of the machine after you have opened the machine door and pinched the spring-loading device (see Fig. 7-40).

8. Now load the vial of medication into the space provided. Be sure to clamp it securely into place and then pinch the drive release mechanism AGAIN by pinching the spring-loaded level and slide it down until it locks into place. It is important to remember that you may hear a "CLICK" once the flange of the injector or syringe locks (see Fig. 7-41). Close the door to the pump and plug it into a safe outlet in the patient's room, unless battery-driven operation is needed.

▼ **Fig. 7-40**

A

B

▼ **Fig. 7-41**

9. Once you are in the patient's room, remove the protective cap from the Y-site of the PCA tubing and connect it (keeping ends sterile) to the distal end of the patient's IV (maintenance fluids for patient) fluid tubing (see Fig. 7-42).

10. You must now prime (clear the tubing of all air) the remainder of the PCA tubing using the roller clamp on the maintenance tubing infusion to control and regulate flow (see Fig. 7-43).

▼ **Fig. 7-42**

▼ **Fig. 7-43**

11. You are now ready to attach the male end of the PCA tubing to the female end of the patient's connector tubing and open all slide clamps on the main IV infusion tubing, PCA tubing, and the patient's connector tubing. In some cases the PCA tubing may fit directly into the patient's angiocath hub site. If you have any questions, consult a procedure manual or contact the IV team for assistance.

12. At this time you may want to press the ON/OFF button on the IV pump. Several messages will appear (see Fig. 7-44A and B) such as DOOR OPEN, VOLUME DELIVERED, CHECK SYRINGE, ALARM (especially if the injector is not positioned or secured properly). FOUR-HOUR DOSE LIMIT will appear once the machine is turned on. Set the FOUR-HOUR DOSE LIMIT as prescribed by the patient's physician. This represents the maximum amount of medication the patient can receive in a 4-hour time period and as prescribed in the designated INCREMENTS of 50 cc (such as 1 cc every 10 minutes or 20 cc limit within 4 hours). If a loading dose has been prescribed by the physician, use the LOCKOUT LIMIT setting and place at 00 minutes. Then, using the DOSE VOLUME setting, dial in the prescribed volume to be delivered and press LOADING DOSE. The volume will appear on the pump's screen. If there is **no** loading dose ordered, use the setting DOSE VOLUME and put in the prescribed amount in tenths of a cc and use the LOCKOUT INTERVAL for the interval between doses given in minutes. Remember that 9 minutes will be designated as 09 and 15 minutes as 15.

13. Once these steps have been implemented, the pump's door is closed and locked securely and agency protocol regarding use of this equipment, documentation, and use of narcotics has been followed, write the time and date when the medication vial was inserted on a piece of tape or provided tag, and place in a visible area of the pump for the benefit of co-workers and for patient safety (document in appropriate notes in the chart and (MAR), as well).

A   B

▼ **Fig. 7-44**

Provide instructions to the patient and attach the handheld control button to the siderail or area of convenient access to the patient. Have the patient do a mock demonstration for you (see Fig. 7-45). A READY message on the pump signals that it is in the patient mode and the first dose is available. Once the patient presses the button, a beep is heard acknowledging request and READY will disappear once the dose is delivered. Reemphasize these points to the patient.

EVALUATION

Once the medication is begun and the patient is using the PCA pump, be sure to constantly assess and reassess the patient for degree of pain (using pain scale); effectiveness of pain control; respiratory rate; rhythm, and depth (monitor for bradypnea or respiratory rate less than 12 breaths per minute and restlessness); blood pressure for hypotension; and other problems indicated by dizziness, nausea, and vomiting. Two-hour (and more frequent if needed) assessments are suggested for the first 24 hours. After 24 hours assessments may be made every four hours for the length of medication usage via PCA pump.

Always document findings and follow all agency protocol for PCA pump infusions and use and storage of narcotics. Use all appropriate chart forms, as well.

▼ **Fig. 7-45**

Administering Oral Medications

ASSESSMENT

Assess for contraindications to patient receiving oral medication, including difficulty in swallowing, nausea or vomiting, bowel inflammation or reduced peristalsis, recent gastrointestinal surgery, reduced or absent bowel sounds, and gastric suction. Also assess for allergies.

Determine patient's preferences and tolerances for fluids.

PLANNING AND IMPLEMENTATION

1. Prepare needed supplies and equipment:
   - Medication cards, record forms, or printout
   - Medication cart or tray
   - Disposable medication cups
   - Glass of water, juice, or preferred liquid
   - Drinking straw
   - Mortar and pestle (optional)
2. Paper towels
   Check accuracy and completeness of each medication card, form, or printout with physician's written medication order. Check patient's name and drug name, dosage, route of administration, and time for administration. Report discrepancy in order to charge nurse or physician. (Three checks to five "rights" of drug administration enhances safety!)

▼ **Fig. 7-46** (From Potter P, Perry A: *Fundamentals of nursing: concepts, process, and practice*, ed 3, 1995, St Louis, Mosby.)

3. Prepare drug and wash hands
   - Arrange medication tray and cups in medicine room or move medication cart to position outside patient's room.
   - Unlock medicine drawer or cart (see Fig. 7-46). (Narcotics are generally stored in double-locked box separate from medicine drawers or carts.)
   - Prepare medications for one patient at a time. Keep medication tickets or forms for each patient together.
   - Select correct drug from stock supply or unit-dose drawer. Compare label of medication with medication form, card, or printout.
   - Calculate correct drug dose. Take time. Double check calculation.
   - To prepare tablet or capsules from bottle, pour required number into bottle cap and transfer to medication cup. Do not touch with fingers. Extra tablets or capsules may be returned to bottle.
   - To prepare unit-dose tablets or capsules, place packaged tablet or capsule directly into medicine cup. (Do not remove wrapper.)
   - Place all tablets or capsules given at the same time in one cup except for those requiring preadministration assessments (e.g., pulse rate or blood pressure).
   - If patient has difficulty swallowing, grind tablets in mortar with pestle. Place tablet in bottom of mortar and grind. Continue to crush fragments until smooth powder remains. Alternative method is to place tablet between two medication cups and grind with blunt instrument. Again, continue to crush fragments until fine powder is achieved. Mix crushed tablet in small amount of soft food, such as custard or applesauce. CAUTION: Do not crush enteric-coated or sustained-action medications.
   - Prepare liquids:
     (1) Remove bottle cap from container and place cap upside down.
     (2) Hold bottle with label against palm of hand while pouring.
     (3) Hold medication cup at eye level and fill to desired level on scale (see Fig. 7-47). (Scale should be even with fluid level at its surface or base of meniscus, not edges.)
     (4) Discard excess liquid in cup into sink. Wipe lip of bottle with paper towel.
     (5) Draw volumes of less than 10 ml in syringe (without needle). To prevent accidental ingestion during administration, never use needle to draw up oral medication.

- When preparing narcotic, check narcotic record for previous drug count, compare with supply available, remove drug, and complete necessary information on narcotic form and sign (see Fig. 7-48).
- Compare medication form, card, or printout with prepared drug and container.
- Return stock containers or unused unit-dose medications to shelf or drawer and reread label.
- Place medications and cards, forms, or printouts together on tray or cart.
- Do not leave drugs unattended.

4. Administer medications:
- Take medications to patient at correct time.
- Identify patient by comparing name on card, form, or printout with name on patient's identification bracelet. Ask client to state full name.

▼ **Fig. 7-47** (From Potter P, Perry A: *Fundamentals of nursing: concepts, process, and practice,* ed 3, 1995, St Louis, Mosby.)

▼ **Fig. 7-48** (From Potter P, Perry A: *Fundamentals of nursing: concepts, process, and practice,* ed 3, 1995, St Louis, Mosby.)

- Perform necessary preadministration assessment for specific medications (e.g., blood pressure or pulse).
- Explain purpose of each medication and its action to patient. Allow patient to ask questions about drugs.
- Assist patient to sitting or side-lying position.
- Administer drugs properly and adhere to Universal Precautions:
  (1) Ask if patient wishes to hold solid medications in hand or cup before placing in mouth.
  (2) Offer full glass of water or juice with drugs to be swallowed.
  (3) For sublingually administered drugs, have patient place medication under tongue and allow it to dissolve completely. Caution patient against swallowing.
  (4) Mix powdered medications with liquids at bedside and give to patient to drink.
  (5) Caution patient against chewing or swallowing lozenges.
  (6) Give effervescent powders and tablets immediately after dissolving.
- If patient is unable to hold medications, place medication cup to lips and gently introduce each drug into mouth, one at a time. Do not rush.
- If tablet or capsule falls to floor, discard it and repeat preparation.
- Stay with patient until each medication has been swallowed. If uncertain whether medication has been swallowed, ask patient to open the mouth.
- For highly acidic medications (e.g., aspirin), offer nonfat snack (e.g., crackers).
- Assist patient in returning to comfortable position.
- Dispose of soiled supplies and wash hands.
- Return medication cards, forms, or printouts to appropriate file for next administration time.
- Replenish stock such as cups and straws, return cart to medicine room, and clean work area.

EVALUATION

1. Record actual time that each drug was administered on medication record or computer. Include initials or signature.
2. Return within 30 minutes to 1 hour to evaluate therapeutic response to medications and any side effects if they have occurred.
3. Constantly monitor patient for side effects or adverse reactions, especially if you've administered a first dose or a new drug.
4. Document.

Instilling Ophthalmic Medications

ASSESSMENT

Prior to instilling opthalmic medications, always check the patient's chart for the order as well as any drug allergies, cautions, and contraindications to use of the medication. Also check the medication for its sterility and for the date of expiration (see Fig. 7-49).

PLANNING AND IMPLEMENTATION

1. Gather medication and all necessary equipment such as a sterile 2 × 2 gauze. Gather gloves.

To Administer Ointment

2. Put on gloves and adhere to Universal Precautions. Position patient in either a sitting or supine position and place the head so that it is slightly tilted back. Remove any secretions from the eye by wiping the area with a sterile 2 × 2 gauze from inner to outer canthus. Have the patient look upward and instill the medication into the conjunctival sac by exerting only gentle traction to keep the conjunctival sac open. Gently squeeze the tube of medication to instill an even strip (about 1 to 2 cm) of medication along the border of the conjunctival sac starting at the inner canthus and working toward the outer canthus.

3. Once the medication is instilled, release the lower lid of the eye and ask the patient to close eye and move it around to help distribute the medication. Remove any excess medication with a sterile 2 × 2 gauze, wiping from inner to outer canthus. Document on appropriate parts of the chart and medication record.

To Instill Eyedrops

■ With dominant hand resting on patient's forehead, hold filled medication eye dropper approximately 1 to 2 cm (½ to ¾ in) above conjunctival sac.

■ Drop prescribed number of drops into conjunctival sac.

■ If patient blinks or closes eye or if drops land on outer lid margins, repeat procedure.

■ When administering drugs that cause systemic effects, protect your finger with clean tissue and apply gentle pressure to patient's nasolacrimal duct for 30 to 60 seconds.

■ After instilling drops, ask patient to close eye gently.

EVALUATION

1. Once instilled, assess and reassess the patient for drug effectiveness and possible adverse reactions or worsening of symptoms.

2. Document.

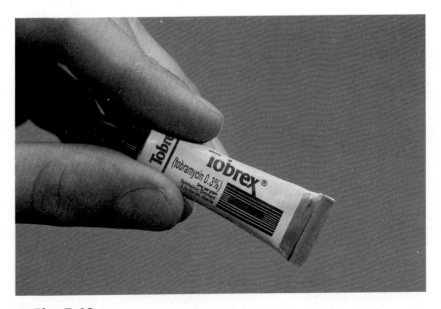

▼ **Fig. 7-49**

Administering Eardrops

ASSESSMENT

1. Review physician's medication order for patient's name, drug name, concentration, time of administration, number of drops to instill, and ear (right or left) to receive medication.
2. Wash hands.

PLANNING AND IMPLEMENTATION

1. Prepare equipment and supplies:
   - Medication bottle and dropper
   - Medication card, form, or printout
   - Cotton-tipped applicator
   - Tissue
   - Cotton ball (optional)
   - Disposable gloves (adhere to Universal Precautions).
2. Apply gloves.
3. Assess condition of external ear structures and canal.
4. Explain procedure to patient.
5. Have patient assume side-lying position with ear to be treated facing up. If cerumen or drainage occludes outermost portion of ear canal, wipe out gently with cotton-tipped applicator. Do *not* force wax inward to block or occlude canal.
6. Straighten ear canal by pulling auricle down and back (children) or upward and outward (adult).
7. Instill prescribed drops holding dropper 1 cm (½ in) above ear canal.
8. Ask patient to remain in side-lying position 2 to 3 minutes. Apply gentle massage or pressure to tragus of ear with finger.
9. At times, physician orders placement of cotton ball into outermost part of canal. Do not press cotton into innermost part of canal.
10. Remove cotton in 15 minutes.
11. Dispose of soiled supplies and gloves and wash hands.
12. Assist client to comfortable position after drops are absorbed. Document and record.

EVALUATION

1. Evaluate condition of external ear between drug instillations, and monitor patient's response.
2. Monitor for side effects and adverse reactions.

Administering Nasal Drops

ASSESSMENT

1. Review physician's medication order for patient's name, drug name, concentration of solution, number of drops, and time of administration. Check for allergies.
2. Refer to medical record to determine which sinus is affected.

PLANNING AND IMPLEMENTATION

1. Wash hands and adhere to Universal Precautions.
2. Prepare equipment and supplies and arrange at bedside:
   - Prepared medication with clean dropper
   - Medication card, form, or printout
   - Facial tissue
   - Small pillow (optional)
   - Washcloth (optional)
   - Disposable gloves
3. Check patient's identification by reading identification bracelet and asking name.
4. Explain procedure regarding positioning and sensations to expect, such as burning or stinging of mucosa or choking sensation as medication trickles into throat.
5. Instruct patient to blow nose unless contraindicated (e.g., risk of increased intracranial pressure or nose bleeds).
6. Administer nasal drops:
   - Assist client to supine position.
   - Position head properly:
     (1) Posterior pharynx—tilt patient's head backward.
     (2) Ethmoid or sphenoid sinus—tilt head back over edge of bed or place pillow under shoulder and tilt head back (see Fig. 7-50A).
     (3) Frontal and maxillary sinus—tilt head back over edge of bed or pillow with head turned toward side treated (see Fig. 7-50B).
     Support patient's head with nondominant hand.
   - Instruct patient to breathe through mouth.
   - Hold dropper 1 cm (½ in) above nares and instill prescribed number of drops toward midline of ethmoid bone.
   - Have client remain in supine position 5 minutes.
   - Offer facial tissue to blot runny nose, but caution against blowing nose for several minutes.
7. Assist patient to a comfortable position after drug has been absorbed.

8. Dispose of soiled supplies in proper container and wash hands.
9. Record medication administration, including drug name, concentration, number of drops, nostril into which drug was instilled, and time of administration.

EVALUATION

1. Observe patient for side effects 15 to 30 minutes after administration. Monitor for possible rebound congestion associated with overuse of decongestant sprays.
2. Monitor for therapeutic effects.

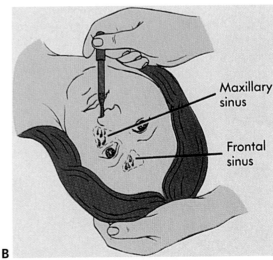

▼ **Fig. 7-50** (From Potter P, Perry A: *Fundamentals of nursing: concepts, process, and practice*, ed 3, 1995, St Louis, Mosby.)

Administering Medications via a Nasogastric Tube

ASSESSMENT

Before administering the medication, follow the 5 "rights" of medication administration and check for any cautions and contraindications regarding use of the medication, including concerns and safety issues for nasogastric tubes.

PLANNING AND IMPLEMENTATION

Gather all equipment needed for the procedure such as a large bulb or piston syringe, an emesis basin, protective blue pad, towels, 30 to 60 cc tap water, and disposable gloves. Adhere to Universal Precautions.

1. Identify your patient and position with head of the bed elevated. Place protective pad under patient's head and on the chest area.
2. FOR SMALL-BORE TUBES, after obtaining and setting-up a piston syringe of at least 30 cc in volume (to minimize pressure and damage the tube) (see Fig. 7-51), confirm placement of tube (confirmed, for the first time by radiology). (*Note:* After the position of nasogastric tube has been confirmed, [see Fig. 7-52] a three-way stopcock may be used to help control flow of solution.)

▼ **Fig. 7-51**

▼ **Fig. 7-52**

Attach the small medication syringe to the tube after it has been uncapped and infuse the medication while applying gentle pressure on the syringe's piston (see Fig. 7-53). Once medication is instilled, flush with approximately 10 cc tap water. Cap the tube with the plug and position patient in a high-Fowler's position or a slightly elevated right side-lying position.

With large-bore NG tubes, leave medication in the medication cup and confirm placement of the tube. With the piston removed from the syringe, uncap the NG tube, pour in 30 cc of water to clear tubing, and pour the medication from the dosage cup into the barrel of the syringe, followed by 30 cc of tap water to ensure that the medication is cleared from the tube. ALWAYS allow any fluid to flow via gravity in the NG tubes—NEVER force any fluid into the tube (see Fig. 7-54).

Once completed, close the tube with the cap and position patient in high-Fowler's position or slightly elevated right side-lying position (see Fig. 7-55).

EVALUATION

1. Once instilled, assess and reassess the patient for drug effectiveness and for possible adverse reactions or worsening of symptoms.
2. Monitor closely for possible aspiration.

▼ **Fig. 7-53**

▼ Fig. 7-54

▼ Fig. 7-55

PART 2

CENTRAL NERVOUS SYSTEM: STUDY SKILLS BRIEFS

VOCABULARY

In any subject matter mastering the vocabulary is essential to mastering the content. But in a complex, technical subject such as nursing pharmacology, if the vocabulary is not mastered, understanding the content will be almost impossible. Each chapter in this text contains a glossary of unfamiliar terms at the beginning and, as an independent learner, you should spend some time and energy on the vocabulary contained in the glossary. Do not expect to completely understand and master the terms from the glossary alone. The terms are further defined and explained in the body of the chapter, and it is when you read the chapter that you should expect to fully master the vocabulary. However, the time you spend working on the glossary will pay off when you read the chapter.

Consider the terms *agonist* and *antagonist* in the Chapter 8 glossary. These terms share a common word part, which means the words are related in meaning. This is an important first step in mastering them. What does "agonist" mean? What is the similarity between "agonist" and "antagonist"? What is the essential difference between the two? Asking these questions as you start to work on Chapter 8 is a valuable technique for beginning to master the language of the content. Do not simply memorize the terms. Learn what they mean, and link relationships between words with com-

mon elements. As you practice this technique it will become easier to retain the meaning.

In the Chapter 8 glossary there is another group of words that should be viewed as a group that shares an important relationship. The first of these words is *pain*. The definition provided is clear and relatively easy to understand, but your focus should be not just on that single word because there are five other words that relate to "pain." The words are *acute*, *chronic*, *somatic*, *superficial*, and *visceral*. Each of these words defines and categorizes "pain" in very specific ways. As you go about setting up vocabulary cards, look at the opening pages in this chapter. You will find that there is considerable discussion of these terms, and that discussion is useful in helping you obtain the fullest understanding of these terms. Again, a reminder. Do not simply focus on a meaning for each term, but also ask what the similarities and/or differences are and how these words relate to one another.

TEXT NOTATION

In Chapter 1 I discussed a method for text underlining. If it is done carefully, this strategy is particularly useful for later review of text material. The object of text underlining is to pick out important terms, ideas, and key information so that you can come back to it at some later point for quick review. There are three key elements in successful text notation. First, you must read the material once before attempting any underlining. Second, you must be acutely aware of the author's language. Finally, you must be highly selective in underlining. The most common fault in underlining is to mark too much material. What follows are two paragraphs from Chapter 8 that I have underlined. My underlining should be viewed as an example of what can be done. Each reader will mark the text somewhat differently based on his/her background and experience. As you study this example, think not only about what I have chosen to underline but also about WHY I chose that material.

To fully understand how analgesics work, it is necessary to know what pain is and what its characteristics are. <u>**Pain**</u> is <u>most commonly defined</u> as an <u>unpleasant sensory and emotional experience</u> associated with either actual or potential tissue damage. It is a very personal and individual experience. Although the mechanisms of pain and the nature of pain pathways are becoming better understood, <u>an individual patient's perception of pain and appreciation of its meaning are complex</u> processes. Pain <u>involves psychologic and emotional processes</u>. Because pain is a very individual experience and cannot be quantified, for a caregiver to effectively manage a patient suffering from pain, it is essential that he or she cultivate a relationship with the patient that is built on trust and faith. There is <u>no single approach to effective pain management</u>. Instead pain management has to be individualized and take into account the cause of the pain, if known, the existence of concurrent medical conditions, the characteristics of the pain, and the psychologic and cultural characteristics of the patient. It also requires ongoing reassessment of the pain and the effectiveness of treatment. Therefore <u>pain</u> is often <u>described as having two elements</u>—a <u>physical element</u> and a <u>psychologic element</u>.

The <u>physical element</u> of pain involves the <u>patient's actual sensation of pain</u>. This involves various nerve pathways and the brain and is often <u>referred to as the</u> <u>**pain threshold**</u>, or the <u>level of stimulus needed to produce the perception of pain</u>. This is a <u>measure of the physiologic response</u> of the nervous system and is therefore <u>similar for most persons</u>. The <u>psychologic element</u> represents the <u>patient's emotional response</u> to the pain. These responses are greatly molded by the patient's age, sex, culture, previous pain experience, and anxiety level. This <u>psychologic element</u> of pain is also <u>called</u> <u>**pain tolerance**</u>, or the <u>amount of pain a patient can endure without its interfering with normal function</u>. Pain tolerance can vary from patient to patient because it is a subjective response to pain not a

physiologic function. As a result, the patient's personality, environment, culture, or ethnic background can separately or collectively alter this response. Relatively speaking, <u>a constant pain threshold exists in all persons under normal circumstances</u>, but <u>pain tolerance</u>, or the point beyond which pain becomes unbearable, <u>varies widely</u> among persons. It can even vary within the patient depending on the circumstance involved. Table 8-1 lists the <u>various conditions</u> that can cause a person's pain threshold to be altered.

LANGUAGE CONVENTIONS

Certain words and phrases are like signal lights at an intersection. They serve to tell the reader that something special, important, or noteworthy is happening. To the attentive, active reader these conventions contribute significantly to understanding what the author is trying to convey. Whether you are highlighting, underlining, doing margin notes, or studying the material using the PURR model, it is important that you become sensitive to these conventions.

The text following the topic heading *NARCOTIC ANALGESICS* contains several examples. The second sentence contains the phrase *classified by*. Whenever an author says that something is being classified it means there are at least two (and perhaps several more) elements of the term or idea that are being classified. This means that you should immediately ask a question about the reading, "What is being classified? How many classifications are there for this?" These questions will help you focus on what to learn and keep your attention firmly fixed on the process of learning.

Another example of this use of classification is found in the next paragraph, "Narcotics broken down into <u>three main classes</u>"; the underlining is my emphasis. This phrase should leap off the page and shout at you, "Here is something I must remember. How many classes? Three!" The author has already set a focus for you in this case. What must you learn and remember? The three main classes of narcotics. As you read this chapter, or any other chapter, try to become aware of words and phrases like these that are intended to draw your attention to something the author especially wanted to emphasize. The more aware of language conventions you become, the easier it will be to become a selective reader. Selective readers do not try to remember everything they read, but are able to select from the mass of information those concepts and/or terms that the writers tried to stress.

Chapter 8

Narcotic Analgesic Agents

Objectives

When you reach the end of this chapter, you will be able to:

1 Discuss the use of narcotics in pain management.

2 Discuss the differences between a narcotic agonist, agonist-antagonist, and antagonist.

3 List the different drugs in groupings of narcotic analgesics.

4 Compare the mechanisms of action, drug effects, therapeutic uses, side effects, adverse effects, and interactions of the narcotic agonists and agonist-antagonists.

5 Develop a comprehensive nursing care plan, including patient education, as it relates to the nursing process and administration of narcotics in the patient experiencing pain.

CHAPTER OUTLINE

Physiology and Psychology of Pain
Narcotic Analgesics
  Chemical structure
  Mechanism of action
  Drug effects
  Therapeutic uses
  Side effects and adverse effects
    Toxicity and overdose
  Interactions
  Dosages
  Laboratory results
Drug Profiles
  ⚓ Morphine sulfate
  Codeine sulfate
  ⚓ Fentanyl
  ⚓ Meperidine hydrochloride
  Methadone hydrochloride
  Propoxyphene hydrochloride/Napsylate
Agonist-Antagonist Narcotics
Narcotic Antagonists
  Naloxone hydrochloride
  Naltrexone hydrochloride

Nursing Process
Assessment
Nursing Diagnoses
Planning
  Outcome criteria
Implementation
Evaluation

Glossary

Acute pain Pain that is sudden in onset and usually subsides when treated. (p. 90)

Adjuvant agent A drug that is not a primary analgesic but has been shown to have independent or additive analgesic properties. (p. 93)

Agonist A substance that binds to a receptor and causes a response. (p. 92)

Agonist-antagonist A substance that binds to a receptor and causes the receptor to be stimulated and a response to occur while simultaneously binding to another receptor, occupying it but not stimulating it. (p. 92)

Analgesics Medications that relieve pain without causing loss of consciousness and sometimes referred to as *painkillers*. (p. 89)

Antagonist An agent that binds to a receptor and prevents a response. (p. 92)

Chronic pain Persistent or recurring pain that is often very difficult to treat. (p. 90)

Gate theory The most common and well-described theory of pain transmission and pain relief: It uses a gate model to explain how impulses from damaged tissues are sensed in the brain. (p. 90)

Narcotic analgesics Very strong and addicting pain relievers. (p. 92)

Narcotic withdrawal (opioid abstinence syndrome) The signs and symptoms associated with the abstinence from or withdrawal of opioid analgesics when the body has become physically dependent on the substance. (p. 94)

Opiate and opioid analgesics Narcotic pain relievers that contain opium, are derived from opium, or are chemically related to opium. (p. 92)

Opioid tolerance A common physiologic result of

long-term opioid use in which larger doses of opioids are required to maintain the same level of analgesia. (p. 94)

Pain An unpleasant sensory and emotional experience associated with actual or potential tissue damage. (p. 89)

Pain threshold The level of stimulus that results in the perception of pain. (p. 89)

Pain tolerance The amount of pain a patient can endure without its interfering with normal function. (p. 90)

Partial agonist A substance that binds to part of a receptor and causes effects similar to but less pronounced than those of a pure agonist. (p. 92)

Physical dependence The physical adaptation of the body to the presence of an opioid or other addicting substance (e.g., barbiturates). (p. 94)

Psychologic dependence (addiction) A pattern of compulsive opioid use characterized by a continuous craving for the substance and the need to use it for effects other than pain relief. (p. 93)

Somatic pain Pain that originates from skeletal muscles, ligaments, or joints. (p. 90)

Superficial pain Pain that originates from the skin or mucous membranes. (p. 90)

Visceral pain Pain that originates from organs or smooth muscles. (p. 90)

Medications that relieve pain without causing loss of consciousness are referred to as **analgesics** but are also often called *painkillers*. There are various classes of analgesics, and these are determined by the chemical structures and the mechanisms of action of the agents. This chapter focuses on those agents commonly used to relieve moderate to severe pain. These agents are called *narcotic analgesics*. The next most common analgesic class consists of the nonsteroidal antiinflammatory drugs (NSAIDs), which are discussed in Chapter 42.

PHYSIOLOGY AND PSYCHOLOGY OF PAIN

To fully understand how analgesics work, it is necessary to know what pain is and what its characteristics are. **Pain** is most commonly defined as an unpleasant sensory and emotional experience associated with either actual or potential tissue damage. It is a very personal and individual experience. Although the mechanisms of pain and the nature of pain pathways are becoming better understood, an individual patient's perception of pain and appreciation of its meaning are complex processes. Pain involves psychologic and emotional processes. Because pain is a very individual experience and cannot be quantified, for a caregiver to effectively manage a patient suffering from pain, it is essential that he or she cultivate a relationship with the patient that is built on trust and faith. There is no single

approach to effective pain management. Instead pain management has to be individualized and take into account the cause of the pain, if known, the existence of concurrent medical conditions, the characteristics of the pain, and the psychologic and cultural characteristics of the patient (see the box below). It also requires ongoing reassessment of the pain and the effectiveness of treatment. Therefore pain is often described as having two elements—a physical element and a psychologic element.

The physical element of pain involves the patient's actual sensation of pain. This involves various nerve pathways and the brain and is often referred to as the **pain threshold,** or the level of stimulus needed to produce the perception of pain. This is a measure of the physiologic response of the nervous system and is therefore similar for most persons. The psychologic element represents the patient's emotional response to

CULTURAL IMPLICATIONS
Pain and Pain Management

- Each culture has its own beliefs, thoughts, and ways of approaching, defining, and managing pain.

- Attitudes, meanings, and perceptions of pain vary with each culture.

- Many African-Americans believe in the power of healers who rely strongly on the religious faith of the people and often use prayer and the laying on of hands.

- Hispanic-Americans believe in prayer, the wearing of amulets, and the use of herbs and spices in maintaining health and states of wellness. Specific herbs are used in teas, and therapies often include religious practices, massage, and "cleansings" such as the passing of herbs over the body.

- The traditional methods of healing for the Chinese include acupuncture, herbal remedies, yin and yang, and cold treatment. Moxibustion is another form of healing and involves placing pulverized wormwood on the skin over specific meridian points.

- For Native Americans, treatments include massage, the application of heat, sweatbaths, herbal remedies, and being in harmony with nature.

- Nurses should be aware of all the cultural influences on health-related behaviors, on patients' attitudes toward medication therapy, and ultimately on its effectiveness. A thorough assessment with questions about the patient's cultural background and practices is important to the effective and individualized delivery of nursing care.

the pain. These responses are greatly molded by the patient's age, sex, culture, previous pain experience, and anxiety level. This psychologic element of pain is also called **pain tolerance**, or the amount of pain a patient can endure without its interfering with normal function. Pain tolerance can vary from patient to patient because it is a subjective response to pain not a physiologic function. As a result, the patient's personality, environment, culture, or ethnic background can separately or collectively alter this response. Relatively speaking, a constant pain threshold exists in all persons under normal circumstances, but pain tolerance, or the point beyond which pain becomes unbearable, varies widely among persons. It can even vary within the patient depending on the circumstance involved. Table 8-1 lists the various conditions that can cause a person's pain threshold to be altered.

Pain can also be further classified in terms of its onset and duration as either acute or chronic. Acute and chronic pain differ not only in their onset and duration but also in how they are treated. They are also associated with various diseases or conditions. **Acute pain** is sudden in onset and usually subsides when treated. **Chronic pain** is persistent or recurring and is often very difficult to treat. Table 8-2 gives the different characteristics of acute and chronic pain and lists various diseases and conditions associated with each.

Pain can be further classified according to its source. The two most commonly mentioned sources of pain are somatic and visceral pain. **Somatic pain** originates from skeletal muscles, ligaments, or joints. **Visceral pain** originates from organs or smooth muscles. Sometimes pain is described as superficial. This type of pain originates from the skin or mucous membranes and is called **superficial pain**. Pain treatment can be more appropriately selected when the source of the pain is known. Visceral and superficial pain usually require narcotics for relief, whereas somatic pain usually responds better to nonnarcotic analgesics like NSAIDs.

There are several theories to explain pain transmission and pain relief. The most common and well described is the **gate theory**. This theory, proposed by Melzack and Wall in 1965, uses the analogy of a gate to describe how impulses from damaged tissues are sensed in the brain. First, the tissue injury causes the release of several substances such as bradykinin, histamine, potassium, prostaglandins, and serotonin. Many of our current pain management strategies are aimed at altering the actions and levels of these substances. Once these substances are released by the damaged tissue, an action potential is initiated. This action potential travels along a sensory nerve fiber and activates a pain receptor. There are two basic types of these nerve fibers—A and C. Table 8-3 summarizes the differences in the size and function in these two types of nerve fibers. The different types of pain experienced are believed to be related to the relative proportions of A and C fibers in a particular area of the body.

These pain fibers, along with other sensory nerve fibers, enter the spinal cord and travel up to the brain. The site where these fibers enter the spinal cord is referred to as the *dorsal (posterior) horn of the spinal cord*. It is here that the so-called gates are located. These gates regulate the flow of sensory impulses. If impulses are stopped by the gate at this junction, no impulses are transmitted to the higher centers of the brain. Because it is at these higher centers where impulses are

Table 8-1	Conditions That Alter Pain Threshold

PAIN THRESHOLD	CONDITIONS
Lowered	Anger, anxiety, depression, discomfort, fear, isolation, chronic pain, sleeplessness, and tiredness
Raised	Diversion, empathy, rest, sympathy, and medications (analgesics, antianxiety agents, and antidepressants)

Table 8-2	Acute versus Chronic Pain		
TYPE OF PAIN	ONSET	DURATION	EXAMPLES
Acute	Sudden (minutes to hours)	Limited (has an end)	Acute myocardial infarction Acute appendicitis Dental procedures Kidney stones Surgical procedures
Chronic	Slow (days to months)	Persistent or recurring (endless)	Arthritis Cancer Lower back pain Peripheral neuropathy

consciously perceived by the patient, in this instance there would be no perception of pain. Figure 8-1 depicts the gate theory of pain transmission.

The opening and closing of this gate are influenced by the relative activation of the large-diameter A-fibers and the small-diameter C-fibers. The closing of the gate seems to be effected by the activation of A-fibers. This causes the inhibition of impulse transmission to the brain and thus no perception of pain. Opening of the gate is effected by stimulation of the C-fibers. This allows impulses to be transmitted to the brain and pain to be perceived. This gate is also connected to (innervated) nerve fibers that originate in the brain as opposed to fibers that originate from the gate and go to the brain. The nerve fibers that go from the brain to the gate allow the brain to have some control over this gate. They enable the brain to evaluate, identify, and localize the pain. Thus the brain can control the gate, either keeping the gate closed or allowing it to open so that the brain is stimulated and pain perceived. The cells that control the gate, called the *T-cells*, have a threshold. Impulses that reach these T-cells must overcome this threshold before an impulse is permitted to travel up to the brain.

The body is equipped with certain endogenous neurotransmitters known as *enkephalins* and *endorphins*. These substances are produced within the body to fight pain and are considered the body's pain killers. They are capable of binding with opioid receptors and inhibiting the transmission of pain impulses by closing the gate. These endogenous analgesic substances are released whenever the body experiences pain. They are responsible for the phenomenon of a runner's high. Figure 8-1 depicts this entire process.

Table 8-3	A and C Nerve Fibers				
TYPE OF FIBER	**MYELIN SHEATH**	**FIBER SIZE**	**CONDUCTION SPEED**	**TRANSMISSION**	**TYPE OF PAIN**
A	Yes	Large	Fast	Inhibited	Sharp and well localized
C	No	Small	Slow	Facilitated	Dull and nonlocalized

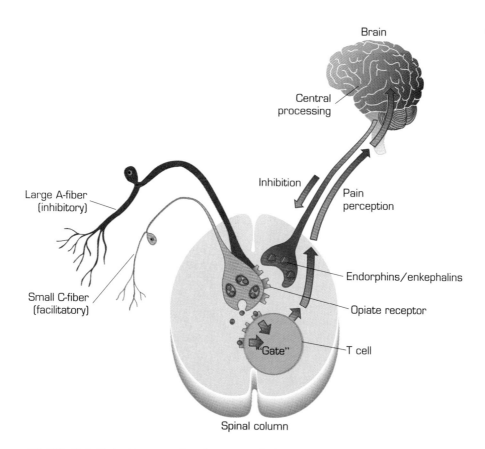

▼ FIG. 8-1 Gate theory of pain transmission.

Another phenomenon of pain relief that can be explained by the gate theory is that of massaging or of applying liniment to a painful area. Typically this reduces pain. When rubbing or applying liniment to an area, large sensory fibers from peripheral receptors carry impulses to the spinal cord. This causes impulse transmission to be inhibited and the gate to be closed. This in turn reduces the recognition of the pain impulses arriving by means of the small fibers. This is the same pathway that the opioid analgesics use to alleviate pain.

NARCOTIC ANALGESICS

Narcotic analgesics are very strong pain relievers. Narcotics can be classified either by their chemical structure or by their action at their respective receptors (i.e., mechanism of action).

Chemical Structure

When classified by their chemical structure, narcotics can be broken down into three main classes: the naturally occurring **opiates**, the semisynthetic opioids, and the synthetic opioids. **Opioid analgesics** are narcotic pain relievers that contain or are derived from opium. Most narcotics are opioids, which are synthetic narcotics with opiate-like activities or with opiate-like effects. Table 8-4 lists the various narcotic analgesics and their respective chemical categories. Many of the undesirable characteristics of the narcotics are directly related to their chemical structure. It is this chemical structure that causes histamine to be released. The naturally occurring opiates cause the most to be released and the synthetic opioids cause the least. It is this histamine release that causes the itching, rash, and hemodynamic changes (e.g., drop in blood pressure and decrease in heart rate). Often if a patient cannot

tolerate a natural opiate like morphine, a switch is made to a synthetic opioid like meperidine to decrease the histamine release and reduce the unwanted side effects.

Mechanism of Action

There are three types of narcotics, agonists, agonist-antagonists, and partial agonists, and these are determined by their action at the receptor. An **agonist** binds to a receptor and causes a response. An **agonist-antagonist** binds to a receptor and causes a response just as a pure agonist does, but it also binds to another type of receptor and blocks a response just as an antagonist does. A **partial agonist** binds to part of a receptor and causes effects similar to, but less pronounced than, those of a true agonist. Besides these three main types of narcotics, there are also substances that reverse the effects of these agents on pain receptors. These agents are referred to as **antagonists**. An antagonist binds to a receptor and prevents a response. Sometimes they may also push an agonist off from its receptor and therefore reverse its response. Sometimes an antagonist competes for the binding site on the opioid receptor. In this event the agent with the greater affinity for the receptor binds to it, either stimulating it or blocking it.

The actual receptors that narcotics bind to to relieve pain are listed and their characteristics summarized in Table 8-5. Five types of opioid receptors have been identified to date: mu, kappa, sigma, delta, and epsilon. Three of these, mu, kappa, and sigma, are the main ones. Many of the characteristics of a particular narcotic, such as its ability to sedate, its potency, or its ability to cause hallucinations, can be attributed to the particular narcotic's affinity for these various receptors.

Table 8-4	Chemical Classification of Narcotics
CHEMICAL CATEGORY	**NARCOTIC AGENTS**
Natural opiates	Codeine, morphine, and opium
Semisynthetic opioids	Buprenorphine (P), hydrocodone, hydromorphone, levorphanol, nalbuphine (A/A), oxycodone, and oxymorphone
Synthetic opioids	Alfentanil, butorphanol (A/A), fentanyl, meperidine, methadone, pentazocine, propoxyphene, and sufentanil

A/A, agonist/antagonist; P, partial agonist.

Table 8-5	Opioid Receptors and Their Characteristics	
RECEPTOR TYPE	**PROTOTYPICAL AGONIST**	**EFFECTS**
Mu	⚓ Morphine	Supraspinal analgesia Respiratory depression Euphoria ++ Sedation
Kappa	Ketocyclazocine	Spinal analgesia ++++ Sedation Miosis
Sigma	SKF 10047	Dysphoria Psychomotor stimulation Hallucinations

Drug Effects

Narcotic analgesics achieve their beneficial effects by their actions in the central nervous system. However, they also act outside the central nervous system, and many of their unwanted effects stem from these actions.

Therapeutic Uses

The main effect of narcotics is to alleviate moderate to severe pain. The degree to which pain is relieved or unwanted side effects occur depends on the specific agent, the receptors it binds to, and its chemical structure. Often drugs from other chemical categories are added to the narcotic regimen as **adjuvant agents**. These assist the primary agents in relieving pain. The NSAIDs are commonly used in this capacity. This allows the use of smaller doses of narcotics, which accomplishes two important functions. First, it diminishes some of the side effects that are more commonly seen with higher doses of narcotics, such as respiratory depression, constipation, and urinary retention. Second, it approaches the pain stimulus from another mechanism and has a resulting synergistic beneficial effect in reducing the pain.

Many narcotics have an affinity for the central nervous system. Once there, they suppress the medullary cough center, which results in cough suppression. The most commonly used narcotic for this is codeine. Hydrocodone has also been used in many cough suppressants either alone or in combination with other agents. Sometimes the narcotic-related cough suppressants have a depressant effect on the central nervous system and cause sedation. To avoid this problem, dextromethorphan, a nonnarcotic cough suppressant, is often given instead.

An unwanted side effect of narcotics, decreased gastrointestinal motility (constipation), is sometimes used therapeutically to treat diarrhea. Some of the most common narcotic-containing antidiarrhea preparations are camphorated opium tincture (paregoric) and diphenoxylate (Lomotil).

Strong narcotic analgesics like fentanyl, sufentanil, and alfentanil are commonly used in combination with anesthetics during surgery. These agents are used not only to relieve pain but to also maintain a balanced state of anesthesia. This practice of using combinations of drugs rather than a single agent to produce anesthesia is referred to as *balanced anesthesia*.

Side Effects and Adverse Effects

As already mentioned, many of the unwanted effects of narcotic analgesics are related to their effects on parts of the body other than the central nervous system. Some of these unwanted effects can be explained by the respective agent's selectivity for the receptors listed in Table 8-5. The various body systems that the narcotics affect and their side effects and adverse effects are summarized in Table 8-6.

Narcotics that have an affinity for both mu and sigma receptors produce euphoria and hallucinations. These are the narcotics that are most likely to be abused and used for recreational use. The person taking them to alter his or her mental status will soon become psychologically dependent on them. **Psychologic dependence (addiction)** is a pattern of compulsive drug use characterized by a continuous craving for a narcotic and the need to use it for effects other than pain relief.

All narcotics cause some histamine release, and it is thought that this histamine release is responsible for many of the unwanted side effects such as itching or pruritus, rash, and hemodynamic changes. The histamine release causes peripheral arteries and veins to dilate, which leads to flushing and orthostatic hypotension. The amount of histamine release that a narcotic analgesic causes is related to its chemical class. The naturally occurring opiates elicit the most histamine release; the synthetic opioids, the least. The various narcotics and their respective chemical class are listed in Table 8-4.

One of the most serious side effects of narcotics is respiratory depression. When narcotics are given, care should be taken to titrate the dose so that the patient's pain is controlled without respiratory function being affected. Individual responses to narcotics vary, and patients may occasionally suffer respiratory compromise or the loss of airway reflexes despite careful dose titration. Respiratory depression can be prevented in part by using agents with very short durations of ac-

Table 8-6	Narcotic-Induced Side Effects and Adverse Effects by Body System
BODY SYSTEM	**SIDE EFFECT OR ADVERSE EFFECT**
Central nervous system	Sedation, disorientation, euphoria, light-headedness, dysphoria, lowered seizure threshold, and tremors
Cardiovascular system	Hypotension, palpitations, and flushing
Respiratory tract	Respiratory depression and aggravation of asthma
Gastrointestinal tract	Nausea, vomiting, constipation, and biliary tract spasm
Genitourinary tract	Urinary retention
Other	Itching, rash, and wheal formation

tion and no active metabolites. It seems to be more common in persons with a preexisting condition causing respiratory compromise such as asthma or chronic obstructive pulmonary disease. Respiratory depression is strongly related to the degree of sedation. Stimulation of the patient may be adequate to reverse mild hypoventilation. If this is unsuccessful, assisted ventilation by bag and mask or if needed by endotracheal intubation may be needed to support respiration. It may also be necessary to administer naloxone, a narcotic reversal agent, to reverse severe respiratory depression. However, keep in mind that naloxone will not only reverse the patient's respiratory depression but will also reverse the pain control. Careful slow titration of naloxone will prevent over-reversal of the narcotic-induced respiratory depression and pain relief. The effects of naloxone are short-lived, usually lasting about 1 hour. With long-acting opioid narcotics the respiratory depressant effects can reappear after the naloxone has worn off, and redosing may be needed.

Gastrointestinal tract side effects are common in patients receiving narcotics. Nausea, vomiting, and constipation are the most common ones associated with the narcotic analgesics. Narcotics irritate the gastrointestinal tract, stimulating the chemoreceptor trigger zone in the central nervous system, which in turn causes nausea and vomiting. Narcotics slow peristalsis and increase water absorption from intestinal contents. These two actions combine to produce constipation. This is more pronounced in a hospitalized patient who is nonambulatory, because lack of daily activity also causes constipation.

Urinary retention, or the inability to void, is another unwanted side effect of narcotic analgesics. They do this by increasing bladder tone. This is sometimes treated with low doses of an opioid agonist-antagonist like nalbuphine or with an opioid antagonist like naloxone.

Severe hypersensitivity or anaphylaxis to narcotic analgesics is rare. Most patients will experience gastro-intestinal tract or histamine-mediated reactions to narcotics and call these "allergic reactions." True anaphylaxis is rare, even with intravenously administered narcotics. Some patients may complain of flushing, itching, or wheal formation at the injection site, but this is usually local and histamine mediated.

Toxicity and Overdose

Narcotic analgesics produce both their beneficial effects and their toxic or unwanted effects by means of receptors. These receptors and the positive and negative effects they bring about are listed in Table 8-5. The narcotic antagonists naloxone and naltrexone bind to and occupy all these receptor sites (mu, kappa, and sigma). They are competitive antagonists with a strong affinity for these binding sites. Therefore they can push off opioids that already occupy the receptor. In doing so they can reverse the adverse effects induced by the narcotic such as respiratory depression. These agents are used in the management of both narcotic overdose and narcotic addiction. The commonly used narcotic antagonists (reversal agents) are listed in Table 8-7.

In the management of narcotic overdose or toxicity, it is important to recognize the signs and symptoms of withdrawal. **Opioid tolerance** is a common physiologic result of long-term narcotic use; patients with opioid tolerance require larger doses of the opioid agent to maintain the same level of analgesia. The physiologic adaptation of the body to the effects of a narcotic is referred to as **physical dependence**. Opioid tolerance and physical dependence are expected in patients undergoing long-term narcotic treatment and should not be confused with psychologic dependence (addiction), manifested by drug abuse behavior. The confusing of these terms in relation to narcotic therapy leads to ineffective pain management and contributes to the problem of undertreatment. Physical dependence on narcotics is seen when an agent is discontinued abruptly or when an opioid antagonist is administered. This physiologic response is referred to as **narcotic withdrawal** or **opioid abstinence syndrome**.

Table 8-7	Narcotic Antagonists (Reversal Agents)		
Generic Name	**Trade Name**	**Dosage**	**Cautions**
Naloxone (IV)	Narcan	0.4-2 mg q2-3/min (<10 mg) IV infusion: 2 mg in 500 ml (titrate to response)	Raised or lowered blood pressure Arrhythmias Pulmonary edema Withdrawal
Naltrexone (PO)	ReVia	25-50 mg qd	Nervousness Headache Nausea/vomiting Pulmonary edema Withdrawal

It is manifested by anxiety, irritability, chills and hot flashes, joint pain, lacrimation, rhinorrhea, diaphoresis, nausea, vomiting, and abdominal cramps and diarrhea.

The timing of the onset of withdrawal symptoms is directly related to the half-life of the narcotic analgesic being used. The withdrawal symptoms resulting from the discontinuance or reversal of short acting opioid therapy (codeine, hydrocodone, morphine, and hydromorphone) will arise within 6 to 12 hours and peak at 24 to 72 hours. The withdrawal symptoms associated with the long half-life agents (methadone, levorphanol, and transdermal fentanyl) may not appear for 24 hours or more after drug discontinuation and may be milder. The appearance of the abstinence syndrome indicates physical dependence on the narcotics, which may occur after just 2 weeks of therapy. It does not, however, imply the existence of psychologic dependence or addiction! Most patients with cancer take narcotic analgesics for more than 2 weeks, and only very rarely do they exhibit the drug abuse behavior and psychologic dependence that characterize addiction.

Interactions

Potential drug interactions with narcotics are significant. See Table 8-8 for a full discussion of the risks associated with the coadministration of other agents.

Dosages

For the recommended dosages of selected agents see the following dosages table.

Table 8-8	Narcotics: Drug Interactions	
Drug	**Mechanism**	**Effect**
Alcohol		
Antihistamines		
Barbiturates	Additive effects	Increased respiratory depression (with barbiturates)
Benzodiazepines		
Phenothiazines		
Other central nervous system depressants		
Monoamine oxidase inhibitor	Unknown	Respiratory depression and hypotension, especially with meperidine

Laboratory Results

Narcotics can cause an abnormal increase in the serum levels of amylase, alanine aminotransferase, alkaline phosphatase, bilirubin, lipase, creatinine kinase, and lactic dehydrogenase. Other abnormal results include a decrease in urinary 17-keto-steroid level and an increase in the urinary alkaloid and glucose concentrations.

DRUG PROFILES

⚓ MORPHINE SULFATE

Morphine is an alkaloid obtained from opium and is the prototype narcotic drug. Opium is the dried juice of the poppy plant *Papaver somniferum* and is a mixture of narcotic and nonnarcotic alkaloids. The potential for the misuse of morphine is high, as is the addiction liability. It is also highly constipating.

The drug is contraindicated in patients showing hypersensitivity to it, and extreme caution is required when administering it to patients with head injuries.

⬡ PHARMACOKINETICS

HALF-LIFE	ONSET	PEAK	DURATION
1.7-4.5 hr	Rapid	IM: 30-60 min	IM: 6-7 hr

CODEINE SULFATE

Codeine sulfate methylmorphine is the second narcotic alkaloid obtained from opium. However, the yield is low, and the high medical consumption of codeine necessitates its synthesis by methylating morphine. Codeine is similar to morphine in terms of its pharmacokinetic and pharmacodynamic properties, but is less effective as an analgesic and is widely used as an antitussive agent in an array of cough preparations. It is currently listed on schedule C-II of controlled substances, which would imply a high addiction liability. However, codeine addiction is theoretical and practically nonexistent.

⬡ PHARMACOKINETICS

HALF-LIFE	ONSET	PEAK	DURATION
2.5-4 hr	15-30 min	35-45 min	4-6 hr

D O S A G E S

SELECTED ANALGESIC AGENTS

AGENT	PHARMACOLOGIC CLASS	DOSAGE RANGE	PURPOSE
⬇Morphine sulfate	Narcotic Opiate Opium alkaloid	*Pediatric* SC: 0.1-0.2 mg/kg dose—do not exceed a 15-mg single dose	Narcotic analgesic
		Adult IM/SC: 5-20 mg q4h; rectal: 10-20 mg q4h; IV: 2.5-15 mg.	Narcotic analgesic
Codeine sulfate	Narcotic Opiate Opium alkaloid	*Pediatric* PO/SC/IM: 2-5 y/o, 2.5-5 mg q4-6h. Do not exceed 30 mg/day	Antitussive
		Adult/Children >12 y/o 10-20 mg q4-6h—do not exceed 120 mg/day	Antitussive
		Pediatric 6-11 y/o, 5-10 mg q4-6h	Antitussive
		Adult 15-60 mg 3-4 times/day	Narcotic analgesic
⬇Meperidine HCl	Narcotic Synthetic opioid	*Pediatric* PO/IM/SC: 0.5-0.8 mg/lb q3-4h prn	Narcotic analgesic
		Adult PO/IM/SC: 50-150 mg q3-4h prn; IM/SC: 50-100 mg; IM/SC: 50-100 mg 30-90 min before anesthesia	Obstetric analgesia, preop sedation
		Pediatric IM/SC: 0.5-1 mg/kg 30-90 min before anesthesia	Preop sedation
Methadone HCl	Narcotic Synthetic opioid	*Adult* PO/IM/SC: 2.5-10 mg q3-4h; ≥40 mg once/day, reduced doses every few days; ≥40-120 mg once/day	Narcotic analgesic, narcotic detoxification, narcotic addiction maintenance
Propoxyphene HCl/ napsylate	Analgesic	*Adult* PO: 65 mg q4h prn—do not exceed 340 mg/day; 100 mg q4h prn—do not exceed 600 mg/day	Analgesic
Naloxone HCl	Narcotic antagonist	*Pediatric* IM/IV/SC: 0.01 mg/kg IV followed by 0.1 mg/kg if needed; 0.005-0.01 mg/kg IV—repeat in 2-3 min intervals	Narcotic overdose, postop reversal
		Adult IM/IV/SC: 0.4-2 mg IV—repeat in 2-8 min if needed; 0.1-0.2 mg/kg IV—repeat in 2-3 min intervals	Narcotic overdose, postop reversal
Naltrexone HCl	Narcotic antagonist	*Adult* PO: 50 mg q24h or 100 mg qod or 150 mg q3h	Maintenance of opioid-free state

y/o, years old.

⚓ FENTANYL

Fentanyl (Durasesic, Fentanyl Oralet, and Sublimaze) is a synthetic opioid narcotic used to treat moderate to severe pain. It is also used as an adjunct to general anesthetics. It is available in several dosage forms: transdermal patches (Durasesic), buccal lozenges (Fentanyl Oralet), and parenteral injections (Sublimaze). It is also available as a combination product called Innovar, in which it is combined with droperidol. Fentanyl is a very potent analgesic. The potencies of some of the more common opioid narcotics as compared with 10 mg of both intramuscular and oral forms of morphine are listed in Table 8-9. Fentanyl at a dose of 100 μg (0.10 mg) given intravenously is equivalent to 10 mg of morphine given intramuscularly.

One of the new ways of administering fentanyl is the transdermal delivery system, or the Durasesic patch. It has been shown to be highly effective in the treatment of various chronic types of pain syndromes such as cancer-induced pain. It is recommended that patients never before exposed to narcotics be started on the lowest-strength patch of 25 μg/h (2.5 mg/10 cm^2). However, prior exposure to narcotics is common in many patients. In these patients it is necessary to know the appropriate dose (the equipotent dose) of transdermal fentanyl) to convert the patient over to. Table 8-10 is provided to aid in this conversion.

The analgesic potency of 10 mg of intramuscular morphine relative to that of 100 μg of intravenous fentanyl was used by the manufacturer to derive the equivalent potency dose of transdermal fentanyl. Thus, a 10-mg intramuscular or 60-mg oral dose of morphine given every 4 hours for 24 hours (60 mg daily intramuscularly or 360 mg daily orally) was considered by the manufacturer to be approximately equivalent to a transdermal fentanyl system that delivered 100 μg/h. The transdermal fentanyl doses that should be used and the estimated daily equivalent doses of morphine are given in Table 8-10. (The table was arranged in this manner so as to avoid having to prepare a table for every dosage range.) To perform the conversion shown in this table, first you should determine the daily (24-hour) narcotic requirement of your patient. Second, if the narcotic is not morphine, you should convert its dose to the equianalgesic dose of morphine using Table 8-9. Finally, the equipotent transdermal fentanyl dose can be calculated using Table 8-10.

Most patients will experience adequate pain control for 72 hours with this method of fentanyl delivery. A new patch should be applied every 72 hours.

Fentanyl is classified as a pregnancy category C agent and is contraindicated in patients who have shown a hypersensitivity reaction to narcotic analgesics and in those with myasthenia gravis. It is available in transdermal doses of 25 μg/h (2.5 mg/10 cm^2), 50 μg/h (5 mg/20 cm^2), 75 μg/h (7.5 mg/30 cm^2), and 100 μg/h (10 mg/40 cm^2); as a buccal lozenge in doses of 200, 300, and 400 μg; as a 50-μg/ml parenteral injection; and as a combination product (Innovar) consisting of 50 μg/ml of fentanyl and 2.5-mg/ml of droperidol. The commonly recommended transdermal dosages are determined on the basis of a patient's prior narcotic use. If a patient has no such history, then a 25-μg patch should be used. If he or she has been treated with other opioids, then Table 8-10 should be used to determine the equivalent transdermal fentanyl dose. This table is conservative in its doses for achieving pain relief, and often supplemental short-acting narcotic analgesics should be added as needed. Dosage

Table 8-9	Equianalgesic Narcotic Potency	
Narcotic Analgesic	**Equianalgesic Dose (mg)**	
	Intramuscular	**Oral**
⚓Morphine	10	60
Codeine	130	200
Hydromorphone	1.5	7.5
⚓Meperidine	75	—
Methadone	10	20
Oxycodone	15	30
Oxymorphone	1	10 (rectal)

Table 8-10	Transdermal Fentanyl Dose	
Oral 24-Hour ⚓Morphine (in mg/day)	**Intramuscular 24-Hour ⚓Morphine (in mg/day)**	**Transdermal ⚓Fentanyl (in μg/h)**
45-134	8-22	25
135-224	23-37	50
225-314	38-52	75
315-404	53-67	100
405-494	68-82	125
495-584	83-97	150
585-674	98-112	175
675-764	113-127	200
765-854	128-142	225
855-944	143-157	250

titration in patients with fentanyl patches should be done as needed every 72 hours.

❖ PHARMACOKINETICS

HALF-LIFE	ONSET	PEAK	DURATION
IV: 1.5-6 hr	Rapid	Minutes	30-60 min
IM: 1.5-6 hr	7-15 min	20-30 min	1-2 hr
Transdermal: 13-40 hr	Delayed	12-24 hr	48-72 hr

⚓ MEPERIDINE HYDROCHLORIDE

Meperidine hydrochloride is a widely used synthetic narcotic analgesic. The misuse potential and addiction liability associated with its use are both high. The drug is contraindicated in patients showing a hypersensitivity to it and in patients currently or recently treated with monoamine oxidase inhibitors. The concurrent use of these inhibitors and meperidine can lead to deep coma and death.

❖ PHARMACOKINETICS

HALF-LIFE	ONSET	PEAK	DURATION
3-5 hr	Rapid	30-60 min	2-4 hr

METHADONE HYDROCHLORIDE

Methadone hydrochloride is a synthetic narcotic analgesic. The potential for misuse and the addiction liability are both high for this agent. It is the narcotic of choice for the detoxification treatment of narcotic addicts. The drug has seen widespread use in the methadone maintenance program. The usual dose for methadone maintenance ranges from 40 to 120 mg or higher, given once daily. Concurrent use of agonist-antagonist narcotics (pentazocine and the like) in heroin-addicted or methadone-maintenance patients can induce significant withdrawal symptoms.

❖ PHARMACOKINETICS

HALF-LIFE	ONSET	PEAK	DURATION
25 hr	30-60 min	1½-2 hr	(22-48 hr)

PROPOXYPHENE HYDROCHLORIDE/NAPSYLATE

Propoxyphene hydrochloride is an analgesic agent that is structurally related to methadone. However, it is not a true narcotic, and its misuse potential and addiction liability are both low. It is used for the relief of mild to moderate pain.

Propoxyphene napsylate is more insoluble than propoxyphene hydrochloride, and this makes for more stable liquid and solid (tablets and the like) dosage formulations.

❖ PHARMACOKINETICS

HALF-LIFE	ONSET	PEAK	DURATION
6-12 hr	.25-1 hr	2-2.5 hr	4-6 hr

AGONIST-ANTAGONIST NARCOTICS

The agonist-antagonist narcotics include buprenorphine, butorphanol, dezocine, nalbuphine, and pentazocine. They are also known as the *partial opiate agonists*. The agonist-antagonist narcotics are very similar to the agonist narcotic agents from the standpoint of their pharmacokinetic and pharmacodynamic properties, and they have the same therapeutic indications. They are potent synthetic analgesics, but their misuse potential and addiction liability are both low.

The antagonistic activity of this group can produce withdrawal symptoms in narcotic-dependent patients. They are also contraindicated in patients who have shown hypersensitivity reactions to the drugs.

NARCOTIC ANTAGONISTS

The narcotic antagonists are synthetic derivatives of oxymorphone, a potent semisynthetic narcotic. They produce their narcotic antagonistic activity by competing with narcotics for central nervous system receptor sites.

NALOXONE HYDROCHLORIDE

Naloxone hydrochloride is a pure narcotic antagonist because it possesses no agonist morphinelike properties. Accordingly, the drug does not produce analgesia or respiratory depression. Naloxone is the drug of choice for the complete or partial reversal of narcotic-induced respiratory depression. It is also indicated in the diagnosis of suspected acute narcotic overdose. If its administration does not significantly reverse the narcotic overdose, this indicates the condition may be due to an overdose of narcotic drugs or a dosing process.

The drug is contraindicated in patients with a history of hypersensitivity.

❖ PHARMACOKINETICS

HALF-LIFE	ONSET	PEAK	DURATION
64 min	<2 min	Rapid	Variable with dose and route

NALTREXONE HYDROCHLORIDE

Naltrexone hydrochloride is a narcotic antagonist used as an adjunct for the maintenance of a narcotic-free state in former narcotic addicts. The drug is contraindicated in patients with acute hepatitis or liver failure, a demonstrated hypersensitivity to the drug, or narcotic dependency in patients currently receiving narcotics; and in patients suffering from acute narcotic withdrawal.

☙ PHARMACOKINETICS

HALF-LIFE	ONSET	PEAK	DURATION
3.9-12.9 hr	Rapid	1 hr	24-72 hr

The most serious adverse effect is dose-related hepatocellular toxicity. Other adverse effects include nasal congestion, nosebleeds, phlebitis, depression, nightmares, and photophobia.

NURSING PROCESS

Patients experiencing pain pose many challenges to the nurse and other health care providers who are involved in their health care. Adequate analgesia, pain relief without complications, and patient teaching are all goals of the health care overseen by the nurse in this context. Nurses need to adequately and accurately assess the nature of the patient's pain as well as evaluate and monitor his or her response to the analgesic, regardless of whether narcotic or nonnarcotic analgesics are used, so as to provide safe and effective nursing care.

ASSESSMENT

Before you administer a narcotic agonist or agonist-antagonist, you must obtain an accurate and thorough medication history. This ensures the safe use of these medications, meaning analgesic treatment that is free of complications or injury to the patient. The nurse should ask about and document information regarding allergies; the use of other narcotics (the use of other narcotics with agonists can lead to toxicity and overdosage; their use with agonist-antagonists can lead to an effect antagonistic to the analgesic); alcohol use; the nature of the pain including its severity (perhaps graded on a scale of 1 to 10, with 10 being the worst);

the type of pain (stabbing, throbbing, dull ache, sharp, diffuse, localized, referred, or knifelike); precipitating and relieving factors; home remedies used and the response to them; and other pain treatments (pharmacologic and nonpharmacologic). Vital signs (blood pressure, pulse, and respirations) should also be noted, determined, and documented. Do not forget that during the acute pain response, the stimulation to the sympathetic nervous system may result in elevated vital sign values (blood pressure, >120/80 mm Hg; pulse, >100 beats/min; respiration, >20 breaths/min) and narcotics will depress vital signs! Always document baseline intake and output measurements and continue to monitor and document these throughout the narcotic treatment because of the associated urinary retention.

Before administering a narcotic agent, it is also essential to check the route and time of the previous analgesic administration and the patient's response. Always check the patient's chart, physician's order, nurses' notes, and medication administration chart before administering any additional doses of an analgesic!

With regard to the administration of the synthetic agonist-antagonist drugs, it is important to determine whether the patient is in an addictive state because the administration of an adjunctive narcotic may well precipitate withdrawal in such patients. Narcotic antagonists such as naloxone hydrochloride and naltrexone have an antagonistic effect on narcotic agonists and are used to reverse their effects in the event of toxicity or overdosage.

Drug interactions (increased effects) with narcotic agonists and agonist-antagonists occur with the following agents: alcohol, other central nervous system depressants, sedative-hypnotics, muscle relaxants, major tranquilizers, and antipsychotic agents. Narcotics are contraindicated in patients with allergies to them, bronchial asthma, narcotic addiction, head injuries, and increased intracranial pressure. Cautious use, meaning close monitoring of the patient's response, reaction, and vital signs during narcotic treatment, is called for in patients with any disease or altered state of the liver or kidneys.

NURSING DIAGNOSES

Nursing diagnoses appropriate for the patient who is taking analgesics include the following:

- Pain related to etiology and need for analgesia
- Pain related to nausea, vomiting, and constipation from side effects of narcotics and other analgesics
- Risk for injury and falls related to decreased sensorium from narcotic
- Risk for constipation related to side effects of analgesics (narcotics)

■ Risk for infection related to bladder retention and narcotics on CNS

■ Knowledge deficit related to unfamiliarity of narcotics, their use, and side effects

PLANNING

Goals appropriate to the use of analgesics include the following:

■ Patient identifies the rationale and therapeutic and side effects associated with the use of analgesics

■ Patient states measures that will enhance the effectiveness of the analgesic.

■ Patient will state measures that will decrease the occurrence of commonly associated side effects.

Outcome Criteria

Outcome criteria related to the use of analgesics are as follows:

■ Patient will experience minimal side effects and complications associated with the use of analgesics such as nausea, vomiting, constipation, and so on.

■ Patient will demonstrate increased comfort levels as seen by decreased use of analgesics, increased activity, and decreased complaints of pain.

■ Patient uses nonpharmacologic measures to enhance comfort such as relaxation therapy, distraction, and music therapy.

■ Patient manages side effects associated wth analgesics through fluid intake and possible antiemetic therapy.

IMPLEMENTATION

If it is time for the patient to receive another dose of a narcotic medication, then you should administer the narcotic, record it in the nurses' notes and medication record, and sign with a full signature. The medication, amount, site, and response should all be documented

---

Narcotics Administration Guidelines

NARCOTIC	NURSING ADMINISTRATION
Buprenorphine and butorphanol	When giving IV, infuse over 3 to 5 minutes; always assess respirations. Give IM butorphanol in deep gluteal muscle mass.
Codeine	Give oral doses with food to minimize gastrointestinal tract upset; ceiling effects with oral codeine.
Dezocine	Mixed agonist-antagonist; short duration of action; IM: deep gluteal muscle mass.
⚓Fentanyl	IM and IV dosages to be administered slowly and per package insert instructions to prevent muscular rigidity and arrest; when administered IV or epidurally, should have resuscitative equipment nearby and naloxone at the bedside; patches come in various strengths, so watch dosing versus order very carefully to prevent overdosage; fentanyl will also soon be available in lozenge form for anesthetic premedication in children and adults.
Hydromorphone	May be given SC, rectally, IV, PO, or IM.
Levorphanol	May be given PO, SC, or IV; IV forms to be given over 5 minutes or adhere to manufacturer guidelines; longer acting (6-8 hours).
⚓Meperidine Methadone	Given by a variety of routes: IV, IM, SC, or PO; highly protein bound, so watch for interactions and toxicity with PO, SC, or IM forms.
⚓Morphine	In a variety of forms: SC, IM, IV, extended and immediate release, and morphine sulfate (Duramorph) for epidural infusion; morphine sulfate (MS Contin) now available in a 200-mg, sustained-release tablet.
Nalbuphine	IV dosages of 10 mg undiluted over 5 minutes.
Naloxone	Antagonist given for narcotic overdose; 0.4 mg usually given IV over 15 seconds or less.
Propoxyphene	Oral dosing only; high abuse potential.
Oxycodone	Often mixed with acetaminophen or aspirin; oral and suppository dosage forms.
Oxymorphone	Oral, IM, IV, SC, and rectal suppository dosage forms.
Pentazocine	SC, IV, and IM forms; mixed agent; 5 mg IV to be given over 1 minute.
Sufentanil	Used as adjunct to anesthesia and so given with oxygen.

(see Chapter 7). When using narcotics, both pure and mixed agents, you must always be sure to medicate patients before the pain becomes severe or when the pain is beginning to return so as to provide adequate analgesia and pain control. It is often recommended that the oral forms of narcotics be taken with food to minimize gastrointestinal tract upset, specifically nausea. Antiemetic therapy may be needed should such nausea and vomiting prove uncontrollable.

Safety measures such as keeping the side rails up and having the call bell within the patient's reach are crucial in preventing falls stemming from possible confusion, hypotension, and decreased sensorium, especially in the elderly patient. When administering morphine, meperidine, and like drugs, you should withhold the dose and contact the physician in the event there is any decline in the patient's condition or if the vital signs are abnormal (see normal values given earlier), especially a respiratory rate of less than 12 breaths/min.

When administering intramuscular injections of analgesics, sites should be adequately and accurately oriented, the site cleansed with an antiseptic, a needle in the proper size and gauge used (see Chapter 7), the injectant aspirated before injection, and the site and other information documented as with any prn medication.

With the intravenous administration of analgesics, always follow the insert instructions regarding the diluent and time over which the amount ordered should be delivered. When patient-controlled analgesia is being used, the amounts and times of dosing should be noted in the appropriate records. When a narcotic is used, *always* check and recheck the narcotic count and immediately report any errors in counting to the charge nurse, nurse manager, or supervisor. Never assume that someone else will report or detect the error!

Another point to remember when administering analgesics is that each medication has a different onset of action, peak, and duration of action, and these differences apply to the route of administration as well. In addition, each patient responds differently. See the box on p. 100 for narcotic administration guidelines.

To reverse a narcotic overdose or narcotic-induced respiratory depression, a narcotic antagonist such as naloxone must be administered. If naloxone is the an-

---

HOME HEALTH POINTS
Points to Remember

- With most narcotics, such as the opiates, the patient's mental and physical abilities may be impaired, so every effort should be made to instruct the patient, family members, and caregivers about the need for safety measures such as not allowing the patient to engage in activities requiring mental alertness, for example, driving a car or operating any type of machinery.

- Remind patients that different narcotics should not be mixed in any form or manner.

- Instruct persons caring for the patient and the patient proper about careful and accurate pain assessment and the need to keep a journal containing information about the patient's pain, precipitating factors, alleviating factors, and the response to pain medication and non-pharmacologic measures.

Narcotics: Points of Interest

Butorphanol	Make sure to give IM in deep gluteal muscle mass.
Codeine	Used for analgesia and cough; caution patient to change positions slowly to prevent postural hypotension.
⚡Fentanyl	Unusual side effect of muscular rigidity; always watch for respiratory depression, bradycardia, and cardiac arrest; not to be used in patients with myasthenia gravis; make sure to remove old patch and wash off residual medicine before applying new transdermal patch; used for relief of chronic pain such as that in cancer patients; advantages include its 72-hour duration.
⚡Meperidine	Assess respirations before administering and withhold if respirations are <12 breaths/min.
Methadone	Longer duration of action to about 6-8 hours.
⚡Morphine	Always assess respirations before administration; IV administration should be done carefully.
Nalbuphine	Assess respirations carefully.
Pentazocine	Mixed agent that can be given IV, IM, and PO.
Propoxyphene	Euphoria produced by medication often results in its misuse; addicting, especially with long-term use.

tagonist used in your unit, 0.4 to 2 mg should be given either intravenously in its undiluted form and administered over 15 seconds, or as ordered, or the dose should be given as an injection diluted in water, 5% dextrose in water, or normal saline solution (see Table 8-7). The guidelines in the package insert should also be followed. Emergency resuscitative equipment should be nearby in the event of respiratory or cardiac arrest. Patient education guidelines are presented in the box below. Other practical points are given in the boxes at right and on the following page.

Patient Teaching TIPS

✔ Encourage the patient to keep a record or journal of their pain experience and all methods of treatment, both pharmacologic and nonpharmacologic.

✔ Patients should follow instructions on the medication vial or bottle regarding the dose, route, and frequency of the medication. Following instructions closely is essential to preventing toxicity or overdose that may result in cardiac or respiratory arrest.

✔ The physician or health care provider should be contacted if emesis occurs while the patient is taking the narcotic, because nausea and vomiting are common side effects; often medication is needed to alleviate the nausea.

✔ Constipation is a common side effect of narcotic use and may be prevented with forced fluids (unless contraindicated) and a high-fiber diet.

✔ The physician should be contacted should the patient show symptoms of allergic reaction such as wheezing, difficulty breathing, itching, hives, or central nervous system changes such as weakness, dizziness, or fainting.

✔ Withdrawal symptoms associated with narcotics include nausea, vomiting, cramps, fainting spells, and fever.

✔ Patients should be instructed to carefully read the directions on the narcotic prescription container as well as on any over-the-counter medications so that they are alerted to possible contraindications or drug interactions.

✔ Side effects patients should be alerted to include gastrointestinal tract upset, constipation, drowsiness, dizziness, headache, sleepiness, tinnitus (ringing of the ears), blurred vision, palpitations, bradycardia, and hypotension.

✔ Patients should be encouraged to change positions slowly to prevent possible orthostatic hypotension.

PEDIATRIC CONSIDERATIONS
Narcotics Administration and Implications

■ Assessment of the pediatric patient is challenging, to say the least, and all types of behavior that may indicate pain, such as muscular rigidity, restlessness, screaming, fear of moving, and withdrawn behavior, have to be carefully considered.

■ Assessment of pain is very important in pediatric patients because they are often undermedicated! Always thoroughly assess the pediatric patient and do not underestimate the child's complaints!

■ When the pediatric patient is to receive narcotics, the nurse should be very careful to recheck dosages against the physician's order and pharmacy references and to double-check the fractions and decimals to minimize and prevent errors.

■ If suppositories are used, be careful to administer the exact dose and do not split, halve, or divide the adult dose into a child's dose, because this may result in the administration of an unknown dose.

■ Always monitor pediatric patients very closely for any unusual behavior or signs and symptoms while they are receiving narcotics.

■ Central nervous system changes such as dizziness, light-headedness, drowsiness, hallucinations, changes in the level of consciousness, and a sluggish pupil reaction should be reported immediately to the physician and no further medication given until further orders are received from the physician.

■ Always monitor and document vital signs before, during, and after the administration of narcotic analgesics. Withhold the medication if respirations are <12 breaths/min or if there are any changes in the level of consciousness.

■ Respiratory status—respiratory rate, rhythm, character, rate, and difficulty—should be carefully assessed in pediatric patients.

■ Generally speaking, smaller doses of narcotics are indicated for the pediatric patient.

■ Keep bed or crib side rails up and the bed in a low position at all times!

■ Meperidine should be used cautiously in patients younger than 18 years.

■ Oral opium derivatives should be given with meals or milk, to decrease gastrointestinal tract distress.

■ With opiates and other forms of narcotics, the therapeutic response is a decrease in pain.

■ Allergic reactions include a rash or urticaria.

■ Withdrawal symptoms include nausea, vomiting, cramps, faintness, fever, and anorexia.

GERIATRIC CONSIDERATIONS
Narcotics Administration and Implications

- Assess patient carefully before administration of narcotics because a dose and interval adjustment may be necessary, depending on the development of undesirable adverse reactions such as confusion, decreased respirations, and excessive central nervous system depression.

- Height and weight should be recorded and noted before the start of narcotic treatment.

- Carefully monitor elderly patients who are receiving narcotics because they are generally more sensitive to these agents. This includes frequent monitoring of vital signs, respiratory function, and central nervous system status. Document any changes.

- Smaller doses of narcotics are generally indicated for the aged patient, and idiosyncratic or unexpected reactions may occur in patients of this age group.

- Polypharmacy is often a problem in the elderly, so it is important to have a complete list of all medications the patient is currently taking.

- Keep side rails up and bed in low position with call bell/light at bedside.

- With possible decreased circulation, the absorption of IM or IV dosage forms will vary, and often result in a slower absorption of parenteral forms of opioids.

- Encourage elderly patients to ask for medications because they often hesitate to ask for pain medication because they do not want to "bother" the nurse or give in to pain.

- Note, report, and document any unusual reactions to the narcotic agents.

EVALUATION

After and during the administration of narcotic or non-narcotic analgesics, it is important to monitor the patient for both therapeutic and side effects. Therapeutic effects include decreased complaints of pain and increased periods of comfort, with improved activities of daily living, appetite, and sense of well-being. Side effects vary with each drug (see earlier discussion in Chapter 8) but often consist of nausea, vomiting, constipation, dizziness, headache, blurred vision, decreased urinary output, headache, drowsiness, lethargy, sedation, palpitations, bradycardia, bradypnea, dyspnea, and hypotension. Should vital signs change, the patient's condition decline, or pain continue, the nurse should contact the physician immediately. Respiratory depression may be manifested by a rate of less than 12 breaths/min, dyspnea, diminished breath sounds, or shallow breathing.

TAKE HOME POINTS

Pain

- Involves senses and emotions that are unpleasant.
- Associated with actual or potential tissue damage.
- Personal and individual experience.
- Many conditions can make it worse or better.

Analgesic

- Relieves pain without causing loss of consciousness.
- Painkillers.

Types of Pain

- Acute (sudden in onset and severe) versus chronic (persistent or recurring pain lasting more than 6 months).
- Somatic (skeletal muscles, ligaments, or joints) versus visceral (organs or smooth muscle).
- Superficial (skin or mucous membranes).

Gate Theory

- Gate in dorsal horn of spinal column allows pain sensation from damaged tissues to travel to brain.
- If sensation gets to brain, we feel pain. If not, we don't.
- Brain can in return send inhibitory signals to gate to turn it down or close it.

Physical versus Psychologic Dependence

- Physical = adaptation of body to narcotic analgesic (expected).
- Psychologic = compulsive drug use with intent to alter mental status (unexpected).

Types of Analgesics

- NSAIDS = nonnarcotic, nonsteroidal analgesics used for acute and chronic pain.
- Narcotics are natural or synthetic agents that either contain or are derived from morphine (opiates) or have opiate-like effects or activities (opioids).

Mechanism of Action

- Agonist = binds to receptor and causes response.
- Agonist-antagonist = acts as an agonist at one type of receptor and as an antagonist at another type of receptor.
- Antagonist = binds to receptor and prevents response.

Nursing Considerations

- Pain must be managed before it gets uncontrollable.
- Nonnarcotic agent used first.
- Stronger analgesics used as the next step to pain control.

Critical Thinking **A C T I V I T I E S**

1. You are assigned to a patient who is in the terminal phases of breast cancer. As a home health care nurse, you have many responsibilities; however, you have not cared for many patients who are in the terminal phases of their illness. In fact, most of your patients are postoperative ones and have only required assessments, dressing changes, and wound care.

Ms. O.D. is 56 years old and underwent bilateral mastectomy 4 years ago. She had lymph node involvement at the time of surgery, and recently metastasis to the bone has been diagnosed. She has been taking Percodan (1 tablet every 6 hours) at home but is not sleeping through the night and is now complaining of increasing pain to the point that her quality of life has decreased significantly. She wants to stay at home during the terminal phases of her illness but needs to have adequate and safe pain control. Her husband of 28 years is very supportive, and they have no children. They are both college graduates and have medical insurance.

Questions

(Provide references from within this chapter for the selection of the specific narcotic agent.)

a. Ms. O.D.'s recent increase in pain has been attributed to bone metastasis in the area of the lumbar spine. At this time the Percodan is not beneficial and you as the home health care nurse need to recommend another pain medication to the physician. What medication would you recommend to relieve the bone pain, and what is your rationale for this recommendation?

b. Identify the patient education guidelines for the specific medication you recommend to the physician.

c. Outline a comprehensive nursing care plan appropriate to the specific agent used or recommended.

2. Ms. M.B. is 67 years old and has recently undergone surgery, chemotherapy, and irradiation for breast cancer. She has been in pain after her therapy, for which she has been taking oxycodone and acetaminophen (Percocet), two tablets PO q3h prn, and extended-release morphine (MS Contin) 30 mg q12h.

She has been taking the Percocet every 3 hours and the morphine sulfate continuously every 12 hours, but is still in pain. Oral thrush has also developed as the result of her chemotherapy, and she can no longer tolerate swallowing. It is decided that her oral medications should be changed. The physician wants to know her total daily dose of narcotics so that this can be converted to the equivalent dose of transdermal fentanyl and to supplement with prn morphine injections.

Questions

a. What is her total daily dose of oxycodone and morphine?

b. What dose of morphine is equivalent to her total daily dose of combined oxycodone and morphine?

c. What dose of transdermal fentanyl should this patient receive?

▲▲

BIBLIOGRAPHY

Albanese J, Nutz P: *Mosby's 1995 nursing drug cards,* St Louis, 1995, Mosby.

Faxstat: New warning, *Facts and Comparisons* 3(4):1, 1994.

Faxstat: New status, *Facts and Comparisons* 3(2):1, 1994.

Johnson KB: *Harriet Lane handbook*, ed 13, St Louis, 1993, Mosby.

Keen JH: *Critical care and emergency drug reference*, St Louis, 1994, Mosby.

Knoben JE, Anderson PO: *Handbook of critical drug data*, ed 6, Hamilton, Ill, 1988, Drug Intelligence Publications.

McEvoy GK: *AHFS drug information*, Bethesda, Md, 1989, American Society of Hospital Pharmacists.

Reed B: Managing postoperative pain . . . controlling pain, *Nursing 94*, 24(8):26, 1994.

Skidmore-Roth L: *Mosby's 1995 nursing drug reference*, St Louis, 1995, Mosby.

Chapter 9

General and Local Anesthetic Agents

Objectives

When you reach the end of this chapter, you will be able to:

1 Define anesthesia.
2 Discuss the similarities of and differences between general and local anesthetics.
3 List the most commonly used general and local anesthetics and associated risk factors.
4 Describe the nursing care required for the different stages of anesthesia.
5 Discuss the nursing care required for the patient receiving general anesthetics.
6 Discuss the nursing care required for the patient receiving local anesthetics.
7 Provide patient education guidelines for the patient receiving an anesthetic.

CHAPTER OUTLINE

Anesthetics

General Anesthetics
  Mechanism of action
  Drug effects
  Therapeutic uses
  Side effects and adverse effects
    Toxicity and management of overdose
  Interactions
  Dosages

Drug Profiles
  Enflurane
  ⚓ Isoforane
  Halothane
  Methoxyflurane
  Nitrous Oxide
Local Anesthetics
  Mechanism of action
  Drug effects
  Therapeutic uses
  Side effects and adverse effects
    Toxicity and management of overdose
  Interactions

Drug Profile
  ⚓ Lidocaine

Nursing Process
Assessment

Nursing Diagnoses
Planning
  Outcome criteria
Implementation
Evaluation

Glossary

Adjunctive agents (ad junk′ tiv) Agents used in combination with anesthetic agents to control the side effects of anesthetics or to help maintain the anesthetic state in the patient. (p. 107)

Anesthesia (an′ es thé zhə) A drug-induced state in which the CNS is altered to produce varying degrees of pain relief, depression of consciousness, skeletal muscle relaxation, and diminished or absent reflexes. (p. 107)

Anesthetics (an′ əs the′ tik) Agents that depress the CNS to produce depression of consciousness, loss of responsiveness to sensory stimulation, or muscle relaxation. (p. 107)

Balanced anesthesia The practice of using combinations of drugs to produce anesthesia rather than using a single agent. Common combinations include a sedative-hypnotic, an antianxiety agent, an analgesic, an antiemetic, and an anticholinergic. (p. 107)

General anesthetics Agents that induce the state of anesthesia. Their effects are global in that they affect the whole body, with loss of consciousness being one of those effects. (p. 107)

Local anesthetics Agents that render a specific portion of the body insensitive to pain without affecting consciousness. Also called *regional anesthetics*. (p. 111)

Overton-Meyer theory A theory that describes the relationship between the lipid solubility of anesthetic agents and their potency. It is often used to explain how anesthetic agents are believed to work. (p. 107)

Parenteral anesthetics (pə ren' tər əl) Agents that can be administered directly into the CNS by various spinal injection techniques. In addition, they can be injected adjacent to main nerves to accomplish anesthesia of the peripheral nervous system. (p. 111)

Topical anesthetics A class of local anesthetics that are applied directly to the skin and mucous membranes. They consist of solutions, ointments, gels, creams, powders, ophthalmic drops, and suppositories. (p. 111)

Anesthetics are agents that depress the central nervous system (CNS), which in turn produces depression of consciousness, loss of responsiveness to sensory stimulation (including pain), or muscle relaxation. This state of depressed CNS activity is called **anesthesia**. There are many mechanisms by which anesthetics accomplish these responses, but in general they all do so by interfering with nerve conduction. Anesthetics can produce one or all of the actions just mentioned, depending on the agent. Anesthetics are most commonly classified as either general anesthetics and local anesthetics, depending on where in the CNS the particular anesthetic agent works.

Anesthetics

GENERAL ANESTHETICS

A **general anesthetic** is an agent that induces a state in which the CNS is altered so that varying degrees of pain relief, depression of consciousness, skeletal muscle relaxation, and reflex reduction are produced. General anesthesia can be achieved by the use of one or a combination of drugs. Often a combination of drugs is used to accomplish general anesthesia, allowing less of each of the agents to be used and a more balanced, controlled state of anesthesia to be achieved. General anesthetic agents are used most commonly to produce deep muscle relaxation and loss of consciousness during surgical procedures.

There are two main categories of general anesthetics, and this is determined by their respective routes of administration. The first group, inhaled anesthetics, are volatile liquids or gases that are vaporized in oxygen and inhaled to induce anesthesia. The second group, injectable anesthetics, are administered

intravenously. The different inhaled gases and volatile liquids used as general anesthetics are listed in Table 9-1.

Intravenously administered anesthetic agents are used to induce or maintain general anesthesia, to induce amnesia, and as an adjunct to inhalation-type anesthetics. These agents are commonly used in combination with **adjunctive agents**, which are sedative-hypnotics, antianxiety agents, opioid and nonopioid analgesics, antiemetics, and anticholinergics that can minimize some of the undesirable after-effects of excessive doses of the inhaled anesthetics. This practice is called **balanced anesthesia**. Some of the after-effects are excessive salivation, bradycardia, and vomiting. This combining of several different agents makes it possible for general anesthesia to be accomplished with smaller amounts of anesthetic gases, thereby lessening the side effects. The intravenous anesthetics, their dosage forms, and the usual doses are given in Table 9-2. A brief list of the adjunctive agents is given in Table 9-3, and these agents are discussed in greater detail in chapters devoted to discussion of the respective classes of agents.

Mechanism of Action

Many theories have been proposed to explain the actual mechanism of action of general anesthetics. However, the agents vary widely in their chemical structure, and therefore their mechanism of action is not easily explained by a structure–receptor relationship. The concentrations required for different anesthetics to produce a given state of anesthesia also differ greatly. The **Overton-Meyer theory** explains some of the properties of anesthetic agents that may make the mechanism of action of these agents easier to understand. This theory states that there is a relationship

Table 9-1	Inhaled General Anesthetics
AGENTS	
GENERIC NAME	**TRADE NAME**
Inhaled gas	
Cyclopropane	(many)
Nitrous oxide	(laughing gas)
Inhaled volatile liquid	
Halothane	Fluothane, Somnothane*
Methoxyflurane	Penthrane
Enflurane	Ethrane
⚓Isoflurane	Forane

*Canadian trade name.

between the lipid solubility of an anesthetic agent and its potency: the greater the solubility of the agent in fat, the greater the effect. Nerve cell membranes have a high lipid content, as does the blood-brain barrier. Anesthetic agents can therefore easily cross this blood-brain barrier and concentrate in nerve cell membranes. Initially this produces a loss of the senses of sight, touch, taste, smell, awareness, and hearing, and usually the patient becomes unconscious. Even though the vital centers responsible for blood pressure and breath-ing, the heart and lungs, are controlled by the medulla, they usually can be spared because the medullary center is depressed last.

Drug Effects

The main effect of the general anesthetics is an orderly and systematic paralysis of the CNS. They produce a progressive depression of cerebral and spinal cord functions. Therapeutic (anesthetic) doses cause minimal depression of the medullary centers that govern vital functions. However, an anesthetic overdose paralyzes the medullary centers, and this can lead to death stemming from circulatory and respiratory failure.

The progressive paralysis of nervous system functions produced by the general anesthetics can be categorized into four distinct stages, summarized in Table 9-4. These stages vary greatly depending on the anesthetics used but are best seen with ether of chloroform.

Therapeutic Uses

The general anesthetics are used to produce unconsciousness and skeletal muscular relaxation for surgical procedures.

Side Effects and Adverse Effects

The adverse effects of the general anesthetics are dose dependent and vary with the individual agents. The heart, peripheral circulation, liver, kidneys, and respiratory tract are the sites primarily affected. Myo-

Table 9-2 Intravenous Anesthetic Agents

AGENT		
GENERIC NAME	TRADE NAME	DOSAGE
Etomidate	Amidate	0.2-0.6 mg/kg IV
Ketamine	Ketalar	1-4.5 mg/kg IV; 6.5-13 mg/kg IM
Methohexital	Brevital, Brietal*	50-120 mg IV (induction); 20-40 mg IV (maintenance)
Propofol	Diprivan	1-2.5 mg/kg IV (induction); 50-200 μg/kg/min IV (maintenance)
Thiamylal	Surital	Titrate to response IV
Thiopental	Pentothal	25-75 mg IV as needed

*Canadian trade name.

Table 9-3 Adjunctive Anesthetic Agents

AGENT	PHARMACOLOGIC CLASS	DOSAGE RANGE	PURPOSE
Alfentanil (Alfenta) Fentanyl (Sublimaze) Sufentanil (Sufenta)	Opioid analgesic	130-245 μg/kg IV 50-100 μg/kg IV 8-30 μg/kg IV	Anesthesia induction
Diazepam (Valium, Meval*) Midazolam (Versed)	Benzodiazepine	2-20 mg PO/IV/IM 0.05-0.35 mg/kg IV	Amnesia and anxiety
Atropine Glycopyrrolate (Robinul) Scopolamine	Anticholinergic	0.1-0.6 mg IM/IV/SC 0.0044 mg/kg IM 0.3-0.6 SC/IM	To dry up excessive secretions
Meperidine (Demerol) Morphine	Opioid analgesic	50-100 mg IM/SC 5-20 mg IM/SC	Pain prevention and pain relief
Hydroxyzine (Atarax, Vistaril, Multipax*) Pentobarbital (Nembutal) Promethazine (Phenergan, Histanil*) Secobarbital (Seconal)	Sedative-hypnotic	25-100 mg IM 150-200 mg IM 25-50 mg IM 100-250 mg IV	Amnesia and sedation

*Canadian trade name.

Table 9-4   Stages of Anesthesia

CNS Effects	Stage 1	Stage 2	Stage 3 Planes — 1	2	3	4	Stage 4
Consciousness	Maintained Analgesia Euphoria Some distortion of perceptions Variable amnesia	Lost	Absent	Absent	Absent	Absent	Absent
Respiration	No alteration, or increased rate with some irregularity	Rapid, irregular	Regular	Regular, but expirations longer than inspirations	Diaphragmatic	Thoracic ceased Diaphragmatic depressed	No respiratory movement Respiratory paralysis
Skeletal muscles	Normal tone	Tone increased	Small muscles relaxed	Large muscles relaxed	Complete relaxation	Complete relaxation	Diaphragm paralyzed
Eyes							
Pupils	Reaction to light	Dilated	Constricted	Mid-dilation	Increasing dilatation	Dilated	Dilated
Movements	Unchanged	Increased	Increased	None	None	None	None
Tear secretion				Decreased	Decreased	Absent	Absent
Reflexes							
Lid	Present	Present	Absent	Absent	Absent	Absent	Absent
Corneal	Present	Present	Present	Absent	Absent	Absent	Absent
Pharyngeal or "gag"			Absent	Absent			
Laryngeal				Absent			
Cough				Absent	Absent in large bronchi	Absent in small bronchi	
Heart rate	Unchanged	Increased	Decreased	Normal	Decreased	Decreased	Decreased
Blood pressure	Unchanged	Increased	Normal				Increased
Venous pressure		Increased	Unchanged				

From McKenry, Salerno: *Mosby's pharmacology in nursing*, ed 19, St Louis, 1995, Mosby.

cardial depression is a common side effect. All of the halogenated anesthetics are capable of causing hepatotoxicity, and methoxyflurane can cause significant respiratory depression.

With the development and use of newer agents, many of the unwanted side effects of the older agents (such as hepatotoxicity and myocardial depression) are now a thing of the past. In addition, many of the bothersome side effects such as nausea, vomiting, and confusion have become less common, as balanced anesthesia has been more widely used. This practice prevents many of the unwanted, dose-dependent side effects and toxicity associated with the anesthetic agents while simultaneously achieving a more balanced general anesthesia.

Toxicity and Management of Overdose

In large doses all anesthetics are potentially life-threatening, with cardiac and respiratory arrest the ultimate causes of death. However, these agents are almost exclusively administered in a very controlled environment by personnel trained in advanced cardiac life support, and these agents are also very quickly metabolized. In addition, the medullary center, which governs the vital centers, is the last area of the brain to be affected by the anesthetics and the first to regain function if it is lost. These factors combined make an anesthetic overdose rare and easily reversible.

Symptomatic and supportive therapy is usually all that is needed in the event of an anesthetic overdose.

Interactions

Because general anesthetics produce both productive and adverse effects on so many body systems, they are associated with a wide array of drug interactions that also vary widely in severity (see Table 9-5). No significant laboratory test interactions have been reported.

Dosages

For the recommended dosages of selected general anesthetic agents, see the dosages table below.

Table 9-5	General Anesthetics: Common Drug Interactions		
DRUG		**MECHANISM**	**RESULTS**
General anesthetics			
Antihypertensives	⎫		Increased hypotension
Beta-blockers	⎬ Additive effect		Increased myocardial depression
Tetracycline	⎭		Increased renal toxicity
Euflurane			
Isoniazid		Liver enzyme induction	Fluoride toxicity

DOSAGES

SELECTED GENERAL ANESTHETIC AGENTS

AGENT	PHARMACOLOGIC CLASS	DOSAGE RANGE	PURPOSE
Enflurane (Ethrane)	Inhalation general anesthetic (Halogenated ether)	0.5%-3% concentration	General anesthesia
Isoflurane (Forane)	Inhalation general anesthetic (Enflurane isomer)	1.5%-3% concentration	General anesthesia
Halothane (Fluothane)	Halogenated inhalation general anesthetic	0.5%-1.5% concentration	General anesthesia
Methoxyflurane (Penthrane)	Inhalation general anesthetic (Halogenated ether)	0.1%-2% concentration with appropriate drugs	General anesthesia
Nitrous oxide ("laughing gas")	Inorganic inhalation general anesthetic	20%-40% with oxygen 70% with 30% oxygen	Analgesia Anesthesia

DRUG PROFILES

All of the agents used for general anesthesia are, of course, prescription-only drugs. Desflurane, enflurane, halothane, isoflurane, and methoxyflurane are all volatile liquids; nitrous oxide is a gas. The dose of each agent depends on the surgical procedure to be performed and the physical characteristics of the patient. All of the general anesthetics have a rapid onset of activity that is maintained for the duration of the surgical procedure by continuous administration of the agent.

ENFLURANE

Enflurane (Ethrane) is a fluorinated ether that produces good muscular relaxation and minimal cardiac sensitivity to catecholamines. The drug can produce seizures in the setting of low carbon dioxide blood levels and should not be used in patients with convulsive disorders. The dosage information is given in the table on the previous page.

ISOFLURANE

Isoflurane (Forane) is very similar to enflurane in its chemical structure. However, the differences in its chemical structure give it some favorable characteristics that distinguish it from its chemical relative. Isoforane has a more rapid onset of action, causes less cardiovascular depression, and overall has been associated with little or no toxicity. The dosage information is given in the table on the previous page.

HALOTHANE

Halothane (Fluothane) is a halogenated hydrocarbon (containing three molecules of fluoride and one each of chlorine and bromine) that is frequently used with nitrous oxide. It causes considerable cardiac sensitivity to catecholamines, it produces poor muscular relaxation when used alone, and its high halogen content can result in significant liver toxicity. The dosage information is given in the table on the previous page.

METHOXYFLURANE

Methoxyflurane (Penthrane) is a fluorinated and chlorinated ether that produces excellent muscular relaxation without causing any significant cardiac sensitivity to catecholamines. However, the biotransformation of this agent produces free halogen ions that can cause significant liver toxicity, and its use is therefore contraindicated in patients with liver disease. In addition, methoxyflurane produces respiratory depression, which limits its use to patients undergoing short operations. The dosage information is given in the table on the previous page.

NITROUS OXIDE

Nitrous oxide, also known as *laughing gas*, is the only inhaled gas currently used as a general anesthetic. It is the weakest of the general anesthetic agents and is primarily used for dental procedures or as a useful supplement to other more potent anesthetics. The dosage information is given in the table on the previous page.

LOCAL ANESTHETICS

Local anesthetics are the second class of anesthetics. They are also called *regional anesthetics* because they render a specific portion of the body insensitive to pain. They do this by interfering with nerve transmission in specific areas of the body, blocking nerve conduction only in the area where they are applied without causing loss of consciousness. They are most commonly used in those clinical settings in which loss of consciousness, whole body muscle relaxation, and loss of responsiveness are either undesirable or unnecessary, for example, during childbirth. Other uses for local anesthetics include dental procedures, the suturing of skin lacerations, spinal anesthesia, and diagnostic procedures such as lumbar puncture or thoracentesis.

The local anesthetics belong to several different groups of organic compounds and are classified as either topical or parenteral anesthetics. **Topical anesthetics** are applied directly to the skin and mucous membranes. They come in the form of solutions, ointments, gels, creams, powders, ophthalmic drops, and suppositories. These agents, the route of administration, and the dosages are listed in Table 9-6. The **parenteral anesthetics** can be administered directly into the CNS by various spinal injection techniques. Anesthesia of specific areas of the peripheral nervous system is accomplished either by injecting the agents adjacent to main nerves, which produces a large body area of anesthesia, or by infiltrating it, for a more limited area of anesthesia. Some of the common types of local anesthesia are described in the box on p. 113. The parenteral anesthetic agents and the pharmacokinetics are summarized in Table 9-7.

Mechanism of Action

The local anesthetics work by rendering a specific portion of the body insensitive to pain, and they do this by interfering with nerve transmission in specific areas of the body. Nerve conduction is blocked only in the area where they are applied without consciousness being lost.

Local anesthetics block both the generation and conduction of impulses through all nerve fibers (sensory, motor, and autonomic) by blocking the movement of certain ions (sodium, potassium, and calcium) important to this process. They do this by making it more difficult for these ions to move in and out of the nerve fiber. For this reason, some of these agents are also described as *membrane stabilizing* because they stabilize the nerve fiber (cell membrane) so that it is less permeable to the free movement of ions.

Drug Effects

The local anesthetics have effects on all nerve fibers: sensory, motor, and autonomic. The membrane-stabilizing effects occur first in the small fibers then in the large fibers. In terms of paralysis, usually autonomic activity is affected first, then pain and other sensory functions are lost, with motor activity the last to be lost. When the effects of the local anesthetics wear off, they do so in reverse order, with the first senses to return being motor activity, then sensory functions, and last autonomic activity.

Other prominent effects of the local anesthetics are their circulatory and respiratory effects. The local anesthetics produce sympathetic blockade, which means that the two neurotransmitters of the sympathetic nervous system, norepinephrine and epinephrine, are blocked. The cardiac drug effects of this sympathetic blockade result in decreased stroke volume, cardiac output, and peripheral resistance. The respiratory drug effects cause normal respiratory function to be interfered with. Tachyphylaxis, or a decrease in response after the repetitive administration of local anesthetics, is another bothersome drug effect.

Table 9-6	Topical Anesthetics	
AGENT	**ROUTE**	**DOSAGE STRENGTH**
Benzocaine (Dermoplast, Lanacaine, Solarcaine)	Topical Aerosol and spray	0.5%-20% ointment or cream
Butamben (Butesin)	Topical	1% ointment
Cocaine	Topical	1%-10% solution, jelly
Dibrecaine (Nupecainal)	Injection and topical	0.5%-1% solution, ointment, or cream
Proparacaine (Alcaine, Ophthetic)	Ophthalmic	0.5% solution
Pramoxine (Tronolane)	Topical	1% jelly, cream, or lotion
Tetracine (Pontocaine)	Injection, topical, and ophthalmic	0.5%-2% solution, ointment, or cream

Table 9-7	Parenteral Anesthetic Agents			
PROPERTIES	**⇩LIDOCAINE**	**MEPIVACAINE**	**PROCAINE**	**TETRACAINE**
Trade name	Xylocaine	Carbocaine	Novocain	Pontocaine
Potency*	2nd	2nd	3rd	1st
Onset	Immediate	<5 min	2-5 min	5-10 min
Duration	60-90 min	120-150 min	30-60 min	90-120 min
Dose	0.5%-4% injection	1%, 1½%, 2%, 3% injection	1%, 2%, 10% injection	0.2%, 0.3%, 1% injection

*Denotes order of potency from the most (1st) to the least (5th) potent.

Types of Local Anesthesia

Infiltration

Small amounts of anesthetic solution are injected into the tissue that surrounds the operative site. This approach to anesthesia is commonly used for such procedures as suturing wounds or dental surgery. Often agents that cause constriction of local blood vessels are also administered to limit the site of action locally.

Nerve Block

Anesthetic solution is injected at the site where a nerve innervates a specific area such as a tissue. This allows large amounts of anesthetic agent to be delivered to a very specific area without affecting the whole body. It is often reserved for more difficult to treat pain syndromes such as those seen in the setting of various cancers.

Spinal

Anesthetic solution is injected into the epidural space or the subarachnoid space that surrounds the spinal cord. Different nerves can be anesthetized depending on the location of the injection. This type of local anesthesia is frequently used for obstetric procedures.

Topical

The anesthetic agent is applied directly onto the surface of the skin, eye, or any other mucous membrane to relieve pain or prevent it from being sensed. It is frequently used for diagnostic eye examinations and suturing of skin.

Therapeutic Uses

Local anesthetics are used for surgical, dental, or diagnostic procedures as well as for the treatment of certain types of pain and are administered by two techniques: infiltration anesthesia and nerve block anesthesia. Infiltration anesthesia is commonly used for minor surgical and dental procedures and involves injecting the local anesthetic solution intradermally, subcutaneously, or submucosally across the path of nerves supplying the area to be anesthetized. The local anesthetic may be administered in a circular pattern around the operative field. Nerve block anesthesia is used for surgical, dental, and diagnostic procedures and in the therapeutic management of pain. It involves injecting the local anesthetic actually into or around the nerve trunks or nerve ganglia that supply the area to be numbed.

Some local anesthetics, for either infiltration or nerve block anesthesia, are combined with vasoconstrictors such as epinephrine, phenylephrine, and norepinephrine to help confine the local anesthetic to the injected area and prevent systemic absorption.

Side Effects and Adverse Effects

The side effects and adverse effects of the local anesthetics are, under most circumstances, limited and of little clinical importance. The undesirable effects usually result from high plasma concentrations of the drug resulting from inadvertent intravascular injection, an excessive dose or rate of injection, slow metabolic breakdown, or injection into a highly vascular tissue. In addition, when a local anesthetic gets absorbed into the circulation, it can result in adverse reactions similar to those produced by general anesthetics.

Toxicity and Management of Overdose

Local anesthetics have little opportunity to cause toxicity under most circumstances. However, as just mentioned, they can become just as toxic as the general anesthetics if they become systemically absorbed. To prevent this from occurring, vasoconstrictors such as epinephrine are coadministered with local anesthetics to keep the anesthetic at its local site of action. Another reason for the lower incidence of toxic effects with local anesthetics is that the doses of local anesthetics are on average much smaller than those of the general anesthetics. One patient population at high risk for suffering toxic effects from local anesthetics are small chil-

Table 9-8	Local Anesthetics: Common Drug Interactions	
LOCAL ANESTHETIC	**INTERACTING DRUG**	**RESULT**
Bupivacaine	Epinephrine, halothane,	Dysrhythmias
Chloroprocaine	Enflurane	
Etidocaine		
↓Lidocaine (basically all local agents)	MAOIs, tricyclic antidepressants, phenothiazines	Hypertension

MAOIs, monoamine oxidase inhibitors.

dren undergoing dental procedures. This is because of their smaller body surface area. If for some reason significant amounts of the locally administered anesthetic get absorbed systemically, cardiovascular and respiratory function may be compromised. Symptomatic and supportive therapy is usually all that is needed to reverse the toxic effects stemming from systemic absorption of the agent.

Interactions

Common drug interactions with the various local anesthetics are listed in Table 9-8. There are few clinically significant drug interactions that occur with the local anesthetics, however, because their site of action is limited to the site of injection.

DRUG PROFILE

Besides lidocaine, described in detail here, other local anesthetics include bupivacaine, chloroprocaine, eti-docaine, mepivacaine, prilocaine, procaine, propoxy-caine, and tetracaine. There are two types of local anesthetics, as determined by their chemical structure: amide and ester. This refers to the type of linkage between the aromatic ring and the amino group of the agent, two of the structural components that make an anesthetic an anesthetic. Lidocaine belongs to the amide type of local anesthetics. Some patients may report that they have allergic or anaphylactic types of reactions to "caines," as they may refer to lidocaine and the other amide agents. In these situations it may be wise to try a local anesthetic of the ester type.

⚓ LIDOCAINE

Lidocaine (Xylocaine) is one of the most commonly used local anesthetics. It comes in several strengths and in many combinations with epinephrine and is used for both infiltration and nerve block anesthesia. It comes as a 0.5%, 1%, 1.5%, 2%, and 4% parenteral injection as well as in a 0.5%, 1%, 1.5%, and 2% concentration in combination with epinephrine in a parenteral injection. Lidocaine is classified as a pregnancy category B agent and is contraindicated in those who have a hypersensitivity to it. Commonly recommended dosages are listed in the table below.

DOSAGES

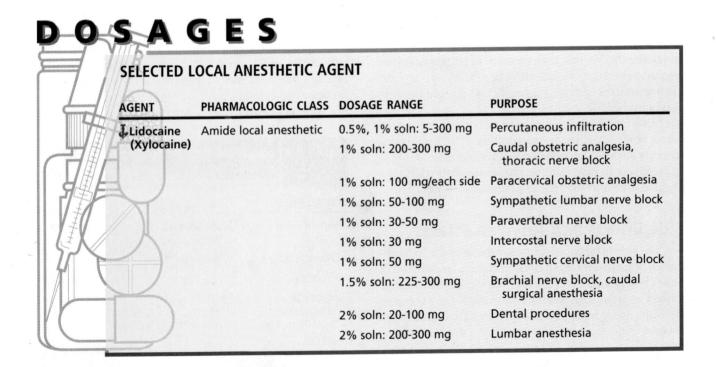

SELECTED LOCAL ANESTHETIC AGENT

AGENT	PHARMACOLOGIC CLASS	DOSAGE RANGE	PURPOSE
⚓ Lidocaine (Xylocaine)	Amide local anesthetic	0.5%, 1% soln: 5-300 mg	Percutaneous infiltration
		1% soln: 200-300 mg	Caudal obstetric analgesia, thoracic nerve block
		1% soln: 100 mg/each side	Paracervical obstetric analgesia
		1% soln: 50-100 mg	Sympathetic lumbar nerve block
		1% soln: 30-50 mg	Paravertebral nerve block
		1% soln: 30 mg	Intercostal nerve block
		1% soln: 50 mg	Sympathetic cervical nerve block
		1.5% soln: 225-300 mg	Brachial nerve block, caudal surgical anesthesia
		2% soln: 20-100 mg	Dental procedures
		2% soln: 200-300 mg	Lumbar anesthesia

Table 9-9	Stages of General Anesthesia: Nursing Responsibilities	
STAGES OF ANESTHESIA	**ASSESSMENT**	**RESPONSIBILITIES**
Stage 1: analgesia	Patient unconscious; HR> and BP> to normal; R> to normal	Assess vital signs; keep environment quiet; safety measures
Stage 2: excitement	Loss of consciousness occurs; VS are increased	Monitor VS; protect patient from injury; quiet to ease induction process
Stage 3: surgical	Patient unconscious	Assess VS; assess environment and patient's safety; reflexes absent; prevent injury
Stage 4: medullary	Do not want patients in this stage; this is a toxic and dangerous phase	Have resuscitative equipment nearby; have emergency drugs nearby for treating respiratory or cardiac arrest

BP, blood pressure; *HR*, heart rate; *R*, respiration; *VS*, vital signs.

NURSING PROCESS

ASSESSMENT

One of the most important responsibilities of the nurse in a patient receiving general anesthesia is to assess the patient's status during the four stages of anesthesia. These responsibilities are summarized in Table 9-9.

After the conclusion of the procedure and the termination of general anesthesia, the nurse's next main concern is summarized by the general rule of ABCs, or airway, breathing, and circulation. Once the patient is quickly assessed from head to toe and all vital signs are checked, the nurse needs to collect data about the specific anesthetic used, the procedure done, the allergies the patient may have, the patient's medical history, and any complications that may have occurred during anesthesia. In addition, the nurse must review current laboratory results and assess the status of any tubes, dressings, intravenous catheters, and equipment. All body systems, including the integumentary system, need to be assessed frequently and thoroughly and the findings documented (see the boxes on the next page for pediatric and geriatric considerations). The intake and output amounts, wound drainage amounts, secretion amounts, and the patient's pain level and level of consciousness are also important data to note. Allergic reactions and either CNS stimulation or depression may occur if access of the agent to the circulation has occurred. Frequent assessments

will help to detect any changes in the patient, no matter how small.

Local anesthesia still carries with it some potential for causing complications such as diminished sensation and motor responses and postural hypotension. However, unlike general anesthesia, the nurse may be the one responsible for administering a topical local anesthetic. In this event, the nurse should be sure to assess whether the patient has any preexisting illnesses and allergies; whether the patient uses OTC medications, alcohol, or any prescriptive medications, and whether the patient is or has been a smoker.

NURSING DIAGNOSES

Nursing diagnoses appropriate to the patient receiving either general or local anesthesia are as follows:
- Risk for injury related to decreased sensorium resulting from general anesthesia or to decreased sensation resulting from local anesthesia.
- Decreased cardiac output related to systemic effects of general anesthesia.
- Decreased gaseous exchange related to CNS depression produced by general anesthesia.
- Anxiety related to the use of an anesthetic and the prospect of surgery.
- Knowledge deficit because of lack of information regarding and experience with anesthesia and surgery.

PLANNING

Goals related to the care of the patient receiving general or local anesthesia are as follows:
- Patient will state the side effects of general or local anesthesia (depending on situation).

PEDIATRIC CONSIDERATIONS
Anesthesia

■ The premature infant, neonate, or pediatric patient is more affected by anesthesia than the young or middle-aged adult patient. All of their body systems are very sensitive to the effects of anesthesia, so the nurse must take all precautions to protect the patient and ensure his or her safety during all phases of surgery and all phases of anesthesia, whether general or regional.

■ The pediatric patient's hepatic, cardiac, respiratory, and renal systems are either not fully developed or they are not yet fully functional, which makes these patients more susceptible to problems such as CNS depression, toxicity, atelectasis, pneumonia, and cardiac abnormalities.

■ It is important to assess for the presence of any disease of the cardiac, renal, hepatic, or respiratory systems and to document any pertinent findings because of the attendant increased risk of complications during anesthesia in such settings. Add to this the risk associated with a very young age or with being a newborn or preemie, and the possible complications of surgery and adverse effects of anesthesia become even more problematic and more likely to occur.

■ The neonate is at a higher risk of upper airway obstruction or laryngospasms during general anesthesia because of the airway physical characteristics in this age group.

■ A more rapid metabolic rate and small airway diameter also put the neonate at greater risk of suffering complications during general anesthesia.

■ Carefully calculated doses must consider the neonate's weight and/or body surface area.

■ Nitrous oxide is commonly used in pediatric patients because of the decreased risk of hepatitis associated with this agent.

■ Resuscitative equipment should be nearby in any neonatal or pediatric unit.

■ Any change in the level of consciousness should be assessed, noted, documented, and reported immediately to a physician, even if it occurs during the postoperative period.

GERIATRIC CONSIDERATONS
Anesthesia

■ The very old patient is more affected by anesthesia than the young or middle-aged adult patient. All of their body systems are very sensitive to the effects of anesthesia, so the nurse must take all precautions to protect the patient and ensure his or her safety during all phases of surgery and all phases of anesthesia, whether general, regional, or local.

■ The elderly patient's hepatic, cardiac, respiratory, and renal systems are all affected by aging, and these age-related changes make the patients more susceptible to problems such as CNS depression, toxicity, atelectasis, pneumonia, and cardiac abnormalities.

■ It is important to assess for the presence of any disease of the cardiac, renal, hepatic, or respiratory systems and to document any pertinent findings because of the increased risk of complications during anesthesia in such settings. Add to this the risk associated with advanced age, and the possible complications of surgery and adverse effects of anesthesia become even more problematic and more likely to occur.

■ Patient will comply with care to decrease the chances of complications after anesthesia.

■ Patient will follow preoperative instructions regarding his or her care during the postoperative period (see the box on the next page for home health points).

■ Patient will verbalize anxiety prn regarding surgery and anesthesia.

Outcome Criteria

Outcome criteria related to the use of general or local anesthesia are as follows:

■ Patient will experience minimal to no side effects of general or local anesthesia such as myocardial depression during operative period.

■ Patient will remain free of complications such as injury, falls, and hepatotoxicity during the perioperative period (preoperative, intraoperative, and postoperative).

■ Patient will be free of or experience minimal anxiety as evidenced by fewer complaints, better relaxation ability, and decreased postoperative pain.

■ Patient will be compliant with all measures and treatments such as turning, coughing, and deep breathing during the perioperative period.

■ Patient will state potential complications of both general and local anesthesia.

■ Patient will experience minimal to no injury related to anesthesia.

■ Patient will describe what to expect during the recovery period of anesthesia.

HOME HEALTH POINTS
Anesthesia

■ Home health care plays an important role in the recovery of any patient being discharged from the hospital to home. Home health care is a resource for all phases of the rehabilitation and recovery process, especially in any aged patient.

■ Community resources are available for the use of all aged patients during their recovery and rehabilitation at home after surgery. Contacting a home health care agency and city-sponsored social service agencies is a starting point to the receipt of these services.

■ Meals on wheels are often available for the elderly patient, and senior citizen resources and agencies are available through most city governments. Elderly patients are also encouraged to contact city-sponsored or church-related transportation services to meet their transportation needs.

▼

Patient Teaching **TIPS**

General Anesthesia

✔ Obtain a listing of all prescription and OTC medications the patient may be taking so that any possible drug interactions can be averted by discontinuance of the medication before surgery. Encourage patient to have a list of all medications currently taken—on person—at all times.

✔ Obesity, smoking, and cardiac or respiratory disease are all factors that heighten the risks associated with anesthesia and should be identified preoperatively so that proper preparations can be made.

✔ Patient teaching about the procedure and the care before, during, and after surgery help to alleviate anxiety and promote recovery.

✔ Explain the rationale for the use of preoperative medications as well as the need to be NPO (to prevent aspiration).

✔ Patient teaching on turning, coughing, and deep breathing is also important for the promotion of healing and recovery.

✔ Patient teaching about postoperative pain control methods is also important to alleviating anxiety and promoting healing.

✔ Explain the rationale for any other treatments, such as the use of drainage tubes, catheters, intravenous lines, and so on.

✔ The importance of frequent vital sign monitoring should be discussed with the patient to minimize anxiety and fear postoperatively.

✔ Always ask patients whether they have any allergies to medications or foods.

✔ Instruct patients about the importance of safety features such as keeping side rails up and using the call light during the postoperative phase.

IMPLEMENTATION

Regardless of the type of anesthesia a patient is receiving, some important points the nurse must consider during this time include close and frequent observation of the patient and all body systems with specific attention to the ABCs of nursing care and vital signs. This should be done as frequently as necessary or in conformance with the protocol. If any sudden elevation in body temperature occurs while a patient is receiving general anesthesia, this should be reported to the anesthesiologist immediately because it may indicate the occurrence of malignant hyperthermia, a potentially fatal complication especially associated with the use of succinylcholine. Malignant hyperthermia is a life-threatening emergency and requires prompt medical attention. Other nursing actions to be carried out after a patient has received general anesthesia include monitoring all aspects of body functions, instituting safety measures, and implementing the physician's orders.

Oxygen is generally administered after a patient has received general anesthesia to compensate for the respiratory depression that occurred during surgery. In addition, hypotension and orthostatic hypotension are a problem after anesthesia because of the vasodilation it produces. In addition, when administering pain medication postoperatively, it is important to remember that the dose of any sedative or analgesic administered after surgery when the patient returns to the room or is in the recovery room is often decreased by one-half to one-fourth so that CNS depression does not occur. For IV anesthesia, all resuscitative equipment should be kept nearby.

In general, any sudden elevation in body temperature immediately postoperatively should be reported to the physician immediately because of the continued risk of malignant hyperthermia associated with general anesthesia that includes succinylcholine. Additional nursing observations during and after general (as well as local and spinal) anesthesia include the status of breath sounds, assessed by auscultation (hypoventilation may be a complication of general anesthesia); any changes in neurologic status (no matter how

Local Anesthesia

✔ Always perform a thorough patient assessment, including questions about allergies, prescribed and OTC medications, and any medical problems.

✔ Make sure patients understand how local anesthetics work, their side effects, and why the specific local agent was selected.

✔ For those patients receiving epidural or spinal anesthesia, vital sign and systems assessments should be done frequently during and after the procedure so as to monitor for and assess any complications. Inform patient of this to help decrease anxiety.

✔ Remind patients about decreased motor and sensory status so they know what to expect.

TAKE HOME POINTS

Anesthesia
- CNS altered so that pain perception and consciousness are lost; also includes skeletal muscle relaxation and loss of reflexes.
- Drug-induced state of altered nerve conduction.
- Can be either general or local.
- Allows exposure to the surgical area so the surgeon can carry out specific and often very sophisticated procedures.

General Anesthetics
- Agents that induce a state of anesthesia.
- Global—affect the whole body.

Balanced Anesthesia
- Combinations of drugs to produce anesthesia.
- Sedative-hypnotic, anxiolytic, analgesic, antiemetic, anticholinergic, and a neuromuscular blocking agent.

Local Anesthetics
- Also called *regional anesthetics*.
- Render specific portion of body insensitive to pain without affecting consciousness.

Topical Anesthetics
- Applied to skin and mucous membranes.
- Solutions, ointments, gels, creams, powders, ophthalmic drops, and suppositories.

Nursing Considerations
- The perioperative phase includes the preoperative, intraoperative, and postoperative stages.
- Each stage calls for a complex and specific plan of care.

minute!); and any changes in sensation in body parts distal to the site of local anesthesia or distal to where the safety restraints were placed during the surgery. Improper positioning during surgery may lead to the damage of arteries and nerves. When caring for a client who has received either general or local anesthesia, all body functions should be monitored and safety measures implemented. Reorientation of the patient to his or her surroundings and implementation of the physician's orders should also be part of the patient's care during the postoperative phase. See Table 9-9 for more information regarding nursing interventions during the stages of anesthesia.

A local anesthetic solution that is cloudy or discolored or that contains any sort of crystalloids should not be used. It is also important to remember that some anesthesiologists mix the solution with sodium bicarbonate to minimize the local pain during infiltration, but this also causes a more rapid onset of action and a longer duration of sensory analgesia. Resuscitative equipment should be kept close by. If an anesthetic ointment or cream is used, thoroughly cleanse the area to be anesthetized and dry it before application. If a suppository is being used, refrigerate it before use, remove the wrapper, moisten the suppository with water or water-soluble lubricant, and then insert it.

If a local anesthetic is being used in the nose or throat, it is important to remember that it may lead to paralysis of the structures of the upper respiratory tract, leading to possible aspiration. Exact amounts of the agent should be used and administered only at the prescribed times. Local anesthetics are not to be swallowed unless the physician has instructed this. If this

is to be done, the nurse should then constantly observe the patient and check his or her gag reflex after administration of the agent, withholding food or drink until the gag reflex has returned.

Local anesthesia produces paralysis of certain areas, such as the area below the waist, so it is important to protect the patient from injury resulting from this loss of sensation. Bed side rails should be kept up, and there should be no untoward pressure on the affected skin area because the body's normal sensation and protective mechanisms have been diminished. After a spinal anesthetic, patients must remain flat in bed for up to 12 hours to prevent a spinal headache. They should also be well hydrated during this period.

Teaching tips important for patients receiving either local or general anesthesia are given in the boxes on p. 117 and 118.

EVALUATION

The therapeutic effects of any general or local anesthetic include loss of sensation during the procedure such as loss of sensation in the eye for the purpose of corneal surgery or loss of consciousness and other reflexes, such as pain, for the purpose of abdominal or other major procedures. The patient who has received general anesthesia should be constantly monitored for the occurrence of adverse effects of the anesthesia. These effects include myocardial depression, convulsions, respiratory depression, allergic rhinitis, and decreased renal or liver functioning. Patients who have received a local anesthetic also need to be constantly monitored for the occurrence of adverse effects of the anesthesia (mostly stemming from the systemic absorption of the specific agent). These effects include bradycardia, myocardial depression, hypotension, and arrhythmias. As mentioned earlier in this chapter, significant overdoses of local agents or direct injection into a blood vessel may result in cardiovascular collapse or cardiac or respiratory depression.

Critical Thinking ACTIVITIES

1. Assessment of a patient during the intraoperative period of surgery would most likely yield which of the following findings:
   a. Alertness and sharp mental acuity during stage 1 of anesthesia.
   b. Stimulation of vital centers during stage 4.
   c. Depression of vital signs during stage 3.
   d. Complete respiratory paralysis during stage 2.

2. Assessment of vital signs immediately postoperatively should occur at least:
   a. Every hour and prn.
   b. Only as needed.
   c. Every 15 minutes and as needed.
   d. Whenever the patient shows significant changes.

3. Major side effects expected as the result of local anesthesia, such as epidural or spinal anesthesia, include which of the following:
   a. Hypotension.
   b. Tachypnea.
   c. Edema.
   d. Dysphagia.

4. One of your patients states, "Well, it really doesn't make a difference. Smoking can't hurt me with surgery. As long as I just get moving, I'll be all right!" How would you respond regarding the effects of smoking on general anesthesia?

BIBLIOGRAPHY

Albanese J, Nutz P: *Mosby's 1995 nursing drug cards*, St Louis, 1995, Mosby.

Hussar DA: New drugs, *Nursing 93*, p 57, May 1993.

Johnson KB: *Harriet Lane handbook*, ed 13, St Louis, 1993, Mosby.

Keen JH: *Critical care and emergency drug reference*, St Louis, 1994, Mosby.

Keeney SA: Nursing care of the postoperative patient receiving epidural analgesia, *Medsurg Nurs* 2(3):191, 1993.

Kendall F: Documenting local anesthesia patient care, *AORN J* 58(4):715, 1993.

Knoben JE, Anderson PO: *Handbook of critical drug data*, ed 6, Hamilton, Ill, 1988, Drug Intelligence Publications.

McEvoy GK: *AHFS drug information*, Bethesda, Md, 1989, American Society of Hospital Pharmacists.

McKenry L, Salerno E: *Mosby's pharmacology in nursing*, ed 19, St Louis, 1995, Mosby.

Polomano RC, Blumenthal NP, Riegler FX: Interpleural analgesia for the management of postoperative pain, *Medsurg Nurs* 2(3):185, 1993.

Skidmore-Roth L: *Mosby's 1995 nursing drug reference*, St Louis, 1995, Mosby.

Chapter 10

Hypnotic and Sedative Agents

Objectives

When you reach the end of this chapter, you will be able to:

1 Differentiate between a sedative and a hypnotic agent.

2 Describe the differences between benzodiazepines and barbiturates as sedative-hypnotic agents.

3 Identify specific benzodiazepine and barbiturate agents.

4 Discuss the nursing process as it relates to the nursing care of patients receiving sedative-hypnotic agents.

5 Understand the importance of using nonpharmacologic approaches to treat sleep disturbances.

6 Develop patient education guidelines for patients receiving sedative-hypnotic agents.

CHAPTER OUTLINE

Sleep
Barbiturates
  Mechanism of action
  Drug effects
  Therapeutic uses
  Side effects and adverse effects
    Toxicity and overdose
  Interactions
    Laboratory test interactions
  Dosages
Drug Profiles
  Phenobarbital
  Aprobarbital
  Butabarbital
  Pentobarbital
  Secobarbital
Benzodiazepines
  Mechanism of action
  Drug effects
  Therapeutic uses
  Side effects and adverse effects
    Toxicity and overdose
  Interactions
    Laboratory test interactions
  Dosages
Drug Profiles
  Estazolam
  Flurazepam

  Quazepam
  Temazepam
  Triazolam
Miscellaneous

Nursing Process
Assessment
Nursing Diagnoses
Planning
  Outcome criteria
Implementation
Evaluation

Glossary

Anxiolytic (ang zi o lit′ ik) A medication that relieves anxiety. (p. 126)

Barbiturates (bahr bich′ ər əts) A class of drugs that are chemical derivatives of barbituric acid, an agent that can induce sedation and sleep. (p. 121)

Benzodiazepines (ben zō di az ə pēn) A chemical category of drugs and the ones most frequently prescribed as sedative-hypnotic and anxiolytic agents. (p. 126)

Gamma-aminobutyric acid (GABA) (ə me no bu tēr′ ik) An inhibitory neurotransmitter found in the brain. (p. 121)

Hypnotics Drugs that when given at low doses calm or soothe the CNS without inducing sleep but when given at high doses may cause sleep. (p. 121)

Non–rapid eye movement (non–REM) One of the stages of the sleep cycle. It characteristically has four stages and precedes rapid eye movement sleep. Most of a normal sleep cycle consists of non–rapid eye movement sleep. (p. 121)

Rapid eye movement (REM) One of the stages of the sleep cycle. One of the characteristics of rapid eye movement sleep is the rapid movement of the eyes, vivid dreams, and irregular breathing. (p. 121)

Sedatives Drugs that have an inhibitory effect on the CNS to the degree that they reduce nervousness, excitability, or irritability without causing sleep. (p. 121)

Sedative-hypnotics Drugs that can act in the body either as a sedative or hypnotic. (p. 121)

Sleep A transient, reversible, and periodic state of rest in which there is a decrease in physical activity and consciousness. (p. 121)

Sleep architecture The various steps involved in the sleep cycle, including normal and abnormal patterns of sleep. (p. 121)

Tachyphylaxis (tak e fe lak sis) The rapid appearance of a progressive decrease in response to a drug after repetitive administration of the drug. (p. 130)

Therapeutic index The level of drug in the blood that provides a therapeutic effect without causing toxicity. (p. 121)

Drugs that have a calming effect or that depress the central nervous system (CNS) are referred to as *sedatives* and *hypnotics*. A drug is classified as either a sedative or a hypnotic agent depending on the degree to which it inhibits the transmission of nerve impulses to the CNS. **Sedatives** reduce nervousness, excitability, and irritability without causing sleep, but a sedative can become a hypnotic if it is given in large enough doses. **Hypnotics** cause sleep. They have a much more potent effect on the CNS than sedatives do. Many drugs can act in the body as either a sedative or a hypnotic, and for this reason are called **sedative-hypnotics**.

Sedative-hypnotics can be classified chemically into three main groups: the barbiturates, the benzodiazepines, and the nonbarbiturates or miscellaneous agents. Before discussing the sedative-hypnotics in depth, it is important that the physiology of normal sleep is understood because of the significant effects these agents can have on normal sleep patterns.

SLEEP

Sleep is defined as a transient, reversible, and periodic state of rest in which there is a decrease in physical activity and consciousness. Normal sleep is cyclic and repetitive, and a person's responses to stimuli are markedly reduced during sleep. During waking hours the body is bombarded with stimuli that provoke the senses of sight, hearing, touch, smell, and taste. These stimuli elicit voluntary and involuntary movements or functions. During sleep a person is no longer aware of the sensory stimuli within his or her immediate environment.

Sleep research involves studying the patterns of sleep, or what is sometimes referred to as **sleep architecture**. The architecture of sleep consists of two basic stages that occur cyclically: **rapid eye movement** sleep **(REM)** and **non–rapid eye movement** sleep **(non–REM)**. The normal cyclic progression of the stages of sleep is summarized in Table 10-1. Various sedative-hypnotics affect different stages of the normal sleep pattern. If usage is prolonged, emotional and psychologic changes can occur. An appreciation of this will help prevent the inappropriate use of long-term sleeping agents.

BARBITURATES

The **barbiturates** were first introduced into clinical use in 1903 and were the standard agents for treating insomnia and producing sedation. Chemically they are derivatives of barbituric acid. Although there are close to 50 different barbiturates approved for clinical use in the United States, only a handful are in common clinical use today. This is in part due to the favorable safety profile and proven efficacy of the class of drugs commonly referred to as the *benzodiazepines*. Barbiturates can produce many unwanted side effects. They are habit-forming and have a narrow **therapeutic index**, which is the dosage range within which the drug is effective but above which it is rapidly toxic. The barbiturates can be classified into four different groups based on their onset and duration of action. Table 10-2 lists the agents within each category and summarizes their pharmacokinetic characteristics (onset and duration of action).

Mechanism of Action

Barbiturates are CNS depressants that act primarily on the brainstem in an area called the *reticular formation*. Their sedative and hypnotic effects are dose related, and they act by reducing the nerve impulses traveling to the area in the brain called the *cerebral cortex*. Their ability to inhibit nerve impulse transmission is in part due to their ability to potentiate an inhibitory amino acid known as **gamma-aminobutyric acid (GABA)**, which is found in high concentrations in the CNS. Barbiturates are capable of raising the convulsive or seizure threshold and are therefore also effective in treating status epilepticus and tetanus- or drug-induced convulsions. In addition, selected barbiturates are used as prophylaxis for epileptic seizures.

Table 10-1	Stages of Sleep	
STAGE	CHARACTERISTICS	AVERAGE TIME IN EACH STAGE (FOR YOUNG ADULT)
Non–REM sleep		
1	Dozing or feelings of drifting off to sleep. Persons can be easily awakened. Insomniacs have longer stage 1 periods than normal.	3%-6%
2	Person is relaxed but can be easily awakened. Has occasional REMs and also slight eye movements.	40%-52%
3	Deep sleep; difficult to wake person up. Respiratory rates, pulse, and blood pressure may decrease.	5%-8%
4	Sleepwalking or bedwetting may occur. Very difficult to wake person up; may be very groggy if done. Dreaming, especially about daily events.	10%-19%
REM sleep		
	REMs occur. Vivid dreams occur. Breathing may be irregular.	23%-34%

Modified from McKenry, Salerno: *Mosby's pharmacology in nursing*, ed 19, St Louis, 1995, Mosby.
REM, rapid eye movement.

Table 10-2	Barbiturates: Onset and Duration		
	PHARMACOKINETICS		
CATEGORY	ONSET	DURATION	BARBITURATES
Ultrashort	IV: <15 min	IV: <2 hr	Mephobexital, thiamylal, thiopental
Short	PO: 15-20 min	PO: 2-4 hr	Pentabarbital, secobarbital
Intermediate	PO: 2-30 min	PO: 4-6 hr	Aprobarbital, butabarbital
Long	PO: 30-60 min	PO: 6-8 hr	Phenobarbital

Drug Effects

In low doses the barbiturates act as sedatives. Increasing the dose produces a hypnotic effect, but this also decreases the respiratory rate. In normal doses they have little effect on the circulation. Barbiturates as a class are notorious enzyme inducers. They stimulate the enzymes in the liver that are responsible for the metabolism or breakdown of drugs. By stimulating these enzymes they cause drugs to be converted more quickly into active substances so that they have a faster onset of action, but the drugs are also broken down more quickly to inactive substances, therefore shortening their duration of effect. Warfarin, theophylline, and phenytoin are three such drugs. They are very commonly prescribed and potentially very dangerous drugs because of this reaction that can occur.

Therapeutic Uses

All barbiturates have the same sedative-hypnotic efficacy but differ in their potency, onset, and duration of action. They are used as hypnotics, sedatives, and anticonvulsants and also for anesthesia during surgical procedures. They are used for the following therapeutic reasons:

Ultrashort: Anesthetic for short surgical procedures, anesthesia induction, control of convulsions, narcoanalysis, and reduction in intracranial pressure in neurosurgical patients.
Short: Sedative-hypnotic and control of convulsive conditions.
Intermediate: Sedative-hypnotic and control of convulsive conditions.

Long: Sedative-hypnotic, epileptic seizure prophylaxis, and treatment of neonatal hyperbilirubinemia.

Side Effects and Adverse Effects

The main side effects of the barbiturates affect the CNS and include drowsiness, lethargy, dizziness, hangover, and paradoxical restlessness or excitement. Their chronic effects on normal sleep architecture can be detrimental. Sleep research has shown that adequate rest from the sleep process is obtained only when there are proper amounts of REM sleep, which is sometimes referred to as *deep sleep*. The barbiturates deprive persons of REM sleep, which can result in agitation and an inability to deal with normal stress. When the barbiturate is stopped and REM sleep once again occurs, a rebound phenomenon can occur. During this rebound the proportion of REM sleep is increased, the patient's dream time constitutes a larger percentage of the total sleep pattern, and the dreams are often nightmares. The adverse effects of barbiturates relative to the body systems affected are listed in Table 10-3.

Toxicity and Overdose

Overdose frequently results in respiratory depression, leading to respiratory arrest. Often this is done therapeutically to induce anesthesia. In this situation, however, the patient is ventilated mechanically and respiration is controlled or assisted mechanically. Another situation in which intentional overdoses are given for therapeutic reasons is in the management of uncontrollable seizures. Such patients are sometimes put into what is called a *phenobarbital coma*. Because of the inhibitory effects of barbiturates on nerve transmission in the brain (possibly GABA mediated), the uncontrollable seizures can be stopped until appropriate drug levels of anticonvulsant drugs are achieved.

An overdose of barbiturates produces CNS depression ranging from sleep to profound coma and death. Respiratory depression progresses to Cheyne-Stokes respiration, hypoventilation, and cyanosis. Affected patients often have cold, clammy skin or are hypothermic or later they can exhibit fever, areflexia, tachycardia, and hypotension. Pupils are usually slightly constricted but may be dilated in the event of severe poisoning.

Treatment of an overdose is mainly symptomatic and supportive. The mainstays of therapy should consist of maintenance of an adequate airway, assisted respiration, and oxygen administration if needed, along with fluid and pressor support as indicated. The multiple-dose (every 4 hours) nasogastric administration of activated charcoal is highly effective in removing

Table 10-3	Barbiturates: Adverse Effects
BODY SYSTEM	**SIDE/ADVERSE EFFECTS**
Nervous system	Drowsiness, lethargy, vertigo, headache, mental depression, and myalgic, neuralgic, or arthralgic pain
Gastrointestinal	Nausea, vomiting, diarrhea, and constipation
Blood	Agranulocytosis, thrombocytopenia, and megaloblastic anemia
Respiratory	Respiratory depression, apnea, laryngospasm, bronchospasm, and coughing
Cardiovascular	Vasodilation and hypotension, especially if given too rapidly
Other	Hypersensitivity reactions: urticaria, angioedema, rash, fever, serum sickness, or Stevens-Johnson syndrome

barbiturates from the stomach as well as the circulation. Barbiturates are highly metabolized by the liver, and they increase enzyme activity there. In an overdose, however, the amount of barbiturate may overwhelm the liver's ability to metabolize it. This is where the activated charcoal may be helpful. This helps pull the drug from the circulation and eliminate it by means of the gastrointestinal system. Some of the barbiturates (phenobarbital, aprobarbital, and mephobarbital) can be eliminated more quickly by the kidneys when the urine is alkalized. This keeps the drug in the urine and prevents it from being resorbed back into the circulation. This, along with forced diuresis, can hasten elimination of the barbiturate.

Interactions

The potential drug interactions with the barbiturates are considerable in their intensity and oftentimes dramatic. The risks encountered in the coadministration of barbiturates and certain agents are summarized in Table 10-4. Most of the drug-drug interactions involving barbiturates are secondary to their effects on the hepatic enzyme system. As mentioned earlier, the barbiturates increase the activity of hepatic microsomal enzymes. This is sometimes called *enzyme induction*. Induction of this enzyme system results in increased drug metabolism and breakdown. However, if

Table 10-4	Barbiturates: Drug Interactions	
DRUG	**MECHANISM**	**RESULTS**
Alcohol		
Antihistamines		
Benzodiazepines	Additive effects	Increased depressant effects
Narcotics		
Tranquilizers		
Monoamine oxidase inhibitors	Inhibit metabolism of barbiturates	Prolonged barbiturate effects
Anticoagulants	Increased metabolism of anticoagulants	Decreased anticoagulant response

the two drugs are competing for the same enzyme system for metabolism, this can lead to inhibited drug metabolism or breakdown.

Laboratory Test Interactions

Barbiturates can also interact with body substances and affect the results of various laboratory tests. Barbiturates can cause an increase in the serum levels of bilirubin, SGPT (serum glutamate pyruvate transaminase), SGOT (serum glutamic-oxaloacetic transaminase), and alkaline phosphatase.

Dosages

As already mentioned, the barbiturates can act as either sedatives or hypnotics depending on their dosage. The various barbiturates and their recommended sedative and hypnotic dosages are listed in the dosages table on p. 125.

DRUG PROFILES

The barbiturates are available in a variety of dosage forms, including tablets, capsules, elixirs, injections, and suppositories. They are all rated as pregnancy category D drugs by the FDA. (Inside the back cover is listed a description of what each pregnancy category means.) All barbiturates are considered prescription-only drugs because of the potential for their being misused and the severe effects that result if they are not used appropriately. From a legal standpoint they are

Table 10-5	Barbiturates: Controlled Substance Schedule
SCHEDULE	**BARBITURATES**
C-II	Secobarbital, pentobarbital
C-III	Aprobarbital, butabarbital
C-IV	Phenobarbital

considered controlled substances. As discussed in Chapter 5, controlled substances are medications that the U.S. Drug Enforcement Administration has identified as drugs that have a high abuse potential. State laws are often more stringent than federal laws in terms of the way in which these drugs are dispensed, so health care providers must be careful to comply with both federal and state laws. A detailed description of schedules I through V can be found in the appendix. The various barbiturates are listed in Table 10-5 according to the controlled substance schedule.

They are contraindicated in patients with known hypersensitivity reactions to them, latent porphyria, significant liver dysfunction, and known previous addiction.

PHENOBARBITAL

Phenobarbital is the most frequently prescribed barbiturate, either alone or in combination with other drugs. It is considered the *prototypical* barbiturate and is classified as a long-acting agent. Phenobarbital is used for the prevention of grand mal seizures and fever-induced convulsions. In addition, it has been useful in the treatment of hyperbilirubinemia in neonates. It has also been used for the treatment of Gil-

D O S A G E S

SELECTED BARBITURATES

AGENT	ONSET AND DURATION	DOSAGE RANGE	PURPOSE
Aprobarbital (Alurate)	Intermediate acting	*Adult* PO: 40 mg tid 40-100 mg HS	Sedation Hypnotic
Butabarbital (Buticaps, Butisol, Butalan)	Intermediate acting	*Pediatric* PO: 2-6 mg/kg before surgery *Adult* PO: 15-30 mg 3-4 times/day 50-100 mg before surgery 50-100 mg HS	Preop sedation Sedation Preop sedation Hypnotic
Pentobarbital (Nembutal)	Short acting	*Pediatric* IM/IV/PO: 2-6 mg/kg Rectal: 2 mo-1 y/o, 30 mg; 1-4 y/o, 30-60 mg; 5-12 y/o, 60 mg; 12-14 y/o, 60-120 mg HS *Adult* PO/rectal: 100-200 mg HS IM: 150-200 mg IV: 150 mg/70 kg	Anticonvulsant, preop sedation, sedation Hypnotic Hypnotic Anticonvulsant, preop sedation, hypnotic Anticonvulsant, preop sedation, hypnotic
Phenobarbital (Solfoton)	Long acting	*Neonate* PO: 5-10 mg/kg/day *Pediatric* PO: 6 mg/kg or 180 mg/m²/day in 3 equally divided doses IM/IV: 1-3 mg/kg *Adult* PO: 30-120 mg/day divided 100-320 mg HS *Adult* IM/IV: 200-200 mg 60-90 min before surgery	Hyperbilirubinemia Sedation Preop sedation Sedation Hypnotic Preop sedation
Secobarbital (Seconal)	Short acting	*Pediatric* PO: 2-6 mg/kg IM: 4-5 mg/kg 2 mg/kg several times/day IM/IV: 3-5 mg/kg *Adult* PO: 100 mg HS 200-300 mg 1-2 hr before surgery IM: 100-200 mg HS 1 mg/kg 10-15 min before surgery IV: 50-250 mg 100-150 mg IM/IV: 5.5 mg/kg	Preop sedation Preop sedation Sedation Anticonvulsant Hypnotic Preop sedation Hypnotic Preop sedation Hypnotic Dental sedation before nerve block Anticonvulsant

bert's syndrome. It is most commonly used, however, as a sedative-hypnotic agent. (See the preceding table for the dosages.) Pregnancy category D.

🦴 P H A R M A C O K I N E T I C S

HALF-LIFE	ONSET	PEAK	DURATION
PO/IV: 53-118 hr	PO: 30 min	PO: 8-12 hr	PO: 10-12 hr
	IV: 5 min	IV: 30 min	IV: 4-10 hr

APROBARBITAL

Aprobarbital is used for routine sedation and as a hypnotic in the short-term treatment of insomnia for periods of up to 2 weeks. The common dosages for achieving the sedative and hypnotic effects of aprobarbital are given in the preceding dosages table. Pregnancy category D.

🦴 P H A R M A C O K I N E T I C S

HALF-LIFE	ONSET	PEAK	DURATION
14-34 hr	30-45 min	3 hr	8-12 hr

BUTABARBITAL

Butabarbital as a single agent is used for routine sedation and as a hypnotic in the short-term management of insomnia. It is also combined with aspirin, acetaminophen, and caffeine in various formulations used to treat migraine headaches. The common dosages of butabarbital that apply when it is administered as a single agent are given in the preceding dosages table. Pregnancy category D.

🦴 P H A R M A C O K I N E T I C S

HALF-LIFE	ONSET	PEAK	DURATION
100 hr	30-45 min	3-4 hr	6-8 hr

PENTOBARBITAL

Pentobarbital is principally used as a hypnotic agent for the short-term management of insomnia. It is also used preoperatively to relieve anxiety and provide sedation. In addition, it is used for sedation and occasionally to control status epilepticus or acute seizure episodes resulting from meningitis, poisons, eclampsia, alcohol withdrawal, tetanus, or chorea. Pentobarbital may also be used to treat withdrawal symptoms in patients who are physically dependent on barbiturates or nonbarbiturate hypnotics. The sedative and hypnotic dosages are given in the preceding dosages table. Pregnancy category D.

🦴 P H A R M A C O K I N E T I C S

HALF-LIFE	ONSET	PEAK	DURATION
PO/IV: 35-50 hr	PO: 15-60 min	PO: 30-60 min	PO: 1-4 hr
	IV: <1 min	IV: <30 min	IV: 15 min

SECOBARBITAL

Secobarbital is used primarily as a hypnotic agent to induce sleep. It may be administered intravenously to control status epilepticus or acute seizures, similar to the way in which pentobarbital is used. It may also be used to maintain a steady state of unconsciousness during general, spinal, or regional anesthesia or to facilitate intubation procedures. The common sedative and hypnotic dosages are given in the preceding dosages table. Pregnancy category D.

🦴 P H A R M A C O K I N E T I C S

HALF-LIFE	ONSET	PEAK	DURATION
PO/IV: 30 hr	PO: 15 min	PO: 2-4 hr	PO: 1-4 hr
	IV: 1-3 min	IV: <30 min	IV: 15 min

BENZODIAZEPINES

The **benzodiazepines** are the most frequently prescribed sedative-hypnotic agents and one of the most commonly prescribed class of drugs. This is directly attributed to their favorable side effect profiles, their efficacy, and their safety. Even when a drug in this class is taken as the sole agent in an overdose (i.e., not with alcohol), it is relatively benign, resulting in little more than sedation. Benzodiazepines are classified as either anxiolytics or sedative-hypnotics depending on their primary usage. An **anxiolytic** relieves anxiety, and the benzodiazepine anxiolytics are discussed in Chapter 13. The benzodiazepines discussed in this chapter, however, are the ones that work primarily to produce sedation or sleep. There are five such agents commonly used as sedative-hypnotics. They are listed in Table 10-6 and can be further classified on the basis of their duration of action as either long acting or short acting.

Mechanism of Action

As mentioned earlier, the sedative and hypnotic action of benzodiazepines is related to their ability to depress activity in the CNS. The specific areas they affect in the CNS appear to be the hypothalamic, thalamic, and limbic systems of the brain. Recent research

Table 10-6	Sedative-Hypnotic Benzodiazepines
GENERIC NAME	TRADE NAME
Long acting	
⚓Flurazepam	Dalmane
Quazepam	Doral
Short acting	
Estazolam	Prosom
Temazepam	Restoril
Triazolam	Halcion

has indicated that there are specific receptors in the brain for benzodiazepines. These receptors are thought to be the same as those of the CNS inhibitory transmitter GABA. If they are not the same, then they are adjacent to the GABA receptors. Their depressant action on the CNS appears to be related to their ability to inhibit stimulation of the brain. They have many favorable effects compared with the barbiturates. They do not suppress REM sleep to the same extent as barbiturates, and their withdrawal does not result in severe rebound REM sleep. They also do not induce hepatic microsomal enzyme activity and are therefore safe to administer to patients who are taking medications that are metabolized by this enzyme system.

Drug Effects

The benzodiazepines have a calming effect on the CNS. This causes the inhibition of hyperexcitable nerves in the CNS that might be responsible for causing seizure activity. Similarly, this calming effect on the CNS makes benzodiazepines useful in controlling agitation and anxiety. It also reduces excessive sensory stimulation and induces sleep. They have also been shown to induce skeletal muscle relaxation. Their receptors in the CNS are in the same area as those that play a role in alcohol addiction. Therefore they are used in the treatment of and prevention of the symptoms of alcohol withdrawal.

Therapeutic Uses

The benzodiazepines have a variety of therapeutic applications. They are most frequently used for sedation, sleep induction, skeletal muscle relaxation, and anxiety relief. They have also been used in the treatment of alcohol withdrawal, agitation, depression, and epilepsy. They are often combined with anesthe-

tics, analgesics, and neuromuscular-blocking agents in what is called *balanced anesthesia*. Their use in this setting is mostly for their amnestic properties, because most persons undergoing surgery would rather not remember the events of their procedure.

Side Effects and Adverse Effects

As a class the benzodiazepines have a relatively safe side effect profile. The side effects and adverse effects associated with their use are mild and infrequently reported, and they primarily involve the CNS. The more commonly reported undesirable effects are headache, drowsiness, paradoxical excitement or nervousness, dizziness or vertigo, and lethargy. Because of the benzodiazepines' effect on the normal sleep cycle, a hangover effect is sometimes reported. Other less common side effects and adverse effects are palpitations, dry mouth, nausea, vomiting, hypokinesia, and occasional nightmares.

Toxicity and Overdose

An overdose of benzodiazepines may result in one or all of the following symptoms: somnolence, confusion, coma, and diminished reflexes. An overdose of just benzodiazepines rarely results in hypotension and respiratory depression. These are more commonly seen when benzodiazepines are coingested with other CNS depressants such as alcohol or barbiturates. The same holds true for their lethal effects. In the absence of the concurrent ingestion of alcohol or other CNS depressants, benzodiazepine overdoses rarely result in death.

The treatment of benzodiazepine intoxication is generally symptomatic and supportive. If ingestion is recent, decontamination of the gastrointestinal system is indicated. As a rule of thumb, the administration of syrup of ipecac (an emetic agent used to induce vomiting in overdoses) to produce gastric decontamination is contraindicated in persons who have ingested medications that cause sedation, the concern being that an unconscious patient induced to vomit could easily aspirate stomach contents. Therefore gastric lavage is generally the best and most effective means of gastric decontamination. Activated charcoal and a saline cathartic may be administered after gastric lavage to remove any remaining drug. Hemodialysis is not useful in the treatment of benzodiazepine overdose.

Flumazenil can be used to acutely reverse the sedative effects of benzodiazepines. It formerly went by the product name Mazicon but was renamed and is now called Romazicon. This was done to prevent its confusion with Mevacron, which is a nondepolarizing neuromuscular-blocking agent used to paralyze patients. Flumazenil antagonizes the action of benzo-

Table 10-7	Flumazenil Treatment Regimen	
INDICATION	**RECOMMENDED REGIMEN**	**DURATION**
Reversal of conscious sedation or general anesthesia	0.2 mg (2 ml) given IV over 15 sec, wait 45 sec, then give 0.2 mg if consciousness does not occur; may be repeated at 60-sec intervals as needed up to four additional times (maximum total dose, 1 mg)	1-4 hr
Management of suspected benzodiazepine overdose	0.2 mg (2 ml) given IV over 30 sec; wait 30 sec, then give 0.3 mg (3 ml) over 30 sec if consciousness does not occur; further doses of 0.5 mg (5 ml) can be given over 30 sec at intervals of 1 min up to a cumulative dose of 3 mg.	1-4 hr

Important note: Flumazenil has a relatively short half-life and duration of effect of 1 to 4 hours; therfore, if using flumazenil to reverse the effects of a long-acting benzodiazepine, the dose of the reversal agent may wear off and the patient may become sedated again, requiring more flumazenil.

Table 10-8	Benzodiazepines: Drug Interactions	
DRUG	**MECHANISM**	**RESULT**
CNS depressants	Additive effects	Increased CNS depression
Cimetidine	Decreased benzodiazepine metabolism	Prolonged benzodiazepine action
Monoamine oxidase inhibitors	Decreased metabolism	Increased benzodiazepine effects

diazepines on the CNS by directly competing with benzodiazepines for binding at the benzodiazepine receptor in the CNS. However, it has a stronger affinity for the receptor and knocks the benzodiazepine off from the receptor, reversing the sedative action of the benzodiazepine. The dosage regimen to be followed for the reversal of conscious sedation or general anesthesia induced by benzodiazepines and the management of suspected benzodiazepine overdose is summarized in Table 10-7.

Interactions

The potential drug interactions with the benzodiazepines are significant in their intensity, particularly when they are taken in combination with other CNS depressants and monoamine oxidase inhibitors. The risks associated with the coadministration of other agents are listed and described in Table 10-8.

Laboratory Test Interactions

There are no laboratory test interactions that occur with the five benzodiazepines that are typically used as either sedatives or hypnotics.

Dosages

The benzodiazepines discussed in this chapter are those that are commonly used to treat insomnia. Therefore the dosage recommendations given in the dosages table on p. 129 are those for achieving hypnotic effects. All agents used for the treatment of insomnia should be limited to a short-term usage of less than 2 to 4 weeks. With long-term usage, rebound insomnia and severe withdrawal can develop. Geriatric patients should also be started on lower doses because they generally experience a more pronounced effect from benzodiazepines.

DRUG PROFILES

The benzodiazepines are all prescription-only drugs, and they are designated as C-IV controlled substances. All five benzodiazepines discussed here have active metabolites, which can accumulate during long-term use, especially in patients who have altered metabolic function (hepatic dysfunction) or altered excretion capabilities (renal dysfunction). There are several other benzodiazepines, but these are more commonly used

DOSAGES

BENZODIAZEPINES: SELECTED HYPNOTIC AGENTS

AGENT	ONSET AND DURATION	DOSAGE RANGE	PURPOSE
Estazolam (Prosom)	Short acting	*Adult* PO: 1-2 mg HS *Geriatric* PO: 0.5 mg or higher HS	
⚓Flurazepam (Dalmane)	Long acting	*Adult* PO: 15-30 mg HS *Geriatric* PO: 15 mg HS	
Quazepam (Doral)	Long acting	*Adult* PO: 7.5 or 15 mg HS *Geriatric* PO: Adult dose 1-2 days then reduce	Hypnotic
Temazepam (Restoril)	Short acting	*Adult* PO: 15-30 mg HS *Geriatric* PO: 7.5 mg or higher HS	
Triazolam (Halcion)	Short acting	*Adult* PO: 0.25-0.5 mg HS *Geriatric* PO: 0.125-0.25 mg HS	

to treat anxiety or agitation, to produce amnesia, and to relax skeletal muscles and are discussed in detail in the appropriate chapters. All benzodiazepines are rated pregnancy category X agents. They are all also contraindicated in patients who have shown a hypersensitivity reaction to them and in pregnant women.

ESTAZOLAM

Estazolam (Prosom) is available in 1- and 2-mg tablets. The usual adult dosage is 1 to 2 mg at bedtime; the geriatric dosage is usually 0.5 mg at bedtime (see the table above). Pregnancy category X.

♥ PHARMACOKINETICS

HALF-LIFE	ONSET	PEAK	DURATION
10-24 hr	20 min	2 hr	24 hr

⚓ FLURAZEPAM

Flurazepam (Dalmane) is available in 15- and 30-mg capsules. It is considered a long-acting hypnotic agent

and is indicated for the short-term treatment of insomnia for periods of up to 4 weeks. Flurazepam has two active metabolites that account for its hypnotic effects. These active metabolites have also been shown to be responsible for inducing a "hangover" effect, causing lethargy or grogginess the morning after the medication has been taken. The recommended dosages for adult and geriatric patients are given in the table above. Pregnancy category X.

♥ PHARMACOKINETICS

HALF-LIFE	ONSET	PEAK	DURATION
50-100 hr	15-45 min	30-60 min	7-8 hr

QUAZEPAM

Quazepam (Doral) is available in 7.5- and 15-mg tablets. Quazepam is considered a long-acting hypnotic agent and is indicated for the short-term treatment of insomnia for periods of up to 4 weeks. The recommended dosages for adult and geriatric patients are given in the table above. Pregnancy category X.

PHARMACOKINETICS

HALF-LIFE	ONSET	PEAK	DURATION
25-41 hr	30 min	2 hr	20 hr

TEMAZEPAM

Temazepam (Restoril) is available in 15- and 30-mg tablets. It is contraindicated in patients who have narrow-angle glaucoma because it can exacerbate the glaucoma. It is indicated for the short-term treatment of insomnia. The common dosages are given in the table on p. 129. Pregnancy category X.

PHARMACOKINETICS

HALF-LIFE	ONSET	PEAK	DURATION
9.5-12.4 hr	30-60 min	2-3 hr	7-8 hr

TRIAZOLAM

Triazolam (Halcion) is available in 0.125- and 0.25-mg tablets, and it is indicated for the short-term treatment of insomnia. The smallest effective dose given for the shortest time needed is generally the best approach to take. The common dosages for adult and geriatric patients are given in the table on p. 129. Pregnancy category X.

PHARMACOKINETICS

HALF-LIFE	ONSET	PEAK	DURATION
2-5 hr	15-30 min	0.5-1.5 hr	6-7 hr

MISCELLANEOUS

There are several other miscellaneous medications that do not fall into the barbiturate or benzodiazepine drug class. These agents include chloral hydrate, glutethimide, methyprylon, ethchlorvynol, and paraldehyde. These are all prescription-only drugs. Of these five sedative-hypnotic agents, chloral hydrate is the one most commonly prescribed because the other four are associated with severe side effects and are extremely toxic if taken inappropriately or in an overdose.

Chloral hydrate (Noctec) is one of the oldest nonbarbiturate sedative-hypnotic agents. It has the favorable characteristic of not suppressing REM sleep at the usual therapeutic doses, and the incidence of hangover effects associated with its use is low because of its relatively short duration of action. One potential disadvantage to its use is that tachyphylaxis can develop rather quickly. **Tachyphylaxis** is the rapid appearance of a progressive decrease in response to a pharmaco-

logically or physiologically active substance after its repetitive administration. This makes chloral hydrate only useful for short-term therapy. High doses lead to dependence and cause gastrointestinal tract irritation. The combination of alcohol and chloral hydrate leads to rapid loss of consciousness. This combination is commonly referred to as a Mickey Finn.

Nonprescription sleeping aids often contain antihistamines, and some may also contain analgesics such as aspirin or acetaminophen. The most common antihistamines contained in over-the-counter sleeping aids are doxylamine, diphenhydramine, and pyrilamine. Besides having antihistaminic effects, these agents are heavily sedating. They have a depressant effect on the CNS. The analgesics are sometimes added to offer some pain relief, if that is a component of the sleep disturbance or insomnia. As with other CNS depressants such as barbiturates and benzodiazepines, patients should avoid the consumption of alcohol when taking them. The combination can result in respiratory depression and death.

NURSING PROCESS

ASSESSMENT

Before administering any hypnotic or sedative agent, be it a barbiturate or benzodiazepine, you need to determine whether the patient has or has had any of the following conditions or disorders: allergies, CNS disorders, sleep disorders (and the previous treatments for these), diabetes, addictive disorders, personality disorders, or thyroid conditions. You also need to find out whether the patient consumes alcohol, takes any other CNS depressants or other prescribed and over-the-counter medications, what his or her renal and liver function status is, the patient's age (because of the increased effects of these agents in elderly persons and small children), the nature of the patient's sleep patterns, the patient's stress level, and his or her respiratory and cardiac status. The drug interactions for both barbiturates and benzodiazepines are discussed earlier in this chapter and summarized in Tables 10-4 and 10-8, respectively. It is a known fact that sedative-hypnotic agents and other drugs affecting the CNS, such as anticonvulsants, neuroleptics, and analgesics, have a 90% chance of causing adverse drug reactions.

In addition, it is important to assess the patient's

Sedative-Hypnotic Agents: Points of Interest

AGENT	POINT
Aprobarbital	Intermediate acting; onset in about 20 minutes; with oral dosing give with meals to decrease nausea and vomiting.
Butabarbital	Effects last about 6-8 hours; cautious use in the elderly; keep tablets in an airtight container.
Pentobarbital	Short acting; can be given PO, by rectal suppository, or IM; IM injection given deep in large muscle mass; as with any of these agents, patients should avoid caffeine intake 4 hours around the time of dosing because of the decreased effectiveness that results.
Secobarbital	Same as for pentobarbital; also given IM, PO, and as suppository; as with any sedative-hypnotic agent, do not mix with alcohol.
Phenobarbital	Long acting (up to a 16 hours' duration); so is in the body longer and thus can react with other medications such as alcohol and other CNS depressants; because of long duration, use cautiously in the elderly patient who has decreased liver and renal function.
Estazolam	Take with food to minimize gastrointestinal upset; *always* make sure patients have swallowed medication.
⚓Flurazepam	Causes less REM rebound versus that caused by the other benzodiazepines; cautious use and smaller doses in the elderly patient; give 15-30 minutes before bedtime.
Quazepam	Give 15 to 30 minutes before bedtime; hangover common in elderly patients.
Temazepam	Induces sleep within 20-40 minutes; give 20-30 minutes before bedtime.
Triazolam	Short-term use only; try other medications in this category, as ordered by a physician; cautious use with elderly and causes confusion, so protect from injury.

vital signs, including the supine and erect blood pressures, especially if the intravenous use of any of these agents is planned. For instance, if diazepam is to be administered, hold the drug if the systolic blood pressure drops 20 mm Hg or more or if the pulse or respiratory rate declines. Also survey the laboratory data, such as the complete blood count and the results of hepatic studies (lactate dehydrogenase, creatine kinase, and bilirubin) and renal studies (blood urea nitrogen and creatinine).

NURSING DIAGNOSES

Nursing diagnoses appropriate to the patient taking sedative-hypnotic agents include:
- Risk for injury or falls related to decreased sensorium.
- Sleep pattern disturbance related to the drug's interference with REM sleep.
- Risk for injury, drug overdose, or adverse reactions related to the combined use of the agent with alcohol or other medications such as tranquilizers and analgesics.
- Risk for injury or addiction related to physical or psychologic dependency.
- Impaired gas exchange related to possible respiratory depression.

- Knowledge deficit related to inadequate information about the drug and non-drug treatment regimen for the sleeping disturbance.

PLANNING

Goals related to the administration of sedative-hypnotic agents are as follows:
- Patient remains free of self injury and falls related to decreased sensorium
- Patient remains free of further sleep deprivation
- Patient experiences little or no rebound insomnia
- Patient remains free of or experiences minimal side effects and toxic effects from sedative-hypnotic agents
- Patient remains free of drug interaction effects
- Patient experiences no problems with addiction
- Patient remains free of respiratory depression
- Patient complies with drug therapy as ordered
- Patient keeps follow-up visits as ordered by the physician.

Outcome Criteria

Outcome criteria related to the administration of sedative-hypnotic agents are as follows:

- Patient states ways to minimize self injury and falls related to decreased sensorium such as changing positions slowly
- Patient will state pharmacologic and nonpharmacologic (relaxation therapy, massage) measures to enhance sleep patterns
- Patient will state risk for REM interference from sedative-hypnotic agents with associated sleep

hangovers and use nonpharmacologic measures as appropriate
- Patient will state the common side effects, toxic effects, and the symptoms to be reported to the physician related to sedative-hypnotic agents such as drowsiness, confusion, and respiratory depression
- Patient minimizes side effects and toxic effects by taking medications as prescribed

Patient Teaching TIPS

Benzodiazepines and Barbiturates

✔ Take medication only as prescribed. If one dose does not work, you should *not* take a double dose. Follow the physician's orders in regard to the dosing of the medication.

✔ Keep a journal of your sleep habits and response to both drug and nondrug therapy.

✔ Avoid driving or operating heavy machinery or equipment and avoid activities requiring mental alertness while on this medication.

✔ Avoid any other type of CNS-altering medications, especially CNS depressants such as tranquilizers, narcotics, and alcohol.

✔ Always try measures other than medications to help you sleep because of the REM rebound they cause, which results in your feeling more tired and not rested or in "hangover" effects the morning after. This hangover effect is more common in elderly patients and is less common with barbiturates.

✔ Keep all medications away from children.

✔ Because of the different characteristics of the benzodiazepines, such as flurazepam, it may take a night or two before you notice an improvement in your sleep patterns.

✔ Always check with your physician first or with the pharmacist before taking any over-the-counter medications because of the many drug interactions associated with sedative-hypnotic agents.

✔ It often takes 2 to 3 weeks for the therapeutic effects (improved sleep) of the oral forms of barbiturates to occur.

✔ Never stop taking these medications abruptly, especially the barbiturates, because of their highly addicting potential and because of the rebound insomnia you may experience.

✔ These agents should not be used every night or for more than a few days at a time (if possible) because of their potential to cause side effects, their interference with REM sleep, and their addicting properties.

TAKE HOME POINTS

Sedatives
- Reduce nervousness, excitability, or irritability by producing a calming effect without causing sleep.
- Can become hypnotic if given in large enough doses—major difference between sedatives and hypnotics.
- Inhibit transmission of nerve impulses to the CNS.

Hypnotics
- Calm or soothe the CNS to the point of sleep.
- More potent effect on inhibition of the CNS than sedatives have.
- Induce sleep.

Benzodiazepines
- Family of drugs that reduce nervousness, excitability, or irritability of CNS.
- Commonly prescribed as sedative-hypnotics and anxiolytics.

Anxiolytics
- Drugs that relieve anxiety (increased nerve stimulation to the brain).
- Calm the CNS.

Sleep Architecture
- Stages in sleep cycle.
- Composed of non–REM and REM sleep.
- Non–REM = 4 stages; REM = vivid dreams occur here.
- The phases of sleep are affected by sedative-hypnotic agents.

Nonpharmacologic Approaches to Inducing Sleep
- Establish set sleep patterns.
- Avoid exercise before bedtime.
- Avoid heavy meals late in the evening.
- Drink warm decaffeinated drinks such as warm milk before bedtime.

■ Patient will state the common drug interactions with alcohol and other medications, such as tranquilizers and analgesics, that may be life-threatening

■ Patient states importance of measures to minimize problems with addiction such as taking medication only as needed

■ Patient, family, or significant other will state need to contact physician about possible complications, such as respiratory depression

■ Patient demonstrates increased knowledge related to inadequate information about treatment, drug and nondrug, and regimen for sleeping disturbance.

IMPLEMENTATION

Benzodiazepines generally have an onset of action of about 30 to 60 minutes (see the pharmacokinetics boxes for respective agents) and must therefore be given 15 to 30 minutes before bedtime so as to maximize their effectiveness in inducing sleep. Most benzodiazepines, with the exception of flurazepam, interfere with REM sleep and produce REM rebound, and all of these agents should be given cautiously in elderly patients. Nondrug therapy such as relaxation, music, and back massage should be encouraged when possible.

Barbiturates differ in their onset of action, duration, and potency. Short-acting barbiturates (secobarbital) should be given 15 to 30 minutes before bedtime, as should some of the intermediate-acting agents (butabarbital). The longer-acting agents such as phenobarbital have an onset of action of 60 minutes. When administering any of these agents by intramuscular injection, the injection should be given deep into a large muscle mass to prevent tissue sloughing.

Regardless of the agent given, for the safety of the patient and the prevention of injury stemming from decreased sensorium, it is crucial to keep the side rails up, to not allow smoking, to assist the patient with ambulation (especially the elderly), and to have the call light at the patient's bedside. Documentation of the dose, route, and time of administration along with the safety measures taken is also important. The patient teaching tips are listed on p. 132.

EVALUATION

Some of the criteria by which to determine a patient's therapeutic response to a sedative-hypnotic agent are on increased ability to sleep at night, fewer awakenings, shorter sleep induction time, few side effects such as hangover effects, and improved sense of well-being because of improved sleep. You must constantly watch for and document the occurrence of any of the side effects of benzodiazepines or barbiturates. The side effects of benzodiazepines include lethargy, confusion, drowsiness, dizziness, lightheadedness, headache, a hangover effect, sedation during the day, nausea, and vomiting. The side effects of barbiturates include paradoxical excitement in children and the elderly, lethargy, confusion, headache, drowsiness, a hangover effect, rash, nausea, vomiting, the Stevens-Johnson syndrome (with agents like phenobarbital), and respiratory depression.

Critical Thinking A C T I V I T Y

1. Mrs. S.L. is a 65-year-old woman who underwent total hip replacement 6 days earlier. She is suffering from a lack of sleep and has tried all the nondrug therapy techniques. The physician has now ordered chloral hydrate, 250 mg at bedtime prn, for sleep.

   ### Questions

   a. What are some of the home health care tips pertinent to the administration of sedative-hypnotic agents in an aged patient?

   b. Why would chloral hydrate be preferred in this patient over the other classes of sedative-hypnotic agents?

2. What instructions should be given to a 31-year-old registered nurse who was found unresponsive after drinking beer all day at a rock concert and who has a 6-year history of grand mal seizures, but these have been adequately controlled with phenytoin and diazepam?

BIBLIOGRAPHY

Albanese J, Nutz P: *Mosby's 1995 nursing drug cards*, St Louis, 1995, Mosby.

Glod CA: Xanax: pros and cons, *J Psychosoc Nurs Ment Health Serv* 30(6):36, 1992.

Johnson KB: *Harriet Lane handbook*, ed 13, St Louis, 1993, Mosby.

Keen JH: *Critical care and emergency drug reference*, St Louis, 1994, Mosby.

Knoben JE, Anderson PO: *Handbook of critical drug data*, ed 6, Hamilton, Ill, 1988, Drug Intelligence Publications.

Lammon CA, Adams AH: Recognizing benzodiazepine overdose, *Nursing* 23(1):33, 1993.

McEvoy GK: *AHFS drug information*, Bethesda, Md, 1989, American Society of Hospital Pharmacists.

News capsules: P&T update: new approvals and dosage forms, *Hosp Formul* 28:207, 1993.

O'Donnell J: Understanding adverse drug reactions, *Nursing 92* 22(8):34, 1992.

Sherman D: Evaluation and treatment of sleep disorders, *Contemp Long-term Care* 14:70, 1991.

Skidmore-Roth L: *Mosby's 1995 nursing drug reference*, St Louis, 1995, Mosby.

Sweetwyne K: Neonatal sedation and analgesia, *Neonat Pharmacol Q* 2:5, 1993.

Tatro DS: Keeping up: drug treatment of panic disorder, *Drug Newslett* 12:85, 1993.

Chapter 11

Antiepileptic Agents

Objectives

When you reach the end of this chapter, you will be able to:

1 Discuss the rationale for the use of the various agents in the treatment of the various forms of epilepsy.

2 List the anticonvulsant agents according to their classification and the drug of choice.

3 Identify the mechanism of action, contraindications, dosages, routes of administration, side effects, and toxic effects associated with the various anticonvulsants.

4 Discuss the importance of patient education and compliance in the control of seizure activity.

5 Develop a comprehensive nursing care plan showing the application of the nursing process as it relates to the nursing care of patients receiving anticonvulsants.

CHAPTER OUTLINE

Epilepsy
Anticonvulsants
  Mechanism of action
  Drug effects
  Therapeutic uses
  Side effects and adverse effects
  Interactions
  Dosages
Drug Profiles
Benzodiazepines
  Clonazepam
  Clorazepate Dipotassium
Other Agents
  Carbamazepine
  ⚓ Ethosuximide
  Phenobarbital
  ⚓ Phenytoin
  Valproic Acid

Nursing Process
Assessment
Nursing Diagnoses
Planning
  Outcome criteria
Implementation
Evaluation

Glossary

Anticonvulsant (an tĭ kən vul′ sənt) A substance or procedure that prevents or reduces the severity of epileptic or other convulsive seizures. (p. 136)

Autoinduction (aw to in dək′ shən) A metabolic process that occurs when a drug increases its own metabolism over time, leading to lower-than-expected drug concentrations. (p. 143)

Convulsion (kən vul′ shən) A type of seizure involving (excessive stimulation of neurons in the brain and characterized by the spasmodic contraction of involuntary muscles. See also seizure. (p. 136)

Epilepsy (ep ĭ lep′ sē) A group of neurologic disorders characterized by recurrent episodes of convulsive seizures, sensory disturbances, abnormal behavior, or loss of consciousness, or any combination of these. (p. 136)

International Classification of Seizures The most extensively used system of classifying seizures. Both the symptoms and characteristics of the various types of seizures are described. (p. 136)

Primary or **idiopathic epilepsy** (id ē o path′ ik) Epilepsy that develops without an apparent cause. More than 50% of cases of epilepsy are of unknown origin. (p. 136)

Secondary epilepsy Epilepsy that has a distinct cause (e.g., trauma). (p. 136)

Seizure (se′ zhər) Excessive stimulation of neurons in the brain leading to a sudden burst of abnormal neuron activity that results in temporary changes in brain function. (p. 136)

Status epilepticus (sta′ təs ep i lep′ tĭ kəs) A medical emergency in which there are continual generalized tonic-clonic convulsions that occur without interruption. (p. 138)

EPILEPSY

A seizure disorder, or what is more commonly referred to as **epilepsy,** is not a specific disease like cancer or diabetes. It is a disorder of the brain that is a symptom of a disease. Most likely it involves the generation of excessive electrical discharges from nerves located in the area of the brain known as the *cerebral cortex.*

The terms *convulsion, seizure,* and *epilepsy* are often used interchangeably, but they do not have the same meaning. A **seizure** is a brief episode of abnormal electrical activity in the nerve cells of the brain. A **convulsion** is characterized by spasmodic contractions of involuntary muscles. Epilepsy is a chronic, recurrent pattern of seizures. These excessive electrical discharges can often be detected by an electroencephalogram (EEG), which is frequently obtained to help diagnose epilepsy. Other diagnostic aids that are helpful in the diagnosis of epilepsy are computed tomography (CT) and magnetic resonance imaging (MRI). The information yielded by these diagnostic aids in conjunction with the common symptoms of the particular seizure disorder help establish the diagnosis. Commonly reported symptoms are abnormal motor function, loss of consciousness, altered sensory awareness, and psychic changes.

The cause of most cases of epilepsy is unknown, and this is true for more than 50% of the cases of epilepsy. That type of epilepsy for which a cause cannot be identified is called **primary** or **idiopathic epilepsy.** Other types of epilepsy have a distinct cause such as trauma, infection, a cerebrovascular disorder, or other illnesses. These types of epilepsy are termed **secondary epilepsy.** The chief causes of secondary epilepsy in children and infants are developmental defects, metabolic disease, or injury at birth. Acquired brain disorders account for the major causes of secondary epilepsy in adults. Some examples are head injury, disease or infection of the brain and spinal cord, a cerebrovascular accident (or stroke), a metabolic disorder, a primary or metastatic brain tumor, or some other recognizable neurologic disease.

The accurate diagnosis of a seizure disorder requires careful patient observation, a reliable patient history, and an EEG. Other diagnostic tests that are often used are CT and MRI, which are superior to the clinical examination, EEG, and routine skull radiographs in revealing structural lesions of the CNS as the cause of the seizure disorder. Of the two (MRI versus CT), MRI is more sensitive than CT and is now preferred in the evaluation of a patient with seizures.

Seizures can be classified into distinct categories based on their characteristics. In traditional classifications, seizures were categorized as grand mal seizures, petit mal seizures, jacksonian epilepsy, and psychomotor attacks. In a newer classification system a more systematic approach is used, which breaks down seizures into two main types: partial seizures and generalized seizures. This system of classification is called the **International Classification of Seizures**. It is the more extensively used one because it more adequately describes the symptoms and characteristics of the various types of seizures. The various types of partial and generalized seizures are listed in the box on the next page.

ANTICONVULSANTS

Anticonvulsants are medications that are used to prevent the seizures typically associated with epilepsy. Anticonvulsant drugs are very commonly referred to as *antiepileptic drugs* (AEDs). This is probably a more appropriate term because many of these medications are indicated for the management of all types of epilepsy, not just convulsions.

The combined goal of AED therapy is to control or prevent seizures while maintaining a reasonable quality of life. Many AEDs have side effects, and balancing seizure control with side effects is often a difficult task. In most cases the therapeutic goal is not to eliminate seizure activity but rather to maximally reduce the incidence of seizures while minimizing drug-induced toxicity. Many patients must take AEDs for their entire life. Treatment may eventually be stopped in some, but others will suffer repeated seizures if constant levels of AEDs are not maintained in their blood. In both children and adults there is only a 40% chance of recurrence after the first partial or generalized seizure; therefore many physicians choose not to initiate treatment after the first seizure. However, it is the consensus that AED therapy should be implemented in patients who have had two or more seizures.

There are several AEDs available. Often only a combination of agents can control the disorder, but most seizure disorders can be controlled. Generally single-drug therapy must fail before two-drug and then multiple-drug therapy is implemented. A patient should always be started on a single AED and the dosage slowly increased until the seizures are controlled or until clinical toxicity occurs. If the first AED does not work, the drug should be tapered slowly while a second AED is introduced. AEDs should never be stopped abruptly unless a severe adverse effect occurs. It is sometimes difficult to control a patient's seizures using a single AED, but monotherapy is likely to result in higher serum drug concentrations, fewer adverse effects, and better control.

Serum drug concentrations are useful guides in assessing the effectiveness of therapy. They should, however, be only guidelines. The goal should be to slowly titrate to the lowest effective serum drug level that controls the seizure disorder. This decreases the risk of

International Classification of Seizures

Partial Seizures

Description
Short alterations in consciousness, repetitive unusual movements (chewing or swallowing movements), psychologic changes, and confusion.

Simple seizures
- No impaired consciousness
- Motor symptoms (most commonly face, arm, or leg)
- Hallucinations of sight, hearing, or taste along with somatosensory changes (tingling)
- Autonomic nervous system responses
- Personality changes

Complex seizures
- Impaired consciousness
- Memory impairment
- Behavioral effects
- Purposeless behaviors
- Aura, chewing and swallowing movements, unreal feelings, bizarre behavior
- Tonic, clonic, or tonic-clonic seizures

Generalized Seizures

Description
Most often seen in children and commonly characterized by temporary lapses in consciousness lasting a few seconds. Staring off into space, daydreaming, and inattentive look are common symptoms. Patients may exhibit rhythmic movements of their eyes, head, or hands but do not convulse. May have several attacks per day.

- Both cerebral hemispheres involved
- Tonic, clonic, myoclonic, or tonic-clonic seizures possible
- Brief loss of consciousness for a few seconds with no confusion
- Head drop or falling-down symptoms

medication-induced adverse effects and interactions. The serum concentrations of phenytoin, phenobarbital, carbamazepine, and primidone correlate better with seizure control and toxicity than do those of valproic acid, ethosuximide, and clonazepam. Emphasis should be placed primarily on the clinical symptoms and patient's history rather than on strict adherence to established drug concentration ranges.

There are six traditional classes of AEDs, and many new agents have been marketed recently. These newer agents were developed with the goal of eliminating many of the drug interactions and side effects associated with the older agents. Successful control of a seizure disorder hinges on selecting the appropriate drug class and drug dosage, the patient complying with the treatment regimen, and limiting toxicity. Maintaining serum drug levels within therapeutic ranges helps not only to control seizures but also to reduce side effects. There are established normal therapeutic ranges for many AEDs, but these are useful only as guidelines. Each patient should be monitored individually and the dosages adjusted based on the individual case. Many patients are maintained successfully below or above the usual therapeutic range.

The underlying cause of most cases of epilepsy is an excessive electrical discharge from nerves within the CNS. The object of AED therapy is to prevent the generation and spread of these excessive discharges while simultaneously protecting surrounding normal cells.

Mechanism of Action

Like many classes of drugs, the exact mechanism of action of the AEDs is not known. The AEDs may act in a couple of ways to control epilepsy. Some researchers believe they act directly on abnormal neurons, decreasing their excitability and responsiveness to abnormal stimuli. Seizure activity may also be reduced by raising the seizure threshold, which is the amount of stimulation needed to stimulate a nerve and cause a response. Others believe that AEDs prevent the spread of abnormal impulses to normal neurons near the area of damaged or abnormal nerves. This may help to limit the seizure activity to a small portion of the brain by confining excessive electrical activity. There is strong evidence, however, showing that they alter the movement of sodium, potassium, calcium, and magnesium ions. The normal conduction of nerve impulses relies heavily on the movement of ions like sodium, potassium, calcium, and magnesium. The changes in the movement of these ions induced by AEDs result in stabilized and less responsive cell membranes. This ion theory may explain how AEDs decrease excitability and responsiveness.

Drug Effects

AEDs stabilize nerve cells and keep them from becoming hyperexcited by preventing hyperactive neuron discharges from being generated in areas of the brain that are dysfunctional. They also prevent the spread of these abnormal impulses to neurons located near the abnormal neurons. The primary pharmacologic effects of AEDs are threefold. First, they increase the threshold of activity in the area of the brain called the *motor cortex*. In other words, they make it more difficult for a nerve to be excited or they reduce the nerve's response to incoming electrical or chemical stimulation. Second, they act to depress or limit the spread of a seizure discharge from its origin. They do this by suppressing the transmission of impulses from one nerve to the next. Third, they can decrease nerve conduction. AEDs may also have effects outside the neuron, indirectly affecting the area in the brain re-

sponsible for the problem by altering, for instance, the blood supply to that area.

Therapeutic Uses

The major therapeutic indication for AEDs is the prevention or control of seizure activity. They are especially useful for maintenance therapy in patients with the chronic recurring type of seizures that are commonly associated with epilepsy. As evidenced by the wide range of seizure disorders listed in the box on the previous page, epilepsy is a very diverse disorder. As a result, no one drug can control all types of epilepsy. Although our understanding of epilepsy is still growing, we have a good idea of the primary causes of many of the various seizure disorders. Each involves a distinct area of dysfunction and has certain characteristics that make certain drugs more effective than others in treating it. Therefore particular drugs are indicated for the control of specific seizures. Some of the AEDs and the seizure disorders they are used to treat are listed in Table 11-1.

AEDs are chiefly used for the long-term maintenance treatment of epilepsy. However, AEDs are also useful for the acute treatment of convulsions and status epilepticus. **Status epilepticus** is a common seizure disorder that is a life-threatening emergency; it is characterized by generalized tonic-clonic convulsions that occur in succession. Affected patients typically do not regain consciousness between the many convulsions. Hypotension, hypoxia, and cardiac dysrhythmias complicate the disorder, and brain damage and death quickly ensue if prompt, appropriate therapy is not started. This typically is done with diazepam (Valium). There are, however, other agents that are also useful

Table 11-1	Antiepileptic Drugs of Choice						
PARTIAL SEIZURES		GENERALIZED SEIZURES					
SIMPLE	COMPLEX	GTC	ABSENCE	MYOCLONIC	CLONIC	TONIC	ATONIC
First choice							
CBZ	CBZ	CBZ	ESX	VPA	VPA	VPA	VPA
PHB	PHB	PHB	PHB				
PHT	PHT	PHT	VPA				
PMD	PMD	PMD					
VPA	VPA	VPA					
Second choice							
CNZ	CNZ	CZM	AZM	CNZ	CNZ	CBZ	CNZ
CRZ	CRZ	CZP	CNZ			CNZ	
						PHT	

AZM, acetazolamide; *CBZ,* carbamazepine; *CNZ,* clonazepam; *CRZ,* clorazepate; *ESX,* ethosuximide; *GTC,* generalized tonic-clonic; *PHB,* phenobarbital; *PHT,* phenytoin; *PMD,* primidone; *VPA,* valproic acid.

for the treatment of status epilepticus. The agents most commonly used are listed in Table 11-2.

Once status epilepticus is controlled, long-term drug therapy is begun with other agents for prevention. Patients who undergo brain surgery or who have suffered severe head injuries may receive prophylactic AED therapy. These patients are at high risk for acquiring a seizure disorder, and frequently severe complications will arise if seizures are not controlled.

Side Effects and Adverse Effects

AEDs are plagued by many side effects, which often limit their usefulness. Agents must be withdrawn from many patients because of some of these effects. Each AED is associated with its own diverse set of side effects, which makes it difficult to categorize all the classes of AEDs according to their common side effects. The various AEDs and their most common side effects are listed in Table 11-3.

Table 11-2	**Antiepileptic Drugs Used for Treatment of Status Epilepticus**			
PROPERTY	**DIAZEPAM**	**LORAZEPAM***	**⚓PHENYTOIN**	**PHENOBARBITAL**
Dose (mg/kg)	0.3-0.5 (<20 mg)	0.05-0.1	15-25	15-20
Onset (min)	3-10	1-20	5-30	10-30
Duration	Minutes	Hours	12-24 hr	Days
Half-life (hr)	35	15	10-60	96
Adverse effects	Hypotension, apnea, somnolence	Hypotension, apnea, somnolence	Cardiac arrhythmias, hypotension	Hypotension, apnea, somnolence

*Nonlabeled use.

Table 11-3	**Antiepileptic Drug Side Effects**	
DRUG OR DRUG CLASS	**SIDE EFFECTS**	
Barbiturates	CNS:	Drowsiness, dizziness, lethargy, paradoxical restlessness, excitement
	GI:	Nausea, vomiting
	Other:	Rash, Stevens-Johnson syndrome, urticaria
Carbamazepine	Blood:	Bone marrow suppression (aplastic anemia, agranulocytosis, thrombocytopenia)
	Skin:	Exfoliative dermatitis, erythema multiforme, Stevens-Johnson syndrome
	Heart:	Arrhythmias, congestive heart failure
	Other:	Thrombophlebitis, vision and hearing disturbances, acute urinary retention, dyspnea, pneumonitis, pneumonia
Divalproex (valproic acid)	Other:	Pancreatitis, irregular menses, secondary amenorrhea, galactorrhea, rare breast enlargement
	Blood:	Thrombocytopenia
Felbamate	GI:	Anorexia, nausea, vomiting
	Other:	Headache, intramenstrual bleeding, respiratory and urinary tract infections
	Pediatric:	Fever, purpura, nervousness, somnolence
Hydantoins	Heart:	Arrhythmias
	Skin:	Exfoliative dermatitis, lupus erythematosus, Stevens-Johnson syndrome
	Blood:	Bone marrow suppression (agranulocytosis, thrombocytopenia, megaloblastic anemia)
	Other:	Neuropathies, gingival hyperplasia
Oxazolidinediones	Blood:	Bone marrow suppression (thrombocytopenia, agranulocytosis, aplastic anemia)
	CNS:	Visual disturbances, drowsiness
	Skin:	Lupus erythematosus, malignant lymphoma syndrome
	Other:	Myasthenia gravis, nephrosis, gingival and vaginal bleeding
Succinimides	Blood:	Agranulocytosis, aplastic anemia, leukopenia, vaginal bleeding
	Skin:	Stevens-Johnson syndrome, lupus erythematosus
	Other:	Drowsiness, headache, swollen tongue, gingival hyperplasia

CNS, central nervous system; *GI*, gastrointestinal.

Table 11-4	Antiepileptic Agents: Drug Interactions	
DRUG	**MECHANISM**	**RESULTS**
Carbamazepine		
Bone marrow depressants	Additive effect	Increased bone marrow toxicity
Doxycycline, phenytoin, theophylline, warfarin	Alters metabolism	Significant decrease in their half-lives
Divalproex (valproic acid)		
Barbiturates	Additive effect	Increased CNS depression
Clonazepam	Not determined	May produce absence status
↓Phenytoin	Not determined	May produce breakthrough seizures
Felbatol		
Carbamazepine	Alters clearance	Decreased Felbatol levels
↓Phenytoin	Inhibits hepatic enzymes	Increased phenytoin levels
Hydantoins		
Disulfiram, isoniazid, valproic acid	Inhibits hepatic enzymes	Increased hydantoin levels
Tricyclic antidepressants	Not determined	Possible seizures
Oxazolidinediones		
Bone marrow depressants	Additive effect	Increased bone marrow toxicity
Phenacemide		
Ethotoin	Not determined	Paranoid symptoms
Succinimides		
Bone marrow depressants	Additive effects	Increased bone marrow toxicity

Interactions

The drug interactions that can occur with the AEDs are many and varied, and these are summarized in Table 11-4. Significant drug interactions for selected agents are listed in Table 11-4.

Dosages

For an overview of dosages, see the table on p. 141.

DRUG PROFILES

The AEDs are prescription-only drugs. These drugs are associated with many characteristics that make it undesirable for patients to be taking them without the supervision of a qualified medical specialist. They are available in many oral, injectable, and rectal formulations. The FDA's pregnancy risk classification of the AEDs is summarized in Table 11-5.

In most children and adults, epilepsy can be controlled with a first-line AED such as carbamazepine,

Table 11-5	Anticonvulsants: FDA Pregnancy Risk Classification
PREGNANCY CLASS	**ANTICONVULSANT**
C	Carbamazepine
D	Barbiturates, paramethadione, valproic acid, Divalproex
Unclassified	Hydantoin, succinimides, trimethadione, primidone, acetazolamide, diazepam, clonazepam, clorazepate

ethosuximide, phenobarbital, primidone, phenytoin, or valproic acid. For patients who do not respond to the first-line AEDs, there are a number of second-line AEDs that are used occasionally, agents such as clonazepam, clorazepate, methsuximide, and acetazolamide. These are considered second-line agents because their efficacy or adverse effect profiles are not as favorable as those of the first-line agents.

Until the 1990s no major new drugs for the treatment of epilepsy had been introduced in the United States since 1978, when valproic acid was introduced. In recent years, at least 22 investigational AEDs have undergone clinical testing. A few of these have already

DOSAGES

SELECTED ANTICONVULSANT AGENTS

AGENT	PHARMACOLOGIC CLASS	DOSAGE RANGE	PURPOSE
Clonazepam (Klonopin)	Benzodiazepine	*Pediatric* PO: ≤10 y/o or 30 kg, 0.1-0.2 mg/kg/ day *Adult* PO: 4-20 mg/day	Lennox-Gastaut; absence, akinetic, and myoclonic seizures
Clorazepate dipotassium	Benzodiazepine	*Pediatric* PO: 9-12 y/o, 15-60 mg/day *Adult/children* PO: >12 y/o, 22-90 mg/day	Partial seizures
Carbamazepine (Tegretol)	Miscellaneous	*Pediatric* PO: 6-12 y/o, 200-800 mg/day *Adult/Pediatric* PO: >12 y/o, 200-1200 mg/day	Partial seizures with complex symptoms; tonic-clonic, mixed seizures; trigeminal-glossopharyngeal neuralgia
⚓Ethosuximide (Zarontin)	Succinimide	*Pediatric* PO: 3-6 y/o, 250 mg/day then adjust; >6 y/o, 500 mg/day then adjust *Adult* PO: 500 mg/day then adjust	Absence seizures
Phenobarbital (Solfoton)	Barbiturate	*Pediatric* PO: 3-5 mg/kg or 125 mg/m^2/day IM/IV: 100-400 mg *Adult* PO: 100-300 mg/day IM/IV: 200-600 mg *Adult/Pediatric* PO: 3-4 mg/kg/day	Partial, tonic-clonic seizures Convulsions Partial, tonic-clonic seizures Convulsions Prophylaxis for febrile convulsions
Primidone (Mysoline)	Barbiturate	*Pediatric* PO: <8 y/o, 125-250 mg tid *Adult/Pediatric* PO: >8 y/o, 250 mg 4-6 times/day	Partial seizures Tonic-clonic seizures
⚓Phenytoin (Dilantin)	Hydantoin	*Pediatric* PO: 4-8 mg/kg/day IV: 15-20 mg/kg *Adult* PO: 300-600 mg/day IV: 10-15 mg/kg	Tonic-clonic, psychomotor seizures Convulsions Tonic-clonic, psychomotor seizures Convulsions
Valproic acid (Depakene, Depakote)	Miscellaneous	*Adult/Pediatric* PO: 15-60 mg/kg/day	Multiple seizures

been recommended for approval by an FDA advisory subcommittee, and others have recently been approved and are being marketed. These new drugs have shown better efficacy and toxicity profiles than the older agents. Of these newer agents, four have shown great promise: felbamate, gabapentin, lamotrigine, and vigabatrin. Two of these have received FDA approval. However, there have been many reports of aplastic anemia and acute liver failure associated with felbamate use, and it is likely to be removed from the market. Gabapentin (Neurontin) has also been approved by the FDA and is faring well. Lamotrigine and vigabatrin are in investigational studies but should be marketed soon.

New formulations of already available AEDs are soon to be marketed. Fosphenytoin is a water-soluble, phosphorylated phenytoin derivative that can be given intramuscularly or intravenously without causing the pain associated with the present product. An intravenous formulation of valproate is also being developed and is soon to be released. A new controlled-release system, called the *osmotically released oral system* (OROS), is now available for another effective first-line AED carbamazepine. This system offers the combined advantage of providing long-duration, steady carbamazepine serum levels and ensuring increased patient compliance.

BENZODIAZEPINES

The benzodiazepines are used as first-line agents in the treatment of status epilepticus and generally as second-line agents for the treatment of epilepsy. The prototypical benzodiazepine for the treatment of status epilepticus is diazepam (Valium), although lorazepam (Ativan) has also been used for this purpose. (See Table 11-2 for a list of all the agents that are commonly used in the treatment of status epilepticus and their important pharmacodynamic and pharmacokinetic properties.) Diazepam remains the drug of choice for the treatment of status epilepticus because of its quick onset. Lorazepam has a longer biologic half-life, approximately 15 hours, and therefore has a longer duration of action. It is less lipophilic and undergoes less extensive distribution than diazepam; consequently it remains in the CNS longer and has a longer duration of action.

CLONAZEPAM

The two benzodiazepines that are primarily used as second-line AEDs are clonazepam and clorazepate (see next section). Clonazepam (Klonopin) is the most widely used oral AED of the benzodiazepine family in the United States. It is used to treat a variety of seizure disorders. Its greatest value is in the treatment of generalized seizures, but it is also effective in reducing the frequency of absence, generalized tonic-clonic, and myoclonic seizures. A major factor limiting its use is the high frequency of toxicity associated with its use. The three most common adverse effects are drowsiness, ataxia, and behavioral and personality changes. The behavioral disturbances can be marked and include hyperactivity, irritability, moodiness, and aggressive behavior. Many of these can be reduced or prevented by using the lowest effective dose. A tolerence to the drug develops in approximately one third of the patients who initially respond to clonazepam, and their seizures recur, usually within 1 to 6 months of starting therapy. Some of these patients respond to an increased dose, but others no longer respond to clonazepam at any dose. It is classified as a pregnancy category C drug. Clonazepam comes in 0.5-, 1-, and 2-mg tablets. There is no oral liquid preparation. It is a prescription-only drug. Recommended dosages are given in the table on p. 141.

PHARMACOKINETICS

HALF-LIFE	ONSET	PEAK	DURATION
20-46 hr	20-60 min	1-4 hr	6-12 hr

CLORAZEPATE DIPOTASSIUM

Clorazepate dipotassium (Tranxene) is a long-acting benzodiazepine anxiolytic used primarily as an add-on drug for patients whose seizures continue despite maximum efforts at treating with a single agent. Clorazepate is a pro-drug that is converted to the active drug *N*-desmethyldiazepam in the liver. It has been shown to be more effective in the treatment of generalized seizures than in the treatment of other types of seizures. Clorazepate is classified as a pregnancy category D agent. It comes in 3.75-, 7.5-, and 15-mg tablets and in 11.25- and 22.5-mg extended-release tablets. It is a prescription-only drug. Recommended dosages are given in the table on p. 141.

PHARMACOKINETICS

HALF-LIFE	ONSET	PEAK	DURATION
55-100 hr	15 min	1-2 hr	4-6 hr

OTHER AGENTS
CARBAMAZEPINE

Carbamazepine (Tegretol) is the second most frequently prescribed AED in the United States, after phenytoin. It was marketed in the late 1960s for the treatment of epilepsy in adults after its efficacy and safety for the treatment of trigeminal neuralgia were proved. It was granted approval for use in pediatric patients in 1976. It is chemically related to the tricyclic antidepressants and is considered a first-line AED for the treatment of simple partial, complex partial, and generalized tonic-clonic seizures. It is contraindicated in patients with absence and myoclonic seizures and those who have shown a hypersensitivity reaction to it in the past. Carbamazepine is available as an oral suspension (100 mg/5 ml), a 200-mg tablet, and a 100-mg chewable tablet. The typical therapeutic serum carbamazepine drug level is 8 to 12 μg/ml, but as with all AEDs, the therapeutic concentrations should be used only as a guideline. Carbamazepine is metabolized to carbamazepine epoxide, which has both anticonvulsant and toxic effects. Carbamazepine undergoes **autoinduction,** which is the process whereby a drug increases its own metabolism over time, leading to lower-than-expected drug concentrations. With carbamazepine this process usually occurs within the first couple months after the start of therapy. Carbamazepine is classified as a pregnancy category C drug. It is a prescription-only drug. The recommended dosages are given in the table on p. 141.

✇ PHARMACOKINETICS

HALF-LIFE	ONSET	PEAK	DURATION
14-16 hr	Slow	4-8 hr	12-24 hr

⚘ ETHOSUXIMIDE

Ethosuximide (Zarontin) is a very safe and effective first-line AED that is used primarily for the treatment of absence seizures. Such seizures occur primarily in childhood. Occasionally when valproate is ineffective in controlling primary generalized epilepsy involving seizure types other than absence attacks, the addition of ethosuximide improves seizure control. It is in this setting that ethosuximide is used mostly in adults. Its common side effects are nausea and abdominal discomfort, drowsiness, anorexia, and headache. In rare cases, behavioral changes may be seen, including psychosis. It is classified as a pregnancy category C agent. Ethosuximide comes in a syrup (250 mg/5 ml) and capsule (250 mg) form. It is a prescription-only drug. Recommended dosages are given in the table on p. 141.

✇ PHARMACOKINETICS

HALF-LIFE	ONSET	PEAK	DURATION
24-70 hr	4-7 days*	1-4 hr	12-24 hr

*4-7 days until reaches steady state.

PHENOBARBITAL

Two of the most commonly used AEDs are the barbiturates phenobarbital (Solfoton) and primidone (Mysoline). Primidone is metabolized in the liver to phenobarbital and phenylethylmalonamide, both of which have anticonvulsant properties. Phenobarbital has been used since 1912, principally for controlling tonic-clonic and partial seizures. Phenobarbital is also a first-line agent for the management of status epilepticus and is an effective prophylactic drug for the control of febrile seizures. By far the most common adverse effect is sedation, but tolerance to this effect usually develops with continued therapy. In pediatric patients the most common adverse effects are irritability, hyperactivity, depression, sleep disorders, and cognitive abnormalities. Therapeutic effects are generally seen at serum drug levels of 15 to 40 μg/ml. It interacts with many drugs because it is a major inducer of hepatic enzymes, causing more rapid clearance of some drugs. Its major advantage is that it has the longest half-life of all the standard AEDs, which allows for once-a-day dosing. This can be a substantial advantage for patients who have a hard time remembering to take their medication or for those who have erratic schedules. A patient may take a dose 12 or even 24 hours too late and may still have therapeutic blood levels at that time. In addition, phenobarbital is the most inexpensive AED, costing only pennies a day compared with several dollars for other AEDs. Phenobarbital is classified as a pregnancy category D agent. It is available for oral administration as capsules (16 mg), tablets (8, 15, 16, 60, 32, 60, 65, 100 mg), and an elixir (15 and 20 mg/ 5 ml). It also comes as an intravenous injection (30, 60, 65, and 130 mg/ml). It is a prescription-only drug. Recommended dosages are given in the table on p. 141.

✇ PHARMACOKINETICS*

HALF-LIFE	ONSET	PEAK	DURATION
53-118 hr	20-60 min	8-12 hr	6-12 hr

*For PO therapy.

⚘ PHENYTOIN

Phenytoin (Dilantin) has been used as a first-line AED for many years. It is primarily indicated for the management of tonic-clonic and partial seizures. Most common side effects are lethargy, abnormal movements, mental confusion, and cognitive changes. Therapeutic drug levels are 5 to 20 μg/dl. At toxic levels, phenytoin can cause nystagmus, ataxia, dysarthria, and encephalopathy. Long-term phenytoin therapy can cause gingival hyperplasia, acne, hirsutism, and hypertrophy of subcutaneous facial tissue, resulting in an appearance known as "Dilantin facies." Scrupulous dental care can help prevent gingival hypertrophy. Another long-term consequence of phenytoin therapy is osteoporosis. Vitamin D therapy may be necessary to prevent this, particularly in women. Phenytoin can interact with other medications, and there are two main reasons for this. First, it is highly bound to plasma proteins and competes with other highly protein-bound medications for binding sites. Second, it inhibits hepatic microsomal enzymes, mainly the cytochrome P-450 system.

Phenytoin has many advantages from the standpoint of long-term therapy. It is usually well tolerated, highly effective, and relatively inexpensive. It can also be given intravenously if needed. Phenytoin's long half-life allows it to be given only twice a day and in some cases, once a day. As stressed earlier, compliance with AED treatment is very important to seizure control. Therefore, if a patient only has to remember to take medication once or twice a day, this will lead to increased compliance and an increased likelihood of therapeutic drug levels being reached, and hence better seizure control. Phenytoin is available in both oral and intravenous forms. Orally administered phenytoin comes as a suspension (30 and 125 mg/5 ml), chewable tablets (50 mg), regular-release tablets (30 and 100 mg), and extended-release tablets (30 and 100 mg). It also comes as a 50-mg/ml injection. Phenytoin is a pregnancy category D agent and it is a prescription-only drug. The recommended dosages are given in the table on p. 141.

⚗ P H A R M A C O K I N E T I C S

HALF-LIFE	ONSET	PEAK	DURATION
10-34 hr	2-24 hr	1.5-2.5 hr	6-12 hr

VALPROIC ACID

Valproic acid (Depakene and Depakote) is used primarily in the treatment of generalized seizures (absence, myoclonic, and tonic-clonic). It has also been shown to be effective for controlling partial seizures. The main side effects are drowsiness; nausea, vomiting, and other gastrointestinal disturbances; tremor; weight gain; and transient hair loss. The most serious ones are fatal—hepatotoxicity and pancreatitis. Valproic acid can interact with many medications, the main reasons for these interactions being protein binding and liver metabolism. It is highly bound to plasma proteins and competes with other highly protein bound medications for binding sites. It also is highly metabolized by hepatic microsomal enzymes and competes for metabolism. Valproic acid is categorized as a pregnancy category D agent. It comes as valproate sodium syrup (250 mg/5 ml), divalproex sodium capsules with sprinkle particles (250 mg), liquid-filled capsules (250 mg), and extended-release divalproex sodium tablets (125, 250, and 500 mg). It is a prescription-only drug. Recommended dosages are given in the table on p. 141.

⚗ P H A R M A C O K I N E T I C S

HALF-LIFE	ONSET	PEAK	DURATION
6-16 hr	15-30 min	1-4 hr	4-6 hr

NURSING PROCESS

It is important to the safe use of the various classes of agents used in the management of seizure disorders to understand the nursing process as it relates to each of these major classes. This discussion will focus on the different groups of the barbiturates, benzodiazepines, hydantoins, and oxazolidinediones. Some of these AEDs, such as the barbiturates and benzodiazepines, were also discussed with the sedative-hypnotic agents (see Chapter 10).

ASSESSMENT

When any AED is to be administered, the nurse should first obtain a thorough health history so that any possible drug interactions (see Table 11-4), drug allergies, and previous unusual or untoward reactions to any of these medications can be known in advance. In addition, the nurse needs to gather any information regarding cardiac, respiratory tract, renal, liver, or CNS disorders because of the precautions that may be called for in the use of AEDs.

NURSING DIAGNOSES

Nursing diagnoses appropriate to the use of anticonvulsants include, but are not limited to, the following:

■ Risk for injury (falls, sedation, or dizziness) related to decreased sensorium stemming from drug effects.
■ Knowledge deficit related to lack of familiarity with and information concerning the use of AEDs.
■ Noncompliance (therapeutic regimen) related to patient's misuse of drugs or lack of understanding about the seizure disorder and its treatment.

PLANNING

The goals of nursing care in a patient taking AEDs are as follows:

- Patient experiences little or no adverse effects associated with noncompliance and/or with overtreatment or undertreatment.
- Patient can identify therapeutic effects of the AEDs.
- Patient remains compliant with therapy and without major harm to self during AED treatment.

Outcome Criteria

Outcome criteria related to the use of AEDs include the following:
- Patient will state the therapeutic drug effects as well as the side effects of the AED such as sedation, confusion, CNS depression.
- Patient (or family members) will state the importance of taking the medication exactly the way it has been prescribed such as the same time every day.
- Patient will state the dangers associated with sudden withdrawal of the medication such as rebound convulsions.
- Patient will maintain a protective environment at home and at work to minimize self-injury.

IMPLEMENTATION

AEDs, specifically the oral agents, should be taken regularly at the same time of day at the recommended dose and with meals to diminish the GI upset often associated with these agents. Oral suspensions should be shaken thoroughly, and capsules should not be crushed, opened, or chewed. Because there are both extended-release and immediate-release forms of oral hydantoins, it is important for the nurse to be sure which agent is being prescribed. The extended-release agents are usually taken once a day. If there are any questions about the medication order or the medication prescribed, the physician should be contacted immediately for clarification.

When given intramuscularly parenteral agents should be given deep in muscles, usually in the gluteal muscles, with rotation of the sites when more than one injection is being given. A 23-gauge, 1½ needle (as used for most intramuscular injections) is recommended, but the nurse should follow the manufacturer's recommendations as well as make decisions on the basis of each patient's situation.

Parenterally administered AEDs should be given with caution to prevent accidental arterial access and possible cardiac or respiratory arrest. If subcutaneous tissue access does occur because of infiltration of the drug at the intravenous site, ischemia and sloughing may occur because of the high alkalinity of some of these agents, specifically the hydantoins. Any of the intravenously administered AEDs, but especially the hydantoins, specifically phenytoin, should be delivered slowly while any changes in the vital signs—usually a decrease in pulse (<60 beats/min), blood pressure (<120/80 mm Hg), and the respiratory rate (<12 breaths/min)—are watched for and monitored. The intravenous site should also be checked for any redness or irritation. When administering phenytoin, always check package inserts or drug handbooks for the number of milligrams per seconds or minutes and do not mix the agent with any other solution because of the attendant risk of precipitate formation. Only normal saline solutions are to be used with phenytoin. Patient teaching tips are given in the previous chapter on sedative-hypnotic agents, with additional comments presented in the box below. See also the box on p. 146 for the pediatric implications.

EVALUATION

A therapeutic response to AEDs does not mean the patient has been cured of the seizures but only that seizure activity is decreased or absent. Any response to the medication should be documented in the nurses' notes. In addition, when monitoring and evaluating the effects of AEDs, the nurse needs to constantly assess the patient's mental status, mood and mood changes, sensorium, behavioral changes or changes in the level of consciousness, affect, eye problems or visual disorders, sore throat, or fever (blood dyscrasia is a side effect of the hydantoins). The occurrence of vomiting, diplopia, cardiovascular collapse, and the Stevens-Johnson syndrome indicates toxicity of the bone marrow, and the physician should be contacted immediately and no further doses administered.

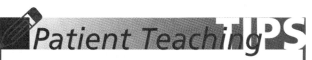

Patient Teaching TIPS

Anticonvulsant Therapy

✔ Patients need to fully understand their seizure disorder and the importance of consistent treatment.

✔ Omissions and any problems with dosing should be reported to the physician immediately!

✔ Patients should carry an ID card or wear a Medic-Alert bracelet or necklace at all times naming the diagnosis, the medications they are taking, and any other pertinent facts.

✔ Patients should avoid driving or engaging in other activities that require alertness when taking any anticonvulsants.

✔ Patients should be encouraged to keep a log or journal recording all seizure activity.

PEDIATRIC CONSIDERATIONS
Anticonvulsant Therapy

- When a skin rash develops in a child or infant taking phenytoin, the drug should be discontinued immediately and the physician notified.
- Chewable dosage forms should **not** be used for once-a-day administration, and IM injections of phenytoin should be avoided.
- Family members, parents, significant others, or caregivers should be encouraged to keep a record of the signs and symptoms, response to therapy, and any adverse reactions.
- Wearing of a Medic-Alert bracelet or necklace should be encouraged and information on this given.
- Suspension forms should always be shaken thoroughly before use and an exact graduated device or oral syringe used for more accurate dosing.
- Pediatric patients are much more sensitive to barbiturates and may respond to lower-than-expected doses, show more profound CNS depressive effects, or exhibit depression, confusion, or excitement (paradoxical reactions).
- Safe response of neonates to the benzodiazepines has not been established. Prolonged CNS depression has been associated with use of these agents in pediatric patients.
- Oral forms of valproic acid should not be given with milk because this may cause them to dissolve early and irritate local mucosa.
- Report excessive sedation, confusion, lethargy, or decreased movement in pediatric patients taking any of the AEDs.

TAKE HOME POINTS

Epilepsy, Seizures, and Convulsions
- These three terms have very different meanings.
- They should not be used interchangeably.
- Epilepsy = disorder of brain manifested as a chronic, recurrent pattern of seizures.
- Seizures = abnormal electrical activity in brain.
- Convulsions = a type of seizure (spasmodic contractions of involuntary muscles).

Classification of Seizures
- Partial = short alterations in consciousness, repetitive unusual movements, psychologic changes, and confusion.
- Generalized = most common in childhood; temporary lapses in consciousness (seconds); rhythmic movement of eyes, head, or hands; does not convulse; and may have several a day.

Status Epilepticus
- Common seizure disorder, life-threatening emergency.
- Characterized by tonic-clonic convulsions.
- Brain damage and death = quick, if not treated.

Nursing Considerations
- Nurse must distinguish between focal, primary, secondary, status, tonic-clonic, grand mal, and petit mal seizures.
- Documentation of any seizure activity and the specific characteristics of the movements in the patient is important to a diagnosis and to adequate treatment.
- Noncompliance is the most notable factor leading to treatment failure.

Critical Thinking A C T I V I T I E S

1. What would the difference be between an allergic reaction and a toxic reaction in a patient taking phenytoin? What is the appropriate nursing action you should take if either of these occur in your patient?

2. M.M. is a 21-year-old woman who was brought to the emergency room in status epilepticus. The physician has decided to treat the woman with intravenous diazepam and phenytoin. He asks you to give a loading dose of 1.5 gm at a rate of 50 mg/min. What rate should you set the pump for (in milliliters per hour)?

BIBLIOGRAPHY

Albanese J, Nutz P: *Mosby's 1995 nursing drug cards*, St Louis, 1995, Mobsy.

Connelly JF: Vigabatrin, *Ann Pharmacother* 27:197, 1993.

Crumrine PK: A trio of pediatric neurologic emergencies, *Emerg Med* 25:103, 1993.

Dichter MA: Deciding to discontinue antiepileptic medication, *Hosp Pract* 27:16, 1993.

Dupuis RE, Miranda-Massari J: Anticonvulsants: pharmacotherapeutic issues in the critically ill patient. *AACN Clin Issues Crit Care Nurs* 2:639, 1991.

Fisher RS: Emerging antiepileptic drugs, *Neurology* 43(suppl 5):S12, 1993.

French J: The long-term therapeutic management of epilepsy, *Ann Intern Med* 120:411, 1994.

Graves NM: Pharmacokinetics and interactions of antiepileptic drugs, *Am J Hosp Pharm* 50(suppl 5):S23, 1993.

Graves NM: Felbamate, *Ann Pharmacother* 27:1073, 1993.

Green MW, Selman JE: Review article: the medical management of trigeminal neuralgia, *Headache* 31:588, 1991.

Haves G, Kootsikas ME: Reassessing the lower end of the phenytoin therapeutic range: a review of the literature, *Ann Pharmacother* 27:1389, 1993.

Holmes GL: Critical issues in the treatment of epilepsy, *Am J Hosp Pharm* 50(suppl 5):S23, 1993.

Jagoda A, Riggio S: Refractory status epilepticus in adults, *Ann Emerg Med* 22:1337, 1993.

Johnson KB: *The Harriet Lane handbook,* ed 13, St Louis, 1993, Mosby.

Keen JH: *Critical care and emergency drug reference,* St Louis, 1994, Mosby.

Kilpatrick CJ, Moulds RF: Anticonvulsants in pregnancy, *Med J Aust* 154:199, 1991.

Knoben JE, Anderson PO: *Handbook of clinical drug data,* ed 6, Hamilton, Ill, 1988, Drug Intelligence Publications.

Legion V: Health education for self-management by people with epilepsy, *J Neurosci Nurs* 23:300, 1991.

Leppik IE, Graves N, Devinsky O: New antiepileptic medications, *Neurol Clin* 11:905, 1993.

Leppik IE, Wolff DL: Antiepileptic medication interactions, *Neurol Clin* 11:905, 1993.

Mattson RH: Current challengers in the treatment of epilepsy, *Neurology* 44(suppl 5):S4, 1994.

McEvoy GK: *AHFS drug information,* Bethesda, Md, 1989, American Society of Hospital Pharmacists.

McLean MJ: Clinical pharmacokinetics of gabapentin, *Neurology* 44(suppl 5):S17, 1994.

Ramsay RE: Clinical efficacy and safety of gabapentin, *Neurology* 44(suppl 5):S23, 1994.

Skidmore-Roth L: *Mosby's 1995 nursing drug reference,* St Louis, 1995, Mosby.

So EL: Update on epilepsy, *Med Clin North Am* 77:203, 1993.

Talwar D: Mechanisms of antiepileptic drug action, *Pediatr Neurol* 6:289, 1990.

Taylor CP: Emerging perspectives on the mechanism of action of gabapentin, *Neurology* 44(suppl 5):S31, 1994.

Zakrzewska JM, Patsalos PN: Drugs used in the management of trigeminal neuralgia, *Oral Surg Oral Med Oral Pathol* 74:439, 1992.

Chapter 12

Antiparkinsonian Agents

Objectives

When you reach the end of this chapter, you will be able to:

1 Identify the different classes of medications used as antiparkinsonian agents.

2 Discuss the mechanism of action, dosages, indications, contraindications, cautions, side effects, and toxic effects associated with the use of each antiparkinsonian agent.

3 Develop a comprehensive nursing care plan as it relates to the nursing process in the administration of antiparkinsonian agents.

4 Develop thorough patient teaching guidelines for the patient receiving antiparkinsonian agents.

CHAPTER OUTLINE

Parkinson's Disease
Neuroprotective Therapy
  Mechanism of action
  Drug effects
  Therapeutic uses
  Side effects and adverse effects
  Interactions
  Dosage
Drug Profile
  Selegiline
Dopaminergic Therapy
  Mechanism of action
  Drug effects
  Therapeutic uses
  Side effects and adverse effects
  Interactions
  Dosages
Drug Profiles
  Levodopa
  ⚓ Levodopa-Carbidopa
  ⚓ Amantadine
  Bromocriptine and Pergolide
Anticholinergic Therapy
  Mechanism of action
  Drug effects
  Therapeutic uses
  Side effects and adverse effects
  Interactions
  Dosages

Drug Profiles
  Benztropine Mesylate
  ⚓ Trihexyphenidyl
Nursing Process
Assessment
Nursing Diagnoses
Planning
  Outcome criteria
Implementation
Evaluation

Glossary

Akinesia (a kĭ ne′ zhə) Motor and psychic hypoactivity or muscular paralysis. (p. 152)

Chorea (kor e′ ə) A condition characterized by involuntary, purposeless, rapid motions such as flexing and extending the fingers, raising and lowering the shoulders, or grimacing. In some forms the person is also irritable, emotionally unstable, weak, restless, and fretful. (p. 150)

Dyskinesia (dis kĭ ne′ zhə) An impaired ability to execute voluntary movements. Tardive dyskinesia is one type and is caused by prolonged use of phenothiazine medications in elderly patients or by brain injury. (p. 150)

Dystonia (dis to′ ne ə) Any impairment of muscle tone. The condition commonly involves the head, neck, and tongue and often occurs as an adverse effect of a medication. (p. 150)

Parkinson's disease (PD) (pahr′ kin sənz) A slowly progressive, degenerative neurologic disorder characterized by resting tremor, pill-rolling of the fingers, a masklike facies, shuffling gait, forward flexion of the trunk, loss of postural reflexes, and muscle rigidity and weakness. It is usually an idiopathic (of no known cause) disease in people over 60 years of age, although it may occur in younger people, especially after acute encephalitis or carbon monoxide or metallic poisoning. (p. 149)

PARKINSON'S DISEASE

Parkinson's disease (PD) is a chronic, progressive, degenerative disorder affecting the dopamine-producing neurons in the brain. Myasthenia gravis, dementia, and Alzheimer's disease are other common CNS-neuromuscular disorders. PD was initially recognized in 1817, at which time it was called "shaking palsy." The symptoms of both the early and advanced stages of the disease along with the treatment options were first described by James Parkinson. It was not until the 1960s, however, that the underlying pathologic defect was discovered. It was postulated then that a dopamine deficit in the area of the brain called the *substantia nigra* was the cause of the disorder.

PD afflicts nearly a million Americans. It is primarily a disease of the elderly, rarely developing in persons under 40 years of age, but the number of patients with PD will only continue to increase as our aged population grows. There is a 2% chance of PD developing in a person during his or her lifetime. In most patients the disease becomes apparent between 45 and 65 years of age, with the mean age at onset being 56 years. Men and women are equally affected. Family history does not seem to be a contributing factor. PD is also a prominent cause of disability because of the frequent accompanying motor complications.

The primary cause of PD is an imbalance in two neurotransmitters—dopamine and acetylcholine—in the area of the brain called the *basal ganglia*. This imbalance is caused by failure of the nerve terminals there to produce the essential neurotransmitter dopamine. Dopamine is an inhibitory neurotransmitter, and acetylcholine is an excitatory neurotransmitter in this area of the brain. A correct balance between these two neurotransmitters is needed for the proper regulation of posture, muscle tone, and voluntary movement. Patients who suffer from PD have an imbalance in these neurotransmitters. Figure 12-1 illustrates the difference in neurotransmitter concentrations in normal persons and patients with PD.

A significant advance in our understanding of the etiology and pathogenesis of PD came in 1983 when the potent neurotoxin MPTP (1-methyl-4-phenyl-1,2,3,6-tetrahydropyridine) and its metabolic breakdown product MPP (1-methyl-4-phenylpyridine) were discovered. MPTP and MPP selectively destroy the substantia nigra, or that area of the brain that is dysfunctional in PD. It has been shown that a parkinso-

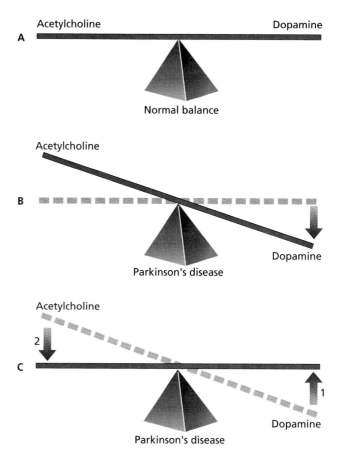

A, Normal balance of acetylcholine and dopamine in the CNS.
B, In Parkinson's disease, a decrease in dopamine results in an imbalance.
C, Drug therapy in Parkinson's disease is aimed at correcting the imbalance between acetylcholine and dopamine. This can be accomplished by either
   1. increasing the supply of dopamine or
   2. blocking or lowering acetylcholine levels.

▼ **FIG. 12-1** The neurotransmitter abnormality of Parkinson's disease.

nian syndrome almost identical to idiopathic PD develops in laboratory animals injected with this neurotoxin. Others theorize that PD is the result of an earlier head injury or of excess iron in the substantia nigra, which undergoes oxidation and causes the generation of toxic free radicals. In still another theory, it is thought that because dopamine levels decrease with age, PD represents a premature aging of the nigrostriatal cells resulting from environmental or intrinsic biochemical factors, or both.

There are no readily available laboratory tests that can detect or confirm PD. Results of computed tomography, magnetic resonance imaging, cerebrospinal fluid analysis, and electroencephalography are usually normal and of little diagnostic value. These may be useful tools for ruling out other possible diseases as causes of the symptoms. Therefore the diagnosis of PD

Table 12-1	Classic Parkinsonian Symptoms
SYMPTOM	**DESCRIPTION**
Bradykinesia	Slowness of movement
Rigidity	"Cogwheel" rigidity, resistance to passive movement
Tremor	Pill-rolling: tremor of the thumb against the forefinger, seen mostly at rest; is less severe during voluntary activity; starts usually on one side then progresses to the other; is the presenting sign in 70% of the cases
Postural instability	Danger of falling, hesitation in gait as patient starts or stops walking

Table 12-2	Antiparkinsonian Agents
DRUG CATEGORY	**AGENTS**
Neuroprotective agents	Selegiline
Dopaminergic agents	Levodopa, levodopa-carbidopa, amantadine, bromocriptine, pergolide
Anticholinergic agents	Benztropine, biperiden, ethopropazine, procyclidine, trihexyphenidyl, diphenylhydramine

is usually made on the basis of the classic symptoms and physical findings. The classic symptoms of PD are listed in Table 12-1.

Symptoms of the disease do not appear until approximately 80% of the dopamine store in the substantia nigra of the basal ganglia has been depleted. This means that by the time PD is diagnosed, only approximately 20% or less of the patient's original nigral dopaminergic terminals are functioning normally.

Nerve terminals can take up substances, store them, and release them for use when needed, and it is this factor that forms the basis for antiparkinsonian treatment. As long as there are functioning nerve terminals that can take up dopamine, the symptoms of PD can be at least partially controlled. However, the blood-brain barrier does not allow exogenously supplied dopamine to enter the brain. It does, nevertheless, allow levodopa, a naturally occurring dopamine precursor, to do so. After levodopa has been taken up by the dopaminergic terminal, it is converted into dopamine and then released as needed. Levodopa therapy can thus correct the neurotransmitter imbalance in patients with early PD who still have functioning nerve terminals.

Unfortunately, PD is a progressive condition. With time the number of surviving dopaminergic terminals that can take up exogenously administered levodopa and convert it into dopamine decrease, and rapid swings in the response to levodopa, known as the on-off phenomenon, occur.

The result is worsening PD when too little dopamine is present or dyskinesias when too much is present. **Dyskinesias** is the difficulty in performing voluntary movements that some patients with PD have. The two most commonly associated with antiparkinsonian therapy are **chorea** (irregular, spasmodic, in-

voluntary movements of the limbs or facial muscles) and **dystonia** (abnormal muscle tone in any tissue).

The first step in the treatment of PD is a full explanation of the disease to the patient and his or her family. Physical therapy and speech therapy are almost always needed when the patient is in the later stages of the disease. As already discussed, drug therapy is aimed at increasing the levels of dopamine as long as there are functioning nerve terminals. It is also aimed at antagonizing or blocking the effects of acetylcholine and slowing the progression of the disease. The agents available for the treatment of PD and their respective categories are listed in Table 12-2.

NEUROPROTECTIVE THERAPY

In recent years there has been an increasing focus on developing treatment strategies to slow the progression of PD. Selegiline, a very potent, irreversible monoamine oxidase B (MAO-B) inhibitor derived from amphetamine, has been one means of accomplishing this end.

As early as 1965, nonselective monoamine oxidase inhibitors (MAOIs) were being used to improve the therapeutic effect of levodopa in patients with PD, but a major adverse effect of MAOIs has been that they interact with tyramine-containing foods (cheese, red wine, beer, and yogurt). This has been termed *the cheese effect*, and the result is severe hypertension. This has considerably restricted their therapeutic use. In 1974 selegiline was introduced as an investigational option for PD. As an MAO-B inhibitor selegiline does not elicit the classic cheese effect at doses of 10 mg or less a day. In the years that followed, many investigational studies were conducted, and in October 1989, selegiline received FDA approval for use in conjunction with levodopa therapy in the treatment of PD. Since then, several small studies and one large study have shown the drug to have a neuroprotective effect.

Mechanism of Action

MAO is one of the two major pathways by which dopamine is degraded. Type B accounts for about 70% of all MAO activity in the brain. One of the current theories advanced to explain the etiology of PD is that the neurotoxicity that causes the destruction of the cells of the substantia nigra is accomplished by MPP, the enzymatically active toxin of MPTP. This enzymatic conversion to MPP is accomplished by MAO-B. By blocking this enzyme with the MAO-B inhibitor selegiline, MPP is prevented from being made and the substantia nigra is spared. Figure 12-2 illustrates this enzymatic inhibition process.

Drug Effects

MAOs are widely distributed throughout the body. The areas where concentrations are high are the liver, kidney, stomach, intestinal wall, and brain. There are two subclasses of MAOs: A and B. Most of the type-B MAO is in the CNS, primarily in the brain. The primary role of MAOs is the catabolism or breakdown of catecholamines such as dopamine, norepinephrine, and epinephrine, as well as the breakdown of serotonin. Therefore an MAO-B inhibitor like selegiline would cause an increase in the levels of catecholamines and serotonin in the CNS. This can be broadly regarded as stimulation of the sympathetic nervous system.

Therapeutic Uses

Selegiline is currently approved for use in combination with levodopa or levodopa-carbidopa. It is an adjunctive agent used when a patient's response to levodopa is fluctuating. It allows the dose of levodopa to be decreased. Improvement in functional ability, and decreased severity of symptoms are common after selegiline is added. However, only approximately 50% to 60% of patients show a positive response.

Selegiline may be somewhat beneficial as a prophylactic agent. Selegiline administration before exposure to the neurotoxin MPTP has been shown to prevent the onset of a PD-like syndrome in laboratory animals, indicating a possible neuroprotective effect. Several studies have shown that selegiline-treated patients required levodopa therapy approximately 1.8 times later than control patients. One problem that patients with PD experience is that as their disease progresses it becomes more and more difficult to control it with levodopa. Ultimately levodopa no longer controls the PD, and the patient is seriously debilitated. This generally occurs between 5 to 10 years after the start of levodopa therapy. Prophylactic selegiline use may delay the development of serious debilitating PD for 9 to 18 years. Because the average age of patients at the onset of PD is between 55 and 65 years, such a delay would mean most patients will die before the functional disability occurs.

Side Effects and Adverse Effects

The most common adverse effects associated with selegiline use are mild and consist of nausea, lightheadedness, dizziness, abdominal pain, insomnia, confusion, and dry mouth. The adverse effects seen with selegiline use as they relate to the various body systems are listed in Table 12-3. Reactions seen when the dosage exceeds 10 mg/day include a hypertensive crisis upon the consumption of tyramine-containing food, memory loss, muscular twitches and jerks, and grinding of the teeth.

Interactions

The number of drugs that selegiline interacts with is relatively small, and the degree of interaction is dose dependent. At recommended doses of 10 mg/day, the

▼ FIG. 12-2 Mechanism of action of selegiline. *MAO-B*, monoamine oxidase type B; *MPP*, 1-methyl-4-phenylpyridine; *MPTP*, 1-methyl-4-phenyl-1,2,3,6-tetrahydropyridine.

Table 12-3	Selegiline: Adverse Effects
BODY SYSTEM	**SIDE/ADVERSE EFFECT**
Cardiovascular	Hypotension, dysrhythmia, tachycardia, palpitations, angina, edema
Central nervous system	Altered sensation, pain, dizziness, drowsiness, irritability, anxiety, extrapyramidal side effects
Gastrointestinal	Nausea, vomiting, constipation, diarrhea, anorexia
Respiratory	Asthma, shortness of breath

drug maintains its selective MAO-B inhibition. However, at doses that exceed 10 mg/day, selegiline becomes a nonselective MAOI, contributing to the development of the cheese effect. Meperidine is contraindicated in patients receiving nonselective MAOIs because this has been associated with the occurrence of fatal hypertensive episodes. It is suggested that meperidine as well as other opioids be avoided in patients taking more than 10 mg/day of selegiline.

Dosage

For the recommended dosage of selegiline see the table below.

DRUG PROFILE

SELEGILINE

Selegiline is an MAO-B inhibitor used as an adjunctive agent along with levodopa to decrease the amount of levodopa needed. It has also been shown to exert a neuroprotective effect when started early in therapy. It is a prescription-only drug that comes only in an oral form as a 5-mg tablet. It is classified as a pregnancy category C agent. Selegiline has three active metabolites whose half-lives are listed in the table below. The

recommended dosage for selegiline is given in the table below.

✚ PHARMACOKINETICS

HALF-LIFE	ONSET	PEAK	DURATION
2 hr	1 hr	0.5-2 hr	1-3 days

*Selegiline has three active metabolites with long half-lives of 18-21 hours.

DOPAMINERGIC THERAPY

Because in PD little or no dopamine is produced, acetylcholine is left as the predominant neurotransmitter. Dopaminergic agents are used to help replace the lost dopamine or enhance the function of the few neurons that are left to produce their own. The dopaminergic agents can be broken down into three categories based on their underlying mechanisms of action: those that release dopamine (indirect acting), those that increase brain levels of dopamine (replacement), and dopaminergic agonists (direct acting). The ultimate goal is to increase the levels of dopamine in the brain. By doing so and creating a balance with acetylcholine, akinesias, the most detrimental complications of PD, can be reversed. **Akinesias** are symptoms such as a masklike facial expression and impaired postural reflexes. They eventually render the patient unable to care for himself or herself.

Mechanism of Action

Levodopa and the combination product levodopa-carbidopa *directly replace* the deficient neurotransmitter

DOSAGES

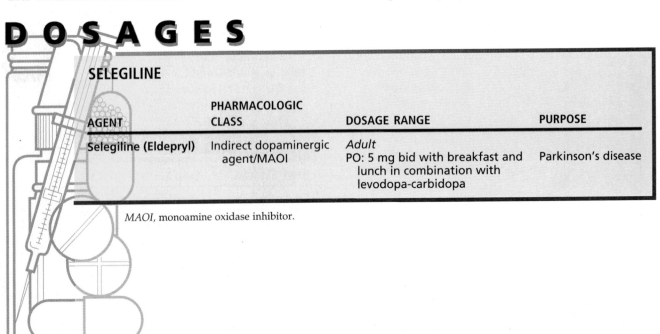

SELEGILINE			
AGENT	PHARMACOLOGIC CLASS	DOSAGE RANGE	PURPOSE
Selegiline (Eldepryl)	Indirect dopaminergic agent/MAOI	*Adult* PO: 5 mg bid with breakfast and lunch in combination with levodopa-carbidopa	Parkinson's disease

MAOI, monoamine oxidase inhibitor.

dopamine in the substantia nigra. They are considered the cornerstone of the treatment of PD. Levodopa is the biologic precursor of dopamine required by the brain for dopamine synthesis. Dopamine must be administered in this form because, as mentioned previously, exogenously administered dopamine cannot pass through the blood-brain barrier, whereas levodopa can. Once it does, it is converted directly into dopamine. Traditionally, very large doses of levodopa had to be administered to get enough dopamine to the brain because much of the levodopa administered was broken down outside the CNS by the enzyme dopa decarboxylase. These large doses resulted in high peripheral levels of dopamine and many unwanted side effects such as confusion, involuntary movements, GI distress, and hypotension. These problems are avoided when levodopa is given with **carbidopa,** a peripheral decarboxylase inhibitor that does not cross the blood-brain barrier. Therefore it prevents levodopa breakdown in the periphery, allowing the levodopa to reach and cross the blood-brain barrier without crossing it itself. Once in the brain, the levodopa is then broken down to dopamine, which can be used directly.

Originally developed and used for the prophylaxis and treatment of viral disorders, amantadine (Symmetrel) has proved to be a valuable adjunct to the traditional antiparkinsonian drugs. Amantadine appears to exert its antiparkinsonian effect by causing the release of dopamine and other catecholamines from their storage sites in the ends of nerves. Amantadine also blocks the reuptake of dopamine into the nerve endings, which allows more dopamine to accumulate both centrally and peripherally. Therefore amantadine's dopaminergic effects are the result of its *indirect actions* on the nerve.

Bromocriptine (Parlodel) and pergolide (Permax) are dopaminergic agonists that directly stimulate the dopamine receptors. Chemically bromocriptine is an ergot alkaloid similar to ergotamine in its chemical structure. Its antiparkinsonian effects are due to its ability to activate dopamine receptors and stimulate the production of more dopamine, helping to correct the imbalance between acetylcholine and dopamine in the CNS. Pergolide, on the other hand, has no effect on dopamine synthesis or dopamine storage sites. It stimulates dopamine receptors in the nigrostiatal area of the brain, the area believed to be defective in patients with PD.

Drug Effects

When broken down in the periphery by dopa decarboxylase, levodopa becomes dopamine. When in the periphery, this dopamine causes involuntary movements, GI distress, and orthostatic hypotension.

It has even been known to cause arrhythmias. When levodopa is given with carbidopa, the enzyme inhibitor, much more levodopa then enters the brain, where it can offset the imbalance between dopamine and acetylcholine.

Therapeutic Uses

The therapeutic effects of the replacement drugs levodopa and levodopa-carbidopa are identical. The only difference is that, as already explained, the combination product is more efficient in increasing the dopamine level in the brain.

The therapeutic effects of the indirect-acting dopaminergic agent amantadine are its antidyskinetic effects (its ability to promote voluntary movements) and its antiviral properties (both the prevention and treatment). The direct-acting dopaminergic agents bromocriptine and pergolide also have antidyskinetic effects. In addition they can inhibit lactation, suppress growth hormone production, and inhibit prolactin production.

Side Effects and Adverse Effects

There are many potential side effects and adverse effects associated with the dopaminergic agents. The most common of these are listed in Table 12-4.

Interactions

The drug interactions involving dopaminergic drugs can cause significant adverse reactions, including a decrease in the efficacy of the dopaminergic drug, a hypertensive crisis, and reversal of the dopaminergic drug's effect. The major drug interactions that occur with the dopaminergic drugs are summarized in Table 12-5.

Dosages

For the recommended dosages of the dopaminergic agents, see the table on p. 154.

DRUG PROFILES

LEVODOPA

As described earlier, the treatment of PD centers around attempts to replace the dopamine deficiency,

Table 12-4	Dopaminergic Agents: Adverse Effects

BODY SYSTEM	SIDE/ADVERSE EFFECT
⚓Levodopa and carbidopa	
Cardiovascular	Palpitations, orthostatic hypotension
Central nervous system	Agitation; anxiety; psychotic and suicidal episodes; choreiform, dystonic, and other involuntary movements; headache and blurred vision
Blood	Hemolytic anemia, agranulocytosis
⚓Amantadine	
Central nervous system	Impaired concentration, dizziness, increased irritability, nervousness, blurred vision
Gastrointestinal	Anorexia, nausea, constipation, vomiting
Other	Purple-red skin spots; dryness of mouth, nose, and throat; increased weakness
Bromocriptine and pergolide	
Cardiovascular	Hypotension
Central nervous system	Drowsiness; headaches; depression; confusion; hallucinations; uncontrolled movement of body, face, tongue, arms, hands, and head
Gastrointestinal	Nausea, diarrhea, constipation, abdominal cramps, anorexia

Table 12-5	Dopaminergic Drugs: Drug Interactions

DRUG	MECHANISM	RESULTS
Hydantoins	Increase levodopa metabolism	Decreased levodopa effects
Haloperidol or phenothiazines	Block dopamine receptors in brain	Decreased levodopa effects
Monoamine oxidase inhibitors	Inhibit metabolism	Hypertensive crisis
Pyridoxine (vitamin B$_6$)	Promotes levodopa breakdown	Reversal of levodopa effects (carbidopa may prevent this)

DOSAGES

SELECTED DOPAMINERGIC AGENTS

AGENT	CATEGORY	DOSAGE RANGE	PURPOSE
⚓Amantadine (Symmetrel)	Indirect acting	*Adult* PO: 100-400 mg/day	Triggers release of dopamine
Bromocriptine (Parlodel)	Direct acting	*Adult* PO: 10-40 mg/day	Dopamine agonist
⚓Levodopa-carbidopa (Sinemet)	Replacement	*Adult* PO: 10/100, 1 tablet 3-8 times/day; 25/100, 1 tablet 3-6 times/day; 25/250, 1 tablet 3-4 times/day CR: 1 tablet bid	Replaces dopamine
Pergolide (Permax)	Direct acting	*Adult* PO: up to 5 mg/day in combination with levodopa-carbidopa	Dopamine agonist

CR, controlled release.

but dopamine does not cross the blood-brain barrier whereas levodopa, a precursor of dopamine, does. However, because levodopa is also converted into dopamine in the rest of the body, the resulting high levels throughout the body cause many unwanted side effects.

Levodopa is a prescription-only drug that is classified as a pregnancy category C medication. It is contraindicated in patients who have shown a hypersensitivity reaction to it, those with narrow-angle glaucoma or a history of melanoma, and those concurrently taking MAOIs. Levodopa is only available in an oral form as 100-, 250-, and 500-mg capsules and tablets. Recommended dosages are given in the table on p. 154.

☣ P H A R M A C O K I N E T I C S

HALF-LIFE	ONSET	PEAK	DURATION
1-3 hr	2-3 wk*	1-3 hr	<5 hr

*Therapeutic effect.

⚓ LEVODOPA-CARBIDOPA

With the addition of the peripheral decarboxylase inhibitor carbidopa, which does not cross the blood-brain barrier, many of the unwanted side effects caused by peripherally broken down levodopa are prevented because more of the levodopa can reach the site of action without being broken down. As a result, much lower daily doses of levodopa are needed. Levodopa-carbidopa (Sinemet and Sinemet CR) has become the cornerstone in the treatment of PD. It also appears to limit the on-off phenomenon that some patients with PD experience. This phenomenon is seen in patients taking levodopa for a long time. Such patients may experience periods when they have good control, the "on" time, and periods when they have bad control or break-through PD, the "off" time. A variety of studies has shown that Sinemet CR increases the "on" time and decreases the "off" time.

Levodopa-carbidopa is a prescription-only drug that is classified as a pregnancy category C medication. It is contraindicated in patients who have shown a hypersensitivity reaction to it, those with narrow-angle glaucoma or a history of melanoma, and those concurrently taking MAOIs. This combination agent is only available orally as tablets with the following proportions of levodopa to carbidopa, respectively: 100 mg to 10 mg, 100 mg to 25 mg, and 250 mg to 25 mg. There are also controlled-release formulations of this combination product consisting of 200 mg of levodopa and 50 mg of carbidopa. Recommended dosages are given in the table on p. 154.

☣ P H A R M A C O K I N E T I C S

HALF-LIFE	ONSET	PEAK	DURATION
1-3 hr	2-3 wk*	1-3 hr	<5 hr

*Therapeutic effect.

⚓ AMANTADINE

Amantadine (Symmetrel) is believed to work in the CNS by eliciting the release of dopamine from nerve endings, causing higher concentrations of dopamine in the CNS. It is most effective in the earlier stages of PD when there are still significant numbers of nerves to act on and dopamine to be released. As the disease progresses, however, the population of functioning nerves diminishes, and so does the amantadine's effect. Amantadine is usually effective for only 6 to 12 months. After amantadine fails to relieve the hypokinesia and rigidity, a dopamine agonist such as bromocriptine or pergolide is usually tried next.

Amantadine is considered a pregnancy category C medication and is a prescription-only drug. It is contraindicated in patients who have shown a hypersensitivity reaction to it in the past, women who are lactating, and children younger than 1 year old (remember that amantadine is also an antiviral agent). Amantadine is only available orally as 100-mg tablets and an oral solution that provides 50 mg per 5 ml of syrup. Recommended dosages are given in the table on p. 154.

☣ P H A R M A C O K I N E T I C S

HALF-LIFE	ONSET	PEAK	DURATION
11-15 hr	48 hr	2-4 hr	6-12 wk

BROMOCRIPTINE AND PERGOLIDE

Once amantadine becomes ineffective, a dopamine agonist like pergolide or bromocriptine (Parlodel) may be prescribed in its place. Bromocriptine differs from pergolide in that it only stimulates the dopamine-2 receptors and antagonizes or blocks the dopamine-1 receptors. Pergolide stimulates or acts as an agonist at both types of receptors. Eventually levodopa-carbidopa is needed to control the patient's symptoms, but by using amantadine until it fails then a dopamine agonist until it fails, the need for levodopa therapy may be postponed for up to 3 years. These two agents may also be given with levodopa-carbidopa so that lower doses of the levodopa are needed. This often results in prolonging the "on" periods, when PD is controlled, and decreasing the "off" periods, when PD is not controlled.

Bromocriptine is only available with a prescription and is categorized as a pregnancy category D medication. It is contraindicated in patients who have shown a hypersensitivity reaction to any of the ergot alkaloids, patients with severe ischemic disease, and those with severe peripheral vascular disease. Bromocriptine is only available orally as 5-mg capsules and as 2.5-mg tablets. Recommended dosages are given in the table on p. 154.

⬡⬡ P H A R M A C O K I N E T I C S

HALF-LIFE	ONSET	PEAK	DURATION
3-5 hr	0.5-1.5 hr	1-3 hr	4-8 hr

Pergolide is only available with a prescription and is listed as a pregnancy category B medication. It is contraindicated in patients who have shown a hypersensitivity reaction to it or to other ergot alkaloids. It comes only in an oral form as 0.05-, 0.25-, and 1-mg tablets. Recommended dosages are given in the table on p. 154.

⬡⬡ P H A R M A C O K I N E T I C S

HALF-LIFE	ONSET	PEAK	DURATION
27 hr	15-30 min	1-3 hr	1-2 days

ANTICHOLINERGIC THERAPY

Anticholinergics, or drugs that block the effects of acetylcholine, are sometimes useful in treating the muscle tremors and muscle rigidity associated with PD. These two symptoms are caused by excessive cholinergic activity. The anticholinergics do little, however, to relieve the bradykinesia (extremely slow movements) associated with PD. The rationale for the use of anticholinergics is to reduce excessive cholinergic activity in the brain. The first agents in this category to be used were the belladonna alkaloids, atropine and scopolamine. However, because the anticholinergic side effects—dry mouth, urinary retention, blurred vision, and others—can be excessive, new synthetic anticholinergics and antihistamines with better side effect profiles were developed, agents such as benztropine and trihexyphenidyl.

Mechanism of Action

All anticholinergics work in some way to block acetylcholine (central cholinergic excitatory pathways). Because of the reduced number of dopamine-producing nerves, the acetylcholine-producing nerves are left unchecked and acetylcholine accumulates. This usually results in muscle tremors and muscle rigidity, which is sometimes described as *cogwheel rigidity*. The muscle tremors are usually worse while the patient is at rest and consist of a pill-rolling movement and bobbing of the head.

Drug Effects

The anticholinergic drugs have either the opposite effect or oppose the effects of the neurotransmitter acetylcholine, which is responsible for causing increased salivation, lacrimation (tearing of the eyes), and urination, as well as diarrhea, increased GI motility, and possibly emesis (vomiting). The acronym SLUDGE is often used to describe these cholinergic-induced effects. With these in mind, effects of anticholinergics would be the opposite of the SLUDGE symptoms, effects such as antisecretory effects (dry mouth or decreased salivation), urinary retention, decreased GI motility (constipation), dilated pupils (mydriasis), and smooth muscle relaxation.

Therapeutic Uses

Anticholinergic agents decrease salivation and relax smooth muscles. They readily cross the blood-brain barrier and therefore can get right to the site of the imbalance in the CNS—the substantia nigra. It is because of their ability to directly relax smooth muscles that the muscle rigidity and akinesia (little or no movement) are reduced. Besides their use as antidyskinetic agents in PD, anticholinergics are also used for the treatment of drug-induced extrapyramidal reactions.

Side Effects and Adverse Effects

The side effects and adverse effects associated with anticholinergic drug use are many, and the most common ones are listed in Table 12-6. They often occur

Table 12-6	Anticholinergic Adverse Effects
BODY SYSTEM	**SIDE/ADVERSE EFFECT**
Central nervous system	Drowsiness, confusion, disorientation, hallucinations
Gastrointestinal	Constipation, nausea, vomiting
Genitourinary	Urinary retention, pain on urination
Other	Blurred vision, dilated pupils (mydriasis), sensitivity to the sun (photophobia), dry skin

more frequently when the agents are given in high doses. Anticholinergic-induced adverse effects are also more common in the elderly. However wise and judicious use of such drugs can lead to very effective treatment free of the unwanted side effects.

Interactions

The interactions that occur between anticholinergic drugs and other drugs and drug classes can be very damaging. These various agents and the results of interactions are listed in Table 12-7.

Dosages

For information on the dosages of benztropine and trihexyphenidyl in the treatment of PD, see the table below.

DRUG PROFILES

The anticholinergics are helpful in alleviating the muscle tremors and rigidity seen in patients with PD. They are not, however, as effective as the other drug classes used in the treatment of PD in correcting the underlying problem, but are very effective for the relief of only minimal symptoms and for the treatment of those patients who cannot tolerate or do not respond to dopamine replacement drugs such as levodopa or the dopaminergics such as amantadine and bromocriptine. They are also useful as adjuncts to these primary

Table 12-7	Anticholinergic Drugs: Drug Interactions	
DRUG	**MECHANISM**	**RESULTS**
Alcohol and CNS depressants		
Amantadine and antihistamines		
Phenothiazines	Additive	Enhanced CNS depressant effects
Tricyclic antidepressants		
Antacids		Reduced absorption and decreased therapeutic effect of anticholinergic

DOSAGES

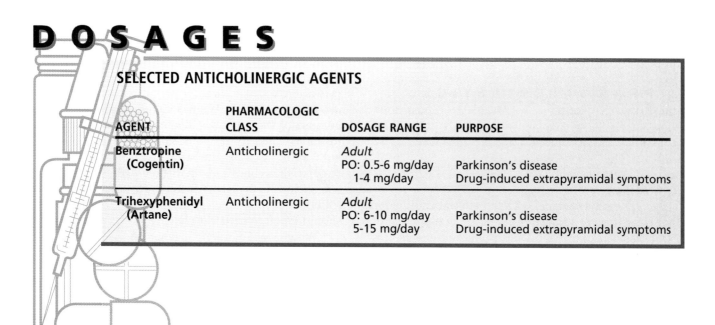

SELECTED ANTICHOLINERGIC AGENTS

AGENT	PHARMACOLOGIC CLASS	DOSAGE RANGE	PURPOSE
Benztropine (Cogentin)	Anticholinergic	*Adult* PO: 0.5-6 mg/day 1-4 mg/day	Parkinson's disease Drug-induced extrapyramidal symptoms
Trihexyphenidyl (Artane)	Anticholinergic	*Adult* PO: 6-10 mg/day 5-15 mg/day	Parkinson's disease Drug-induced extrapyramidal symptoms

drugs. Treatment is usually started with small doses, which are gradually increased until the benefits or side effects appear. Some of the more commonly used agents are trihexyphenidyl (Artane), ethopropazine (Parsidol), diphenhydramine (Benadryl), and benztropine mesylate (Cogentin). They must be used cautiously in the elderly because significant side effects such as confusion, urinary retention, visual blurring, palpitations, and increased intraocular pressure can develop. The most commonly used agents are the synthetic anticholinergics, which are associated with fewer of the side effects commonly seen with the belladonna alkaloid derivatives such as atropine and scopolamine.

BENZTROPINE MESYLATE

Benztropine (Cogentin) is a synthetic anticholinergic agent that resembles both atropine and diphenhydramine in its chemical structure. **Biperiden** (Akineton) is also a synthetic anticholinergic agent used in the treatment of PD. They both have anticholinergic, antihistaminic, and local anesthetic properties and are primarily used as adjuncts in the treatment of all forms of PD. They are also useful in the treatment of phenothiazine-induced extrapyramidal reactions. Benztropine is only available with a prescription and comes in an oral form as 0.5-, 1-, and 2-mg tablets and as an intravenous injection delivering 1 mg/ml. It is rated as a pregnancy category C agent. Its use is contraindicated in patients who have shown a hypersensitivity reaction to it; in those who have narrow-angle glaucoma, myasthenia gravis, urinary retention, a history of peptic ulcer disease, megacolon, or prostate hypertrophy; and in children under 3 years of age. Recommended dosages are given in the table on p. 157.

P H A R M A C O K I N E T I C S

HALF-LIFE	ONSET	PEAK	DURATION
≈ 4-8 hr	≈ 1 hr	2-4 hr	1-2 days

TRIHEXYPHENIDYL

Trihexyphenidyl (Artane) is a synthetic anticholinergic that is used as an adjunctive agent in the treatment of PD. It has weak peripheral anticholinergic effects. It is contraindicated in patients who have shown a hypersensitivity reaction to it and in patients with any of the conditions listed as contraindications to benztropine treatment. It is also considered a pregnancy category C agent. Trihexyphenidyl is only available in oral forms as a 5-mg extended-release capsule, a 2-mg/5 ml elixir, and a 2- and 5-mg tablet. Recommended dosages are given in the table on p. 157.

P H A R M A C O K I N E T I C S

HALF-LIFE	ONSET	PEAK	DURATION
3-4 hr	<1 hr	2-3 hr	6-12 hr

NURSING PROCESS

ASSESSMENT

After patients are first confronted with the diagnosis of PD, they soon learn how the disease can affect their every movement and alter activities of daily living (ADL). Before any medication is administered, you must perform a thorough assessment and take a thorough nursing history so that the symptoms and the ways in which the disease has affected the patients' ADL are documented and possible contraindications and cautions are identified.

The thorough nursing history should include questions about the following activities and body systems: CNS: ADL, gait, balance, tremors, weakness, lethargy, and level of consciousness; gastrointestinal and genitourinary: appetite and bladder and bowel patterns; psychological and emotional: mood, affect, depression, and personality changes.

When an anticholinergic agent such as benztropine or trihexyphenidyl is prescribed, you should assess the patient carefully to determine whether he or she has a history of urinary retention, bladder difficulties or obstruction, myasthenia gravis, or acute narrow-angle glaucoma (mydriasis leads to an increase in intraocular pressure), because these are contraindications to the use of these agents. Age is a significant factor as well because of the increased likelihood of side effects or toxicity related to the physiologic changes associated with aging (see the geriatric box on the following page). Other conditions that these agents can exacerbate include tachycardia, benign prostatic hypertrophy (BPH), and peptic ulcer disease, so these patients should be monitored closely.

When dopaminergic agents such as levodopa, amantadine, or levodopa-carbidopa are prescribed, the patient should be asked whether he or she has a seizure disorder, hypotension, peptic ulcer disease, a renal or hepatic disorder, asthma, a history of myocardial infarction, BPH, or an anemia, or suffers from psychosis or some other affective disorder, because these are all contraindications to their use. Drugs that can interact with these agents include MAOIs and fu-

GERIATRIC CONSIDERATIONS
Antiparkinsonian Agents

- Elderly patients taking the anticholinergics often used for PD are at risk for the development of health problems associated with the side effects of these medications, such as dry mouth, constipation, urinary retention—especially in men with benign prostatic hypertrophy, and impaired thought processes.

- The anticholinergics are contraindicated in patients with narrow-angle glaucoma or with a history of urinary retention.

- Some aged patients taking anticholinergic agents experience paradoxical reactions, such as excitement, confusion, or irritability.

- Overheating is a problem in patients taking anticholinergics, so the aged should especially avoid excessive exercise during the warm weather and avoid excessive heat exposure.

- Levodopa should be used cautiously, with close monitoring of the aged, especially if there is a history of cardiac, renal, hepatic, endocrine, pulmonary, ulcer, or psychiatric disease.

- The elderly patient taking levodopa is at an increased risk for suffering side effects, especially confusion.

- Levodopa-carbidopa is often started at a low dose because of the increased sensitivity of the aged patient to these medications.

▼

Patient Teaching TIPS
Anticholinergics

✔ Patients should be instructed to take medication with or after meals to minimize GI upset.

✔ Patients should drink lots of fluids, at least 2000 ml per day, unless otherwise instructed by their physician or not allowed this amount of fluid.

✔ Medications should be taken exactly as prescribed and at bedtime to prevent drowsiness during the day.

✔ Patients should understand the importance of not discontinuing medications suddenly.

✔ Patients should avoid taking any OTC medications unless physician has okayed this first.

✔ Patients should avoid operating heavy machinery or driving if they feel sedated or drowsy from the medication.

✔ Patients should be instructed to change positions slowly to prevent falling or fainting because of the postural hypotension (drop in blood pressure with position changes) produced by these agents.

---

razolidone. Given in combination with the dopaminergic medications, these drugs may result in a hypertensive crisis.

NURSING DIAGNOSES

Nursing diagnoses appropriate to the patient with PD taking antiparkinsonian agents include:

- Impaired mobility decreased as related to the muscle tremors and rigidity.
- Potential for body image disturbance because of the pathophysiologic changes associated with PD.
- Risk for constipation as related to PD.
- Risk for altered urinary elimination and retention as related to PD.
- Risk for injury and falls stemming from the physical disabilities produced by PD.
- Altered nutritional status (less than body requirements) as related to PD.
- Knowledge deficit related to pharmacotherapy and its therapeutic and side effects.

PLANNING

Goals of nursing care related to the administration of antiparkinsonian agents include:

- Patient remains free of self-injury.
- Patient states the purpose of the specific medications prescribed for the disease.
- Patient states the side effects and toxic effects of medications.
- Patient regains as normal as possible bowel and bladder elimination patterns.
- Patient maintains adequate nutritional status.
- Patient remains as independent as possible.
- Patient will be less anxious and fearful.
- Patient regains a positive self-concept.
- Patient remains compliant to therapy.

Outcome Criteria

Outcome criteria related to the administration of antiparkinsonian agents include:

- Patient (and significant others) will state ways of preventing self-injury such as use of assistive devices.
- Patient will state purposes, side effects, and toxic effects associated with the specific antiparkinso-

Patient Teaching TIPS

Dopaminergics

✔ Patients should change positions slowly because of the postural hypotension (drop in blood pressure with position changes) that can occur. Patients should take their time changing positions from lying to sitting and then gradually standing.

✔ Make sure patients know to report to their physician any of the following side effects that may indicate an overdose: excessive twitching, drooling, eye spasms.

✔ Patients should always take their medication exactly as prescribed and should not omit or double a dose. If an omission or error occurs in the administration of these (or any) medications, the physician should be notified immediately.

✔ Avoid sudden withdrawal of medication.

✔ Levodopa preparations may darken the patient's urine and sweat.

✔ Patients should be instructed to avoid taking vitamin B_6 supplements and eating vitamin-fortified foods. (Specific food examples [meats, poultry, fish, eggs, sweet potatoes, lima beans, and whole grain cereals] should be given to patients before they undertake home management or are discharged from the hospital.)

✔ These medications should be taken with juice and a low-protein snack or after meals so as to prevent interactions with pyridoxine (vitamin B_6) in food.

✔ Encourage patients to keep a journal of their progress and problems.

TAKE HOME POINTS

Neurotransmitter Abnormality in PD
■ Chronic, progressive, degenerative disorder of dopamine-producing neurons in brain.
■ Normal subject = balance between acetylcholine and dopamine levels in the CNS.
■ Patient with PD = raised acetylcholine and lowered dopamine levels.
■ Drug therapy = lower acetylcholine level and raise dopamine level.

Classic PD Symptoms
■ Bradykinesia (slow movements), rigidity (cogwheel), tremor (pill-rolling), and postural instability.
■ Dyskinesias = difficulty performing voluntary movements (two common ones = chorea and dystonias).
■ Chorea = irregular, spasmodic, involuntary movements of limbs or facial muscles.
■ Dystonias = abnormal muscle tone in any tissue.

Drug Therapy for PD
■ Neuroprotective, dopaminergic, and anticholinergic.
■ Neuroprotective = selegiline—may slow progression of PD.
■ Dopaminergic = indirect- and direct-acting and replacement drugs.
■ Indirect = release dopamine; direct = stimulate dopamine receptors (agonists); replacement = raise brain dopamine level.

Cornerstone = Levodopa
■ Levodopa and levodopa-carbidopa replace deficient dopamine in brain.
■ Levodopa = biologic precursor of dopamine.
■ Levodopa can pass through blood-brain barrier to get to site of action in the brain; dopamine cannot.

Carbidopa
■ Peripheral decarboxylase inhibitor.
■ Does not cross blood-brain barrier; prevents levodopa breakdown in periphery.

Patient Considerations
■ Require long-term care because of progressive and debilitating nature of illness.
■ Require much support and education.

nian medications such as emesis, nausea, instability, and palpitations.

■ Patient will state ways to prevent some of the side effects and toxic effects of antiparkinsonian medications such as frequent mouth care and increased fluids.

■ Patient will discuss ways to minimize problems associated with drug-induced alterations in bowel and bladder elimination patterns through changes in diet and fluid intake.

■ Patient will discuss measures to ensure an adequate nutritional status with possible antiemetic therapy.

■ Patient will begin to perform ADL more independently.

■ Patient will openly verbalize fears, anxieties, and changes in self-image with members of the health care team and supportive staff.

Critical Thinking **A C T I V I T I E S**

1. Mrs. Brad has been diagnosed with PD and has been prescribed levodopa. Her most distressing side effect is the dizziness and lightheadedness caused by the medication. What intervention would you, as her nurse, suggest and why?

2. Classic Parkinsonian symptoms include:
   a. bradykinesia
   b. postural stability
   c. flaccidity
   d. tremor with activity

▲▲

IMPLEMENTATION

Nursing actions related to the administration of the various antiparkinsonian agents focus primarily on safe drug administration and patient education. When patients are receiving anticholinergic agents, you should give oral doses after meals with single daily doses administered at bedtime. Fluid intake and frequent mouth care should be encouraged because of the dryness of mouth. Any intravenously administered medications, such as benztropine mesylate, should be given slowly, with the patient remaining in bed for an hour afterward. Patient teaching tips are presented on p. 159.

During the start of dopaminergic agent therapy, patients should be assisted when walking because of the dizziness caused by these agents. Oral doses should be given with food to help minimize GI upset. It is also important to remember that pyridoxine (vitamin B$_6$) in doses greater than 10 mg will reverse the effects of levodopa. Foods high in vitamin B$_6$ should therefore also be avoided. Patients should be encouraged to force fluids, unless contraindicated, drinking at least 2000 ml per day, as well as consume an adequate amount of food high in roughage and fiber. A hypertensive crisis may result if levodopa preparations are taken with MAOIs, so these drugs are generally not administered concurrently and at least 2 weeks should be allowed to elapse between the use of these medications. It is also important to remember that the dopaminergic agents are generally titrated to the patient's response. Patient teaching tips are presented on p. 160.

EVALUATION

Monitoring the patient's response to any of the antiparkinsonian medications is crucial to documenting treatment success or failure. Therapeutic responses to the antiparkinsonian agents include an improved sense of well-being; improved mental status; increase in appetite; ability to perform ADL, to concentrate and

to think clearly; and less intense parkinsonism manifestations such as less tremor, shuffling of gait, muscle rigidity, and involuntary movements. In addition to monitoring for therapeutic responses, you must also watch for the occurrence of side effects, such as confusion, anxiety, irritability, depression, paranoia, headache, weakness, lethargy, nausea, vomiting, anorexia, palpitations, postural hypotension, tachycardia, dry mouth, constipation, urinary retention, blurred vision, dark urine, difficulty swallowing, and nightmares.

BIBLIOGRAPHY

Ahlskog JE: Treatment of Parkinson's disease: from theory to practice, *Postgrad Med* 95 (5):52-4, 57-8, 61-4, 1994.

Albanese J, Nutz P: *Mosby's 1995 nursing drug cards*, St Louis, 1995, Mosby.

Cumming JL: Behavioral complications of drug treatment of Parkinson's disease, *J Am Geriatr Soc* 39:708, 1991.

Goetz CG et al: Update on Parkinson's disease, *Patient Care* 26:172, 1992.

Hodges LC: New drugs for Parkinson's disease, *J Neurosci Nursing* 22:254, 1990.

Johnson KB: *Harriet Lane handbook*, ed 13, St Louis, 1993, Mosby.

Keen JH: *Critical care and emergency drug reference*, St Louis, 1994, Mosby.

Knoben JE, Anderson PO: *Handbook of critical drug data*, ed 6, Hamilton, Ill, 1988, Drug Intelligence Publications.

Lieberman A: An integrated approach to patient management in Parkinson's disease, *Neurol Clin* 10:553, 1992.

McEvoy GK: *AHFS drug information*, Bethesda, Md, 1989, American Society of Hospital Pharmacists.

Pleet AB: Newly-diagnosed Parkinson's disease: a therapeutic update, *Geriatrics* 47:24, 1992.

Saint-Cyr JA: Neuropsychological and psychiatric side effects in the treatment of Parkinson's disease, *Neurology* 43(suppl 6):S47, 1993.

Skidmore-Roth L: *Mosby's 1995 nursing drug reference*, St Louis, 1995, Mosby.

Varon J, Jacobs MB: Treating the progressive stages of Parkinson's disease, *Postgrad Med* 90:63, 69, 1991.

Chapter 13

Psychotherapeutic Agents

Objectives

When you reach the end of this chapter, you will be able to:

1 Identify the various drugs in the following classes of psychotherapeutic agents: antianxiety agents, antidepressants, antimanic agents, and antipsychotics.

2 Discuss the mechanism of action, indications, therapeutic effects, side effects, toxic effects, drug interactions, contraindications, and cautions associated with the various psychotherapeutic agents.

3 Develop a nursing care plan as it relates to the nursing process and administration of the various psychotherapeutic agents.

4 Develop patient education guidelines for patients who are receiving psychotherapeutic drugs.

CHAPTER OUTLINE

Psychosis, Affective Disorders, and Anxiety

Antianxiety Agents
  Mechanism of action
  Drug effects
  Therapeutic uses
  Side effects and adverse effects
    Toxicity and management of overdose
  Interactions
  Dosages
Drug Profiles
Benzodiazepines
    Alprazolam
    Chlordiazepoxide
    Diazepam
    ⚓ Lorazepam
Miscellaneous Agents
    Meprobamate
    Hydroxyzine

Drugs Used to Treat Affective Disorders

Antidepressant Agents
  Cyclic antidepressants
    Mechanism of action
    Drug effects
    Therapeutic uses
    Side effects and adverse effects
      Toxicity and management of overdose
    Interactions
    Dosages

Drug Profiles
    Amoxapine
    ⚓ Amitriptyline
    Nortriptyline
Monoamine Oxidase Inhibitors
  Mechanism of action
  Drug effects
  Therapeutic uses
  Side effects and adverse effects
    Toxicity and management of overdose
  Interactions
  Dosages

Drug Profiles
    Phenelzine
    Tranylcypromine
Second-Generation Antidepressants
  Mechanism of action
  Drug effects
  Therapeutic uses
  Side effects and adverse effects
  Interactions
  Dosages

Drug Profiles
    Bupropion
    Trazodone
    ⚓ Fluoxetine
    Paroxetine
    Sertraline
Antimanic Agents

continued

Antipsychotic Agents
  Mechanism of action
  Drug effects
  Therapeutic uses
  Side effects and adverse effects
  Interactions
  Dosages
Drug Profiles
Phenothiazines
    Chlorpromazine
    Fluphenazine
Thioxanthenes
    Thiothixene
Butyrophenones
  ⚓ Haloperidol
Dihydroindolones
    Molindone
Dibenzoxazepines
    Loxapine
Dibenzodiazepines
  ⚓ Clozapine
Nursing Process
Assessment
Nursing Diagnoses
Planning
  Outcome criteria
Implementation
Evaluation

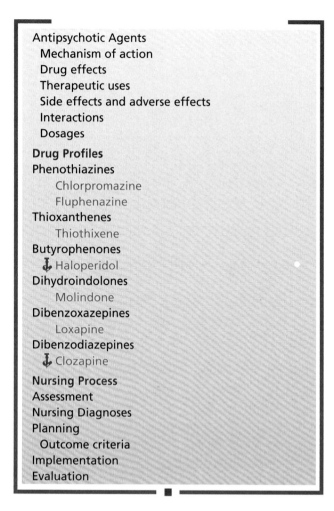

Glossary

Affective disorders (a fec′ tiv) Those emotional disorders that are characterized by changes in mood. (p. 164)

Agoraphobia (a gə rə fō bēə) Fear of leaving the familiar setting of home. (p. 164)

Antihistamine (-his tə mēn) Any substance capable of reducing the physiologic and pharmacologic effects of histamine, including a wide variety of drugs that block histamine receptors. (p. 165)

Antipsychotic (-sī kä tik) Of or pertaining to a substance or procedure that counteracts or diminishes symptoms of serious mental illness. (p. 180)

Anxiety The unpleasant state of mind in which unreal or imagined dangers are anticipated. (p. 164)

Barbiturates (bar bi chə rət) One of the oldest drug classes used to treat anxiety. (p. 165)

Benzodiazepine (bən zō dī a′ zə pen) One of a group of psychotropic agents prescribed to alleviate anxiety. (p. 165)

Biogenic amine hypothesis (BAH) Theory suggesting that depression and mania are due to alterations in neu-

ronal and synaptic catecholamine concentrations. (p. 170)

Bipolar affective disorder (BAD) A major psychologic disorder characterized by episodes of mania, depression, or mixed mood. (p. 164)

Buspirone (BuSpar) (boo spi rōn) An oral antianxiety drug. (p. 165)

Carbamates (kahr bə māt) One of the oldest drug classes used to treat anxiety. (p. 165)

Depression (de presh′ ən) An abnormal emotional state characterized by exaggerated feelings of sadness, melancholy, dejection, worthlessness, emptiness, and hopelessness that are inappropriate and out of proportion to reality. (p. 164)

Diazepam (di az′ ə pam) A benzodiazepam sedative and tranquilizer. (p. 165)

Dysregulation hypothesis Views depression and affective disorders as not simply decreased or increased catecholamine activity, but as failures of the regulation of these systems. (p. 170)

Flumazenil (Romazicon) (floo ma′ zə nil) A benzodiazepine receptor blocker that directly opposes the actions of the benzodiazepines. (p. 166)

Gamma-aminobutyric acid (GABA) An inhibitory amino acid in the brain that functions to inhibit nerve transmission in the central nervous system. (p. 165)

Lorazepam (lor az′ ə pam) A benzodiazepine tranquilizer. (p. 165)

Mania (mā ne ə) A state characterized by an expansive emotional state, extreme excitement, excessive elation, hyperactivity, agitation, overtalkativeness, flight of ideas, increased psychomotor activity, fleeting attention, and sometimes violent, destructive, and self-destructive behavior. (p. 164)

Midazolam (mid a′ zo lam) A parenteral central nervous system depressant. (p. 165)

Monoamine oxidase inhibitor (MAOI) (mon o′ ə mēn ok′ sĭ dās) Any of a heterogeneous group of drugs used primarily in the treatment of depression. These drugs also exert an antianxiety effect, especially anxiety associated with phobia. (p. 165)

Permissive hypothesis Implicates reduced concentrations of serotonin (5-HT) as the predisposing factor in individuals with affective disorders. (p. 170)

Psychosis (sī ko′ sis) Term used to describe a major emotional disorder that impairs the mental function of the affected individual to the point that the individual cannot participate in everyday life. (p. 164)

Psychotherapeutics (sī kō ther ə pu′ tiks) Refers to the therapy of emotional and mental disorders. (p. 164)

Tetracyclic (tet rə sik′ lik) Antidepressant agent used to treat anxiety disorders. (p. 165)

Tricyclic (trī sik′ lik) Antidepressant agents, such as amitryptyline and imipramine hydrochloride, that block reuptake of amine neurotransmitters, but the exact mechanism of antidepressant action of these drugs is unknown. (p. 165)

The treatment of emotional and mental disorders is called **psychotherapeutics.** When a person's ability to cope with his or her environment—to carry out the activities of daily living and to interact with others—is seriously impaired, a psychotropic drug may be a treatment option. These drugs are among the most commonly prescribed drugs in the United States today. To understand better the nature and goals of this treatment, the types and definitions of these various disorders are first presented.

Psychosis, Affective Disorders, and Anxiety

Most people experience emotions such as anxiety, depression, and grief. They are normal human emotions. However, the effect of these emotions on one's ability to engage in normal daily activities and to interact with others can vary considerably, and the duration and intensity of these emotions can range from occasional depression or anxiety to a state of constant emotional distress that interferes with one's ability to carry on normal activities of daily living.

There are three main emotional and mental disorders: psychoses, affective disorders, and anxiety. A **psychosis** is a major emotional disorder that impairs mental functioning to the point where the person cannot participate in everyday life. A hallmark of psychosis is a loss of contact with reality. These behavioral problems or psychotic disorders include depressive and drug-induced psychoses, schizophrenia, and autism.

Affective disorders are characterized by changes in mood and range from **mania** (abnormally pronounced emotions) to **depression** (abnormally reduced emotions). Some patients may exhibit both mania and depression, experiencing periodic swings in emotions, from extremely reduced emotions to very intense, hyperactive emotions, and this is referred to as a **bipolar affective disorder** (BAD).

Anxiety is the unpleasant state of mind in which unreal or imagined dangers are anticipated. It is divided into several distinct disorders and these have been classified by the American Psychiatric Association and the classification published in the *Diagnostic and Statistical Manual for Mental Disorders*, third edition, revised (DSM-III-R). This reference delineates the demographic features and diagnostic criteria for the major psychiatric disorders and has categorized anxiety into the following disorders:

- Obsessive-compulsive disorder
- Posttraumatic stress disorder
- Generalized anxiety disorder
- Panic disorder
- Social phobia
- Simple phobia

Anxiety is a normal physiologic emotion, but the results of epidemiologic studies show that 2% to 6% of adults suffer from a generalized anxiety disorder, 1% from a panic disorder, and 4% to 5% from **agoraphobia,** or fear of leaving the familiar setting of home. The obsessive-compulsive disorder was thought to be rare but is now observed to be twice as common as schizophrenia or panic disorders in the general population. Anxiety may occur as a result of a wide range of medical illnesses (e.g., cardiovascular or pulmonary disease, hypothyroidism, hyperthyroidism, pheochromocytoma, and hypoglycemia). Many of the anxiety disorders are situational. They arise because of a specific event and subside with time. The treatment of these should be limited to psychotherapy. However, when the anxiety disorder markedly affects one's quality of life and relationships or interferes with one's ability to function normally, pharmacotherapy, or drug treatment, in conjunction with psychotherapy becomes desirable, and both should be instituted.

The exact causes of mental disorders are not fully understood. Many theories have been advanced in an attempt to explain the causes and pathophysiology of mental dysfunction. In the biochemical imbalance concept, mental disorders are thought to arise as the result of abnormal levels of endogenous chemicals in the brain such as neurotransmitters. There is strong evidence indicating that the brain levels of the catecholamines (especially dopamine) and the indolamines (serotonin and histamine) play an important role in maintaining mental health. Other biochemicals that seem necessary for the maintenance of normal mental function are gamma-aminobutyric acid (GABA), acetylcholine, and various inorganic ions such as lithium. A knowledge of these various etiologies, especially the biochemical imbalance theory, can aid in an understanding of psychotherapeutic drug action because many of the agents used to treat psychoses, affective disorders, and anxiety block or stimulate the release of these endogenous mediators.

ANTIANXIETY AGENTS

Medications are only one of the many therapeutic options in persons afflicted with the various anxiety disorders. Although the benzodiazepines are generally the first-line drug treatment for anxiety disorders, there are other classes of drugs that are also effective. The efficacy of certain classes of medications in the

Table 13-1	Various Anxiety Disorders: Drugs of Choice			
DISORDER	**TCA**	**BENZO-DIAZEPINE**	**MAOI**	**BUSPIRONE**
Panic disorder	+++	++++	+++	0
Generalized anxiety disorder	+	++++	?++	+++
Obsessive-compulsive disorder	+++	?+	?+	0
Posttraumatic stress disorder	+	?+	+	?+
Simple phobia	0	+	0	0
Social phobia	+	+	+	0

TCA, tricyclic and tetracyclic antidepressants; *MAOI,* monoamine oxidase inhibitors; ? = has shown some efficacy but limited use; +, limited use and efficacy; ++, some use and efficacy; +++, frequent use, good efficacy; ++++, most frequent use, best efficacy; 0, no efficacy or use.

treatment of certain anxiety disorders and their superiority over other drug classes have been documented. These various drug classes are listed in Table 13-1 according to the anxiety disorders they are effective in treating.

Mechanism of Action

Of the several drug classes shown to be effective in the treatment of anxiety disorders, all reduce anxiety by reducing overactivity in the CNS. There are, however, differences among the various drug classes.

The **benzodiazepines** seem to exert their anxiolytic effects by depressing activity in the areas of the brain called the *brainstem* and the *limbic system.* Benzodiazepines are believed to accomplish this by increasing the action of **GABA,** an inhibitory amino acid in the brain that functions to inhibit nerve transmission in the CNS. The benzodiazepines have binding sites in the same channels that govern the release of GABA. The binding of benzodiazepines with these sites produces not only an anxiolytic effect but also sedation and muscle relaxation.

There are several other drug classes used for the treatment of anxiety disorders. The **barbiturates** and **carbamates** are probably the oldest such drug classes. Their anxiolytic properties are related to their ability to depress CNS activity and cause sedation. These

agents have many undesirable side effects that make them poor drugs for the long-term treatment of anxiety. They are heavily sedating, they interact with many other drugs, and they interfere with normal sleep patterns (suppress rapid eye movement sleep). Meprobamate is one of the more frequently prescribed carbamates used to relieve anxiety.

Antihistamines are also used as anxiolytics because of their ability to depress the CNS by sedating the patient. The antihistamine most commonly used for the relief of anxiety is hydroxyzine. It has few antihistaminic properties but is very sedating. There are two salt forms of hydroxyzine: hydroxyzine hydrochloride (Atarax) and hydroxyzine pamoate (Vistaril), both of which are effective anxiolytics.

Monoamine oxidase inhibitors (MAOI), **buspirone** (BuSpar), and **tricyclic** and **tetracyclic** antidepressants have also been used to treat anxiety disorders. These agents are discussed in greater detail in the section of this chapter, Antidepressant Agents. They relieve anxiety by decreasing overactivity in the CNS.

Drug Effects

Beside their anxiolytic effects just mentioned, the drugs produce several other effects throughout the body. These are sedative, hypnotic, appetite stimulating, analgesic, and anticonvulsant effects. Because of their wide range of effects, they are used for a variety of indications.

Therapeutic Uses

The carbamates such as meprobamate are not only used as anxiolytics but also as sedative-hypnotics. The barbiturates such as phenobarbital are also used in the treatment of seizures, insomnia, hyperbilirubinemia, and chronic cholestasis and for their sedative effects. The antihistamines are used to treat anxiety because of their sedative side effects, but their actual intended therapeutic effect is to block the actions of histamine released in the setting of allergies. The tricyclic antidepressants and the selective serotonin-reuptake inhibitors such as fluoxetine are also indicated for the treatment of depression.

However, it is the benzodiazepines that are the largest and most commonly prescribed anxiolytic drug class because they offer several advantages over these other drug classes used to treat anxiety. At therapeutic doses they have little effect on consciousness, they are very safe from the standpoint of their side effect profile, and they do not interact with many other drugs. Three very commonly prescribed anxiolytic benzodiazepines are **diazepam** (Valium), **lorazepam** (Ativan), and **midazolam** (Versed). They also have a wide va-

Table 13-2	Benzodiazepines: Approved Indications

APPROVED INDICATIONS	BENZODIAZEPINES
Alcohol withdrawal	Chlordiazepoxide, diazepam, lorazepam, oxazepam
Anxiety	Alprazolam, chlordiazepoxide, clorazepate, diazepam, halazepam, ↓lorazepam, oxazepam, prazepam
Depression	Alprazolam, oxazepam
Muscle spasm	Diazepam
Preoperative sedation	Chlordiazepoxide, diazepam, ↓lorazepam
Seizure disorders	Clorazepate, diazepam

Table 13-3	Benzodiazepines: Common Adverse Effects

BODY SYSTEM	SIDE/ADVERSE EFFECTS
Central nervous system	Drowsiness, sedation, loss of coordination, dizziness, blurred vision, headaches, paradoxical reactions (insomnia, increased excitability, hallucinations)
Gastrointestinal	Nausea, vomiting, constipation, dry mouth, abdominal cramping
Other	Pruritus, skin rash

riety of therapeutic applications. They are used to relieve anxiety, sedate, produce muscle relaxation, control seizures, treat depression, and treat alcohol withdrawal, to cite just a few of the many therapeutic applications of this very safe and effective drug class. The benzodiazepines commonly used as sedative-hypnotics are described in Chapter 10 and have slightly different therapeutic actions from those of the benzodiazepines used to treat anxiety. The commonly used anxiolytic benzodiazepines and their approved indications are listed in Table 13-2.

Side Effects and Adverse Effects

The most common undesirable effect of the anxiolytic drugs is an overexpression of their therapeutic effects. All these classes of drugs decrease CNS activity, and many of the unwanted effects of these agents are related directly to this action. The most common side effects and adverse effects of the benzodiazepines are listed in Table 13-3.

Toxicity and Management of Overdose

There is a potential for the benzodiazepines to cause serious life-threatening toxicities, but when taken in normal doses in otherwise healthy persons, they are very safe, effective anxiolytics. When taken along with other sedating medications or with alcohol, life-threatening respiratory depression or arrest can occur. This serious consequence can also occur in persons whose metabolism or elimination capabilities are impaired because of liver or kidney dysfunction. In such settings the benzodiazepines can accumulate and not be eliminated. This further accentuates their therapeu-

tic and toxic actions. An overdose of benzodiazepines may result in one or any combination of the following symptoms: somnolence, confusion, coma, or respiratory depression.

The treatment of benzodiazepine intoxication is generally symptomatic and supportive. If ingestion is recent, decontamination of the gastrointestinal system is indicated. As a rule of thumb, gastric decontamination using syrup of ipecac (an agent used to induce vomiting in overdose) is contraindicated in persons who have ingested medications that cause sedation because of the risk of aspiration of the stomach contents. Therefore gastric lavage is generally the best and most effective means of gastric decontamination. Activated charcoal and a saline cathartic may be administered after gastric lavage to remove any remaining drug. Hemodialysis is not useful in the treatment of benzodiazepine overdose.

Many of the benzodiazepines' therapeutic and toxic effects are mediated by receptors in the CNS. Therefore **Flumazenil** (Romazicon), a benzodiazepine receptor blocker (antagonist), is used to reverse the effects of benzodiazepine overdose. It directly opposes the actions of the benzodiazepines by directly competing with benzodiazepines for binding at the benzodiazepine receptors in the CNS. It has a stronger affinity for the receptor and thus knocks the benzodiazepine off from the receptor, reversing the sedative action of the benzodiazepine. The treatment regimen for the reversal of benzodiazepine overdose is summarized in Table 13-4.

Interactions

There are a wide variety of drug interactions that occur with the use of the anxiolytics, particularly the benzodiazepines. The most significant of these are listed in the Table 13-5.

Table 13-4	Flumazenil Treatment Regimen	
RECOMMENDED REGIMEN		**DURATION**
0.2 mg (2 ml) given IV over 30 sec; wait 30 sec; if still no response, give 0.2 mg (2 ml); may repeat at 60-sec intervals as needed up to four additional times (maximum total dose, 1 mg)		1-4 hr

Important note: Flumazenil has a relatively short half-life and duration of effect of 1 to 4 hr; therefore, if the intent is to reverse a long-acting benzodiazepine, the effects of the flumazenil may wear off and the effects of the benzodiazepine may reappear.

Table 13-5	Benzodiazepines: Drug Interactions	
DRUG	**MECHANISM**	**RESULTS**
Alcohol CNS depressants	Additive effect	Increased depression
Cimetidine Disulfiram MAOIs Tobacco	Decreased metabolism	

D O S A G E S

SELECTED ANTIANXIETY AGENTS

AGENT	PHARMACOLOGIC CLASS	DOSAGE RANGE	PURPOSE
Alprazolam (Xanax)	Benzodiazepine	*Adult* PO: 0.25-0.5 mg tid. Do not exceed 4 mg/day *Geriatric* PO: 0.25 mg 2-3 times/day	Anxiolytic Anxiolytic
Chlordiazepoxide (Librium)	Benzodiazepine	*Pediatric* PO: >6 y/o, 5 mg 2-4 times/day *Adult* PO: 5-25 mg 3-4 times/day IM/IV: 50-100 mg; then 25 mg 3-4 times/day for severe anxiety 50-100 mg q2-4h prn for alcoholism 50-100 mg IM before surgery	Anxiolytic Preop sedation
Diazepam (Valium)	Benzodiazepine	*Pediatric* PO: >6 mo: 1.25 mg 3-4 times/day *Adult* PO: 2-10 mg 2-4 times/day *Geriatric* PO: 2-2.5 mg 1-2 times/day *Pediatric* IM/IV: > 30 days: 1-2 mg repeated in 3-4 hr prn ≥5 y/o: 5-10 mg repeated in 3-4 hr prn >30 days: 0.2-0.5 mg q2-5 min to a maximum of 5 mg ≥5 y/o: 1 mg q2-5 min to a maximum of 10 mg *Adult* IM/IV: 2-10 mg repeated in 3-4 hr prn 10 mg followed by 5-10 mg in 3-4 hr prn 5-10 mg IV w/in 5-10 min before procedure 10 mg IM before surgery 5-10 mg repeated in 3-4 hr prn 5-10 mg repeated at 10- to 15-min intervals to a maximum of 30 mg. Repeat in 3-4 hr prn.	Anxiety, alcoholism, muscle spasm, convulsive disorders Tetanus Tetanus Status epilepticus Status epilepticus Anxiety Alcoholism Cardioversion Preop sedation Muscle spasm Status epilepticus

continued

SELECTED ANTIANXIETY AGENTS—cont'd

AGENT	PHARMACOLOGIC CLASS	DOSAGE RANGE	PURPOSE
⚓Lorazepam (Ativan)	Benzodiazepine	*Adult* PO: 2-6 mg/day divided PO: 2-4 mg HS IM: 0.05 mg/kg to a maximum of 4 mg IV: 2-4 mg	Anxiolytic Hypnotic Preop sedation Preop sedation
Meprobamate (Equanil, Miltown)	Carbamate	*Pediatric* 6-12 y/o PO: 100-200 mg 2-3 times/day *Adult* PO: 1.2-1.6 d/d in 3-4 divided doses	Anxiolytic Anxiolytic
Hydroxyzine (Atarax, Vistaril)	Antihistamine	*Pediatric* <6 y/o PO: 50 mg/day divided ≥6 y/o: PO: 50-100 mg/day divided PO: 0.6 mg/kg IM: 1.1 mg/kg *Adult* PO: 50-100 mg qid IM: 50-100 mg q4-6h PO: 25 mg 3-4 times/day PO: 50-100 mg IM: 25-100 mg IM: 25-100 mg	Anxiolytic/pruritus Pre/postop sedation Nausea vomiting Anxiolytic Anxiolytic Pruritus Pre/postpartum sedation Nausea/vomiting Nausea/vomiting

Dosages

For the recommended dosages of selected antianxiety agents, see the dosages table on p. 167.

DRUG PROFILES

BENZODIAZEPINES

Benzodiazepines are contraindicated in patients who have shown a hypersensitivity reaction to them and in patients who have narrow-angle glaucoma. They are all prescription-only drugs, and they are all FDA pregnancy category D agents. They are also all scheduled drugs: chlorazepate is a schedule II drug, and the rest are schedule IV drugs.

ALPRAZOLAM

Alprazolam (Xanax) is most commonly used as an anxiolytic and for the treatment of depression. It is only available for oral administration as a 0.25-, 0.5-, and 1-mg tablet. The 0.25-mg tablet is the dose recommended for the geriatric patient. The commonly recommended dosages are given in the table on p. 167.

� PHARMACOKINETICS

HALF-LIFE	ONSET	PEAK	Duration
11-16 hr	<1 hr	1-2 hr	6-12 hr

CHLORDIAZEPOXIDE

Chlordiazepoxide (Librium) is used for many indications but is most frequently used for the treatment of alcohol withdrawal, for the relief of anxiety, and as a preoperative sedative agent. Chlordiazepoxide combined with the antimuscarinic drug clidinium is Librax, and this is used as an adjunct in the treatment of peptic ulcer disease. It is available orally as a 5-, 10-, and 25-mg capsule and intravenously as a 20-mg/ml injection. The commonly recommended dosages are given in the table on p. 167.

� PHARMACOKINETICS

HALF-LIFE	ONSET	PEAK	DURATION
9-34 hr	30-60 min	0.5-4 hr	12-24 hr

DIAZEPAM

Diazepam (Valium) is the most frequently prescribed benzodiazepine. It is indicated for the relief of anxiety, alcohol withdrawal, and seizure disorders like status epilepticus, for sedation, and as an adjunct for the relief of skeletal muscle spasms. Diazepam has active metabolites that can accumulate in patients who have renal or hepatic dysfunction, and this can result in additive, cumulative effects that may be manifested as prolonged sedation, respiratory depression, or coma. It is available orally as a 2-, 5-, and 10-mg tablet and intravenously as a 5-mg/ml injection. The commonly recommended dosages are given in the table on p. 167.

✸ PHARMACOKINETICS

HALF-LIFE	ONSET	PEAK	DURATION
20-50 hr	30-60 min	1-2 hr	12-24 hr

⚓ LORAZEPAM

Lorazepam (Ativan) is a widely used benzodiazepine. It is currently approved for use in the management of anxiety disorders, for the short-term relief of anxiety, and as a preoperative medication to provide sedation and light anesthesia and to diminish patient recall (amnesia). It has also shown good efficacy in the prevention and treatment of chemotherapy-related nausea and vomiting and of the symptoms of acute alcohol withdrawal. It is available orally as a 0.5-, 1-, and 2-mg tablet and intravenously as a 2- or 4-mg/ml injection. It may also be administered sublingually. When administered in this fashion, its onset of action is similar to that associated with intravenous administration but without the inconveniences. The commonly recommended dosages are given in the table on p. 168.

✸ PHARMACOKINETICS

HALF-LIFE	ONSET	PEAK	DURATION
IV: 12-16 hr	IV: rapid	IV: 15-20 min	IV: 4 hr
PO: 12-16 hr	PO: 15-45 min	PO: 2 hr	PO: 12-24 hr

MISCELLANEOUS AGENTS

There are several categories of drugs that can be used in the treatment of anxiety disorders. Although the benzodiazepines are by far the most widely prescribed anxiolytics, often drugs in other categories may be prescribed because of certain advantages they offer. Some of the more commonly used drugs are described in the following sections. The efficacy of the carbamates in treating anxiety disorders, with meprobamate the prototype, has been shown. The antihistamine hydroxyzine and the nonbenzodiazepine anxiolytic buspirone are also very effective antianxiety agents.

MEPROBAMATE

Meprobamate (Equanil, Miltown) is a carbamate-derivative anxiolytic agent. It is the most frequently prescribed carbamate drug for the treatment of anxiety disorders. It is not as frequently prescribed as the benzodiazepines because of its high tendency to cause sedation and interfere with motor coordination, and because tolerance rapidly develops in patients taking it. It is contraindicated in patients who have shown a hypersensitivity reaction to carbamates. Meprobamate is similar to the benzodiazepines in that it is also a schedule IV controlled substance and is considered a pregnancy category D drug. It is only available orally as a 200-, 400-, and 600-mg tablet. The commonly recommended dosages are given in the table on p. 168.

✸ PHARMACOKINETICS

HALF-LIFE	ONSET	PEAK	DURATION
PO: 6-16 hr	<1 hr	1-3 hr	6-12 hr
PO sus rel: 6-16 hr	Unknown	Unknown	Up to 12 hr

HYDROXYZINE

Hydroxyzine is available in two different salt forms: the hydrochloride salt (Atarax) and the pamoate salt (Vistaril). Both forms are used to treat anxiety disorders. Hydroxyzine is an antihistamine that suppresses activity in the CNS, which makes it useful as both an anxiolytic and antiemetic agent. It is available orally as a 10-mg/5 ml solution; a 25-mg/5 ml suspension; a 10-, 25-, 50-, and 100-mg tablet and capsule; and a 10-, 25-, and 50-mg film-coated tablet. It is also available as a 25- and 50-mg/ml intramuscular injection. The commonly recommended dosages are given in the table on p. 168. Pregnancy category C.

✸ PHARMACOKINETICS

HALF-LIFE	ONSET	PEAK	DURATION
3 hr	15-30 hr	30-60 min	4-6 hr

Drugs Used to Treat Affective Disorders

Several classes of drugs are used in the treatment of the affective disorders. The two main drug categories are the antidepressants and the antimanic agents.

ANTIDEPRESSANT AGENTS

Antidepressants are the pharmacologic treatment of choice for major depressive disorders. Not only are they very effective in treating depression, they are also useful for treating other disorders, such as dysthymia, schizophrenia, eating disorders, and personality disorders. These agents are also commonly used in the treatment of various medical conditions, including migraine headaches, chronic pain syndromes, peptic ulcer disease, and sleep disorders.

Many of the drugs currently used to treat affective disorders increase neurotransmitter concentrations in the CNS. This is based on the belief that alterations in the levels of certain neurotransmitters in the CNS are responsible for causing depression. One of the most widely held hypotheses advanced to explain depression in these terms is the **biogenic amine hypothesis (BAH).** Specifically, it postulates that depression results from a deficiency of neuronal and synaptic catecholamines (primarily norepinephrine) and mania from an excess of amines at the adrenergic receptor sites in the brain. This hypothesis is illustrated in Fig. 13-1.

Another hypothesis advanced to explain the etiology of affective disorders is the **permissive hypothesis.** It implicates reduced concentrations of serotonin as the predisposing factor in patients with affective disorders. While depression results from decreases in both the serotonin and catecholamine levels, mania results from increased catecholamine but decreased serotonin levels. The permissive hypothesis is illustrated in Fig. 13-2.

A new leading theory attempting to explain the etiology of affective disorders is the **dysregulation hypothesis.** It is essentially a reformulation of the biogenic amine hypothesis. It views depression and affective disorders not simply in terms of decreased or increased catecholamine activity but as a failure of the regulation of these systems.

The drug categories most commonly used in the treatment of affective disorders are the tricyclic and tetracyclic antidepressants, the selective serotonin-reuptake inhibitors (SSRIs), and the monoamine oxidase inhibitors (MAOIs).

Cyclic Antidepressants

Within the cyclic antidepressant drug class there are agents that have a tricyclic chemical structure and those that have a tetracyclic structure. Although they are different structurally, they are similar pharmacologically and therapeutically.

Mechanism of Action

The cyclic antidepressants (tricyclics and tetracyclics) are believed to work by correcting the imbalance in the neurotransmitter concentrations at the nerve endings in the CNS (the biogenic amine hypothesis). This is accomplished by blocking the reuptake of the neurotransmitters and thus causing these neurotransmitters to accumulate at the nerve endings. (It stands to reason that if depression is the result of abnormally low concentrations of these neurotransmitters, then an agent like a cyclic antidepressant that causes the concentrations of neurotransmitters to increase at nerve endings should alleviate the depression.) Some also believe that these agents may help regulate malfunctioning nerves (the dysregulation hypothesis).

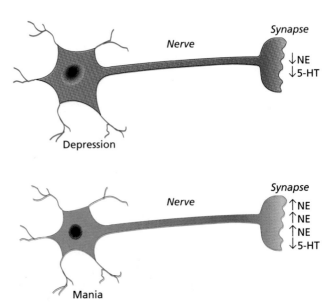

▼ FIG. 13-1 Biogenic amine hypothesis. *NE,* norepinephrine.

▼ FIG. 13-2 The permissive hypothesis. *NE,* norepinephrine; *5-HT,* serotonin.

Table 13-6	Cyclic Antidepressants: Therapeutic and Undesirable Drug Effects by Receptor Site
BLOCKADE OF:	**DRUG EFFECT***
Norepinephrine reuptake	*Antidepressant,* tremors, tachycardia, additive pressor effects with sympathomimetic drugs
Serotonin reuptake	*Antidepressant,* nausea, headache, anxiety
Muscarinic receptors	Dry mouth, constipation, blurred vision, tachycardia, urinary retention
Histaminergic receptors	Sedation, weight gain, hypotension
Adrenergic receptors	Orthostatic hypotension, antihypertensive effects
Dopaminergic receptors	Extrapyramidal and endocrine side effects
Serotonergic receptors	*Alleviation of rhinitis,* hypotension

*Italicized effects are the desirable ones.

Table 13-7	Cyclic Antidepressants: Adverse Effects
BODY SYSTEM	**SIDE/ADVERSE EFFECTS**
Cardiovascular	Tremors, tachycardia, orthostatic hypotension, dysrhythmias
Central nervous system	Anxiety, confusion, extrapyramidal effects, sedation
Gastrointestinal	Nausea, constipation, dry mouth
Other	Blurred vision, urinary retention, weight gain, impotence

Drug Effects

The cyclic antidepressants have several advantageous therapeutic effects, but their use is also associated with many adverse effects. Both these advantageous and adverse effects can be explained by the functions of the various receptors these agents affect. As already mentioned, the cyclic antidepressants' therapeutic effects result from their ability to inhibit the reuptake of norepinephrine and serotonin at the nerve endings, but they also block muscarinic, histaminergic, adrenergic, dopaminergic, and serotonergic receptors, and this is responsible for their adverse effects. The therapeutic and undesirable effects as they relate to the receptors affected are presented in Table 13-6.

Therapeutic Uses

The cyclic antidepressants are considered to be the first-line agents in the pharmacologic treatment of depression. The tricyclic antidepressants (TCAs) have been available for more than 40 years and are widely prescribed. Overall they have demonstrated a remarkable efficacy, and their side effect profiles are well established. They are also considerably less expensive than most of the newer agents, with many of them available in generic formulations. Imipramine and desipramine are probably the most widely prescribed of the TCAs. In addition, imipramine is used as an adjunct in the treatment of childhood enuresis (bed wetting), and clomipramine is useful in the treatment of obsessive-compulsive disorders. Besides their bene-

ficial antidepressant effects, the TCAs are useful as adjunctive analgesics. TCAs have also been used in the treatment of trigeminal neuralgia. Their therapeutic effects are given in Table 13-6.

Side Effects and Adverse Effects

The most frequent undesirable effects of the cyclic antidepressants are due to their effects on various receptors, mostly the muscarinic receptors. Blockade of these receptors by TCAs results in many undesirable anticholinergic side effects and adverse effects, the most common ones being sedation, anticholinergic effects, impotence, and orthostatic hypotension. The various undesirable effects as they relate to body systems are listed in Table 13-7.

Toxicity and Management of Overdose. TCA overdoses are notoriously lethal. It is estimated that 70% to 80% of those who die of TCA overdose do so before reaching the hospital. The primary organ systems affected are the CNS and cardiovascular system, and death usually results from either seizures or arrhythmias. There is no specific antidote for TCA poisoning. Management efforts are aimed at decreasing drug absorption through the administration of multiple doses of activated charcoal; speeding up elimination by alkalinizing the urine to a pH of greater than 7.55; minimizing damage resulting from CNS and cardiovascular events by giving diazepam for the control seizures or antiarrhythmics for the control of arrhythmias; and providing basic life support.

Interactions

There are a wide variety of drug interactions that occur with the cyclic antidepressants; the most significant ones are listed in Table 13-8.

Dosages

For the recommended dosages for selected tricyclic antidepressant agents, see the dosages table on the next page.

Table 13-8	Cyclic Antidepressants: Drug Interactions	
DRUG	**MECHANISM**	**RESULTS**
Adrenergics (e.g., norepinephrine, epinephrine)		Increased sympathetic stimulation
Anticholinergics		
Chlorpromazine	Additive	Increased atropine-like effects
CNS depressants		Increased CNS depression
MAOIs		Increased therapeutic and toxic effects
Warfarin	Inhibits metabolism	Increased anticoagulation effect

DOSAGES

SELECTED CYCLIC ANTIDEPRESSANTS

AGENT	PHARMACOLOGIC CLASS	DOSAGE RANGE	PURPOSE
Amoxapine (Asendin)	Tetracyclic antidepressant	*Adult* PO: 150-300 mg/day divided *Geriatric* PO: 100-150 mg/day divided	
Amitriptyline (Elavil, Endep)	Tricyclic antidepressant	*Adolescent/Geriatric* PO: 10 mg tid, 20 mg HS *Adult* PO: 75-300 mg/day divided *Adult* IM: 20-30 mg qid	Depression
Nortriptyline (Aventyl, Pamelor)	Tricyclic antidepressant	*Adolescent/Geriatric* PO: 30-50 mg/day divided *Adult* PO: 25-100 mg/day divided	

DRUG PROFILES

The cyclic antidepressants are very effective agents in the treatment of various affective disorders, but they are also associated with serious side effects, and thus patients taking them need to be monitored closely. For this reason all the antidepressants are only available with a prescription. Virtually all are rated as pregnancy category C agents, except maprotiline, which is classified as a category B agent.

There are many drugs in the cyclic antidepressant drug class. Within the drug category there are the tertiary and secondary TCAs and the tetracyclic antidepressants. These are also sometimes referred to as the *first-generation antidepressants* because they were the first agents within the cyclic antidepressant drug class to be developed for this purpose. Following is a list of the various cyclic antidepressants according to their respective categories.

Tertiary TCAs	Secondary TCAs	Tetracyclic antidepressants
Amitriptyline	Desipramine	Amoxapine
Doxepin	Nortriptyline	Maprotiline
Imipramine	Protriptyline	
Trimipramine		

AMOXAPINE

Amoxapine (Asendin) is structurally similar to the neuroleptic drug loxapine and is one of the tetracyclic antidepressants. It offers some advantages over older drugs within the cyclic antidepressant class in that it primarily inhibits norepinephrine uptake and is less sedating than other TCAs. Disadvantages to its use are that it causes some of the side effects associated with the neuroleptics, such as extrapyramidal side effects, tardive dyskinesia, and the neuroleptic malignant syndrome. Amoxapine is only available orally as a 10-, 25-, 50-, 75-, 100-, and 150-mg tablet. The commonly recommended dosages are given in the table on p. 172.

❂ P H A R M A C O K I N E T I C S

HALF-LIFE	ONSET	PEAK	DURATION
8-30 hr	1-2 wk	2-6 wk	6-12 hr

⚓ AMITRIPTYLINE

Amitriptyline (Elavil, Endep) is one of the oldest and most widely used of all the TCAs. It is the prototypical tertiary-amine TCA and is also used in the treatment of various pain disorders such as trigeminal neuralgia. It has very potent anticholinergic properties, which can lead to many adverse effects such as dry mouth, constipation, blurred vision, urinary retention, and arrhythmias. There are two combination products that contain amitriptyline: Limbitrol, which also contains chlordiazepoxide, and Eltrafon or Triavil, which also contains perphenazine. Amitriptyline is available orally as a 10-, 25-, 50-, 75-, 100-, and 150-mg tablet and intravenously as a 10-mg/ml injection. The commonly recommended dosages are given in the table on p. 172.

❂ P H A R M A C O K I N E T I C S

HALF-LIFE	ONSET	PEAK	DURATION
10-50 hr	45 min	2-12 hr	6-12 hr

NORTRIPTYLINE

Nortriptyline (Aventyl, Pamelor) is one of the prototypical secondary-amine TCAs. It is only available orally as either a 10-mg/5 ml solution or as a 10-, 25-, 50-, and 75-mg tablet. The commonly recommended dosages are given in the table on p. 172.

❂ P H A R M A C O K I N E T I C S

HALF-LIFE	ONSET	PEAK	DURATION
18-90 hr	1-2 hr	7-8.5 hr	Variable

MONOAMINE OXIDASE INHIBITORS

The MAOIs are highly effective antidepressants. They are useful clinically for the treatment of any type of depression but are especially useful for the atypical types such as those characterized by reverse vegetative symptoms (increased sleep and appetite) or by marked panic, phobic, or other anxiety symptoms. In general they are considered second-line agents for the treatment of depression that is not responsive to other pharmacologic therapies such as the TCAs. Although MAOIs are effective in the treatment of these disorders, a serious disadvantage to their use is their potential to cause a hypertensive crisis when taken with a substance containing tyramine.

The available MAOI antidepressants phenelzine (Nardil) and tranylcypromine (Parnate) are nonselective inhibitors of both types A and B MAO. Type A is the predominant type of MAO in nerve endings. It preferentially metabolizes serotonin and norepinephrine. On the other hand, type B MAO is the primary type of MAO in the gastrointestinal tract and platelets. It metabolizes phenylethylamine and benzylamine. Dopamine and tyramine are metabolized by both types of MAO.

Mechanism of Action

The MAOIs work by inhibiting the enzyme MAO, which is widely distributed in the body, especially in nerves, the liver, and lung tissue. MAO is responsible for inactivating many of the important neurotransmitters in our nervous system, in particular the biogenic amines dopamine, epinephrine, norepinephrine, and serotonin. The antidepressant activity of the MAOs appears to be related to their inhibition of the MAO system, which in turn results in increased levels of epinephrine, norepinephrine, and serotonin at their storage sites in the nerves. The increased levels of these monoamines in the brain leads to a reduction in depression.

Drug Effects

By inhibiting the MAO enzyme system in the CNS of patients suffering from depression, amines such as dopamine, serotonin, and norepinephrine are not broken down and therefore higher levels occur, which in turn alleviates the symptoms of depression. The MAOIs were discovered by chance. Research for new chemical derivatives of isoniazid for the treatment of tuberculosis revealed a group of new agents that had antitubercular activity. During clinical trials with these new derivatives, a consistant mood elevation in depressed patients with tuberculosis was noted. So besides their antidepressant effects, some of the older MAOIs have antibacterial effects as well.

Therapeutic Uses

As mentioned already, the MAOIs may be used for the treatment of any type of depression, but they are especially useful for the atypical types including for the treatment of depression that is not responsive to other therapies. However, because of their ability to cause a hypertensive crisis when they are taken with a substance containing tyramine, the MAOIs are generally considered second-line agents. This dangerous and potentially life-threatening condition is discussed with the MAOI interactions.

Side Effects and Adverse Effects

The MAOIs are better than the TCAs from the standpoint of undesirable effects in that they produce very few serious effects. The most common cardiovascular effect is orthostatic hypotension. The various side effects and adverse effects that can occur with MAOIs are listed in Table 13-9.

Toxicity and Management of Overdose

Clinical symptoms of MAOI overdose generally do not appear until about 12 hours after ingestion. The primary signs and symptoms are cardiovascular and neurologic in nature. The most serious cardiovascular effects are tachycardia and circulatory collapse, and the neurologic symptoms of major concern are seizures and coma. Hyperthermia and miosis are also generally present in overdose. The recommended treatment is aimed at eliminating the ingested toxin and protecting the organ systems at greatest risk of damage—the brain and heart. Recommended treatments are gastric lavage, urine acidification to a pH of 5, and hemodialysis.

Interactions

There is a wide variety of drug interactions that occur with the MAOIs. The most frequent and significant of these interactions are listed in Table 13-10.

The MAOIs are one of the few drug classes that are capable of interacting with food and leading to a severe reaction. In this case food containing the amino acid tyramine is the primary culprit, and a hypertensive crisis is the reaction. It is essential for both the patient and the nurse to know the various foods and drinks that should be avoided, and these are listed in Table 13-11. The sympathomimetic agents can also interact with the MAOIs and together cause a hypertensive crisis.

A hypertensive crisis occurs in approximately 8% of the patients on MAOIs. It is believed to occur when MAO inactivates gastrointestinal and liver tyramine, which then enters the bloodstream. (Tyramine is normally degraded by MAO in the intestines). This tyramine displaces presynaptic norepinephrine, and this norepinephrine in conjunction with the increase in the norepinephrine stored and released from nerve terminals through the actions of the MAOIs becomes too much, and hypertension ensues. The chief complaints

Table 13-9	MAOIs: Adverse Effects
BODY SYSTEM	**SIDE/ADVERSE EFFECTS**
Cardiovascular	Orthostatic hypotension, tachycardia, palpitations, edema
Central nervous system	Dizziness, drowsiness, restlessness, insomnia, headache
Gastrointestinal	Anorexia, abdominal cramps, nausea
Other	Blurred vision, impotence, skin rashes

Table 13-10	MAOIs: Drug Interactions	
DRUG	**MECHANISM**	**RESULTS**
Sympathomimetics (e.g., amphetamine, ephedrine, phenylpropanolamine)	Release of catecholamine stores	Increased blood pressure, hypertensive crisis
Meperidine	Interferes with meperidine metabolism	Agitation, hyperpyrexia, circulatory collapse
Tricyclic antidepressants	Additive effects	Increased therapeutic and toxic effects

Table 13-11	Food and Drink to Avoid When Taking MAOIs

FOOD/DRINK	EXAMPLES
High Tyramine Content—Not Permitted	
Aged mature cheeses	Cheddar, blue, Swiss
Smoked/pickled meats, fish, or poultry	Herring, sausage, corned beef, salami, pepperoni
Aged/fermented meats, fish, or poultry	Chicken or beef-liver pate, game
Yeast extracts	Brewer's yeast
Red wines	Chianti, burgundy, sherry, vermouth
Italian broad beans	Fava beans
Moderate Tyramine Content—Limited Amounts Allowed	
Meat extracts	Bouillon, consomme
Pasteurized light and pale beer	
Ripe avocado	
Low Tyramine Content—Permissible	
Distilled spirits (in moderation)	Vodka, gin, rye, scotch
American and mozzarella cheese	Cottage cheese, cream cheese
Chocolate and caffeine beverages	
Fruit	Figs, raisins, grapes, pineapple, oranges
Soy sauce	
Yogurt, sour cream	

in such patients are severe occipital headache, stiff neck, flushing, palpitations, diaphoresis, nausea and vomiting, and elevated systolic and diastolic blood pressure. The blood pressure may increase abruptly and dramatically, usually within minutes of ingesting the food, beverage, or restricted medication (sympathomimetic agent). This may lead to hyperpyrexia (increased body temperature) and potentially to cerebral hemorrhage, stroke, coma, or death.

Once ingestion occurs, it is considered a medical emergency and immediate treatment should be sought. Patients should be given phentolamine, chlorpromazine, or nifedipine (Procardia), 10 mg sublingually. This is such a sudden and severe reaction that often patients are told they should always have nifedipine available in the event of inadvertent tyramine ingestion.

Dosages

For recommended dosages for selected MAOIs, see the table on the following page.

DRUG PROFILES

The MAOIs are contraindicated in patients with the following conditions: cerebrovascular or cardiovascular disorders, pheochromocytoma, a known hypersensitivity reaction to them, and liver or renal dysfunction. The MAOIs should also not be used in combination with adrenergic agents, tyramine-rich foods, or meperidine. All the MAOIs are classified as pregnancy category C agents. Of the agents prescribed for the treatment of depression, phenelzine tends to be prescribed more frequently and tranylcypromine may be more activating (perhaps because of its structural similarity to amphetamine). They are equally effective, although most physicians lean toward a favorite.

Before the start of treatment with any of the MAOIs, it is recommended that the baseline platelet MAO activity be determined. Subsequent measurements obtained after the patient has been started on the MAOI should then be compared with it to determine the change in activity. Measuring the percentage of inhibition during MAOI therapy helps in establishing a therapeutic dose. To achieve maximum benefit, the goal should be 85% to 90% inhibition.

Occasionally a TCA is combined with an MAOI in the treatment of depression refractory to treatment with a TCA alone or with some other agent. Typically this is done by giving an MAOI to a patient already taking a TCA or the two may be started together at 50% of the usual dose of each. If a patient's depression is stabilized on an MAOI but the physician wishes to add a TCA, then there must be at least a 2-week washout period before the start of TCA treatment. Without this washout period, the patient might experience hyperthermia, delirium, convulsions, and coma.

PHENELZINE

Phenelzine (Nardil) is also an MAOI that has been used for the treatment of affective disorders such as depression. In investigational studies it has also shown some effectiveness in the treatment of panic disorders. It is only available orally as 15-mg tablets. The commonly recommended dosages are given in the following dosages table.

DOSAGES

MAOIs: SELECTED ANTIDEPRESSANT AGENTS

AGENT	PHARMACOLOGIC CLASS	DOSAGE RANGE	PURPOSE
Phenelzine (Nardil)	Monoamine oxidase inhibitor	*Adult* PO: initial dose, 45-90 mg/day divided, followed by 15 mg/day or qod	Depression
Tranylcypromine (Parnate)		*Adult* PO: 30-60 mg/day divided	

❖ PHARMACOKINETICS

HALF-LIFE	ONSET	PEAK	DURATION
Variable	2 wk*	<6 wk	2 wk*

*Therapeutic effect.

TRANYLCYPROMINE

Tranylcypromine (Parnate) is an MAOI used for the treatment of depression. It is structurally similar to amphetamine. It is only available orally as 10-mg tablets. The commonly recommended dosages are given in the table above.

❖ PHARMACOKINETICS

HALF-LIFE	ONSET	PEAK	DURATION
2-3 hr	<2 hr	1.5-3 hr	3-10 days*

*To reach therapeutic effect.

SECOND-GENERATION ANTIDEPRESSANTS

The second-generation antidepressants are a group of newer antidepressant drugs that are generally considered superior to TCAs in terms of their side effect profiles, but not from the standpoint of their overall efficacy or onset of action. The individual antidepressants that make up this group of agents are trazodone (Desyrel), bupropion (Wellbutrin), and the selective serotonin-reuptake inhibitors (SSRIs) fluoxetine (Prozac), paroxetine (Paxil), and sertraline (Zoloft). The inhibition of serotonin reuptake seems to be the common mechanism of action for trazodone and the SSRIs. Bupropion also seems to inhibit reuptake of serotonin and possibly norepinephrine. These newer antidepressants offer several attractive advantages over the traditional TCAs and MAOIs. They are associated with significantly less severe and fewer systemic side effects and adverse effects, especially those that the elderly have little tolerance to—the anticholinergic and cardiovascular side effects. They are very safe and have very few drug-drug or drug-food interactions. It does, however, take approximately the same amount of time for them to reach maximum clinical effectiveness, approximately 4 to 6 weeks, as it does for the TCAs and MAOIs.

The SSRIs were developed to slow or inhibit the reuptake of serotonin into presynaptic terminals (nerve endings) and thus to increase the levels of serotonin at the nerve endings. Sertraline in the most selective of the three agents in inhibiting serotonin as opposed to norepinephrine reuptake, and fluoxetine is the least selective. Fluoxetine is the only one of the three that has an active metabolite. Fluoxetine along with its active metabolite has an elimination half-life of 2 to 4 days as opposed to a 1-day half-life for sertraline and paroxetine.

Mechanism of Action

A common feature of the second-generation antidepressants is their ability to selectively inhibit serotonin reuptake while having little if any effect on norepinephrine or dopamine reuptake. There are some slight differences between trazodone, bupropion, and the SSRIs. Trazodone, marketed in 1982, was the first of these agents to become available. It selectively inhibits serotonin reuptake and has negligible effects on norepinephrine reuptake. Bupropion seems to possess novel pharmacologic actions. It has very weak effects on norepinephrine and serotonin reuptake and also weakly inhibits dopamine reuptake. The SSRIs are specific and potent inhibitors of presynaptic serotonin reuptake (reuptake of serotonin into the nerve endings).

Drug Effects

The increase in serotonin reuptake causes increased concentrations of serotonin at nerve endings in the CNS, resulting in numerous functional changes associated with enhanced serotoninergic neurotransmission. This increased serotonin concentration in the CNS seems to lead to a decrease in rapid eye movement sleep. It also has a potentiating effect when given with narcotic analgesics in that the increased serotonin concentration at nerve endings appears to work synergistically with the narcotic analgesic in relieving pain.

A main advantage of the SSRIs over the TCAs and MAOIs is that they have little or no effect on the cardiovascular system. The absence of substantial anticholinergic activity, alpha₁ adrenergic blocking activity, catecholamine-potentiating effects, and quinidine-like cardiotoxic effects appears to be the principal reason for the general lack of cardiovascular effects associated with the SSRIs. They also seem to have very little if any effect on the cardiac conduction system. The SSRIs also possess anorectic activity, and this appetite-inhibiting action may result from the blocking of serotonin reuptake and the attendant increase in the serotonin concentration at the nerve endings.

Therapeutic Uses

The second-generation agents (trazodone, bupropion, and the SSRIs) have been used to treat many of the affective disorders. Depression, the bipolar affective disorder, obesity, eating disorders, obsessive-compulsive disorder, panic attacks or disorders, and myoclonus are only some of the many disorders that this highly effective drug class can be used to treat. The second-generation antidepressants have shown some beneficial effects in the treatment of various substance abuse problems such as alcohol dependence.

Side Effects and Adverse Effects

The second-generation antidepressants offer an advantage over the TCAs and MAOIs in that their side effect and adverse effect profiles are very clean. The

Table 13-12	Second-Generation Antidepressants: Adverse Effects
BODY SYSTEM	**SIDE/ADVERSE EFFECT**
Central nervous system	Headache, dizziness, tremor, nervousness, insomnia, fatigue
Gastrointestinal	Nausea, diarrhea, constipation, dry mouth
Other	Sweating, male sexual dysfunction

second-generation antidepressants and especially the SSRIs are associated with very few serious undesirable effects. The various side effects and adverse effects that can occur in patients taking second-generation antidepressants are listed in Table 13-12.

Interactions

The second-generation antidepressants are highly bound to plasma proteins such as albumin. When given with other drugs that are also highly bound to protein (warfarin and dilantin), both compete for binding sites on the surface of albumin. This results in more free, unbound drug and therefore a greater, more pronounced drug effect.

The SSRIs have the capacity to inhibit cytochrome P-450. The cytochrome P-450 system is an enzyme system in the liver that is responsible for the metabolism of several drugs. Inhibition of this enzyme system results in higher levels of drugs because they accumulate rather than getting broken down to their inactive metabolites. This also prolongs the action of drugs metabolized by the cytochrome P-450 system. The two SSRIs fluoxetine and paroxetine seem to be more potent inhibitors of this enzyme system than sertraline. There is still much controversy over whether the cytochrome P-450 system is inhibited. Many studies have shown that this event is minimal or even nonexistent. The most frequent and significant drug interactions are listed in Table 13-13.

Because of the potentially fatal pharmacodynamic interactions that can occur between SSRIs and the MAOIs, to prevent this it is recommended that the SSRI be washed out (discontinued) for at least 5 weeks before the start of fluoxetine treatment and for 2 weeks before the start of sertraline or paroxetine treatment.

Dosages

For dosage information for selected second-generation antidepressants, see the table on p. 178.

Table 13-13	Second-Generation Antidepressants: Drug Interactions	
DRUG	MECHANISM	RESULTS
MAOIs	Enhances serotonin activity	Hyperthermia, diaphoresis, shivering, tremor, seizures, ataxia, autonomic instability
TCAs	Increases TCA toxicity	Sedation, decreased energy, lightheadedness, dry mouth, constipation, elevated TCA levels
Carbamazepine	Decreases carbamazepine metabolism	Increased carbamazepine levels, carbamazepine toxicity, ocular changes, vertigo, tremor
Warfarin	Warfarin displaced from protein-binding sites	Increased warfarin effects

DOSAGES

SELECTED SECOND-GENERATION ANTIDEPRESSANTS

AGENT	PHARMACOLOGIC CLASS	DOSAGE RANGE	PURPOSE
Bupropion (Wellbutrin)		*Adult* PO: 200-400 mg/day divided	
Trazodone (Desyrel)		*Adult* PO: 150-600 mg/day divided	
⚓Fluoxetine (Prozac)	Antidepressant	*Adult* PO: 20-80 mg/day divided	Depression
Paroxetine (Paxil)		*Adult* PO: 20-50 mg/day divided	
Sertraline (Zoloft)		*Adult* PO: 50-200 mg taken once/day	
Lithium (Eskalith, Lithane, Cibalith-S)	Antimanic agent	*Adult* PO: 600-1200 mg/day divided	

DRUG PROFILES

The second-generation antidepressants trazodone, bupropion, and the SSRIs have proved to be valuable additions to the antidepressant armamentarium. They are highly effective as antidepressants and are associated with very few serious side effects and adverse effects. They are considered first-line agents in the treatment of depression with symptoms of anxiety, and depression with suicidal ideations, and also in patients unable to tolerate adverse reactions to other agents.

BUPROPION

Bupropion (Wellbutrin) was originally approved by the FDA in 1985 but was withdrawn by the manufacturer because of its apparently high potential for inducing seizures in nondepressed patients being treated for bulimia. Subsequent investigations revealed the overall estimated frequency of seizures was approximately 0.4%, and the drug was reintroduced in 1989. Bupropion is a unique antidepressant in terms of both its structure and mechanism of action. It has no appreciable effect either on the uptake of serotonin or norepinephrine or on the activity of MAO. It does, however, have a modest effect on the blockade of dopamine reuptake.

Bupropion is contraindicated in patients who have shown a hypersensitivity reaction to the drug, those with a seizure disorder or who currently or in the past have suffered from anorexia nervosa or bulimia, and those currently on MAOI treatment. It is considered a pregnancy category B agent. It is only available orally as 75- and 100-mg tablets. The commonly recommended dosages are given in the table on the previous page.

☠ P H A R M A C O K I N E T I C S

HALF-LIFE	ONSET	PEAK	DURATION
10-14 hr	up to 4 wk*	3 hr	wk to mo

*Therapeutic effect.

TRAZODONE

Trazodone (Desyrel) was marketed in the United States in 1982. It was the first of the second-generation antidepressants that could selectively inhibit serotonin reuptake but that negligibly affected norepinephrine reuptake. One advantage of trazodone over the TCAs is its minimal adverse effect on the cardiovascular system. It is, however, very sedating and this can be severe and impair cognitive function in the elderly. Trazodone has also rarely been associated with transient nonsexual prolonged erection. This is reportedly the result of alpha-adrenergic blockade.

Trazodone's use is contraindicated in patients who have shown a hypersensitivity reaction to it. It is only available orally as 50-, 100-, 150-, and 300-mg tablets. The commonly recommended dosages are given in the table on the previous page. Pregnancy category C.

☠ P H A R M A C O K I N E T I C S

HALF-LIFE	ONSET	PEAK	DURATION
6-9 hr	1-2 wk*	2-4 wk*	wk*

*Therapeutic effect.

⚓ FLUOXETINE

Fluoxetine (Prozac) was the first SSRI marketed for the treatment of depression, becoming commercially available in 1988. Since that time, it has become the number one prescribed antidepressant in the United States and one of the most frequently prescribed of all drugs. It is contraindicated in patients who have shown a hypersensitivity reaction to it and in those taking MAOIs. Fluoxetine is available orally as a 20-mg capsule and as a 20-mg/5 ml solution. The commonly recommended dosages are given in the table on the previous page. Pregnancy category B.

☠ P H A R M A C O K I N E T I C S

HALF-LIFE	ONSET	PEAK	DURATION
1-3 days	1-4 wk*	6-8 hr	Unknown

*Therapeutic effect.

PAROXETINE

Paroxetine (Paxil) is another SSRI antidepressant agent and is the newest of the SSRIs. It is contraindicated in patients who have shown a hypersensitivity reaction to them and those taking MAOIs. Paroxetine is available orally as a 20- and 30-mg film-coated tablet. The commonly recommended dosages are given in the table on the previous page. Pregnancy category B.

☠ P H A R M A C O K I N E T I C S

HALF-LIFE	ONSET	PEAK	DURATION
14 hr	1-4 wk*	5-8 hr	Unknown

*Therapeutic effect.

SERTRALINE

Sertraline (Zoloft) is another SSRI antidepressant agent. Of the three SSRIs discussed here, sertraline is the most selective in inhibiting serotonin reuptake and has very little effect on the inhibition of the cytochrome P-450 enzyme system in the liver. It also has no metabolites with clinically significant activity. It is contraindicated in patients who have shown a hypersensitivity to it and those taking MAOIs. Sertraline is available orally as 50- and 100-mg tablets. The commonly recommended dosages are given in the table on the previous page. Pregnancy category B.

☠ P H A R M A C O K I N E T I C S

HALF-LIFE	ONSET	PEAK	DURATION
24 hr	1-8 wk*	6-8 hr	Unknown

*Therapeutic effect.

ANTIMANIC AGENTS

Clinical evidence indicates that the catecholamines, dopamine and norepinephrine, play an important pathophysiologic role in the development of mania. Serotonin also appears to be involved. The only drugs currently available that can effectively alleviate the major symptoms of mania are the lithium salts.

The antimanic effect of lithium is not fully understood. Results of studies indicate that lithium ions alter sodium ion transport in nerve cells, resulting in a shift in catecholamine metabolism. The therapeutic levels of lithium that are required are close to the toxic levels, but there is increasingly greater tolerance to these toxic levels during acute manic phases. For the management of acute mania a lithium serum level of 1.0 to 1.5 mEq/L is usually required. Desirable long-term maintenance levels range between 0.6 and 1.2 mEq/L.

There are no absolute contraindications to lithium therapy, and the side effects and adverse effects are dependent on the serum levels. Levels exceeding 2.0

to 2.5 mEq/L produce moderate to severe toxicity. The most serious adverse effect is cardiac arrhythmias. Other effects include drowsiness, slurred speech, epileptic-type seizures, choreoathetotic movements, and hypotension. Long-term treatment may cause hypothyroidism.

The concurrent use of thiazides, angiotensin-converting enzyme type I, and calcium channel blockers increase lithium toxicity. Use with haloperidol can result in irreversible brain damage. The recommended dosages of lithium are given in the table on p. 178.

ANTIPSYCHOTIC AGENTS

Antipsychotic drugs are used to treat serious mental illness such as the bipolar affective disorder, depressive and drug-induced psychoses, schizophrenia, and autism. Antipsychotics are also used to treat extreme mania, certain movement disorders (e.g., Tourette's syndrome), and some medical conditions (nausea and intractable hiccups). The antipsychotics are also referred to as *tranquilizers or neuroleptics* because they produce a state of tranquility and work on abnormally functioning nerves.

Constituting about two thirds of all antipsychotics,

the phenothiazines are the largest group of antipsychotic drugs, but like many drug discoveries, were discovered by chance, in this case during research for new antihistamines. In 1951 chlorpromazine was the first of the phenothiazines to be discovered in this way. The phenothiazines are associated with a high incidence of anticholinergic side effects because they are so closely related to the antihistamines. Since the early 1950s, therefore, researchers have been working on developing phenothiazines with few side effects. Although the phenothiazines can provide much relief to the mentally ill patient, they can also cause many undesirable side effects.

The phenothiazines can be divided into three groups based on structural differences: aliphatic, piperidine, and piperazine phenothiazines. Besides the phenothiazine antipsychotics there are four other categories of drugs that are commonly used to treat mental illness: the thioxanthenes, butyrophenones, dihydroindolones, and dibenzoxazepines. The available neuroleptics or antipsychotics are listed in Table 13-14 according to their respective drug categories and comparative properties. Many of the therapeutic and toxic effects of the antipsychotics are the consequence of their chemical structures.

Table 13-14	Antipsychotic Agents and Their Comparative Properties					
DRUG NAME	**ANTIPSYCHOTIC POTENCY**	**MG:MG RATIO***	**SEDATION**	**ANTICHOLINERGIC**	**CARDIOVASCULAR**	**EXTRAPYRAMIDAL SYMPTOMS**
Phenothiazines						
Aliphatic						
Chlorpromazine	Low	1:1	High	High	High	Low
Triflupromazine	High	1:20	Low	Low	Low	High
Piperidine						
Mesoridazine	Low	1:2	High	High	High	Low
Thioridazine	Low	1:1	High	High	High	Low
Piperizine						
Fluphenazine	High	1:50	Low	Low	Low	High
Perphenazine	High	1:15	Low	Low	Low	High
Prochlorperazine	High	1:10	Low	Low	Low	High
Trifluoperazine	High	1:20	Low	Low	Low	High
Thioxanthenes						
Chlorprothixene	Low	1:2	High	High	High	Low
Thiothixene	High	1:50	Low	Low	Low	High
Butyrophenones						
⚓Haloperidol	High	1:50	Low	Low	Low	High
Dihydroindolone						
Molindone	Inter	1:100	Inter	Inter	Inter	Inter
Dibenzoxazepine						
Loxapine	Inter	1:10	Inter	Inter	Inter	High

Low, low incidence; *Inter,* intermediate incidence; *High,* high incidence.
*Compared with chlorpromazine.

Table 13-15	Major Dopamine Systems in the Brain	
DA SYSTEM	**DA-RELATED FUNCTION**	**EFFECTS OF DA RECEPTOR BLOCKADE**
Nigrostriatal	Mediates function of the extrapyramidal motor system (EPS movement)	*Reversible:* Dystonia, pseudoparkinsonism, akathisia *Irreversible:* Tardive dyskinesia (must catch early to reverse!)
Mesolimbic	Regulates stereotypical and other behaviors	Therapeutic antipsychotic effects
Mesocortical	Regulates behavior	Therapeutic antipsychotic effects
Hypothalamic-pituitary	Regulates prolactin secretion, temperature, appetite, emesis	Increased prolactin levels resulting in galactorrhea, amenorrhea, and decreased libido; loss of temperature regulation, increased appetite, and antiemetic effects

DA, dopamine; *EPS,* extrapyramidal symptoms.

There is very little difference between antipsychotics in their mechanism of actions; therefore selection of an antipsychotic is based primarily on the least undesirable drug side effect and the patient's type of psychosis. Of the currently available antipsychotic agents, no single drug stands out as being either more or less effective in the treatment of the symptoms of psychosis. It should also be stressed that antipsychotic drug therapy does not provide a cure for mental illness but is only a way of chemically controlling the symptoms of the illness. These agents represent a significant advance in our treatment of mental illnesses, as borne out by the fact that the early treatment of mental illnesses, that before the 1950s, consisted of such extreme measures as isolation, physical restraint, shock therapy, and even lobotomy.

Mechanism of Action

All antipsychotics are believed to have a common mechanism of action. They are believed to block dopamine receptors in the brain and thus to decrease the dopamine concentration in the CNS. Specifically, the phenothiazines block the receptors that dopamine normally binds to postsynaptically in certain areas of the CNS, such as the limbic system and the basal ganglia. These are the areas associated with emotions, cognitive functioning, and motor functions. This results in a tranquilizing effect in psychotic patients. Both the therapeutic and toxic effects of these agents are the direct result of the dopamine blockade in these areas.

Drug Effects

The antipsychotics have many effects throughout the body. Besides blocking the dopamine receptors in the CNS, they also block alpha receptors, which results in hypotension and other cardiovascular effects. Many

of the adverse effects of these drugs stem from their ability to block histamine receptors—anticholinergic effects. They also block serotonin. This in combination with their ability to block dopamine receptors in the chemoreceptor trigger zone and peripherally, along with their ability to inhibit the vagus nerve in the gastrointestinal tract, accounts for the ability of certain antipsychotics to function as antiemetics. By blocking dopamine receptors in the brainstem reticular system they also have antianxiety effects. Most phenothiazines and haloperidol can also augment prolactin release, which can result in swelling of the breasts and milk secretion in women taking these agents.

Therapeutic Uses

As just mentioned, the major therapeutic effect of the antipsychotic agents is the result of blockade of the dopamine receptors in certain areas of the CNS. These are the areas where regulation of dopamine activity tends to be dysfunctional, and this is one possible explanation for mental illness. There are certain areas of the brain where dopamine activity is abnormally increased and others where it is abnormally decreased. The antipsychotics attempt to reestablish dopamine pathways and other neurotransmitter systems and restore normal activity. The various areas within the CNS where antipsychotics have a major effect are listed in Table 13-15.

Side Effects and Adverse Effects

The side effects of the individual antipsychotic drugs are many and are important to remember. The antipsychotic agent with the least desirable side-effect profile is often the agent that is used. This may vary from patient to patient. The common side effects caused by blockade of the dopamine, muscarinic, his-

Table 13-16	Antipsychotics: Receptor-Related Side Effects	
RECEPTOR	**SIDE/ADVERSE EFFECT**	**DRUG CATEGORY**
Dopamine	Extrapyramidal movement disorders, dystonia, parkinsonism, akathisia, tardive dyskinesia	High-potency drugs
Endocrine	Prolactin secretion (galactorrhea, gynecomastia), menstrual changes, sexual dysfunction	Low-potency drugs
Muscarinic	Blurred vision, worsening of narrow-angle glaucoma, dry mouth, tachycardia, constipation, urinary retention, decreased sweating	Low-potency drugs
Histamine	Sedation, drowsiness, hypotension, weight gain	Low-potency drugs
Alpha-adre-nergic	Postural hypotension, lightheadedness, re-flex tachycardia	Low-potency drugs

Table 13-17	Antipsychotics: Adverse Effects
BODY SYSTEM	**SIDE/ADVERSE EFFECT**
Central nervous system	Sedation, delirium, neuroleptic malignant syndrome
Cardiovascular	Orthostatic hypotension, syncope, dizziness, ECG changes, conduction abnormalities
Gastrointestinal	Dry mouth, constipation, paralytic ileus, hepatotoxicity
Genitourinary	Urinary hesitancy, urinary retention, impaired erection, priapism, ejaculatory problems
Hematologic	Leukopenia and agranulocytosis
Dermatologic	Photosensitivity, hyper-pigmentation, rash, pruritus
Metabolic and endocrine	Galactorrhea, irregular menses, amenorrhea, decreased libido, increased appetite, polydipsia, impaired temperature regulation

Table 13-18	Antipsychotics: Drug Interactions	
DRUG	**MECHANISM**	**RESULTS**
Antacids	Decreased absorption	Reduced absorption of phenothiazines
Antihypertensives	Antagonism	May potentiate hypotension
CNS depressants	Additive effects	Increased CNS depression

tamine, and alpha-adrenergic receptors are listed in Table 13-16.

These undesirable effects can also be classified according to the body system affected. Some of the most significant antipsychotic-induced reactions are agranulocytosis, hemolytic anemia, exfoliative dermatitis, and the neuroleptic malignant syndromes. CNS effects include drowsiness, extrapyramidal reactions, and tardive dyskinesia. Ocular adverse effects include blurred vision, corneal lens changes, epithelial keratopathy, and pigmentary retinopathy. Cardiovascular effects include postural hypotension and changes in the electrocardiogram. The common side effects and adverse effects caused by antipsychotic drugs are listed in Table 13-17.

Interactions

The antipsychotics have a variety of interactions with other drugs, the most common of which are listed in Table 13-18.

Dosages

For recommended dosages for selected antipsychotic agents, see the table on p. 184.

DRUG PROFILES

The antipsychotics, or neuroleptics, are prescription-only medications that are indicated for the treatment of various psychotic disorders. Of the currently available agents, no single drug has stood out as being either more or less effective in the treatment of the symptoms of psychosis. All antipsychotics work through the same mechanism—blocking brain dopamine receptors. Some of the factors that should be considered before selecting an antipsychotic agent are the patient's history of a prior response to an agent and the desired side-effect profile. It is also important to start with the lowest possible dose of an orally administered drug. There are many classes of drugs used to treat mental illness, but, as mentioned earlier, the largest class and the agents most frequently prescribed are the phenothiazines.

PHENOTHIAZINES
CHLORPROMAZINE

Chlorpromazine (Thorazine) has strong anticholinergic and sedative effects and is a strong antiemetic. It is considered a low-potency neuroleptic agent and therefore the associated incidence of extrapyramidal symptoms is low. The incidence of sedative, anticholinergic, and cardiovascular side effects is high, however. It is indicated for the symptomatic relief of nausea, vomiting, hiccups, and porphyria; for preoperative sedation; and for the treatment of psychotic disorders.

Chlorpromazine is contraindicated in patients who have shown a hypersensitivity reaction to phenothiazines and in those suffering from circulatory collapse, liver dysfunction, blood dyscrasias, coma, bone marrow depression, or alcohol or barbiturate withdrawal. It is classified as a pregnancy category C agent. It is available in oral, rectal, and intravenous dosage formulations. In the oral form it is available as 30-, 75-, and 150-mg extended-release capsules; 10-, 25-, 50-, 100-, and 200-mg tablets; a 10-mg/5 ml solution; and a 30- and 100-mg/ml concentrated solution. In its rectal formulation it comes as 25- and 100-mg suppositories. The parental form of chlorpromazine comes as a 25-mg/ml injection. The commonly recommended dosages are given in the table on the next page.

✷ PHARMACOKINETICS

HALF-LIFE	ONSET	PEAK	DURATION
PO: 6 hr	PO: 30-60 min	PO: unknown	PO: 4-6 hr
PO-ER: 6 hr	PO-ER: 30-60 min	PO-ER: unknown	PO-ER: 10-12 hr
Rectal: 6 hr	Rectal: 1-2 hr	Rectal: unknown	Rectal: 3-4 hr
IM: 6 hr	IM: unknown	IM: unknown	IM: 4-8 hr
IV: 6 hr	IV: rapid	IV: unknown	IV: unknown

FLUPHENAZINE

Fluphenazine (Prolixin) is available in three different salt forms, which give it varying degrees of antipsychotic potency. The decanoate and enanthate salt forms have the longest durations of action, and the hydrochloride salt form is fairly short in duration. Flu-

phenazine has the greatest potency of all the phenothiazines: 1 mg of the drug has the antipsychotic potency of 200 mg of chlorphenazine. It is primarily used to treat psychotic disorders and schizophrenia. It is considered a high-potency neuroleptic and is therefore associated with a high incidence of extrapyramidal symptoms, but the associated incidence of sedative, anticholinergic, and cardiovascular effects is low. It is contraindicated in patients who have shown a hypersensitivity reaction to phenothiazines and in those suffering from circulatory collapse, liver dysfunction, blood dyscrasias, coma, bone marrow depression, or alcohol or barbiturate withdrawal. It is classified as a pregnancy category C agent. The two long-acting salt forms, decanoate and enanthate, are available as 25-mg/ml intravenous injections. The hydrochloride salt form is available orally as a 2.5-mg/5 ml elixir; a 5-mg/ml solution; and 1-, 2.5-, 5-, and 10-mg tablets. It is also available as a 2.5-mg/ml intravenous injection. The commonly recommended dosages are given in the table on the next page.

✷ PHARMACOKINETICS

HALF-LIFE	ONSET	PEAK	DURATION
PO: 15-16 hr*	PO (hydrochloride): 1 hr	PO (hydrochloride): 1.5-2 hr	PO (hydrochloride): 6-8 hr
IM: up to 2 wk†	IM (hydrochloride): 1 hr	IM (hydrochloride): 0.5 hr	IM (hydrochloride): 6-8 hr
	IM (enanthate): 24-72 hr	IM (enanthate): unknown	IM (enanthate): 1-3 wk
	IM (decanoate): 24-72 hr	IM (decanoate): unknown	IM (decanoate): ≥4 wk

*Following single dose.
†Following multiple IM injections.

THIOXANTHENES
THIOTHIXENE

Thiothixene (Navane) is a high-potency neuroleptic agent. Its use is associated with a high incidence of extrapyramidal symptoms but a low incidence of sedative, anticholinergic, and cardiovascular side effects. Thiothixene is primarily used for the treatment of psychotic disorders, schizophrenia, and acute agitation. It is contraindicated in patients who have shown a hypersensitivity reaction to it and in those suffering from circulatory collapse, liver dysfunction, blood dyscrasias, bone marrow depression, coma, narrow-angle glaucoma, or alcoholism. It is classified as a pregnancy category C agent. Thiothixene is available orally as 1-, 2-, 5-, 10-, and 20-mg capsules and as a 5-mg/ml solution. It is also available as a 10- or 2-mg/ml intra-

DOSAGES

SELECTED ANTIPSYCHOTIC AGENTS

AGENT	PHARMACOLOGIC CLASS	DOSAGE RANGE	PURPOSE
Chlorpromazine (Thorazine)	Phenothiazine antipsychotic	*Adult* PO: 30-1000 mg or more/day divided IM: 25 mg followed by 25-50 mg in 1 hr *Pediatric* PO: 50-200 mg/day divided IM: ≤5 y/o, 40 mg/day divided 5-12 y/o, 75 mg/day divided	Psychotic disorders, mania, schizophrenia
Fluphenazine (Prolixin)	Phenothiazine antipsychotic	*Adult* PO: 0.5-20 mg/day divided IM: 2.5-10 mg/day divided *Geriatric* PO: 1-2.5 mg/day divided	Psychotic disorders, schizophrenia
Thiothixene (Navane)	Thioxanthene antipsychotic	*Adult* PO: 6-30 mg/day divided IM: 4 mg 2-4 times/day	Psychotic disorders, schizophrenia, acute agitation
⚓Haloperidol (Haldol)	Butyrophenone antipsychotic	*Pediatric* PO: ≥3 y/o, 0.05-0.15 mg/kg/day divided *Adult* PO: 2-100 mg/day divided IM: 2-5 mg for prompt control	Psychotic disorders, control of tics, vocal utterances in Gilles de la Tourette syndrome, short-term treatment of hyperactive children showing excessive motor activity, prolonged parenteral therapy in chronic schizophrenia
Molindone (Moban)	Dihydroindolone antipsychotic	*Adult* PO: 50-225 mg/day divided	Psychotic disorders
Loxapine (Loxitane)	Dibenzoxazepine antipsychotic	*Adult* PO: 20-250 mg/day divided	Psychotic disorders
⚓Clozapine (Clozaril)	Dibenzodiazepine antipsychotic	*Adult* PO: 330-900 mg/day divided	Management of psychotic symptoms in schizophrenic patients for whom other antipsychotics have failed

muscular injection. The commonly recommended dosages are given in the table above.

⚡PHARMACOKINETICS

HALF-LIFE	ONSET	PEAK	DURATION
PO: 34 hr	PO: days-wk	PO: unknown	PO: unknown
IM: 34 hr	IM: 1-6 hr	IM: unknown	IM: unknown

BUTYROPHENONES

⚓ HALOPERIDOL

Haloperidol (Haldol) is structurally different from the thioxanthenes and the phenothiazines but has similar antipsychotic properties. It is a high-potency neuroleptic agent that has a favorable cardiovascular, anticholinergic, and sedative side effect profile but can often cause extrapyramidal symptoms. Haloperidol is available in three different salt forms: the base, decanoate, and lactate salt. Haloperidol decanoate has an extremely long duration of effect. It is used primarily for the long-term treatment of psychosis and is especially useful in patients who are noncompliant with their drug treatment. It is contraindicated in patients who have shown a hypersensitivity reaction to it, those in a comatose state, those taking large amounts of CNS depressants, and those with Parkinson's disease. It is classified as a pregnancy category C agent. It is available in an oral form as 0.5-, 1-, 2-, 5-, 10-, and 20-mg tablets and as a 2-mg/ml solution and an intravenous form in two injections for intramuscular use: one, the long-acting decanoate salt, comes as a 50- or 100-mg/ml injection; the other, the lactate salt, comes as a 5-mg/ml injection. The commonly recommended dosages are given in the preceding table.

✤ PHARMACOKINETICS *

HALF-LIFE	ONSET	PEAK	DURATION
PO, IM: 13-35 hr x̄ = 21 hr	PO: 2 hr	PO: 2-6 hr	PO: 8-12 hr
	IM: 20-30 min	IM: 30-45 min	IM: 4-8 hr
	IM: 3-9 days	IM: unknown	IM: 1 mo

*Decanoate salt form.

DIHYDROINDOLONES
MOLINDONE

Molindone (Moban) is a high-potency neuroleptic agent that is approximately a hundred times more potent than chlorpromazine. Molindone, like the phenothiazines, blocks dopamine receptors in the brain. It is primarily used in the treatment of psychotic disorders and schizophrenia. Molindone is only available in an oral form as a 20-mg/ml solution and as 5-, 10-, 25-, 50-, and 100-mg tablets. It is a pregnancy category C drug. Its use is contraindicated in patients who have shown a hypersensitivity reaction to it, those in coma, and children. The commonly recommended dosages are given in the table on the previous page.

✤ PHARMACOKINETICS

HALF-LIFE	ONSET	PEAK	DURATION
Variable	30-60 min	1.5 hr	24-36 hr

DIBENZOXAZEPINES
LOXAPINE

Loxapine (Loxitane) is a tricyclic dibenzoxazepine-derivative antipsychotic agent. Like the phenothiazines, it is indicated for the treatment of psychotic disorders and schizophrenia. Loxapine is available for oral administration as a 25-mg/ml solution and as 5-, 10-, 25-, and 50-mg tablets. It is a pregnancy category C drug. Its use is contraindicated in patients who have shown a hypersensitivity reaction to it and those suffering from circulatory collapse, liver dysfunction, blood dyscrasias, bone marrow depression, coma, narrow-angle glaucoma, or alcoholism. The commonly recommended dosages are given in the table on the previous page.

✤ PHARMACOKINETICS

HALF-LIFE	ONSET	PEAK	DURATION
PO: 4 hr	PO: 30 min	PO: 1.5-3 hr	PO: 12 hr
IM: 12 hr	IM: unknown	IM: 5 hr	IM: unknown

DIBENZODIAZEPINES
⚕ CLOZAPINE

Clozapine (Clozaril) is a unique antipsychotic agent. It is similar to loxapine in its chemical structure in that it is a piperazine-substituted tricyclic antipsychotic, but pharmacologically it is different from all the currently available antipsychotics in terms of its mechanism of action. Because of these pharmacologic differences, clozapine is considered an atypical antipsychotic agent. Clozapine is believed to work on the serotoninergic, adrenergic, and cholinergic neurotransmitter systems in the brain. It also more selectively blocks the dopaminergic receptors in the mesolimbic system. Other antipsychotic agents block dopamine receptors in an area of the brain called the *neostriatum*, but blockade in this area of the brain is believed to give rise to the unwanted extrapyramidal symptoms. Because clozapine has very weak dopamine-blocking abilities in this area, it is associated with minor or no extrapyramidal symptoms.

Clozapine has been extremely useful for the treatment of patients who have failed treatment with other antipsychotic agents, especially those with schizophrenia. Patients taking clozapine must be monitored very closely for the development of agranulocytosis, which is a dangerous drug-induced blood disorder. The risk of agranulocytosis developing as the result of clozapine therapy is 1% to 2% after the first year; this compares with a risk of 0.1% to 1% for the phenothiazines. Clozapine is only available in an oral form as 25- and 100-mg tablets. It is a pregnancy category B drug. Its use is contraindicated in patients who have shown a hypersensitivity reaction to it and in those with myeloproliferative disorders, severe granulocytopenia, CNS depression, coma, or narrow-angle glaucoma.

The commonly recommended dosages are given in the table on p. 184.

PHARMACOKINETICS

HALF-LIFE	ONSET	PEAK	DURATION
6 hr	PO: 1-6 hr	wk	4-12 hr

NURSING PROCESS

ASSESSMENT

Both the physical and emotional status of patients taking psychotherapeutic drugs needs to be assessed. Often patients are so mentally distressed that their physical needs go unmet, and this results in a complexity of problems. Before therapy with any of the psychotherapeutic agents is initiated, the baseline values of all vital signs need to be documented. This includes postural (lying and standing) blood pressure readings so that the degree of a drop in blood pressure caused by medication effects can be identified and documented. It is also important to have liver and renal function studies performed before and during psychotropic drug therapy, and these are especially important in patients on long-term therapy so that complications and potential toxicity can be prevented or identified early. The patient's level of consciousness, mental alertness, and potential for injury to self and others also need to be assessed and documented.

With any of these agents, the nurse should always check the patient's mouth to make sure he or she has swallowed oral doses. This can prevent possible hiding or hoarding of medications, which may lead to toxicity, overdose, or noncompliance. Use of liquid preparations, when available, may minimize such problems.

Appetite, sleeping patterns, addictive behaviors,

PEDIATRIC CONSIDERATIONS
Psychotherapeutic Agents

■ Pediatric patients are at a higher risk for suffering side effects from psychotropic agents, especially extrapyramidal symptoms. Always closely monitor pediatric patients taking psychotropic agents!

■ The incidence of Reye's syndrome and other adverse reactions is greater in pediatric patients taking psychotropic agents who have had chickenpox, CNS infections, measles, acute illnesses, or dehydration.

■ Lithium may lead to decreased bone density or bone formation in children, so children receiving it should be closely monitored for signs and symptoms of lithium toxicity and bone disorders.

■ TCAs are generally not prescribed for patients under 12 years of age. Some antidepressants are used, though, in children with enuresis, attention deficit disorders, and major depressive disorders and may be associated with adverse reactions such as changes in the ECG, nervousness, sleep disorders, fatigue, elevated blood pressure, and GI upset. Pediatric patients are generally more sensitive to the effects of most drugs, and this group of agents is no exception. Be aware of the toxicity risk, which can be fatal. Should confusion, lethargy, visual disturbances, insomnia, tremors, palpitations, constipation, or eye pain occur, report this to the physician immediately.

GERIATRIC CONSIDERATIONS
Psychotherapeutic Agents

■ Elderly patients have higher serum levels of psychotherapeutic agents because of changes in the drug distribution metabolism processes, less serum albumin, decreased lean body mass, less water in tissues, and increased body fat. Because of these changes, elderly patients generally require lower doses of antipsychotic and antidepressant agents.

■ Orthostatic hypotension, anticholinergic side effects, sedation, and extrapyramidal symptoms are more common in elderly patients taking psychotherapeutic agents. Careful evaluation and documentation of baseline values and neurologic findings is therefore important to the safe use of these agents.

■ Increased anxiety is often associated with the use of tricyclic antidepressants. Patients with a history of cardiac disease may be at a higher risk of experiencing arrhythmias, tachycardia, stroke, myocardial infarction, or congestive heart failure.

■ Lithium is more toxic in elderly patients, and lower doses are often necessary, but close monitoring is important to its safe use in this age group. CNS toxicity, lithium-induced goiter, and hypothyroidism are more frequent in the aged patient.

elimination difficulties, hypersensitivity, and other conditions and complaints also need to be watched for and documented.

When administering any of the antianxiety agents, first check to make sure the patient has no history of a hypersensitivity reaction to the agent, especially to the benzodiazepines, or of chemical abuse; if a woman, she is not pregnant; the patient does not have narrow-angle glaucoma; and if a child, he or she is not below 12 years of age (see p. 186). All of these situations are contraindications to the use of antianxiety agents (see Chapter 10). Patients receiving these medications who have liver or renal disease or who are aged or in a debilitated state should be observed closely (see box, p. 186). If patients are deemed elderly, weak, or debilitated, it is critical to document these findings and make safety a top priority in their nursing care. Laboratory studies that should be done before the start of anxiolytic therapy include CBC and lactate dehydrogenase, creatinine, alkaline phosphatase, and BUN measurements. In addition, if you identify a drop in systolic blood pressure of 20 mm Hg or greater, you must inform the physician of this immediately. Drug interactions for all categories of psychotherapeutic agents are given in Tables 13-5, 13-8, 13-10, 13-13, and 13-18.

The antidepressant agents most commonly used are either TCAs or MAOIs. TCAs are contraindicated in patients who have shown a hypersensitivity reaction to them, who are actively suicidal, or who are recovering from a myocardial infarction. Cautious administration is recommended for patients with a history of benign prostatic hypertrophy, urinary retention, anemia, a seizure disorder, psychosis, suicidal thoughts, narrow-angle glaucoma, liver dysfunction, renal disease, thyroid disease, or heart block, as well as in the elderly and children younger than 12 years. Patients with cardiac disease and the elderly may be at risk for cardiac disturbances associated with toxicity or overdose.

There are many cautions, contraindications, and interactions pertaining to the use of MAOIs (see Table 13-13 for drug interactions). Contraindications include hypersensitivity reactions, elderly age, and severe cardiac, renal, or hepatic disease. Patients receiving MAOIs who have a history of suicide attempts or suicidal ideations, or who have seizure disorders, hyperactivity, diabetes, or psychosis should also be closely monitored. This pertains to pregnant women taking them, too. Foods and beverages high in tyramine, such as cheese, beer, wine (especially red wines), soy sauce, meat tenderizer, figs, chicken liver, beef liver, bananas, avocados, yogurt, sour cream, and sherry, should be avoided because sudden and severe hypertension can occur when these are taken with an MAOI (see Table 13-9). Caffeinated beverages should also be avoided

because of the hypertension and arrhythmias that can develop.

Phenothiazines are the major group of antipsychotic agents and differ in their potency and side effects. Haloperidol is similar to other "high-potency" neuroleptics in that its sedating effects are low but the incidence of extrapyramidal symptoms is high; these include tremors and muscle twitching and result from the blockade of the dopamine receptors, which has an inhibitory effect on specific movements in the musculoskeletal system. Extrapyramidal movement disorders are manifested as parkinsonism-like motor disturbances and are very irritating and uncomfortable for the person experiencing them. For home health care tips see the box below.

Loxapine, molindone, and thiothixene (nonphenothiazine antipsychotic agents) are miscellaneous agents.

HOME HEALTH POINTS
Phenothiazines

- Tell patients that, if they experience dizziness, lightheadedness, or palpitations, they should inform the physician of this, and the problem should then be assessed. These symptoms may be indicative of postural hypotension and may be prevented by changing positions slowly, especially lying to sitting or standing. Encourage patients to sit on the side of the bed for a few minutes before standing.
- Patients should be informed that it may take up to 3 weeks before a therapeutic response occurs.
- Patients need to protect themselves from exposure to sun and avoid the use of tanning beds. Sunscreen should be used whenever there is a possibility for exposure to the sun, such as when going for a walk outdoors or working in the yard. This is to prevent "solar" erythema.
- Patients need to understand the importance of good and regular dental care to prevent infections and oral candidiasis related to drug-induced dry mouth.
- Patients should avoid temperature extremes such as swimming in cold water, walking in hot weather, and soaking in hot tubs because of the increased risk of hyperthermia leading to heat prostration or of hypothermia.
- Alcohol and alcohol-containing products, such as cough syrups, must be avoided because of the increased risk of CNS depression.
- Follow-up medical visits, therapy sessions, and follow-up laboratory studies to monitor therapeutic drug levels are to be encouraged and patients frequently reminded of this.

RESEARCH

Detecting depression among primary care patients

In a study supported in part by the Agency for Health Care Policy and Research (HS06802), 40% of psychiatric patients compared with about 26% of other patients had double depression (a major depression and mild depression and anxiety lasting longer than 2 years), meaning that the most severely depressed patients are treated by psychiatrists, less depressed patients by psychologists or nonphysician therapists, and least depressed patients by primary care physicians in both prepaid and fee-for-service systems of care. Furthermore, patients of primary care physicians were sick enough to warrant treatment and had an average of 13 different symptoms of depression in the year prior to the study; 75% had recurrent depression. Patients whose depression was diagnosed by general practitioners were only slightly more depressed (characterized by one symptom) than those whose depression was not diagnosed. This study reinforces the importance of improving clinical detection of depressive disorders by general practitioners, especially by primary care providers who serve as referral "gatekeepers" to specialty care in prepaid systems of health care.

Wells M, Burnham A, Camp P: Severity of depression in prepaid and fee-for-service general medical and mental health specialty practices, *Med Care* 33(4): 350-364, 1995.

Each is associated with contraindications, cautions, and drug interactions (see Table 13-18). Thioridazine is contraindicated in patients who have shown a hypersensitivity reaction to it, in those with blood dyscrasias or bone marrow depression, and in children below the age of 2 years. It should be used with caution and the effects in patients showing adverse reactions, in women who are pregnant or lactating, and in patients with seizure disorders, high blood pressure, or hepatic or cardiac disease should be closely monitored. It is important to assess the patient's history carefully regarding cardiac disease because of the orthostatic hypotension and tachycardia these agents can induce, which are potentially life-threatening in the elderly patient. The patient's medication history and the current medications being taken should also be carefully noted because of the possible drug interactions that can occur.

There are also several important contraindications to and cautions concerning the use of the nonphenothiazine agents such as loxapine and haloperidol. Loxapine and such agents are contraindicated in patients who have shown hypersensitivity reactions to them; in those suffering from blood dyscrasias, brain damage, bone marrow depression, or alcohol or barbiturate withdrawal; and in children. They should be used cautiously in pregnant or lactating women; patients with cardiac, seizure, or liver disorders; men with benign prostatic hypertrophy; and patients younger than 16 years of age. Besides the same situations cited for loxapine, haloperidol is also contraindicated in patients with Parkinson's disease, angina, urinary retention, or narrow-angle glaucoma. They should be used cautiously in patients with any of the conditions listed for loxapine.

It takes about 3 weeks before therapeutic blood levels of lithium are reached, so patients should be closely watched before and during this time and given supportive care. Lithium is contraindicated in patients who have shown a hypersensitivity reaction to it; in those with renal disease, liver disease, organic brain syndrome, brain trauma, schizophrenia, severe dehydration, or cardiac disease; in pregnant or lactating women; and in children below the age of 12 years. Cautious use is recommended in the elderly, in patients with endocrine disorders such as diabetes mellitus and thyroid disorders, and in those with a seizure disorder or urinary retention. Baseline urine laboratory studies should include measurement of the albumin, uric acid, and glucose levels and of the specific gravity. Baseline assessment of sodium intake and skin turgor is important because decreased sodium and fluid intake may lead to lithium toxicity whereas increased sodium and fluid intake may lead to lithium loss. A baseline assessment of neuromotor functioning is also important because poor coordination, tremors, and weakness that arise after the start of therapy can be symptoms of toxicity.

NURSING DIAGNOSES

Nursing diagnoses appropriate to the nursing care of patients receiving any of the psychotherapeutic agents include:

■ Alteration in thought processes, impaired because of mental state.

■ Alteration in social interaction, impaired because of disease state.

■ Risk for injury related to disease process or side effects of medications.

■ Risk for alteration in nutrition, less than body requirements—related to physiologic impact of mental disorder.

■ Risk for alteration in sleep patterns, deficit or excess—related to disease process or drug effects.

■ Risk for alteration in self-image, decreased because of disease process and side effects of medications.

■ Risk for alteration in urinary elimination patterns, retention as the result of drug side effects.

■ Knowledge deficit related to lack of information about the specific psychotherapeutic drugs and their side effects.

PLANNING

Goals related to the administration of psychotherapeutic medications include:

- Patient experiences no further deterioration in thought processes.
- Patient will not sustain injury while on medication.
- Patient exhibits improved nutritional status.
- Patient regains normal sleep patterns.
- Patient exhibits (overtly and covertly) a more positive self-image.
- Patient remains free of any alterations in urinary elimination patterns.
- Patient remains compliant with therapy.
- Patient will be free of complications associated with the drug and with food and drug interactions.

Outcome Criteria

Outcome criteria related to the aforementioned goals include:

- Patient will demonstrate improved or no deterioration in thought processes and will be less hostile, withdrawn, and delusional once medication has reached steady state.
- Patient will demonstrate more open and appropriate behavior and communication with health care team and significant others.
- Patient will be free from falls, dizziness, and fainting attributable to side effects.
- Patient will show healthy nutrition habits with appropriate weight gain and a diet that includes foods from all four food groups.
- Patient will report improved sleep patterns and feeling more rested.
- Patient will openly discuss feelings of poor self-image and self-concept with staff.
- Patient will report any problems with urinary retention.
- Patient will state the importance of taking medications exactly as prescribed at the same time every day and without omissions.
- Patient will state the importance of appointments with the physician or other health care providers to follow improvement and monitor therapy.
- Patient will state the common side effects of the medication as well as those adverse effects (e.g., confusion and changes in LOC) to be reported to the physician.
- Patient will list those medications and foods to be avoided while taking any psychotherapeutic medication.

IMPLEMENTATION

Regardless of the psychotherapeutic agent prescribed, several general nursing actions are important to the safe administration of these agents. First and foremost is a firm (unless the patient is confrontational or aggressive) but patient attitude. Simple explanations about the drug and its effects as well as the length of time before therapeutic effects can be expected should be given. Vital signs should be monitored during therapy, especially in the elderly and patients with a history of cardiac disease. The name of the drug, the dosage and route of administration, and more specifically, the patient's response should all be documented. Abrupt withdrawal of any of these medications should be avoided.

More specific nursing actions in patients taking anxiolytics include frequent checks of the vital signs because of the orthostatic hypotension that can occur. Patients may be told to wear elastic compression stockings should orthostatic hypotension be problematic. Advise patients to change positions slowly, especially from a sitting or reclining position, and to avoid operating heavy equipment or machinery should sedation or drowsiness occur. The combination of psychotherapy and drug therapy is emphasized because patients need to learn and acquire more effective coping skills. Drug therapy alone is not as effective as it is when combined with psychotherapy. Patients should be reminded to keep anxiolytics and other medications out of the reach of children, and only small amounts of medications should be dispensed at any one time to minimize the risk of suicidal attempts. Even though these agents have a wide safety margin, their simultaneous use with alcohol or other CNS depressants can prove fatal. When administering hydroxyzine intramuscularly, it is important to use a Z-track method to prevent tissue injury at the site of injection. Lorazepam is often administered intravenously as an adjunct to anesthesia; in this setting it should be administered with the proper diluent in equal amounts and infused at a rate of 2 mg or less over 1 minute. Lorazepam given intramuscularly should be given deep into a large muscle mass, such as the gluteus maximus. Patient teaching tips are presented in the box on p. 190.

Antidepressants must be administered carefully per the physician's order, and it is important for patients to realize that it often takes 1 to 3 and often 4 weeks before the therapeutic effects are evident. Careful monitoring of the patient and the provision of supportive care and therapy are important during this time. Make sure the patient understands this and continues to take the medication as prescribed. You may administer the oral forms with meals to prevent gastrointestinal upset. Sedation often occurs in patients taking tricyclic antidepressants. If this lasts more than 2 weeks and interferes with normal activities, the physician should be notified of the problem. When administering an antidepressant for the first time, especially to elderly or weakened patients, assist them with ambulation and other activities during which falls may occur as a result of drowsiness or postural hypoten-

Patient Teaching TIPS

Anxiolytics and Antidepressants

✔ Take your medication exactly as prescribed by your physician. Do not skip or omit any doses and do not double up on the medication. If you remember you have not taken your medication and it is within an hour or 2 hours of the time you would have taken it, than go ahead and take the dose. If it is more than 2 hours after this time, skip that dose and take the medication at the next scheduled time.

✔ Keep medications out of reach of children.

✔ Change positions slowly to avoid fainting or dizziness. Call your physician immediately should you experience any fainting episodes while taking these medications.

✔ Do not suddenly stop taking this medication.

✔ If you experience drowsiness and sedating effects, do not operate heavy equipment or machinery.

✔ Avoid consuming alcohol and taking other CNS depressants.

✔ Do not take over-the-counter medication or any other medication without checking with your physician first to make sure this is okay.

✔ You may experience more drowsiness during the beginning of treatment. With the TCAs this should decrease after the first few weeks of therapy.

✔ You may take the oral forms of these medications with meals to decrease GI upset.

✔ You should contact your physician should you experience sores in the mouth, fever, sore throat, hallucinations, confusion, disorientation, shortness of breath, difficulty in breathing, yellow discoloration of the skin or eyes, or irritability.

✔ Caffeine and caffeinated beverages such as cola, tea, and coffee as well as cigarette smoking decrease the effectiveness of your medication.

✔ Keep all appointments and follow-up visits with your physician and other health care providers.

✔ Always carry or have about you a Medic-Alert tag or bracelet naming the medication you are taking.

✔ The therapeutic effects of MAOIs may not occur for up to 4 weeks. Therefore do not alter your dosing if you are not feeling better before this time. Remember a hypertensive crisis may occur if you consume foods high in tyramine, foods such as cheese, beer, wine, avocados, bananas, and liver. Caffeinated beverages should also be avoided. Remember that the drug will remain in the body for up to 2 weeks after discontinuing the medication. Contact your physician should you experience chest pain, a severe throbbing headache, rapid pulse, or nausea.

---

sion. Encourage the patient to consume at least 2000 ml of water or other fluids a day and to increase his or her intake of bulk to try and counteract constipation. Sucking on hard candy or chewing gum are helpful for relieving the discomfort of dry mouth.

If a patient who has been taking TCAs is scheduled to undergo a surgical procedure, it is important to wean him or her off the medication a few days beforehand so that an interaction with the anesthesic agents does not occur; however, this is only done with a physician's order. During TCA treatment, it is important to recognize and document the occurrence of blurred vision, excessive drowsiness or sleepiness, urinary retention, or constipation and to consult and discuss this with the physician. It is also important to emphasize the need for the patient on long-term therapy to wear a medication ID bracelet or tag naming the agent being taken.

MAOIs are very potent antidepressants and are reserved for those patients who do not respond to TCA or other modes of therapy. The side effects of these agents are often severe, and these include orthostatic

hypotension, arrhythmias, ataxia, hallucinations, seizures, tremors, dry mouth, and impotence, to name just a few. Patients should be told to contact their physician should any of these occur. In addition, tachycardia, seizures, respiratory depression, mental confusion, and restlessness may occur as a result of overdose and can persist for up to several weeks. The onset of any of these symptoms should be reported to and discussed immediately with the physician. The desired antidepressant effects of MAOIs do not usually occur before 1 to 4 weeks after the start of therapy. Patients should be weaned carefully from these medications a few weeks before any surgical procedure.

The antipsychotic agents, mainly the phenothiazines, can be administered orally or parenterally. The oral forms are well absorbed and will cause less GI upset if taken with food or a full glass of water. Hard candy or gum may be used to relieve dry mouth. Perspiration may be increased, so patients should be warned about engaging in excessive activity or being exposed to hot or humid climates because excessive sweating could lead to dehydration and then drug toxicity. You should contact the physician immediately should the patient exhibit tremors, uncontrollable movements of the tongue, muscle spasms, sore throat, or fever.

Haloperidol is another antipsychotic agent that may take up to 3 weeks for the full therapeutic effects to occur. It may be given orally or intramuscularly. Its high protein binding characteristic may lead to toxicity as the result of slower metabolism and excretion. Patient teaching tips are presented in the box below.

Lithium is used mainly for patients who are in manic states, but its exact mechanism of action is unknown. Crucial to its safe use, however, is keeping the patient adequately hydrated and in a state of electrolyte balance because its excretion is decreased (therefore leading to increased serum levels) in the setting of hyponatremia. Patients who are dehydrated may also experience lithium toxicity. Patient teaching tips are presented in the box below right.

EVALUATION

Both the therapeutic effects of psychotropic medications and the patient's progress within the treatment regimen must be monitored. Mental alertness, cognition, affect, mood, the ability to carry out activities of daily living, appetite, and sleep patterns are all areas that need to be closely monitored and documented. In concert with the drug therapy, the patient must acquire more effective coping skills. Psychotherapy, relaxation therapy, and an increase in exercise can all help in this regard.

The therapeutic effects of anxiolytics are evidenced by improved mental alertness, cognition, and mood; fewer anxiety and panic attacks; improved sleep patterns and appetite; more interest in self and others; less tension and irritability; and less feeling of fear, impending doom, and stress. Adverse effects to watch for in patients taking anxiolytic agents include hypotension, lethargy, fatigue, drowsiness, confusion, constipation, dry mouth, blood dyscrasias, lightheadedness, and insomnia.

Evidence of the therapeutic effects of antidepressants, which may take 1 to 4 weeks before appearing, include improved sleep patterns and nutrition, increased feelings of self-esteem, less feeling of hopelessness, increased interest in self and appearance, increased interest in daily activities, and less depressive manifestations or suicidal thoughts and ideations. Adverse reactions consist of drowsiness, dry mouth, con-

Patient Teaching TIPS

Phenothiazines and Haloperidol

✔ Take all medications exactly as prescribed. Do not double, omit, or skip doses. Remember, it may be several weeks before an improvement is experienced.

✔ Phenothiazines may cause drowsiness, dizziness, or fainting, so change positions slowly.

✔ You should wear sunscreen when taking phenothiazines because of the photosensitivity they cause.

✔ Avoid taking antacids or antidiarrheal preparations within 1 hour of a dose of a phenothiazine.

✔ Notify your physician immediately should you note fever, sore throat, yellow discoloration of the skin, or uncontrollable movements of the tongue while taking a phenothiazine.

✔ Do not take phenothiazines or haloperidol with alcohol or with any other CNS depressant.

✔ Long-term haloperidol therapy may result in tremors, nausea, vomiting, or uncontrollable shaking of small muscle groups, and any of these symptoms should be reported to your physician.

Patient Teaching TIPS

Lithium

✔ Take your medication exactly as prescribed. Do not double, skip, or omit doses.

✔ It may take several weeks before you notice any improvement related to the drug therapy.

✔ You make take your medicine with meals to decrease gastrointestinal upset.

✔ If you become ill with vomiting or diarrhea or are unable to eat or drink, it is important that you notify your physician of this immediately. Dehydration of any type, even as the result of excessive sweating, may result in drug toxicity.

✔ Many of the side effects of lithium will disappear with time; however, you should contact your physician should you experience any excessive vomiting, tremors, weakness, or any involuntary movements.

✔ Make sure to keep your appointments, especially ones when blood is drawn to determine the serum lithium levels.

✔ Always wear a Medic-Alert tag naming the agent you are taking.

✔ Keep the medication out of the reach of children.

stipation, dizziness, postural hypotension, sedation, blood dyscrasias, and tremors. Overdose is evidenced by irritability, agitation, CNS irritability, seizures, and then progression to CNS depression with respiratory or cardiac depression.

MAOIs are very potent antidepressants but therapeutic effects do not occur for up to 4 weeks after the start of therapy. These effects are similar to the ones produced by the TCAs. Adverse effects include sedation, dry mouth, constipation, postural hypotension, blurred vision, seizures, and tremors. Toxic reactions are manifested by confusion or hypotension and possibly by respiratory or cardiac distress. The potential for drug-food interactions cannot be overemphasized because of the violent hypertension that can result when these agents are taken with foods and beverages high in tyramine.

The therapeutic effects of antipsychotic drugs should include improvement in mood and affect and alleviation of the psychotic symptoms and episodes. Emotional instability, hallucinations, paranoia, delusions, garbled speech, and inability to cope should begin to abate once the patient has been on the medication for several weeks. It is also critical to carefully monitor a patient's potential to injure himself or herself or others during the delay between the start of therapy and symptomatic improvement. It is also important to watch the patient for the development of adverse reactions to the phenothiazines. These include dizziness and syncope stemming from orthostatic hypotension, tachycardia, confusion, drowsiness, insomnia, hyperglycemia, blood dyscrasias, and dry mouth. Overdose is manifested by excessive CNS depression, severe hypotension, and extrapyramidal symptoms such as dyskinesias and tremors. These symptoms should be reported immediately to the physician.

TAKE HOME POINTS

Psychosis
- Major emotional disorder; impairs mental function; person cannot participate in everyday life.
- Hallmark = loss of contact with reality.

Affective Disorders
- Emotional disorder characterized by changes in mood.
- Range from mania (abnormally elevated emotions) to depression (abnormally reduced emotions).

Anxiety
- A normal physiologic emotion.
- Five main types: obsessive-compulsive disorder, posttraumatic stress disorder, generalized anxiety disorder, panic disorder, social phobia, and simple phobia.
- Situational; arise because of specific events.
- Treat with drugs when markedly affects quality of life, relationships, or normal functioning.

Benzodiazepines
- Drug of choice.
- Most commonly prescribed; several advantages over other categories of drugs.
- Little effect on consciousness; very safe; do not interact with many other drugs.
- Most common ones are diazepam and lorazepam.

Flumazenil = Benzodiazepine Antagonist
- Blocks the benzodiazepine receptor; directly opposes the actions of the benzodiazepines.
- Used to reverse the sedative effects of benzodiazepines.

Selective Serotonin-Reuptake Inhibitors
- Second-generation antidepressants; newer antidepressants.
- Generally considered superior to TCAs in terms of side effect profiles.
- Specifically and potently inhibit presynaptic serotonin reuptake.

Antipsychotics, Tranquilizers, or Neuroleptics
- All terms used to refer to the drugs commonly used to treat serious mental illness.
- Used for bipolar affective disorder, psychoses, schizophrenia, and autism.
- Called *tranquilizers* because produce a state of tranquility.
- Called *neuroleptics* because they work on abnormal functioning nerves.

Nursing Considerations
- Assessment of medication and drug history or use is critical to patient safety.
- All medications, including psychotherapeutic agents, must be taken *exactly* as prescribed.
- Avoiding alcohol and other CNS depressants is important to patient safety.

The therapeutic effects of haloperidol, another antipsychotic agent, are similar to those of the other agents, but you should monitor your patient for adverse reactions particular to haloperidol. These include sedation; ticlike, trembling movements of the hands, face, neck, and head; hypotension; and dry mouth. Overdose is manifested by severe sedation, hypotension, respiratory depression, and coma. It takes approximately 3 weeks for the therapeutic effects of haloperidol to appear, but it is still important to watch the patient for possible dyskinesia and trembling during this time. Should these occur, the nurse should consult the physician immediately to discuss possible actions.

Lithium's therapeutic effects are characterized by less mania, and it is during the manic phase that lithium is better tolerated by the patient. Therapeutic levels of lithium range from 1.0 to 1.5 mEq/L and should be determined frequently, every few days initially and then at least every few months while the patient is on the drug. You should also monitor the patient's mood, affect, and emotional stability. Adverse reactions to lithium include arrhythymias, hypotension, sedation, slurred speech, slowed motor abilities, and weight gain. Gastrointestinal symptoms such as diarrhea and vomiting, drowsiness, weakness, and unsteady gait are indicative of overdose. The physician should be consulted immediately if these occur.

Critical Thinking A C T I V I T I E S

1. What conditions would be responsible for decreasing the excretion of lithium from the body? Explain the impact of this decrease on the patient.

2. Mrs. Biggs has inadvertently been given too much lorazepam and is experiencing respiratory arrest. You have identified that use of the benzodiazepine reversal agent flumazenil is indicated. The dose called for is 0.2 mg delivered over 15 seconds, then another 0.2 mg if consciousness does not occur after 45 seconds. This is to be repeated at 60-second intervals as needed up to four additional times for a maximum total dose of 1 mg. Flumazenil (Romazicon) comes as a 0.1-mg/ml vial. What dose should you draw up into the needle to deliver 0.2 mg each time?

3. Mr. Hatchet has a psychotic disorder that has been controlled on chlorpromazine therapy (50 mg q4h) until recently, when severe anticholinergic side effects from the chlorpromazine a low-potency antipsychotic, have necessitated his being switched to haloperidol, a high-potency antipsychotic. The physician would like to know what the equivalent daily dose of haloperidol would be. What is the equivalent daily dose of haloperidol?

▲▲▲

BIBLIOGRAPHY

Albanese J, Nutz P: *Mosby's 1995 nursing drug cards*, St Louis, 1995, Mosby.

Dyer J: A missing link between psychotropics and MI? *Am J Nurs* April 1993, p 65.

Glod CA: Psychopharmacology and clinical practice, *Nurs Clin North Am* 26:375, 1991.

Johnson KB: *Harriet Lane handbook*, ed 13, St Louis, 1993, Mosby.

Keen JH: *Critical care and emergency drug reference*, St Louis, 1994, Mosby.

Knoben JE, Anderson PO: *Handbook of critical drug data*, ed 6, Hamilton, Ill, 1988, Drug Intelligence Publications.

Maletta G et al: Guidelines for prescribing psychoactive drugs in the elderly: Part 1, *Geriatrics* 46(9):40, 1991.

Maletta G et al: Guidelines for prescribing psychoactive drugs in the elderly: Part 2, *Geriatrics* 46(9):52, 1991.

McEvoy GK: *AHFS drug information*, Bethesda, Md, 1989, American Society of Hospital Pharmacists.

Mendels J: Clinical management of the depressed geriatric patient: current therapeutic options, *Am J Med* 94(suppl 5A): 13S, 1993.

Preskorn SH: Recent pharmacologic advances in antidepressant therapy for the elderly, *Am J Med* 94(suppl 5A): 2S, 1993.

Skidmore-Roth L: *Mosby's 1995 nursing drug reference*, St Louis, 1995, Mosby.

Chapter 14

Central Nervous System Stimulant Agents

Objectives

When you reach the end of this chapter, you will be able to:

1 Identify the various CNS stimulants.

2 Define the following terms: analeptic, CNS stimulant, and methylxanthines.

3 Discuss the mechanism of action, indications, contraindications, cautions, side effects, and toxic effects of CNS stimulants.

4 Develop a nursing care plan, including patient education, as it relates to the nursing process in patients receiving CNS stimulants.

CHAPTER OUTLINE

CNS Stimulants
  Mechanism of action
  Drug effects
  Therapeutic uses
  Side effects and adverse effects
  Interactions
  Dosages
Drug Profiles
Analeptics
  Caffeine
  Doxapram
Anorexiants
  Benzphetamine
  Diethylpropion
  Fenfluramine
  Phenylpropanolamine
Amphetamines
  Amphetamine
  ⚓ Methylphenidate hydrochloride

Nursing Process
Assessment
Nursing Diagnoses
Planning
  Outcome criteria
Implementation
Evaluation

Glossary

Amphetamines (am fet′ ə mēnz) CNS stimulants that produce mood elevation or euphoria, increase mental alertness and capacity to work, decrease fatigue and drowsiness, and prolong wakefulness. (p. 195)

Analeptics (an′ ə lep tik) CNS stimulants that have generalized effects on the brainstem and spinal cord, which in turn produces an increase in responsiveness to external stimuli and stimulates respiration. (p. 195)

Anorexiants (an′ o rek se ənt) Drugs used to control or suppress appetite. These also stimulate the CNS. (p. 195)

Attention deficit disorder (ADD) Syndrome affecting children, adolescents, and rarely adults. It is characterized by learning disabilities and behavioral problems. (p. 195)

CNS stimulants Drugs that stimulate a specific area of the brain or spinal cord. (p. 195)

Narcolepsy (nahr′ ko lep sē) Syndrome characterized by sudden sleep attacks, cataplexy, sleep paralysis, and visual or auditory hallucinations at the onset of sleep. (p. 196)

Sympathomimetic agents (sim′ pə tho mi met′ ik) Another name for CNS stimulants. (p. 195)

CNS STIMULANTS

CNS stimulants are drugs that stimulate a specific area of the brain or spinal cord. Many of the actions mimic those of the sympathetic nervous system neurotransmitters norepinephrine and epinephrine, and for this reason they are sometimes referred to as **sympathomimetic agents.** The CNS stimulants elevate mood, produce a sense of increased energy and alertness, decrease appetite, and enhance the performance of tasks impaired by fatigue or boredom. Two of the oldest known stimulants are cocaine and amphetamine. These are also the prototypical agents. Cocaine is a natural alkaloid that was first extracted from the plant *Erythroxylon coca* in the mid-19th century but had been used by natives of the Andes for its stimulant effects for centuries before. Caffeine, which is contained in coffee and tea, is another plant-derived CNS stimulant.

CNS activity is regulated by a checks-and-balances system, and this consists of both excitatory and inhibitory systems. CNS stimulation can result from either excessive stimulation of the excitatory neurons or blockade of the inhibitory neurons, but most CNS stimulants act by stimulating the excitatory neurons in the brain. There are many such drugs, but only a few have therapeutic properties.

There are two ways of classifying these therapeutic CNS stimulants. The first is according to their location of action in the CNS, and hence the site where they produce their therapeutic effects. The agents are listed in this way in Table 14-1. CNS stimulants may also be classified on the basis of structural similarities and are listed in this way in Table 14-2. However the CNS stimulants are classified, their therapeutic applications are limited to four areas. They can be used as analeptics or as appetite suppressants and for the treatment of **attention deficit disorder** (ADD) or narcolepsy.

The **amphetamines** produce mood elevation or euphoria, increase mental alertness and the capacity for work, decrease fatigue and drowsiness, and prolong wakefulness. They are used to treat narcolepsy and ADD. The amphetamines produce tolerance and psychologic dependence. They are associated with a high abuse potential and are therefore classified as schedule II drugs under the Controlled Substances Act. Because of this high abuse potential, this class of CNS stimulants is used more frequently for nonmedical (recreational) purposes than for therapeutic ones.

The **analeptics** were used primarily to stimulate respiration when the natural reflex was lost. However, their use has waned as modern techniques of respiratory therapy have come available that can adequately ventilate a patient by mechanical means. In addition, respiratory paralysis caused by overdoses of narcotics, alcohol, barbiturates, and general anesthetics can now be appropriately treated with reversal agents or by

Table 14-1	CNS Stimulants: Site of Action
SITE OF ACTION	**CNS STIMULANT**
Cerebral cortex	Amphetamines
Medulla and brainstem	Analeptics
Hypothalamic and limbic regions	Anorexiants

Table 14-2	Structurally Related CNS Stimulants
CHEMICAL CATEGORY	**CNS STIMULANT**
Amphetamines	Amphetamine, dextroamphetamine, methamphetamine, methylphenidate, pemoline
Sympathomimetics	Phenylpropanolamine
Xanthines	Caffeine, theophylline

more reliable and effective methods of mechanical assistance.

The **anorexiants** suppress appetite and are used in the treatment of exogenous obesity.

Mechanism of Action

CNS stimulants have varying mechanisms of actions, and their effects on the CNS are many. The analeptics (aminophylline, theophylline, caffeine, and doxapram) have generalized effects on the brainstem and spinal cord and, as just pointed out, tend to stimulate respiration. The methylxanthines analeptics (caffeine, aminophylline, and theophylline) work by inhibiting the enzyme phosphodiesterase. This enzyme breaks down a substance called *cyclic adenosine monophosphate* (cAMP). When the breakdown of cAMP is blocked, it accumulates. This results in the relaxation of smooth muscle in the respiratory tract, the dilation of pulmonary arterioles, and stimulation of the CNS. Caffeine can stimulate the CNS at almost any level depending on the dose. Its ability to stimulate areas in the CNS is greater than that of the other two methylxanthines. Doxapram's mechanism of action is similar to that of the three methylxanthines, but it has a greater affinity for the area of the brain that senses carbon dioxide content. When the carbon dioxide content of the blood is high, this stimulates the respiratory center in the brain to induce deeper and faster breathing in an attempt to exchange more oxygen for carbon dioxide.

The anorexiants are believed to work by suppressing appetite control centers in the brain, although this has yet to be proved scientifically. There are some minor differences between these agents in terms of their individual actions. Benzphetamine and mazindol resemble the amphetamines from the standpoint of their activity in the CNS, but diethylpropion has little effect on the cardiovascular system. Fenfluramine actually depresses the CNS while suppressing the appetite center in the brain. Phentermine has very little effect on mood but does cause some cardiovascular stimulation. The only appetite suppressant available without a prescription, phenylpropanolamine, mildly suppresses appetite but also causes generalized CNS stimulation.

As already mentioned, amphetamines are used to treat the attention deficit disorder and narcolepsy. These are very potent stimulators of the CNS, and therefore the abuse potential associated with their use is very high. The amphetamines increase the amount and the duration of effect of catecholamine neurotransmitters in the CNS responsible for stimulation, mainly norepinephrine and dopamine. The drugs used to treat ADD and narcolepsy cause an increase in the release of these neurotransmitters and block their reuptake. As a result of this blockade, norepinephrine and dopamine are in contact with their receptors longer and therefore their duration of action and effectiveness are prolonged.

Drug Effects

Many of the effects of the CNS stimulants are dose related. Their pharmacologic actions are similar to the actions of the sympathetic nervous system, in that the CNS and the respiratory system are the primary body systems affected. The CNS effects most frequently noted are increased motor activity and mental alertness, diminished sense of fatigue, emotional or mood elevation, and mild euphoria; the respiratory effects most commonly seen are relaxation of bronchial smooth muscle, increased respiration, and dilation of pulmonary arteries. Other body systems can also be affected by CNS stimulants, and these include the cardiovascular, gastrointestinal, genitourinary, and endocrine systems. Often stimulation of these other body systems results in the unwanted effects, as discussed later.

Therapeutic Uses

The therapeutic effects of the CNS stimulants are varied and best discussed from the standpoint of the individual drug category. The therapeutic effects of the analeptics are limited to the relaxation of smooth muscle in the respiratory tract, the dilation of pulmonary arterioles, and the stimulation of areas within the CNS that control respiration, mainly the medulla and spinal cord.

The anorexiants primarily work by broadly stimulating the CNS. As mentioned earlier, it is believed that their action specifically targets the appetite control centers in the brain, but this has yet to be proved. Some evidence points toward increased fat mobilization, decreased absorption of dietary fat, and increased cellular glucose uptake as other possible therapeutic effects.

The agents used to treat ADD stimulate the areas of the brain responsible for mental alertness and attentiveness—the cerebral cortex and subcortical structures such as the thalamus. This results in increased motor activity and mental alertness and a diminished sense of fatigue.

Narcolepsy is a condition in which patients unexpectedly fall asleep in the middle of normal activity. Therefore an agent that can increase mental alertness would be most beneficial in treating a condition such as this, and that is what the amphetamines, the primary agents used to treat narcolepsy, do. The amphetamines main sites of action in the CNS appear to be the cerebral cortex and possibly the reticular activating system. Stimulation of these areas also results in increased motor activity and a diminished sense of fatigue.

Other therapeutic effects are seen with CNS stimulants such as caffeine. Caffeine may induce diuresis and is a helpful agent in the treatment of migraines when coadministered with other drugs. It does this by increasing blood flow to the kidneys and decreasing the resorption of sodium and water. The constriction of the cerebral blood vessels that caffeine may induce also potentiates the action of the other agents given in combination with it.

Side Effects and Adverse Effects

The CNS stimulants have a wide range of adverse effects, and these most often arise when these agents are administered at doses higher than the therapeutic doses. The most common undesirable effects associated with the administration of CNS stimulants are listed in Table 14-3 according to the body system affected.

Interactions

The drug interactions associated with the CNS stimulants vary greatly from class to class. The drug interactions that occur with the analeptics and ano-rexiants differ from those seen for the amphetamines. Those drug interactions most commonly encountered for the three classes of CNS stimulants are listed in Table 14-4.

Dosages

The recommended dosages for selected CNS stimulants are given in the table on the following page.

Table 14-3	CNS Stimulants: Common Adverse Effects
BODY SYSTEM	**SIDE/ADVERSE EFFECTS**
Cardiovascular	Palpitations, tachycardia, hypertension, angina, arrhythmias
Central nervous system	Nervousness, restlessness, jitteriness, anxiety, insomnia, headache, tremor, blurred vision
Gastrointestinal	Nausea, vomiting, diarrhea, abdominal pain, dry mouth
Genitourinary	Increased urinary frequency, diuresis
Endocrine*	Hypoglycemia, hyperglycemia, increased metabolic rate

*Apply to methylxanthines, such as theophylline, only.

DRUG PROFILES

ANALEPTICS

Although most of the analeptic CNS stimulants are highly toxic and have a high abuse potential, and are therefore only available with a prescription, caffeine and phenylpropanolamine are the two exceptions. Both of these agents are available at low doses in OTC preparations. The profiles for aminophylline and theophylline can be found in Unit VII on respiratory system drugs.

CAFFEINE

Caffeine (Nö-Döz) is a CNS stimulant that can be found in OTC drugs and combination-prescription drugs. It is also contained in many beverages and foods. Just a few of the many foods and drugs that contain caffeine are listed in the box on p. 199. Caffeine is contraindicated in patients with a known hypersensitivity to the drug and should be used with caution in patients who have a history of peptic ulcers or cardiac arrhythmias or who have recently suffered a myocardial infarction. Caffeine is available orally as 200- and 250-mg extended-release capsules and as

Table 14-4	CNS Stimulants: Common Drug Interactions	
DRUG	**MECHANISM**	**RESULT**
Amphetamines		
Tricyclic antidepressants	Additive toxicities	Cardiovascular adverse effects (dysrhythmias, tachycardia, hypertension)
CNS stimulants	Additive toxicities	Cardiovascular adverse effects, nervousness, insomnia, convulsions
Digoxin	Additive toxicity	Increased risk of dysrhythmias
MAOIs	Increase release of catecholamines	Headaches, dysrhythmias, severe hypertension
Beta-blockers	Increase alpha-adrenergic effects	Hypertension, bradycardia, dysrhythmias, heart block
Anorexiants and analeptics		
CNS stimulants	Additive toxicities	Nervousness, irritability, insomnia, dysrhythmias, seizures
MAOIs	Increase release of catecholamines	Headaches, dysrhythmias, severe hypertension

DOSAGES

SELECTED CNS STIMULANTS

AGENT	PHARMACOLOGIC CLASS	DOSAGE RANGE	PURPOSE
Caffeine (Nö-Döz)	Xanthine cerebral stimulant	*Adult* PO: 100-200 mg q3-4h	Aids in staying awake
Doxapram (Dopram)	Respiratory stimulant (analeptic)	*Adult/Pediatric >12 y/o* 0.5-1 mg/kg IV as a single injection not to exceed 1.5 mg/kg, or infusion of 5 mg/min until desired effect, then reduced to 1-3 mg/min	Postanesthetic respiratory depression
		1-2 mg IV given twice at 5-min intervals then repeated at 1-2 hr intervals prn	Drug-induced respiratory depression
		Infusion 1-2 mg/min for up to 2 hr	Acute hypercapnia
Benzphetamine (Didrex)	CNS stimulant (anorexiant)	*Adult* PO: 25-50 mg 1-3 times daily	Appetite control in obesity
Diethylpropion (Tenuate)	CNS stimulant (anorexiant)	*Adult* PO: 25 mg tid 1 hr ac or extended-release 75-mg tablet in AM or mid-AM	Appetite control in obesity
Fenfluramine (Pondimin)	CNS stimulant (anorexiant)	*Adult* PO: 20 mg tid ac	Appetite control in obesity
Phenylpropanolamine (Dexatrim, Acutrim)	CNS stimulant (anorexiant)	*Adult* PO: 25 mg tid ½ hr ac or one 75-mg extended-release capsule or tablet in AM	Appetite control in obesity
Amphetamine	CNS stimulant	*Pediatric 3-5 y/o* PO: 2.5 mg/day and increased weekly until desired effect	Attention deficit disorder
		Pediatric ≥6 y/o PO: 5 mg 1-2 times/day and increased weekly until desired effect to a daily maximum of 40 mg	Attention deficit disorder
		Adult PO: 5-10 mg tid ½-1 hr ac	Appetite control in obesity
⚓Methylphenidate (Ritalin)	CNS stimulant	*Pediatric ≥6 y/o* PO: 5 mg twice daily before breakfast and lunch and increased weekly until desired effect to a daily maximum of 60 mg	Attention deficit disorder
		Adult PO: 20-60 mg/day divided in 2-3 doses 30-45 min ac	Narcolepsy

Caffeine-Containing Foods and Drugs	
Medications	
Nonprescription medications	
Analgesics	
Anacin	32 mg/tablet
Excedrin	65 mg/tablet
Cold medications	
Dristan AF	16.2 mg/tablet
Stimulants	
NöDöz	100 mg/tablet
Vivarin	200 mg/tablet
Prescription medications (for migraines)	
Fioricet	40 mg/tablet
Esgic	40 mg/tablet
Cafergot	100 mg/tablet
Beverages	
Coffee (brewed)	80-150 mg/5-oz cup
Coffee (instant)	85-100 mg/5-oz cup
Coffee (decaffeinated)	2-4 mg/5-oz cup
Tea (brewed)	30-75 mg/5-oz cup
Soft drinks	35-60 mg/12-oz drink
Cocoa	5-40 mg/5-oz cup

100-, 150-, and 200-mg regular-release tablets. It is available parenterally as a 250-mg/ml injection. Caffeine is considered a pregnancy category B drug. For the recommended adult and neonate dosages, refer to the table on the previous page.

✱ PHARMACOKINETICS

HALF-LIFE	ONSET	PEAK	DURATION
3-4 hr	15-45 min	50-75 min	<6 hr

DOXAPRAM

Doxapram (Dopram) is another analeptic that is commonly used in conjunction with supportive measures to hasten arousal and to treat the respiratory depression associated with an overdose of CNS depressants (e.g., barbiturates, opioid analgesics, and general anesthetics), the acute respiratory insufficiency associated with chronic obstructive pulmonary disease, or respiratory depression in the postoperative recovery period that is not caused by skeletal muscle relaxants.

Doxapram is contraindicated in newborns because of the benzyl alcohol in the injectable formulation of the drug. It is also contraindicated in patients with epilepsy or other convulsive disorders, those who have shown a hypersensitivity reaction to the drug, those showing evidence of head injury, those suffering from cardiovascular impairment or severe hypertension,

and patients who have had a cerebrovascular accident. It is only available parenterally as a 20-mg/ml injection. Doxapram is considered a pregnancy category B drug. For the recommended dosages, refer to the table on the previous page.

✱ PHARMACOKINETICS

HALF-LIFE	ONSET	PEAK	DURATION
2-4 hr*	<30 sec	<2 min	5-12 min

*Metabolites: 4-8 hr.

ANOREXIANTS

As mentioned earlier, the anorexiants are CNS stimulants that control or suppress appetite. There are only some minor differences among the agents in terms of their actions.

BENZPHETAMINE

Benzphetamine (Didrex) is a CNS stimulant that is primarily used as an adjunct to diet in the short-term treatment (a few weeks) of exogenous obesity. Structurally it very closely resembles amphetamine, and it is believed to produce its anorexiant effects secondary to CNS stimulation. Under the Federal Controlled Substances Act of 1970, benzphetamine is classified as a schedule III (C-III) drug. It has been clearly demonstrated to cause fetal harm, and possible risk to the fetus outweighs any possible benefit to pregnant women taking the drug; therefore it is classified as a pregnancy category X agent. It is contraindicated in patients with advanced arteriosclerosis, hyperthyroidism, moderate to severe hypertension, symptomatic cardiovascular disease, glaucoma, or a known hypersensitivity or idiosyncrasy to sympathomimetic amines; in those in agitated states; and in those with a history of drug abuse. In addition, the drug is contraindicated during or within 14 days of the administration of monoamine oxidase inhibitors. Benzphetamine is only available orally as 25- and 50-mg tablets. For the recommended dosages, refer to the table on p. 198.

✱ PHARMACOKINETICS

HALF-LIFE	ONSET	PEAK	DURATION
7-14 hr	15 min	<2 hr	4 hr

*pH <6.6.

DIETHYLPROPION

Diethylpropion (Tenuate) is primarily used as an adjunct to diet in the short-term treatment (a few weeks) of exogenous obesity. It is also structurally similar to amphetamine. It differs from benzphetamine in that it has little effect on the cardiovascular system but it is like benzphetamine in that it is also harmful to the fetus and should not be used in pregnant women. It is therefore also classified as a pregnancy category X drug. The contraindications to diethylpropion use are the same as those that apply to benzphetamine use. It is only available orally as a 25-mg regular-release tablet and 75-mg extended-release tablet. For the recommended dosages, refer to the table on p. 198.

✸ PHARMACOKINETICS

HALF-LIFE	ONSET	PEAK	DURATION
8 hr	1 hr*	2 wk*	4 hr*

*Therapeutic effect.

FENFLURAMINE

Fenfluramine (Pondimin) is used as an adjunct to diet in the short-term treatment (a few weeks) of exogenous obesity. It is also structurally similar to amphetamine. Fenfluramine actually depresses the CNS while suppressing the appetite center in the brain. It is classified as a pregnancy category X drug and the contraindications to its use are the same as those that apply to benzphetamine use. It is only available orally as 20-mg tablets. For the recommended dosages, refer to the table on p. 198.

✸ PHARMACOKINETICS

HALF-LIFE	ONSET	PEAK	DURATION
20 hr	1-2 hr	2-4 hr	4-6 hr

PHENYLPROPANOLAMINE

Phenylpropanolamine (Dexatrim, Acutrim, and others) is the only anorexiant that can be obtained without a prescription. It is structurally related to ephedrine and amphetamine and is chemically classified as a sympathomimetic. Specifically, its actions mimic those of the sympathetic nervous system neurotransmitters norepinephrine and epinephrine. The CNS stimulation and anorexiant effect of phenylpropanolamine are much weaker than those of the amphetamines. Its use is contraindicated in patients with glaucoma, prostatic hypertrophy, or diabetes, as well as in those with the contraindications that apply to the rest of the anorexiants. Extensive uncontrolled clinical experience with the drug has not revealed any evidence of its causing harm to the fetus during pregnancy, but its absolute safety cannot be assured. It is only available orally in many tablet and capsule preparations and in many different strengths. For the recommended dosages, refer to the table on p. 198. Safety for use during pregnancy has not been established.

✸ PHARMACOKINETICS

HALF-LIFE	ONSET	PEAK	DURATION
3-4 hr	30 min	1 hr	4-6 hr

AMPHETAMINES

As mentioned earlier, the class of CNS stimulants used to treat ADD and narcolepsy are the amphetamines, and they do so by increasing the amount and the duration of effect of the catecholamine neurotransmitters. The overall response is global CNS excitement and stimulation, with improved mental alertness and attentiveness the therapeutic effect.

AMPHETAMINE

Amphetamine is the prototypical CNS stimulant used to treat ADD, narcolepsy, and obesity. When used in the treatment of these conditions, it is only as an adjunct to psychologic, educational, and social therapies. Its use is associated with a wide array of CNS effects, many of which are undesirable or unintended. It is for these reasons that many of the other anorexiants and the other drugs used to treat narcolepsy and ADD were developed. Amphetamine is contraindicated in patients who have shown a hypersensitivity reaction to it as well as those with the contraindications that apply to the other CNS stimulants. It is available orally as 6.25- and 10-mg capsules and 5- and 10-mg tablets. It, like many of the other CNS stimulants, is rated as a pregnancy category X drug, and therefore its use should be avoided during pregnancy. For recommended dosages, refer to the table on p. 198.

✸ PHARMACOKINETICS

HALF-LIFE	ONSET	PEAK	DURATION
7-14 hr*	30-60 min	<2 hr	10 hr

*pH <6.6.

⚓ METHYLPHENIDATE HYDROCHLORIDE

Methylphenidate (Ritalin) has become the drug of choice for the treatment of ADD and narcolepsy. Much attention of late has been focused on this CNS stimulant because of its dramatic effect in the treatment of ADD, a condition that may affect adults as well as children. However, this heightened interest may have more to do with the better diagnosis and a growing awareness of the disorder than with the drug's particular attributes. Like the other CNS stimulants, its use should be considered adjunctive to psychologic, educational, social, and other remedial measures in the treatment of ADD, narcolepsy, and weight loss. The side effect profile of methylphenidate is much less unfavorable than that of many of the other CNS stimulants. As a result of its relative safety, it can be used in more patients without as much concern regarding some of the more severe toxicities seen with other CNS stimulants. Overstimulation of the CNS (severe cardiovascular and nervous system complications) can still occur, but this is a much less common event. Methylphenidate is contraindicated in patients with a history of marked anxiety, tension, and agitation. It is also contraindicated in patients with glaucoma and in those with a known hypersensitivity to it. Methylphenidate is classified as a pregnancy category C drug. It is available orally as 5-, 10-, and 20-mg tablets and 20-mg extended-release tablets. For recommended dosages, refer to the table on p. 198.

P H A R M A C O K I N E T I C S

HALF-LIFE	ONSET	PEAK	DURATION
1-3 hr	30-60 min	1-3 hr	4-6 hr

Nursing Process

ASSESSMENT

CNS stimulants are most often used for the treatment of drug-induced or postanesthetic respiratory depression. These agents are also used for the treatment of ADD with hyperactivity, as well as for the treatment of narcolepsy and exogenous obesity. Before administering these agents, you must carefully assess the patient and gather data from their nursing history regarding potential contraindications, cautions, and drug interactions. Contraindications to the use of these medications include a hypersensitivity to them, seizure disorders, and liver dysfunction. Contraindications to doxapram include all of the foregoing plus hypertension and severe cardiac disorders. Vital signs, especially blood pressure in patients with a history of cardiac disease, should be assessed and the findings recorded for baseline purposes. The height and weight

of children who are taking methylphenidate should be measured and recorded before therapy is initiated and their growth rate should be plotted during therapy because this agent may retard growth. Patients need to be questioned about other medications they are taking, specifically whether they are taking MAOIs or vasopressors, antihypertensive agents, oral anticoagulants, tricyclic antidepressants, or anticonvulsants.

NURSING DIAGNOSES

Nursing diagnoses appropriate to patients taking CNS stimulants include:
- Altered nutrition (less than body requirements) related to drug effects.
- Altered sleep patterns (decreased sleep) related to drug effects.
- Risk for altered cardiac output (decreased) related to possible palpitations and tachycardia.
- Altered self-image (decreased) related to possible growth retardation in children.
- Anxiety related to drug effects.
- Knowledge deficit related to lack of information about drug regimen.

PLANNING

Goals associated with the use of CNS stimulants include:
- Patient maintains normal body weight and height.
- Patient continues normal growth and development while on medications.
- Patient experiences minimal sleep deprivation.
- Patient will be free of cardiac symptoms and associated complications of drug therapy.
- Patient maintains positive self-esteem.
- Patient appears less anxious.
- Patient remains compliant to drug therapy.

Outcome Criteria

Outcome criteria related to the nursing care of patients receiving CNS stimulants include the following:
- Patient maintains normal body weight and height and, if pediatric patient, will continue normal growth and development patterns, with weight and height falling within normal limits on growth chart, while taking CNS stimulants.
- Patient shows improved sensorium and level of consciousness with increased attentiveness.
- Patient experiences more restful sleep using nonpharmacologic measures.
- Patient's vital signs, specifically blood pressure and pulse, will be within normal limits.

Patient Teaching TIPS

CNS Stimulants

✔ Patients should avoid other sources of CNS stimulants such as caffeine, which is found in coffee, tea, cola products, and chocolate.

✔ Patients should take their medication exactly as prescribed by their physician. They should not skip, omit, or double-up on doses.

✔ Patients should avoid taking OTC preparations unless they are approved by their physician.

✔ Patients should not drink alcohol or consume any products that contain alcohol.

✔ Patients should keep a log of their daily activities.

✔ Patients should not stop taking these medications abruptly.

✔ Patients should take medication at least 6 hours before bedtime so as to decrease insomnia.

✔ If taking medication for treatment of obesity, patients should take it 30 to 45 minutes before meals.

✔ Patients should suck on hard candy, chew gum, or sip fluids to minimize dry mouth.

■ Patient communicates feelings of self-image, self-esteem, anxiety, and anger as needed and openly.

■ Patient states symptoms (e.g., palpitations, chest pain) to report to the physician immediately.

Implementation

Doxapram is administered intravenously (see the dosages table on p. 198) but at different doses (not to exceed 1.5 mg/kg) depending on the purpose. These infusions should be administered at the rate of approximately 1 to 3 mg/min for the reversal of anesthesia-induced respiratory depression and should not be mixed in alkaline solutions that include theophylline, thiopental sodium, and bicarbonate. 5% Dextrose in water is usually the diluent used with doxapram, and these solutions should be infused by means of an intravenous pump. Because patients' sensorium is generally diminished in this situation, placing them in a Sims' or semi-Fowler's position is necessary to prevent possible aspiration. If side effects occur, the infusion should be discontinued immediately and the physician notified.

Methylphenidate should be administered at least 6 hours before bedtime so as to diminish the insomnia it causes. Methylphenidate should also be given ap-

TAKE HOME POINTS

CNS Stimulants
■ Drugs that stimulate the brain or spinal cord (e.g., cocaine and caffeine).
■ Actions mimic those of the sympathetic nervous system neurotransmitters norepinephrine and epinephrine.
■ Also called *sympathomimetic agents* because they mimic the sympathetic nervous system neurotransmitters.

Amphetamines, Analeptics, and Anorexiants
■ Family of CNS stimulants.
■ Therapeutic uses: analeptics, appetite control, ADD, and narcolepsy.

Amphetamines
■ Elevate mood or produce euphoria; increase mental alertness and capacity for work.
■ Decrease fatigue and drowsiness; prolong wakefulness.
■ Treat narcolepsy and ADD.

Analeptics
■ Generalized effects on brainstem and spinal cord.
■ Increase responsiveness to external stimuli and stimulate respiration.
■ Treat respiratory paralysis caused by overdose of narcotics, alcohol, barbiturates, and general anesthetic agents.

Anorexiants
■ Control or suppress appetite; may also be used to stimulate the CNS.
■ Work by suppressing appetite control centers in brain.
■ Contraindications to use of CNS stimulants in a patient's history include hypersensitivity, seizure activity, convulsive disorders, and liver dysfunction.

Nursing Considerations
■ Children who take methylphenidate should always have baseline height and weight recorded before initiating drug therapy and should continue to plot their height and weight in a journal during therapy.
■ Therapeutic responses to agents used in treatment of hyperkinesia include decreased hyperactivity, increased attention span and concentration, and improved behavior patterns.
■ Side effects to monitor for in individuals taking CNS stimulants include changes in mental status or sensorium, mood, affect, and sleep patterns; physical dependency, and irritability.

proximately 45 minutes before meals. Because dry mouth is an expected side effect, the patient should perform frequent mouth care, and sucking on hard candy or frequently sipping fluids may provide some relief. If the patient is taking the CNS stimulant for the treatment of obesity, a holistic approach should be used that includes exercise and dietary teaching, all under the supervision of a physician. See the patient teaching tips on p. 202.

EVALUATION

Therapeutic responses to agents used in the management of hyperkinesia include decreased hyperactivity, increased attention span and concentration, and improved behavior. The therapeutic response to agents used for the management of narcolepsy would be the ability to remain awake. Anorexiants should cause the patient's appetite to decrease and weight loss to occur. You also need to monitor the patient for the development of adverse effects to these medications; these included mental status changes and changes in sensorium, mood, affect, and sleep patterns; physical dependency; irritability; and withdrawal symptoms such as headache, nausea, and vomiting.

Critical Thinking A C T I V I T I E S

1. H.F. is a 67-year-old man who has not resumed spontaneous breathing after surgery despite reversal of the nondepolarizing muscle relaxant given to him for the procedure. The anesthesiologist asks you to administer a 1.5-mg/kg bolus of doxapram followed by an infusion delivered at a rate of 2 mg/min. H.F. weighs 78 kg. The pharmacist delivers a 20-mg/ml vial of doxapram for injection and a 250-ml bag of doxapram for infusion, the concentration of which is 1 mg/ml.
   a. Calculate how many milliliters of the injection the patient should be given to accomplish the 1.5-mg/kg dose.
   b. What rate (ml/hr) should you set the pump at to deliver the 2-mg/min infusion of doxapram?
2. Narcolepsy has been diagnosed in Ms. Potter, a 68-year-old retired nurse and she has been on a CNS stimulant for the past 6 months. Formulate a list of questions to ask her caregiver that will help to determine the effectiveness of her drug therapy.

▲▲▲

BIBLIOGRAPHY

Albanese J, Nutz P: *Mosby's 1995 nursing drug cards*, St Louis, 1995, Mosby.

Johnson KB: *Harriet Lane handbook*, ed 13, St Louis, 1993, Mosby.

Keen JH: *Critical care and emergency drug reference*, St Louis, 1994, Mosby.

Knoben JE, Anderson PO: *Handbook of critical drug data*, ed 6, Hamilton, Ill, 1988, Drug Intelligence Publications.

McEvoy GK: *AHFS drug information*, Bethesda, Md, 1994, American Society of Hospital Pharmacists.

Skidmore-Roth L: *Mosby's 1995 Nursing drug reference*, St Louis, 1995, Mosby.

Smitherman, CH: A drug to ease attention-deficit hyperactivity disorder, *MCN* 15(6): 362, 1990.

PART 3

AUTONOMIC NERVOUS SYSTEM: STUDY SKILLS BRIEF

PURR APPLICATION
Planning for the PART

The basic explanation provided for the PURR model in Chapter 1 demonstrates the application process as it relates to individual chapters. There is another application for the PURR model that can be very useful. That application encourages the learner to take a broader view of the assignment. In the case of this text you have noticed that the chapters are grouped together into multiple chapter blocks called PARTS. Part organization is not some random process applied by the author to further complicate the subject. Part organization is a carefully thought out process to put content together in a fashion that is logical and meaningful. Since the author has spent considerable time trying to link the chapters together in the most logical pattern, it is to your advantage as a student to learn to take advantage of the work already done for you.

Part Title

Begin the process of Part planning by looking at the part title, "Autonomic Nervous System." Then look at the part structure. There are five chapters contained in Part 3. All these chapters must be concerned with the autonomic nervous system. Even before you have done any reading in any chapter, you are beginning to look for the links that will establish the relationship not only for the ideas in individual chapters, but also the broader link that connects the five chapters in this part with each other and with the ideas that have come in earlier parts and will follow in later parts.

There is a clear example in this part of the way in which parts relate to one another. Look back at Part 2,

"Central Nervous System." Clearly that part deals with some aspect of the nervous system as does this part. One learning objective you should establish for yourself is the relationship between these two parts. You must be able to define and explain central nervous system and autonomic nervous system. However, defining these and going no further limits the learning you can achieve. Ask yourself some additional questions that will help you to establish a connection between these parts. "What is the difference in functions of the central and the autonomic nervous systems?" "Are there pharmacologic agents that have application in both the central and autonomic nervous systems?" The principle is to keep stressing the links that must exist throughout all the parts and chapters you are studying. The normal study pattern that most students apply is one that focuses on the individual chapters, but it is essential that the broader scope of chapter and part be maintained.

Part Chapters

After considering the Part title and looking for relationships between the new part and past parts studied, the next step in applying the Plan step of PURR to a part is to spend a few minutes studying the chapter title and looking for the relationships that must exist. Part 3 has five chapters, and there is a clear pattern in these chapters. Chapters 15 and 16 both contain the term "adrenergic." Clearly the two chapters are dealing with the same broad topic. However, Chapter 15 covers adrenergic agents and Chapter 16 covers adrenergic-blocking agents. Apply questioning strategies at this point. "What does adrenergic mean?" "What is an adrenergic agent?" These two questions are essential in mastering the content of Chapter 15, and should be questions that you ask yourself almost without thinking. However, the next step is one that can greatly enhance your understanding when you start to read the material. This is a step that is easily overlooked. Notice that Chapter 15 deals with agents and Chapter 16 deals with blocking agents. There must a difference between an agent and a blocking agent. Focus now with a few questions that will keep you aware that the content in Chapter 15 has a direct relationship to the content in Chapter 16. "What is the difference between an agent and a blocking agent? When is the pharmacologic application of an agent appropriate? Under what conditions should a blocking agent be chosen?" Then ask a question to help maintain the focus on the concept of the entire part. "What aspects of the autonomic nervous system are related to the adrenergic agents and blocking agents?"

Chapters 17 and 18

Once you begin to focus on the relationship of chapters within a part, certain things will begin to become apparent. Chapters 17 and 18 cover agents and blocking agents. These two chapters develop the concept as related to cholinergics, rather than adrenergics. But the same questions you used as a focus for Chapters 15 and 16 can be recycled in setting up the study of Chapters 17 and 18. Simply replace the term adrenergic with cholinergic and you are ready to begin reading these two chapters with a clear personal learning objective.

Chapter 19

When you look at Chapter 19 the first thing that stands out is the absence of a chapter devoted to gan-

glionic agents. There is only one chapter on ganglionic agents, and it focuses on blocking agents. The first question that comes to mind as I look at this chapter is, "Why are there no ganglionic agents? Adrenergic and cholinergic have agents and blocking agents. What is there that is different about ganglions that we need to be informed only about the blocking agents?"

Active Questioning

This is the key concept to master in working through the process for planning your learning for an entire part rather than for single chapters. The idea is to view the part as a whole rather than seeing only the content of individual chapters. In the preceding discussion I have provided a number of sample questions to help you begin the process. These questions should not be seen as the only questions you should ask, but rather as samples to help you develop a questioning process.

Keep in mind that you may ask questions that seem useful and appropriate when you are using only the chapter titles as the question stimulus. Some of the questions will prove to be very useful when reading the chapter. On the other hand some of the initial questions you generate may have little or no application as you read and understand the content of an individual chapter. Do not worry about the quality of the questions when planning on the part level. Questions can (and sometimes should) be revised or discarded when the details of the chapter become clearer. The important point is that you begin the part with some questions to help you focus your own reading and learning. Also, you will find that the more you apply active questioning as a part of your learning strategy the better your questions will become.

Chapter 15

Adrenergic Agents

Objectives

When you reach the end of this chapter, you will be able to:

1 Briefly discuss the normal anatomy and physiology of the autonomic nervous system, including the events that take place during synaptic transmission within the sympathetic and parasympathetic divisions.

2 List the various adrenergic agonists, or sympathomimetics.

3 Discuss the mechanism of action, therapeutic effects, uses, and adverse and toxic effects of adrenergic agonists, as well as the antidotes to overdose and to the unwanted effects.

4 Develop a nursing care plan that includes expected outcomes and patient teaching tips as it relates to the administration of the various adrenergic agents and the treatment of side effects and overdose or toxicity stemming from the use of these agents.

5 Identify the drug interactions associated with the use of adrenergic agonists.

6 Evaluate the therapeutic versus the side effects of the different adrenergic agonists.

CHAPTER OUTLINE

Sympathetic Nervous System
Adrenergic Drugs
  Mechanism of action
  Drug effects
  Therapeutic uses
  Side effects and adverse effects
    Toxicity and management of overdose
  Interactions
    Laboratory test interactions
  Dosages
Drug Profiles
Anorexiants
    Dextroamphetamine sulfate
  ⬇ Methylphenidate hydrochloride
Bronchodilators
  ⬇ Albuterol sulfate
  ⬇ Epinephrine
    Isoproterenol hydrochloride
Nasal Decongestants
    Pseudoephedrine hydrochloride
Ophthalmic Decongestants
    Tetrahydrozoline
Vasoactive Adrenergics
  ⬇ Dobutamine
    Dopamine

  ⬇ Epinephrine
    Isoproterenol
    Norepinephrine
    Phenylephrine
Nursing Process
Assessment
Nursing Diagnoses
Planning
  Outcome criteria
Implementation
Evaluation

Glossary

Adrenergics (ad' ren ər' jik) Drugs that stimulate the sympathetic nervous system. They are also referred to as *adrenergic agonists* or *sympathomimetics* because they mimic the effects of the sympathetic neurotransmitters norepinephrine and epinephrine. (p. 207)

Adrenergic receptors Receptor sites for the sympathetic neurotransmitters norepinephrine and epinephrine. (p. 208)

Alpha-adrenergic receptors (al' fə) Adrenergic receptors that are further divided into alpha$_1$- and alpha$_2$-adrenergic receptors and are differentiated by their location on nerves. (p. 208)

Anorexiants (an' o rek' se ənt) Agents used as adjuncts to diet in the short-term management of obesity. (p. 210)

Beta-adrenergic receptors (bāt′ ə) Located on post-synaptic effector cells—the cells, muscles, and organs that the nerves stimulate. Beta$_1$-adrenergic receptors differ from beta$_2$-adrenergic receptors in that they are primarily in the heart; beta$_2$-adrenergic receptors are located in the smooth muscle of the bronchioles and arterioles and in visceral organs. (p. 208)

Catecholamines (kat′ ə kol′ ə mēnz) Substances that can produce a sympathomimetic response. They are either endogenous catecholamines; such as epinephrine, norepinephrine, and dopamine, or synthetic catecholamines, such as isoproterenol and dobutamine. (p. 207)

Dopaminergic receptors (do′ pə mēn er′ jik) Adrenergic receptors that, when stimulated by dopamine, cause the renal, mesenteric, coronary, and cerebral arteries to dilate and the flow of blood to increase. (p. 209)

Ophthalmics (of thal′ mikz) Topically applied eye medications. (p. 211)

Positive chronotropic effect (kron′ ō trop′ ik) Refers to an increased heart rate. (p. 210)

Positive dromotropic effect (drom′ o trop′ ik) Causes an increase in conduction through the atrioventricular node. (p. 210)

Positive inotropic effect (in ō trop′ ik) Refers to an increased force of contraction. (p. 210)

Synaptic cleft (sĭ nap′ tik) **or the neuroeffector junction** (noor′ ō ə fek′ tər) The space between the nerve ending and the effector organ. (p. 209)

Adrenergics are a large group of both exogenous (synthetic) and endogenous (naturally occurring) substances. They have a wide variety of therapeutic uses depending on their site of action and their effect on receptors. Adrenergics stimulate the sympathetic nervous system (SNS) and are also called adrenergic agonists or sympathomimetics because they mimic the effects of the SNS neurotransmitters norepinephrine (NE) and epinephrine (EPI), which are referred to chemically as **catecholamines.** In describing the adrenergic class of medications, it is helpful to understand how the SNS operates in relation to the rest of the nervous system.

SYMPATHETIC NERVOUS SYSTEM

Figure 15-1 depicts the divisions of the nervous system, showing the relationship of the SNS to the entire nervous system. The SNS is the counterpart to the parasympathetic nervous system; together they make up the autonomic nervous system. They provide a checks-and-balances system for maintaining the normal homeostasis of the autonomic functions of the human body.

Throughout the body there are receptor sites for catecholamines NE and EPI. These are referred to as

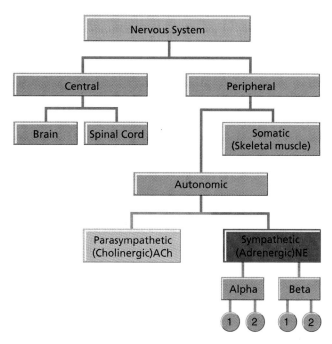

▼ **FIG. 15-1** The sympathetic nervous system in relationship to the entire nervous system.

Table 15-1	Adrenergic Receptor Responses to Stimulation	
LOCATION	**RECEPTOR**	**RESPONSE**
Cardiovascular		
Blood vessels	Alpha$_1$/beta$_2$	Constriction/dilation
Cardiac muscle	Beta$_1$	Increased contractility
Atrioventricular node	Beta$_1$	Increased conduction
Sinoatrial node	Beta$_1$	Increased heart rate
Gastrointestinal		
Muscle	Alpha/beta	Increased motility
Sphincters	Alpha$_1$	Constriction
Genitourinary		
Bladder sphincter	Alpha$_1$	Constriction
Penis	Alpha$_1$	Ejaculation
Uterus	Alpha$_1$/beta$_2$	Contraction/relaxation
Respiratory		
Bronchial muscles	Beta$_2$	Dilation

the **adrenergic receptors,** and these are the sites where adrenergic drugs bind and produce their effects. The adrenergic receptors are located at many anatomical sites, and many physiologic responses are produced when they are stimulated or blocked. The adrenergic receptors are further divided into **alpha-adrenergic** and **beta-adrenergic receptors,** depending on whether they respond to NE or EPI, respectively. Both types of adrenergic receptors have subtypes, designated 1 and 2, and these provide a further means of checks and balances that control stimulation and blockade, constriction and dilation, and the increased and decreased production of a substance.

Alpha$_1$- and alpha$_2$-adrenergic receptors are differentiated by their location on nerves. Alpha$_1$-adrenergic receptors are located on the cell, muscle, or organ that the nerve stimulates, the postsynaptic effector

cells. Alpha$_2$-adrenergic receptors are located on the presynaptic nerve terminals, actually on the nerve that stimulates the effector cells. They control the release of neurotransmitters. The predominant alpha-adrenergic agonist response is vasoconstriction and CNS stimulation.

Beta-adrenergic receptors are all located on postsynaptic effector cells—the cells, muscles, or organs that the nerves stimulate. Beta$_1$-adrenergic receptors are different from beta$_2$-adrenergic receptors in that they are primarily located in the heart; the beta$_2$-adrenergic receptors are located in the smooth muscle of the bronchioles, arterioles, and visceral organs. A beta-adrenergic agonist response results in bronchial, gastrointestinal, and uterine smooth muscle relaxation; glycogenolysis; and cardiac stimulation. Table 15-1 contains a more detailed listing of the adrenergic re-

▼ **FIG. 15-2** The mechanism by which stimulation of a nerve fiber results in a physiologic process; adrenergic drugs mimic this same process.

ceptors and the responses elicited when they are stimulated by a neurotransmitter or a drug that acts like a neurotransmitter. (See also Fig. 15-2.)

There is another adrenergic receptor besides the alpha- and beta-adrenergic receptors called the **dopaminergic receptor.** When stimulated by dopamine, these receptors cause the vessels of the renal, mesenteric, coronary, and cerebral arteries to dilate and the flow of blood to increase. Dopamine is the only substance that can stimulate these receptors.

The catecholamines are produced by the SNS and are stored in vesicles or granules located in the ends of nerves. Here the transmitter waits until the nerve is stimulated, whereupon the vesicles move to the nerve ending and release their contents into the space between the nerve ending and the effector organ called the **synaptic cleft.** The released contents of the vesicle, the catecholamine, then have the opportunity to bind to the receptor sites located all along the effector organ. This area is also referred to as the *neuroeffector junction.* Once the neurotransmitter binds to the receptors, the effector organ responds. Depending on the function of the particular organ, this elicits smooth muscle contraction, an increased heart rate, the increased production of a substance, or contraction of a blood vessel. This process is stopped by the action of enzymes and by reuptake of the neurotransmitter. The catecholamines are specifically metabolized by two enzymes, monoamine oxidase (MAO) and catechol *O*-methyltransferase (COMT). Each enzyme breaks down the catecholamine but is responsible for doing it in a different area. MAO breaks down the catecholamine that is freely floating around in the nerve ending, and COMT breaks down the catecholamine that is outside the nerve ending at the synaptic cleft. The neurotransmitter is also actively taken back up into the nerve ending by a pump. This restores the catecholamine to the vesicle and provides another means of maintaining an adequate supply of the substance. This process is illustrated in Fig. 15-2.

ADRENERGIC DRUGS

Drugs that have effects similar to or that mimic the effects of the SNS neurotransmitters NE, EPI, and dopamine are referred to as adrenergics and, as mentioned earlier, these neurotransmitters are referred to as *catecholamines.* However, this term refers specifically to an adrenergic drug that has a basic chemical structure similar to that of NE, EPI, or dopamine. Catecholamines produce a sympathomimetic response and are either endogenous substances such as EPI, NE, and dopamine or synthetic substances such as isoproterenol, dobutamine, and phenylephrine.

The catecholamines that are used therapeutically produce the same end result as the endogenous ones,

but without the need to stimulate the nerve to release the neurotransmitter. Instead, when epinephrine, dobutamine, or any of the adrenergic drugs are given, they bathe the area between the nerve and the effector organ, the synaptic cleft. Once there, they have the opportunity to induce a response. This can be accomplished in one of three ways: direct stimulation, indirect stimulation, or a mixture of the two.

A direct-acting sympathomimetic binds directly to the receptor and causes a physiologic response (Fig. 15-3). Phenylephrine is an example of such an agent. An indirect-acting sympathomimetic is an adrenergic drug that when given causes the release of the catecholamine from the storage sites (vesicles) in the nerve endings, which then binds to the receptors and causes a physiologic response (Fig. 15-4). Amphetamine and other related anorexiants are examples of such agents. A mixed-acting sympathomimetic both directly stimulates the receptor by binding to it and indirectly stimulates the receptor by causing the release of the neurotransmitter stored in vesicles at the nerve endings

▼ **FIG. 15-3** Mechanism of physiologic response by direct-acting sympathomimetics.

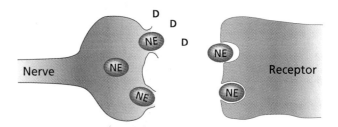

▼ **FIG. 15-4** Mechanism of physiologic response by indirect-acting sympathomimetics.

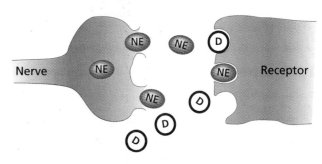

▼ **FIG. 15-5** Mechanism of physiologic response by mixed-acting sympathomimetics.

Table 15-2	Catecholamines and Their Dose-Response Relationship	
DRUG	**DOSAGE**	**RECEPTOR**
Dopamine (Intropin)	Low: 0.5-2 μg/kg/min Moderate: 2-4 or <10 μg/kg/min High: >10 μg/kg/min	Dopaminergic Beta$_1$ Alpha$_1$
Dobutamine (Dobutrex)	Maintenance: 2-10 μg/kg/min High: 40 μg/kg/min	Beta$_1$ >> beta$_2$ > alpha$_1$
Epinephrine (Adrenalin)	Low: 1-4 μg/min High: 4-40 μg/min	Beta$_1$ > beta$_2$ >> alpha$_1$ Alpha$_1$ ≥ beta$_1$

(Fig. 15-5). Ephedrine is an example of a mixed-adrenergic drug.

There are also noncatecholamine adrenergic drugs such as phenylephrine, metaproterenol, and albuterol. In general these drugs have a longer duration of action than either the endogenous or synthetic catecholamines.

Catecholamines and noncatecholamines can act at very specific receptors, they can act at different receptors depending on their dose, or they can act at several different receptors all at once. Examples of a few of the catecholamines and the dose-specific selectivity of these agents for various adrenergic receptors are given in Table 15-2.

Although adrenergics work primarily at postganglionic receptors, the receptors that immediately innervate the effector organ, gland, muscle, and so on, certain agents are also capable of working centrally.

The two most common ways of classifying the adrenergics are either by the specific receptors they affect or by the indications for their use.

Mechanism of Action

To fully understand the mechanism of action of adrenergics it is necessary to have a working knowledge of normal adrenergic transmission, which takes place at the junction between the nerve (the postganglionic sympathetic neuron) and the innervated organ (effector organ or the receptor site). The process of SNS stimulation is illustrated in Fig. 15-2 and discussed earlier in the chapter.

Drug Effects

When alpha-adrenergic receptor sites located on smooth muscles are stimulated by adrenergic drugs, this produces vasoconstriction. There are many areas of the body covered by smooth muscles with alpha-adrenergic receptors on them. The binding of adrenergic drugs to these alpha-adrenergic receptors on the smooth muscle of blood vessels, for instance, causes vasoconstriction; at other sites, this causes the relaxation of gastrointestinal smooth muscle, contraction of the uterus and bladder, male ejaculation, decreased insulin release, and contraction of the ciliary muscles of the eye, causing them to dilate.

Activation of beta$_1$-adrenergic receptors by adrenergic drugs produces relaxation of the bronchi (bronchodilation), gastrointestinal relaxation, uterine relaxation, relaxation of the detrusor muscle in the urinary bladder, and glycogenolysis. Beta$_1$-adrenergic receptor stimulation also causes cardiac stimulation. There are beta$_1$-adrenergic receptors on the myocardium and in the conduction system of the heart, the sinoatrial (SA) node and the atrioventricular (AV) node. When these beta$_1$-adrenergic receptors are stimulated by an adrenergic drug, this results in an increased force of contraction, or a **positive inotropic effect;** an increased heart rate, or a **positive chronotropic effect;** and an increase in conduction through the AV node, or a **positive dromotropic effect.** Beta$_2$-adrenergic receptor stimulation in the liver causes glycogenolysis and in the kidney causes an increase in renin secretion.

Therapeutic Uses

The adrenergics, or sympathomimetics, are employed in the treatment of a wide variety of illnesses and conditions. Their selectivity for either alpha- or beta-adrenergic receptors and their affinity for certain tissues or organs determines the settings in which they are most commonly used. Some adrenergics are used as adjuncts to diet in the short-term treatment of obesity. Although there is much controversy over their usage in this context, there are still a few agents used to help patients lose weight. As with any weight loss program, patients must also be taught to control overeating, to consume a well-balanced diet, and to exercise. Agents used as adjuncts to diet in the short-term management of obesity are referred to as **anorexiants,** and these include:

■ Benzphetamine
■ Dextroamphetamine
■ Diethylpropion
■ Phentermine

- Phenylpropanolamine
- Dexedrine

Certain adrenergic drugs have an affinity for the adrenergic receptors located in the respiratory system and are classified as bronchodilators. They tend to preferentially stimulate the beta-adrenergic receptors rather than the alpha-adrenergic receptors. Of the two subtypes of beta-adrenergic receptors, these adrenergics are more attracted to the beta$_2$-adrenergic receptors on the bronchial, uterine, and vascular smooth muscles than the beta$_1$-adrenergic receptors on the heart. Following are some common bronchodilators that are beta-adrenergics:

- Albuterol
- Bitolteral
- Ephedrine
- Epinephrine
- Ethylnorepinephrine
- Isoetharine
- Isoproterenol
- Metaproterenol
- Terbutaline

Adrenergics can also be used to reduce intraocular pressure and dilate pupils (mydriasis), properties that make them useful in the treatment of open-angle glaucoma. They accomplish these tasks by stimulating alpha- or beta$_2$-adrenergic receptors, or both. The two adrenergics used for this purpose are epinephrine and dipivefrin.

The intranasal application of certain adrenergics can cause the constriction of dilated arterioles and a reduction in nasal blood flow, thus decreasing congestion. These adrenergic drugs work by stimulating alpha-adrenergic receptors and have little or no effect on beta-adrenergic receptors. Following is a list of these nasal decongestants:

- Epinephrine
- Ephedrine
- Naphazoline
- Oxymetazoline
- Phenylephrine
- Phenylpropanolamine
- Pseudoephedrine
- Tetrahydrolzoline

In another topical application, some adrenergics can be applied to the surface of the eye. These are called **ophthalmics** and work much the same way as nasal decongestants except that they affect the vasculature of the eye. When administered, they stimulate alpha-adrenergic receptors located on small arterioles in the eye and temporarily relieve conjunctival congestion. Following is a list of these ophthalmic adrenergics:

- Epinephrine
- Naphazoline
- Phenylephrine
- Tetrahydrozoline

The final group of adrenergics are sometimes referred to as *vasoactive sympathomimetics, pressors, inotropes,* or *cardioselective sympathomimetics* because they are used to support the heart during cardiac failure or shock. These agents have a variety of effects on the various alpha- and beta-adrenergic receptors, and these effects can also be related to the specific dose of the adrenergic agent. Following is a list of the common vasoactive adrenergic agents:

- Dobutamine
- Dopamine
- Ephedrine
- Epinephrine
- Isoproterenol
- Metaraminol
- Methoxamine
- Norepinephrine
- Phenylephrine

Side Effects and Adverse Effects

Some of the most frequent unwanted CNS effects of the alpha-adrenergic agents include headache, restlessness, excitement, insomnia, and euphoria. The cardiovascular effects of the alpha-adrenergics include palpitations or dysrhythmias, tachycardia, vasoconstriction, and hypertension. Effects on other body systems include anorexia or loss of appetite, dry mouth, nausea, vomiting, and rarely taste changes.

The beta-adrenergic agents can adversely affect the CNS, causing mild tremors, headache, nervousness, and dizziness. Beta-adrenergic agents can also have unwanted effects on the cardiovascular system, and these effects include increased heart rate (positive chronotrope), palpitations (dysrhythmias), and fluctuations in blood pressure. Other significant effects include sweating, nausea, vomiting, and muscle cramps.

Toxicity and Management of Overdose

The toxic effect or effects seen as the result of an overdose of the adrenergic drugs are mainly an extension of their common adverse effects (e.g., seizures, hypotension or hypertension, arrhythmias, palpitation, nervousness, dizziness, fatigue, malaise, insomnia, headache, tremor, dry mouth, and nausea). The two most life-threatening toxic effects involve the CNS and cardiovascular system. In the acute setting, seizures can be effectively managed with diazepam. Intracranial bleeding can also occur, often as a result of extremely elevated blood pressures. These elevated blood pressures not only run the risk of precipitating hemorrhage in the brain but elsewhere in the body as well. The best and most effective treatment in this situation is lowering the blood pressure using a rapid-acting alpha-adrenergic–blocking drug. This can directly reverse the adrenergic-induced state.

Table 15-3	Adrenergics: Drug Interactions	
DRUG	**MECHANISM**	**RESULT**
Alpha- and beta-adrenergic agents	Antagonism	Reduced therapeutic effects
Urinary alkalizers	Reduce excretion	Increased drug effects
Anesthetic agents		Increased risk of cardiac arrhythmias
OTC cold preparations		Overdose of adrenergic agents with cardiac and CNS effects, some of which may be life-threatening
Digitalis		Increased ectopic beats with arrhythmias

Antidepressants
    Tricyclic
    MAOIs
	Reduce metabolism	Increased vasopressor effects
		Acute hypertensive crisis and possible respiratory depression and cardiac arrhythmias

Antihistamines		Increased vasopressor effects
Thyroid preparations		Increased adrenergic effects
Antihypertensive agents	Antagonism	Reduced effects of adrenergic agents
Beta-blockers		Decreased bronchodilating effects of adrenergic agents
Antipsychotic agents		Vasopressor effects of adrenergic agents blocked

Many of the adrenergic drugs are either synthetic analogues of our own naturally occurring neurotransmitters (NE, EPI, and dopamine) or are the actual endogenous adrenergic compound. Therefore, when these drugs are taken in an overdose or signs and symptoms of toxicity develop, reversing these effects takes a relatively short time. The large majority of these compounds have very short half-lives and therefore their effects are relatively short-lived. Much of the recommended treatment of overdoses is symptomatic and supportive. Stopping the drug should quickly cause the toxic symptoms to subside. If death occurs, it is usually the result of either respiratory failure or cardiac arrest. The treatment of an overdose should be aimed at the support of these body systems.

Interactions

The potential drug interactions that can occur with adrenergic agents are significant. Although many of the interactions only result in a diminished adrenergic effect because of direct antagonism at and competition for receptor sites, some reactions can be life-threatening. The various drug interactions and the results of the interaction are summarized in Table 15-3.

Laboratory Test Interactions

Alpha-adrenergic agents can cause the serum levels of corticosteriods to be increased and the glucose levels to be decreased. Therefore interpretations of these laboratory results should be done with caution in patients taking these medications. The alpha-adren-

ergic agents can cause the plasma cortisol and corticotropin concentrations to be elevated.

Dosages

For the recommended dosages of various adrenergic agents, see the following dosages tables.

DRUG PROFILES

The adrenergics are used in the treatment of a variety of illnesses and there are many indications for their use. Their selectivity for either alpha- or beta-adrenergic receptors and their affinity for various tissues or organs defines the settings in which they are most commonly used.

ANOREXIANTS

The anorexiants are indirect alpha-adrenergic agents, and the class can be subdivided into amphetamines and amphetamine-like drugs. The precise mechanism responsible for producing appetite suppression is unknown. Results from animal studies indicate that this may result from stimulation of the hypothalamus, an

D O S A G E S

SELECTED AMPHETAMINE ADRENERGIC–INTERACTING AGENTS

AGENT	PHARMACOLOGIC CLASS	DOSAGE RANGE	PURPOSE
Amphetamine (many trade names)	Alpha-adrenergic anorexiant	*Adult* PO: 5-10 mg tid ½-1 hr ac	Appetite control in obesity
Benzphetamine (Didrex)	Alpha-adrenergic anorexiant	*Adult* PO: 25-50 mg 1-3 times/day	Appetite control in obesity
Dextroamphetamine (Dexedrine)	Alpha-adrenergic anorexiant/ CNS stimulant	*Pediatric* PO: 3-5 y/o: 2.5 mg/day and increase weekly until desired effect ≥6 y/o: 5 mg bid and increase weekly until desired effect to a maximum of 40 mg/day *Adult/Pediatric ≥12 y/o* PO: 10-30 mg/day divided	Attention deficit disorder Appetite control in obesity
		Adult/Pediatric ≥12 y/o PO: 5-60 mg/day as a single dose or divided into 2-3 doses	Narcolepsy
Fenfluramine (Pondimin)	Amphetamine-like anorexiant	*Adult* PO: 20 mg tid ac to a daily maximum of 40 mg tid	Appetite control in obesity
Methamphetamine (Desoxyn)	Alpha-adrenergic anorexiant/ CNS stimulant	*Pediatric* PO: 3-5 y/o: 0.1-0.5 mg/kg/day in AM ≥6 y/o: 5 mg bid and increased to 40 mg/day	Attention deficit disorder
		Adult/Pediatric 6-12 y/o PO: 5-60 mg/day divided	Narcolepsy
		Adult/Pediatric ≥12 y/o PO: 2.5-5 mg tid 30-60 min ac	Appetite control in obesity
⚓**Methylphenidate (Ritalin)**	Amphetamine-like CNS stimulant	*Pediatric ≥6 y/o* PO: 5 mg bid before breakfast and lunch and increased weekly until desired effect to a maximum of 60 mg	Attention deficit disorder
		Adult PO: 20-60 mg/day divided in 2-3 doses 30-45 min ac	Narcolepsy

area within the brain. However, it has not been firmly established whether their pharmacologic action principally stems from appetite suppression, other CNS actions, or metabolic effects. This is often used as the basis for arguments against their use.

The use of amphetamines for other indications such as the treatment of narcolepsy and of attention deficit disorders in children stems from their ability to stimulate the CNS. These agents are prescription-only drugs and have a controlled drug status of C-II. The amphetamines consist of amphetamine complex, amphetamine sulfate, dextroamphetamine sulfate, and methamphetamine sulfate. The amphetamine-like drugs are very similar to the amphetamines in their actions but vary in their chemical structure. This subclass of drugs consists of benzphetamine, phendimetrazine, fenfluramine, phentermine, methylphenidate, and phenylpropanolamine.

DOSAGES

SELECTED BRONCHODILATOR ADRENERGICS

AGENT	PHARMACOLOGIC CLASS	DOSAGE RANGE	PURPOSE
↓Albuterol (Proventil, Ventolin, Volmax)	Beta$_2$-adrenergic	*Adult/Pediatric ≥4 y/o* Aerosol: 2 inhal. (180 μg) q4-6h *Pediatric 2-6 y/o* PO: 2 mg 3-4 times/day *Adult/Pediatric ≥12 y/o* PO: 2-4 mg 3-4 times/day *Adult/Pediatric ≥12 y/o* Solution: 2.5 mg 3-4 times/day by nebulization *Adult/Pediatric ≥12 y/o* Powder: 200 μg q4-6h by rotohaler device	
Bitolteral (Tornalate)	Beta$_2$-adrenergic	*Adult/Pediatric ≥12 y/o* Aerosol: 2 inhal. (0.74 mg) given at 1-3 min intervals; a third dose may be given if required.	
↓Epinephrine (Primatene, Bronkaid, others)	Alpha-beta–adrenergic	*Adult/Pediatric ≥4 y/o* Aerosol: 160-250 μg q3h or more *Adult/Pediatric ≥4 y/o* Solution: 8-15 gtts of a 1%, 2%, 2.25% solution by nebulizations q3h or more	
Isoetharine (Arm-a-med, Bronkometer, Beta-2, and others)	Beta$_2$-adrenergic	*Adult* Aerosol: 1-2 inhal. (340-680 μg) q4h or more *Adult* Solution: 0.25-0.5 ml of 1% solution diluted 1:3 by oxygen aerosolization or IPPB; or 3-7 inhal. of undiluted 1% solution by hand nebulizer. Consult package insert for % solutions dosages	Bronchodilation
Isoproterenol (Medihaler-Iso, others)	Beta-adrenergic	*Adult/Pediatric* Aerosol: 1-2 inhal. (120-262 μg); do not exceed 6 doses in 24 hr *Pediatric* SL tablets: 5-10 mg; do not exceed 30 mg/day *Adult* SL tablets: 10-20 mg; do not exceed 60 mg/day *Adult/Pediatric* Solution: 1:100 solution: 3-7 deep inhal. by hand nebulizer up to 5 times/day 1:200 solution: 5-15 deep inhal. up to 5 times/day	
Terbutaline (Brethine, Brethaire, Bricanyl)	Beta$_2$-adrenergic	*Adults/Pediatric ≥12 y/o* Aerosol: 2 inhal. (400 μg) q4-6h *Pediatric* SC: 3.5-5 μg/kg *Adult* SC: 0.25 mg; do not exceed 0.5 mg in 4-hr period *Pediatric 12-15 y/o* PO: 2.5 mg tid; do not exceed 7.5 mg/day *Adult* PO: 5 mg q6h tid; do not exceed 15 mg/day	

IPPB, intermittent positive-pressure breathing.

DOSAGES

SELECTED NASAL DECONGESTANT ADRENERGICS

AGENT	PHARMACOLOGIC CLASS	DOSAGE RANGE	PURPOSE
Tetrahydro-zoline (Tyzine Pediatric, Tyzine)	Alpha-adrenergic	*Pediatric 2-6 y/o* 2-3 gtts of 0.05% solution into nostril q4-6h *Adult/Pediatric ≥6 y/o* 2-4 gtts or 3-4 sprays of 0.1% solution into nostril q4h	Nasal decongestant
Pseudo-ephedrine (Sudafed, Afrin, Pediacare drops, others)	Alpha-beta adrenergic	*Pediatric 3-6 mo* PO drops: 3 gtts/kg q4-6h for 4 doses *Pediatric 1-2 y/o* PO drops: 7 gtts/kg q4-6h for 4 doses *Pediatric 2-5 y/o* PO: 15 mg q4-6h. Do not exceed 60 mg/day *Pediatric 6-12 y/o* 30 mg q4-6h. Do not exceed 120 mg/day *Adult/Pediatric ≥ 12 y/o* 60 mg q4-6h. Do not exceed 240 mg/day	Nasal decongestant

DEXTROAMPHETAMINE SULFATE

Dextroamphetamine sulfate (Dexedrine) is one of the most widely prescribed amphetamines and is used as an appetite suppressant as well as for the control of narcolepsy and attention deficit disorder. It is contraindicated in patients who have shown a hypersensitivity reaction to it, and in those with advanced arterial sclerosis, significant hypertension, hypothyroidism, and glaucoma. A severe hypertensive crisis can result if it is taken with MAOIs. The MAOI must have been discontinued for more than 2 weeks before it is safe to start dextroamphetamine therapy. Dextroamphetamine is available in 5-mg tablets and in 5-, 10-, and 15-mg Spansules (sustained-release tablets). See the table on p. 213 for common dosages. Pregnancy category C.

☙ PHARMACOKINETICS

HALF-LIFE	ONSET	PEAK	DURATION
10-30 hr	30 min	1-3 hr	4-20 hr

♃ METHYLPHENIDATE HYDROCHLORIDE

The use of methylphenidate (Ritalin) has grown rapidly over the past 5 years as researchers have learned more about various behavioral problems in children, particularly the attention deficient disorder. Not only has this emotional and behavioral disorder been diagnosed in more and more children but it has been diagnosed in more and more adults as well. Narcolepsy is another condition in which methylphenidate has been shown to be very effective. It is contraindicated in patients who have shown a hypersensitivity reaction to it, in those suffering from anxiety, glaucoma, Gilles de la Tourette's syndrome, and in children under 6 years of age. The various recommended dosages for these indications are given in the table on p. 213. (See also discussion in Chapter 14 about this agent.) Pregnancy category C.

☙ PHARMACOKINETICS

HALF-LIFE	ONSET	PEAK	DURATION
PO: 1-3 hr	30-60 min	1-3 hr	4-6 hr
PO sus rel: 1-3 hr	2 hr	4 hr	6-8 hr

BRONCHODILATORS

The bronchodilating adrenergic agents are mostly beta-adrenergic in their actions. They are very effective as antiasthmatic agents and are used in the treatment of acute attacks because of their rapid onset of action

DOSAGES

SELECTED VASOACTIVE ADRENERGICS

AGENT	PHARMACOLOGIC CLASS	DOSAGE RANGE	PURPOSE
⇩Dobutamine (Dobutrex)	Beta$_1$-adrenergic	*Adult* IV infusion: 2.5-40 µg/kg/min	Cardiac decompensation
Dopamine (Intropin)	Beta$_1$-adrenergic	*Adult* IV infusion: initiate at 1-5 µg/kg/min and increase if needed; for severe cases, initiate at 5 µg/kg/min and gradually increase in 5-10 µg/min increments to 20-50 µg/kg/min if needed.	Shock syndrome
⇩Epinephrine (Adrenalin)	Alpha-beta–adrenergic	*Pediatric* SC: 10 µg/kg repeated every 20 min if required *Adult* SC: 0.1-0.5 mg repeated every 10-15 min if required	}Anaphylaxis
		Neonatal IV: 10-30 µg/kg every 3-5 min if required *Pediatric* IV: 10 µg/kg every 3-5 min if required *Adult* IV: 0.5-1 mg every 3-5 min if required	}Cardiopulmonary resuscitation
Isoproterenol (Isuprel)	Beta-adrenergic	*Adult* IV infusion: 0.5-5 µg/min	Shock
		Intracardiac: 0.02 mg IM: 0.2 mg; subsequently 0.02-1 mg IV: 0.02-0.06 mg; subsequently 0.01-0.2 mg Infusion: 5 µg/min range, 2-20 µg/min SC: 0.2 mg; subsequently 0.15-0.2 mg	}Heart block/ arrhythmias
Norepinephrine (Levophed)	Alpha-beta–adrenergic	*Pediatric* IV infusion: usual rate, 2 µg/min *Adult* IV infusion: usual rate, 8-12 µg/min	}Hypotensive states
Phenylephrine (Neosynephrine)	Alpha-adrenergic	*Adult* IM/SC: 1-10 mg; do not exceed initial dose of 5 mg.	Hypotension
		IV infusion: 10 mg/100 ml solution; initial rate, 100-180 gtts/min; maintenance dose, 40-60 gtts/min.	Severe hypotension
		IV: 0.5 mg in 15-20 sec; subsequent dose, 0.1-0.2 mg	Paroxysmal supraventricular tachycardia

and efficacy. Ephedrine, ethylnorepinephrine, and EPI also possess alpha-adrenergic activity. Although most of these agents are prescription-only drugs, a few are available as OTC medications.

Activation of the beta$_2$-adrenergic receptors causes the bronchi to dilate. The beta$_2$-adrenergics are the pre-ferred bronchodilators because they produce fewer cardiac-related side effects than the nonselective beta agents. These drugs are pregnancy category C agents, except terbutaline, which is listed as a pregnancy category B drug (see inside cover). These drugs are available in oral, aerosol, and injection forms.

⚓ ALBUTEROL SULFATE

Albuterol (Proventil, Salbutamol, Ventolin, and Volmax) is a selective beta$_2$-adrenergic bronchodilator. It is contraindicated in patients with a known hypersensitivity to it. It can be administered by inhalation, orally, and by injection. It is available as an inhaler or as 2- and 4-mg tablets. See the table on p. 214 for dosage information.

⬡ P H A R M A C O K I N E T I C S

HALF-LIFE	ONSET	PEAK	DURATION
PO: 2.5 hr	PO: 30 min	PO: 2.5 hr	PO: 4-6 hr
Inhaler: 4 hr	Inhaler: 5-15 min	Inhaler: 1-1.5 hr	Inhaler: 4-6 hr

⚓ EPINEPHRINE

EPI (Adrenalin) is a naturally occurring catecholamine produced by the adrenal medulla. It is a very potent alpha-beta–adrenergic agent that produces vasoconstriction, increased blood pressure, cardiac stimulation, and dilatation of the bronchioles. It is the drug of choice for the relief of acute asthma attacks and for the treatment of anaphylaxis. In addition, EPI is used to treat open-angle glaucoma, to restore cardiac rhythm in cardiac arrest, and to control bleeding (a hemostatic agent). It is also used as an ophthalmic agent and a nasal decongestant and to prolong the activity of infiltrated local anesthetics. Its use is contraindicated in many settings, including hypersensitivity, narrow-angle glaucoma, shock due to trauma, halogenated general anesthetics, coronary insufficiency, and labor. In addition, its use with local anesthetics administered in the toes or fingers is not recommended. See the table on p. 214 for dosage information.

⬡ P H A R M A C O K I N E T I C S

HALF-LIFE	ONSET	PEAK	DURATION
Variable (min)	SC: 5-10 min	SC: 20 min	SC: 20 min
	PO inhalation, IV: 1 min	PO inhalation, IV: <20 min	PO inhalation, IV: <30 min

ISOPROTERENOL HYDROCHLORIDE

Isoproterenol (Isupri) is a nonselective beta-sympathomimetic (beta$_1$-beta$_2$) antiasthmatic agent. The beta$_1$-adrenergic activity results in a positive inotropic and chronotropic cardiac effect with a corresponding increase in the stroke volume and oxygen consumption. Beta$_2$-adrenergic activation produces bronchial, GI tract, and uterine smooth muscle relaxation. Isoproterenol is indicated for the treatment of acute and chronic forms of asthma, bronchitis, and bronchiectasis. Other indications include cardiac arrest, Adams-Stokes syndrome, and ventricular arrhythmias due to atrioventricular block.

Isoproterenol is contraindicated in patients with a known hypersensitivity to it and in those suffering from digitalis-induced tachycardia or with preexisting cardiac arrhythmias. See the table on p. 214 for dosage information.

⬡ P H A R M A C O K I N E T I C S

HALF-LIFE	ONSET	PEAK	DURATION
IV: 2 min	IV: immediate	IV: <15 min	IV: <1 hr
Inhalation: 2 min	Inhalation: immediate	Inhalation rapid	Inhalation: 1 hr
SL: 2 min	SL: 30 min	SL: varies	SL: 2 hr

NASAL DECONGESTANTS

The sympathomimetic agents used as nasal decongestants consist of both alpha- and alpha-beta–adrenergic agents. The alpha-adrenergic activity of these agents is responsible for causing vasoconstriction in the nasal mucosa. This produces shrinkage of the mucosa, which promotes easier nasal breathing. However, excessive use of nasal decongestants can lead to greater congestion because of a rebound phenomenon that occurs. The decongestants are administered topically with nasal drops, which are instilled into each nostril. The ephedrine salts, phenylephrine hydrochloride and pseudoephedrine, can produce nasal decongestion when taken orally, either as sole agents or in combination with allergy, cold, cough, and sinus relief preparations.

The contraindications to the use of the systemically administered nasal decongestants are the same for all of the agents and include hypersensitivity, heart diabetes, hypertension, thyroid disorders, and enlargement of the prostate gland.

PSEUDOEPHEDRINE HYDROCHLORIDE

Pseudoephedrine (Sudafed and Afrin) is a natural plant alkaloid that is obtained from the *Ephedra* plant. It is a stereoisomer of ephedrine and is a widely used orally administered decongestant. See the table on p. 215 for the recommended dosages. Pregnancy category B.

⬡ P H A R M A C O K I N E T I C S

HALF-LIFE	ONSET	PEAK	DURATION
Variable (min)*	15-30 min	30-60 min	4-6 hr SR: 8-12 hr

*Half-life is pH-dependent; pH of 5.5-6 = 9-16 hr.

OPHTHALMIC DECONGESTANTS

Ophthalmic decongestants are adrenergics that are applied topically to the eye. When instilled into the eye, they stimulate alpha-adrenergic receptors located on the small arterioles in the eye. This results in constriction and relieves conjunctival congestion, thus decreasing redness in the eye. Although EPI, phenylephrine, and naphazoline are all used as ophthalmic decongestants, tetrahydrozoline is the one most widely used.

TETRAHYDROZOLINE

Tetrahydrozoline (Murine, Visine, and others) is applied topically to the eye to temporarily relieve congestion, itching, and minor irritation in patients with red and irritated eyes. It causes constriction of the blood vessels of the eye and is sometimes also used during some diagnostic eye procedures. It is the active ingredient in such OTC products as Visine, Soothe, and Murine Plus eyedrops. It is contraindicated in patients with a hypersensitivity reaction to it and in those with narrow-angle glaucoma. The recommended dosages are given in the table on p. 215. Pregnancy category C.

♣ PHARMACOKINETICS

HALF-LIFE	ONSET	PEAK	DURATION
Variable (min)	<3 min	Short (min)	4-8 hr

VASOACTIVE ADRENERGICS

The adrenergics that have primarily cardioselective effects are referred to as *vasoactive adrenergics*. They are used to support a failing heart or one that is in shock. These agents have a wide range of effects on alpha- and beta-adrenergic receptors, depending on the dose. The vasoactive adrenergics are very potent, quick-acting injectable drugs. They are listed by the FDA as pregnancy category C agents (see inside cover). Although dosage recommendations are given in the table on p. 216, all of these drugs are titrated to the desired physiologic response. All of the vasoactive adrenergics are rapid in onset, and their effects very quickly cease when they are stopped. Therefore careful titration and monitoring are required in patients receiving them.

♣ DOBUTAMINE

Dobutamine (Dobutrex) is a $beta_1$-selective vasoactive adrenergic drug that is structurally similar to the naturally occurring catecholamine dopamine. By stimulating the $beta_1$ receptors on the heart (myocardium), it increases cardiac output by increasing contractility (positive inotrope) and increases the stroke volume, especially in patients with congestive heart failure. The recommended dosages are listed in the table on p. 216.

♣ PHARMACOKINETICS

HALF-LIFE	ONSET	PEAK	DURATION
2-5 min	<2 min	<10 min	<10 min

DOPAMINE

Dopamine (Intropin) is a naturally occurring catecholamine neurotransmitter in the SNS. It has potent dopaminergic and $beta_1$- and $alpha_1$-adrenergic receptor activity, depending on the dose. Dopamine is used to treat cardiogenic shock, septic shock, myocardial infarction, cardiac decompensation after open heart surgery, and poor blood flow to the kidneys during renal failure. The drug is contraindicated in patients who have a tumor that secretes catecholamines, a pheochromocytoma. It is available as an intravenously injectable drug. The recommended vasoactive dosages are given in the table on p. 216.

♣ PHARMACOKINETICS

HALF-LIFE	ONSET	PEAK	DURATION
<2 min	2-5 min	Rapid	10 min

♣ EPINEPHRINE

EPI (Adrenalin) is also an endogenous vasoactive catecholamine. It acts directly on both the alpha- and beta-adrenergic receptors of tissues innervated by the SNS. It is used in emergency situations and is one of the primary vasoactive drugs used in many advanced cardiac life support (ACLS) protocols. The physiologic response it elicits is dose related. At low dosages it stimulates mostly beta-adrenergic receptors, increasing the force of contraction and heart rate, but at high dosages it stimulates mostly alpha-adrenergic receptors, causing vasoconstriction. The dosages recommended for the treatment of various disorders are given in the table on p. 216.

♣ PHARMACOKINETICS

HALF-LIFE	ONSET	PEAK	DURATION
<5 min	<2 min	Rapid	5-30 min

ISOPROTERENOL

Isoproterenol (Isuprel) acts directly on the beta-adrenergic receptors. In normal doses it has little or no effect on alpha-adrenergic receptors. The main effects of therapeutic doses of isoproterenol are relaxation of smooth muscle of the bronchial tree, cardiac stimulation, and peripheral vasodilation. It can also relax GI and uterine smooth muscle by stimulating the $beta_2$-adrenergic receptors. In addition, isoproterenol inhibits the anaphylaxis-induced release of histamine and may be used to treat patients experiencing an anaphylactic reaction. Common dosages are given in the table on p. 216.

⬡ PHARMACOKINETICS

HALF-LIFE	ONSET	PEAK	DURATION
<2 min	Immediate	<15 min	8-50 min

NOREPINEPHRINE

NE (Levophed) acts predominantly by directly stimulating alpha-adrenergic receptors. It also has some direct-stimulating beta-adrenergic effects on the heart ($beta_1$-adrenergic receptors) but none on the lung ($beta_2$-adrenergic receptors). The most evident effects, however, are those on the alpha-adrenergic receptors, which leads to vasoconstriction. NE is directly metabolized to dopamine and is primarily used in the treatment of hypotension and shock. Common dosages are given in the table on p. 216.

⬡ PHARMACOKINETICS

HALF-LIFE	ONSET	PEAK	DURATION
<5 min	Immediate	1-2 min	1-2 min

PHENYLEPHRINE

Phenylephrine (Neosynephrine) works almost exclusively on the alpha-adrenergic receptors. It is also believed to act indirectly by causing the release of NE from its storage sites. It is primarily used as a short-term agent to augment blood pressure in patients in shock, to control some arrhythmias (supraventricular tachycardias), and to produce vasoconstriction with regional anesthesia. It is also used as an ophthalmic agent and administered topically as a nasal decongestant. Common vasoactive dosages are listed in the table on p. 216.

⬡ PHARMACOKINETICS

HALF-LIFE	ONSET	PEAK	DURATION
<5 min*	Immediate*	Rapid*	15-20 min*

*IV use.

NURSING PROCESS

ASSESSMENT

Adrenergic, or sympathomimetic, drugs have a variety of effects depending on the receptors they stimulate. Stimulation of the alpha-adrenergic receptors results in vasoconstriction, stimulation of $beta_1$-adrenergic receptors produces cardiac stimulation, and stimulation of the $beta_2$-adrenergic receptors results in bronchodilation. Because of these properties, the use of adrenergics requires careful patient assessment to minimize the possible side effects and maximize the therapeutic effects.

In a thorough assessment, the nurse should first gather information about the patient's allergies and past and present medical conditions. A system overview and a thorough medication history should also form part of this assessment. Some pertinent questions to ask the patient include: Are you allergic to any medication, food, topical products, environmental products, and so on? Are you asthmatic and if so how frequent and severe are the attacks? What are their manifestations and precipitating factors? What previous treatment have you received for the asthma and has it been successful or failed? Do you have a history of hypertension, cardiac arrhythmias, or any other cardiovascular disease?

Adrenergic drugs may precipitate tachycardia, hypertension, myocardial infarction, or heart failure, so they should be given cautiously in patients receiving them who have these later disorders and such patients should be closely monitored. The drug interactions to assess for before administering adrenergic agents are listed in Table 15-3.

NURSING DIAGNOSES

Nursing diagnoses associated with the use of adrenergic agonists include, but are not limited to:
- Pain (chest discomfort) related to side effects of tachycardia and palpitations.
- Knowledge deficit regarding therapeutic regimen, side effects, drug interactions, and precautions related to use of sympathomimetics.
- Risk for injury related to possible side effects (nervousness, vertigo, hypertension, or tremors).
- Altered sleep patterns, insomnia, related to CNS stimulation caused by adrenergic agents.
- Risk for noncompliance with therapy related to

lack of information about the importance of the medication.

■ Altered cardiac output (decreased) related to cardiovascular side effects consisting of palpitations, hypertension, tachycardia, and anginal pain.

PLANNING

Goals for the patient receiving sympathomimetics include:

■ Patient will take drugs as ordered and follow directions explicitly.

■ Patient's symptoms will be relieved.

■ Patient remains compliant with the drug therapy.

■ Patient demonstrates an adequate knowledge about the use of the specific medications.

Outcome Criteria

Outcome criteria related to the administration of adrenergic agonists include:

■ Patient will state the importance of pharmacologic and nonpharmacologic treatment of the respiratory or other disorder that is present, such as asthma.

■ Patient states the importance of compliance with the therapy and the risks and complications associated with overuse of the medication such as excessive CNS stimulation, insomnia, tachycardia.

■ Patient states conditions and side effects that should be reported to the physician such as chest pain, restlessness, insomnia.

■ Patient states the importance of scheduling and keeping follow-up appointments with the physician to monitor effectiveness of drug therapy.

■ Patient improves in his or her condition once on the medication regimen with decreased signs and symptoms, such as decreased coughing or wheezing.

IMPLEMENTATION

There are several nursing interventions that can maximize the therapeutic effects of adrenergic agents and minimize the side effects. Always check the packaging inserts concerning dilutional agents and the amount, and use a TB syringe when giving these agents subcutaneously so that accurate, small doses are administered. When these agents are to be administered by an inhaler or nebulizer, teach the patient how to correctly administer the agent and how to properly cleanse the equipment. Be careful not to administer two adrenergic agents such as EPI and isoproterenol at the same time because of the high risk of the precipitating side effects such as tachycardia and hypertension. At least 4 hours should elapse between doses of these medications to prevent serious cardiac arrhyth-

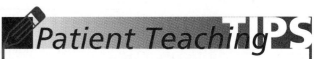

Patient Teaching TIPS

Adrenergics

✔ Patients should always take medications as prescribed, as excessive dosing may cause CNS and cardiovascular stimulation.

✔ When taking inhaled forms of medication for metered-dose administration, patients should shake the container thoroughly, exhale through nose, and administer medication by aerosol while inhaling or breathing in deeply through mouthpiece of inhaler. Patients should hold their breath for a few seconds and exhale slowly. When using the inhaler for more than one breath application, patients should wait 2 minutes between inhalations of the agent and *only* take amount ordered!

✔ If patients have a history of diabetes mellitus, hypertension, hyperthyroidism, arrhythmias, chest pain, or seizures, they should make sure their physician knows of these and of any other medications they may be taking for these conditions. Because of the CNS and cardiovascular stimulation produced by adrenergic agents, these medical conditions need to be very closely monitored and the agents must be carefully used to prevent worsening of the preexisting CNS or cardiac disorder.

✔ Patients should not take OTC medication or any other medications without their physician's approval.

✔ If patients' respiratory difficulties increase with use of these medications, they should contact their physician immediately because of the possible tolerance to their actions this may represent.

✔ Patients taking inhaled forms of isoproterenol (Isuprel), should be told not to be alarmed if their sputum or saliva turns pink; this is caused by the medication.

✔ Sublingual forms of these medications must be held under your tongue, and *not* swallowed until they are completely dissolved. Patients should rinse out their mouths afterward so as to prevent dental problems such as tooth decay.

mias from occurring. Often these medications are used in combination with other agents in the management of asthma because of their synergistic effects.

When administering IV infusions of these agents, only use clear solutions, mix in 5% dextrose in water, administer with an infusion device such as an IV pump in conjunction with cardiac monitoring, and infuse the agent slowly so as to not precipitate drastic and possibly dangerous cardiovascular changes, such as in the patient's blood pressure or pulse rate. If giving as an

PEDIATRIC IMPLICATIONS
Beta-Adrenergic Agonist Administration

■ Children are usually more sensitive to medications, and these are no exception; watch child closely for excessive cardiac or CNS stimulation.

■ Terbutaline is generally not used in children 12 years old and under.

■ Other medications, including OTC medications, should not be used unless physician okays.

■ Monitor closely for cardiovascular adverse reactions such as palpitations and chest pain.

▼

GERIATRIC IMPLICATIONS
Beta-Adrenergic Agonist Administration

■ Older persons are more sensitive to medications, and these are no exception.

■ Because of the possible presence of other medical conditions such as hypertension, peripheral vascular disease, and cardiovascular disease, elderly patients need to be monitored carefully before, during, and after the use of these medications.

■ Immediately report any chest pain, palpitations, blurred vision, headache, seizures, or hallucinations.

■ Cautious use is recommended with OTC and other medications, so contact the physician for further instructions if the patient is taking any other medications.

■ Monitor vital signs, especially blood pressure and pulse rate.

▼

TAKE HOME POINTS

Adrenergics
■ Drugs that stimulate the sympathetic nervous system; also called *adrenergic agonists* and *sympathomimetics.*

■ Mimic the CNS neurotransmitters NE and EPI.

Dopaminergic Receptors
■ Predominant response when stimulated = vasodilation.

■ Located on *postsynaptic* effector cells, blood vessels, and organs.

■ Primary site: renal, mesenteric, coronary, and cerebral arteries.

Catecholamines
■ Substances that produce a sympathomimetic response (stimulate the SNS).

■ Endogenous (natural) catecholamines = EPI, NE, and dopamine.

■ Exogenous (synthetic) catecholamines = isoproterenol and dobutamine.

Nursing Considerations
■ Patients should avoid respiratory irritants and patients with infections should try to minimize situations that require the use of the adrenergic agonists.

■ Patients should avoid any OTC or other prescribed medications because of possible drug interactions.

■ Rebound nasal congestion or ulcerations of the nasal mucosa may occur if drugs are overused. Educate patient to use only as directed.

■ Medications should be used only as directed.

■ Overuse of inhalant agents can lead to toxicity.

ophthalmic preparation, do not let the eye dropper touch the eye so that the remaining solution in the dropper and container is not contaminated, and drop the solution into the conjunctival sac.

Patients with chronic lung disease who are receiving an adrenergic agent should avoid any of the factors that can exacerbate their condition (e.g., allergens, foods, and cigarette smoking) and implement those measures that can help diminish the risk of respiratory infection. Fluid intake of up to 3000 ml per day should be encouraged, unless contraindicated, and patients should be encouraged to keep a journal of their symptoms and any improvement or worsening in their condition. Patient teaching tips are listed in the box on p.

220. Special considerations to be borne in mind for aged or pediatric patients taking beta-adrenergics are presented in the boxes above.

EVALUATION

Therapeutic effects to monitor for in patients receiving adrenergic agents for the treatment of hypotension, shock, or cardiac arrest include less edema; increased urinary output; return to normal vital signs (blood pressure, ≥120/80 mm Hg or increase in mm Hg blood pressure with each reading; pulse, >60 but <120 beats/min; respiratory rate, >12 but <20 breaths/min); improved skin color (pallor to pink) and temperature (cool to warm); and increased level of consciousness. Improvement in the condition of patients with bronchial asthma would be evidenced by return to a normal respiratory rate (r >12 but <20 breaths/ >12 breaths/min); improved breath sounds throughout the lung fields with less rales; increased air exchange, including that in the lung bases; decreased to no cough; less dyspnea; improved blood gas levels; and increased tolerance of activity. If these agents are used for nasal congestion, the patient should report less congestion and a better ability to breathe.

You must also look for possible side effects of these medications in your patient. These include, but are not limited to, cardiac arrhythmias, hypertension, tachycardia, nervousness, anxiety, tremors, insomnia, and restlessness. Rebound nasal congestion, rhinitis, and nasal mucosa ulcerations are possible adverse effects of the nasal decongestants.

Critical Thinking **ACTIVITIES**

Sample Test Questions

1. Which of the following conditions, situations, or medications would be considered a contraindication to the use of an adrenergic agonist?
   a. Aminophylline.
   b. Dehydration.
   c. Polyuria.
   d. MAOIs.

2. For patients receiving adrenergic agonist agents, common side effects include which of the following?
   a. Hypotension.
   b. Sedation.
   c. Insomnia.
   d. Dysphagia.

3. Which one of the following medications is specifically known to be a renal blood vessel dilator when given in low doses and thus used to prevent renal failure in patients with compromised renal perfusion:
   a. Epinephrine.
   b. Ephedrine.
   c. Dopamine.
   d. Norepinephrine.

4. A 55-year-old man is brought to the emergency room by rescue personnel after his involvement in a motor vehicle accident. His pulse is weak and thready and the rate is 168 beats/min. Blood pressure is 58/38 mm Hg. Respirations are labored and rate is 36 breaths/min. His condition worsens, and he now has no pulse and is in cardiac arrest. The drug that would most likely be used at this point to treat the patient would be:
   a. Dopamine, 1:10,000 concentration IV.
   b. Ephedrine, 1:100 concentration IV.
   c. Benadryl, 1:1000 concentration IV.
   d. Epinephrine, 1:10,000 concentration IV.

5. W.T. is a 76-year-old woman who has undergone coronary artery bypass grafting 1 day earlier. Her cardiac and urine output are both low. She is beginning to show signs of heart failure and pulmonary congestion. You have already given her two doses of furosemide but with no resulting diuresis. The physician says to start the patient on a dopamine infusion at 2 μg/kg/min. She weighs 60 kg, and your standard dopamine concentration is 800 μg/ml.
   a. Calculate the rate (ml/hr) at which the infusion should be run.
   b. If the same patient becomes volume restricted and the physician says to switch the dopamine to quad strength, at what infusion rate (ml/hr) should the dopamine be delivered now?

BIBLIOGRAPHY

Albanese J, Nutz P: *Mosby's 1995 nursing drug cards,* St Louis, 1995, Mosby.

Johnson KB: *Harriet Lane handbook,* ed 13, St Louis, 1993, Mosby.

Keen JH: *Critical care and emergency drug reference,* St Louis, 1994, Mosby.

Knoben JE, Anderson PO: *Handbook of Critical Drug Data,* ed 6, Hamilton, Ill, 1988, Drug Intelligence Publications.

McEvoy GK: *AHFS drug information,* Bethesda, Md, 1989, American Society of Hospital Pharmacists.

Skidmore-Roth L: *Mosby's 1995 nursing drug reference,* St Louis, 1995, Mosby.

Chapter 16

Adrenergic-Blocking Agents

Objectives

When you reach the end of this chapter, you will be able to:

1 Be familiar with the normal anatomy and physiology of the autonomic nervous system as it pertains to beta-adrenergic blocking agents.

2 Provide examples of the various adrenergic antagonists.

3 Discuss the mechanism of action, therapeutic effects, uses, and adverse and toxic effects of adrenergic antagonists.

4 Be familiar with the antidotes used to treat adrenergic-blocking agent overdose.

5 Develop a nursing care plan that includes expected outcomes as it relates to the administration of the various adrenergic antagonists and the treatment of side effects and overdose or toxicity stemming from use of these agents.

6 Identify the drug interactions associated with the use of adrenergic antagonists, or sympatholytics.

7 Evaluate the therapeutic versus the side effects of the different adrenergic antagonists.

CHAPTER OUTLINE

Alpha-Blockers
  Mechanism of action
  Drug effects
  Therapeutic uses
  Side effects and adverse effects
    Toxicity and management of overdose
  Interactions
  Dosages

Drug Profiles
  Ergotamine tartrate
  Phenoxybenzamine hydrochloride
  Phentolamine
  Tolazoline
  Prazosin

Beta-Blockers
  Mechanism of action
  Drug effects
  Therapeutic uses
  Side effects and adverse effects
    Toxicity and management of overdose
  Interactions
  Dosages

Drug Profiles
  Acebutolol
  ⚓ Propranolol
  Atenolol
  Esmolol
  Labetalol
  ⚓ Metoprolol
  ⚓ Sotalol
  Newer beta-blockers

Nursing Process
Assessment
Nursing Diagnoses
Planning
  Outcome criteria
Implementation
Evaluation

Glossary

Agonists (ag' ə nists) Drugs with a specific cellular affinity that produces a predictable response. (p. 225)

Angina (an ji' nə) Paroxysmal chest pain caused by anoxia of the myocardium. (p. 231)

Antagonists (an tag' ə nists) Adrenergic blockers that bind to adrenergic receptors but inhibit or block stimulation of the CNS. (p. 225)

Arrhythmias (ə rith' me əz) Irregular heartbeats. (p. 231)

Blood-brain barrier Semipermeable membrane that selectively allows substances with specific characteristics to pass into the brain. (p. 230)

Cardioprotective The characteristic of beta-blockers to inhibit stimulation by circulating catecholamines. (p. 231)

Cardioselective beta-blockers Beta-blocking drugs that are selective for beta$_1$-adrenergic receptors. Also called *beta$_1$-blocking agents.* (p. 230)

Extravasation (ek strav' ə sa' shən) Passage or escape into the tissues, usually of blood, serum, or lymph. (p. 227)

Glycogenolysis (gli' ko jə nol' ə sis) Process that occurs in the heart when beta-blockers reduce or block the production of glucose from glycogen. (p. 230)

Intrinsic sympathomimetic activity (ISA) (in trin' zik \ sim' pə tho' mi met ik) Action of agents within the beta-blocking class. (p. 230)

Lipolysis (lĭ pol' ə-sis) The decomposition or splitting up of fat. (p. 230)

Lipophylicity (lip' o fil is ət ē) Attraction to lipid or fat. (p. 231)

Nonspecific beta-blockers Beta-blocking drugs that block both beta$_1$- and beta$_2$-adrenergic receptors. (p. 230)

Orthostatic hypotension (or tho' stat' ik \ hi' po ten' shən) Abnormally low blood pressure occurring when a person assumes the standing position. (p. 229)

Oxytocics (ok' sĭ to' sikz) Drugs used to treat postpartum and postabortion bleeding caused by uterine relaxation and enlargement. They stimulate the smooth muscle of the uterus to contract. (p. 226)

Pheochromocytoma (fe' o kro' mo si to' mə) Vascular tumor that secretes norepinephrine and stimulates the CNS. (p. 227)

Sympatholytics Another name for antagonists. (p. 225)

Vaughan Williams classification System of classifying antiarrhythmic agents. (p. 231)

The autonomic nervous system consists of the parasympathetic and sympathetic nervous systems. The class of drugs discussed in this chapter works primarily on the sympathetic nervous system (SNS). As discussed in Chapter 15, the adrenergic drugs stimulate the SNS, and these drugs are also called **agonists** because they bind to receptors and cause a response. The adrenergic blockers have the opposite effect and are therefore referred to as **antagonists**. They also bind to adrenergic receptors but in doing so inhibit or block stimulation of the SNS. They are also referred to as **sympatholytics** because they "lyse," or inhibit, SNS stimulation.

Throughout the body there are receptor sites for the sympathetic neurotransmitters norepinephrine (NE) and epinephrine (EPI). These are called the *adrenergic receptors,* and there are two basic types—alpha and beta. There are subtypes of both the alpha- and beta-adrenergic receptors, designated 1 and 2. Alpha$_1$- and alpha$_2$-adrenergic receptors are differentiated by their location on nerves. Alpha$_1$-adrenergic receptors are located on the cell, muscle, or organ that the nerve is stimulating (postsynaptic effector cells). The alpha$_2$-adrenergic receptors are located on the actual nerves that stimulate the effector cells. Beta$_1$-adrenergic receptors are located primarily on the heart. Beta$_2$-adrenergic receptors are located primarily on the smooth muscles of the bronchioles and blood vessels. It is at these receptors that adrenergic blockers work, and these agents are classified by the type of adrenergic receptor they block—alpha or beta. Hence they are called *alpha-blockers* and *beta-blockers.*

ALPHA-BLOCKERS

Alpha-adrenergic–blocking agents, or alpha-blockers, interrupt or block the stimulation of the SNS at the alpha-adrenergic receptor. Various physiologic responses occur when the stimulation of the alpha-adrenergic receptors is inhibited. Adrenergic blockade at the alpha-adrenergic receptors leads to vasodilation, decreased blood pressure, miosis or constriction of the pupil, or suppressed ejaculation. The ergot alkaloids dihydroergotamine mesylate, ergoloid mesylate, ergotamine tartrate and ergonovine maleate are alpha-blockers that are used mainly for their vasoconstrictor properties. The alpha-blockers doxazosin, prazosin, and terazosin are used as antihypertensive agents because they cause vasodilation. Each of these two groups of agents block alpha-adrenergic receptors, but they have an affinity for different sites in the body, and therefore the resultant effects differ. Other alpha-blockers are phenoxybenzamine, phentolamine, reserpine, and tolazoline.

Mechanism of Action

As already mentioned, the alpha-blockers work by blocking or inhibiting the normal stimulation of the SNS. They do this either by directly competing with the SNS neurotransmitter NE or by a noncompetitive process. Most alpha-blockers are competitive in their actions. They have a higher affinity for the alpha-adrenergic receptor than the NE and occupy the receptor before the neurotransmitter can do so. Once this competitive alpha-blocker binds to the receptor, it prevents the cell from being stimulated by the nerve. Noncompetitive alpha-blockers work in a different fashion. They also bind to the alpha-adrenergic receptors, but this type of bond (a covalent bond) causes the receptor to be less responsive to the neurotransmitters NE and EPI. Regardless of which way the blockade is accomplished, the result is a decreased response to stimulation of the SNS. Figure 16-1 illustrates these two mechanisms.

Drug Effects

The alpha-blockers have many effects on the normal physiologic functions of the body. The effects of

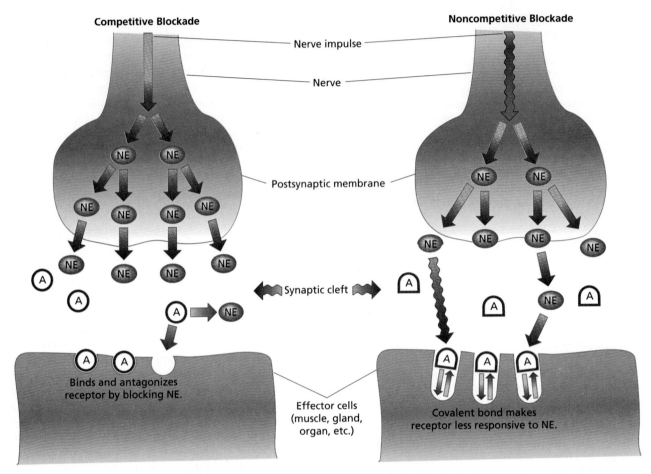

▼ FIG. 16-1 Alpha-blockers mechanisms for alpha-adrenergic competitive and noncompetitive blockade.

each agent differ depending on the agent's selectivity for particular tissues or cells in the body. The ergot alkaloids can cause peripheral vasoconstriction as well as the constriction of dilated arteries. Certain alpha-blockers can stimulate uterine contractions. Others can block alpha-adrenergic receptors on both vascular and nonvascular smooth muscle. The vascular smooth muscle that these alpha-blockers have an affinity for is that in the bladder and its sphincters, the GI tract and its sphincters, the prostate, and the ureters. The nonvascular smooth muscle these agents have an affinity for is in the CNS, liver, and kidneys. Unlike the ergot alkaloids, some alpha-blockers can induce arterial and venous dilation and thus decrease peripheral vascular resistance and blood pressure. Alpha-blockers can also affect certain concentrations of neurotransmitters, causing a depletion of catecholamines such as NE and EPI. Others can directly block a neurotransmitter such as serotonin (5-hydroxytryptamine) or indirectly cause it to be depleted.

Therapeutic Uses

The alpha-blockers have many therapeutic effects, but these effects differ greatly depending on the par-

ticular agent. The ergot alkaloids constrict the dilated arteries going to the brain (the carotid arteries) that are responsible for causing vascular headaches such as migraines. The vasoconstriction of these dilated arteries relieves the headache and other symptoms. They are also used as **oxytocics,** agents used to control postpartum and postabortion bleeding caused by uterine relaxation and enlargement. These agents increase the intensity of uterine contractions and induce local vasoconstriction.

Alpha-blockers such as doxazosin, prazosin, and terazosin cause both arterial and venous dilation. This reduces peripheral vascular resistance and blood pressure; thus these agents are used to treat hypertension. Alpha-adrenergic receptors are also present on the prostate and bladder, and for this reason alpha-blockers are used in patients with benign prostatic hyperplasia (BPH) to decrease resistance to urinary outflow. This reduces urinary obstruction and relieves some of the effects of BPH.

Other alpha-blockers can inhibit excitatory responses to adrenergic stimulation. These agents noncompetitively block alpha-adrenergic receptors on smooth muscle and various exocrine glands. Because of this action, these alpha-blockers are very useful in controlling or preventing hypertension in patients who have a **pheochromocytoma,** a tumor that forms on top of the adrenal glands on top of the kidneys and secretes NE, thus causing SNS stimulation. Alpha-blockers are also useful in the treatment of patients who have increased alpha-adrenergic activity. Three such conditions are Raynaud's disease, acrocyanosis, and frostbite. Phenoxybenzamine is an alpha-blocker useful for the treatment of these syndromes.

Other alpha-blockers are more effective at antagonizing responses to circulating EPI and NE. This causes peripheral vasodilation and decreases peripheral resistance as a result of direct relaxation of vascular smooth muscle. They can also be used to treat pheochromocytomas. Because of their potent vasodilating properties and their fast onset of action, they are also used to prevent skin necrosis and sloughing after the **extravasation** of vasopressors such as NE or EPI. When these drugs extravasate, or leak out of the blood vessel into the surrounding tissue, this causes vasoconstriction and ultimately tissue death, or necrosis. If the vasoconstriction is not reversed quickly, the whole limb can be lost. Phentolamine, an alpha-blocker, can reverse this potent vasoconstriction and restore blood flow to the ischemic, vasoconstricted area.

Side Effects and Adverse Effects

The primary side effects and adverse effects of alpha-blockers are those related to their effects on the vasculature. The alpha-blockers' primary side effects and adverse effects are listed by body system in Table 16-1.

Toxicity and Management of Overdose

In an acute overdose, the person's stomach should be emptied immediately either by inducing emesis with syrup of ipecac or by gastric lavage. After this, activated charcoal should be administered to bind to the drug and remove it from the stomach and the circulation. To hasten elimination of the drug bound to the activated charcoal, the first dose should be given with a cathartic such as sorbitol. Symptomatic and supportive measures should be instituted as needed. Blood pressure support with the administration of fluids, volume expanders, and vasopressor agents and the administration of anticonvulsants such as diazepam for the control of seizures are examples of such measures.

Interactions

The most severe of the drug interactions with the alpha-blockers are the ones that potentiate the alpha-

Table 16-1	Alpha-Blockers: Adverse Effects
BODY SYSTEM	**SIDE/ADVERSE EFFECTS**
Cardiovascular	Palpitations, orthostatic hypotension, tachycardia, edema, dysrhythmias, chest pain
Central nervous system	Dizziness, headache, drowsiness, anxiety, depression, vertigo, weakness, numbness, fatigue
Gastrointestinal	Nausea, vomiting, diarrhea, constipation, abdominal pain
Other	Incontinence, nose bleeding, tinnitus, dry mouth, pharyngitis, rhinitis

blockers' effects. The alpha-blockers as a whole are very highly protein bound and compete for binding sites with other drugs that are highly protein bound. With limited sites for binding on protein and increased competition for these sites, the end result is that more drug is not bound and therefore more drug circulates freely in the bloodstream. Because drug that is not bound to protein is active, the end result is a more pronounced drug effect. Some of the common drugs that interact with alpha-blockers and the results of these interactions are given in Table 16-2.

Dosages

For the recommended dosages of alpha-blockers, see the table on p. 229.

*D*RUG PROFILES

The alpha-blockers are prescription-only drugs that are available in many dosage forms. The oral forms include tablets, capsules, solutions, and sublingual tablets. Parenteral formulations include intravenous, intramuscular, and subcutaneous injections. They also come as rectal suppositories. Most alpha-blockers are rated as pregnancy category C agents by the (FDA). The ergot alkaloids, however, are rated as pregnancy category X drugs. (See the inside cover for the definition of these pregnancy categories.)

Table 16-2	Alpha-Blockers: Common Drug Interactions	
DRUG	**MECHANISM**	**RESULTS**
Beta-blockers Calcium channel blockers Diuretics	Additive effects	Profound hypotension
Protein-bound drugs	Compete for binding	Increased effect

ERGOTAMINE TARTRATE

Ergotamine (Ergostat) is an ergot alkaloid. All these ergot alkaloids are obtained from a fungus called *Claviceps purpurea* that grows on rye. It causes dilated blood vessels in the brain, the carotid arteries, to constrict. These dilated arteries are responsible for causing vascular headaches such as migraines and cluster headaches. Ergotamine is contraindicated in patients with peripheral vascular disease, coronary artery disease, sepsis, impaired hepatic or renal function, and severe hypertension, as well as in pregnant women. It is available as a sublingual 2-mg tablet, an aerosolized inhaler, and as a rectal suppository that contains 2 mg of ergotamine and 100 mg of caffeine. There are also several combination-drug preparations available in oral tablet form. These combinations vary; some of the other agents combined with ergotamine in these preparations are belladonna alkaloids, phenobarbital, and caffeine. The dosages table on the next page contains the dosing information for the 2-mg sublingual tablets as well as the aerosol preparation.

❖❖ PHARMACOKINETICS

HALF-LIFE	ONSET	PEAK	DURATION
21 hr	30 min-2 hr	30 min-3 hr	3-4 hr

PHENOXYBENZAMINE HYDROCHLORIDE

Phenoxybenzamine (Dibenzyline) is an alpha-blocker that reduces blood pressure by reducing peripheral vascular resistance. It is used to treat the hypertension caused by pheochromocytoma. Phenoxybenzamine is also useful in the treatment of vascular disorders such as frostbite, Raynaud's disease, and acrocyanosis, which have as an underlying cause increased alpha-adrenergic activity. Phenoxybenzamine directly blocks the alpha-adrenergic receptors and is therefore very useful in the treatment of these vasospastic disorders. The drug is contraindicated in patients who have

shown a hypersensitivity reaction to it or who have conditions in which hypotension is undesirable. It is available as a 10-mg capsule. The recommended dosage is given in the table on p. 229.

❖❖ PHARMACOKINETICS

HALF-LIFE	ONSET	PEAK	DURATION
24 hr	<2 hr	4-6 hr	3-4 days

PHENTOLAMINE

Phentolamine (Regitine) is an alpha-blocker that reduces peripheral vascular resistance and is also used to treat hypertension. Unlike phenoxybenzamine, it can be used to help establish the diagnosis of pheochromocytoma as well as treat the high blood pressure caused by this catecholamine-secreting tumor. To diagnose pheochromocytoma using phentolamine, a single intravenous dose of the drug is given to the hypertensive patient who is suspected of having the tumor. If the blood pressure declines rapidly, it is highly likely the patient has a pheochromocytoma. It is only available as an intravenous preparation, but this confers some advantages because it can then be used to treat the extravasation of vasoconstricting IV drugs such as NE, EPI, and dopamine, which when given IV can leak out of the vein, especially if the IV tube is not correctly positioned. If the drug is allowed to extravasate into the surrounding tissue, this leads to intense vasoconstriction, decreased blood flow, necrosis, and potential loss of the limb. When phentolamine is injected subcutaneously in a circular fashion around the extravasation site, this causes alpha-adrenergic receptor blockade and vasodilation, which in turn increases blood flow to the ischemic tissue, thus preventing permanent damage. It is contraindicated in patients who have shown a hypersensitivity to it, those who have suffered a myocardial infarction, and those with coronary artery disease. The recommended dosage are given in the table on p. 229.

❖❖ PHARMACOKINETICS

HALF-LIFE	ONSET	PEAK	DURATION
19 min	Immediate	2 min	15-30 min

TOLAZOLINE

Tolazoline (Priscoline) is an alpha-blocker that causes peripheral vasodilation and decreases peripheral resistance. It does this primarily by directly relaxating vascular smooth muscle through the competitive blockade of alpha-adrenergic receptors. It is primarily used for the treatment of hypertension in neonates when the hypertension causes the oxygen level in the neonates' bloodstream to decrease and the usual supportive measures are not able to compensate for this.

DOSAGES

SELECTED ALPHA-ADRENERGIC BLOCKING AGENTS

AGENT	PHARMACOLOGIC CLASS	DOSAGE RANGE	PURPOSE
Ergotamine tartrate (Ergostat)	Alpha-blocker	*Adult* Aerosol: one inhalation (0.36 mg) repeated at ≥5-min intervals; do not exceed 6 doses/day or 15/wk. SL tablets: 2 mg; repeat at ½-hr intervals; do not exceed 6 mg/day or 10 mg/wk.	Vascular headache
Phenoxybenzamine hydrochloride (Dibenzyline)	Alpha-blocker	*Adult* PO: initial dose of 10 mg bid; usual range 20-40 mg 2-3 times/day	Hypertension
Phentolamine (Regitine)	Alpha-blocker	*Pediatric* IM/IV: 1 mg 1-2 hr preop and 1 mg prn during surgery	Control/prevention of hypertension during surgery
		Adult IM/IV: 5 mg 1-2 hr preop and 5 mg prn during surgery	
		Adult IV: 5-15 mg	Hypertensive crises
		Adult/Pediatric 5-10 mg into extravasation site	Treatment of NE dermal necrosis
Prazosin (Minipress)	Alpha₁-blocker	*Adult* PO: 1 mg 2-3/day; maintenance range, 6-15 mg/day divided	Hypertension
Tolazoline (Priscoline)	Alpha-blocker	*Neonatal* IV: 1-2 mg/kg via scalp vein, followed by 1-2 mg/kg/hr infusion	Neonatal pulmonary hypertension

Tolazoline is contraindicated in patients who have had hypersensitivity reactions to it and in patients with known or suspected coronary artery disease. It is also contraindicated in patients who have suffered a cerebrovascular accident. It is available only as a parenteral (IV, IM, or SC) injection. The normal dosages are given in the table above.

⬡ PHARMACOKINETICS

HALF-LIFE	ONSET	PEAK	DURATION
3-10 hr	<30 min	30-60 min	3-4 hr

PRAZOSIN

Prazosin (Minipress) is an alpha₁-adrenergic–blocking agent primarily used to treat hypertension and to reduce urinary obstruction in men with BPH. Other drugs that are chemically and pharmacologically re-

lated to prazosin are doxazosin (Cardura) and terazosin (Hytrin). Its primary antihypertensive effects are related to its selective and competitive inhibition of alpha₁-adrenergic receptors. In men with BPH, prazosin relieves the impaired urinary flow and urinary frequency by relaxing and dilating the vasculature and smooth muscle in the area surrounding the prostate. It also rather dramatically lowers blood pressure. A patient's ability to tolerate this drop in blood pressure must be taken into consideration when prescribing alpha-blockers for the treatment of BPH. Often when patients are first started on the drug, they become very lightheaded and may even pass out when standing up after sitting or lying down. This is referred to as **orthostatic hypotension.** Although it is a fairly common problem specific to the alpha₁-blockers prazosin, doxazosin, and terazosin, patients quickly acquire a tolerance to it, most after the first dose. Often patients taking their first dose are told to take it at bedtime to circumvent the problem. Prazosin is contraindicated in patients who have shown hypersensitivity reactions to it. It is available as a 1-, 2-, and 5-mg capsule and as a combination product containing the diuretic polythiazide. This preparation is called Minizide. The normally recommended dosages of prazosin are given in the table on p. 229.

▼ P H A R M A C O K I N E T I C S

HALF-LIFE	ONSET	PEAK	DURATION
2-3 hr	2 hr	1-3 hr	6-12 hr

BETA-BLOCKERS

Beta-adrenergic–blocking agents, beta-blockers, block SNS stimulation of the beta-adrenergic receptors by competing with the endogenous catecholamines NE and EPI. Beta-blockers can be either selective or nonselective, depending on the type of beta-adrenergic receptors they antagonize or block. As mentioned earlier, beta₁-adrenergic receptors are located primarily on the heart. Beta-blockers selective for these receptors are sometimes called **cardioselective beta-blockers,** or beta₁-blocking agents. Other beta-blockers block both beta₁- and beta₂-adrenergic receptors, the latter located primarily on the smooth muscles of the bronchioles and blood vessels. Beta-blockers that block both types of beta-adrenergic receptors are referred to as **nonspecific beta-blockers.** The agents within the beta-blocker class can be further categorized according to whether they have **intrinsic sympathomimetic activity (ISA).** Agents with ISA (acebutolol, penbutolol, and timolol) not only block beta-adrenergic receptors but also partially stimulate them. This was initially believed to be an advantageous characteristic, but clinical use has not borne this out. Following are the currently available beta-blockers:

Nonspecific beta-blockers:
- Carteolol (Cartrol)
- Nadolol (Corgard)
- Penbutolol (Levatol)
- Pindolol (Visken)
- Propranolol (Inderal)
- Sotalol (Betapace)
- Timolol (Blocadren)

Cardioselective beta-blockers:
- Acebutolol (Sectral)
- Atenolol (Tenormin)
- Betaxolol (Kerlone)
- Bisoprolol (Zebta)
- Esmolol (Brevibloc)
- Metoprolol (Lopressor and Toprol XL)
- Labetalol* (Normodyne and Trandate)

*Blocks both alpha- and beta-adrenergic receptors.

Mechanism of Action

Because the beta-blockers compete with and block NE and EPI at the beta-adrenergic receptors located throughout the body, the beta-adrenergic receptor sites can then no longer be stimulated by the neurotransmitters and SNS stimulation is blocked. Although beta-adrenergic receptors are located throughout the body, the most important ones in terms of these agents are the ones located on the surface of the heart, the smooth muscle of the bronchi, and the smooth muscle of blood vessels. The cardioselective beta₁-blockers block the beta₁-adrenergic receptors on the surface of the heart. This decreases heart rate, slows conduction through the atrioventricular (AV) node, prolongs sinoatrial (SA) node recovery, and decreases myocardial oxygen demand by decreasing myocardial contractility. The nonspecific beta-blockers also have this effect on the heart, but they block beta₂-adrenergic receptors on the smooth muscle of the bronchioles and blood vessels as well. This can cause the bronchioles to constrict, which in turn leads to narrowing of the airways and shortness of breath. The nonspecific beta-blockers can also constrict blood vessels by blocking beta₂-adrenergic receptors on the smooth muscle of blood vessels.

Drug Effects

When the beta-adrenergic receptors of the SNS on the heart are blocked, myocardial stimulation is blocked. This results in both decreased contractile force and decreased myocardial oxygen consumption. The smooth muscle that surrounds blood vessels controls the size of the blood vessels and can cause them to dilate or constrict depending on whether the alpha- or beta-adrenergic receptors are stimulated. When SNS stimulation at these smooth muscles is blocked by a beta-blocker, the muscles are then stimulated by the alpha-adrenergic receptors and contract. This causes increased peripheral vascular resistance.

Beta-blockers also affect the conduction cells in the SA and AV nodes. They tend to slow conduction through these cells and to decrease heart rate and contractility. Within the heart, beta-blockers reduce or block the production of glucose from glycogen, a process called **glycogenolysis.** They also elicit the breakdown of fat, a process called **lipolysis.**

Smooth muscle also surrounds the airways in the lungs called *bronchioles.* When beta₂-adrenergic receptors are blocked on these, the smooth muscle contracts, causing these airways to narrow.

Many of the beta-blockers that are lipid soluble can cross the **blood-brain barrier,** a semipermeable membrane that selectively allows substances with certain characteristics such as lipid solubility to pass into the brain. Lipid-soluble beta-blockers that can as a result cross into the brain produce weakness, lethargy, and fatigue.

Therapeutic Uses

The drug effects mentioned in the preceding section vary from beta-blocker to beta-blocker depending on the specific chemical characteristics of the agent. Some of the beta-blockers are used primarily in the treatment of **angina** or chest pain. These work by decreasing demand for myocardial energy and oxygen consumption, which helps shift the supply-and-demand ratio to the supply side and allows more oxygen to get to the heart muscle. This in turn helps relieve the pain in the heart muscle caused by the lack of oxygen.

Other beta-blockers are considered **cardioprotective** because they inhibit stimulation by the circulating catecholamines. Catecholamines are released during muscle damage such as that caused by a myocardial infarction (MI), or heart attack. When a beta-blocker occupies their receptors, the circulating catecholamines cannot then bind to the receptors. Thus, the beta-blockers "protect" the heart from being stimulated by these catecholamines, which would only further increase the heart rate and the contractile force, thereby increasing myocardial oxygen demand. As a result, beta-blockers are frequently given to patients after they have suffered an MI to protect the heart from the effects of these released catecholamines.

As mentioned earlier, beta-blockers also have a profound effect on the conduction system of the heart. The AV node normally receives impulse stimulation from the SA node and slows it down so that the ventricles have time to fill before they are stimulated to contract. Conduction in the SA node, which spontaneously depolarizes at the most frequent rate, is further slowed by beta-blockers, resulting in a decreased heart rate. They also slow conduction through the AV node. These effects of beta-blockers on the conduction system of the heart make them useful agents in the treatment of various types of irregular heartbeats called **arrhythmias.** In the **Vaughan Williams classification** of antiarrhythmic drugs, the beta-blockers are in the class II category.

By blocking peripheral adrenergic receptors and decreasing stimulation from the SNS, beta-blockers are useful in treating hypertension. Although beta-blockers have been shown to worsen congestive heart failure (CHF), certain types of CHF respond favorably to beta-blockers. That form of CHF that has a diastolic dysfunction component responds favorably to beta-blockers.

Because of their **lipophylicity** (attraction to lipid or fat), other beta-blockers can easily gain entry into the CNS and brain. These beta-blockers are used to treat migraine headaches. The topical application of beta-blockers on the eye has also been very effective in treating ocular disorders such as glaucoma.

Side Effects and Adverse Effects

The side effects and adverse effects of beta-blockers are primarily extensions of their pharmacologic activity. Most such effects are mild and diminish with time. Some of the most serious undesirable effects can be caused by acute withdrawal of the drug. This may, for instance, exacerbate the underlying angina they are being used to treat or precipitate an MI. Beta-blocker–induced side effects and adverse effects are listed by body site in Table 16-3.

Toxicity and Management of Overdose

After the acute ingestion of an overdose of a beta-blocker, the stomach should be emptied immediately either by inducing emesis or by gastric lavage. Treatment primarily consists of symptomatic and supportive care. Atropine may be given IV for the management of bradycardia. If the bradycardia persists despite atropine treatment, isoproterenol may be administered. If the bradycardia still persists, placement of a transvenous cardiac pacemaker should be considered. For the treatment of severe hypotension, vasopressors should be titrated until the desired blood pressure and heart rate are achieved. Intravenously administered diazepam may be useful for the treatment of seizures. Most beta-blockers are dialyzable; therefore hemodialysis may be useful in enhancing elimination in the event of severe overdose.

Table 16-3	Beta-Blockers: Common Adverse Effects
BODY SYSTEM	**SIDE/ADVERSE EFFECTS**
Cardiovascular	AV block, bradycardia, congestive heart failure, peripheral vascular insufficiency
Central nervous system	Dizziness, mental depression, lethargy, hallucinations
Gastrointestinal	Nausea, dry mouth, vomiting, diarrhea, cramps, ischemic colitis
Blood	Agranulocytosis, thrombocytopenia
Other	Impotence, rash, alopecia, bronchospasms

Interactions

Most of the drug interactions with beta-blockers result either from the additive effects of the coadministered medications, ones with similar mechanisms of action, or from the antagonistic effects of the agents. Some of the common drugs that interact with beta-blockers and the results of this are given in Table 16-4.

Dosages

For information on the recommended dosages for selected beta-blockers, see the table on the next page.

DRUG PROFILES

Beta-blockers are prescription-only drugs that are available in oral preparations as tablets and capsules and parenteral forms as intermittent injections or continuous intravenous infusions. Topically administered forms are also available. Beta-blocker eyedrops are used in the treatment of glaucoma. All beta-blockers except for acebutolol are rated as pregnancy category C agents. Acebutolol is a pregnancy category B agent.

ACEBUTOLOL

Acebutolol (Sectral) is a cardioselective beta$_1$-blocker used for the treatment of hypertension, ventricular and supraventricular arrhythmias, and angina, and in patients in the immediate period after an MI. It is commonly used alone as an antihypertensive agent or in combination with a diuretic for the additive antihypertensive effects. It is one of the few beta-blockers that possess ISA. It is contraindicated in patients who have

had a hypersensitivity reaction to it; in those with severe bradycardia, heart block greater than first degree, Raynaud's disease, or malignant hypertension; and in those in cardiogenic shock or cardiac failure. It is available as 200- and 400-mg capsules. The commonly recommended dosages are given in the table on p. 233.

♥ PHARMACOKINETICS

HALF-LIFE	ONSET	PEAK	DURATION
3-4 hr	1.5-8 hr	3 hr	10-24 hr

⚓ PROPRANOLOL

Propranolol (Inderal) is the prototypical nonspecific beta$_1$- and beta$_2$-blocking agent. It was one of the very first beta-blockers to be used. The lengthy experience with it has yielded many uses for it. Besides the indications mentioned for acebutolol, propranolol has also been used in the treatment of the tachyarrhythmias associated with cardiac glycoside intoxication and for the treatment of hypertrophic subaortic stenosis, pheochromocytoma, thyrotoxicosis, migraine headaches, and essential tremors, as well as many other conditions. The same contraindications that apply to the cardioselective beta-blockers (cited in the discussion on acebutolol) apply to it as well. In addition, it is contraindicated in patients with bronchial asthma. It is available as an IV injection, as 60-, 80-, 120-, and 160-mg oral long-acting capsules, and 10-, 20-, 40-, 60-, and 80-mg tablets. The recommended dosages are given in the table on p. 233.

♥ PHARMACOKINETICS

HALF-LIFE	ONSET	PEAK	DURATION
3-4 hr	<30 min	1-1.5 hr	8-12 hr

ATENOLOL

Atenolol (Tenormin) is a cardioselective beta-blocker that is commonly used in patients who have an MI to

Table 16-4	Beta-Blockers: Drug Interactions	
DRUG	**MECHANISM**	**RESULT**
Antacids (aluminum hydroxide type)	Decrease absorption	Decreased beta-blocker activity
Antimuscarinics/anticholinergics	Antagonism	Reduced beta-blocker effects
Diuretics and cardiovascular drugs	Additive effect	Additive hypotensive effects
Neuromuscular blocking agents	Additive effect	Prolonged neuromuscular blockade
Oral hypoglycemic agents	Antagonism	Decreased hypoglycemic effects

DOSAGES

SELECTED BETA-ADRENERGIC AGENTS

AGENT	PHARMACOLOGIC CLASS	DOSAGE RANGE	PURPOSE
Acebutolol (Sectral)	Beta$_1$-blocker	*Adult* PO: 400-800 mg/day divided 600-1200 mg/day divided	Hypertension Premature ventricular beats
⚓**Propranolol (Inderal)**	Beta-blocker	*Adult* PO: 80-320 mg/day divided 120-240 mg/day divided 10-30 mg 3-5 times/day 180-240 mg/day divided 20-40 mg 3-4 times/day 120-320 mg/day divided 160-240 mg/day divided 60 mg/day divided for 3 days before surgery with an alpha-blocker IV: 1-3 mg	Angina Hypertension Arrhythmias Prevention of myocardial infarction Hypertrophic subaortic stenosis Essential tremor Migraine Pheochromocytoma surgery Serious arrhythmias
Atenolol (Tenormin)	Beta$_1$-blocker	*Adult* PO: 50-100 mg/day divided 50-200 mg/day divided IV: 5 mg over 5 min followed by 5 mg over 10 min	Hypertension Angina Acute myocardial infarction
Esmolol (Brevibloc)	Beta$_1$-blocker	*Adult* IV: Bolus of 500 μg/kg/min followed by 4 min of 50 μg/kg/min and evaluate IV: 80 mg bolus over 30 min followed by 150 μg/kg/min infusion if needed	Supraventricular tachyarrhythmias Intraoperative-postop/hypertension
Labetalol (Normodyne, Trandate)	Alpha$_1$-beta blocker	*Adult* PO: 200-800 mg/day divided IV: 20 mg with additional doses of 40-80 mg at 10-min intervals until desired effect or a total dose of 300 mg is injected; maintenance infusion of 2 mg/min	Hypertension Severe hypertension
⚓**Metoprolol (Lopressor, Toprol XL)**	Beta$_1$-blocker	*Adult* PO: 100-450 mg/day divided 100 mg bid IV/PO: 3 bolus injections of 5 mg at 2-min intervals followed in 15 min by 50 mg PO q6h for 48 h; thereafter 100 mg bid	Hypertension Late myocardial infarction Early myocardial infarction
⚓**Sotalol (Betapace)**	Beta-blocker	*Adult* PO: 160-320 mg/day divided	Life-threatening ventricular arrhythmias

prevent future MIs and in the treatment of hypertension and angina. It is available as an 0.5-mg/ml injection and as 25-, 50-, and 100-mg tablets. See the table on p. 233 for the recommended dosages.

PHARMACOKINETICS

HALF-LIFE	ONSET	PEAK	DURATION
6-7 hr	IV: immediate PO: <30 min	IV: <5 min PO: 2-4 hr	IV: <12 hr PO: 24 hr

ESMOLOL

Esmolol (Brevibloc) is a very potent, short-acting, beta$_1$-blocker. It is primarily used in acute situations to provide rapid, temporary control of the ventricular rate in patients with supraventricular tachyarrhythmias (SVTs). Because of its very short half-life, it is only given as an intravenous infusion and the serum levels titrated to control the patient's symptoms. It comes as a 250-mg/ml concentrate for injection and as a 10-mg/ml injection. Recommended dosages are given in the table on p. 233.

PHARMACOKINETICS

HALF-LIFE	ONSET	PEAK	DURATION
9 min	Immediate	6 min	15-20 min

LABETALOL

Labetalol (Normodyne, Trandate) is unusual in that it can block both alpha- and beta-adrenergic receptors. It is used in the treatment of severe hypertension and hypertensive emergencies to quickly lower the blood pressure before permanent damage is done. It is available both parenterally as a 5-mg/ml IV injection and in oral forms as 100-, 200-, and 300-mg tablets. The normal dosages are given in the table on p. 233.

PHARMACOKINETICS

HALF-LIFE	ONSET	PEAK	DURATION
6-8 hr	IV: 2-5 min PO: 20-120 min	IV: 5-15 min PO: 1-4 hr	IV: 2-4 hr PO: 8-24 hr

METOPROLOL

Metoprolol (Lopressor, Toprol XL) is a beta$_1$-blocker that has become very popular for use in the post-MI patient. Recent studies of metoprolol have shown increased survival in patients given the agent after they have suffered an MI. It is available as 1-mg/ml injection or as 50-, 100-, and 200-mg tablets (Lopressor) and 47.5-, 95-, and 190-mg extended-release tablets (Toprol XL). It is also available in combination with the diuretic

hydrochlorothiazide (Lopressor HCT). Commonly recommended dosages are given in the table on p. 233.

PHARMACOKINETICS

HALF-LIFE	ONSET	PEAK	DURATION
3-4 hr	IV: immediate PO: 10 min	IV: 10 min PO: 1.5-4 hr	IV: 5-8 hr PO: 24 hr

SOTALOL

Sotalol (Betapace) is a nonspecific beta-blocker that has very potent antiarrhythmic properties. It is commonly used for the management of difficult-to-treat arrhythmias. Often these arrhythmias are life-threatening ventricular arrhythmias such as sustained ventricular tachycardia. Because it is a nonspecific beta-blocker, it causes some of the unwanted side effects typical of these agents. It is available in oral tablet form in 80-, 160-, and 240-mg amounts. Commonly recommended dosages are given in the table on p. 233.

PHARMACOKINETICS

HALF-LIFE	ONSET	PEAK	DURATION
12 hr	<1 hr	2.5-4 hr	2-3 days

Newer Beta-Blockers

Many of the newer beta-blockers are cardioselective beta$_1$-blockers that only need to be taken once a day. The advantage to them is that they do not produce some of the unwanted side effects associated with the nonspecific beta-blockers, effects such as bronchiole constriction and increased peripheral vascular resistance. The once-a-day dosing is another advantage. This helps promote patient compliance, which is very important for the patient taking several other medications to control their hypertension and possibly other diseases as well. Examples of some of these agents are betaxolol and bisoprolol.

NURSING PROCESS

ASSESSMENT

Adrenergic-blocking agents, or sympatholytics, produce a variety of effects on the patient, depending on the type of receptor blocked. Because of the clinical impact all of these agents have on mainly the cardiac and respiratory systems, their use requires careful assessment of the patient to minimize the side effects and maximize the therapeutic effects. To begin a thorough assessment, information should be gathered about the patient's allergies and past and present medical conditions. A system overview and a thorough medication history should form part of this process. Some pertinent questions to pose to the patient who is to receive an adrenergic blocking agent might include: Are you allergic to any medications or foods? Do you have a history of a chronic obstructive pulmonary disease such as emphysema, asthma, or chronic bronchitis? Do you have a history of hypotension, cardiac arrhythmias, bradycardia, CHF, or any other cardiovascular disease? These questions are important because alpha-blockers may precipitate hypotension whereas beta-blockers may precipitate bradycardia, hypotension, heart block, CHF, and bronchoconstriction or increased airway resistance so any preexisting condition that might be exacerbated by the use of these agents might be a contraindication to their use.

Patients should be asked whether they are taking any of the drugs that can interact with the adrenergic-blocking agent that has been prescribed for them. These include alpha-blockers (ergotamines); beta-blockers, which could cause vasoconstriction, especially propranolol, and the other agents listed in Table 16-4. The contraindications to the use of these medications are related to their receptor-blocking effects and resulting cardiovascular actions, so these drugs are contraindicated in patients with peripheral vascular disease, CHF, or bradyarrhythmias.

NURSING DIAGNOSES

Nursing diagnoses related to the use of adrenergic antagonists, or sympatholytics, include, but are not limited to:
- Knowledge deficit related to therapeutic regimen, side effects, drug interactions, and precautions to be taken.
- Risk for injury related to possible side effects of adrenergic antagonistics (numbness and tingling of fingers and toes and so on).
- Altered nutritional status (less than body requirements because of nausea and vomiting) related to use of adrenergic blockers.
- Altered tissue perfusion (decreased) related to cardiovascular side effects of hypertension.

PLANNING

Goals for the patient receiving sympatholytics include, but are not limited to:
- Patient takes medication exactly as prescribed.
- Patient experiences relief of the symptoms for which the medication was prescribed.

Beta-Blockers

✔ Encourage patients to always take medication as prescribed, no more and no less.

✔ Tell patients to never abruptly stop taking the medication.

✔ Encourage patients to contact their physician should they become ill and unable to take the prescribed doses. Rebound hypertension or chest pain may occur if this medication is discontinued abruptly.

✔ Patients should report any weight gain of more than 2 pounds (1 kg) within a week as well as any problems with fluid buildup or edema of the feet or ankles, any shortness of breath, or excessive fatigue or weakness.

✔ Patients should notify their physician if they experience any syncope or dizziness.

✔ Inform patients that they may notice a decrease in their tolerance to exercise, and dizziness or fainting may occur with increased activity. Patients should be encouraged to change positions slowly and to contact their physician if any of the above problems occur.

✔ Patients should be warned not to take OTC medications without the approval of their physician!

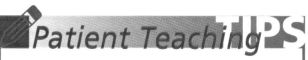

Alpha-Blockers

✔ Encourage patients to take medication as prescribed and to never abruptly stop taking medication.

✔ Patients should avoid OTC medications because of drug interactions.

✔ Keep these and all other medications out of the reach of children.

✔ Patients should notify their physician if palpitations, dyspnea, nausea, or vomiting occur.

✔ Patients should avoid caffeine because of excessive irritability.

✔ Patients should avoid alcohol ingestion and should not engage in hazardous activities until stable blood levels are achieved.

■ Patient remains compliant with the drug therapy.
■ Patient demonstrates an adequate knowledge concerning the use of the specific medications, the side effects, and the appropriate dosing routine to be followed at home.
■ Patient will be free of injury to self as the result of adverse effects of the medications.

Outcome Criteria

Outcome criteria related to the administration of adrenergic blockers include:
■ Patient states the importance of both the pharmacologic and nonpharmacologic treatment of his or her migraine headaches, hypertension, or other reason for drug therapy.
■ Patient states reasons for compliance with the medication therapy and the risks and complications such as syncope, dizziness, and hypotension arising as a result of overuse of the medication.
■ Patient demonstrates the correct method of taking blood pressure with self-taking digital cuff or by using community resources.

■ Patient taking these medications for the treatment of migraine headaches will state the importance of remaining in a quiet, calm, and dark room during a headache.
■ Patient states those conditions which may occur that the physician should be informed immediately of such as palpitations, chest pain, insomnia, and excessive agitation.
■ Patient keeps all follow-up appointments with the physician so as to maintain safe therapy.
■ Patient follows instructions regarding the avoidance of sudden withdrawal of hypertensive agents to avoid rebound hypertensive crises and experiences minimal complications.

IMPLEMENTATION

There are several nursing interventions that can maximize the therapeutic effects of adrenergic-blocking agents and minimize the side effects. Thorough patient education is a must in ensuring good compliance, and the teaching tips are presented on the previous page. Patients taking alpha-blockers should be encouraged

TAKE HOME POINTS

Alpha-Blockers
■ Block stimulation of the alpha$_1$- and alpha$_2$-adrenergic receptors by NE or EPI.
■ Cause a variety of physiologic responses depending on what receptors are blocked.
■ Some agents may stimulate the alpha-adrenergic receptors at regular doses and block them at high doses.

Alpha$_1$-Blockers
■ Predominant response when blocked = vasodilation and relaxation.
■ Block postsynaptic alpha-adrenergic receptors from the stimulatory actions of NE and EPI.
■ Drugs such as prazosin, doxazosin, and terazosin.
■ Vasodilation—drop in blood pressure; reduces urinary obstruction, which leads to increased urinary flow rates.

Beta-Blockers
■ Block stimulation of beta-adrenergic receptors by SNS neurotransmitters NE and EPI as well as dopamine.
■ Predominant response when blocked = constriction and cardiac depression.
■ Have both selective and nonselective beta-blockers.

■ Located on postsynaptic effector cells (cells, muscles, and organs that nerves stimulate).

Cardioselective Beta-Blockers
■ Block just beta$_1$-adrenergic receptors on the heart.
■ Beneficial effects = decreased heart rate, cardiac conduction, and myocardial contractility.

Nonselective Beta-Blockers
■ Block both beta$_1$- and beta$_2$-adrenergic receptors; affect heart and smooth muscle.
■ Have beneficial effects of the selective agents.
■ Have detrimental effects of nonselective agents (constriction of bronchioles and blood vessels).

Nursing Considerations
■ Patients should avoid sudden changes in position because of possible postural hypotension.
■ Patients should report constipation or the development of any urinary hesitancy or bladder distention.
■ Confusion, depression, hallucinations, nightmares, palpitations, and dizziness should be reported to the physician.

to change positions slowly so as to prevent or minimize postural hypotension. When using beta-blockers, patients should know to take their apical pulse for one full minute as well as their blood pressure because of the cardiac depression that can occur with these agents. They should be told to contact the physician if the systolic blood pressure decreases to less than 100 mm Hg or the pulse decreases to less than 60 beats/min. The physician should also be notified if the blood pressure continues to decrease, even by a few millimeters mercury. Patients should also know to report any weight gain, especially more than 2 pounds (1 kg) in a week, weakness, shortness of breath, and edema to their physician immediately. Make sure that patients are weaned off these medications slowly, if this is indicated, because of the possible rebound hypertension or chest pain rapid withdrawal can precipitate.

EVALUATION

Therapeutic effects to monitor for in patients receiving adrenergic-blocking agents include, but are not limited to, a decrease in blood pressure, pulse rate, and palpitations in patients with a pheochromocytoma; alleviation of the symptoms of Raynaud's disease; return to normal blood pressure and pulse with lowering of the blood pressure toward 120/80 mm Hg or the pulse to within normal limits (<100 but >60 beats/min), and a decrease in chest pain in patients with angina.

Patients must also be monitored for the occurrence of the side effects of these medications, which include, but are not limited to, hypotension, tachycardia (alpha-blockers), bradycardia, heart block, CHF, increased airway resistance, fatigue, lethargy, depression, insomnia, and vivid nightmares.

Critical Thinking **A C T I V I T I E S**

1. Essay question: Develop patient teaching for the use of the following medications:
   a. Ergotamine tartrate (Ergostat)
   b. Prazosine (Minipress)
   c. Atenolol (Tenormin)

2. One of your patients, a 46-year-old mother of two adolescent children, is now taking propranolol for the control of tachycardia and hypertension. What instructions should you give her if she says: "Well, if it doesn't work after a month or two, I'll just quit taking it!"

3. You have just come on your shift and are taking over for a nurse who already has your patient's heart rate controlled on an esmolol infusion. It is running at a rate of 54 ml/hr. The physician is making rounds and asks you how many μg/kg/min of esmolol the patient is controlled on. The patient weighs 90 kg and the normal concentration of esmolol is 10 mg/ml. How many μg/kg/min of esmolol is the patient receiving?

▲▲▲

BIBLIOGRAPHY

Albanese J, Nutz P: *Mosby's 1995 nursing drug cards,* St Louis, Mosby, 1995.

Johnson KB: *Harriet Lane handbook,* ed 13, St Louis, 1993, Mosby.

Keen JH: *Critical care and emergency drug reference,* St Louis, 1994, Mosby.

Knoben JE, Anderson PO: *Handbook of critical drug data,* ed 6, Hamilton, Ill, 1988, Drug Intelligence Publications.

McEvoy GK: *AHFS drug information,* Bethesda, Md, 1989, American Society of Hospital Pharmacists.

Saul L: Arrythmia mimics, *AJN* 91(3): 40, 1991.

Saul L. Arrythmia mimics: Part II, *AJN* 91(5): 41, 1991.

Skidmore-Roth L: *Mosby's 1995 nursing drug reference,* St Louis, 1995, Mosby.

Zuckerman IH: Therapeutic management of chronic cardiovascular disease, *US Pharmacist* 15(6): 31, 1990.

Chapter 17

Cholinergic Agents

Objectives

When you reach the end of this chapter, you will be able to:

1 Briefly discuss the normal anatomy and physiology of the autonomic nervous system, including the events that occur during synaptic transmission within the sympathetic and parasympathetic divisions.

2 Cite various examples of the cholinergic drugs.

3 Discuss the mechanism of action, therapeutic effects, uses, and adverse and toxic effects of the cholinergic drugs as well as the antidotes to overdose and to the unwanted effects.

4 Develop a nursing care plan that includes expected outcomes as it relates to the administration of the various cholinergic agents and the treatment of side effects and overdose or toxicity stemming from use of these agents.

5 Identify the drug interactions associated with the use of cholinergics.

6 Evaluate the therapeutic versus the side effects of the different cholinergics.

CHAPTER OUTLINE

Parasympathetic Nervous System
Cholinergic Agents
  Mechanism of action
  Drug effects
  Therapeutic uses
  Side effects and adverse effects
    Toxicity and management of overdose
  Interactions
  Dosages
Drug Profiles
  Bethanechol
 Physostigmine
  Pyridostigmine
Nursing Process
Assessment
Nursing Diagnoses
Planning
  Outcome criteria
Implementation
Evaluation

Glossary

Acetylcholine (as′ ə təl ko lēn) Neurotransmitter responsible for transmission of nerve impulses to effector cells in the parasympathetic nervous system. (p. 239)

Cholinergic agents (ko′ lin ər′ jik) Drugs that stimulate the parasympathetic nervous system. (p. 240)

Cholinesterase (ko′ lin es tər ās) Enzyme responsible for the breakdown of acetylcholine. (p. 240)

Direct-acting agonists Agents that bind to cholinergic receptors to activate them. (p. 240)

Indirect-acting agonists Agents that make more acetylcholine available at the receptor site. (p. 240)

Irreversible cholinesterase inhibitors Agents that form a permanent covalent bond with cholinesterase. (p. 240)

Muscarinic receptors (mus′ kə rin ik) Cholinergic receptors located postsynaptically in the smooth muscle, cardiac muscle, and glands of the parasympathetic fibers and in the effector organs of the cholinergic sympathetic fibers; can be stimulated by the alkaloid muscarine. (p. 239)

Nicotinic receptors (nik′ o tin ik) Cholinergic receptors located in the ganglia of both the parasympathetic and sympathetic nervous systems; can be stimulated by the alkaloid nicotine. (p. 239)

Parasympathomimetics Another name for cholinergic agents that mimic the effects of acetylcholine. (p. 240)

Reversible cholinesterase inhibitors Agents that bind to cholinesterase for minutes to hours but do not form a permanent bond. (p. 240)

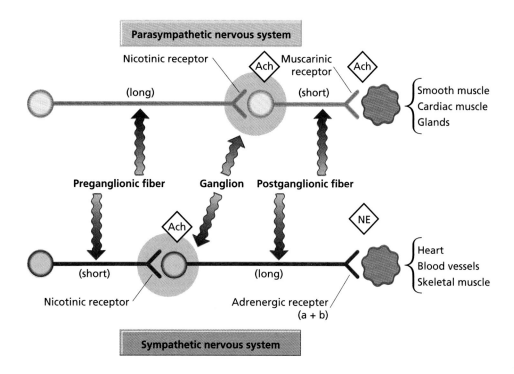

▼ **FIG. 17-1** The parasympathetic and sympathetic nervous systems and their relationship to one another.

Cholinergics, cholinergic agonists, and parasympathomimetics are all terms that refer to the class of drugs that stimulate the parasympathetic nervous system (PSNS). To better understand how these agents work, it is helpful to know how the PSNS operates in relation to the rest of the nervous system.

PARASYMPATHETIC NERVOUS SYSTEM

The PSNS is the opposing system to the sympathetic nervous system in the autonomic nervous system (Fig. 17-1). The neurotransmitter responsible for the transmission of nerve impulses to effector cells in the PSNS is **acetylcholine**. The receptor that binds the acetylcholine and mediates its actions is called a *cholinergic receptor*. These cholinergic receptors consist of two types, as determined by their location and their action once stimulated. **Nicotinic receptors** are located in the ganglia of both the parasympathetic and sympathetic nervous systems. They are called *nicotinic* because they can be stimulated by the alkaloid nicotine. The other cholinergic receptors are the **muscarinic receptors**. These receptors are located postsynaptically in the smooth muscle, cardiac muscle, and glands of the parasympathetic fibers and in the effector organs of the cholinergic sympathetic fibers. They are called *muscarinic* because they are stimulated by the alkaloid mus-

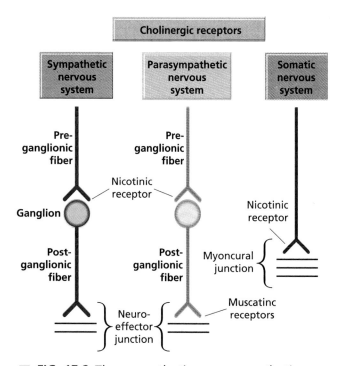

▼ **FIG. 17-2** The sympathetic, parasympathetic (PSNS), and somatic nervous systems. Note the location of the nicotinic and muscarinic receptors within the PSNS.

carine, a substance isolated from mushrooms. Figure 17-2 shows how the nicotinic and muscarinic receptors are arranged in the PSNS.

CHOLINERGIC AGENTS

The **cholinergic agents** mimic the effects of acetylcholine and are therefore sometimes referred to as **parasympathomimetics**. These drugs can stimulate their receptors either directly or indirectly. **Direct-acting** cholinergic agonists bind to cholinergic receptors and activate them. **Indirect-acting** cholinergic drugs act by making more acetylcholine available at the receptor site, thereby allowing the acetylcholine to bind to and stimulate the receptor. They do this by inhibiting **cholinesterase**, the enzyme responsible for breaking down acetylcholine. The indirect-acting cholinergic agents bind to the cholinesterase in one of two ways—reversibly or irreversibly. **Reversible cholinesterase** inhibitors bind to cholinesterase for a period of from minutes to hours; **irreversible cholinesterase** inhibitors bind to cholinesterase and form a permanent covalent bond. The body must then generate new enzyme to override the effects of the irreversible agents.

Following is a list of the direct- and indirect-acting cholinergics:

- Direct-acting agents
  Acetylcholine
  Carbachol
  Bethanechol
  Pilocarpine
- Indirect-acting agents
  Ambenonium
  Demecarium
  Physostigmine
  Echothiophate
  Isoflurophate
  Pyridostigmine
  Edrophonium
  Neostigmine
  Methacholine

These agents are used primarily to reduce intraocular pressure in patients with glaucoma or in those undergoing ocular surgery, to treat various gastrointestinal and bladder disorders, and to diagnose and treat myasthenia gravis.

Mechanism of Action

As described, the cholinergic drugs all work by stimulating the PSNS. The direct-acting cholinergics act as an agonist at the receptor, directly binding to the acetylcholine receptors and causing stimulation. The indirect-acting agents protect acetylcholine from being broken down by acetylcholinesterase, making more of this neurotransmitter available to act directly with the receptor. When the acetylcholine directly binds to its receptor, stimulation occurs. Once binding occurs on the effector cells, the cell membranes of the target organs, the permeability of the cells changes and calcium and sodium are permitted to flow into the cells. This depolarizes the cell membrane and stimulates the muscle.

Drug Effects

The effects of direct- and indirect-acting cholinergics are those that are generally seen when the PSNS is stimulated. There are many ways to remember these effects. A way used by some is to think of the PSNS as the "rest-and-digest" system. One way of remembering the effects of cholinergic poisoning is by using the acronym SLUDGE, which stands for salivation, lacrimation, urinary incontinence, diarrhea, gastrointestinal cramps, and emesis.

Cholinergic drugs stimulate the intestine and bladder, resulting in increased gastric secretions and gastrointestinal motility and increased urinary frequency. They also stimulate the pupil to constrict, causing miosis. This helps to decrease intraocular pressure. In addition, stimulation of the PSNS by the parasympathomimetics causes increased salivation and sweating. The cardiovascular effects are decreased heart rate and vasodilation. These agents also cause the bronchi of the lungs to constrict and the airways to narrow.

At recommended doses the cholinergics primarily affect the muscarinic receptors, but at high doses the nicotinic receptors can also be stimulated. The desired effects come from muscarinic receptor stimulation; many of the undesirable effects are due to nicotinic receptor stimulation. The various beneficial and undesirable effects of the cholinergic agents are listed in Table 17-1 according to the receptors stimulated.

Therapeutic Uses

Most of the direct-acting agents, acetylcholine, carbachol, and pilocarpine, are used topically to reduce intraocular pressure in patients with glaucoma or in those undergoing ocular surgery. They are poorly absorbed orally because they have large quaternary amines in their chemical structure. This is what limits their use to mostly topical application. One exception is the direct-acting cholinergic drug bethanechol, which can be administered orally or as a subcutaneous injection. It primarily affects the detrusor muscle of the urinary bladder and the smooth muscle of the gastrointestinal tract. When given, it causes increased bladder and gastrointestinal tract tone and motility, thereby increasing the movement of contents through these areas. It also causes the sphincters in the bladder and the gastrointestinal tract to relax, allowing them to empty. It is therefore used to treat atony of the bladder and gastrointestinal tract, which sometimes occurs after a surgical procedure.

Table 17-1	Cholinergic Agents: Drug Effects		
		RESPONSE TO STIMULATION	
BODY TISSUE	MUSCARINIC		NICOTINIC
Bronchi (lung)	None		Increased secretion, constriction
Cardiovascular			
Blood vessels	Dilation		Constriction
Heart rate	Slowed		Increased
Blood pressure	Decreased		Increased
Eye	Pupil constriction, decreased accommodation		None
Gastrointestinal			
Tone	Increased		Increased
Motility	Increased		Increased
Sphincters	Relaxed		None
Genitourinary			
Tone	Increased		Increased
Motility	Increased		Increased
Sphincter	Relaxed		Relaxed
Glandular secretions	Increased intestinal, lacrimal, salivary, and sweat gland secretion		Decreased bronchial and salivary secretion
Skeletal muscle	—		Increased contraction

The indirect-acting agents work by increasing acetylcholine concentrations at the receptor sites stimulating the effector cells. They cause skeletal muscle contraction and are therefore used for the diagnosis and treatment of myasthenia gravis. Their ability to inhibit acetylcholinesterase also makes them useful for the reversal of neuromuscular blockade produced either by neuromuscular blocking agents or by anticholinergic poisoning. For this reason, physostigmine is considered the antidote for anticholinergic poisoning.

Side Effects and Adverse Effects

The primary side effects and adverse effects of cholinergic agents are the consequence of overstimulation of the PSNS. They are extensions of the cholinergic reactions that affect many body functions. The major such effects are listed by body system in Table 17-2.

Toxicity and Management of Overdose

There is very little systemic absorption of the typically administered agents and therefore little systemic toxicity. When administered locally in the eye, they can cause temporary ocular changes that can be bothersome changes such as transient blurring and dimming of vision. Systemic toxicity with topically applied cholinergics is seen most commonly when longer-acting agents are given frequently for a long time. This can result in overstimulation of the PSNS and in all the

Table 17-2	Cholinergic Agents: Adverse Effects
BODY SYSTEM	SIDE/ADVERSE EFFECT
Cardiovascular	Bradycardia, hypotension, conduction abnormalities (atrioventricular block and cardiac arrest)
Central nervous system	Headache, dizziness, convulsions
Gastrointestinal	Abdominal cramps, increased GI secretions, nausea, vomiting
Respiratory	Increased bronchial secretions, bronchospasms
Other	Lacrimation, sweating, salivation, loss of binocular accommodation, miosis

attendant responses. Treatment is generally symptomatic and supportive, and the administration of a reversal agent is rarely required.

The likelihood of toxicity is greater for cholinergics that are given orally or intravenously. The most severe consequence of an overdose of a cholinergic agent is a cholinergic crisis. The symptoms of such a reaction may include circulatory collapse, hypotension, bloody diarrhea, shock, and cardiac arrest. Early signs include abdominal cramps, salivation, flushing of the skin, nausea, and vomiting. Transient syncope, transient complete heart block, dyspnea, and orthostatic hypotension may also occur. These can be reversed promptly by the administration of atropine. Severe cardiovascular reactions or bronchoconstriction may be alleviated by epinephrine.

Interactions

The potential drug interactions that can occur with the cholinergics are significant. The various categories of drugs that interact with the cholinergics, the mechanism by which the interaction occurs, and the result of the interaction are given in Table 17-3.

Table 17-3	**Cholinergic Agents: Drug Interactions**	
DRUG	**MECHANISM**	**RESULT**
Anticholinergics Antihistamines Sympathomimetics	Antagonism	Decreased response

Dosages

For the recommended dosages of the cholinergic agents, see the dosages table below.

DRUG PROFILES

Of the direct-acting cholinergic agents, bethanechol is the only agent that is administered orally. Acetylcholine, carbachol, and pilocarpine are applied topically to the eye for the treatment of glaucoma or for a reduction in intraocular pressure during ocular surgery and are discussed in greater detail in Chapter 56, as are the indirect-acting cholinergics echothiophate, demecarium, and isoflurophate, which are used primarily for the treatment of eye disorders or for surgical purposes. The cholinergics are available orally as tablets and syrups, topically as eyedrops, and paren-

DOSAGES

SELECTED CHOLINERGIC AGENTS

AGENT	PHARMACOLOGIC CLASS	DOSAGE RANGE	PURPOSE
Bethanechol (Urecholine)	Direct-acting muscarinic	*Adult* PO: 10-50 mg 3-4 times/day SC: 2.5-5 mg	Postop and postpartum functional urinary retention
↓Physostigmine (Antilirium)	Anticholinesterase (indirect-acting)	*Pediatric* IM/IV: 0.02 mg/kg repeated at 5-10 min intervals until desired effect or a dose of 2 mg is reached *Adult* IM/IV: 0.5-2 mg repeated every 20 min if needed	Anticholinergic and tricyclic antidepressant antidote
Pyridostigmine (Mestinon)	Anticholinesterase (indirect-acting)	*Pediatric* PO: 7 mg/kg/day divided into 5-6 doses *Adult* PO: 60-1500 mg/day divided to provide maximum therapeutic effect	Myasthenia gravis Myasthenia gravis
		IV: 10-20 mg with a suitable anticholinergic	Reversal of postop nondepolarizing neuromuscular blocking agents

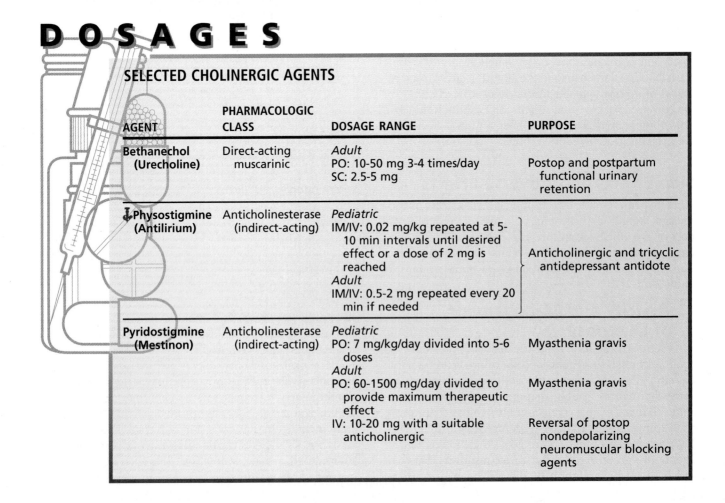

terally as intravenously and subcutaneous injections. The cholinergics are all prescription-only drugs. Most of the cholinergics are rated pregnancy category C agents by the FDA. (See inside cover for the definitions of pregnancy categories.)

BETHANECHOL

Bethanechol (urecholine) is a direct-acting cholinergic agonist that stimulates the cholinergic receptors located on the smooth muscle of the bladder. This stimulation results in increased bladder tone, increased motility, and relaxation of the sphincter of the bladder. It is used in the treatment of acute postoperative and postpartum nonobstructive urinary retention as well as for the management of neurogenic atony of the bladder with retention. It has also been used to prevent and treat the side effects of other classes of drugs such as phenothiazine- and tricyclic antidepressant–induced bladder dysfunction. In addition, it is used in the treatment of postoperative GI atony and gastric retention, chronic refractory heartburn, and familial dysautonomia as well as in the diagnostic test for infantile cystic fibrosis. IM and IV use are contraindicated. It is also contraindicated in patients with hyperthyroidism, peptic ulcer, active bronchial asthma, cardiac disease or coronary artery disease, epilepsy, and parkinsonism. Its use should also be avoided in patients with conditions in which the strength or integrity of the GI tract or bladder wall is questionable or with conditions in which increased muscular activity could prove harmful. Commonly recommended dosages are given in the table on p. 242. Pregnancy category C.

PHARMACOKINETICS

HALF-LIFE	ONSET	PEAK	DURATION
Variable	30-90 min	<30 min	1-6 hr

☧ PHYSOSTIGMINE

Physostigmine (antilirium) is a synthetic quaternary ammonium compound that is very similar in structure to edrophonium, pyridostigmine, neostigmine, and ambenonium. It is an indirect-acting cholinergic agent that has been shown to improve muscle strength and is therefore used in the symptomatic treatment of myasthenia gravis. It is also useful for reversing the effects of nondepolarizing neuromuscular blocking agents after surgery. It is contraindicated in patients who have shown a hypersensitivity or severe cholinergic reaction to the drug. It should be used with caution in patients with epilepsy, bronchial asthma, bradycardia, recent coronary artery occlusion, hyperthyroidism, cardiac arrhythmias, or peptic ulcer. It is available parenterally as an intravenously administered injection and topically as an ophthalmic solution and oint-

ment. Recommended dosages are given in the table on p. 242. Pregnancy category C.

PHARMACOKINETICS

HALF-LIFE	ONSET	PEAK	DURATION
15-40 min	<5 min	5 min	30-60 min

PYRIDOSTIGMINE

Pyridostigmine (Mestinon) is also a synthetic quaternary ammonium compound that is very similar structurally to edrophonium, neostigmine, and ambenonium. It is an indirect-acting cholinergic agent and is used in the symptomatic treatment of myasthenia gravis. It is also useful for reversing the effects of nondepolarizing neuromuscular blocking agents after surgery. It is contraindicated in patients who have shown a hypersensitivity or severe cholinergic reaction to it. It should be used with caution in patients with epilepsy, bronchial asthma, bradycardia, recent coronary artery occlusion, hyperthyroidism, cardiac arrhythmias, or peptic ulcer. It is available orally as a regular and extended-release tablet and as a solution. It is also available as a parenteral preparation. Recommended dosages are given in the table on p. 242. Pregnancy category C.

PHARMACOKINETICS

HALF-LIFE	ONSET	PEAK	DURATION
Variable	PO: 30-45 min IV: 2-5 min	PO: <30 min IV: <5 min	PO: 3-6 hr IV: 2-4 hr

NURSING PROCESS

ASSESSMENT

Cholinergic drugs, or parasympathomimetics, produce a variety of effects stemming from their ability to stimulate the PSNS and mimic the action of acetylcholine. Because these agents decrease heart rate, increase gastrointestinal and genitourinary tone and contractility by stimulating smooth muscle, increase the contractility and tone of bronchial smooth muscle, increase respiratory secretions, and produce miosis, patients who are to receive a cholinergic agent need to be assessed to determine whether they suffer from gastrointestinal or genitourinary obstruction, asthma, peptic ulcer disease, or coronary artery disease because of the potential for these agents to exacerbate these problems. Information about the patient's allergies and past and present medical conditions should also be gathered. In addition, a system overview and a thorough medication history should form part of this assessment so that possible drug interactions or contraindications to use of the cholinergic agent can be identified in advance.

NURSING DIAGNOSES

Nursing diagnoses associated with the use of cholinergics include, but are not limited to:

- Pain (abdominal) as the result of nausea, vomiting, or increased peristalsis.
- Knowledge deficit regarding therapeutic regimen, side effects, drug interactions, and precautions related to the use of cholinergic agents.
- Risk for injury related to possible side effects of cholinergic agents (bradycardia and hypotension).
- Altered cardiac output (decreased) related to the cardiovascular side effects of arrhythmias, hypotension, and bradycardia.

PLANNING

Goals for the patient receiving cholinergic agents include, but are not limited to:

- Patient receives or takes medications as prescribed.
- Patient experiences relief of the symptoms for which the medication was prescribed.

- Patient remains compliant with the drug therapy regimen.
- Patient demonstrates an adequate knowledge concerning the use of the specific medication, its side effects, and the appropriate dosing at home.
- Patient remains free of self-injury resulting from adverse effects of the medication.

TAKE HOME POINTS

Cholinergics, Cholinergic Agonists, and Parasympathomimetics

- Names for the class of drugs that stimulate the PSNS.
- PSNS: branch of CNS that opposes the SNS.
- Neurotransmitter of PSNS: acetylcholine.
- Drugs that mimic acetylcholine: parasympathomimetics.

Nicotinic Receptors

- One of the two types of cholinergic receptors.
- Called *nicotinic* because they are stimulated by nicotine.
- Located on postganglionic nerve fiber in both PSNS and SNS.

Muscarinic Receptors

- One of the two types of cholinergic receptors.
- Called *muscarinic* because they are stimulated by muscarine.
- Located on postsynaptic cells, muscles, and glands (not on nerve!).

Cholinesterase

- Enzyme responsible for the breakdown of acetylcholine.
- Indirect-acting cholinergics act by inhibiting this enzyme.
- These agents can either reversibly or irreversibly bind to this enzyme.

Nursing Considerations

- Cholinergics should be given as directed and the patient carefully monitored.
- Bradycardia, hypotension, headache, dizziness, respiratory depression, or bronchospasms occurring in a patient taking cholinergics should be reported immediately to the physician, and the patient monitored carefully.
- Always encourage patients taking cholinergics to change positions slowly to avoid dizziness and fainting resulting from postural hypotension.

Patient Teaching TIPS

Cholinergic Agents (parasympathomimetics)

✔ Patients should always take the medication as ordered because an overdose can cause life-threatening problems.

✔ It is often more effective to space the doses of these medications evenly apart to optimize the effects of the medication. Make sure patients understand this before discharge.

✔ Encourage patients to call their physician should they experience increased muscle weakness, abdominal cramps, diarrhea, or difficulty breathing.

✔ Inform patients that if they are taking the medications for the treatment of myasthenia gravis, symptoms associated with the disease should abate; that is, he or she should experience less ptosis (eyelid drooping), less diplopia (double vision), less difficulty swallowing and chewing, and less weakness.

Outcome Criteria

Outcome criteria related to the administration of cholinergic agents include:

- Patient will state the importance of both the pharmacologic and nonpharmacologic treatment of their gastrointestinal or genitourinary disorder or glaucoma in achieving good health.
- Patient will state reasons for compliance with the medication therapy and the risks associated with noncompliance as well as the complications associated with overuse of the medication such as bronchospasms, increased abdominal cramping, decreased pulse and blood pressure, etc.
- Patient will state conditions under which to contact the physician such as wheezing, bradycardia, and increased abdominal pain.
- Patient will state the importance of scheduling and keeping follow-up appointments with the physician as related to management of disorder for which medication has been prescribed.

IMPLEMENTATION

There are several nursing interventions that can be implemented to maximize the therapeutic effects of cholinergic agents and minimize their side effects. One is to always make sure patients who have undergone an operation ambulate as early as possible as ordered after their procedure to help minimize or prevent gastric and urinary retention and maximize the effects of these medications. The packaging inserts should always be checked for instructions concerning dilutional agents and the route of administration; for example, bethanechol is administered *only* subcutaneously. Atropine is the antidote to the cholinergics, so this medication should be taped to the wall next to the patient's bed or it should be available somewhere in the patient's room. Patient teaching tips are presented in the box on p. 244.

EVALUATION

Following are some of the therapeutic effects to monitor for in patients receiving cholinergic agents. In patients with myasthenia gravis, the signs and symptoms of the disease should be alleviated (see patient teaching tips on p. 244). In patients suffering a decrease in GI peristalsis postoperatively, there should be an increase in bowel sounds, the passage of flatus, and the occurrence of bowel movements that indicate increased GI peristalsis. In patients suffering from a hypotonic bladder with urinary retention, micturition should occur within about 60 minutes of the administration of bethanecol.

You must also be alert to the occurrence of the side effects of these medications; these include increased respiratory secretions, bronchospasms, difficulty breathing, nausea, vomiting, diarrhea, abdominal cramping, arrhythmias, hypotension, bradycardia, increased sweating, and an increase in the frequency and urgency of the voiding patterns.

Critical Thinking **A C T I V I T Y**

1. Your patient has undergone bladder resection 3 days earlier and is having difficulty urinating. The physician orders bethanechol, starting with 10 mg orally, tid. What should you do at this time regarding the use of bethanechol in this patient?

BIBLIOGRAPHY

Albanese J, Nutz P: *Mosby's 1995 nursing drug cards,* St Louis, 1995, Mosby.

Hickey J: Myasthenia crisis: your assessment counts, *RN* 54(5):54, 1991.

Johnson KB: *Harriet Lane handbook,* ed 13, St Louis, 1993, Mosby.

Keen JH: *Critical care and emergency drug reference,* St Louis, 1994, Mosby.

Knoben JE, Anderson PO: *Handbook of critical drug data,* ed 6, Hamilton, Ill, 1988, Drug Intelligence Publications.

McEvoy GK: *AHFS drug information,* Bethesda, Md, 1994, American Society of Hospital Pharmacists.

Skidmore-Roth, L: *Mosby's 1995 nursing drug reference,* St Louis, 1995, Mosby.

United States Pharmacopeial Convention: *USP DI: Drug information for the health care professional,* ed 13, Bethesda, Md, 1993, United States Pharmacopeial Convention.

Vinik AI, Vinik E: The diabetes complication no one talks about, *Diabet Forecast* 45(7):70, 1992.

Chapter 18

Cholinergic-Blocking Agents

Objectives

When you reach the end of this chapter, you will be able to:

1 Briefly discuss the normal anatomy and physiology of the autonomic nervous system, including the events that are blocked with the use of anticholinergic agents.

2 List examples of the various anticholinergic drugs.

3 Discuss the mechanism of action, therapeutic effects, uses, and adverse and toxic effects of the anticholinergic drugs and the antidotes to overdose and to the unwanted effects.

4 Develop a nursing care plan that includes expected outcomes as it relates to the administration of the various anticholinergic agents and the treatment of side effects and overdose or toxicity stemming from the use of these various agents.

5 Identify the drug interactions associated with the use of anticholinergics.

6 Evaluate the therapeutic versus the side effects of the different anticholinergics.

CHAPTER OUTLINE

Mechanism of action
Drug effects
Therapeutic uses
Side effects and adverse effects
  Toxicity and management of overdose
Interactions
Dosages

Drug Profiles
  Atropine
  ⚓ Scopolamine
  Dicyclomine
  Glycopyrrolate

Nursing Process
Assessment
Nursing Diagnoses
Planning
  Outcome criteria
Implementation
Evaluation

Glossary

Anticholinergics (an ti kō lə nər' jik) Another name for a cholinergic-blocking agent. (p. 247)

Cholinergic-blocking agent Any agent that blocks the action of acetylcholine and substances similar to acetylcholine at receptor sites in the synapse. Such agents in effect block the action of cholinergic nerves that transmit impulses through the release of acetylcholine at their synapses. (p. 247)

Competitive antagonist A drug or other substance that is an antagonist or that resembles a normal human metabolite and interferes with its function in the body, usually by competing for the metabolite's receptors or enzymes. Also called an *antimetabolite*. (p. 247)

Mydriasis (mĭ drī' ə sis) Dilation of the pupil of the eye caused by contraction of the dilator muscle of the iris. (p. 247)

Narrow therapeutic index The therapeutic index is the difference between the minimum therapeutic and minimum toxic concentrations of a drug. If the index is narrow, the range between the therapeutic and toxic drug concentrations is small. (p. 249)

Preganglionic fiber — Ganglion — Postganglionic fiber

▼ FIG. 18-1 Site of action of cholinergic blockers within the PSNS.

Cholinergic blockers, anticholinergics, parasympatholytics, and *antimuscarinic agents* are all terms for the class of drugs that block or inhibit the actions of acetylcholine in the parasympathetic nervous system (PSNS). **Cholinergic-blocking agents** block the action of the neurotransmitter acetylcholine at the muscarinic receptors in the PSNS. Acetylcholine released from the stimulated nerve fiber is then unable to bind to the receptor site and fails to produce a cholinergic effect. This is why the cholinergic blockers are also referred to as **anticholinergics**. Blocking the parasympathetic nerves allows the sympathetic (adrenergic) nervous system to dominate. Because of this, cholinergic blockers have many of the same effects as the adrenergics. Figure 18-1 illustrates the site of action of the cholinergic blockers within the PSNS.

The cholinergic blockers have many important therapeutic uses; they are one of the oldest group of therapeutic agents. Originally they were derived from various plant sources, but today these naturally occurring substances are only part of a larger group of cholinergic blockers that include both synthetic and semisynthetic agents. Following is a list of the currently available cholinergic blockers grouped according to their chemical class.

Natural agents
- Atropine
- Belladonna
- Hyoscocyamine
- Scopolamine

Synthetic and semisynthetic agents
- Anisotropine
- Clidinium
- Dicyclomine
- Glycopyrrolate
- Hexocyclium
- Homatropine
- Isopropamide
- Methscopolamine
- Mepenzolate
- Methantheline
- Oxyphencyclimine
- Propantheline
- Tridihexethyl

Mechanism of Action

The cholinergic blockers are largely **competitive antagonists**. They compete with acetylcholine for binding at the muscarinic receptors of the PSNS, and once they have bound to the receptor, they inhibit nerve transmission at these receptors. This generally occurs at the neuroeffector junction of smooth muscle, cardiac muscle, and exocrine glands. The cholinergic blockers have little effect at the nicotinic receptors, though at high doses they can have partial blocking effects.

Drug Effects

The major sites of action of the anticholinergics are the heart, respiratory tract, gastrointestinal tract, urinary bladder, eye, and exocrine glands. In general the anticholinergics have effects opposite those of the cholinergics at these sites of action.

The blockade of acetylcholine by cholinergic blockers causes the pupils to dilate and increases intraocular pressure. This can occur because the ciliary muscles and the sphincter muscle of the iris are innervated by cholinergic nerve fibers. Cholinergic blockers can therefore keep the sphincter muscle of the iris from contracting and allow unopposed radial muscle stimulation. This results in a dilated pupil **(mydriasis)** and a relaxed eye (cycloplegia). However, this can be detrimental to patients with glaucoma because it results in increased intraocular pressure.

In the gastrointestinal tract, cholinergic blockers cause a decrease in gastrointestinal motility, gastroin-

Table 18-1 Cholinergic Blockers: Drug Effects

Body System	Cholinergic Blocker Effects
Central nervous system	Decrease muscle rigidity and tremors *High doses:* drowsiness, disorientation, hallucinations
Eye	Dilate pupils (mydriasis), decrease accommodation by paralyzing ciliary muscles (cycloplegia)
Cardiovascular	*Small doses:* decrease heart rate *Large doses:* increase heart rate
Respiratory	Decrease bronchial secretions, dilate bronchial airways
Gastrointestinal tract	Relax smooth muscle tone of GI tract, decrease intestinal and gastric secretions, decrease motility and peristalsis
Genitourinary	Relax detrusor muscle of bladder, increase constriction of internal sphincter; these two may result in urinary retention.
Glandular	Decrease bronchial secretions, salivation, sweating

testinal secretions, and salivation. In the cardiovascular system these agents cause an increased heart rate. In the genitourinary system, anticholinergics lead to decreased bladder contraction, which can result in urinary retention. In the skin they reduce sweating, and in the respiratory system they dry mucous membranes and cause bronchial dilation. These effects are listed according to body system in Table 18-1.

Therapeutic Uses

The CNS effects of cholinergic blockers have the therapeutic effect of decreasing muscle rigidity and diminishing tremors. This is of benefit in the treatment of both Parkinson's disease and drug-induced extrapyramidal reactions. The therapeutic cardiovascular effects of anticholinergics are related to their cholinergic-blocking effects on the heart's conduction system. At low doses the anticholinergics slow the heart rate by means of their effects on the cardiac center in the portion of the brain called the *medulla.* At large doses cholinergic blockers block the inhibitory vagal effects on the pacemaker cells of the sinoatrial and atrioventricular nodes and accelerate the heart rate. Atropine is primarily used in the setting of cardiovascular disorders, such as for the diagnosis of sinus node dysfunction, the treatment of patients with symptomatic second-degree atrioventricular block, and

advanced life support in the treatment of sinus bradycardia that is accompanied by hemodynamic compromise.

As already mentioned, when the cholinergic stimulation of the PSNS is blocked by cholinergic blockers, the sympathetic nervous system effects go unopposed. In the respiratory tract this results in decreased secretions from the nose, mouth, pharynx, and bronchi. It also causes relaxation of the smooth muscles in the bronchi and bronchioles, which results in decreased airway resistance and bronchodilation. Because of this, the cholinergic blockers have proved beneficial in treating exercise-induced bronchospasms, chronic bronchitis, asthma, and chronic obstructive pulmonary disease.

Gastric secretions as well as the smooth muscle responsible for producing gastric motility are both under the control of the PSNS, which is primarily under the control of muscarinic receptors. The cholinergic blockers antagonize these receptors, causing decreased secretions, the relaxation of smooth muscle, and decreased GI motility and peristalsis. For these reasons cholinergic blockers are commonly used in the treatment of peptic ulcer disease, irritable bowel disease, and GI hypersecretory states. The effects that anticholinergics have on the bladder have made them useful in the treatment of such genitourinary tract disorders as reflex neurogenic bladder and incontinence. They relax the detrusor muscles of the bladder and increase constriction of the internal sphincter. The cholinergic blockers' ability to decrease glandular secretions also make them potentially useful agents for reducing gastric and pancreatic secretions in patients with acute pancreatitis.

Side Effects and Adverse Effects

Many body systems are affected adversely by the cholinergic blockers, and this is a function of the cholinergic blockers' site of action. The muscarinic receptors are located in a variety of tissues, organs, glands, and cells throughout the body. Therefore blockade of these receptors by the anticholinergics produces a wide range of effects, some desirable, as described in the previous section, and some not so desirable. The various side effects and adverse effects of cholinergic blockers are listed by body system in Table 18-2.

Other factors contributing to the wide variety of possible adverse effects of cholinergic blockers are the affinity of the muscarinic receptors for specific drugs and the drug dose. There are also certain patient populations that are more susceptible to the effects of these drugs. These include infants, the elderly, fair-skinned children with Down's syndrome, and children with spastic paralysis or brain damage.

Table 18-2	Cholinergic Blockers: Adverse Effects
BODY SYSTEM	**CHOLINERGIC-BLOCKING EFFECTS**
Central nervous system	CNS excitation, restlessness, irritability, disorientation, hallucinations, delirium
Eye	Dilated pupils, decreased visual accommodation, increased intraocular pressure
Cardiovascular	Increased heart rate, arrhythmias
Respiratory	Decreased bronchial secretions
Gastrointestinal	Decreased salivation, gastric secretions, and motility
Genitourinary	Urinary retention
Glandular	Decreased sweating

Table 18-3	Cholinergic Blockers: Drug Interactions	
DRUG	**MECHANISM**	**RESULT**
Antihistamines Anticholinergics Phenothiazines	Additive effects	Increased effects
Tricyclic antide- pressants MAOIs		
Orally adminis- tered medica- tions	Increased gastrointestinal absorption	

Toxicity and Management of Overdose

The dose of cholinergic blockers is particularly important because there is a very narrow difference between therapeutic and toxic doses. This drug characteristic is commonly referred to as a **narrow therapeutic index**. The treatment of cholinergic blocker overdose consists of symptomatic and supportive therapy. The patient should be hospitalized, and close, continuous monitoring including continuous ECG monitoring should be initiated. The stomach should be emptied by whichever route is most appropriate, inducing emesis with syrup of ipecac if the patient is awake and not convulsing or performing lavage if this not the case. Activated charcoal has proved very effective in removing drug that is already absorbed.

Fluid therapy and other standard measures used for the treatment of shock should be instituted as needed. Delirium, hallucinations, coma, and cardiac arrhythmias respond favorably to physostigmine treatment. Its routine use as an antidote for cholinergic blocker overdose is controversial, however. It has the potential for producing severe adverse effects such as seizures and asystole and should therefore be reserved for the treatment of patients showing extreme delirium or agitation who could inflict injury on themselves.

Interactions

The potential drug interactions that can occur with the cholinergic blockers are significant. Knowledge of the broad categories of drugs that should not be coadministered with the cholinergic blockers can help prevent potentially serious consequences. These various drugs and the mechanism and result of interaction are summarized in Table 18-3. Isopropamide can also alter the results of thyroid function tests.

Dosages

For the recommended dosages of selected cholinergic blockers, see the table on the next page.

DRUG PROFILES

All cholinergic blockers are prescription-only drugs. They are available in many dosage formulations: oral, topical, and injectable. Most of the cholinergic blockers are classified as pregnancy category C agents; dicyclomine and mephenzolate are classified as pregnancy category B agents.

One of the oldest and best known naturally occurring cholinergic blockers are the belladonna alkaloids, and it is the belladonna alkaloid contained in these agents that is responsible for their therapeutic effects. Of these, atropine is the prototypical agent. It has been in use for hundreds of years and continues to be widely used because of its effectiveness. Besides atropine, scopolamine is the other major naturally occurring drug. These drugs come from a variety of plants within the potato family (Solanaceae). Some examples are *Atropa belladonna* (deadly nightshade), *Hyoscyamus niger* (henbane), and *Datura stramonium* (jimson weed or thorn apple).

Of the semisynthetic and synthetic cholinergic blockers, there are many therapeutically useful agents. These agents are used in the treatment of a variety of

DOSAGES

SELECTED CHOLINERGIC-BLOCKING AGENTS

AGENT	PHARMACOLOGIC CLASS	DOSAGE RANGE	PURPOSE
Atropine		*Pediatric* PO/IM/IV/SC: 0.01 mg/kg q4-6h	Therapeutic anticho-linergic effect
		IM: 3 kg, 0.1 mg; 7-9 kg, 0.2 mg; 12-16 kg, 0.3mg; 20-27 kg, 0.4 mg; 32 kg, 0.5 mg; 41 kg, 0.6 mg	Preop
		IV: 0.02 mg/kg	Bradycardia
		IV: 0.05 mg/kg repeated every 10-30 min if required	Anticholinesterase (insecticide) antidote
		Adult PO: 0.1-1.2 mg q4-6h IM/IV/SC: 0.3-1.2 mg q4-6h	
		IM: 1 mg	Hypotonic radiography
		IV: 0.5-1 mg	Bradycardia
		1-2 mg followed by 2 mg IM/IV q5-60 min prn	Anticholinesterase (Infecticide anti-dote)
⚓**Scopolamine (Transderm Scop)**	Anticholinergic	*Pediatric* IM/IV/SC: 0.006 mg/kg	Adjunct to anesthesia
		Adult IM/IV/SC: 0.3-0.65 mg	Adjunct to anesthesia
		Transdermal: 1 patch (1.5 mg) delivers 0.5 mg/day for 3 days	Prevention of motion sickness
Dicyclomine (Bentyl)		*Adult* PO: start with 20 mg qid and slowly increase to the most effective dose, which is 40 mg qid	Irritable bowel syndrome
Glycopyrrolate (Robinul)		*Pediatric 1 mo-12 y/o* IM/IV: 0.002 mg/lb 30-60 min before surgery; a higher dose of 0.004 mg/1b may be required for children 1 mo-2 y/o	Preanesthetic inhibi-tion of secretions and intraoperatively for control of vagal cardiac irregularities
		Adult IM: 0.1-0.2 mg 3-4 times/day	Peptic ulcer
		IV: 0.1 mg repeated as needed every 2-3 min	Preanesthetic
		Adult/pediatric ≥12 y/o PO: 1 mg tid or 2 mg 2-3 times/day	Peptic ulcer
		Adult/pediatric IV: 0.2 mg for each 1 mg of neo-stigmine or 5 mg of pyridostigmine	Reversal of neuromus-cular blockade

illnesses and conditions ranging from peptic ulcer disease and irritable bowel syndrome to the symptoms of the common cold, as well as preoperatively to dry up secretions. They are the synthetic derivatives of the plant-derived belladonna alkaloids and are generally more specific in binding predominantly with muscarinic receptors. They may also be associated with fewer side effects.

ATROPINE

Atropine is a naturally occurring antimuscarinic. It may be prepared synthetically but is usually obtained by extraction from various members of the Solanaceae family of plants (deadly nightshade or jimson weed). In general, atropine is more potent than scopolamine in its cholinergic-blocking effects on the heart and in its effects on the smooth muscles of the bronchi and intestines. Atropine is effective in the treatment of many of the conditions listed in the section Therapeutic Uses. It is contraindicated in patients with angle-closure glaucoma, adhesions between the iris and lens, certain types of asthma (not cholinergic associated), advanced hepatic and renal dysfunction, hiatal hernia associated with reflux esophagitis, intestinal atony, obstructive GI or urinary conditions, and severe ulcerative colitis. It is available as a parenteral injection in several concentrations and strengths, as a solution to be mixed with normal saline solution and inhaled, as a 0.4-mg tablet, or in combination with phenobarbital as an oral solution. The recommended dosages are given in the table on p. 250. Pregnancy category C.

⚛ PHARMACOKINETICS

HALF-LIFE	ONSET	PEAK	DURATION
IV: 2.5 hr	Immediate	2-4 min	4-6 hr

⚓ SCOPOLAMINE

Scopolamine (Transderm Scop) is another naturally occurring cholinergic blocker and one of the principal belladonna alkaloids. It appears to be the most potent antimuscarinic for the prevention of motion sickness and seems to accomplish this by correcting the imbalance between acetylcholine and norepinephrine in the higher centers in the brain, particularly in the vomiting center, responsible for the symptoms of motion sickness. It is available in several different delivery systems that make it very useful for various indications. For the prevention of motion sickness it comes in a convenient transdermal delivery system, a patch that can be applied just behind the ear 4 to 5 hours before travel. It also comes in several parenteral formulations for injection by various routes: intravenous, intramuscular, and subcutaneous. It is also available as a topical preparation for ocular indications and as a 0.25-mg capsule. The contraindications that apply to atropine apply to it as well. The recommended dosages for various indications can be found in the table on p. 250. Pregnancy category C.

⚛ PHARMACOKINETICS

HALF-LIFE	ONSET	PEAK	DURATION
Variable	IV: 30-60 min	IV: 30-45 min	IV: 4 hr
	Patch: 4-5 hr	Patch: 6 hr	Patch: 72 hr

DICYCLOMINE

Dicyclomine (Bentyl, and others) is a synthetic antispasmodic cholinergic blocker primarily used in the treatment of functional disturbances of gastrointestinal motility such as irritable bowel syndrome. It has also been used alone and in combination with phenobarbital for the treatment of colic and enterocolitis in in-

fants. It is most commonly administered orally as either a 10-mg capsule or a 20-mg capsule or tablet. It is also available as an orally administered syrup that contains 10 mg/5 ml of the drug. As a parenteral preparation it comes as a 10-mg/ml intramuscular injection. Intravenous administration is not recommended. It is contraindicated in patients who have a known hypersensitivity to anticholinergics and in those with narrow-angle glaucoma, GI obstruction, myasthenia gravis, paralytic ileus, GI atony, or toxic megacolon. The recommended dosages can be found in the table on p. 250. Pregnancy category B.

⚛ PHARMACOKINETICS

HALF-LIFE	ONSET	PEAK	DURATION
9-10 hr	1-2 hr	1-1.5 hr	3-4 hr

GLYCOPYRROLATE

Glycopyrrolate (Robinul) is a synthetic antimuscarinic agent that blocks receptor sites in the autonomic nervous system which control the production of secretions and the concentration of free acids in the stomach. It is most commonly used as an adjunct in the treatment of peptic ulcer disease and as a preoperative medication to reduce salivation and excessive secretions in the respiratory and GI tract. It is contraindicated in patients who have a hypersensitivity to it and in those with narrow-angle glaucoma, myasthenia gravis, gastrointestinal or genitourinary obstruction, tachycardia, myocardial ischemia, hepatic disease, ulcerative colitis, and toxic megacolon. It should also not be given to children younger than 3 years. Glycopyrrolate is available orally as a 1- and 2-mg tablet and parenterally as a 0.2-mg/ml intramuscular or intravenous injection. The normal recommended dosages are given in the table on p. 250. Pregnancy category C.

⚛ PHARMACOKINETICS

HALF-LIFE	ONSET	PEAK	DURATION
Variable	IV: 1 min	IV: 10-15 min	IV: 4 hr
	PO: <45 min	PO: 1 hr	PO: 6 hr

NURSING PROCESS

ASSESSMENT

Anticholinergic drugs, or parasympatholytics, produce a variety of effects resulting from the blocking of acetylcholine in the PSNS. Because of their various effects at different body sites, such as smooth muscle relaxation, increased glandular secretion, and mydriasis, the nurse must take a thorough medical and medication history so that any of the following contraindications to the use of cholinergic-blocking agents can be revealed: benign prostatic hypertrophy, glaucoma, tachycardia, myocardial infarction, congestive heart failure, and hiatal hernia. In general the cholinergic blockers should not be used in patients with gastrointestinal or genitourinary obstruction and in children under the age of 3 years. Drug interactions are discussed earlier in this chapter.

NURSING DIAGNOSES

Nursing diagnoses associated with the use of cholinergic-blocking agents include, but are not limited to:

■ Altered tissue perfusion (decreased) as the result of tachycardia and preexisting cardiac disorders.
■ Risk for injury related to possible excessive CNS stimulation that results in tremors, confusion, sedation, and amnesia.
■ Pain related to side effects of dry mouth.
■ Altered gaseous exchange (decreased) stemming from thickened respiratory secretions.
■ Altered urinary elimination patterns (retention) resulting from loss of bladder tone caused by medications.
■ Risk for self-injury (heat stroke) stemming from decreased sweating and loss of normal heat-regulating mechanisms (especially in the elderly and in those who engage in excessive exercise or who are in high environmental temperatures).
■ Risk for injury to self (falls) as the result of changes in vision stemming from the mydriatic effects of the medication.
■ Knowledge deficit related to the therapeutic regimen, side effects, drug interactions, and precautions related to the use of anticholinergic agents.

PLANNING

Goals for the patient receiving cholinergic blockers include, but are not limited to:

■ Patient will self-administer medications as prescribed.
■ Patient experiences relief of symptoms for which the medication was prescribed.
■ Patient remains compliant with the drug therapy.
■ Patient demonstrates an adequate knowledge about the use of the specific medications, its side effects, and the appropriate dosing at home.
■ Patient will be free of injury to self stemming from adverse effects of the medication.

Outcome Criteria

Outcome criteria include:

■ Patient will state rationale for the use of cholinergic blockers in preoperative preparation such as decreasing the risk of complications associated with anesthesia.

Patient Teaching TIPS

Anticholinergics

✔ Patients should always take their medication as ordered because an overdose can cause life-threatening problems.

✔ Dry mouth is a common side effect of these medications, so patients taking them on a long-term basis should regularly brush their teeth to combat dental cavities. Patients can chew gum or suck on hard candy to relieve dryness, if these foods are allowed.

✔ Patients should know to be careful when engaging in various activities such as driving a car or operating machinery because of the blurred vision that commonly occurs with these medications.

✔ Patients may experience sensitivity to light and may therefore want to wear dark glasses or sunglasses.

✔ Patients should always get the okay of their physician before taking any other medication, including OTC medications.

✔ If patients are elderly and taking an anticholinergic, they should be reminded that they are at particular risk for suffering heat stroke because of the effects of these agents on the heat-regulating mechanisms in the body. They should therefore avoid exposure to high temperatures as well as strenuous exercise. They should limit physical exertion and always remember the importance of adequate fluid and salt intake, if this is allowed. Also they should use fans, air conditioners, and adequate ventilation to prevent overheating.

✔ Patients should be told to contact their physician should they experience urinary urgency or frequency, constipation, palpitations, tremors, confusion, sedation or amnesia, excessive dry mouth dryness (especially if they have chronic lung infections or chronic lung disease), or fever.

✔ Encourage patients with peptic ulcer disease to adhere to dietary modifications (e.g., no alcohol, caffeine, gas-forming foods, and so on as prescribed) and to use stress reduction techniques.

- Patient states importance of compliance with medication regimen such as avoiding complications of Parkinson's disease.
- Patient states the importance of taking the medication as prescribed and not suddenly withdrawing the medication due to risk of increasing symptomatology.
- Patient states those conditions that the physician should be notified immediately of (e.g., palpitations, arrhythmias, chest pain), if they occur.
- Patient keeps follow-up appointments with the physician to avoid unnecessary adverse effects of complications of treatment or noncompliance.

IMPLEMENTATION

Preventive nursing care is important to the effective use of these medications, especially teaching patients how to decrease their need for these medications, such as those with peptic ulcers. There are several nursing interventions that can also serve to maximize the therapeutic effects of anticholinergics and minimize the side effects. For example, always encourage patients to take the medications as prescribed, especially those with Parkinson's disease or with parkinsonian symptoms produced by certain medications such as the phenothiazines and major antipsychotic agents. As another example, patients taking these medications for the treatment of peptic ulcer disease, should be told to take the larger doses at bedtime because this often helps decrease the ulcer pain, which can be a source of frequent awakenings during the night.

Because atropine is compatible with some of the other commonly used preoperative medications such as meperidine (Demerol), morphine, and promethazine (Phenergan), it can be combined with these agents in the same syringe for preoperative administration. However, whenever mixing several medications together in one syringe, always calculate the doses very carefully. When administering optical solutions to produce mydriasis, always check the concentration of medication and apply pressure to the inner canthus to prevent more systemic absorption. Remember that the antidote to atropine is physostigmine salicylate (Antilirium) given slowly intravenously. Patient teaching tips are presented in the box on the previous page.

EVALUATION

Following are some of the therapeutic effects to look for in patients receiving anticholinergics. Patients with Parkinson's disease should experience fewer problems with tremors, salivation, and drooling. Patients taking these medications for the relief of peptic ulcer disease should experience less abdominal pain. You must also evaluate your patient to determine whether any of the side effects of these medications are occurring, side effects such as constipation, tachycardia, tremors, confusion, hallucinations, CNS depression (which occurs with large doses of atropine), sedation, urinary retention, hot and dry skin, and fever.

TAKE HOME POINTS

Cholinergic Blockers, Anticholinergics, Parasympatholytics, Antimuscarinics

- All names for the drugs that block or inhibit the actions of acetylcholine in the PSNS.
- Block the action of acetylcholine *at the muscarinic receptor.*
- Allow the SNS to dominate; therefore these agents have actions similar to those of the adrenergics.

Chemical Classification

- Natural, semisynthetic, and synthetic anticholinergics.

Receptor Action

- Competitive antagonists (blockers).
- Compete with acetylcholine at the muscarinic receptors; high doses = partial blocking actions at nicotinic receptors.
- Bind to and block acetylcholine at muscarinic receptors located on the cells that the nerve stimulates.
- Contraindications to the use of cholinergic blocking agents include patients with a history of BPH, glaucoma, tachycardia, myocardial infarction, CHF, and hiatal hernia.
- Cautious use of the anticholinergic (cholinergic blocking drugs) include patients with GI or GU obstruction or in children under 3 years of age.
- Parkinsonian symptoms may occur with certain medications such as phenothiazines. Anticholinergics help to prevent their side effects *but* compliance is key to the therapeutic effect.

Nursing Considerations

- Check compatibility of medication in syringe when administering preoperatively.
- Apply pressure to inner canthus for a few seconds after ophthalmic use for mydriasis.
- The antidote for atropine is physostigmine salicylate.

Critical Thinking A C T I V I T I E S

1. You are getting ready to administer preoperative medications to a 75-year-old woman undergoing minor surgery. She has a history of smoking, congestive heart failure, and open-angle glaucoma. What is the rationale for why you do not administer the atropine preoperatively to this patient, as ordered? Also, what is your rationale for contacting the physician about this drug interaction and your subsequent action?

2. The cholinergic blockers are competitive antagonists and work by _____ with acetylcholine at the _____ receptors in the _____ nervous system.
   a. competing / muscarinic / parasympathetic
   b. acting / nicotinic / sympathetic
   c. competing / muscarinic / sympathetic
   d. acting / adrenergic / sympathetic

3. You are caring for a patient that has just coded in the cardiac care unit. The patient is in second-degree heart block, has sinus bradycardia with a heart rate of 30, and has passed out. You recommend that the cholinergic blocker _____ be given to _____ the heart rate.

   1. belladona   2. esmolol   3. atropine
   4. increase   5. decrease   6. slow

   a. 1 and 6   b. 2 and 6   c. 3 and 4   d. 3 and 5

4. Before surgery a patient is given a cholinergic blocker, glycophyrrolate. What is the most likely reason for this _____?
   a. to increase secretions   b. to decrease secretions
   c. to increase heart rate   d. to increase muscle rigidity

5. You are chaperoning a group of eight year olds on a deep-sea fishing trip. One of the parents of these children is an anesthesiologist. She has given all the children a medication to take that is supposed to keep them from getting sick while at sea. Three hours into the fishing expedition you notice that your group of eight year olds are disoriented, hallucinating, irritable, and cannot sit still. You put two and two together and realize the children are suffering from _____ side effects from the cholinergic blocker _____.

   1. central nervous system   2. cardiovascular   3. respiratory
   4. belladonna   5. pilocarpine   6. scopolamine

   a. 1 and 6   b. 2 and 4   c. 3 and 5   d. 1 and 5

6. In question number 3 you are asked to give 0.5 mg of atropine to your patient. The vial concentration is 1 mg/ml. In the haste of this emergency situation, 5 ml of atropine is given. How many milligrams of atropine was given to your patient?

7. If the sympathetic nervous system is for mobilizing the organism in times of stress or during emergency situations, what is the importance of the parasympathetic nervous system? Why are patients at risk for hyperthermia when taking drugs such as atropine?

▲▲

BIBLIOGRAPHY

Albanese J, Nutz P: *Mosby's 1995 nursing drug cards,* St Louis, 1995, Mosby.

Brasitus TA, Foster ES: Peptic ulcer update: approaches to treatment, *Physician's Assis* 12(4): 71, 1988.

Johnson KB: *Harriet Lane handbook,* ed 13, St Louis, 1993, Mosby.

Keen JH: *Critical care and emergency drug reference,* St Louis, 1994, Mosby.

Knoben JE, Anderson PO: *Handbook of critical drug data,* ed 6, Hamilton, Ill, 1988, Drug Intelligence Publications.

McEvoy GK: *AHFS drug information,* Bethesda, Md, 1994, American Society of Hospital Pharmacists.

Skidmore-Roth L: *Mosby's 1995 nursing drug reference,* St Louis, 1995, Mosby.

Smith S: Drugs and the parasympthetic nervous system, *Nurs Times* 83(24): 36, 1987.

Chapter 19

Ganglionic-Blocking Agents

Objectives

When you reach the end of this chapter, you will be able to:

1 Briefly discuss the normal anatomy and physiology of the autonomic nervous system, including the events that take place during synaptic transmission within the sympathetic and parasympathetic divisions.

2 Provide examples of the various ganglionic-blocking agents.

3 Discuss the mechanism of action, therapeutic effects, uses, and adverse and toxic effects of the ganglionic-blocking agents.

4 Develop a nursing care plan that includes expected outcomes as it relates to the administration of the various ganglionic-blocking agents and the treatment of side effects and overdose or toxicity stemming from use of the various agents.

5 Identify the drug interactions associated with the use of ganglionic-blocking agents.

6 Evaluate the therapeutic versus the side effects of the different ganglionic-blocking agents.

CHAPTER OUTLINE

The Nicotinic Receptor
Ganglionic Blockers
  Mechanism of action
  Drug effects
  Therapeutic uses
  Side effects and adverse effects
    Toxicity and management of overdose
  Interactions
  Dosages
Drug Profiles
    Mecamylamine
    Trimethaphan

Nursing Process
Assessment
Nursing Diagnoses
Planning
  Outcome criteria
Implementation
Evaluation

Glossary

Ganglionic-blocking agents (ganglionic blockers) (gang' gle on' ik) Agents that prevent nerves from responding to the action of acetylcholine by occupying the receptor sites for acetylcholine (i.e., the nicotinic receptors) on sympathetic and parasympathetic nerve endings. (p. 256)

Nicotinic receptor (nik' ō tin' ik) The receptor and site of action for acetycholine in both the parasympathetic and sympathetic nervous systems. (p. 256)

THE NICOTINIC RECEPTOR

The stimulation of the two divisions of the autonomic nervous system, the parasympathetic (PSNS) and sympathetic (SNS) nervous systems, is controlled by the neurotransmitter acetylcholine. The receptor for acetylcholine in both systems is the **nicotinic receptor**. It gets its name from the fact that it was the administration of the ganglionic stimulant nicotine that first revealed its existence.

In the SNS this receptor is located between the preganglionic and postganglionic fibers. In the PSNS, however, the receptor is located not only between the preganglionic and postganglionic fibers but also between the postganglionic fibers and the effector cells. Figure 19-1 shows how these nicotinic receptors are arranged in both the PSNS and SNS.

GANGLIONIC BLOCKERS

The nicotinic receptors are the site of action for the **ganglionic blockers**, which either antagonize or bind to and block the actions of acetylcholine at these receptors. This blockade of acetylcholine in the PSNS and SNS inhibits stimulation of the autonomic nervous system. The ganglionic blockers comprise a rather small group of drugs that includes mecamylamine hydrochloride and trimethaphan camsylate. These drugs are older agents and have a rather limited use because of their somewhat nonspecific action. Their effects on the nicotinic receptors in both the PSNS and SNS result in

many side effects. Their primary use is in the treatment of severe or malignant hypertension. The newer antihypertensive drugs that produce fewer side effects and have more selective actions have replaced them for the ongoing treatment of hypertension.

Mechanism of Action

The actions of the ganglionic blockers are believed to result from their inhibition of nerve transmission at the nicotinic receptors (see Fig. 19-1). Ganglionic blockers work by blocking transmission of impulses at both sympathetic and parasympathetic nicotinic receptors. As just mentioned, they do this by competing with acetylcholine for binding, and when acetylcholine cannot bind to its receptor, no impulse can be transmitted to the next nerve fiber or to the organ.

Drug Effects

The inhibition of acetylcholine at nicotinic receptors (ganglionic blockade) results in significant changes in the cardiovascular system, gastrointestinal system, urinary tract, vision, and other vital functions. Ganglionic blockers in particular block SNS stimulation of the adrenal medulla, which is located just above the kidney and is responsible for regulating the release of epinephrine and norepinephrine into the systemic circulation. Thus this inhibition blocks the release of these SNS neurotransmitters. As mentioned earlier,

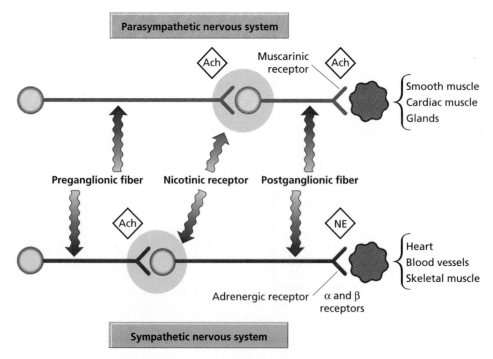

▼ **FIG. 19-1** Location of the nicotinic receptors within the parasympathetic and sympathetic nervous systems.

ganglionic blockers also prevent acetylcholine from binding to effector cells by competing for binding at nicotinic receptors. This also causes a reduction in the levels of circulating catecholamines (norepinephrine and epinephrine). Whether this reduction is produced by the competitive binding or the antagonistic effects of the agents, the body responds by decreasing vascular tone, which causes vasodilation and decreased blood pressure.

Many secretory glands are innervated by the PSNS. By inhibiting the stimulation of nicotinic receptors in the PSNS, ganglionic blockers cause a decrease in the volume and acidity of gastric secretions and inhibit pancreatic, salivary gland, and sweat gland secretions. Ganglionic blockers also cause the loss of smooth muscle tone in the gastrointestinal tract and urinary bladder. This can result in a major slowing down of these two systems, resulting in paralytic ileus and urinary retention. Mydriasis, or dilated pupils, can also result from the administration of ganglionic blockers.

Therapeutic Uses

The ganglionic-blocking agents are very potent antihypertensives but are nonselective in their action. Their use is therefore limited to the treatment of hypertensive emergencies, pulmonary edema resulting from pulmonary hypertension, and uncomplicated malignant hypertension, and to the provision of controlled hypotension during surgical procedures, such as those for brain tumors, cerebral aneurysms, arteriovenous fistulas, aortic grafts, transplants, and coarctations.

Side Effects and Adverse Effects

Because the ganglionic-blocking agents selectively inhibit the autonomic ganglia at the nicotinic receptors, resulting in massive nonselective inhibition of both the PSNS and SNS, many potentially adverse effects can result. The most pronounced ones are the consequence of the parasympathetic blockade. Effects on the gastrointestinal tract include paralytic ileus, dry mouth, constipation, anorexia, nausea, and diarrhea. Other adverse effects consist of urinary retention, impotence, cycloplegia, mydriasis, occasional pulmonary edema, tremor, and inhibition of sweating. Significant cardiovascular adverse effects include tachycardia and orthostatic hypotension. The commonly encountered side effects associated with the use of ganglionic blockers are listed in Table 19-1.

Toxicity and Management of Overdose

Toxicity or an overdose of ganglionic blockers results in overexpression of the agents' therapeutic effects. Profound hypotension, angina, dizziness, and shock can be expected, along with apnea and respiratory arrest. The management of toxicity or overdose involves supporting breathing as needed with the administration of supplemental oxygen, mechanical ventilation, or both. Fluids, positioning that promotes cardiovascular functioning, and vasopressors (e.g., dopamine and norepinephrine) are recommended for cardiovascular support.

Interactions

The drug interactions involving ganglionic blockers can cause significant adverse reactions, including hypotension and respiratory depression. The major drug interactions that occur with the ganglionic blockers are summarized in Table 19-2.

Table 19-1	Ganglionic Blockers: Adverse Effects
BODY SYSTEM	**SIDE/ADVERSE EFFECT**
Cardiovascular	Tachycardia, orthostatic hypotension, dysrhythmias, shock, angina
Gastrointestinal	Paralytic ileus, dry mouth, constipation, nausea, vomiting, diarrhea
Other	Urinary retention, impotence, mydriasis, pulmonary edema, dry mouth

Table 19-2	Ganglionic Blockers: Drug Interactions	
DRUG	**MECHANISM**	**RESULTS**
Diuretics and hypotensive agents	Additive effects	Hypotension
Anesthetics		
Neuromuscular blocking agents	Increases neuromuscular blockade	Prolonged paralysis
Urinary alkalizers	Enhances effects	Increased toxicity of mecamylamine

DOSAGES

SELECTED GANGLIONIC BLOCKING AGENTS

AGENT	PHARMACOLOGIC CLASS	DOSAGE RANGE	PURPOSE
Mecamylamine (Inversine)	Nondepolarizing ganglionic blocking agent	*Adult* PO: Initiate with 2.5 mg bid and adjust in 2.5-mg increments at 2-day or more intervals. Usual maintenance dose is 2.5 mg in 3 divided doses pc	Hypertension and uncomplicated malignant hypertension
Trimethaphan (Arfonad)	Nondepolarizing ganglionic blocking agent	*Adult* IV: 0.3-6 mg/min	Hypertensive emergencies and controlled surgical hypotension

Dosages

For recommended dosages of the ganglionic blockers, see the table above.

*D*RUG PROFILES

The ganglionic blockers are prescription-only drugs that are primarily used to lower blood pressure in emergency situations. One reason they are seldom used today is that tachyphylaxis develops in 24 to 72 hours. They are available in oral preparations as tablets and in a parenteral formulation as an intravenous infusion. Mecamylamine, an oral agent, is a pregnancy category C drug, and trimethaphan, an intravenous agent, is rated as a pregnancy category D drug.

MECAMYLAMINE

The ganglionic blocker mecamylamine (Inversine) is indicated for the treatment of severe hypertension and uncomplicated malignant hypertension. There are many contraindications to the use of this drug, and these include coronary insufficiency, glaucoma, hyper-

sensitivity to it, mild to moderate or labile hypertension, pyloric stenosis, and uremia. In addition, its use with antibiotics or sulfonamides is generally not recommended. Mecamylamine is available in 2.5-mg tablets. Commonly recommended dosages are given in the table above.

▼ PHARMACOKINETICS

HALF-LIFE	ONSET	PEAK	DURATION
24 hr	0.5-2 hr	3-5 hr	6-12 hr

TRIMETHAPHAN

Trimethaphan camsylate (Arfonad) is used for the immediate reduction of blood pressure in patients suffering from hypertensive emergencies. Trimethaphan produces a very quick drop in blood pressure, but its duration of effect is also brief. Therefore other hypotensive agents should be administered as soon as the blood pressure is under control. Contraindications to the use of this drug are the same as those for mecamylamine. Trimethaphan is available as an intravenous infusion. Commonly recommended dosages are given in the table above.

▼ PHARMACOKINETICS

HALF-LIFE	ONSET	PEAK	DURATION
Unknown	Immediate	5-10 min	10-30 min

NURSING PROCESS

ASSESSMENT

The cholinergic blockers are generally used as potent antihypertensive agents, but because they are so potent and nonselective in inhibiting the PSNS, they are used infrequently. Patients who are to receive these medi-

cations should be assessed for the existence of contra-indications, such as a recent myocardial infarction and chronic renal disease. These agents are used very cautiously (with close monitoring) in patients suffering from renal insufficiency or glaucoma. Drugs that interact with them include other antihypertensive agents, diuretics, anesthetics, and neuromuscular blocking agents.

NURSING DIAGNOSES

Nursing diagnoses associated with the use of ganglionic-blocking agents include:

- Altered tissue perfusion (decreased) as the result of orthostatic hypotension.
- Risk for self-injury related to possible excessive CNS effects such as paresthesias, sedation, tremors, weakness, and seizures.
- Risk for injury to mucous membranes related to dry mouth effects of drug.
- Altered urinary elimination patterns (retention) stemming from loss of bladder tone from medication or preexisting benign prostatic hypertrophy.
- Altered nutritional intake (less than body requirements) because of the GI side effects anorexia, nausea, and vomiting.
- Altered body image (decreased) related to side effects (e.g., impotence) or medication.
- Knowledge deficit related to the therapy, side effects, drug interactions, and precautions related to use of ganglionic-blocking agents.

PLANNING

Goals for the patient receiving ganglionic-blocking agents include, but are not limited to:

- Patient takes the drug exactly as prescribed.
- Patient experiences relief of symptoms for which the medication was prescribed.
- Patient remains compliant with drug therapy.
- Patient will demonstrate an adequate knowledge about the use of the specific medications, its side effects, and the appropriate dosing at home.
- Patient will be free of self-injury resulting from adverse effects of the medications.

Outcome Criteria

Outcome criteria related to the administration of ganglionic-blocking agents include:

- Patient will state the importance of the pharmacologic management of moderate to severe hypertension and the necessity to take medication as prescribed to prevent complications of disease and drug therapy.

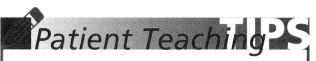

Patient Teaching TIPS

Ganglionic Blockers

✔ Patients should always take the medication as ordered because an overdose can cause life-threatening problems.

✔ Dry mouth is a common side effect of these medications so patients taking them on a long-term basis should regularly brush their teeth to combat dental cavities. Patients can chew gum or suck hard candy to relieve dryness, if these foods are allowed.

✔ Patients should know to be careful when engaging in various activities such as driving a car or operating machinery because of the blurred vision that commonly occurs with these medications.

✔ Patients should always get the okay of their physician before taking any other medication, including OTC medications.

✔ If patients are elderly and taking ganglionic blockers, they should be reminded that they are at particular risk for suffering heat stroke because of the effects of these agents on the heat regulating mechanisms in the body. They should therefore avoid exposure to high temperatures as well as strenuous exercise. They should limit physical exertion and always remember the importance of adequate fluid and salt intake, if this is allowed. Also they should use fans, air conditioners, and adequate ventilation to prevent overheating.

✔ Patients should be told to contact their physician should they experience urinary urgency or frequency; constipation; palpitations, tremors, confusion; sedation or amnesia; excessive dry mouth (especially if they have chronic lung infections or chronic lung disease) or fever.

- Patient will state the importance of complying with the medication regimen because of risk of complications if not taken as directed.
- Patient will state the risks and complications of potent antihypertensive agents such as tremors, decreased sweating, tachycardia, and hypotension.
- Patient will state conditions that may occur that the physician should be notified of such as syncope and chest pain.
- Patient will monitor blood pressure and keep follow-up appointments with the physician.

IMPLEMENTATION

These medications are generally used for the control of hypertension during surgery and for the management of hypertensive emergencies. It is important to remember that these drugs should not be withdrawn abruptly because this may trigger a rebound hypertensive crisis, which could precipitate a cerebrovascular accident. Oral forms should be given with meals so that absorption of the drug is more gradual and effective. IV forms should be given with extreme caution and using an IV pump. For patient education, see the patient teaching tips on p. 259.

EVALUATION

A therapeutic effect to monitor for in patients receiving ganglionic blockers is an improvement in blood pressure to within normal limits with diastolic readings <90 mm Hg. Monitoring for side effects associated with these medications (see Table 19-1) is also important during evaluation.

Critical Thinking **A C T I V I T I E S**

1. The ganglionic blockers _____ the action of _____ at the _____ receptors.

   1. antagonize   2. stimulate   3. increase
   4. norepinephrine   5. epinephrine   6. acetylcholine
   7. alpha and beta   8. nicotinic   9. adrenergic

   a. 2, 4, and 9   b. 1, 6, and 8   c. 3, 5, and 7   d. 1, 4, and 7

2. The ganglionic blockers mecamylamine and trimethaphan are used mainly for what two indications?
   a. hypotensive emergencies and pulmonary hypertension
   b. hypertensive emergencies and pulmonary hypotension
   c. hypertensive emergencies and pulmonary edema
   d. hypotensive crisis and pulmonary edema

3. You are caring for a patient that needs rapid reduction of blood pressure and is in a hypertensive crisis. The patient cannot tolerate sodium nitroprusside, the preferred agent in this situation. Instead trimethaphan (Arfonad) is ordered. You are to start your patient on a 1-mg/min infusion and titrate to maintain a systolic blood pressure between 100-120 mm Hg. Assuming 1 mg/min achieves your desired endpoint, how long will a 500 mg/250 ml bag of Arfonad last?

4. During the administration of trimethaphan for the treatment of a hypertensive emergency, what is important to do while the patient is receiving the medication? Explain your answer.

5. The physician has ordered trimethaphan camsylate to be administered prn for your patient who is in a hypertensive crisis. There is one other antihypertensive drug with a longer duration of action and onset of action ordered. What about this order would you question and why?

BIBLIOGRAPHY

Albanese J, Nutz P: *Mosby's 1995 nursing drug cards,* St Louis, 1995, Mosby.

Johnson KB: *Harriet Lane handbook,* ed 13, St Louis, 1993, Mosby.

Keen JH: *Critical care and emergency drug reference,* St Louis, 1994, Mosby.

Knoben JE, Anderson PO: *Handbook of critical drug data,* ed 6, Hamilton, Ill, 1988, Drug Intelligence Publications.

McEvoy GK: *AHFS drug information,* Bethesda, Md, 1994, American Society of Hospital Pharmacists.

Schrieber TR: The autonomic nervous system and anesthesia, *AANA* 55(5), 441, 477, 1987.

Skidmore-Roth L: *Mosby's 1995 nursing drug reference,* St Louis, 1995, Mosby.

PART 4

CARDIOVASCULAR SYSTEM: STUDY SKILLS BRIEF

LINKING LEARNING

The Part 3 Study Model stressed the importance of planning for the part as a whole. With that in mind, what is the focus of Part 4? The part title is "Cardiovascular System." What is the first question you think you should ask about this part? I would begin by asking, "What is the cardiovascular system?" This is a very obvious question and might seem to be so basic that it need not be asked, but the next six chapters will all develop around this part title. Asking the obvious question sometimes is exactly the thing that should be done to get started.

Chapter Structure

Just as there is a structure to each part in the text, which is constant from one part to the next, there is also a structure in the chapters. This structure is a repeating model that was created by the authors in an attempt to organize the material and present it in the clearest way possible. The chapter structure is a valuable learning asset for those who make use of it. In order to use chapter structure effectively you must understand the structure.

Chapter Objectives

Each chapter begins with a set of objectives. These are established by the authors and serve to tell you what it is that they expect you will know and be able to do when you have completed the chapter. It is sometimes tempting to ignore the objectives and get right on with the task of reading the chapter. Do not give in to that temptation. Read the objectives and spend some

time thinking about what they reveal about the content of the chapter.

Example Based on Chapter 20 Objectives

Objective 1. Define inotropic, chronotropic, dromotropic, digitalization, and digitalis toxicity.

What can you learn from this objective? First, there is the vocabulary. This objective makes it clear that you have some terms to learn. This means that you may want to have some blank note cards available to start setting up vocabulary cards for this chapter. In fact, you should write each of the terms in objective 1 on a separate card and be ready to complete the card as the terms are introduced and explained in the chapter.

The next thing that stands out in this first objective is that three of the terms contain a common element, tropic. This should bring active questioning into play. What does the suffix "tropic" mean? Asking this question now is a way of noting that these three terms do have some common meaning. Also it serves to provide an immediate focus for personal learning when you begin to read the chapter.

Objective 2. Briefly discuss the effect of digitalis on a failing heart.

Objective 1 introduced "digitalis toxicity" and objective 2 also relates to digitalis. The second objective establishes that digitalis has an effect on the heart. From this comes the potential for a new question relating to the first objective. What do inotropic, chronotropic, and dromotropic have to do with either digitalis and/or the heart? Just as it is essential to see the relationship between parts and chapters, it is also essential to see relationships within the chapters. These first two objectives should cause you to consider those relationships and make your own learning much more active.

Chapter Outline

The next chapter structure to consider in this process is the outline that immediately follows the objectives. The first thing to note is the arrangement of the outline. Chapter 20 has the major sections: Cardiac Glycosides and Nursing Process. What is the importance of this structure? It tells you that the authors will focus on the pharmacologic aspects first and then explain how this relates to nursing. This does not tell the learner a great deal about what to anticipate in terms of chapter content, but it does make clear a structure that is consistent in most of the chapters in this text.

Cardiac glycosides is broken down into subsections in this chapter. Spend several minutes considering the organization of these subsections. The first subtopic to be treated is "Mechanism of Action." What is meant by mechanism of action? How do cardiac glycosides act? On what? It does not matter that you cannot answer these questions at this point. What is important is that you ask them as a means of fostering an active and participatory learning attitude when you begin to read the chapter. Think, question, anticipate, then read. This sequence will enhance your learning.

Continue this process of looking at the subtopics and thinking ahead to what will be explained in the chapter. These subsections are the same in every chapter, and this thinking process should become automatic very quickly.

Glossary

The next chapter structure is one that I have already stressed in previous part study models, and it is one that is essential to learning. The glossary is a mini-dictionary for each chapter. Words that have not been introduced earlier in the text and that are central to the content of this chapter are presented here. The listing is in alphabetic order, which means that the glossary terms will not necessarily occur in the same order in the body of the chapter.

As you read terms as presented in the glossary, be aware of the nature of the definition. A glossary definition is specific and brief. It is a very useful place to begin to learn the new terms in the chapter, but the definition presented may not be enough for full understanding. You will find that full understanding will come after reading the chapter and encountering the term within the fuller context of sentences and paragraphs of text that explain not only the term but how it applies in the particular situation.

Glossary and Text Relationship

Use a term in Chapter 20 glossary as an example. The term *inotropic agent* is defined in the glossary. As I read it I understand that inotropic has to do with force or energy of muscle contractions. Since this chapter is titled Cardiac Glycosides, I assume the muscle under consideration is the heart. Further, the glossary states that an inotropic agent is a drug that increases myocardial contractility. Some of this information is clear, and some of it is still somewhat hazy. It should become clearer when connected with the chapter text. The first paragraph of the chapter introduces "**inotropic agents**." "Drugs that increase the force of myocardial contraction are called positive inotropic agents, and such drugs have a beneficial role in the treatment of a failing heart muscle."

With this sentence I find I have a much clearer understanding of what is meant by inotropic agents, and have the added benefit of knowing that there are positive inotropic drugs. This is what must happen to fully master the content specific vocabulary. You must see the core definition as presented in the glossary, but you must also read to determine how that core definition is expanded and exemplified in the body of the text.

When preparing vocabulary cards it is not a good idea to simply copy the definition from the glossary and assume that definition will serve your purpose. Wait to fill out the card until after you encounter the same term in the body of the chapter, and then pick and choose the information from the glossary and the body that will provide you with the clearest understanding of the term. Also, when placing information on vocabulary cards, it is always useful to include chapter number and page number(s) so that you can locate the source of your definition quickly should you find it necessary later.

These chapter structures can provide you with a clear picture of what you are expected to learn and the organizational pattern in which the material will be presented. Being aware of the structures and making use of them in this way will improve your concentration when you begin to read the chapter for understanding and memory. The time spent working with chapter structure is not wasted and does not significantly increase the study time of the chapter. In fact, the time you spend working with the objectives, outline, and glossary will generally save time when you are doing intensive reading and study.

Chapter 20

Cardiac Glycosides

Objectives

When you reach the end of the chapter, you will be able to:

1 Define inotrophic, chronotropic, dromotropic, digitalization, and digitalis toxicity.

2 Briefly discuss the effect of digitalis on a failing heart.

3 Explain the digitalizing process, especially the differences between rapid and slow digitalization.

4 Discuss the nursing care required for patients undergoing digitalization and the specific problems associated with rapid and slow digitalization.

5 Discuss the peak onset, duration of action, metabolism, and excretion of cardiac glycosides.

6 Formulate a nursing care plan based on actual and potential problems that can occur in the patient receiving a digitalis preparation, including outcome criteria and patient education.

7 Identify significant drug, laboratory test, and food interactions associated with digitalis.

8 Explain why specific diseases or conditions (i.e., elderly age and myocardial infarction) are considered "cautions" against or contraindications to the use of a digitalis preparation.

9 Discuss the nurse's responsibility in patients experiencing digitalis toxicity as well as his or her responsibilities to patients receiving Digibind.

CHAPTER OUTLINE

Congestive Heart Failure and Cardiac Arrhythmias
Cardiac Glycosides
  Mechanism of action
  Drug effects
  Therapeutic uses
  Side effects and adverse effects
    Toxicity and management of overdose
   Interactions
  Dosages
Drug Profiles
  ⚓ Digoxin
  Digoxin Immune Fab

Nursing Process
Assessment
Nursing Diagnoses
Planning
  Outcome criteria
Implementation
Evaluation

Glossary

Automaticity (aw tō mə tis i tē) A property of specialized excitable tissue that allows self-activation through the spontaneous development of an action potential, as in the pacemaker cells of the heart. (p. 265)

Cardiac glycoside (glī' ko sīd) A glycoside is any of several carbohydrates that yield a sugar and a nonsugar as the result of hydrolysis. The plant *Digitalis purpurea* yields a glycoside used in the treatment of heart disease; these glycosides are called *cardiac glycosides*. (p. 265)

Chronotropic agent (krōn' ō trōpik) An agent that influences the rate of the heartbeat. A positive chronotropic agent increases the heart rate. (p. 265)

Congestive heart failure An abnormal condition in which cardiac pumping is impaired as the result of myocardial infarction, ischemic heart disease, or cardiomyopathy. Failure of the ventricle to eject blood efficiently results in volume overload, chamber dilatation, and elevated intracardiac pressure. The retrograde transmission of increased hydrostatic pressure from the left ventricle leads to pulmonary congestion; elevated right ventricular pressure leads to systemic venous congestion and peripheral edema. (p. 265)

Dromotropic agent (drōm' ō trōpik) An agent that influences the conduction of electrical impulses. A positive dromotropic agent enhances the conduction of electrical impulses in the heart. (p. 265)

Ejection fraction The proportion of blood that is ejected during each ventricular contraction compared with the total ventricular filling volume. It is an index of left ventricular function, and the normal fraction is 65% (0.65). (p. 265).

Inotropic agents (in' ō trop' ik) *Inotropic* refers to the force or energy of muscular contractions, particularly contraction of the heart muscle. A positive inotropic agent is a drug that increases myocardial contractility. (p. 265)

Left ventricular end-diastolic volume (ven trik' u lər\dī' ə stol' ik) Ventricular diastole begins with the onset of the second heart sound and ends with the first heart sound. The *left ventricular end-diastolic volume* is the total amount of blood in the ventricle before it contracts, or the preload. (p. 265)

Refractory period The period during which a pulse generator (e.g., the heart) is unresponsive to an input signal of specified amplitude and during which it is impossible for the myocardium to respond. This is the period when the cardiac cell is readjusting its sodium and potassium levels and the cardiac cell cannot be depolarized again. (p. 265)

Therapeutic window The drug level range in the blood that is considered beneficial, as opposed to toxic. (p. 267)

Drugs that increase the force of myocardial contraction are called positive **inotropic agents**, and such drugs have a beneficial role in the treatment of a failing heart muscle. A drug that increases the rate at which the heart beats is called a positive **chronotropic agent**. Drugs may also affect how quickly electrical impulses travel through the conduction system of the heart (the sinoatrial [SA] node, atrioventricular [AV] node, bundle of His, and the Purkinje fibers). Drugs that accelerate conduction are referred to as positive **dromotropic agents**. This chapter focuses on one of the main classes of positive inotropic agents, the **cardiac glycosides**, and specifically digoxin.

It has been estimated that close to 2 million office and 1.5 million hospital visits a year are necessitated by exacerbations of congestive heart failure (CHF). Findings yielded by one of the largest and most frequently cited studies involving patients with CHF, the Framingham Study, show that the 5-year survival rate in patients with CHF is approximately 50%. Therefore any drug that could lengthen survival in affected patients or help the failing heart perform its essential duties would be extremely valuable. The glycosides are a prime example.

CONGESTIVE HEART FAILURE AND CARDIAC ARRHYTHMIAS

In patients with **congestive heart failure**, the overworked, failing heart cannot meet the demands placed on it and blood is not ejected efficiently from the ventricles. This occurs because the **ejection fraction** (the amount of blood ejected with each contraction) compared with the total amount of blood in the ventricle just before contraction (the **left ventricular end-diastolic volume**) is decreased. (Normally the ejection fraction is approximately 65% [0.65] of the total volume in the ventricle.) As more blood accumulates in the right and left ventricles, more pressure builds up in the blood vessels leading to the heart. The retrograde transmission of this increased hydrostatic pressure from the left ventricle leads to pulmonary congestion, whereas elevated right ventricular pressure causes systemic venous congestion and peripheral edema.

Because the heart cannot then meet the increased demands placed on it, the blood supply to certain organs is reduced. The organs most dependent on blood supply, the brain and the heart, are the last to be deprived of blood. As an organ that is relatively less dependent on blood supply, the kidney has its blood supply shunted away. Therefore the filtration of fluids and removal of waste products is impaired. When these fluids and waste products accumulate, the patient experiences such symptoms as pulmonary edema and shortness of breath, with kidney failure the end result.

The physical defects producing CHF are of two types: (1) a cardiac defect (myocardial deficiency such as myocardial infarction or valve insufficiency), which leads to inadequate cardiac contractility and filling, and (2) a defect outside the heart (systemic defect such as coronary artery disease or diabetes), which results in an overload on an otherwise normal heart. Either or both of these defects may be present in the same patient. Common causes of myocardial deficiency and systemic defects are listed in the box on p. 266.

In patients with the supraventricular arrhythmias, atrial fibrillation, or atrial flutter, the top aspects of the heart, the atria, are contracting several hundred times a minute. Not only are the atria contracting frequently, but several areas in the atria besides the sinoatrial (SA) node are then acting as the pacemaker of the heart. Normally the atrioventricular (AV) node controls how slowly or quickly impulses arrive in the ventricles, and it also has the ability to receive all these depolarizations and to allow only a certain number to pass through the ventricles. This keeps the patient from going into ventricular fibrillation, which is fatal, and it also allows the ventricles time to fill with blood, an equally important aspect. Even during atrial fibrillation or flutter, patients may show symptoms such as congestive heart failure, however.

All cells in the heart can depolarize spontaneously, a property called **automaticity**. The **refractory period** is the time when the cardiac cells are readjusting their sodium and potassium levels, and during this time, the cardiac cells cannot depolarize again. It is the sodium-potassium ATPase pump that is responsible for the

Myocardial Deficiency and Increased Work Load: Common Causes

Myocardial Deficiency

Inadequate contractility
Myocardial infarction
Coronary artery disease
Cardiomyopathy
Infection
Inadequate filling
Infection
Tamponade
Ischemia

Increased Work Load

Pressure overload
Hypertension
Outflow obstruction
Volume overload
Hypervolemia
Congenital abnormalities
Anemia
Thyroid disease

movement of potassium ions in and sodium ions out of the cardiac cells after they have depolarized, an action potential has been generated, and the electrical impulse has been generated. In patients with either atrial fibrillation or flutter, the AV node is circumvented and the impulses arrive in the ventricle before the refractory period is over. The resultant slow spread of impulses from the atrium through refractory muscle results in continuous atrial excitation—the atrial fibrillation or flutter. (The cardiac conduction system and the abnormalities responsible for causing arrhythmias are described in greater detail in Chapter 21.)

CARDIAC GLYCOSIDES

As the survival statistics cited earlier attest to, any drug that can lengthen survival in patients with CHF by helping the failing heart perform its essential duties would be extremely valuable. The glycosides are a prime example of such a drug. They are one of the oldest and most effective groups of drugs. Not only do they have beneficial effects in the failing heart but they also help restore the heart in atrial fibrillation or flutter to a normal sinus rhythm. They were originally obtained from either the *Digitalis purpurea* or the *Digitalis lanata* plant, both commonly referred to as *foxglove*. The cardiac glycosides have been the mainstay of therapy for CHF for more than 200 years, and they continue to be one of the most frequently used positive inotropic agents. Digoxin and digitoxin are the most commonly prescribed digitalis preparations. The widespread and enduring popularity of digitalis is the result of its unequaled efficacy in the treatment of CHF. Critically ill patients can be restored to near-normal states within hours after digitalization.

Mechanism of Action

The primary beneficial effect of digitalis is thought to be an increase in myocardial contractility. This occurs secondarily to the inhibition of the sodium pump. By inhibiting this enzyme complex, the cellular sodium concentration and subsequently calcium concentration increases. The overall result is enhanced myocardial contraction. Digitalis also augments vagal tone, resulting in increased diastolic filling.

The cardiac glycosides also change the electrical conduction properties of the heart, and this markedly affects the conduction system and cardiac automaticity. The glycosides decrease the velocity (rate) of electrical conduction and prolong the refractory period in the conduction system. The particular area of the conduction system where this occurs is between the atria and the ventricles (SA node to AV node through the ventricles). The cardiac cell remains in a state of depolarization and is unable to start another electrical impulse.

Drug Effects

The cardiac glycosides, especially digitoxin and digoxin, are almost identical in their ability to treat CHF and arrhythmias. The two glycosides vary, however, in terms of their water solubility, half-life, and excretion, and the clinical profile of the patient determines which glycoside is selected. All cardiac glycosides produce dramatic inotropic, chronotropic, and dromotropic cardiac effects. (*Inotropic* refers to the force or energy of muscular contractions; *chronotropic* refers to the rate of the heart beat; and *dromotropic* refers to the conduction of electrical impulses.). These effects include:

- A *positive inotropic* effect resulting in an increase in the force and velocity of myocardial contraction without a corresponding increase in oxygen consumption.
- A *negative chronotropic* effect producing a reduced heart rate.
- A *negative dromotropic* effect that decreases automaticity at the SA node, reduces conductivity at the bundle of His, and prolongs the atrial and ventricular refractory periods.
- An increase in stroke volume.
- A reduction in heart size during diastole.
- A decrease in venous blood pressure and vein engorgement.

- An increase in coronary circulation.
- Promotion of diuresis as the result of improved blood circulation.
- Palliation of exertional and paroxysmal nocturnal dyspnea, cough, and cyanosis.

Therapeutic Uses

The cardiac glycosides are primarily used in the treatment of CHF and supraventricular arrhythmias. In CHF the therapeutic effects of digoxin are secondary to its ability to increase the force of contraction, its positive inotropic action. There are many therapeutic benefits to this. Increasing the force of contraction increases the ejection fraction compared with the left ventricular end-diastolic volume, or preload. As more blood is ejected with each contraction of the heart, there is less blood remaining in the ventricle and thus less pressure that builds up. With this the symptoms of pulmonary edema, pulmonary hypertension, and right-sided ventricular failure subside.

Another benefit of this positive inotropic action is that it promotes diuresis by ensuring that adequate blood is supplied to the kidneys. As a result, fluids are filtered and waste products removed, with relief of shortness of breath and pulmonary edema the end result.

Cardiac glycosides are also effective in the treatment of arrhythmias such as atrial fibrillation and atrial flutter because of their negative chronotropic (decreased heart rate) and negative dromotropic (slowed conduction velocity) actions. Automaticity, conduction velocity, and the refractory period are all affected. Digoxin can slow the depolarization of the SA node and other areas of the atria that may be acting as pacemakers. Thus the glycosides such as digoxin directly slow conduction through the AV node and increase the vagal action on the heart. In addition, the cardiac glycosides lengthen the refractory period, which allows the correct levels of sodium and potassium ions to be reached prior to depolarization.

Side Effects and Adverse Effects

The side effects and adverse effects associated with cardiac glycoside use can be very serious. The primary cardiac glycoside in use today is digoxin, and close monitoring of patients' clinical response to it and the possible development of toxic symptoms is essential. Digoxin has a very narrow **therapeutic window**, or the range of the drug level in the blood that is considered therapeutic. Frequent monitoring of patients' digoxin levels is important until the drug reaches a steady state in the blood. Low potassium levels increase its toxicity, so frequent serum electrolyte level checks are also important. It has been estimated that as much as 20% of the patients taking digitalis exhibit toxic symptoms. The common undesirable effects associated with cardiac glycoside use are listed in Table 20-1.

Toxicity and Management of Overdose

The treatment strategies for digoxin toxicity depend on the severity of the symptoms. These strategies can range from simply withholding the next dose to instituting aggressive therapies. The steps usually taken in the management of cardiac glycoside toxicity are listed in Table 20-2.

When significant toxicity develops as a result of cardiac glycoside therapy, the administration of Digibind (digoxin immune Fab) may be indicated. Digibind is an antibody that recognizes the digoxin as an antigen and forms an antibody-antigen complex thus inactivating the free digoxin. Digibind therapy is not

Table 20-1 | Cardiac Glycosides: Common Adverse Effects

Body System	Side/Adverse Effect
Cardiovascular	Any type of arrhythmia and bradycardia or tachycardia
Gastrointestinal	Anorexia, nausea, vomiting, diarrhea
Central nervous system	Headache, fatigue, malaise, confusion, convulsions
Visual	Colored vision (i.e., green, yellow, or purple), halo vision, or flickering lights

Table 20-2 | Digoxin Toxicity: Step Management

Step	Management
1	Discontinue drug
2	Determine digoxin and electrolyte levels
3	Administer potassium supplements for hypokalemia
4	Institute supportive therapy for gastrointestinal symptoms (nausea, vomiting, or diarrhea)
5	Start electrocardiographic monitoring for cardiac arrhythmias; administer appropriate antiarrhythmic drugs (lidocaine or phenytoin)
6	Administer digibind for severe overdose

indicated in every patient who is showing signs of digoxin toxicity. Following are the clinical settings in which its use may be indicated:

- Hyperkalemia (serum potassium level, >5 mEq/L) in a digitalis-toxic patient.
- Life-threatening cardiac arrhythmias, sustained ventricular tachycardia or fibrillation, and severe sinus bradycardia or heart block unresponsive to atropine treatment or cardiac pacing.
- Life-threatening digoxin or digitoxin overdose: >10 mg of digoxin in adults; >4 mg of digoxin in children.

Interactions

There are a number of significant drug interactions that are possible with the cardiac glycosides. The common ones are listed in Table 20-3. One food interaction, bran in large amounts, may decrease the absorption of oral digitalis drugs.

Dosages

For dosage information on the cardiac glycosides, see in the table on p. 269.

DRUG PROFILES

The cardiac glycosides get their name from their chemical structures. Glycosides are complex steroidlike structures linked to sugar molecules. Because the particular drugs derived from the *digitalis* plant have potent actions on the heart, they are referred to as *cardiac glycosides*, with digoxin by far the most commonly prescribed digitalis preparation. Deslanoside and digi-

Table 20-3	Cardiac Glycosides: Drug Interactions		
DRUG	**MECHANISM**	**RESULT**	
Adrenergics Reserpine Succinylcholine	Increase cardiac irritability	Increased digoxin toxicity	
Amphotericin-B Chlorthalidone Ethacrynic acid Ethoxzolamide Furosemide Laxatives Steroids (adrenal) Thiazide diuretics	Hypokalemia	Increased digoxin toxicity	
Antacids Antidiarrheics Cholestyramine Colistipol	Decrease po absorption	Reduced therapeutic effect	
Anticholinergics	Increase po absorption	Increased therapeutic effect	
Barbiturates Oxyphenbutazone Phenylbutazone	Enzyme inducer	Reduced therapeutic effect	
Quinidine Verapamil Amiodarone	Increase digoxin absorption	Increased digoxin levels (2×); digoxin dose should be reduced 50%	

A digoxin preparation can also interfere with the results of several laboratory tests. It can cause the plasma levels of estrone to be raised and the levels of lactate dehydrogenase and testosterone to be lowered. It can also cause the erythrocyte sodium concentration to be increased and the erythrocyte potassium concentration to be reduced.

In addition to the drug and laboratory test interactions, digoxin can also interact with certain foods. The consumption of excessive amounts of potassium-rich food can decrease its therapeutic effect, whereas the consumption of excessive amounts of licorice can increase digoxin toxicity as the result of the hypokalemia produced.

DOSAGES

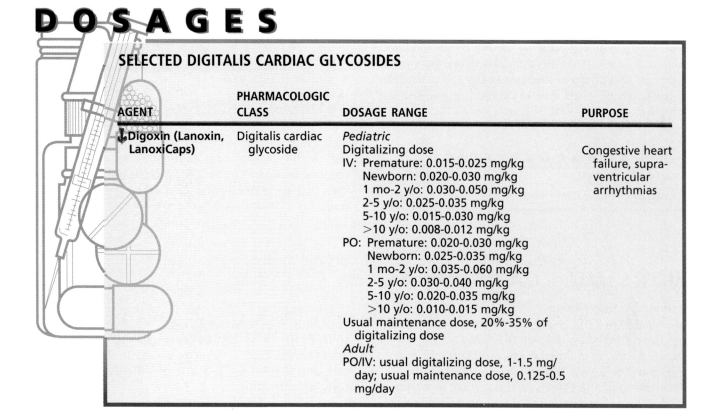

SELECTED DIGITALIS CARDIAC GLYCOSIDES

AGENT	PHARMACOLOGIC CLASS	DOSAGE RANGE	PURPOSE
⚓Digoxin (Lanoxin, LanoxiCaps)	Digitalis cardiac glycoside	*Pediatric* Digitalizing dose IV: Premature: 0.015-0.025 mg/kg 　　Newborn: 0.020-0.030 mg/kg 　　1 mo-2 y/o: 0.030-0.050 mg/kg 　　2-5 y/o: 0.025-0.035 mg/kg 　　5-10 y/o: 0.015-0.030 mg/kg 　　>10 y/o: 0.008-0.012 mg/kg PO: Premature: 0.020-0.030 mg/kg 　　Newborn: 0.025-0.035 mg/kg 　　1 mo-2 y/o: 0.035-0.060 mg/kg 　　2-5 y/o: 0.030-0.040 mg/kg 　　5-10 y/o: 0.020-0.035 mg/kg 　　>10 y/o: 0.010-0.015 mg/kg Usual maintenance dose, 20%-35% of 　digitalizing dose *Adult* PO/IV: usual digitalizing dose, 1-1.5 mg/ 　day; usual maintenance dose, 0.125-0.5 　mg/day	Congestive heart failure, supra-ventricular arrhythmias

toxin are other less commonly prescribed ones. The widespread and long-standing popularity of digitalis preparations is the result of its unequaled efficacy in the treatment of CHF. The cardiac glycosides are prescription-only drugs and are classified as pregnancy category C agents.

⚓ DIGOXIN

As just mentioned, digoxin (Lanoxin, LanoxiCaps) is by far the most commonly prescribed digitalis glycoside. It is a highly effective agent for the treatment of both CHF and atrial fibrillation and flutter. It may also be used clinically to improve myocardial contractility and thus reverse cardiogenic shock or other low cardiac output states. Digoxin is contraindicated in patients who have shown a hypersensitivity to it, and in those with ventricular tachycardia and fibrillation, beriberi heart disease, or the hypersensitive carotid sinus syndrome. Orally digoxin comes as a 50-µg/ml elixir, a 50-, 100-, and 200-µg liquid-filled capsule, and a 125-, 250-, and 500-µg tablet. Parenterally it comes as a 100- and 200-µg/ml intravenous injection. Because of digoxin's fairly long duration of action and half-life, a loading, or "digitalizing," dose is often given to bring serum levels of the drug up to a desirable therapeutic level quicker. See the table above for the recommended digitalizing doses and the daily oral and intravenous adult and pediatric dosages.

☿ PHARMACOKINETICS

HALF-LIFE	ONSET	PEAK	DURATION
33-44 hr	30-120 min	2-6 hr	2-4 days

DIGOXIN IMMUNE Fab

Digoxin immune Fab (Digibind) is the antidote for severe digoxin overdose and is indicated for the reversal of such life-threatening cardiotoxic effects as severe bradycardia, advanced heart block, ventricular tachycardia or fibrillation, and severe hyperkalemia. It has a unique mechanism of action, and as already mentioned, it is believed to work by binding to free (unbound) digoxin, which then blocks or reverses all the drug effects and symptoms of toxicity. Digibind is contraindicated in patients who have shown a hypersensitivity to it. It is only available parenterally as a 40-mg vial. Digibind is dosed either in milligrams or by the number of vials, depending on the dose calculation method or the reference chart used. It is commonly dosed based on the patient's serum digoxin level in conjunction with his or her weight. The recommended dosages vary according to the amount of cardiac glycoside ingested. Each milligram can neutralize 15 µg of digoxin or digitoxin. For recommended dosages consult the manufacturer's latest dosage table recommendations. It is important to bear in mind that after Digibind is given, all subsequent digoxin serum levels will be elevated for days to weeks because of the presence of both the free (unbound) digoxin (toxic digoxin) and the digoxin that has been bound by the Digibind (nontoxic digoxin). At this point, therefore, the clinical signs and symptoms of digoxin toxicity rather than the digoxin serum levels should be used to monitor the effectiveness of reversal therapy.

⬡ PHARMACOKINETICS

HALF-LIFE	ONSET	PEAK	DURATION
14-20 hr	Immediate	Immediate	Days to weeks

NURSING PROCESS

Because of the high incidence of CHF, an understanding of the nursing implications associated with its medical treatment is critical to the safe and effective care of patients receiving cardiac glycosides as the mainstay of treatment. Owing to the narrow therapeu-

NURSING ▪ CARE ▪ PLAN

Congestive Heart Failure

Mr. E.D. a 72-year-old man admitted with CHF, has been started on digoxin 0.125 mg for maintenance doses. He will be on your nursing unit for the next 1 to 2 days and will require frequent monitoring of the effects of the cardiac glycoside. Vital parameters are as follows upon admission to

your unit: confused in early PM, UO about 240 cc/shift, P110, RR 33, BP 100/56, 1+pitting pedal edema, SOB, DOE, < energy levels, unable to dress self, and skin intact. Lab studies show normal H&H, BUN, urinalysis, but K+ at 3.4.

Assessment with nursing diagnoses	Planning with goals and outcome criteria	Implementation with patient education	Evaluation
Subjective Complaints of SOB, DOE, pedal edema **Objective** Rales lower bases wt >2 lb in 5 days RR 32, P102 BP 100/60 **Nursing Diagnoses** Altered tissue perfusion, cardiopulmonary due to tachycardia pathology associated with CHF	**Goals** Patient will show improved tissue perfusion within 48 hr of treatment **Outcomes** Patient will have increased tissue perfusion, cardiopulmonary within 8 hr as evidenced by: Urinary output Rales P>60<100 RR 16-20 Pedal edema Weight	Take patient's vital sign q4h and prn, including apical pulse I&O q8h Daily weights Monitor digitalis levels as ordered Monitor serum electrolytes Take apical pulse for 1 full min and notify physician if P<60; hold drug until further orders Breath sounds q4h and as needed Elevate head of bed Keep feet elevated at all times Passive ROM	Patient will show the following therapeutic responses to digitalis treatment: <Weight Ease of breathing >UO <Edema Less SOB/DOE >Ability to perform ADL Vital signs within normal limits Patient will be monitored for (and experience minimal) side effects associated with digitalis therapy such as bradycardia, headache, GI symptoms, blurred vision, anorexia

H&H, hematocrit and hemoglobin; *SOB*, shortness of breath; *DOE*, dyspnea on exertion, *UO*, urinary output; *ROM*, range of motion.

Table 20-4	Conditions Predisposing to Digitalis Toxicity
CONDITION/DISEASE	**SIGNIFICANCE**
Cardiac pacemakers	Patients with these devices may exhibit digitalis toxicity at lower-than-usual doses.
Hypokalemia	Increases a patient's risk of serious arrhythmias and renders him or her more predisposed to digitalis toxicity.
Hypercalcemia	Places the patient at higher risk of suffering sinus bradycardia, arrhythmias, and heart block.
Atrioventricular block	Heart block may worsen with increasing levels of digitalis.
Arrhythmias	Arrhythmias may occur that did not exist before digitalis use, and thus could be related to digitalis toxicity.
Hypothyroid, respiratory, or renal disease	Patients with these disorders require lower doses because of the resultant delayed drug excretion they cause.
Elderly age	Because of decreased renal function and the resultant diminished drug excretion along with decreased body mass in this patient population, a lower-than-usual dose is needed to prevent toxicity. The practice of polypharmacy may also lead to toxicity.
Acute myocardial infarction	Increased oxygen demands resulting from increased contractility stemming from the effects of the digitalis preparation may worsen the cardiac ischemia.
Ventricular fibrillation	Ventricular rate may actually increase with digitalis use.

cautious use of the agent or even contraindicate its use (Table 20-4).

Before initiating digitalis therapy, and even during maintenance therapy, several clinical parameters need to be assessed. These include blood pressure, the apical pulse for 1 full minute, heart sounds, breath sounds, weight, intake and output amounts, electrocardiograms, renal function laboratory values (BUN and creatinine), and liver function values (SGOT, SGPT, creatine phosphokinase, lactate dehydrogenase, and alkaline phosphatase). The baseline status of any edema, confusion, nausea, vomiting, anorexia, or diarrhea also needs to be documented. In addition, to assess for possible drug or food interactions, the patient's medication record or a list of the current medications being taken by the patient and his or dietary habits needs to be compiled and recorded. The use of thyroid preparations may result in decreased digitalis levels. One important food interaction to assess for is whether the patient consumes large amounts of bran, which will decrease the absorption of oral digitalis drugs.

NURSING DIAGNOSES

Appropriate nursing diagnoses in patients who are to receive digitalis include, but are not limited to:

- Altered tissue perfusion (cardiopulmonary) related to pathophysiologic impact of CHF.
- Knowledge deficit related to first-time use of a cardiac glycoside and lack of information on CHF and its treatment.
- Risk for injury, self, related to pathologic impact of CHF and potential side effects of medication therapy.
- Altered nutritional status (less than body requirements) related to GI side effects and potential digitalis toxicity.
- Altered tissue perfusion (cardiopulmonary) related to digitalis-induced arrhythmias.
- Noncompliance related to lack of information and to side effects of digitalis drugs.

PLANNING

Goals of care related to the administration of cardiac glycosides include:

- Patient will exhibit improved cardiac output once digitalis therapy initiated.
- Patient will state use, action, side effects, and toxic effects of digitalis therapy.
- Patient will be free from injury related to medication therapy.
- Patient's appetite will be improved or he or she will be free of anorexia while on digitalis.
  In planning for the administration of these prep-

tic index of the cardiac glycosides, the nurse needs to constantly assess the patient, update the plans of care, intervene appropriately, and evaluate or monitor the therapeutic and adverse effects of the drug.

ASSESSMENT

Before the administration of a cardiac glycoside, data must be collected concerning the patient's medication history (past and present over-the-counter, prescription, illegal drugs used) and any drug allergies he or she may have. An assessment of the patient's medical history, including both diseases and conditions, is also crucial and may yield findings that dictate either very

Patient Teaching TIPS

Patients on Digitalis

✔ Patients should be told to take medication at the same time every day and exactly as ordered.

✔ Patients should be warned to never double up on a dose and never skip a dose unless told to do so by physician.

✔ Patients should use only the dropper supplied with the elixir form of digitalis to administer the medication.

✔ Patients should be warned to not change brands of digitalis when refilling prescriptions.

✔ Patients should be told to get the okay of their physician before taking any other medication with the digitalis preparation, be it a prescribed or OTC medication.

✔ Patients should know to notify their physician if their radial pulse is less than 60 or more than 120 beats/min or if it is erratic and also if they are experiencing anorexia, nausea, vomiting, diarrhea, or blurred vision, or seeing green or yellow halos around objects. In the event of any of these problems, patients should withhold the dose.

✔ Patients should inform the physician if they experience a weight gain of 2 lbs or greater (about 1 kg) per day.

✔ It is important for patients to wear a Medic-Alert bracelet or necklace naming the medication, or medications, they are taking and their cardiac condition as well as to carry an alert card on their person. Patients should be told to contact their local emergency medical services department to find out how to post or supply information in their home regarding their cardiac condition and the medications they are taking.

✔ Patients taking antacids or eating ice cream, milk products, yogurt, or cheeses should be told to take their dose 2 hours before or after they take these medications or foods.

✔ Family members must also be taught the side effects and the importance of taking the patient's pulse before giving the drug as well as the signs and symptoms of toxicity.

✔ Patients should be encouraged to consume foods high in potassium, especially if they are also taking a potassium-depleting diuretic. They should report any signs and symptoms of weakness, fatigue, or lethargy.

✔ Patients should know that anorexia is an early manifestation of toxicity.

✔ Patients should weigh themselves daily before breakfast to check for possible weight loss or gain resulting from fluid overload or loss and report immediately 1- to 2-lb weight increase that occurs within 1 day.

✔ Patients should be told to never withdraw or discontinue the drug abruptly.

---

arations, it important to check the dosage when administering either digoxin or digitoxin because of the difference in the pharmacokinetic properties of these drugs; for example, 80% of digoxin is excreted by the kidneys and 90% of digitoxin is first metabolized by the liver. These differences, in conjunction with the patient's particular medical history, often determine whether the physician prescribes digoxin (preferred in patients with impaired liver function) or digitoxin (preferred in patients with impaired renal function).

Outcome Criteria

Outcome criteria in patients receiving a digitalis preparation include :

■ Patient will have improved to strong peripheral pulses, increased endurance for activity, decreased fatigue, and pink, warm extremities.

■ Patient will have increased urinary output resulting from therapeutic effects of digitalis.

■ Patient will have improved heart and lung sounds with decreased arrythmias and rales.

■ Patient's skin and mucous membranes (color and temperature) will be improved to pink and warm.

■ Patient will maintain appetite while on digitalis therapy and report anorexia, nausea, and vomiting immediately to physician.

■ Patient will be free of digitalis toxicity as evidenced by no complaints of bradycardia.

■ Patient will demonstrate proper technique for taking radial pulse for 1 full minute prior to taking medication.

■ Patient will be able to cite those digitalis-related problems the physician should be notified of such as palpitations, arrhythmias, chest pain, and pulse less than 60 beats/min.

PEDIATRIC IMPLICATIONS
Cardiac Glycosides

- Digoxin should be given according to a regular time schedule 1 hour before or 2 hours after the child's or infant's feeding.
- Make sure that the dosing of these agents is accompanied by close monitoring and individualized dosing and nursing care. Calculating dosages is of great importance to safe and cautious nursing care—caution, caution, and more caution is needed, as a one-decimal-point placement error may result in a tenfold dosage error, which would be fatal! All medication calculations should be double-checked by another registered nurse or by a pharmacist or physician because of this narrow margin of error.
- Toxicity is manifested in children by nausea, vomiting, bradycardia, anorexia, and arrhythmias.
- The physician should be notified immediately should the following symptoms indicative of CHF develop: increased fatigue, sudden weight gain (2 lbs or greater in 1 week), respiratory distress, or profuse scalp sweating.

IMPLEMENTATION

Before administering any dose of a cardiac glycoside, the nurse should count the patient's apical pulse and auscultate the heart beat for 1 full minute. If the pulse is 60 beats/min or less or greater than 120 beats/min, then the dose should be withheld and the physician notified of the problem. In addition, the physician should be contacted if the patient experiences any of the following manifestations of toxicity: anorexia, nausea, vomiting or diarrhea, and visual disturbances such as blurred vision or the perception of green or yellow halos around objects.

Other nursing interventions include checking the dosage form and amounts *carefully* as well as the physician's order to make sure the specific drug ordered has been dispensed (such as digitoxin versus digoxin). Digitalis preparations may be administered with meals but not with foods high in fiber because the fiber will bind to the digitalis and this will make less drug available for absorption. If the medication is to be given intravenously, the following interventions are critical: administer undiluted IV forms at around 0.25 mg/min or over more than 5 minutes. The administration of IM forms of cardiac glycosides is extremely painful and is not indicated or recommended because of the tissue necrosis and erratic absorption that may ensue. Di-

HOME HEALTH POINTS
Digitalis Preparations

- Patients should be instructed on how to take radial pulse before each dose of digitalis preparation. For the elderly and physically or mentally challenged it is important to have home health care personnel supervise the medication regimen, as these individuals will be at risk for possible interactions with other medications or for possible toxicity.
- Patients should keep a journal at home in reference to the following: date, day, time of dose, amount of medication taken, dietary intake, any unusual side effects or changes in condition, and pulse rate. The following is an example of a chart-type journal, which may help to identify therapeutic as well as side effects and toxicity associated with the medication administration at home (see below):

- Patients should be encouraged to contact the physician or health care provider with any unusual complaints or if the pulse is *below* 60 beats/min or erratic, or if they are experiencing anorexia, nausea, or vomiting. Any changes in visual acuity should also be reported to their health care provider or home health care nurse.
- Patients taking digitalis preparations should be encouraged to wear a Medic-Alert ID band, and have one ordered before discharge from the hospital.
- A weight gain of 1 or 2 lb a day or 5 lb or more in a week should be reported to the health care provider or to the home health care nurse.

Drug dose	Date and time	Apical pulse rate	Weight	Side effects	Diet intake	Any changes or unusual complaints	Misc.

goxin and digitoxin are incompatible with any other medication in solution or syringe. It is important to remember that, regardless of the dosage form, if the patient's apical pulse is less than 60 or more than 120 beats/min, the dose should be withheld, the physician notified of the problem, the vital signs monitored, and all interventions documented. Should toxicity become life-threatening, Digibind, the antidote to digoxin or digitoxin toxicity, should be administered over 30 minutes or given as an IV bolus if cardiac arrest is imminent. See the boxes on patient teaching tips on p. 272 and pediatric implications on p. 273.

The nursing interventions called for in patients undergoing digitalization need to be considered separately. Although not commonly used in contemporary practice, digitalization may still be done in some areas of practice for the management of CHF. Rapid digitalization (to get faster action) is generally reserved for patients with CHF who are in acute distress. Such patients are hospitalized because digitalis toxicities can appear quickly in this setting and are directly correlated to the high drug concentrations used. Should the

patient undergoing rapid digitalization exhibit *any* of the manifestations of toxicity, the physician should be contacted immediately. Such patients should be observed constantly and serum digoxin or digitoxin levels measured frequently. Slow digitalization is generally performed in an outpatient setting in patients with CHF who are not in such acute distress. In this context it takes longer for toxic effects to appear (depending on the specific drug's half-life) than it does for the toxic effects stemming from rapid digitalization. The main advantages of slow digitalization are that it can be done on an outpatient basis and with oral dosage forms and it is safer than rapid digitalization. Disadvantages are that it takes longer for the therapeutic effects to occur and the symptoms of toxicity are more gradual, and therefore more insidious, in onset.

EVALUATION

Monitoring patients after the administration of cardiac glycosides is crucial for identifying therapeutic effects as opposed to side effects. Because cardiac glycosides

---

TAKE HOME POINTS

Inotropic
- Refers to the force of myocardial contraction.
- Positive inotropic agents increase the force of contractions (e.g., digoxin).
- Negative inotropic agents decrease force of contraction (e.g., beta-blockers, calcium channel blockers).

Chronotropic
- Refers to the rate at which the heart beats (beats/min).
- Positive chronotropic agents increase the heart rate (e.g., epinephrine, atropine).

Dromotropic
- Refers to the conduction of electrical impulses through the water.
- Positive dromotropic agents increase the speed of the electrical impulse through the heart.
- Cardiac conduction = start in SA node and goes to AV node, then down bundle of His to Purkinje fibers.

Cardiac Glycosides
- One of the oldest and most effective group of drugs obtained from a plant source.
- Originally obtained from *digitalis* plant, commonly referred to as *foxglove*.
- Mainstay of CHF treatment for over 200 years.

Ejection Fraction
- Amount of blood ejected at each contraction over amount of blood in heart before contraction.
- Normally around 65% (0.65).
- Patients with CHF have low ejection fractions because their hearts are failing as pumps.

Nursing Considerations
- Contraindications to the use of digitalis products include patients with a history of allergy to the medication(s), ventricular tachycardia ad fibrillations, beriberi heart disease and hypersensitive carotid sinus syndrome.
- Predisposers to digitalis toxicity include hypokalemia, hypercalcemia, hypothyroid states, and elderly.
- Taking an apical pulse for 1 full minute is a standard of care expected when administering digitalis drugs.
- A physician should be notified at the first signs of anorexia, nausea, vomiting, or for bradycardia with a pulse below 60 beats per minute.

increase the force of myocardial contractility (positive inotropic effect), alter electrophysiologic properties (decrease rate—negative chronotropic effect), and decrease AV node conduction (negative dromotropic effect), the therapeutic effects include increased urinary output; decreased edema; decreased shortness of breath, dyspnea, and rales; decreased fatigue; resolving of the paroxysmal nocturnal dyspnea; and improved peripheral pulses, skin color, and temperature. While monitoring for the therapeutic effects, it is essential, because of the low therapeutic index of digitalis preparations, to assess patients for the development of side effects such as anorexia, nausea, vomiting, diarrhea, ventricular arrhythmias, heart block, bradycardia, and confusion. Monitoring laboratory values such as the serum creatinine, potassium, calcium, sodium, and chloride levels as well as the digoxin (0.5-2 ng/ml) and digitoxin (13-25 ng/ml) therapeutic levels will also help ensure the delivery of safe and efficacious treatment.

Critical Thinking **A C T I V I T I E S**

1. Atrial fibrillation develops in the patient you are caring for. The patient is not currently on any agent to treat this and is becoming quite symptomatic. The physician prescribes digoxin at a dosage of 0.5 mg IV stat, followed by 0.25 mg IV every 6 hours for two doses. How much digoxin (in milliliters) should you give each time?

2. Your patient, a 78-year-old-man, has a potassium level of 3.0 mEq/L. He states that he has been nauseous and without an appetite and has experienced some diarrhea. He has been taking digoxin for the past few weeks for the treatment of recently diagnosed CHF. Discuss the implication of hypokalemia in a patient who is on digitalis preparations.

BIBLIOGRAPHY

Clayton BD, Stock YN: *Basic pharmacology for nurses,* ed 10, St Louis, 1993, Mosby.

Edmunds MW: *Introduction to clinical pharmacology,* ed 2, St Louis, 1995, Mosby.

Johnson KB: *Harriet Lane handbook,* ed 13, St Louis, 1993, Mosby.

Keen JH: *Critical care and emergency drug reference,* St Louis, 1994, Mosby.

Knoben JE, Anderson PO: *Handbook of critical drug data,* ed 6, Hamilton, Ill, 1988, Drug Intelligence Publications.

McEvoy GK: *AHFS drug information,* Besthesda, Md, 1994, American Society of Hospital Pharmacists.

McKenry LM, Salerno E: *Mosby's pharmacology in nursing,* ed 19, St Louis, 1995, Mosby.

Skidmore-Roth L: *Mosby's 1995 nursing drug reference,* St Louis, 1995, Mosby.

Chapter 21

Antidysrhythmic Agents

Objectives

When you reach the end of this chapter, you will be able to:

1 Define the most commonly encountered dysrhythmias.
2 Describe normal cardiac function.
3 Identify the various classes of antidysrythmics as determined by their mechanism of action.
4 Provide examples of specific drugs within each class of antidysrythmic agents.
5 Discuss the mechanism of action, therapeutic effects, and adverse effects of the various antidysrythmics and the various uses for these agents.
6 Develop a nursing care plan with expected outcomes as it relates to the administration of the various antidysrythmics and the treatment of overdose or toxicity.
7 Identify the various drug interactions associated with the antidysrhythmic agents.
8 Evaluate the therapeutic versus toxic effects of the different antidysrhythmic agents.

CHAPTER OUTLINE

Dysrhythmias and Normal Cardiac
   Electrophysiology
Antidysrhythmic Agents
  Mechanism of action
  Drug effects
  Therapeutic uses
  Side effects and adverse effects
    Toxicity and management of overdose
  Interactions
  Dosages
Drug Profiles
Class Ia Drugs
  ⚓ Quinidine
  Procainamide
  Disopyramide
Class Ib Drugs
  ⚓ Lidocaine
  Tocainide
  Mexiletine
Class Ic Drugs
  Encainide and Flecainide
  Propafenone
Class II Drugs
  Atenolol
  ⚓ Esmolol
  Metoprolol

  Propranolol
  Sotalol
Class III Drugs
  Bretylium
  ⚓ Amiodarone
Class IV Drugs
  Diltiazem
  ⚓ Verapamil
Unclassified Antidysrhythmics
  Adenosine
Nursing Process
Class I Drugs

Assessment
Nursing Diagnoses
Planning
  Outcome criteria
Implementation
Evaluation

Class II Drugs

Assessment
Nursing Diagnoses
Planning and Outcome Criteria
Implementation
Evaluation

Class III Drugs

Assessment

continued

Nursing Diagnoses

Planning and Outcome Criteria

Implementation

Evaluation

Class IV Drugs

Assessment

Nursing Diagnoses

Planning and Outcome Criteria

Implementation

Evaluation

Glossary

Action potential An electrical impulse consisting of a self-propagating series of polarizations and depolarizations that is transmitted across the cell membranes of a nerve fiber during the transmission of a nerve impulse and across the cell membranes of a muscle cell during contraction or other activity of the cell. (p. 277)

Action potential duration The interval during which a cell is repolarizing to its baseline membrane potential. (p. 279)

Arrhythmia (ə rith′ me ə) In the most literal sense, this means the absence of a rhythmic pattern. A term also commonly used to refer to any deviation from the normal pattern of the heartbeat, or dysrhythmia. (p. 277)

Cardiac Arrhythmia Suppression Trial (CAST) The name of the major research study conducted by the National Heart, Lung, and Blood Institute to investigate the possibility of eliminating sudden cardiac death in patients with asymptomatic, non–life-threatening ectopy that has arisen after a myocardial infarction. (p. 288)

Dysrhythmia (dis rith′ me ə) Any disturbance or abnormality in a normal rhythmic pattern. (p. 277)

Effective refractory period The period after the firing of an impulse during which a cell may respond to a stimulus but the response will not be passed along or continued. (p. 279)

Fast channels, sodium channels Other terms for *fast-response channels*. These cells can rapidly conduct electrical impulses. (p. 278)

Internodal pathways, Bachmann's bundle Special pathways in the atria that carry electrical impulses which are spontaneously generated by the sinoatrial node. These impulses cause the heart to beat. (p. 279)

Relative refractory period The time during which a depressed response to a strong stimulus is possible. (p. 279)

Resting membrane potential The transmembrane voltage that exists when the heart muscle is at rest. (p. 277)

Sodium-potassium ATPase pump A mechanism for transporting sodium and potassium ions across cell membranes against an opposing concentration gradient. Energy for this transport system is obtained from the hydrolysis of adenosine triphosphate by means of an enzyme called *adenosine triphosphatase* (ATPase). (p. 277)

Sudden cardiac death Unexplained cessation, or death, of cardiac function. (p. 289)

Threshold potential The spontaneous depolarization of cells after a critical state of electrical tension is reached. (p. 279)

Vaughan Williams classification The most commonly used system used to classify antidysrhythmic drugs. (p. 280; see also Table 21-2, p. 280)

DYSRHYTHMIAS AND NORMAL CARDIAC ELECTROPHYSIOLOGY

A **dysrhythmia** is any deviation from the normal rhythm of the heart. The term **arrhythmia**, which is also used to refer to these deviations, literally means 'no rhythm,' which implies asystole or no heartbeat at all. Thus the more accurate term for an irregular heart rhythm is *dysrhythmia* because a patient who has no cardiac rhythm is in asystole, or dead. There are many conditions in which dysrhythmias can develop. Some of the more common arise after a myocardial infarction (MI) or cardiac surgery or as the result of coronary artery disease. These dysrhythmias are usually serious and require treatment with an antidysrhythmic agent, though not all have to be treated.

The disturbances in cardiac rhythm are the result of abnormally functioning cardiac cells. Therefore, to help understand the pathologic mechanism responsible for dysrhythmias, it is first necessary to review the electrical properties of cardiac cells. Figure 21-1 illustrates the process from the standpoint of a single cardiac cell. Inside a cardiac cell there exists a net negative charge relative to the outside of the cell. This difference in the electronegative charge exists in all types of cardiac cells and is referred to as the **resting membrane potential** (RMP). The RMP results from an uneven distribution of ions (sodium, potassium, and calcium) across the cell membrane. To maintain this uneven distribution of ions requires the **sodium-potassium ATPase pump**, an energy-requiring ionic pump. Cardiac cells become excited when there is a change in this distribution of ions across its membrane, and this movement of ions across the cardiac cell's membrane results in the propagation of an electrical impulse and the subsequent contraction of the myocardial muscle. This is called an **action potential** and it consists of four phases. Phase 1 of the action potential starts when the fast sodium channel closes and a period of rapid repolarization begins. During phase 2, calcium ion influx occurs through the slow channels. This causes a plateau phase during which the membrane potential changes only slightly. Over time potassium ions flow outward and the cell is repolarized to its baseline level (phase 3). To restore the cell to its original state, the energy-dependent, sodium-potassium ATPase pump, or sodium pump, moves sodium

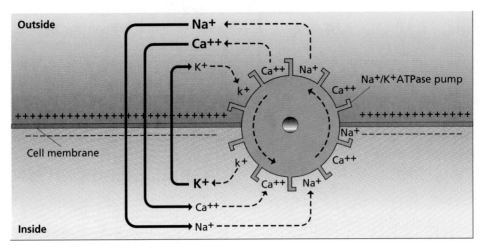

▼ FIG. 21-1 Resting membrane potential of a cardiac cell.

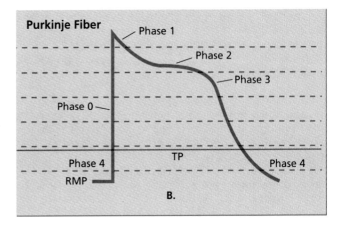

▼ FIG. 21-2 action potentials. *RMP,* resting membrane potential; *SA,* sinoatrial; *TP,* threshold potential.

ions out and potassium ions into the cell. Phase 4 is the RMP.

The movement of ions across the cardiac cell's membranes (action potential) varies in speed from one area to another in the heart's conduction system. Figure 21-2 illustrates the action potentials in two different types of cells found in the conduction system of the heart. The action potential of the specialized electrical conducting cells in the sinoatrial (SA) node is shown in Fig. 21-2, *A,* and the action potential of a Purkinje cell (fiber) located in the specialized electrical conducting system is depicted in Fig. 21-2, *B.* Figure 21-3 also illustrates the movement of sodium, potassium, and calcium ions into and out of a Purkinje cell during the four phases of the action potential. There are several important differences in the action potentials of the SA node and Purkinje cell. The RMP in the Purkinje cell is approximately −80 to −90 mV compared with −50 to −60 mV in the SA nodal cell, and the level of the RMP (phase 4) is an important determinant of the

rate of impulse conduction to other cells. The less negative the RMP at the onset of phase 0, the slower the upstroke velocity of phase 0. The slope or rate of rise of phase 0 is directly related to the impulse conduction velocity or speed. If the slope of phase 0 is steep such as it is in the Purkinje cells, this means that electrical conduction through these cells is fast.

The action potential of the Purkinje cells illustrated in Fig. 21-2, *B,* has a rapid rate of rise of phase 0, and therefore electrical impulses are conducted quickly. These cells are referred to as *fast-response* or *fast-channel cells.* During this phase, channels open, permitting a rapid influx of sodium ions into the cell. The terms **fast channels** and **sodium channels** both refer to these fast-response channels. Many antidysrhythmic agents affect the RMP and sodium channels, which in turn affects the rate of impulse conduction.

Because the cells of the SA or AV nodes have RMPs of −50 to −60 mV, they have a much slower upstroke velocity, or a slower phase 0. This slow rate of rise in

Phase 1 Phase 2

▼ FIG. 21-3 Purkinje fiber action potential.

phase 0 of the SA and AV nodes is primarily dependent on the entry of calcium ions through the slow channel. These cells are therefore called *slow-channel tissue* or *calcium channels,* and conduction in these cells is slower than that in the myocardial or other electrical conduction tissue. Drugs that affect calcium ion movement into or out of these cells tend to have significant effects on the SA and AV nodal conduction rates.

The time interval between phase 0 and phase 4 when the cell is repolarizing and returning to its RMP is called the **action potential duration** (APD). The period between phase 0 and midway through phase 3 is called the absolute or **effective refractory period** (ERP). During the ERP the cardiac cell cannot be stimulated to depolarize and conduct electricity. During the remainder of phase 3 until the return to the RMP (phase 4), the cardiac cell is vulnerable to depolarization if it receives an impulse. This period is referred to as the **relative refractory period** (RRP), and during it a strong stimulus can initiate a premature depolarization. If a cardiac cell receives a strong enough stimulus during the RRP, it will be when the cell is at a lower membrane potential (less negative) and this will result in slow impulse conduction. Figure 21-4 illustrates these various aspects of an action potential.

The RMP of certain cardiac cells gradually and spontaneously decreases (becomes less negative) over time, and this is probably secondary to small changes in the flux of sodium and potassium ions. Depolarization eventually occurs when a certain critical voltage is reached, the **threshold potential** (TP). This process of spontaneous depolarization is referred to as *automaticity* (or *pacemaker activity*). It is normal when it occurs in the SA node, AV node, and His-Purkinje system. When tissues besides these assume the property of spontaneous depolarization, dysrhythmias occur.

The SA node, AV node, and His-Purkinje cells all

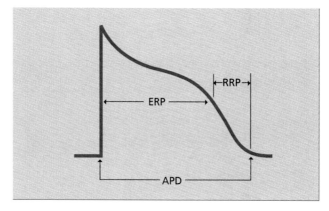

▼ FIG. 21-4 aspects of an action potential. *APD,* action potential duration; *ERP,* effective refractory period; *RRP,* relative refractory period.

possess automaticity, but the SA node is the pacemaker of the heart because it spontaneously depolarizes the fastest. The SA node has an intrinsic rate of 60 to 100 depolarizations *or* beats per minute, that of the AV node is 40 to 60 beats per minute, and that of the ventricular Purkinje fibers is 40 or less beats per minute. The action potentials in different areas of the heart along with other characteristics of the cells in these different areas are compared in Table 21-1.

As the pacemaker of the heart, the SA node, which is located near the top of the right atrium, generates the electrical impulse needed to produce the heartbeat. This impulse then travels through the atria via specialized pathways called the **internodal pathways** and **Bachmann's bundle**. While the impulse is traveling through these specialized pathways, it is causing the myocardial muscle in the atria to contract. This impulse is then received by the AV node, which is located near the bottom of the right atrium. The AV node slows this very fast moving electrical impulse just long enough to allow the ventricles to accept the blood that the atria have just squeezed into them. If the AV node did not slow the impulse, the ventricles would contract almost at the same time as the atria, resulting in a smaller volume of blood being injected (decreased cardiac output).

Upon stimulation, the AV node generates an electrical impulse that passes into the bundle of His, a band of cardiac muscle fibers located between both the right and left ventricles in what is called the *ventricular septum.* The bundle of His distributes the impulse into both ventricles via the right and left bundle branch. Each branch terminates in the Purkinje fibers that are located in the myocardium of the ventricles. The stimulation of the Purkinje fibers causes ventricular contraction and blood to leave the ventricles, going to the lungs from the right ventricle and to the rest of the body from the left ventricle.

Any abnormality in cardiac automaticity or impulse conduction will result in some type of dysrhythmia.

ANTIDYSRHYTHMIC AGENTS

There are numerous drugs available to treat dysrhythmias, and these are classified based on where and how they affect cardiac cells. The most commonly used system is the **Vaughan Williams classification,** and it uses as its basis the effect produced by the particular agent on the action potential. This approach has yielded four major groups of agents. Class I antidysrhythmics are considered membrane-stabilizing agents, but they are further divided into Ia, Ib, and Ic agents, depending on the magnitude of their effects on phase 0, the APD, and the ERP. Class II drugs are beta-blockers that depress phase 4 depolarization. Class III drugs primarily prolong repolarization during phase 3. Class IV drugs depress phase 4 depolarization and prolong repolar-

Table 21-1 Comparison of Action Potentials in Different Cardiac Tissue

Tissue	Action Potential Wave	Speed of Response	Threshold Potential (mV)	Conduction Velocity (m/sec)
SA node		Slow	−60	<0.05
Atrium		Fast	−90	−1
AV node		Slow	−60	<0.05
His-Purkinje		Fast	−95	3
Ventricle		Fast	−90	1

Table 21-2 Vaughan Williams Classification of Antidysrhythmic Drugs

Functional Class	Drugs
Class I: Membrane-stabilizing agents; fast sodium channel blockers	
Ia: ↑ blockade of sodium channel, delay repolarization, ↑ APD	↓Quinidine, disopyramide, procainamide
Ib: ↑ blockade of sodium channel, accelerate repolarization, ↓ APD	Tocainide, mexiletine, phenytoin, lidocaine
Ic: ↑ ↑ ↑ blockade of sodium channel, ± on repolarization	Flecainide, encainide, propafenone
Class II: Beta-blocking agents	All beta-blockers
Class III: Principal effect on cardiac tissue is to ↑ APD	↓Amiodarone, bretylium, sotalol
Class IV: Calcium channel blockers	All calcium channel blockers
Other: Antidysrhythmic drugs that have the properties of several classes and therefore cannot be placed in one particular class	Digoxin, adenosine, moricizine

APD, action potential duration; ↑, increase; ↓, decrease; ±, .

ization during phases 1 and 2. The calcium channel blockers (slow channel blockers) like verapamil belong to class IV. The various agents in these four classes are listed in Table 21-2. Several of the antidysrhythmics exert more than one type of effect on the action potential. Moricizine is such an agent, but it is classified most commonly by itself in class I because it exhibits the properties of class Ia, Ib, and Ic agents.

Mechanism of Action

The antidysrhythmic drugs can correct abnormal cardiac electrophysiologic functioning by various mechanisms of action. As the membrane-stabilizing agents, class I drugs exert their actions on the sodium (fast) channels, but as already noted, there are some slight differences in the actions of the agents within this class, resulting in three subgroups of agents. The class Ia agents (quinidine, procainamide, and disopyramide) block sodium channels; more specifically they delay repolarization and increase the APD. The class Ib agents (tocainide, mexiletine, phenytoin, and lidocaine) block the sodium channels, but unlike the class Ia agents, they accelerate repolarization and decrease the APD. The class Ic agents (flecainide, encainide, and propafenone) have a more pronounced effect on the blockade of sodium channels but have little effect on repolarization or the APD. As previously mentioned, moricizine is most frequently classified simply as a class I drug with no subclass specifications because it has characteristics of all three subclasses.

The class II agents are the beta-blockers. They work by reducing or blocking sympathetic nervous system stimulation to the heart and, as a result, the transmission of impulses in the heart's conduction system. This results in depression of phase 4 depolarization. These drugs mostly affect slow tissue.

The class III agents (amiodarone, bretylium, and sotalol) increase the APD by prolonging repolarization

in phase 3. They affect fast tissue and are most commonly used to manage difficult to treat dysrhythmias.

The class IV agents are the calcium channel blockers, and as their name implies, they work by inhibiting the slow-channel pathways, or the calcium-dependent channels. By doing this, they depress phase 4 depolarization.

The mechanisms of action of the major classes of antidysrhythmics are summarized in Table 21-3.

Drug Effects

The antidysrhythmic drugs primarily alter cardiac electrophysiology. These effects include changes in the SA node and ectopic pacemakers, AV node, conduction velocity, autonomic nervous system innervation, ERPs, and various segments of the ECG. The effects can be summarized for the various classes of agents, as follows:

Class I: moricizine
1. Prolongs AV node conduction velocity.
2. Prolongs bundle of His and Purkinje cell conduction velocity.
3. Prolongs the PR and QRS complex intervals of the ECG.
4. Eliminates or reduces ectopic foci stimulation.
5. Minimal effect on the SA node and automaticity.

Class Ia: disopyramide, procainamide, quinidine
1. Depress myocardial excitability.
2. Prolong the ERP.
3. Eliminate or reduce ectopic foci stimulation.
4. Decrease inotropic effect.
5. Anticholinergic (vagolytic).

Class Ib: lidocaine, mexiletine, phenytoin, tocainide
1. Decrease myocardial excitability in the ventricles.

Table 21-3	Antidysrhythmics: Mechanisms of Action			
Vaughan Williams class	I	II	III	IV
Action	Blocks sodium channels, affects phase 0	Increases spontaneous depolarization, affects phase 4	Prolongs APD	Blocks slow calcium channels
Tissue	Fast	Slow	Fast	Slow
Effect on action potential				

APD, action potential duration.

2. Eliminate or reduce ectopic foci stimulation in the ventricles.
3. Minimal effect on the SA node and automaticity.
4. Minimal effect on the AV node and conduction.
5. Minimal anticholinergic (vagolytic) activity.

Class Ic: Flecainide, propafenone, encainide

1. Dose-related depression of cardiac conduction, especially in the bundle of His–Purkinje system.
2. Minimal effect on atrial conduction.
3. Eliminate or reduce ectopic foci stimulation in the ventricles.
4. Minimal anticholinergic (vagolytic) activity.

Class II: Acebutolol, esmolol, propranolol, sotalol*

1. Block beta-adrenergic cardiac stimulation.
2. Reduce SA node activity.
3. Eliminate or reduce atrial ectopic foci stimulation.
4. Reduce ventricular contraction rate.
5. Reduce cardiac output and blood pressure.

Class III: Amiodarone, bretylium

1. Prolong the ERP.
2. Prolong myocardial action potential.
3. Block both alpha- and beta-adrenergic cardiac stimulation.

Class IV: adenosine, (natural endogenous cellular chemical) verapamil, diltiazem

1. Prolong AV node ERP.
2. Reduce AV node conduction.
3. Reduce rapid ventricular conduction due to atrial flutter.

Therapeutic Uses

The antidysrhythmic agents are affective in treating a variety of cardiac dysrhythmias. The antidysrhythmic drugs and the most common indications for their use are listed in Table 21-4.

Side Effects and Adverse Effects

Side effects and adverse effects common to most antidysrhythmics include hypersensitivity reactions, nausea, vomiting, and diarrhea. Other common effects include dizziness, headache, and blurred vision. In addition, any antidysrhythmic is capable of producing a proarrhythmic (dysrhythmic) effect. This occurs most

---

*Sotalol has both class II and class III properties because of its chemical structure. It is a racemic mixture of both dextro- and levoenantiomers. The dextroenantiomer has class III properties while the levoenantiomer has class II properties.

frequently in association with amiodarone, moricizine, or propafenone therapy.

Toxicity and Management of Overdose

The main toxic effects of the antidysrhythmics involve the heart, circulation, and CNS. Specific antidotes are not available, and the management of an overdose involves maintaining adequate circulation

Table 21-4	Antidysrhythmic Drugs: Indications
DRUG	**INDICATIONS**
Class Ia	
Quinidine Procainamide Disopyramide	Atrial fibrillation, premature atrial contractions, premature ventricular contractions, ventricular tachycardia, Wolff-Parkinson-White syndrome
Class Ib	
Lidocaine Tocainide Mexiletine	Ventricular arrhythmias only (premature ventricular contractions, ventricular tachycardia, ventricular fibrillation)
Class Ic	
Encainide Flecainide Propafenone	Severe ventricular dysrhythmias only
Class I	
Moricizine	Symptomatic ventricular and life-threatening dysrhythmias
Class II	
Beta-blockers Atenolol Esmolol Metaprolol Propranolol Sotalol	General myocardial depressants for both supraventricular and ventricular dysrhythmias
Class III	
Amiodarone Bretylium Sotalol	Life-threatening ventricular tachycardia or fibrillation resistant to other drugs; also sustained ventricular tachycardia Ventricular tachycardia or fibrillation Same as amiodarone's
Class IV	
Calcium channel blockers Diltiazem Verapamil	Paroxysmal supraventricular tachycardia; rate control for atrial fibrillation and flutter

Table 21-5 Antidysrhythmics: Management of Overdose

DRUG	TOXIC EFFECT	MANAGEMENT
Acebutolol	Bradycardia Bronchospasm Cardiac failure Hypotension	1-3 mg IV atropine divided Beta$_2$-adrenergic or theophylline Digitalization Vasopressor
Adenosine	Usually self-limiting due to very short half-life	Competitive antagonists caffeine or theophylline
⇩Amiodarone	Bradycardia Hypotension	Beta-adrenergic agent Positive inotropic agent or vasopressor
Bretylium	Hypertension Hypotension	Nitroprusside Dopamine or norepinephrine and fluid therapy
Disopyramide	Loss of consciousness, cardiac and respiratory arrest	Neostigmine for anticholinergic effects, induced emesis, activated charcoal, and hemodialysis
⇩Esmolol		Same as acebutolol's
Flecainide	Reduced heart rate	Dopamine or dobutamine; acidify very alkaline urine
⇩Lidocaine	Convulsions	Diazepam or thiopental
Mexiletine	Bradycardia, hypotension	Atropine; acidify urine to promote excretion
Moricizine	Hypotension, CHF, and MI	Gastric evacuation and advanced life support systems
Phenytoin	Circulatory and respiratory arrest, convulsions	Life support systems when required
Procainamide	Cardiac depression	IV pressor agents and supportive measures
Propafenone	Convulsions	Diazepam and mechanical assisted respiration
Propranolol		Same as acebutolol's
⇩Quinidine	Cardiac dysrhythmias	Sodium lactate reduces toxicity except in alkalosis; lidocaine
Sotalol		Same as acebutolol's
Tocainide	Convulsions	Diazepam or short-acting barbiturate
⇩Verapamil	Bradycardia Cardiac failure Conduction problems Hypotension	Atropine Dopamine or dobutamine Cardiac pacing Vasopressors, 10% calcium chloride solution

and respiration using general support measures and any required symptomatic treatment (see Table 21-5).

Interactions

The antidysrhythmics can interact with many different categories of drugs. The most serious drug interactions are the ones that can result in dysrhythmias, hypotension or hypertension, respiratory distress, or a summation of either the therapeutic or toxic effects. See Table 21-6 for a summary of the drug interactions.)

Dosages

For information on the dosages of the various antidysrhythmics see the dosages table on p. 285.

DRUG PROFILES

CLASS Ia DRUGS

The group Ia drugs are considered membrane-stabilizing drugs because they possess local anesthetic properties. They stabilize the membrane and have depressant effects on phase 0 of the action potential. All the class Ia agents are classified as pregnancy category C agents.

Table 21-6	Antidysrhythmics: Drug Interactions	
DRUG	**MECHANISM**	**RESULT**
Antidysrhyth-mics	Additive	Proarrythmic, may cause dysrhythmias
Anticoagu-lants	Anticoagulant dis-placed from protein-binding sites	More pronounced anticoagulant effects
Phenytoin	Phenytoin dis-placed from protein-binding sites	More pronounced phenytoin ef-fects
Sulfonylurea compounds	Sulfonylurea dis-placed from protein-binding sites	More pronounced sulfonylurea ef-fects

⚓ QUINIDINE

Quinidine (Quinidex, Cardioquin, Quinaglute, Dura-Tab) has both a direct action on the electrical activity of the heart and an indirect (anticholinergic) effect. Its anticholinergic action results in inhibition of the para-sympathetic nervous system and allows sympathetic nervous system activity to go unopposed. This accel-erates the rate of electrical impulse formation and con-duction. Significant adverse effects of the agent include cardiac asystole, atrial embolism, and ventricular ec-topic beats. Contraindications to use of the drug in-clude hypersensitivity to it, thrombocytopenic pur-pura resulting from previous therapy, AV block, intraventricular conduction defects, and abnormal rhythms (proarrhythmic effects). Quinidine is avail-able both orally and parenterally and in three different salt forms. The oral preparations consist of 324-mg ex-tended-release quinidine gluconate tablets, 275-mg quinidine polygalacturonate tablets, and 200- and 300-mg regular-release and 300-mg extended-release quin-idine sulfate tablets. Parenterally quinidine gluconate comes as an 80-mg/ml injection. Common dosages are listed in the dosages table. Pregnancy category C.

⬡ PHARMACOKINETICS

HALF-LIFE	ONSET	PEAK	DURATION
PO: 6-7 hr	1-3 hr	PO: 0.5-6 hr	PO: 6-8 hr

PROCAINAMIDE

The electrophysiologic effect of procainamide (Prones-tyl, Pronestyl-SR, Procan SR) is similar to that of quin-idine, but it differs from quinidine in that its indirect effect (anticholinergic action) is weaker. Procainamide is useful in the management of atrial and ventricular tachydysrhythmias. It is reported to be more effective in the treatment of ventricular disturbances, especially in suppressing premature ventricular contractions and preventing the recurrence of ventricular tachycardia. The intravenous form of procainamide is generally preferred over that of quinidine. Procainamide is chemically related to the local anesthetic procaine. Sig-nificant adverse effects of the agent include ventricular dysrhythmias and blood disorders. It can cause a lupus erythematosus–like syndrome, and this occurs in about 30% of patients on long-term therapy. It can also cause gastrointestinal effects such as nausea, vomiting, and diarrhea, but these are less intense than those of quinidine. Other side effects include fever, leukopenia, a maculopapular rash, urticaria, pruritus, flushing, and torsades de pointes resulting from prolongation of the QT interval.

Procainamide is contraindicated in patients who have shown hypersensitivity reactions to it and in those with complete heart block, lupus erythematosus, and second- or third-degree heart block. It is available in three different oral forms: 250-, 375-, and 500-mg capsules; 500-, 750-, and 1000-mg extended-release, film-coated tablets; and 250-, 375-, and 500-mg film-coated tablets. Parenterally procainamide comes as a 100- and 500-mg/ml injection. Common dosages are listed in the dosages table. Pregnancy category C.

⬡ PHARMACOKINETICS

HALF-LIFE	ONSET	PEAK	DURATION
IV/IM: 3 hr	IV/IM: 10-30 min	IV/IM: 10-60 min	IV/IM: 3 hr
PO: 3 hr	PO: 0.5-1 hr	PO: 1-2 hr	PO: 3 hr*

*8-hr extended.

DISOPYRAMIDE

Disopyramide (Norpace, Norpace CR) is used primar-ily for the treatment of ventricular dysrhythmias. Its therapeutic efficacy is comparable to that of quinidine and procainamide, but it can produce significant side effects, including anticholinergic effects, ventricular dysrhythmias, and particularly cardiovascular depres-sion. For these reasons its use is limited, especially in patients with poor left ventricular (LV) function.

Significant adverse reactions from it are hypoten-sion and widening of the QRS interval on the ECG, as well as those mentioned for quinidine and procain-amide. The incidence of systemic lupus erythematosus associated with its use is less than that associated with

D O S A G E S

SELECTED ANTIDYSRHYTHMIC AGENTS

AGENT	PHARMACOLOGIC CLASS	DOSAGE RANGE	PURPOSE
⚓Quinidine (Quinidex [sulfate], Cardioquin [polygalacturonate], Quinaglute Dura-Tab [gluconate]	Class Ia antidysrhythmic	*Adult* Gluconate PO: 324-648 mg q8-12h IM: 600 mg followed by 400 mg q2h or more if needed IV: 330-750 mg Polygalacturonate: PO: 275 mg 3-4 times/day Sulfate PO: 0.2 g q2-3h for 5-8 doses with daily increases until sinus rhythm is restored or toxic effects occur 0.2-0.3 g 3-4 times/day	Atrial dysrhythmias Atrial dysrhythmias Conversion of a trial fibrillation Atrial dysrhythmias
Procainamide (Pronestyl, Pronestyl-SR, Procan SR)	Class Ia antidysrhythmic	*Adult* PO:0.5-1 g q4-6h 50 mg/kg/day divided IM:50 mg/kg/day divided 100-500 mg IV: 50-100 mg every 5 min up to 500 mg with a maintenance infusion of 1-6 mg/min	Atrial dysrhythmias Ventricular dysrhythmias Alternate PO dosage Dysrhythmias during surgery Rapid dysrhythmia control
Disopyramide (Norpace, Norpace CR)	Class Ia antidysrhythmic	*Adult* PO: 150 mg q6h; CR: 300 mg q12h with a daily range of 400-800 mg divided	Ventricular dysrhythmias
⚓Lidocaine (Xylocaine)	Class Ib antidysrhythmic	*Pediatric* IV: suggested bolus dose, 0.5-1 mg/kg; usual maintenance infusion rate, 10-50 µg/kg/min *Adult* IM: 4.3 mg/kg; may be repeated after 60-90 min IV: bolus dose, 50-100 mg; may be repeated in 5 min. Do not exceed 200-300 mg over 1 hr. Usual maintenance infusion rate, 1-4 mg/min	Ventricular dysrhythmias
Tocainide (Tonocard)	Class Ib antidysrhythmic	*Adult* PO: initial dose, 400 mg q8h with a daily range of 1200-1800 mg in 3 doses with a maximum of ≥2400 mg/day	Ventricular dysrhythmias
Mexiletine (Mexitil)	Class Ib antidysrhythmic	*Adult* PO: start with 200 mg q8h. A minimum of 2-3 days is required between dosage adjustments, which are 50- or 100-mg increments up or down. For rapid control, 400 mg followed by 200 mg in 8 hr. Stabilized patients may be put on a 12-hr schedule with a maximum dose of 450 mg q12h	Ventricular dysrhythmias

continued

SELECTED ANTIDYSRHYTHMIC AGENTS—cont'd

AGENT	PHARMACOLOGIC CLASS	DOSAGE RANGE	PURPOSE
Encainide (Enkaid)	Class Ic antidysrhythmic	*Adult* PO: Start with 25 mg tid. If required, raise dosage to 35 mg tid after 3-5 days. Some patients may require 50 mg qid or 75 mg qid. Dose increment requires an interval of 3-5 days and 75 mg is the maximum single dose	Life-threatening dysrhythmias
Flecainide (Tambocor)	Class Ic antidysrhythmic	*Adult* PO: 50 mg q12h can be increased by 50 mg bid every 4 days until desired effect with a daily maximum of 300 mg for PSVT. 100 mg q12h with increment of 50 mg bid every 4 days if needed; usual dose, 150 mg q12h with daily maximum of 300 mg	Paroxysmal supra-ventricular tachycardia–par-oxysmal atrial flutter/fibrillation Sustained ventricular tachycardia
Propafenone (Rythmol)	Class Ic antidysrhythmic	*Adult* PO: start with 150 mg q8h and increase every 3-4 days; usual range, 450-900 mg/day divided	Ventricular dysrhythmias
Atenolol (Tenormin)	Beta$_1$-blocker (class II antidysrhythmic)	*Adult* IV: 5 mg over 5 min followed by 5 mg over 10 min followed by 50 mg PO 10 min after last IV injection and another 50 mg 12 hr later, then 100 mg/day for a further 6-9 days	Acute MI
⚓Esmolol (Brevibloc)	Beta$_1$-blocker (class II antidysrhythmic)	*Adult* IV: bolus dose of 500 μg/kg/min followed by 4 min of 50 μg/kg/min and evaluate	Supraventricular tachyarrhythmias
Metoprolol (Lopressor)	Beta$_1$-blocker	*Adult* IV/PO: 3 bolus injections of 5 mg at 2-min intervals followed by 50 mg PO every 6 hr for 48 hr, thereafter 100 mg bid PO: 100 mg bid	Early MI Late MI
Propranolol (Inderal)	Beta-blocker (class II antidysrhythmic)	*Adult* IV: 1-3 mg; if needed, repeated in 2 min and additional doses if needed q ≥ 4h. Switch to PO as soon as possible	Serious dysrhythmias
Sotalol (Betapace)	Beta-blocker	*Adult* PO: 160-320 mg/day divided	Life-threatening dysrhythmias
Bretylium (Bretylol)	Class III antidysrhythmic	*Adult* IM/IV: 5-10 mg/kg repeated at 5-30 min intervals if needed to a total dose of 30-35 mg/kg	Ventricular dysrhythmias

continued

SELECTED ANTIDYSRHYTHMIC AGENTS—cont'd

AGENT	PHARMACOLOGIC CLASS	DOSAGE RANGE	PURPOSE
⚓Amiodarone (Cordarone)	Class III antidysrhythmic	*Adult* PO: 800-1600 mg/day for 1-3 wk and reduced to 600-800 mg/day for 5 wk: usual maintenance dose, 400 mg/day	Ventricular dysrhythmias
Diltiazem (Cardizem)	Calcium channel blocker	*Adult* IV: bolus dose, 0.25 mg/kg over 2 min; second dose, 0.35 mg/kg over 2 min after 15 min prn; then 5-10 mg/hr or higher by continuous infusion	Supraventricular dysrhythmias
⚓Verapamil (Calan, Isoptin, Verelan)	Calcium channel blocker (class IV antidysrhythmic)	*Pediatric* IV: ≤1 y/o: 0.1-0.2 mg/kg bolus over 2 min; repeat dose after 30 min IV: 1-15 y/o: 0.1-0.3 mg/kg bolus over 2 min. Do not exceed 5-mg dose. Repeat dose not exceeding 10 mg may be given after 30 min. *Adult* PO: Start with 80 mg 3-4 times/ day; daily range, 240-480 mg IV: 5-10 mg bolus over 2 min; repeat dose of ≤10 mg may be given after 30 min.	Supraventricular tachyarrhythmias
Adenosine (Adenocard)	Class IV antidysrhythmic	*Adult* IV: 6-mg bolus over 1-2 sec. If needed, a second rapid bolus of 12 mg, which may be repeated a second time if required	Supraventricular tachycardia, conversion to normal sinus rhythm

the use of procainamide. Contraindications to its use are similar to those of quinidine and procainamide. Disopyramide is only available orally as 100- and 150-mg regular-release and extended-release capsules. Common dosages are listed in the dosages table. Pregnancy category C.

🐝 PHARMACOKINETICS

HALF-LIFE	ONSET	PEAK	DURATION
PO: 4-10 hr	PO: 30 min-3.5 hr	PO: 30 min-3 hr x̄: 2.5 hr	PO: 6-12 hr

CLASS Ib DRUGS

The class Ib drugs share many characteristics with the class Ia agents but are grouped together because they act preferentially on ischemic myocardial tissue. They have little effect on conduction velocity in normal tis-

sue. The class Ib agents have a weak depressive effect on phase 0 depolarization, the APD, and the ERP. They include lidocaine, tocainide, and mexiletine. Mexiletine and tocainide are classified as pregnancy category C agents, and lidocaine is classified as a pregnancy category B agent.

⚓ LIDOCAINE

Lidocaine (Xylocaine) is the prototypical Ib agent. It is one of the most effective drugs for the treatment of ventricular dysrhythmias, but it can only be administered intravenously because it has an extensive first-pass effect, that is, when taken orally, the liver metabolizes most of it to inactive metabolites.

Lidocaine exerts its effects on the conduction system of the heart by making it difficult for the ventricles to develop a dysrhythmia, an action called *raising the ventricular fibrillation threshold*. It does this by decreasing the sensitivity of the cardiac cell membrane to impulses and decreasing the cell's ability to depolarize on its own (decreasing automaticity). Many of these effects are accomplished by blockade of fast sodium channels.

Lidocaine is the drug of choice for treating the acute ventricular dysrhythmias associated with MI. Significant adverse effects include CNS toxicities such as twitching, convulsions, and confusion; respiratory depression or arrest; and the cardiovascular effects hypotension, bradycardia, and dysrhythmias. It is contraindicated in patients who are hypersensitive to its use, have severe SA or AV intraventricular block, or have the Stokes-Adams or Wolff-Parkinson-White syndrome. Lidocaine is only available parenterally for intramuscular or intravenous administration. It comes as a 100-mg/ml IM injection and as a 10-, 20-, 40-, 100-, and 200-mg/ml IV injection. Common dosages are listed in the dosages table. Pregnancy category B.

☙ PHARMACOKINETICS

HALF-LIFE	ONSET	PEAK	DURATION
IV/IM: 8 min, 1-2 hr (terminal)	IV/IM: 2-15 min	IV/IM: 5-10 min	IV/IM: 20 min-1½ hr

TOCAINIDE

Tocainide (Tonocard) is an orally active chemical derivative of lidocaine. However, in only about 60% of those patients whose dysrhythmia is stabilized on lidocaine will tocainide have the same success. Conversely, if lidocaine does not control the dysrhythmia, it is unlikely tocainide will do so. Tocainide does not undergo extensive first-pass metabolism, and so therefore it can be administered orally. It is useful for the treatment of various ventricular dysrhythmias. Its efficacy is probably due to its relatively long half-life of approximately 15 hours. It effectively suppresses the frequency of premature ventricular contractions (PVCs) but is less effective than the other class I agents in preventing chronic, recurrent ventricular tachycardia or fibrillation.

The most frequent side effects include dizziness, paresthesias (tingling), and tremor. Other complaints include nausea and vomiting, which can be minimized by taking the medication with food or an antacid. The most serious side effects are hematologic in nature and include agranulocytosis, leukopenia, and thrombocytopenia. Pulmonary disorders such as pulmonary fibrosis, interstitial pneumonitis, pulmonary edema, and pneumonia may also occur.

Tocainide is contraindicated in patients with a known hypersensitivity to it and in those with second- or third-degree heart block. It is available orally as 400- and 600-mg film-coated tablets. Common dosages are listed in the dosages table. Pregnancy category C.

☙ PHARMACOKINETICS

HALF-LIFE	ONSET	PEAK	DURATION
PO: 10-17 hr	Unknown	PO: 0.5-3 hr	8 hr

MEXILETINE

Mexiletine (Mexitil) is structurally and pharmacologically similar to lidocaine, and its effects on the conduction system of the heart are also very similar. As with tocainide, a response to parenteral lidocaine does not predict a response to mexiletine. Mexiletine effectively suppresses PVCs in patients suffering from an acute MI, chronic coronary artery disease, or digitalis toxicity, and in those undergoing cardiac surgery. It has proved particularly useful when taken in combination with selected class Ia or Ic agents or with beta-blockers.

The most frequent adverse effects are nausea, vomiting, dizziness, and tremor. These reactions are usually not serious, however, and are dose related and minimized by taking the drug with food or an antacid. Contraindications to its use include hypersensitivity, cardiogenic shock, and second- or third-degree AV block. It is available orally only as 150-, 200-, and 250-mg capsules. Common dosages are listed in the dosages table. Pregnancy category C.

☙ PHARMACOKINETICS

HALF-LIFE	ONSET	PEAK	DURATION
PO: 12 hr	Unknown	PO: 2-3 hr	Unknown

CLASS Ic DRUGS

The class Ic drugs (flecainide, encainide, and propafenone) have a more pronounced effect on sodium channel blockade than the Ia and Ib agents but have little effect on repolarization or the APD. These drugs markedly slow conduction in the atria, AV node, and ventricles. Because of their marked effect on conduction, these drugs strongly suppress PVCs, reducing or eliminating them in a large number of patients. All class Ic drugs are classified as pregnancy category C agents.

ENCAINIDE AND FLECAINIDE

Encainide (Enkaid) and flecainide (Tambocor) have many similar characteristics, and they are both chemical analogues of procainamide, with flecainide a fluorinated local anesthetic analogue of procainamide. Encainide decreases cardiac contractility and cardiac output less than does flecainide. A large, multicenter double-blind, placebo-controlled study, called the **Cardiac Arrhythmia Suppression Trial**, was conducted by the National Heart, Lung, and Blood Institute to determine whether the incidence of **sudden cardiac death** rate could be reduced in post-MI patients with asymptomatic non–life-threatening ectopy through the use of either encainide or flecainide. The findings showed that the excessive mortality and nonfatal cardiac arrest rates in patients treated with flecainide or encainide were actually comparable to or worse than those seen in patients who received placebo. Because of these findings, the FDA required that the labeling for flecainide and encainide be revised to indicate that their use should be limited to the treatment of documented life-threatening ventricular dysrhythmias such as sustained ventricular tachycardia. Treatment with either agent should be initiated in the hospital. These drugs are not indicated for the management of less severe dysrhythmias such as nonsustained ventricular tachycardia or frequent PVCs.

Although flecainide and encainide are better tolerated than quinidine or procainamide and more effective than mexiletine or tocainide, they are more proarrhythmic, and it is this proarrhythmic potential that limits their use to the management of life-threatening dysrhythmias. Flecainide has a negative inotropic effect and depresses LV function. Unlike flecainide, encainide is less likely to significantly depress LV function. Less serious, but more frequent noncardiac adverse effects include dizziness, visual disturbances, and dyspnea. Contraindications to their use include hypersensitivity, cardiogenic shock, second- or third-degree AV block, and non–life-threatening dysrhythmias.

Encainide and flecainide are both available as oral preparations. Encainide comes as 25-, 35-, and 50-mg capsules and flecainide as 50-, 100-, and 150-mg tablets. Common dosages are listed in the dosages table. Encainide is a pregnancy category B agent. Flecainide is a pregnancy category C agent.

⬡ PHARMACOKINETICS

HALF-LIFE	ONSET	PEAK	DURATION
Encainide 1-2 hr	Unknown	0.5-1.5 hr	Unknown
Flecainide; PO: 12-27 hr	Unknown	PO: 3 hr	Unknown

PROPAFENONE

Propafenone (Rythmol) is similar in action to flecainide and encainide. It reduces the fast inward sodium current in Purkinje fibers and to a lesser extent in myocardial fibers as well. Unlike other class I drugs, propafenone has mild beta-blocking effects. This may contribute to its overall effects on the conduction system. It is also believed to have calcium channel–blocking effects, which may contribute to propafenone's mild negative inotropic effects.

Like flecainide and encainide, propafenone's use is limited to the treatment of documented life-threatening ventricular dysrhythmias such as sustained ventricular tachycardia. Treatment should also be started while the patient is in the hospital. Unlike encainide and flecainide, however, propafenone can be used in patients with depressed LV function. It may be a better antidysrhythmic agent than disopyramide, procainamide, and quinidine in these patients. It should be used with caution in patients with congestive heart failure (CHF) because of its beta-blocking actions and its dose-dependent negative inotropic effects.

Propafenone is generally well tolerated. The most frequently reported adverse reaction is dizziness. Patients may also complain of a metallic taste, constipation, and headache, along with nausea and vomiting. These GI side effects may be reduced by taking the propafenone with food. Propafenone is contraindicated in patients with a known hypersensitivity to it, and in those with bradycardia, bronchial asthma, significant hypotension, uncontrolled CHF, cardiogenic shock, or various conduction disorders. It is available orally as 150- and 300-mg film-coated tablets. Common dosages are listed in the dosages table. Pregnancy category C.

⬡ PHARMACOKINETICS

HALF-LIFE	ONSET	PEAK	DURATION
2-10 hr	Unknown	3-5 hr	Unknown

CLASS II DRUGS

The class II antidysrhythmics are also known as the beta-blockers. These agents work by reducing or blocking sympathetic nervous system stimulation to the heart and the heart's conduction system. By doing this the beta-blockers prevent catecholamine-mediated actions on the heart. The resulting cardiovascular effects include a reduced heart rate, delayed AV node conduction, reduced myocardial contractility, and decreased myocardial automaticity. The pharmacologically induced effects of the beta-blockers are especially beneficial after an MI because of the many catecholamines released at this time, making the heart hyperirritable and predisposed to many types of dysrhythmias. The beta-blockers offer protection from these potentially very dangerous complications. Several studies have demonstrated a significant reduction in the incidence of sudden cardiac death after MI in patients treated with beta-blockers on an ongoing basis. This reduction is on the average of 25%.

Although there are several beta-blockers, only a handful are commonly used as antidysrhythmic drugs, and these are the ones described in the following drug profiles. The class II agents are classified as pregnancy category C agents.

ATENOLOL

Atenolol (Tenormin) is a cardioselective beta-blocker, which means that it preferentially blocks the beta$_1$-adrenergic receptors that are primarily located on the heart. Noncardioselective beta blockers not only block the beta$_1$-adrenergic receptors on the heart but also the beta$_2$-adrenergic receptors in the lungs, and could therefore exacerbate a preexisting case of asthma or chronic obstructive pulmonary disease. Besides atenolol's class II antidysrhythmic properties, it is also useful in the treatment of hypertension and angina.

Atenolol is contraindicated in patients with severe bradycardia, second- or third-degree heart block, CHF, cardiogenic shock, or a known hypersensitivity to it. Orally atenolol comes as 25-, 50-, and 100-mg tablets. Parenterally it comes as 0.5-mg/ml intravenous injections. Common dosages are listed in the dosages table. Pregnancy category C.

✹ PHARMACOKINETICS

HALF-LIFE	ONSET	PEAK	DURATION
PO: 6-7 hr	PO: 1 hr	PO: 2-4 hr	PO: ≥24 hr

⚓ ESMOLOL

Esmolol (Brevibloc) is a short-acting beta-blocker with pharmacologic and electrophysiologic effects on the heart's conduction system similar to those of atenolol. Esmolol is also a cardioselective beta-blocker that primarily and preferentially blocks the beta$_1$-adrenergic receptors on the heart. It is used in the acute treatment of supraventricular tachyarrhythmias or dysrhythmias that originate above the ventricles and are fast instead of slow. It is also used to control hypertension and tachyarrhythmias that develop after an acute MI.

Esmolol is contraindicated in patients with severe bradycardia, second- or third-degree heart block, CHF, cardiogenic shock, severe asthma, or a known hypersensitivity to it. Esmolol is only available parenterally as a concentrated 250-mg/ml injection for intravenous infusion and a 10-mg/ml intravenous injection. Common dosages are listed in the dosages table. Pregnancy category C.

✹ PHARMACOKINETICS

HALF-LIFE	ONSET	PEAK	DURATION
IV: 9 min	IV: very rapid	IV: rapid	IV: short

METOPROLOL

Metoprolol (Lopressor) is another cardioselective beta-blocker commonly given after an MI to reduce the risk of sudden cardiac death. It is also used in the treatment of hypertension and angina. It is available orally as 50-, 100-, and 200-mg extended-release tablets; and as 50- and 100-mg regular-release tablets. Parenterally it comes as a 1-mg/ml intravenous injection. In the treatment of hypertension it is combined with the thiazide diuretic hydrochlorothiazide in a product called *Lopressor HCT*. The contraindications to metoprolol use are the same as those of both atenolol and esmolol. Common dosages are listed in the dosages table. Pregnancy category C.

✹ PHARMACOKINETICS

HALF-LIFE	ONSET	PEAK	DURATION
PO: 3-4 hr	PO: 1 hr	PO: 2-4 hr	PO: 13-19 hr

PROPRANOLOL

Propranolol (Inderal) was one of the very first beta-blockers introduced into clinical practice, and this occurred in 1967. It was then primarily used in the treatment of dysrhythmias. Propranolol is a nonspecific beta-blocker that blocks both beta$_1$- and beta$_2$-adrenergic receptors on the heart and lungs. Its primary effect on the conduction system of the heart is the blockade of cardiac beta$_1$-adrenergic receptors, thereby preventing catecholamine-mediated stimulation of the heart. The resulting cardiovascular effects are a reduced heart rate, delayed AV node conduction, reduced myocardial contractility, and decreased myocardial automaticity. Propranolol is also believed to have membrane-stabilizing properties that may play a small role in its overall antidysrhythmic effect.

Because propranolol is the oldest of this class of drugs, there are now many indications for its use. Hypertension, angina, supraventricular dysrhythmias, ventricular tachycardia, the tachyarrhythmias associated with cardiac glycoside toxicity, hypertrophic subaortic stenosis, pheochromocytoma, thyrotoxicosis, migraines, post-MI, and essential tremor are just some of these. The contraindications to propranolol use are the same as atenolol's. It is available in both oral and parenteral dosage forms. Orally it is comes as 60-, 80-, 120-, and 160-mg extended-release capsules; 10-, 20-, 40-, 60-, 80-, and 90-mg tablets; and a 20–mg/5 ml and a 40–mg/5 ml oral solution. Parenterally propranolol comes as a 1-mg/ml injection. Common dosages are listed in the dosages table. Pregnancy category C.

PHARMACOKINETICS

HALF-LIFE	ONSET	PEAK	DURATION
IV: immediate release: 3-5 hr; sustained release: 8-11 hr	IV: 2 min PO: 30 min	IV: 15 min PO: 1-1½ hr	IV: 3-6 hr

SOTALOL

Sotalol (Betapace) is another nonselective beta-blocker that is used to treat dysrhythmias. It is unique in that it possesses antidysrhythmic properties similar to those of the class III agents such as amiodarone while simultaneously exerting beta-blocker or class II effects on the conduction system of the heart. In addition, sotalol has proarrhythmic properties similar to those of the class Ic agents, which means that while patients are taking sotalol, it can cause serious dysrhythmias such as torsades de pointes or a new ventricular tachycardia or fibriliation. For this reason, sotalol is usually reserved for the treatment of documented life-threatening ventricular dysrhythmias such as sustained ventricular tachycardia.

Contraindications to sotalol use include hypersensitivity to it, bronchial asthma, cardiogenic shock, and sinus bradycardia. Sotalol is available only orally as 80-, 160-, and 240-mg tablets. Common dosages are listed in the dosages table. Pregnancy category C.

PHARMACOKINETICS

HALF-LIFE	ONSET	PEAK	DURATION
PO: 12 hr	PO: 1-2 hr	PO: 2-4 hr	PO: 8-12 hr

CLASS III DRUGS

The class III agents consist of amiodarone and bretylium. These agents control dysrhythmias by inhibiting repolarization and markedly prolonging refractoriness and the APD. They are indicated for the management of life-threatening ventricular tachycardia or ventricular fibrillation that is resistant to other drug therapy. They have also been very effective in the treatment of sustained ventricular tachycardias. Both of these agents are classified as pregnancy category C agents.

BRETYLIUM

Bretylium (Bretylol) was initially marketed as an antihypertensive agent, but not much later its effects on the conduction system were noted. It has both a direct and an indirect effect on cardiac conduction. The direct effect prolongs the APD of the Purkinje fibers and ventricular myocardium and the ERP. The indirect effect is due to an adrenergic-blocking effect, in that bretylium accumulates in the nerve endings of the sympathetic nervous system, where it displaces norepinephrine. This results in a short-term rise in blood pressure, but after this, the further release of norepinephrine is blocked and ultimately the reuptake of norepinephrine is inhibited.

Bretylium is only available parenterally. It is used for the treatment of serious dysrhythmias such as life-threatening ventricular tachycardia or fibrillation. Therefore bretylium is most commonly used in intensive care unit settings in patients who do not respond to lidocaine, quinidine, procainamide, or disopyramide treatment. The major adverse effect associated with its use is postural hypotension, occurring in about 50% of patients. Other common side effects include nausea and vomiting. However, all of these side effects can be reduced by administering it by slow intravenous infusion. Bretylium is contraindicated in patients with a known hypersensitivity to it. It is only available parenterally as a 2- and 4-mg/ml injection for intravenous infusions and as a 50-mg/ml bolus injection. Common dosages are listed in the dosages table. Pregnancy category C.

PHARMACOKINETICS

HALF-LIFE	ONSET	PEAK	DURATION
4-17 hr	IV: 5 min	IV: rapid (<1 hr)	IV: 6-24 hr

AMIODARONE

Amiodarone (Cordarone) markedly prolongs the APD and the ERP in all cardiac tissues. Besides these dramatic effects it is also known to block both the alpha- and beta-adrenergic receptors of the sympathetic nervous system. Clinically it is one of the most effective antidysrhythmic agents for controlling supraventricular and ventricular dysrhythmias. It is indicated for the management of sustained ventricular tachycardia, ventricular fibrillation, and nonsustained ventricular tachycardia. It is reported to be effective in 40% to 60% of all patients with ventricular tachycardia. Recently it has shown promise in the management of difficult-to-treat or resistant atrial dysrhythmias.

Amiodarone has many unwanted adverse effects, and many of these can be attributed to its chemical properties. Amiodarone is very lipophilic, or "fat loving." Therefore it can penetrate and concentrate in the adipose tissue of any organ in the body, where it may cause unwanted effects. It also has iodine in its chemical structure. One organ that sequesters iodine from our diets is the thyroid gland. As a result amiodarone can cause either hypothyroidism or hyperthyroidism. Adverse reactions occur in approximately 75% of the patients treated with the agent, but the incidence and severity of these are more common in association with higher doses (those exceeding 400 mg/day) and prolonged therapy. The most common reaction is corneal microdeposits, which may cause visual halos, photophobia, and dry eyes. This occurs in virtually all adults who take the drug for more than 6 months.

The most serious adverse effect is pulmonary toxicity, which is fatal in about 10% of patients and involves a clinical syndrome of progressive dyspnea and cough accompanied by damage to the alveoli. The end result can be pulmonary fibrosis. Another serious complication of amiodarone therapy is that it too may not only treat the dysrhythmias but may also provoke them.

Amiodarone has an exceptionally long half-life, approaching many days. As a result, the therapeutic as well as any adverse effects of amiodarone may linger long after the drug has been discontinued. In fact, it may take as long as 2 to 3 months after the drug has been discontinued for some side effects to subside. For all these reasons, although very effective, amiodarone is typically considered a drug of last resort. Therapy is typically started in the hospital and closely monitored until the serum levels are within a therapeutic range.

Amiodarone is contraindicated in patients who have a known hypersensitivity to it, as well as in those with severe sinus bradycardia or second- or third-degree heart block. Amiodarone is currently only available orally as 200-mg tablets, but a parenteral formulation should be available in 1995. Common dosages are listed in the dosages table. Pregnancy category C.

❦ PHARMACOKINETICS

HALF-LIFE	ONSET	PEAK	DURATION
PO: 15-100 days	PO: 1-3 wk	PO: 2-10 hr	PO: 10-150 days

CLASS IV DRUGS

The class IV antidysrhythmic drugs are the calcium channel blockers (CCBs). Although there are more than nine such agents currently available, only a few are commonly used as antidysrhythmics. Besides their effectiveness as antidysrhythmics, the CCBs are effective in the treatment of hypertension and angina.

Verapamil and diltiazem are the two CCBs most commonly utilized for the treatment of dysrhythmias, specifically those that arise above the ventricles—paroxysmal supraventricular tachycardia (PSVT), and for controlling the ventricular response to atrial fibrillation and flutter by slowing conduction and prolonging refractoriness of the AV node (i.e., not allowing the ventricles to beat as fast). These agents block the slow inward flow of calcium ions into the slow (calcium) channels in cardiac conduction tissue. The conduction effects of these agents are limited to the atria and the AV node, where conduction is prolonged and the tissues are made more refractory to stimulation. These agents have little effect on the ventricular tissues.

DILTIAZEM

Diltiazem (Cardizem) is primarily indicated for the temporary control of a rapid ventricular response in a patient with atrial fibrillation or flutter and PSVT. Its use is contraindicated in the settings of hypersensitivity, acute MI, pulmonary congestion, Wolff-Parkinson-White syndrome, severe hypotension, cardiogenic shock, sick sinus syndrome, or second- or third-degree AV block. Diltiazem is available both orally and parenterally. Orally diltiazem comes as 30-, 60-, 90-, and 120-mg tablets; 60-, 90-, and 120-mg sustained-release, twice-a-day capsules; and 120-, 180-, 240-, and 300-mg controlled-delivery, once-a-day capsules. Parenterally diltiazem is available as a 5-mg/ml injection. Common dosages are listed in the dosages table. Pregnancy category C.

❦ PHARMACOKINETICS

HALF-LIFE	ONSET	PEAK	DURATION
3½-9 hr	30-60 min	2-3 hr	4-8 hr 12 hr*

*For extended-release product.

♃ VERAPAMIL

Verapamil (Calan, Isoptin, Verelan) has actions similar to those of diltiazem in that it also inhibits calcium ion influx across the slow calcium channels in cardiac conduction tissue. This results in dramatic effects on the AV node. Verapamil is used to prevent recurrent PSVT and to treat atrial flutter or fibrillation. It can also temporarily control a rapid ventricular response to these frequent atrial stimulations, usually decreasing the heart rate by at least 20%. Besides its use for the management of various dysrhythmias, verapamil is also used to treat angina, hypertension, and hypertrophic cardiomyopathy.

The contraindications that apply to diltiazem apply to verapamil as well, and it is also available both orally and parenterally. Orally it comes as 40-, 80-, and 120-mg film-coated tablets and 120-, 180-, and 240-mg extended-release tablets and capsules. Parenterally it comes as a 2.5-mg/ml injection for intravenous administration. Common dosages are listed in the dosages table. Pregnancy category C.

❋ PHARMACOKINETICS

HALF-LIFE	ONSET	PEAK	DURATION
2-3 hr	PO: 30 min	1-2 hr	8-40 hr
	IV: 3-5 min	Unknown	2 hr

UNCLASSIFIED ANTIDYSRHYTHMICS
ADENOSINE

Adenosine (Adenocard) is an unclassified antidysrhythmic agent. It is a naturally occurring nucleoside that slows the electrical conduction time through the AV node and is indicated for the conversion of PSVT to sinus rhythm. It is particularly useful for the treatment of PSVT that has failed to respond to verapamil or when a patient has coexisting conditions such as CHF, hypotension, or LV dysfunction that limit the use of verapamil. It is contraindicated in patients with second- or third-degree heart block, sick sinus syndrome, atrial flutter or fibrillation, or ventricular tachycardia, as well as in those with a known hypersensitivity to it. It is has an extremely short half-life of less than 10 seconds. For this reason, it is only administered intravenously and only as a fast IV push. It will frequently cause asystole for a period of seconds. All other side effects are minimal because of its very short duration of action. It is only available parenterally as a 3-mg/ml injection. Common dosages are listed in the dosages table. Pregnancy category C.

❋ PHARMACOKINETICS

HALF-LIFE	ONSET	PEAK	DURATION
<10 sec	1 min	Immediate	Very short

*N*URSING PROCESS

Because the four classes of antidysrhythmics produce a variety of effects on the action potential of the cardiac cell, they exert a major effect on cardiac electrophysiologic function. This diversity of therapeutic effect and the attendant side effects pose a special challenge to the nurse, who is responsible for ensuring the safe and efficacious use of these agents. Because the nursing process that applies to the administration of these agents varies for each of the four classes of agents, each process is discussed separately.

Class I Drugs

ASSESSMENT

Before administering any of the class I antidysrhythmics to a patient, the nurse must obtain a thorough drug and medical history. Contraindications to the administration of these drugs include a known hypersensitivity to them, CHF, complete heart block, hypotension, myasthenia gravis, urinary retention, hepatic or renal insufficiency, a congenitally prolonged QT interval (class Ia agents); second- or third-degree heart block, hypersensitivity to the local anesthetics lidocaine and tocainide, cardiogenic shock, and hypokalemia (class Ic agent).

Class Ia agents should be administered cautiously in patients with electrolyte imbalances, especially hypokalemia. Class Ib agents should be administered cautiously in patients with hepatic or renal disease, CHF, bradycardia, a markedly altered urinary pH (affects excretion), and weights of less than 50 kg (111 lbs), as well as in the elderly. The cautious administration of class Ic agents is required in patients with severe renal or liver disease, CHF, prolonged QT intervals, and blood dyscrasias.

Drugs that interact with the class I antidysrhythmics include the neuromuscular blockers, which interact with quinidine, procainamide, and disopyramide, resulting in increased skeletal muscle relaxation; the anticholinergic drugs, which results in an enhanced anticholinergic effect; coumarin anticoagulants, which interact with quinidine, resulting in hypothrombinemia; digoxin and quinidine, which results in increased serum digoxin levels; nifedipine, which interacts with quinidine, resulting in decreased serum quinidine levels; cimetidine, which interacts with quinidine, resulting in increased serum quinidine; anticonvulsants, which interact with quinidine or disopyramide, resulting in increased metabolism of these antidysrhythmics; and cimetidine, which interacts with procainamide, resulting in increased levels of the procainamide. In addition, an increased urinary pH will cause the serum levels of quinidine to be elevated.

Class Ib antidysrhythmic drugs interact with other antidysrhythmics and with lidocaine. Lidocaine toxicity may result from the concurrent administration of propranolol or cimetidine.

Class Ic agents interact with digoxin, which leads to an increase in the serum digoxin levels and digoxin toxicity, and with flecainide and alkalinizing drugs, which leads to a decrease in the urinary excretion of flecainide. (See Table 21-6 for a summary of the drug interactions that occur with the antidysrhythmics.)

NURSING DIAGNOSES

Nursing diagnoses related to the administration of type I antidysrhythmics include:

■ Altered tissue perfusion (decreased cardiac and pulmonary) related to the dysrhythmia.

■ Risk for injury to self related to side effects of the medications.

■ Knowledge deficit concerning disease and medication therapy.

PLANNING

Therapeutic goals appropriate for patients receiving class I antidysrhythmic agents include:

■ Patient will be free of further symptoms related to cardiac dysrythymias once therapy is initiated.

■ Patient will have improved tolerance to activity and improved general sense of well-being.

■ Patient will be free of complications associated with noncompliance or with sudden withdrawal of medication.

■ Patient will report any increase in the symptoms of the dysrhythmia.

■ Patient will demonstrate adequate knowledge of drug therapy and its side effects.

Outcome Criteria

Outcome criteria in patients receiving class I antidysrhythmics include:

■ Patient's dysrhythmia symptoms such as shortness of breath and chest pain will be alleviated by the medication therapy.

■ Patient will exhibit signs and symptoms of improved cardiac output, as evidenced by regular apical and radial pulses; vital signs within normal limits; and a decrease in weight, edema, crackles, and shortness of breath attributable to compliance with therapy.

■ Patient will state the importance of complying with the medication regimen and of coming in for follow-up visits with the physician (i.e., decreasing complications and manifestations of dysrhythmias).

■ Patient will state the common side effects of the medication such as constipation, dry mouth, and so on.

IMPLEMENTATION

The administration of class I antidysrhythmics requires some very specific nursing interventions. Initially the ECG and vital signs must be monitored closely in patients who are receiving these medications because, if the QT interval is prolonged by more than

50%, this may precipitate a variety of conduction disturbances. An IV pump is needed when administering procainamide intravenously, and when switching from IV to oral forms, the infusion should be continued for 2 hours after the start of the oral agent, or as prescribed. Solutions of lidocaine containing epinephrine should not be used except as a local anesthetic. See the teaching tips (below) and the box on home health care tips (following page) for patients receiving these agents.

Patient Teaching TIPS

Class I Antidysrhythmics

✔ Patients should be told to take medication without omissions but not to double up on doses to make up for missed doses. Patients should contact their physician if uncertain about what to do in the event of any missed or skipped doses.

✔ Patients should not crush or chew any of the oral sustained-release preparations.

✔ If patients should notice a tablet or capsule in their stool, they should know that this is usually just the wax matrix of the preparation that has not been absorbed and that the medication has been extracted in the intestines.

✔ Adverse reactions associated with the class Ia antidysrhythmics that patients should be aware of include ringing of the ears, anticholinergic effects such as dryness of the mouth and constipation, GI upset, headache, fever, light-headedness, blurred vision, and cinchonism, which results from a reaction to the source of quinidine, *Cinchona,* and includes headache, fever, and light-headedness. Class Ia antidysrhythmic toxicity is manifested by cardiac or respiratory arrest or by loss of consciousness, so careful administration at home is important and should be monitored with a calendar or some other means of dose identification.

✔ Adverse reactions associated with class Ib agents include confusion, tremors (shakiness), convulsions, light-headedness, hypotension, dizziness, tinnitus, double vision, lethargy, and sensations of cold. Class Ib toxicity is manifested by confusion or convulsions.

✔ Adverse reactions associated with class Ic agents include dizziness, headaches, fatigue, shakiness, CHF (shortness of breath, lethargy, decreased urine output, swelling of feet, and weight gain of 2 lbs [1 kg] or more in a week), GI upset, edema, and chest pain. Class Ic toxicity is manifested by bradycardia.

EVALUATION

Monitoring patients receiving class I antidysrhythmics is important in identifying the therapeutic as opposed to the adverse and toxic effects. The therapeutic effects include improved cardiac output, decreased chest discomfort, decreased fatigue, and improved vital signs, skin color, and urinary output and improvement in irregularities to normal rhythm. Adverse effects include bradycardia, dizziness, headache, cinchonism, chest pain, CHF, and peripheral edema. Toxic effects range from cardiac failure and bradycardia to CNS-related effects such as confusion or convulsions.

Class II Drugs

ASSESSMENT

Before administering any of the class II antidysrhythmics, the nurse needs to obtain a thorough drug and medical history. Contraindications to the administration of these drugs include a known hypersensitivity to them, asthma and other forms of chronic obstructive pulmonary disease, sinus bradycardia, second- or third-degree heart block, diabetes mellitus, and peripheral vascular disease. Drugs that interact with the class II agents propranolol and acebutolol hydrochloride include phenothiazines and antihypertensive agents, with hypotension the effect. Propranolol also interacts with cimetidine, resulting in decreased metabolism of the propranolol.

NURSING DIAGNOSES

Nursing diagnoses related to the administration of type II antidysrhythmics include:

- Altered tissue perfusion (cardiac and pulmonary) related to the dysrhythmias.
- Risk for injury to self related to side effects of the medications.
- Impaired gaseous exchange related to adverse reaction to the medications.
- Knowledge deficit concerning disease and medication therapy.

HOME HEALTH POINTS
Antidysrhythmics

- Patients taking antidysrhythmics at home need to be closely monitored by the home health care nurse or by the physician or other health care provider. This should include frequent measurements of the blood levels of the medication as well as frequent monitoring of the blood pressure and pulse. These measures are important, especially in the elderly, because of the toxic effects these agents can have.

- Patient education using pamphlets, posters, journals, and other printed, video, or audio (often available free of charge from pharmaceutical companies) material is encouraged. The patient should be given as much reference material as possible. It is important to provide education and supportive material and resources because of the toxic effects of the medicines, the often seriousness of the disease, and the polypharmacy that is frequently a part of the clinical picture in these patients.

- Make sure patients know to notify the physician or other health care provider of any worsening of their dysrhythmia, as well as any shortness of breath, edema, chest pain, dizziness, or syncope. They should also know to report any of the adverse reactions or possible signs of toxicity of the particular agent they are taking.

Patient Teaching TIPS

Class II Antidysrhythmics

✔ Patients should be told to take medication without omissions but not to double up on doses to make up for missed doses. Patients should contact their physician if uncertain about what to do in the event of any missed or skipped doses.

✔ Patients should not crush or chew any of the oral sustained-release preparations.

✔ Propranolol toxicity is manifested by bradycardia, bronchospasms, heart failure, and hypotension, and patients should report increased lethargy and shortness of breath, edema, a weight gain of 2 lbs or more in a week, cough, decreased urinary output, dizziness, syncopal (fainting) spells, or heart palpitations to their physician.

✔ Oral forms of propranolol hydrochloride should be taken before meals and at bedtime, as ordered by the physician (i.e., if taken 3-4 times a day).

✔ Patients should always take the drug after counting their radial pulse for 1 full minute. If the pulse is less than 60 beats/min, they should notify their physician.

PLANNING AND OUTCOME CRITERIA

The therapeutic goals and outcome criteria in patients receiving any of the class II antidysrhythmic agents are the same as those cited for the class I agents.

IMPLEMENTATION

The administration of any of the class II antidysrhythmics requires some very specific nursing interventions. Initially the ECG and vital signs must be closely monitored in patients receiving these medications because of the cardiovascular adverse effects, such as hypotension, bradycardia, and AV blocks, they can precipitate. These problems usually occur when the drug is first given. Patients taking propranolol should be cautioned to report the appearance of any shortness of breath or skin rash. Should the parenteral solution of any of these drugs appear discolored or contain particulate matter, it should be discarded. IV solutions should be administered over a 3-minute period, especially in elderly patients, so as to minimize the risk of adverse effects. Patients should also be cautioned not to skip doses. For more patient teaching tips, see p. 295. Home health care tips have also been given on p. 295.

EVALUATION

The monitoring of patients receiving any of the class II antidysrhythmics is important in identifying both the therapeutic effects and the adverse and toxic effects. The therapeutic effects include improved cardiac output, decreased chest discomfort, decreased fatigue, regular pulse rate or improvement in irregularities, and improved vital signs, skin color, and urinary output. Adverse effects include bradycardia, dizziness, headache, and peripheral edema. Toxic effects consist of cardiac failure, bradycardia, bronchospasms, hypotension, and conduction problems.

Class III Drugs

ASSESSMENT

Before administering either of the class III antidysrhythmic agents, bretylium and amiodarone, the nurse should collect data regarding the patient's medication history, present and past medical history, drug allergies, and specific laboratory test results. A very thorough assessment is crucial to the safe use of these antidysrhythmics because of the adverse reactions patients can have to them. In fact, it is because of these severe adverse reactions that they are not the first choice for antidysrhythmic therapy. Amiodarone must be administered cautiously in patients who have preexisting bradycardia, conduction or sinus node disorders, severely depressed or compromised ventricular function, or marked cardiomegaly. Bretylium must be administered cautiously in patients with aortic stenosis, pulmonary hypertension, or digitalis-induced dysrhythmias. Drugs they can interact with include digoxin, which results in increased digoxin levels, and warfarin, which results in increased clotting times with hypoprothrombinemia.

NURSING DIAGNOSES

Nursing diagnoses related to the administration of type III antidysrhythmics include:
- Altered tissue perfusion (decreased cardiac and pulmonary) related to the dysrhythmia.
- Risk for injury to self related to side effects of the medications.
- Impaired gaseous exchange related to adverse reaction to the medications.
- Diarrhea related to adverse reaction to the medications.
- Knowledge deficit concerning disease and medication therapy.

PLANNING AND OUTCOME CRITERIA

The therapeutic goals and outcome criteria in patients receiving either of the class III antidysrhythmic agents are the same as those cited for the class I agents.

IMPLEMENTATION

There are some very specific nursing interventions called for in patients receiving either of the class III antidysrhythmics. The ECG should be monitored in patients who are initially receiving these medications or having their doses altered. In addition, blood pressure and other vital signs need to be monitored frequently, especially in those receiving bretylium. Emergency resuscitation equipment should be available during therapy because of the severe hypotension, bradycardia, and other types of dysrhythmias that can arise. IV doses of bretylium are given as an IV push delivered over 1 minute. For patient teaching tips see p. 297. Home health care tips have been given on p. 295.

EVALUATION

Monitoring patients receiving class III antidysrhythmics is important for identifying both the therapeutic effects and the side and toxic effects. The therapeutic effects include improved cardiac output, more regular rhythm, decreased chest discomfort, decreased fatigue, and improved vital signs, skin color, and urinary output. Adverse effects include peripheral neuropathies, extrapyramidal symptoms, headache, fatigue, lethargy, dizziness (bretylium use only), bradycardia, hypotension, dysrhythmias, severe orthostatic hypotension (bretylium use only), microdeposits on the cornea with visual disturbances, hypothyroidism or hyperthyroidism, nausea, vomiting, constipation, hepatic dysfunction with abnormal liver enzyme activity, electrolyte imbalances, photosensitivity, blue-gray skin color changes, severe pulmonary changes with development of pneumonitis, alveolitis with high doses, pulmonary fibrosis, and pulmonary muscle weakness. Patients' thyroid function should be monitored carefully during therapy so that abnormal function can be

identified before any further adverse effects appear. Toxic effects include hypotension or hypertension and bradycardia.

Class IV Drugs

ASSESSMENT

Before administering the class IV antidysrhythmic agents verapamil and diltiazem, the nurse should collect data on the patient's medication history, present and past medical history, drug allergies, and specific laboratory results. Cautious administration of this agent is warranted in patients with hypotension, CHF, sick sinus syndrome, AV conduction disturbances, or hepatic impairment. Indications for its use include PSVT with rapid ventricular response rates. Drugs that interact with it include other antidysrhythmics and antihypertensive agents, which enhance the risk of hypotension and heart failure; digoxin, which increases the digoxin levels and causes digitalis toxicity; and highly protein bound drugs such as hydantoin, aspirin, sulfonamide antibiotics, and sulfonylureas, which result in the adverse effects of either the verapamil, the diltiazem, or the other medication.

Patient Teaching TIPS

Class III Antidysrhythmics

✔ Patients should be told to take medication without omissions but to not double up on doses to make up for missed doses. They should contact their physician if uncertain about what to do in the event of any missed or skipped doses.

✔ Patients should use sunscreen products when out in the sun because of the photosensitivity (increased risk of sunburn with minimal exposure) these agents cause. They should report any unusual tingling of the skin that is followed by blistering or erythematous (reddening) reactions.

✔ Patients should contact their physician should they exhibit any of the following signs and symptoms while receiving amiodarone: lethargy, weight gain, cool and dry skin, bradycardia, hypotension, or intolerance to cold (indicative of hypothyroidism associated with the therapy); or nervousness, palpitations, weight loss, warm and moist skin, and tachycardia (indicative of the hyperthyroidism associated with the therapy).

✔ Side effects of these drugs include numbness and tingling of the extremities, uncontrolled shaking of the head and hands, headache, weakness, fatigue and loss of energy, dizziness, fainting spells (especially with changes of position from lying to standing or sitting to standing or sudden position changes such as stooping over), visual problems, nausea, vomiting, constipation, sunburn (even with very limited sun exposure), blue-gray skin discoloration, or cough.

Patient Teaching TIPS

Class IV Antidysrhythmics

✔ Patients should be told to take medication without omissions but to not double up on doses to make up for missed doses. They should contact their physician if uncertain about what to do in the event of any missed or skipped doses.

✔ Patients should know the various drugs that interact with class IV agents: digoxin, antihypertensives, other antidysrhythmics, sulfonamides (i.e., Septra, Bactrim), sulfonylureas (oral antidiabetic agents), aspirin-containing drugs or aspirin products, phenytoin, coumarin.

✔ Patients should be aware of the adverse effects of diltiazem: dizziness, fatigue, headache, transient hypotension, heart failure (edema or swelling, shortness of breath, cough, palpitations, decreased urine output, and lethargy), and constipation. Signs and symptoms of toxicity include bradycardia (pulse, <60 beats min), heart failure, palpitations and skipped heartbeats, and hypotension.

TAKE HOME POINTS

Dysrhythmias and Dysrhythmic Agents

- Any disturbance or abnormality in a normal pattern of the heartbeat.
- Antidysrhythmic drugs are used to correct dysrhythmias.
- Antidysrhythmics may cause dysrhythmias and for this reason are called *proarrhythmic*.

Mechanisms of Antidysrhythmic Agents

- *Class I:* Membrane-stabilizing agents.
- *Class II:* Beta-adrenergic blockers; depress phase 4 depolarization.
- *Class III:* Prolong repolarization in phase 3.
- *Class IV:* Depress phase 4 depolarization and prolong repolarization of phases 1 and 2.

Vaughan Williams Classification

- Most commonly used system to classify antidysrhythmic drugs.
- Groups drugs according to where and how they affect cardiac cells.
- Broken down into four main classes: class Ia (quinidine), Ib (lidocaine), and Ic (flecainide); class II (beta-blockers); class III (bretylium, amiodarone, and sotalol), and class IV (calcium channel blockers).

Sodium-Potassium ATPase Pump

- Mechanism for transporting sodium and potassium ions across cell membranes against an opposing concentration gradient.
- Energy for this transport system is obtained from the hydrolysis of adenosine triphosphate by means of an enzyme called *adenosine triphosphatase* (ATPase).
- Cardiac glycosides (digoxin) work by inhibiting this pump.

Conduction System of the Heart

- SA (sinoatrial) node → AV (atrioventricular) node → His-Purkinje cells.
- All cells in these areas have what is known as *automaticity* (they can depolarize spontaneously).

- The SA node is the pacemaker because it can spontaneously depolarize easier and faster than the others.

Action Potential

- An electrical impulse consisting of a self-propagating series of polarizations and depolarizations.
- Caused by ions (sodium and potassium) leaking into or out of a cardiac cell.
- Responsible for the release of calcium into the myocardial actin and myosin.
- Therefore responsible for coupling excitation with contraction.
- An electrical phenomenon (depolarization) coupled with a physiologic phenomenon (heart muscle contraction).

Nursing Considerations

- Some of the classes of antidysrhythmics are more toxic than others, but astute nursing assessment and close monitoring are required for all.
- Close monitoring requires ECGs, but heart rate, blood pressure, heart rhythms, general well-being, skin color, temperature, and heart and breath sounds are also important factors.
- It is important to assess the plasma drug levels and to check for possible drug interactions and certain medical conditions before the use of antidysrhythmics.
- Serum potassium levels should be measured before the initiation of therapy.
- Blood pressure, pulse rate, and intake and output amounts should all be measured and documented before the initiation of therapy.
- The therapeutic response to antidysrhythmics includes a decrease in blood pressure in hypertensive patients, a decrease in edema, and a regular pulse rate or pulse rate without major irregularities or improved regularity as opposed to the irregularity that existed before therapy.
- Patient education about the dosage schedule and the side effects to report to the physician is important to safe and effective therapy.

NURSING DIAGNOSES

Nursing diagnoses related to the administration of type IV antidysrhythmics include:

- Altered tissue perfusion (decreased cardiac and pulmonary) related to the dysrhythmias.
- Risk for injury to self related to side effects of the medications.
- Imparied gaseous exchange related to adverse reaction to the medications.

- Diarrhea related to adverse reaction to the medications.
- Altered body image related to changes in body and sexual integrity related to adverse reactions to the medications.
- Knowledge deficit concerning disease and medication therapy.

PLANNING AND OUTCOME CRITERIA

The therapeutic goals and outcome criteria in patients receiving a class IV antidysrhythmic agent are the same as those cited for the class I agents.

IMPLEMENTATION

As with the other classes of antidysrhythmics, there are some very specific nursing interventions called for in patients receiving a class IV antidysrhythmic. Patients who are receiving such an agent initially or having their doses altered must be monitored by ECG. In addition, blood pressure and other vital signs need to be monitored frequently. IV bolus doses should be administered over a 2-minute period, but this should be done over 3 minutes in elderly patients to minimize the adverse effects that can arise in these patients. It is crucial to remember that verapamil and beta-blockers cannot be administered intravenously at the same time or within a few hours of each other. See p. 297 for patient teaching tips. Home health care tips have been given on p. 295.

EVALUATION

It is important to monitor patients receiving a class IV antidysrhythmic to identify both the therapeutic effects and the side and toxic effects. The therapeutic effects include improved cardiac output, decreased chest discomfort, decreased fatigue, and improved vital signs, skin color, and urinary output. The adverse effects include bradycardia, CHF, hypotension, AV conduction disorders, ventricular asystole, peripheral edema, and constipation. Toxic effects include hypotension, bradycardia, heart failure, and conduction disorders.

Critical Thinking ACTIVITIES

1. J.K. is a 68-year-old man who has undergone coronary artery bypass grafting 1 day before. Some irregular heartbeats (dysrhythmias) have developed, and he has been put on procainamide, infused at a rate of 4 mg/min. The nephrologist is concerned about the total volume your patient is receiving because his urine output is very low and asks you to determine how much fluid the patient is receiving a day from his procainamide infusion. The standard procainamide concentration at your hospital is 1 mg/ml.
   a. How many milliliters of fluid is J.K. receiving from his procainamide infusion per day?
   b. The nephrologist would like to keep J.K.'s fluid intake to less than 1000 ml/day. What concentration will accomplish this: 1, 2, 4, or 8 mg/ml?
2. What is the nature of the therapeutic response you would expect in a patient prescribed a diuretic and antidysrhythmic to treat CHF? Explain your answer.

BIBLIOGRAPHY

Albanese J, Nutz P: *Mosby's 1995 nursing drug cards*, St Louis, 1995, Mosby.

Berry SL, Schleicher CA: Adjusting the beat: what to teach about antiarrhythmics, *Am J Nurs* 92:28, 1992.

Cardiovascular supplement, *US Pharm* 16(3), 1991.

Donnelly AJ: Part I: antiarrhythmic agents use in the surgical patient [Pharmacist's corner], *AORN J* 53:1261, 1991.

Fleg JL, Marcus FI, Podrid PJ: Managing arrhythmias in the elderly, *Patient Care* 24(7):31, 43, 53, 1990.

Grant AO: On the mechanism of action of antiarrhythmic agents, *Am Heart J* 123:1130, 1992.

Johnson KB: *Harriet Lane handbook*, ed 13, St Louis, 1993, Mosby.

Keen JH: *Mosby's Critical care and emergency drug reference*, St Louis, 1994, Mosby.

Knoben JE, Anderson PO: *Handbook of critical drug data*, ed 6, Hamilton, Ill, 1988, Drug Intelligence Publications.

McEvoy GK: *AHFS drug information*, Bethesda, Md, 1994, American Society of Hospital Pharmacists.

Nattel S: Comparative mechanisms of action of antiarrhythmic drugs, *Am J Cardiol* 72(16):13F, 1993.

Ravid S: Antiarrhythmic drug therapy in congestive heart failure: indications and complications, *Postgrad Med* 90(8):99, 1991.

Weiner B: Hemodynamic effects of antidysrhythmic drugs, *J Cardiovasc Nurs* 5(4):39, 1991.

Chapter 22

Antianginal Agents

Objectives

When you reach the end of this chapter, you will be able to:

1 Define angina.

2 Explain how cellular ischemia is responsible for causing angina.

3 Discuss how antianginal agents such as nitrates, beta-blockers, and calcium channel blockers decrease anginal pain.

4 Identify the various dosage forms of nitrates, beta-blockers, and calcium channel blockers, along with their indications, advantages, and cautions.

5 Develop a nursing care plan with patient education guidelines and expected outcomes as it relates to the administration and treatment of angina with nitrates, nitrites, beta-blockers, and calcium channel blockers.

6 Evaluate the therapeutic versus the adverse and toxic effects of the different antianginal agents.

CHAPTER OUTLINE

Angina and Coronary Artery Disease

Antianginal Drugs

Nitrates/Nitrites
   Mechanism of action
   Drug effects
   Therapeutic uses
   Side effects and adverse effects
   Interactions
   Dosages

Drug Profiles
   ⬇ Nitroglycerin
   Isosorbide Dinitrate
   Isosorbide Mononitrate
   Pentaerythrital Tetranitrate

Beta-blockers
   Mechanism of action
   Drug effects
   Therapeutic uses
   Side effects and adverse effects
   Interactions
   Dosages

Drug Profiles
   Atenolol
   ⬇ Metoprolol
   Nadolol
   Propranolol

Calcium Channel Blockers
   Mechanism of action
   Drug effects
   Therapeutic uses
   Side effects and adverse effects
   Interactions
   Dosages

Drug Profiles
   Diltiazem
   ⬇ Nifedipine
   Verapamil

Nursing Process
Assessment
Nursing Diagnoses
Planning
   Outcome criteria
Implementation
Evaluation

Glossary

Angina pectoris (an ji′nə, an′jə nə\pek to′ ris) Chest pain occurring when the level of oxygen and energy-rich nutrients in blood is insufficient to meet the demands of the heart. (p. 301)

Chronic stable angina Chest pain that has as its primary cause atherosclerosis. (p. 301)

Coronary arteries Arteries that deliver oxygen to the heart muscle. (p. 301)

Coronary artery disease Any one of the abnormal conditions that can affect the arteries of the heart and produce various pathologic effects, especially a reduced supply of oxygen and nutrients to the myocardium. (p. 301)

Ischemia (is ke′ me ə) Poor blood supply to an organ. (p. 301)

Ischemic heart disease Poor blood supply to the heart. (p. 301)

Reflex tachycardia (tak′ ĭ kahr′ de ə) A rapid heart sinus rhythm caused by a variety of autonomic nervous system effects, such as blood pressure changes, fever, or emotional stress. (p. 303)

Unstable angina Early stage of progressive coronary artery disease. (p. 301)

Vasospastic angina (vas′ o spas′ tik) Ischemia-induced myocardial chest pain caused by spasms of the coronary arteries. (p. 301)

Angina and Coronary Artery Disease

The heart is a very efficient organ but a very demanding one in an aerobic sense because it requires a large supply of oxygen to meet the incredible demand placed on it. Pumping blood to all the tissues and organs of the body is a large job. The heart's much-needed oxygen supply is delivered to the heart muscle by means of the **coronary arteries**. However, when the supply of oxygen and energy-rich nutrients in blood is insufficient to meet the demands of the heart, the heart muscle, or myocardium, aches. This is called **angina pectoris** or chest pain. Poor blood supply to an organ is referred to as **ischemia**. When the organ involved is the heart, the condition is called **ischemic heart disease**.

Ischemic heart disease is the number one killer in the population of the United States today, and the primary cause is disease of the coronary arteries resulting from atherosclerosis. When atherosclerotic plaques form in the lumens (i.e., channels) of these vessels, they become narrow and the amount of oxygen and energy-rich nutrients needed for the heart to meet the demands placed on it is decreased. This disorder is called coronary artery disease, and the final result of **coronary artery disease**, and of ischemic heart disease, is a myocardial infarction, or heart attack. It occurs when blood flow through the coronary arteries to the myocardium is completely blocked, so that the heart muscle cannot receive any of the substances necessary for normal function. If this process is not reversed immediately, that area of the heart will die and become necrotic and nonfunctioning.

The rate at which the heart pumps and the strength of each heart beat (contractility) also place oxygen demands on this organ. There are many substances and situations that can increase heart rate and contractility and thus increase oxygen demand. Some of these substances are caffeine, exercise, and stress. These substances or situations result in stimulation of the sympathetic nervous system (SNS), which results in increased heart rate and contractility. In an already overburdened heart such as one in a patient with coronary artery disease, this can worsen the balance between myocardial oxygen supply and demand and result in angina. Some drugs that are used to treat angina are aimed at correcting the imbalance between myocardial oxygen supply and demand by decreasing heart rate and contractility. Beta blockers and calcium channel blockers are two examples.

The pain of angina results from the following process. Under ischemic conditions when the myocardium is deprived of oxygen, the heart shifts to anaerobic metabolism to meet its energy needs. One of the by-products of anaerobic metabolism is lactic acid. The accumulation of lactic acid and other metabolic by-products causes the pain receptors surrounding the heart to be stimulated, producing the heart pain known as angina. It is the same pathophysiologic mechanism responsible for causing the soreness in skeletal muscles after vigorous exercise.

There are three classic types of chest pain, or angina pectoris. **Chronic stable angina** has as its primary cause atherosclerosis. *Classic angina* and *effort angina* are other names for it. Chronic stable angina can be triggered by either exertion or stress (cold, fear, or emotions). Smoking or the consumption of alcohol, coffee, or drugs that stimulate the sympathetic nervous system can exacerbate it. The pain of chronic stable angina is commonly intense but subsides within 15 minutes with either rest or drug therapy. **Unstable angina** is usually the early stage of progressive coronary artery disease. It often culminates in myocardial infarction in subsequent years, and for this reason, unstable angina is also called *preinfarction angina*. Another term for this type of angina is *crescendo angina* because the pain increases in severity and in the frequency of attacks. In the later stages, pain may even occur while the patient is at rest. **Vasospastic angina** results from spasms of the layer of smooth muscle that surrounds the atherosclerotic coronary arteries. This pain often happens at rest and without any precipitating cause. It does, however, seem to follow a regular pattern, usually occurring at the same time of day. This type of angina is also called *Prinzmetal's angina* or *variant angina*. Dysrhythmias and ECG changes often accompany these anginal attacks.

Table 22-1 | Antianginal Agents: Therapeutic Effects

THERAPEUTIC EFFECT	NITRATES	BETA-BLOCKERS*	CALCIUM CHANNEL BLOCKERS		
			NIFEDIPINE	VERAPAMIL	DILTIAZEM
Supply					
Ischemia	↓↓	↑	↓↓↓	↓↓↓	↓↓↓
Contractility	↓↓↓	↑	↓↓	0↑	0
Duration of diastole	0	↑↑↑	0↑	↑↑↑	↑↑
Demand					
Preload†	↓↓↓	↑	↓0	0	0↓
Afterload	↓	↓	↓↓↓	↓↓	↓↓
Contractility	0	↓↓↓	↓↓↓	↓↓	↓
Heart rate	0	↓↓↓	0	↓↓	↓↓

↓ = decrease; ↑ = increase; 0 = little or no effect.
*In particular those that are cardioselective and do not have intrinsic sympathomimetic activity (ISA).
†*Preload* is pressure in the heart caused by blood volume. The nitrates effectively move part of this blood out of the heart and into blood vessels thereby decreasing preload or filling pressure.

Antianginal Drugs

Recent advances in pharmacotherapy have resulted in the development of a host of new antianginal agents that have been approved for clinical use. The three main classes of drugs used to treat angina pectoris are the nitrates/nitrites, the beta-blockers, and the calcium channel blockers, and their various therapeutic effects are summarized in Table 22-1. There are three main therapeutic objectives of antianginal drug therapy. It must (1) minimize the frequency of attacks and decrease the duration and intensity of the anginal pain; (2) improve the patient's functional capacity with as few side effects as possible; and (3) prevent or delay the worst possible outcome, myocardial infarction. The object of antianginal drug therapy is to increase blood flow to ischemic myocardium or to decrease myocardial oxygen demand, or to accomplish both. Figure 22-1 illustrates how drug therapy works to alleviate angina.

NITRATES/NITRITES

Nitrates, and in particular nitroglycerin, have long been the mainstay of both the prophylaxis and treatment for angina and other cardiac problems. This class of antianginal agents was first discovered by Sir Thomas Lauder Brunton in England, who noted that amyl nitrite was just as effective as venesection in the management of angina. A few years later, a chemically related substance, glyceryl trinitrate (nitroglycerin),

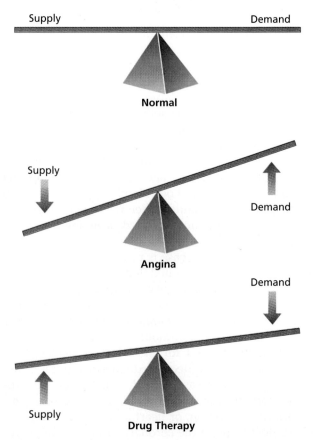

▼ **FIG. 22-1** Benefit of drug therapy for angina with increasing oxygen supply and decreasing oxygen demands.

was successfully isolated and used for this purpose. Today there are several chemical derivatives of these early precursors, all of which are organic nitrate esters. They are available in a wide variety of preparations, including sublingual, buccal, chewable, and oral tablets; capsules; ointments; patches; inhalable sprays; and intravenous solutions. Following is a list of the rapid- and long-acting nitrates available for clinical use:

> Rapid-acting agents
>   Amyl nitrite
>   Nitroglycerin
> Long-acting agents
>   Erythrityl tetranitrate
>   Pentaerythrital tetranitrate
>   Isosorbide dinitrate
>   Isosorbide mononitrate

Mechanism of Action

The nitrates dilate all blood vessels, but they primarily affect the blood vessels of the venous circulation, though at low doses they do have slight arterial vasodilator properties. This venodilation is the result of relaxation of the smooth muscle that surrounds veins. Nitrates also have a potent dilating effect on the coronary arteries.

Drug Effects

If the nitrate-induced venodilation just described occurs rapidly, this causes the cardiovascular system to overcompensate and increase its heart rate, a condition referred to as **reflex tachycardia**. This occurs because the venodilation causes most of the blood to be in the venous circulation and out of the heart, with the result that the heart falsely senses there has been a dramatic loss of blood volume. If this were true, it would be appropriate for the heart to accelerate its rate to move the smaller volume of blood more quickly throughout the body. The heart soon realizes, however, that there has not been a loss of blood volume but that the volume of blood missing in the heart is now in the periphery (e.g., venous system) and slows its rate back to normal.

Therapeutic Uses

The nitrate-induced vasodilation, and hence the reflex tachycardia that leads to slowing of the heart rate, produces many therapeutic effects (see Table 22-1). By causing venodilation, the nitrates bring about a decrease in venous return and in turn a lower left ventricular end-diastolic volume (preload) and pressure. Left ventricular systolic wall tension is also reduced, and myocardial oxygen demand is thereby lowered.

The nitrates cause both large and small coronary vessels to dilate. Often this causes blood to be redistributed and therefore oxygen to be delivered to previously ischemic tissue (myocardium). The nitrates also alleviate coronary artery spasms (vasospastic angina). In addition, coronary arteries that are diseased and have been narrowed by atherosclerosis can also be dilated as long as there is smooth muscle surrounding the coronary artery. Exercise-induced constriction or spasms of atherosclerotic coronary arteries can be reversed or even prevented by nitrates.

Side Effects and Adverse Effects

The nitrates are well tolerated and most side effects are usually transient and involve the cardiovascular system. The most frequent undesirable effect is headache, which usually diminishes in intensity and frequency soon after the start of therapy. Other cardiovascular effects include tachycardia and postural hypotension. Methemoglobinemia is an extremely rare adverse effect and usually occurs in patients with an inherited genetic propensity for the condition. Topical nitrate dosage forms can produce various contact dermatitides, but these are actually reactions to the dosage delivery system and not to the drug (nitroglycerin).

Tolerance to the nitrates' antianginal effects can occur in some patients.

Interactions

Nitrate antianginal drugs can produce additive hypotensive effects when taken in combination with alcohol, beta-blockers, calcium channel blockers, or phenothiazines.

Dosages

The organic nitrates are available in an array of forms and doses. See the dosages table on the following page for more information.

DRUG PROFILES

⚓ NITROGLYCERIN

Nitroglycerin is the prototypical nitrate and is made by many pharmaceutical companies, so it goes by many trade names, some of which are Nitro-Bid, Nitrostat, and Nitrong. It has traditionally been the most

DOSAGES

SELECTED ANTIANGINAL NITRATE CORONARY VASODILATORS

AGENT	PHARMACOLOGIC CLASS	DOSAGE RANGE	PURPOSE
⚓Nitroglycerin (Nitro-Bid, Nitrostat, Nitrong, others)		*Adult* Ointment: 1-5 in ribbon q8h PO: 2.5-6.5 mg q8-12h Sublingual: 0.15-0.6 mg prn Transdermal: apply one patch q24h	
Isosorbide dinitrate (Isordil, Sorbitrate, Dilatrate SR)	Antianginal nitrate coronary vasodilator	*Adult* Chewable/sublingual: 2.5-10 mg prn PO: 5-30 mg 3-4/day or more and 40-80 mg q8-12h for sustained-release formulations	Angina
Isosorbide mononitrate (Imdur, Monoket, ISMO)		*Adult* PO: 20 mg bid given 7 hr apart and 60-120 mg/day for sustained-release formulations	
Pentaerythrital tetranitrate (Peritrate)		*Adult* PO: 10-40 mg 3-4 times/day and 30-45 mg once/day for sustained-release formulations	

important drug used in the symptomatic treatment of ischemic heart conditions such as angina. Nitroglycerin is contraindicated in patients with a known hypersensitivity to it, and in those suffering from increased intracranial pressure, inadequate cerebral perfusion, constrictive pericarditis, pericardial tamponade, severe hypotension, or severe anemia. It is classified as a pregnancy category C agent.

When nitroglycerin is given orally, it goes to the liver to be metabolized before it can be active in the body. During this process a very large amount of the nitroglycerin is removed from the circulation. This is called a large first-pass effect. For this reason, nitroglycerin is administered by many other routes to bypass the first-pass effect. It also comes in many different formulations and has proved useful for the treatment of a variety of cardiovascular conditions. The sublingual and buccal routes of administration are employed for the treatment of chest pain or angina of acute onset or for the prevention of angina when patients find themselves in situations likely to provoke an attack. These routes are advantageous for ameliorating these acute conditions because the area under the tongue and inside the cheek is highly vascular, which means that the nitroglycerin is absorbed quickly and directly into the bloodstream and hence its therapeutic effects occur rapidly. Sublingual nitroglycerin is available as 0.3-, 0.4-, 0.6-mg tablets. Buccal extended-release tablets are available in 1-, 2-, and 3-mg doses. Nitroglycerin also comes as a 0.4–mg/per metered dose aerosol that is sprayed under the tongue.

Nitroglycerin is available in an intravenous form that is used for blood pressure control in the perioperative hypertensive patient as well as for the treatment of ischemic pain, congestive heart failure (CHF), or the pulmonary edema associated with acute myocardial infarction. These intravenous infusions come in concentrations of 0.5 or 5 mg/ml. Oral and topical dosage formulations are used for the long-term prophylactic management of angina pectoris. The oral forms are available as 2.5-, 6.5-, 9-, and 13-mg extended-release capsules and as 2.6- and 6.5-mg extended-release tablets. Topical formulations offer the same advantages as the sublingual and buccal formulations in that they also bypass the liver and the first-pass effect. They also allow for the continuous slow delivery of nitroglycerin, which supplies a steady dose of nitroglycerin to the patient. The topical delivery forms come as a 2% ointment or as 0.1-, 0.2-, 0.3-, 0.4- and 0.6-mg/hr patches that supply 24 hours' worth of nitroglycerin. See the dosages table above for the recommended dosages.

⬡ PHARMACOKINETICS

HALF-LIFE	ONSET	PEAK	DURATION
1-4 min	2-3 min	Unknown	30-60 min

ISOSORBIDE DINITRATE

Isosorbide dinitrate (Isordil, Sorbitrate, Dilatrate SR) is an organic nitrate and therefore a powerful explosive.

It exerts the same effects as the other nitrates. When isosorbide dinitrate is metabolized in the liver, it is broken down into two active metabolites, both of which have the same therapeutic actions as the isosorbide dinitrate itself. Isosorbide dinitrate is used for the acute relief of angina pectoris, for prophylaxis in situations likely to provoke angina attacks (e.g., exercise), and for the long-term prophylaxis of angina pectoris. The contraindications to isosorbide dinitrate use are the same as nitroglycerin's, and it is also a pregnancy category C agent. Isosorbide dinitrate is only available orally as 40-mg extended-release capsules and tablets; 5-, 10-, 20-, 30-, and 40-mg tablets; 5- and 10-mg chewable tablets; and 2.5-, 5-, and 10-mg sublingual tablets. Refer to the dosages table on the previous page for the recommended dosages.

PHARMACOKINETICS

HALF-LIFE	ONSET	PEAK	DURATION
Variable	1 hr	Unknown	4-6 hr

ISOSORBIDE MONONITRATE

Isosorbide mononitrate (Imdur, Monoket, ISMO) is one of the two active metabolites of isosorbide dinitrate, but it has no active metabolites. As a result of these qualities, it produces a more consistent, steady therapeutic response, with less variation in the response within the same patient and between patients. Its contraindications are the same as nitroglycerin's, and it is also a pregnancy category C agent. It is only available in oral formulations: two regular-release products, ISMO and Monoket, and a sustained-release form, Indur. The ISMO and Monoket are taken twice a day, with 7 hours the recommended interval between the first and second dose. This 7-hour interval is believed to delay the development of nitrate tolerance, a limitation to long-term nitrate therapy. ISMO is available as 20-mg tablets and Monoket as 10- and 20-mg tablets. Imdur is available as a 60-mg tablet and is taken only once a day. Refer to the dosages table on the previous page for the dosage recommendations.

PHARMACOKINETICS

HALF-LIFE	ONSET	PEAK	DURATION
5 hr	15-30 min	30-60 min	Unknown

PENTAERYTHRITAL TETRANITRATE

Pentaerythrital tetranitrate (Peritrate) is metabolized to several active metabolites and is recommended only for the long-term prophylactic management of angina. It is not effective for the acute treatment of anginal attacks. It must be taken three to four times a day, and patient response varies considerably. For these reasons it and erythrityl tetranitrate are seldom used. They offer few benefits compared with the newer nitrate formulations, which have comparatively reliable pharmacodynamic characteristics and only need to be taken once or twice a day. Extended-release formulations of pentaerythrital tetranitrate are available, but these still do not confer the pharmacodynamic advantages of the mononitrates. Contraindications to its use are similar to those of the other nitrates, and it is also a pregnancy category C agent. It is available in oral forms as 10-, 20-, and 40-mg regular-release tablets; 30-, 45-, and 80-mg extended-release capsules; and 80-mg extended release tablets. Refer to the dosages table on the previous page for dosage recommendations.

PHARMACOKINETICS

HALF-LIFE	ONSET	PEAK	DURATION
Unknown	30 min	Unknown	4-5 hr

BETA-BLOCKERS

Beta-adrenergic blockers, more commonly referred to as *beta-blockers,* have become the mainstay in the treatment of a wide range of cardiovascular diseases. Most available beta-blockers demonstrate antianginal efficacy, although not all have been approved for this use. Those beta-blockers approved as antianginal agents are atenolol, metoprolol, nadolol, and propranolol.

The beta-blockers' main beneficial effect in the treatment of angina is slowing the heart rate and decreasing contractility. These two effects have two very favorable physiologic results. First, decreasing the heart rate decreases myocardial oxygen demand, because a rapidly beating heart requires more energy and oxygen than a slowly or normally beating heart. In addition, this increases oxygen delivery to the myocardium. Second, by decreasing contractility, the beta-blockers help conserve energy, or decrease demand. As mentioned in previous chapters, beta-blockers bind to and thus block the beta-adrenergic receptors, which would otherwise bind to the sympathetic nervous system neurotransmitters epinephrine and norepinephrine. These catecholamines would ordinarily be released in greater quantities in the setting of exercise or stress to stimulate the heart muscle to contract further, and the physiologic act of contractility requires energy in the form of ATP (adenosine triphosphate), oxygen, and many other vital substances. Therefore any decrease in the energy demands on the heart would be beneficial in alleviating conditions such as angina, in which the supply of these substances is already deficient because of the ischemia.

Beta-blockers are most effective in the treatment of typical exertional angina, as the usual physiologic increase in the heart rate and systolic blood pressure that occurs during exercise or stress is blunted, thereby decreasing the myocardial oxygen demand.

One drawback to the use of beta-blockers is their negative effect on physical performance. Fatigue and lethargy are the most common patient complaints and may be due to either a decreased cardiac output or a direct CNS effect.

There are a number of contraindications to the use of beta-blockers, and these include bronchial asthma, CHF, and serious conduction disturbances. Additionally, several common yet sometimes subtle conditions in elderly patients may be exacerbated by beta-blockers. These include mental depression and peripheral vascular disease. The decision to initiate antiischemic therapy with a beta-blocker in any patient should therefore be made carefully, weighing both the risks and the benefits.

Mechanism of Action

As just mentioned, the beta-blockers are effective in the treatment of angina because they slow the heart rate and decrease contractility, which they accomplish by binding to and blocking the beta-adrenergic receptors located on the heart's conduction system and throughout the myocardium. This has the ultimate effect of decreasing the work load of the heart.

Slowing the heart rate is very beneficial in a patient with ischemic heart disease because the coronary arteries have more time to fill with oxygen-rich and nutrient-rich blood when the heart is relaxed during diastole and to deliver these vital substances to the myocardium. At a normal heart rate of 60 to 80 beats/min, the heart spends 60% to 70% of the time in diastole. As the heart rate increases in the setting of stress or exercise, however, the heart spends more and more time in systole and less and less time in diastole. The physiologic consequence is that the coronary arteries receive increasingly less blood and eventually the myocardium becomes ischemic.

In an ischemic heart the increased demand of increasing contractility also leads to more ischemia and chest pain. By blocking this mechanism, a beta-blocker causes contractility and hence the energy needs to be decreased. This shifts the supply-and-demand ratio back toward a more balanced ratio.

Drug Effects

The primary drug effects of the beta-blockers are related to the cardiovascular system. As covered in previous chapters, the predominant beta-adrenergic receptors in the heart are the beta$_1$-adrenergic receptors. They are responsible for the conduction effects of the conduction system. When they are blocked by beta-blockers, the rate at which the pacemaker, the sinoatrial (SA) node, fires decreases and the time it takes for the node to recover increases. The end result is a decrease in heart rate. Beta-blockers slow conduction through the atrioventricular (AV) node as well, which contributes to slowing the heart rate.

Beta-blockers may also suppress renin activity and the renin-aldosterone-angiotensin system. Renin is a potent vasoconstrictor that the kidneys release when they sense they are not being adequately perfused and receiving enough blood. When beta-blockers inhibit its release, this causes the blood vessels to and in the kidney to dilate, which decreases blood pressure.

Therapeutic Uses

The primary therapeutic effects of the beta-blockers are their antihypertensive, antianginal, and cardioprotective effects, the latter of value after a myocardial infarction.

There are three possible ways in which beta-blockers produce their antihypertensive effects: by blocking both peripheral and cardiac beta-adrenergic receptors, by decreasing sympathetic outflow from the CNS, or by suppressing renal renin release, or by a combination of these processes.

The antianginal effects of the beta-blockers are related to the supply-and-demand imbalance present in the setting of ischemic heart disease and angina. In this condition blood supply is decreased because the blood vessels have been narrowed by atherosclerosis or vasospasm. This has the overall effect of increasing the work load of the heart (increased demand). The two alone or together cause an imbalance between the needed oxygen supply and demand, which the beta-blockers rectify by slowing the heart rate and decreasing contractility.

The therapeutic effects of beta-blockers after a myocardial infarction are many. After a patient has suffered a myocardial infarction, there is a high level of circulating catecholamines (norepinephrine and epinephrine), the release of which has been triggered by the myocardial damage resulting from the infarction. These catecholamines will produce several harmful consequences if their actions go unopposed. They essentially irritate the heart. They cause the heart rate to increase, causing a further imbalance in the supply-and-demand ratio, and they irritate the conduction system of the heart to the point where dysrhythmias may ensue that can be fatal. The beta-blockers block all these harmful effects and have been shown to improve the chances for survival in such patients. They should be given to all patients in the acute stages after a myocardial infarction, unless contraindicated for some reason.

Side Effects and Adverse Effects

The side effects of the beta-blockers are related to their ability to block beta-adrenergic receptors in areas where they are not intended to. For example, the smooth muscle that surrounds many blood vessels throughout the circulation as well as the airways in the lungs has beta$_2$-adrenergic receptors on its surface. When these beta$_2$-adrenergic receptors are stimulated, they cause the smooth muscle to relax. When this occurs in blood vessels, they dilate and blood pressure decreases. When this occurs in the airways of the lungs, they dilate and oxygen delivery increases. A beta-blocker that blocks beta$_2$-adrenergic receptors thus causes the opposite of these physiologic actions, such that blood vessels constrict and hypertension occurs or the airways constrict and the delivery of oxygen decreases. This may in turn exacerbate a patient's underlying asthma or chronic obstructive pulmonary disease. The most common beta-blocker–related side effects and adverse effects are listed in Table 22-2.

Interactions

There are many important drug interactions that involve the beta-blockers. The more common and important of these are listed in Table 22-3.

Table 22-2	Beta-Blocker: Adverse Effects
BODY SYSTEM	**SIDE/ADVERSE EFFECTS**
Cardiovascular	Bradycardia, hypotension, second- or third-degree heart block
Central nervous system	Dizziness, fatigue, mental depression, lethargy, drowsiness, unusual dreams
Other	Wheezing, dyspnea, impotence

Table 22-3	Beta-Blockers: Drug Interactions	
DRUG	**MECHANISM**	**RESULT**
Phenothiazine	Additive hypotensive effects	Hypotension and cardiac arrest
Anticholinergics	Antagonize	Decrease beta-blocker effectiveness
Diuretics and antihypertensives	Additive	Hypotension

Dosages

For information on the dosages of selected beta-blockers used for the treatment of angina, see the dosages table on p. 308.

DRUG PROFILES

As pointed out earlier, beta-blockers are the mainstay in the treatment of a wide range of cardiovascular diseases, mainly hypertension, angina, and the acute stages of myocardial infarction. The beta-blockers are all classified as pregnancy category C agents. Contraindications to their use include hypersensitivity to the particular agent, cardiac failure or shock, second- or third-degree heart block, bronchospastic disease (primarily pertains to use of nonspecific beta-blockers), hypotension, and CHF.

ATENOLOL

Atenolol (Tenormin) is a cardioselective beta$_1$-adrenergic receptor blocker and is indicated for the prophylactic treatment of angina pectoris. Atenolol's use after a myocardial infarction has been shown to lead to a decrease in mortality. It is available in a parenteral form, which is an advantage because often during and immediately after a myocardial infarction, blood flow to the gastrointestinal tract is poor and patients may be intubated, which rules out enteral administration of an agent. In its parenteral form atenolol comes as a 0.5-mg/ml injection. It is also available orally as 25-, 50-, and 100-mg tablets. Refer to the dosages table on p. 308 for the recommended dosages. Pregnancy category C.

PHARMACOKINETICS

HALF-LIFE	ONSET	PEAK	DURATION
6-7 hr	1 hr	2-4 hr	24 hr

⚓ METOPROLOL

Metoprolol (Lopressor) is also a cardioselective beta$_1$-adrenergic receptor blocker that is used for the prophylactic treatment of angina and has many of the same characteristics as atenolol. It has shown similar efficacy in reducing mortality in the victims of myocardial infarction and in treating angina. It is available both orally and parenterally. Orally it comes as 50- and

100-mg tablets and as 50-, 100-, and 200-mg extended-release tablets. Parenterally it comes as a 1-mg/ml injection. Refer to the dosages table below for recommended dosages. Pregnancy category C.

⬡ PHARMACOKINETICS

HALF-LIFE	ONSET	PEAK	DURATION
3-7 hr	1 hr	1 hr	10-12 hr

NADOLOL

Nadolol (Corgard) is a nonselective beta-blocker indicated for the prophylactic treatment of angina and hypertension. It is the most hydrophilic of all the beta-blockers, which may be a beneficial characteristic in elderly patients because as we age we lose muscle mass and gain fat. As a result, the proportion of our bodies composed of fat increases. Pharmacologically the relevance of this physiologic change is that drugs that are more lipophilic (fat soluble) will concentrate to a greater extent in older patients and have a greater effect. Water-soluble drugs such as nadolol will have a more consistent and reliable effect. Nadolol is only available orally as 20-, 40-, 80-, 120-, and 160-mg tablets. Refer to the dosages table below for recommended dosages. Pregnancy category C.

⬡ PHARMACOKINETICS

HALF-LIFE	ONSET	PEAK	DURATION
20-24 hr	Unknown	3-4 hr	10-24 hr

PROPRANOLOL

Propranolol (Inderal) is also a nonselective beta-blocker, thus it can block both beta$_1$- and beta$_2$-adrenergic receptors throughout the body. Unlike nadolol, propranolol is the most lipophilic, or 'fat-loving,' beta-blocker. As a result, it can penetrate into many organs, one of which is the brain. This is why propranolol is used sometimes in the treatment of migraines and essential tremors. It has been around the longest. It comes in many oral as well as a parenteral dosage forms. Orally propranolol is available as 10-, 20-, 40-, 60-, 80-, and 90-mg tablets; 60-, 80-, 120-, and 160-mg extended-release capsules; a 20- and 40-mg/5 ml oral solution; and an 80-mg/ml concentrated solution. Parenterally propranolol is available as a 1-mg/ml injection. Refer to the dosages table below for recommended dosages. Pregnancy category C.

⬡ PHARMACOKINETICS

HALF-LIFE	ONSET	PEAK	DURATION
3.5-6 hr	30 min	1-1½ hr	Up to 12 hr*

*With extended dosage forms.

CALCIUM CHANNEL BLOCKERS

The calcium channel blockers are the most recent antianginal drugs to come available. There are three main classes of calcium channel blockers, phenylalkylamine, benzothiazepine, and dihydropyridine, traditionally represented by verapamil, diltiazem, and nifedipine, respectively. Although they all block calcium channels, their chemical structures and therefore their mecha-

DOSAGES

SELECTED BETA-BLOCKER ANTIANGINAL AGENTS

AGENT	PHARMACOLOGIC CLASS	DOSAGE RANGE	PURPOSE
Atenolol (Tenormin)	Beta$_1$-blocker	*Adult* PO: 50-200 mg/day as a single dose	
⚓Metoprolol (Lopressor)	Beta$_1$-blocker	*Adult* PO: 100-400 mg/day in 2 divided doses	
Nadolol (Corgard)	Beta-blocker	*Adult* PO: 80-240 mg/day as a single dose	Angina
Propranolol (Inderal)	Beta-blocker	*Adult* PO: 80-320 mg/day divided or 80 mg once daily in sustained-release formation	

nisms of action differ slightly. There are more than nine calcium channel blockers available today, with more on the way. Those that are used for the treatment of chronic stable angina are diltiazem, nicardipine, nifedipine, verapamil, and bepridil.

Calcium channel blockers affect both myocardial oxygen demand and supply. They decrease myocardial oxygen demand by causing peripheral arterial vasodilation and by a negative inotropic action (i.e., reduced myocardial contractility). The calcium channel blockers may be particularly effective for the treatment of coronary artery spasms secondary to the relaxation of the smooth muscles in the vessel walls. However, they may not be as effective as beta-blockers in blunting exercise-induced elevations in heart rate and blood pressure.

Mechanism of Action

The cardiovascular effects of calcium channel blockers include depressing the automaticity of and conduction through the SA and AV nodes, decreasing myocardial contractility, and decreasing peripheral and coronary artery tone. Their most dramatic antianginal effects, however, are secondary to their effects on myocardial contractility and the smooth muscle tone of peripheral and coronary arteries.

Calcium plays an important role in the excitation-contraction coupling process that occurs in the heart and vascular smooth muscle cells. It is a vital component in the contraction of any muscle, whether it is smooth muscle or skeletal muscle. Preventing calcium from entering into and interacting in the contraction process therefore prevents muscle contraction, and the result is relaxation. Relaxation of the smooth muscles that surround the coronary arteries cause them to dilate, and this increases blood flow to the heart, which in turn increases the oxygen supply and helps shift the supply-and-demand ratio back to normal. This also occurs in the arteries throughout the body, with the result that the force (systemic vascular resistance) that the heart has to exert itself against when delivering blood to the body, or the afterload, is decreased. Decreasing afterload reduces the work load of the heart and therefore reduces myocardial oxygen demand. This is the primary beneficial antianginal effect of the dihydropyridine calcium channel blockers, and of nifedipine in particular.

Both diltiazem and verapamil have dramatic effects on the cells of the cardiac conduction system, or calcium channels, which are discussed in depth in Chapter 21. It is these channels that are blocked when these calcium channel blockers are given. The electrophysiologic effect of this blockade is a slowing of AV node conduction and a prolonging of the refractory period, also discussed in Chapter 21. This is very beneficial, especially in the setting of atrial fibrillation or flutter, because if these rapidly firing impulses are allowed to pass unhindered to the ventricles, the end result could be life-threatening ventricular fibrillation or tachycardia.

Drug Effects

The effects of the calcium channel blockers are mostly limited to the cardiovascular system. They are a very safe and effective class of drugs with little if any extracardiovascular effects. As already mentioned, by relaxing vascular smooth muscle, they cause a decrease in systemic vascular resistance and in turn a decrease in afterload. They also affect the cardiac conduction system by slowing AV node conduction and prolonging the effective refractory period. This helps the AV node function better as a filter that catches all the electrical impulses from the atria and slows them down.

Therapeutic Uses

The therapeutic benefits of the calcium channel blockers are numerous. Because of their very acceptable side effect and safety profile, they are considered first-line agents for the treatment of such conditions as angina, hypertension, and supraventricular tachycardia. They are also used for the short-term management of atrial fibrillation and flutter, migraines, Raynaud's disease, and subarachnoid hemorrhage. (Their use in these other conditions is described in the appropriate chapters.)

Side Effects and Adverse Effects

The side effects of the calcium channel blockers are very limited and primarily related to overexpression of their therapeutic effects. The most common of the calcium channel blocker–related adverse effects are listed in Table 22-4.

Table 22-4	Calcium Channel Blocker: Adverse Effects
BODY SYSTEM	**SIDE/ADVERSE EFFECT**
Cardiovascular	Hypotension, palpitations, tachycardia
Gastrointestinal	Constipation, nausea
Other	Dermatitis, dyspnea, rash, flushing, peripheral edema, wheezing

310   CHAPTER 22 ▼ Antianginal Agents

Interactions

The drug interactions that can occur with calcium channel blockers vary with the particular agent, though there are not actually many such interactions. One of particular note because of its beneficial effect is the interaction that occurs between cyclosporin and diltiazem. Because diltiazem interferes with the metabolism and elimination of cyclosporin, and thus it is not broken down as quickly, smaller doses of the cyclosporin are needed. This is advantageous because one of cyclosporin's most frequent and devastating effects is that it can destroy the kidney and cause renal failure. Other important drug interactions that involve the calcium channel blockers are listed in Table 22-5.

Table 22-5	Calcium Channel Blockers: Drug Interactions	
DRUG	**MECHANISM**	**RESULT**
Digoxin	Interferes with elimination of digoxin	Can increase digoxin levels
Beta-blockers	Additive effects	Bradycardia and AV block
H₂ blockers	Decrease clearance	Elevated levels of calcium channel blockers

Dosages

For information on the dosages of selected calcium channel blockers, see the dosages table below.

DRUG PROFILES

The calcium channel blockers are beneficial, highly effective agents used to treat angina. Because they have a greater affinity for the peripheral vascular smooth muscle, the dihydropyridines are therefore more suited for the treatment of the hypertension that occurs in the setting of exertional angina. This class of calcium channel blockers has grown enormously. As a class they are very safe and effective calcium channel blockers that have a strong affinity for peripheral vascular smooth muscle. Because of these potent peripheral vasodilating properties, they have a greater propensity to cause peripheral edema and reflex tachycardia, however. They are effective in the treatment of angina because they are potent decreasers of afterload. The benzothiazepines and phenylalkylamines have a greater affinity for the cells of the conduction system and the coronary arteries, making them more suited for the management of dysrhythmias and for the di-

DOSAGES

SELECTED CALCIUM CHANNEL–BLOCKING ANTIANGINAL AGENTS

AGENT	PHARMACOLOGIC CLASS	DOSAGE RANGE	PURPOSE
Diltiazem (Cardizem, Dilacor)		*Adult* PO: initial dose, 30 mg qid ac and hs; range, 180-360 mg divided in 3-4 doses; or 1 daily for the CD (extended-release) capsule. Dosages of 480 mg/day may be needed.	
↓Nifedipine (Adalat, Procardia)	Antianginal slow channel blocker	*Adult* PO: initial dose, 10 mg tid; range, 10-20 mg tid. Do not exceed 30 mg/dose or 180 mg/day.	Angina
Verapamil (Calan, Isoptin, Verelan)		*Adult* PO: initial dose, 80-120 mg tid; range, 240-480 mg/day divided. Do not exceed 480 mg/day.	

Table 22-6	Classification of Calcium Channel Blockers	
GENERIC NAME	**TRADE NAME**	**AVAILABLE ROUTES**
Dihydropyridines		
Amlodipine	Norvasc	PO
Bepridil	Vascor	PO
Felodipine	Plendil	PO
Isradipine	DynaCirc	PO
Nicardipine	Cardene	PO/IV
⬇Nifedipine	Adalat, Procardia	PO
Nimodipine	Nimotop	PO
Benzothiazepines		
Diltiazem	Cardizem, Dilacor	PO/IV
Phenylalkylamines		
Verapamil	Calan, Isoptin, Verelan	PO/IV

lation of atherosclerotic coronary arteries. The various agents are listed in Table 22-6 according to their respective chemical category, though not all of the agents are used as antianginal drugs even though they all have antianginal effects.

The calcium channel blockers are very safe and effective drugs with few contraindications. Some of the contraindications are hypersensitivity to them, second- or third-degree AV block, hypotension, acute myocardial infarction, and cardiogenic shock. They are all classified as pregnancy category C agents.

DILTIAZEM

Diltiazem (Cardizem, Dilacor) is the only benzothiazepine calcium channel blocker. It has a particular affinity for the cardiac conduction system and is very effective for the oral treatment of angina pectoris resulting from coronary insufficiency and hypertension. It is one of the few calcium channel blockers that is also available parenterally, for which it is used for the treatment of atrial fibrillation and flutter along with paroxysmal supraventricular tachycardia. There are two sustained-delivery formulations of diltiazem, which can be confused with each other. There is a Cardizem SR, which is taken twice a day, and Cardizem CD, which is taken once a day. A competing pharmaceutical company makes another once-a-day diltiazem preparation called Dilacor XR. Oral forms of diltiazem come as 30-, 60-, 90-, and 120-mg tablets; 60-, 90-, and 120-mg extended-release capsules; and 120-, 180-, 240-, and 300-mg dual-release capsules and tablets. Refer to

the preceding dosages table for recommended dosages. Pregnancy category C.

⬢ PHARMACOKINETICS

HALF-LIFE	ONSET	PEAK	DURATION
3.5-9 hr	30 min	2-3 hr	Up to 24 hr*

*With extended dosage forms.

⚓ NIFEDIPINE

Nifedipine (Adalat, Procardia) was the first of the dihydropyridine calcium channel blockers to be developed and introduced into clinical use. It is often given sublingually, and for this purpose it comes in liquid-filled capsules that can be squeezed so that the liquid contents are released under the tongue. This route of administration is often used for the acute treatment of hypertension. Nifedipine is only available orally as 10- and 20-mg liquid-filled capsules and as 30-, 60-, and 90-mg extended-release, film-coated tablets. Refer to the preceding dosages table for recommended dosages. Pregnancy category C.

⬢ PHARMACOKINETICS

HALF-LIFE	ONSET	PEAK	DURATION
2-5 hr	20 min	30-60 min	Unknown

VERAPAMIL

Verapamil (Calan, Isoptin, Verelan) is the only phenylalkylamine calcium channel blocker. Like diltiazem, it has a greater affinity for the conduction system of the heart than the dihydropyridine calcium channel blockers such as nifedipine and is therefore effective in treating such rhythm disturbances as paroxysmal supraventricular tachycardias. Verapamil is also used for the treatment of angina, hypertension, and hypertrophic cardiomyopathy. The most common side effect of verapamil is constipation, occurring in less than 9% of patients.

Verapamil comes in many oral dosage formulations and is also available in a parenteral preparation. Verapamil comes as a 40-, 80-, and 120-mg film-coated tablet and as a 120-, 180-, 240-mg extended-release capsule and film-coated, extended-release tablet. Parenterally verapamil is available as a 2.5-mg/ml injection. Refer to the preceding dosages table for recommended dosages. Pregnancy category C.

⬢ PHARMACOKINETICS

HALF-LIFE	ONSET	PEAK	DURATION
4.5-12 hr	0.5-2 hr	1-2 hr	Unknown

NURSING PROCESS

In patients with coronary artery disease, the clinical symptoms result from a lack or inadequate delivery of blood, and the attendant oxygen and nutrients, to the heart, which results in ischemic heart disease. Antianginal agents such as nitrates, nitrites, beta-blockers, and calcium channel blockers are used to reduce ischemia by increasing the delivery of oxygen- and nutrient-rich blood to cardiac tissues or by reducing oxygen consumption by the coronary vessels. Either of these mechanisms can reduce ischemia and lead to a decrease in anginal pain. Nitrates and nitrites work mainly by decreasing venous return to the heart (preload) and decreasing systemic vascular resistance (afterload). Calcium channel blockers decrease calcium influx into the smooth muscle, and this causes vascular relaxation, thus either reversing or preventing the spasms of coronary vessels that cause the anginal pain associated with Prinzmetal's or vasospastic angina and with chronic anginal pain. Beta-blockers help by slowing the heart rate and decreasing contractility thereby decreasing oxygen demands. Even though these groups of drugs have similar clinical effects, the nursing process required for each is somewhat specific in terms of the characteristics and effects of the agents and the indications for and contraindications to their use.

ASSESSMENT

Before administering any of the nitrates or nitrites, a complete health history must be obtained to determine whether the patient has any past or present medical conditions or diseases that would either be a contraindication to the use of these agents or call for cautious use. Other drugs being taken by the patient should also be documented. Patients should be encouraged to describe their anginal attacks because this will help in the selection of the appropriate therapy. Contraindications to the use of nitrates and nitrites include hypersensitivity to these agents, severe anemia, acute myocardial infarction, increased intracranial pressure, hypertension, and cerebral hemorrhage. Cautious use is called for in patients suffering from head injuries or postural hypotension as well as in women who are pregnant or lactating. It is also necessary to assess a patient's vital signs, including respiratory patterns and rate, before and during therapy. Drugs that interact with these agents include beta-blockers, narcotics, diuretics, an-

tihypertensives, anticoagulants, alcohol (results in increased hypotension and even cardiovascular collapse), sympathomimetics (may antagonize the effects of nitrates and nitrites), and tricyclic antidepressants (their effect is enhanced when they are taken with nitrates). Cold temperature and tobacco use can reduce the effectiveness of nitrates. It is also important to remember that cross-tolerance may develop when nitrates and nitrites are taken together.

Before administering calcium channel blockers as an antianginal agent, the nurse should check to make sure the patient has no conditions that are contraindications, conditions such as sick sinus syndrome, second- or third-degree heart block, hypotension with a systolic blood pressure of less than 90 mm Hg, or cardiogenic shock. Cautious use is called for in pregnant or lactating women, children, and patients with renal or liver disease, hypotension, or CHF. Drugs that interact with the calcium channel blockers include theophylline, beta-blockers, antihypertensives, digitalis, cimetidine, lithium, and quinidine, so these drugs should be used cautiously in conjunction with a calcium channel blocker. Contraindications to the use of beta-blockers include patients with asthma, CHF, or serious conduction disturbances. Cautious use is recommended in the elderly.

NURSING DIAGNOSES

Nursing diagnoses related to the administration of antianginal agents include:
- Pain (chest pain) related to pathologic impact of angina.
- Activity intolerance related to angina.
- Knowledge deficit related to first-time use of antianginals.
- Risk for injury related to side effects of antianginals.

PLANNING

Goals of nursing care related to the administration of antianginals include:
- Patient experiences fewer episodes of chest pain with appropriate use of antianginals.
- Patient is able to perform activities of daily living with increasing comfort and less chest pain.
- Patient tolerates moderate, supervised exercise.
- Patient states actions to take when chest pain is unrelieved.
- Patient states side effects of therapy to report.

Outcome Criteria

Outcome criteria related to the administration of antianginals include:

NURSING ▪ CARE ▪ PLAN

Chest Pain

Mr. L.L., a 59-year-old high school principal, was admitted to the ER with complaints of chest pain after a high school basketball game, which he attended after a 12-hour day at work. He experienced chest pain and was taken by ambulance to a local chest pain center where the following were completed: 12 lead ECG and serum enzyme studies to rule out possible MI. Over the next 24 hours he was observed and monitored in the chest pain unit. All studies were negative, and there were no further complaints of chest pain. He was discharged on SL nitroglycerine and is scheduled for an ultrasound and stress test with thallium scan in 1 week.

Assessment with nursing diagnoses	Planning with goals and outcome criteria	Implementation with patient education	Evaluation

Subjective
 	
Complaints of chest pain and palpitations
 	
Objective
 	
Smoker × 20 yr of 2 packs/day
Occasional wine drinker
Principal of high school
Family history of MI
History of hypertension × 2 yr
Minimal exercise and does not watch diet for fat intake
 	
Nursing diagnoses
 	
Knowledge deficit related to:
  Use of sublingual nitroglycerine
  Weight within normal limits for height
	Goals
	
	Patient will verbalize dosing, importance of compliance, side effects, and drug interactions to nitroglycerin, before discharge
	
	Outcome criteria
	
	Patient will be able to demonstrate understanding of medication regimen by being able to accurately verbalize the following:
	  Use of nitroglycerin
	  Side effects of medication
	  Drug interactions
	  Symptoms and side effects to report to the physician immediately
	  When to call 911
	  How to minimize side effects
		SL nitroglycerine is taken to abort acute attacks of angina with an onset of action in 1-3 min, and lasts only 30 min; therefore, it is important to follow these guidelines:
		Place SL tab under the tongue, DO NOT CHEW, let dissolve, and DO NOT SWALLOW until dissolved; take SL tabs at ONE tab every 5 min until chest pain relieved, but no more than 3 tabs with 15 min, and if chest pain unrelieved then activate EMS by calling 911!! These instructions are very important to the effectiveness of the drug
		
		Avoid alcohol and OTC meds with this medication and avoid OTC medications as well
		
		A headache may occur with the dose of drug, and you may develop tolerance to the headache as time goes on; however, a nonnarcotic analgesic is recommended
		
		If the drug stings when in contact with the mucous membranes, it is still potent
		
		The drug loses potency in about 6 mo; always have fresh refills available
			Patient shows therapeutic response to nitroglycerin therapy as evidenced by:
			  Decreased occurrence of chest pain
			
			Patient is monitored for and reports minimal side effects such as:
			  Headache
			  Dizziness
			  Nausea
			  Vomiting
			  Pallor
			  Sweating
			  Hypotension
			  Tachycardia
			  Fainting
			  Flushing of the face

continued

NURSING ▪ CARE ▪ PLAN—cont'd

Assessment with nursing diagnoses	Planning with goals and outcome criteria	Implementation with patient education	Evaluation
		Keep the SL nitroglycerin container away from light, heat, and moisture because these decrease the drug's effectiveness	
		Once you take the nitroglycerin, lay down and be sure to change positions slowly to avoid falling or fainting	
		You may be instructed by the physician to take this medication prior to stressful activities such as exercise or sexual activity to prevent angina	
		Be sure to take the medication exactly as prescribed	

- Patient will have increased comfort related to therapeutic effects of antianginals with fewer precipitating events and episodes.
- Patient will experience increased tolerance for activity while on antianginals with less chest pain with increasing exercise.
- Patient states those symptoms to report to the physician, such as syncope, excessive dizziness, severe headache, or chest pain to the physician.

IMPLEMENTATION

When patients first begin antianginal therapy, it is crucial for the nurse to review the patient's baseline vital signs as well as any documentation of their anginal pain and precipitating factors. If the patient is taking sublingual forms, he or she should be told to take the nitroglycerin at the first sign of angina and should be lying down to prevent or decrease dizziness and fainting resulting from drug-induced hypotension, which may last for up to a half hour. When administering nitroglycerin intravenously, it must be diluted in 5% dextrose in water or 0.9% sodium chloride and must not be given with any other drugs or solutions. Intravenously administered nitroglycerin must be contained in glass IV bottles, with the rate of administration set at the one specified by the manufacturer. Because IV filters or volume-control chambers will absorb the drug, these should not be used for its administration. In addition, intravenous forms of nitroglycerin are only stable for 96 hours after preparation.

Infusion pumps must be used, and aluminum foil should be wrapped around the bottle and tubing, unless packaging inserts instruct otherwise. Any parenteral solution that is discolored blue, green, or dark red should be discarded. If the patient is on long-term treatment with sodium nitroprusside (only administered intravenously and in a hypertensive crisis), his or her thiocyanate levels should be monitored daily. In addition, it is important to remember that amyl nitrite is highly flammable and should be kept away from flames or smoking materials. Because the active ingredient in nitroglycerin is easily destroyed, nitrates and nitrites should be stored in an airtight, cotton filler–free, dark glass bottle with a metal cap.

It is important to remember that the rapid-acting agents (amyl nitrite, sublingual nitroglycerin, and sublingual or chewable isosorbide dinitrate) are indicated for the relief of acute angina attacks. The longer-acting nitrates, along with the topical, transdermal, transmucosal, and oral sustained-release forms, are used

Patient Teaching TIPS

Nitrate Antianginal Agents

✔ When suffering from an acute anginal attack, patients should know to take one SL tablet as soon as possible after the pain begins, then to lie down and rest. If there is no relief after three SL nitrates taken every 5 minutes for 15 minutes, then 911 should be called and emergency rescue personnel told to respond.

✔ Patients should never chew or swallow the SL forms, because this will interfere with the action and effectiveness of the nitrate. SL forms should be placed under the tongue and allowed to dissolve before swallowing it. If they cause a burning sensation under the tongue, the patients should know this shows the drug is still potent.

✔ Transmucosal nitroglycerin tablets should also not be chewed, crushed, or swallowed and should be placed inside the cheek or under the lip and allowed to dissolve slowly.

✔ Patients should be instructed to always keep a fresh supply of nitroglycerin on hand, because even under the best circumstances it loses its strength in about 3 months after the bottle has been opened.

✔ Patients should be aware of the adverse effects of nitrates: flushing of the face, dizziness, fainting, brief throbbing headache, increase in heart rate, and light-headedness. The headaches usually last no longer than 20 minutes and are usually relieved with analgesics.

✔ Medications should be kept out of the reach of children.

✔ Patients should keep a record of the frequency and the characteristics of their anginal attacks, any precipitating factors, the number of pills taken, and adverse effects. Any therapeutic response to any of the antianginal agents should also be recorded in this journal, as well as a description of any symptoms of the medications.

✔ Remember that in addition to certain medications, patients should know to avoid those activities or factors that precipitate angina, such as stress, loss of sleep, overeating, heavy exercise, or the excessive intake of stimulants such as those contained in coffee, tea, chocolate, soft drinks, and cigarettes or other tobacco products.

✔ Alcohol consumption and hot baths plus spending time in jacuzzis, hot tubs, or saunas will result in vessel dilation, with a resultant increase in the chance of hypotension, and thus fainting.

✔ Nitrate topical ointments should be spread in a thin layer on the applicator paper provided with the product. Patients should always use the appropriate applicator paper because the various ointment preparations and applicator papers are not interchangeable. Ointments should not be rubbed or massaged into the skin. Any residue from the old site should be washed off before new ointment is applied. Ointments can be applied to any nonhairy site on the patient's body, not necessarily on the chest or over the heart. The ointment should be covered with either plastic wrap or the application papers to prevent staining or inadvertent removal of the medication.

✔ Rotation of sites is encouraged, and the old ointment or patch should be removed before another application.

✔ Transdermal patches should be applied to a hairless part of the body only after the old patch has been removed and the old site cleansed. These patches can be worn while swimming or bathing, but if one does come off, patients should cleanse the old site and apply a new patch.

✔ Resistance or tolerance to the nitrates may occur, so the patient should contact the physician if anginal symptoms recur.

✔ In general nitrates should be taken at the first hint of anginal pain.

✔ Patients should be encouraged to change positions slowly at all times to prevent a further drop in their blood pressure or fainting.

✔ The physician should be notified if the patient experiences blurred vision, a persistent headache, or dry mouth.

✔ Caution is encouraged whenever the patient engages in hazardous activities because of the dizziness that can occur.

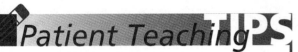

Patient Teaching TIPS

Calcium Channel Blockers

✔ Patients need to take their calcium channel blocker the same time every day and to be careful to take it as prescribed.

✔ Patients should avoid hazardous activities until the drug effects have stabilized and dizziness is no longer a problem.

✔ Patients need to know how to monitor their pulse rate before taking each dose and to record pulse rates and a description of any anginal pain.

✔ Patients should be encouraged to limit their caffeine intake (coffee, caffeinated soft drinks, tea, excess chocolate).

✔ Patients should be instructed to not take OTC medications unless otherwise instructed by their physician.

Patient Teaching TIPS

Beta Blockers

✔ Beta blockers are used for long-term prevention of angina, and patients should be aware that they are not for immediate relief or to abort an attack.

✔ Constipation is a common problem with beta blockers. Forcing fluids and eating a diet high in fiber (fresh figs, prunes, raisins, bran, wheat germ) is recommended unless contraindicated.

✔ These medications should never be discontinued abruptly due to risk of a rebound hypertensive crisis.

✔ Patients should take this medication exactly as prescribed.

✔ Alcohol intake, heat, hot baths, and spending time in jacuzzis, hot tubs, or saunas will result in vasodilation and resultant hypotension and risk for fainting and injury.

✔ Patients should report chest pain, palpitations, excessive dizziness, fainting episodes, pulse rates < 60 bpm, edema, and any dyspnea to their physician.

prophylactically to prevent anginal attacks or decrease their frequency and severity as well as to prevent predictable anginal episodes. Skin exposure to ointment forms of nitrates should be avoided because of the possible absorption of the drug. Patient and family instructions are included in the patient teaching tips on p. 315.

When administering oral calcium channel blockers, the agents should be taken before meals and as ordered. Some of the agents, such as diltiazem, must be stored in a tight container and at room temperature. See the patient teaching tips boxes above for calcium channel blockers and beta blockers. Beta-blockers should be given or taken as ordered. Measures to decrease constipation such as a high-fiber diet and forcing fluids.

EVALUATION

Patients taking antianginal agents must be monitored carefully for the occurrence of an allergic reaction, which may be manifested by dyspnea, swelling of the face, or hives. In addition, the patient needs to be monitored for adverse reactions such as headache, lightheadedness, decreased blood pressure, or dizziness, which may indicate the need for a decreased dose. The patient's journal on his or her angina (its duration, time of onset, activity being performed, and the character)

should be reviewed continuously. If the patient is receiving IV nitrates, it is important to look for the development of pedal edema, skin turgor, nausea, vomiting, rales, dyspnea, or orthopnea. Vital signs should be monitored frequently during acute exacerbations of the angina and during IV administration.

In addition, patients should be monitored for the therapeutic effects of the agents, such as relief of the angina or decreased blood pressure, or both. If the patient is experiencing blurred vision or dry mouth, the drug should be discontinued and the physician notified. If patients report that parts of the sustained-release forms of antianginal medication are appearing in their stool, then the medication is possibly moving too fast through the GI tract and patients may need to be switched to another dosage form. It is important to monitor the blood levels of calcium channel blockers to make sure they are therapeutic (e.g., diltiazem; 0.025-0.1 μg/ml). Patients taking beta-blockers should monitor pulse rate daily and report any rate lower than 60 beats per minute. Dizziness or fainting should also be reported.

TAKE HOME POINTS

Angina

- Angina pectoris or chest pain occurs because of a mismatch between the oxygen supply and oxygen demand.
- Either too much oxygen demand or too little oxygen delivery.
- The heart is a very aerobic or oxygen-requiring muscle.
- When it does not receive enough oxygen, it becomes ischemic; this produces pain.
- Coronary arteries deliver oxygen to the heart muscle; they can become blocked = heart attack.

Coronary Artery Disease

- Abnormal condition of the arteries (blood vessels) that deliver oxygen to the heart muscle.
- Become narrowed, resulting in reduced flow of oxygen and nutrients to the myocardium.
- Nitrates, calcium channel blockers, and beta-blockers may be used to treat the symptoms.

Nitrates

- Nitroglycerin is the prototypical nitrate.
- Dilate constricted coronary arteries, helping to increase oxygen and nutrient supply to the heart muscle.
- Isosorbide dinitrates were the first group of oral agents used for angina.
- Isosorbide mononitrates are the new and improved nitrates for angina.
- Nitroglycerin is the main intravenous nitrate used for angina.
- Dilate coronary arteries, and thus *increase oxygen supply.*

Calcium Channel Blockers

- Relieve angina by reducing afterload (the force the ventricles must push against to eject their blood).
- By reducing afterload they reduce the work load of the heart and therefore the oxygen demand on the heart.

- So they *reduce oxygen demand.*
- Relax the smooth muscle surrounding the blood vessels, causing them to dilate and blood pressure to drop.
- Some may dilate coronary arteries and therefore *increase oxygen supply* as well.

Beta-Blockers

- Relieve angina by slowing the heart rate.
- Slowing the heart rate reduces the work load of the heart.
- This *decreases the oxygen demand* on the heart.

Nursing Considerations

- Contraindications to the use of antianginals include allergies, severe anemia, acute myocardial infarction, increased intracranial pressure, hypertension, and cerebral hemorrhage.
- Cautious use is called for in patients with head injuries or postural hypotension, and in pregnant or lactating women.
- Calcium channel blockers are often used as antianginals and are contraindicated in patients who have sick sinus syndrome, second- or third-degree heart block, hypotension, or cardiogenic shock.
- The IV administration of nitrates should be done in accordance with manufacturer guidelines and institutional policies.
- The various dosage forms of nitrates cannot be used interchangeably.
- Beta-blockers are contraindicated in patients with CHF or second- or third-degree heart block.
- Beta-blockers may exacerbate conditions in patients with respiratory disease such as chronic obstructive pulmonary disease.

Critical Thinking **A C T I V I T I E S**

1. M.J. is a 45-year-old man with stable angina who has recently been prescribed sublingual nitroglycerin tablets for the relief of his anginal attacks. He asks you how many milligrams of nitroglycerin are in his tablets. All the bottle says is "1/150 gr tablets." How many milligrams of nitroglycerin are in M.J.'s 1/150 gr tablets?

2. Your patient has been switched from sublingual nitroglycerin to a transdermal form. What instructions do you need to give him regarding the difference in his therapeutic regimen?

3. You are caring for a patient who has just suffered a myocardial infarction, for which he has received a thrombolytic agent, aspirin, heparin, oxygen, and now a nitroglycerin infusion. The infusion is running at a rate of 33 μg/min, and the concentration of the infusion is 200 μg/ml. At what rate should the infusion pump be set in milliliters per hour?

4. What are the three classes of drugs used to treat angina?
   1. Angiotensin-converting enzyme inhibitors
   2. Beta-blockers
   3. Diuretics
   4. Calcium channel blockers
   5. Nitrates
   6. Adrenergics
      a. 2, 4, and 5
      b. 1, 3, and 6
      c. 1, 3, and 5
      d. 4, 5, and 6

5. What is the prototypical nitrate?
   a. Isosorbide dinitrate
   b. Nifedipine
   c. Isosorbide mononitrate
   d. Nitroglycerin

6. The isosorbide mononitrates have _____ active metabolites.
   a. No
   b. One
   c. Two
   d. Three

BIBLIOGRAPHY

Albanese J, Nutz P: *Mosby's 1995 nursing drug cards,* St Louis, 1995, Mosby.

Anderson KA: A practical guide to nitrate use, *Postgrad Med* 89(1):67, 1991.

Blank CA, Irwin GH: Peripheral vascular disorders: assessment and intervention, *Nurs Clin North Am* 25(4):777, 1990.

Gleeson B: Loosening the grip of anginal pain, *Nursing* 21(1):33, 1991.

Gold ME: Pharmacology of the nitrovasodilators: antianginal, antihypertensive, and antiplatelet actions, *Nurs Clin North Am* 26(2):437, 1991.

Johnson KB: *Harriet Lane handbook,* ed 13, St Louis, 1993, Mosby.

Keen JH: *Mosby's critical care and emergency drug reference,* St Louis, 1994, Mosby.

Knoben JE, Anderson PO: *Handbook of critical drug data,* ed 6, Hamilton, Ill, 1988, Drug Intelligence Publications.

Lazar EJ, Lazar JM, Frishman W et al: Angina pectoris and silent ischemia in the elderly: a management update, *Geriatrics* 47(7):24, 1992.

McEvoy GK: *AHFS drug information,* Bethesda, Md, 1994, American Society of Hospital Pharmacists.

Rising JB: A review of calcium-channel blockers, *US Pharm* 15(12):37, 1990.

Rutherford JD: Pharmacologic management of angina and acute myocardial infarction, *Am J Cardiol* 72:16C, 1993.

Shub C: Stable angina pectoris: 3. Medical treatment, *Mayo Clin Proc* 65:256, 1990.

Skidmore-Roth L: *Mosby's 1995 nursing drug reference,* St Louis, 1995, Mosby.

Zuckerman IH: Therapeutic management of chronic cardiovascular diseases, *US Pharm* 15(6):31, 1990.

Chapter 23

Antihypertensive Agents

Objectives

When you reach the end of this chapter, you will be able to:

1 Define hypertension.
2 Describe the different forms of hypertension.
3 Discuss the rationale for using a stepped-care approach in the management of hypertension.
4 Identify the various classes of drugs used in the treatment of hypertension.
5 Describe the actions of the different classes of drugs used to treat hypertension.
6 Identify the contraindications to and cautions pertaining to the various antihypertensive agents, as well as their side effects and toxic effects.
7 Develop a nursing care plan with patient education guidelines for patients receiving antihypertensive agents.

CHAPTER OUTLINE

Hypertension

Antihypertensive Agents

Adrenergic Agents
  Mechanism of action
  Drug effects
  Therapeutic uses
  Side effects and adverse effects
  Interactions
  Dosages

Drug Profiles
Centrally Acting Agents
  ⚓ Clonidine
Peripherally Acting Adrenergics
  Guanadrel and Guanethidine
  ⚓ Reserpine
Alpha₁-blockers
  ⚓ Prazosin
Angiotensin-converting Enzyme Inhibitors
  Mechanism of action
  Drug effects
  Therapeutic effects
  Side effects and adverse effects
    Toxicity and management of overdose
  Interactions
  Dosages

Drug Profiles
  ⚓ Captopril
  Enalapril

Calcium Channel Blockers
Diuretics
Vasodilators
  Mechanism of action
  Drug effects
  Therapeutic uses
  Side effects and adverse effects
    Toxicity and management of overdose
  Interactions
  Dosages

Drug Profiles
  Diazoxide
  Hydralazine hydrochloride
  Minoxidil
  Sodium nitroprusside

Nursing Process
Assessment
Nursing Diagnoses
Planning
  Outcome criteria
Implementation
Evaluation

Glossary

Alpha₁-blockers Drugs that primarily cause arterial and venous dilation. (p. 323)

Antihypertensives Medications used to treat hypertension. (p. 320)

Cardiac output Amount of blood ejected from the left ventricle and measured in liters per minute. (p. 321)

Centrally acting adrenergic agents Drugs that modify the function of the sympathetic nervous system. (p. 322)

Essential hypertension An elevated systemic arterial pressure for which no cause can be found and that is often the only significant clinical finding. (p. 321)

Hypertension A common, often asymptomatic disorder in which blood pressure persistently exceeds 140/90 mm Hg. (p. 320)

Idiopathic hypertension (id' e o path' ik) High blood pressure that develops without an apparent or known cause. (p. 321)

Orthostatic hypotension (ortho' stat' ik) Common side effect of adrenergic drugs involving a sudden drop in blood pressure when patients change position. (p. 324)

Peripherally acting adrenergic agents Drugs that modify the function of the cardiovascular system. (p. 323)

Primary hypertension Elevated systemic arterial pressure for which no cause can be found and that is often the only significant finding. (p. 321)

Prodrug Drug that is inactive in its present form and must be biotransformed in the liver to its active form. (p. 328)

Rauwolfia alkaloid (rou wool fi ə al'kə loid) Any one of more than 20 alkaloids derived from the root of a climbing shrub, *Rauwolfia serpentina;* used in the treatment of hypertension. (p. 326)

Secondary hypertension High blood pressure associated with several primary diseases, such as renal, pulmonary, endocrine, and vascular diseases. (p. 321)

Step-care approach Antihypertensive treatment program sponsored by National High Blood Pressure Coordinating Committee (NHBPCC) and established to encourage health professionals to use combinations of medications in a systematic fashion with a scientific basis. (p. 320)

Significant advancements have been made in the detection, evaluation, and treatment of high blood pressure, or **hypertension**. Over the past 40 years the development of new medications to treat hypertension **(antihypertensives)** has had an enormous impact on the quality of life of affected persons by reducing the incidence of the various complications associated with high blood pressure. Drug therapy for hypertension first came available in the early 1950s with the introduction of the ganglionic-blocking agents (see Chapter 19). However, side effects and inconsistent effects were common problems with these agents. Then in 1953 the vasodilator hydralazine was introduced and in 1958 the thiazide diuretics. These agents offered important advantages over the existing antihypertensive drug therapies. In addition, with the discovery of these newer drugs came a better understanding of the disease process itself. Now, a myriad of antihypertensive drugs are available, the newer ones commonly being more effective, more versatile, and better tolerated

than the older agents. These agents can be used either alone or in combination with other antihypertensive agents, and the classes of drugs that can be employed are the diuretics, beta-blockers, angiotensin-converting enzyme inhibitors (ACE inhibitors), and calcium channel blockers.

Hypertension

As many as 50 million people in the United States have some form of hypertension, making it the most common disease in the population of the Western Hemisphere. Not only does hypertension affect a large portion of our society, it has many severe consequences if left untreated because hypertension is a major risk factor for coronary artery disease, cardiovascular disease, and death resulting from cardiovascular causes. It is the most important risk factor for stroke and congestive heart failure (CHF), and it is also a major risk factor for renal failure and peripheral vascular disease.

The diagnosis and treatment of hypertension have varied considerably over the years, which has resulted in a great deal of misunderstanding. The National High Blood Pressure Coordinating Committee (NHBPCC), which is associated with the National Institutes of Health, is a leading group that reviews data on hypertension and makes recommendations concerning its diagnosis and treatment. The original mission of the NHBPCC was to foster nationwide efforts to detect, treat, and control hypertension through the education of both the health care professionals and the general public to its existence and dire consequences if left untreated. As part of the treatment efforts, practicing health care professionals were encouraged to use medication combinations in a systematic fashion with a scientific basis, or the **step-care approach**. In this regimen the patient was started off on a small dose of an antihypertensive drug, then the dose was increased and drugs from different classes, or "steps," were added sequentially as needed to achieve and maintain the blood pressure at less than 140/90 mm Hg. Included in this approach were definitions of mild, moderate, and severe hypertension.

There were many misconceptions inherent in this system, however, the most damaging of which was that a person with mild hypertension was only mildly sick and therefore did not need close monitoring or therapy. However, experience showed that there is no such thing as mild hypertension and that it is actually a serious risk factor for cardiovascular disease and death. A new and stricter definition of hypertension was therefore called for because of the overwhelming evidence that raised blood pressure, espe-

RESEARCH

The Joint National Committee on the Detection, Evaluation, and Treatment of High Blood Pressure (Fifth report, 1992) introduced changes that directly affect the way we detect, evaluate, and treat hypertension. One change was the introduction of a more "individualized" therapy, as compared to the traditional stepped-care approach, because it could address specific patient considerations, including pharmacologic alternatives. Health care providers are therefore encouraged to adopt an individualized approach to the planning of drug therapy for hypertension that considers quality of life, use of concurrent therapies, demographic concerns, and presence of concomitant diseases.

Table 23-1 Classification of Blood Pressure

Category*	Systolic Blood Pressure (mm Hg)	Diastolic Blood Pressure (mm Hg)
Normal	<130	<85
High normal	130-139	85-89
Hypertension		
Stage 1	140-159	90-99
Stage 2	160-179	100-109
Stage 3	180-209	110-119
Stage 4	≥210	≥120

*When systolic and diastolic blood pressures fall into different categories, the blood pressure should be classified according to the higher category. For example, a diastolic blood pressure of <90 mm Hg and a systolic blood pressure of >140 mm Hg are classified as isolated systolic hypertension. A blood pressure of 186/70 mm Hg would be stage 3 isolated systolic hypertension.

cially the systolic pressure, represents a significant risk regardless of the degree and should be actively treated.

The NHBPCC has now been in existence for more than 20 years and during this period has developed numerous programs and educational materials for the use of health care professionals and the public. One of the most prominent features of the program has been the consensus reports issued every 4 years by the Joint National Committee on the Detection, Evaluation, and Treatment of High Blood Pressure. In its fifth report released in October 1992, several important changes were introduced that directly affect the way we detect, evaluate, and treat hypertension (see box above).

One of the major changes was a new classification system for blood pressure because of the realization that the term *mild hypertension* did not adequately reflect the serious nature of this condition. This became evident when it was found that even though the vast majority of the 50 million Americans with hypertension have the so-called mild hypertension, most of the morbidity and mortality actually occurs in this group. In addition, many practitioners thought that the stepped-care approach to the treatment of hypertension no longer adequately reflected the current scope of pharmacologic alternatives or furnished the type of care dictated by the then thorough scientific understanding of the disorder. In this report individualized therapy was proposed as a more appropriate treatment strategy than stepped care because it could address specific patient circumstances, including pharmacologic alternatives. Healthcare providers are therefore now encouraged to adopt an individualized approach to the planning of drug therapy that takes into consideration the demographic concerns of their patient, the presence of concomitant diseases, the use of concurrent therapies, and the patient's quality of life.

The new classification scheme categorizes the degrees of blood pressure according to four stages, rather than as "mild," "moderate," and "severe," which can be misleading, and this classification scheme is presented in Table 23-1.

Hypertension can also be defined by its cause. When the specific cause for hypertension is unknown, it may be called **essential, idiopathic,** or **primary hypertension**. Ninety percent of the cases of hypertension are of this type. **Secondary hypertension** makes up the other 10%. It is most commonly the result of another disease such as pheochromocytoma, the eclampsia of pregnancy, or renal artery disease. It may also result from the use of certain medications. If the cause of the secondary hypertension is eliminated, the blood pressure usually returns to normal.

A person's blood pressure is determined by the product of cardiac output and systemic vascular resistance (SVR). **Cardiac output** is the amount of blood that is ejected from the left ventricle and is measured in liters per minute. Normal cardiac output is 4 to 8 L/min. SVR is the force (resistance) the left ventricle has to overcome to eject its volume of blood. Numerous factors interact to regulate these two major variables and keep the blood pressure within normal limits, and these are illustrated in Fig. 23-1. These are the same factors that can be responsible for causing high blood pressure and are the sites of action of many of the antihypertensive drugs.

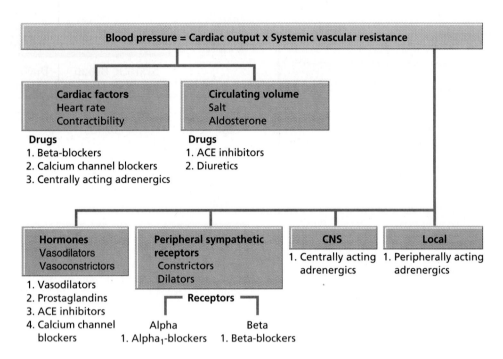

▼ **Fig. 23-1** Normal regulation of blood pressure.

Antihypertensive Agents

As already mentioned, the drug therapy for hypertension should be individualized to accommodate or complement the specific needs or concerns of the patient. Important considerations in planning drug therapy are whether the patient has concomitant medical problems and what the impact of drug therapy on the patient's quality of life will be. Demographic factors, cultural implications (see box at right), the ease of medication administration (e.g., a once-a-day dosing schedule and transdermal administration), and cost are other important considerations.

There are essentially five main categories of pharmacologic agents: diuretics, adrenergic agents, vasodilators, ACE inhibitors, and calcium channel blockers. These may be used either alone or in combination, and the various antihypertensive agents in each category are listed in the box on p. 323. The diuretics are discussed in detail in Chapter 26, and therefore are not discussed here.

ADRENERGIC AGENTS

The adrenergic agents are a large group of antihypertensive agents, as shown in the box on p. 323. The beta-blockers and combined alpha-beta blockers have been discussed in detail in Chapter 16. The centrally and peripherally acting adrenergic agents along with the alpha$_1$-blockers are discussed in this chapter. These

CULTURAL IMPLICATIONS

Levy (1993) reported some interesting findings regarding response of ethnic-racial groups to selected antihypertensive agents. He reported that African-Americans, as compared to whites, were less responsive to beta-blockers, especially propranolol. Chinese individuals, as compared to whites, were twice as sensitive to propranolol's effects on blood pressure and pulse rate.

How might these findings affect antihypertensive therapy for African-Americans and Chinese individuals?

From Levy RA: *Ethnic and racial differences in response to medicine: preserving individualized therapy in managed pharmaceutical programs,* Reston, Va, 1993, National Pharmaceutical Council.

adrenergic agents have different sites where they exert their antihypertensive action. The centrally and peripherally acting adrenergic agents, which are older agents, are not used as frequently now as the newer alpha$_1$-blockers because of the intolerable side effects they produce. The various centrally and peripherally acting adrenergic agents as well as the alpha$_1$-blockers are listed in the box on p. 323.

Mechanism of Action

The **centrally acting adrenergic agents** (clonidine, guanabenz, guanfacine, and methyldopa) all act by

Categories and Subcategories of Antihypertensive Drugs

Diuretics
Thiazides
Loop diuretics
Potassium-sparing diuretics

Adrenergic Agents
Beta-blockers (cardioselective and nonselective)
Alpha₁-blockers
Combined alpha-beta blockers
Centrally acting alpha-blockers
Peripheral acting adrenergic agents

Vasodilators

Angiotensin-Converting Enzyme Inhibitors

Calcium Channel Blockers
Dihydropyridines
Benzothiazepines
Phenylalkylamines

Adrenergic Antihypertensives

Centrally Acting (Alpha₂-Adrenergic Receptor Stimulator)
Clonidine
Guanabenz
Guanfacine
Methyldopa

Peripherally Acting (Adrenergic Receptor Blocker)
Guanadrel
Guanethidine
Reserpine

Adrenergic (Alpha₁-Adrenergic Receptor Blocker)
Doxazosin
Prazosin
Terazosin

modifying the function of the sympathetic nervous system. Because sympathetic nervous system stimulation leads to an increased heart rate and force of contraction, the constriction of blood vessels, and the release of renin from the kidney, the end result is hypertension.

Sympathetic nervous system stimulation is increased when its alpha₁-adrenergic receptors are stimulated and is decreased when its alpha₂-adrenergic receptors are stimulated. Therefore there are two ways to decrease sympathetic nervous system stimulation by means of these receptors and ultimately to decrease blood pressure. The first is by stimulating the alpha₂-adrenergic receptors, and the second is by blocking alpha₁-adrenergic receptors. The centrally acting adrenergic agents decrease blood pressure by stimulating the alpha₂-adrenergic receptors.

The **peripherally acting adrenergic agents** guanadrel, guanethidine, and reserpine also act by modifying the function of the sympathetic nervous system, but they do so by depleting the stores of norepinephrine, the neurotransmitter of the sympathetic nervous system. Without it the sympathetic nervous system cannot stimulate certain organs such as the heart, with the overall result a decrease in blood pressure.

The **alpha₁-blockers** doxazosin, prazosin, and terazosin have a similar mechanism of action to that of the centrally and peripherally acting adrenergic agents in that they also modify the function of the sympathetic nervous system. However, they do so by blocking the alpha₁-adrenergic receptors, which when stimulated produce increased blood pressure. Thus when these receptors are blocked, blood pressure is decreased.

Drug Effects

The drug effects of the centrally acting adrenergic agents are many and varied. The cardiovascular effects are decreased blood pressure and heart rate. The stimulation of the alpha₂-adrenergic receptors by the centrally acting alpha adrenergics also affects the kidneys by reducing the activity of renin, a potent vasoconstrictor. Growth hormone release is also stimulated by alpha-agonists in both adults and children, but the effects are short-lived. The centrally acting adrenergics are also known to decrease gastrointestinal motility and increase the absorption of sodium and water. In addition, they decrease the production of aqueous humor, which results in decreased intraocular pressure. The signs and symptoms of opioid withdrawal in persons physically dependent on it are reduced by the centrally acting adrenergic agent clonidine.

The drug effects of the peripherally acting adrenergic agents are primarily cardiovascular. These agents cause a decrease in blood pressure and the heart rate. Venous dilation and the peripheral pooling of blood may also occur, and slight decreases in SVR usually occur. Postural and postexercise hypotension are common. In addition, peripherally acting adrenergics cause the retention of sodium and water and expansion of blood volume, which may result in tolerance to their hypotensive effect during prolonged therapy, especially if a diuretic is not administered concurrently.

The drug effects of the alpha₁-blockers are primarily related to their ability to dilate arteries and veins, with reduced peripheral vascular resistance and blood pressure the cardiovascular effects. This produces a marked decrease in the systemic and pulmonary venous pressures and an increase in cardiac output. These dilative effects can be useful in patients who have symptomatic benign prostatic hyperplasia (BPH). By virtue of their dilating properties the alpha₁-blockers can reduce the urinary obstruction and relieve urinary hesitancy or urgency.

Therapeutic Uses

The centrally acting adrenergic agents clonidine, guanabenz, guanfacine, and methyldopa are mainly used for the treatment of hypertension, either alone or in combination with other antihypertensive agents. Particular centrally acting adrenergics may also be used prophylactically to prevent migraine headaches and for the treatment of severe dysmenorrhea or menopausal flushing. Clonidine is also useful in the management of withdrawal symptoms in opioid- or nicotine-dependent persons. Various forms of glaucoma may also respond to treatment with certain centrally acting adrenergics.

The peripherally acting adrenergic agents guanadrel, guanethidine, and reserpine used in the treatment of hypertension are commonly administered along with other agents such as diuretics to increase their effectiveness and prevent resistance to their antihypertensive effects. Various forms of glaucoma may also respond to treatment with certain peripherally acting adrenergics.

The therapeutic effects of the alpha$_1$-blockers doxazosin, prazosin, and terazosin are related to their ability to dilate arteries and veins. They have been used in the treatment of hypertension and to relieve the symptoms associated with BPH. They have also proved effective in the management of severe CHF when used in conjunction with cardiac glycosides and diuretics.

Side Effects and Adverse Effects

As with all drug classes, adrenergic drugs can cause side effects and adverse effects. The most common ones are dry mouth, drowsiness and sedation, and constipation, and these are possible side effects of all these agents. Other effects include headaches, sleep disturbances, nausea, rash, and cardiac disturbances such as palpitations. There is also a high incidence of **orthostatic hypotension** in patients taking them, a condition in which there is a sudden drop in blood pressure during changes in position.

Interactions

The adrenergic agents interact primarily with CNS depressants such as alcohol, barbiturates, and narcot-

Table 23-2	Adrenergics: Drug Interactions		
DRUG	**INTERACTS WITH**	**MECHANISM**	**RESULT**
⚓Clonidine	Narcotics Sedatives Hypnotics Anesthetics Alcohol	Additive	Increased CNS depression
	Tricyclic antidepressants MAOIs Appetite suppressants Amphetamines	Opposing actions	Decreased hypotensive effects
	Diuretics Nitrates Other antihypertensive agents	Additive	Increases hypotensive effects
Guanadrel	Diuretics Other antihypertensives	Additive	Increased hypotension
	Tricyclic antidepressants Phenothiazines Ephedreine Phenylpropanolamine	Opposing effects	Decreased hypotensive effect
Reserpine	Diuretics, beta-blockers, other antihypertensives	Additive	Increased hypotension
	Quinidine Procainamide	Additive	Increased cardiac depression
	Barbiturates Alcohol	Additive	CNS depression
	MAOIs	Additive	Excitation and hypertension
⚓Prasozin	Diuretics, other hypotensive agents	Additive	Increased hypotension

ics. The additive effects of these combinations of agents increase CNS depression. Otherwise they are relatively free of drug and laboratory test interactions, although their coadministration with beta-blockers as well as the combination of phenoxybenzamine with epinephrine can both have additive effects and increase hypotension. Terazosin can produce a reduced hematocrit reading. The drug interactions that can occur with certain adrenergic agents are summarized in Table 23-2.

Dosages

For information on the dosages of selected adrenergic antihypertensive agents, see the dosages table below.

DRUG PROFILES

CENTRALLY ACTING AGENTS

Of the four centrally acting adrenergics, clonidine, guanabenz, guanfacine, and methyldopa, clonidine is by far the most commonly used and the prototype. Methyldopa is also widely used in the treatment of hypertension. However, these agents are not typically prescribed as first-line antihypertensive agents be-

cause their use is associated with a high incidence of unwanted side effects such as orthostatic hypotension, fatigue, and dizziness. They may be used as adjunct agents in the therapy for hypertension after other agents have failed or may be used in conjunction with other antihypertensives such as diuretics.

⚓ CLONIDINE

Clonidine (Catapres) is primarily used for its ability to decrease blood pressure. As already noted, clonidine is also useful in the management of opioid withdrawal.

It has a better safety profile than the other centrally acting adrenergics and has the advantage of being available in several dosage formulations, both topical and oral preparations. Topically clonidine comes as a patch that administers a dose of 0.1, 0.2, and 0.3 mg/ 24 hours. Orally clonidine comes as 0.1, 0.2-, and 0.3-mg tablets. Its use is contraindicated in patients who have shown hypersensitivity reactions to it and is classified as a pregnancy category C agent. See the dosages table below for recommended dosages.

⬡ PHARMACOKINETICS

HALF-LIFE	ONSET	PEAK	DURATION
6-20 hr	30-60 min	3-5 hr	8 hr

PERIPHERALLY ACTING ADRENERGICS

The peripherally acting adrenergics are guanadrel, guanethidine, and reserpine. These agents, like the

DOSAGES

SELECTED ANTIHYPERTENSIVE AGENTS: ADRENERGIC/ANTIADRENERGIC AGENT

AGENT	PHARMACOLOGIC CLASS	DOSAGE RANGE	PURPOSE
⚓Clonidine (Catapres)	Alpha$_2$-adrenergic	*Adult* PO: 0.2-0.8 mg/day divided, to a maximum of 2.4 mg/day	
Guanadrel (Hylorel)	Peripherally acting sympatholytic (antiadrenergic)	*Adult* PO: 20-75 mg/day divided in 2-4 doses	Hypertension
Reserpine	Peripherally acting sympatholytic (antiadrenergic)	*Adult* PO: 0.1-0.25 mg/day divided or as a single daily dose	
⚓Prazosin (Minipress)	Alpha$_1$-blocker	*Adult* PO: 3-20 mg/day divided	

centrally acting adrenergics, are seldom used because of their frequent side effects and limited effectiveness. Reserpine does have the advantage, however, of being very inexpensive and has a very long half-life and duration of action, but its antihypertensive effects are diminished at high doses and mental depression develops in many patients taking it.

GUANADREL AND GUANETHIDINE

Guanadrel (Hylorel) is very similar in many aspects to guanethidine (Ismelin). They are both very old antihypertensive agents and their clinical use is limited today. They are now primarily used as adjunctive antihypertensive agents when single-drug therapy has failed to produce a response. They are both only available as oral preparations and are both classified as pregnancy category B agents. Contraindications to their use include hypersensitivity to them, pheochromocytoma, recent MI, CHF, cardiac failure, and sinus bradycardia. Guanadrel is available as 10- and 25-mg oral tablets. For the recommended dosages of guanadrel, see the dosages table on the previous page.

❦ PHARMACOKINETICS

HALF-LIFE	ONSET	PEAK	DURATION
10-12 hr	0.5-2 hr	4-6 hr	4-14 hr

RESERPINE

Reserpine is slightly different from guanadrel and guanethidine in that it is one of the **rauwolfia alkaloids**. Others of these plant-derived alkaloids are *Rauwolfia serpentina*, alseroxylon, and deserpidine, but reserpine is the most commonly used of the focuet. Because these alkaloids promote sodium and water resorption, their antihypertensive effects may diminish with continued use. This is why these drugs are often combined with diuretics in an attempt to offset this effect.

Reserpine is classified as a pregnancy category D drug and is contraindicated in patients suffering from mental depression, active peptic ulcers, or ulcerative colitis, and in those who have shown a hypersensitivity to it. It is only available in oral forms as 0.1- and 0.25-mg tablets. There are many combination products containing reserpine and various diuretics. Recommended dosages are given in the dosages table on the previous page.

❦ PHARMACOKINETICS

HALF-LIFE	ONSET	PEAK	DURATION
4-5 hr -12 days	Very slow	2-3 wk	Unknown

ALPHA₁-BLOCKERS

The alpha₁-blockers are doxazosin, prazosin, and terazosin. They are the newest of the adrenergics and have the best safety and efficacy profiles, but they are not free of adverse effects. They are contraindicated in patients who have shown a hypersensitivity to them and are classified as pregnancy category C agents. They are only available in oral preparations.

⚓ PRAZOSIN

Prazosin (Minipress) is the oldest of the alpha₁-blockers and the prototype. It reduces both peripheral vascular resistance and blood pressure by dilating both arterial and venous blood vessels. It has been shown beneficial in the treatment of hypertension, the relief of the symptoms of obstructive BPH, and as an adjunct to cardiac glycosides and diuretics in the treatment of severe CHF. Prazosin comes as 1-, 2-, and 5-mg capsules and is also available in combination with the diuretic polythiazide. Recommended dosages are given in the dosages table on the previous page.

❦ PHARMACOKINETICS

HALF-LIFE	ONSET	PEAK	DURATION
2-4 hr	2 hr	2-4 hr	<24 hr

ANGIOTENSIN-CONVERTING ENZYME INHIBITORS

The ACE inhibitors represent a large group of antihypertensive agents. There are currently more than seven agents available for clinical use and many more combination agents in which a thiazide diuretic is combined with the parent ACE inhibitor. These agents are very safe and efficacious and are often utilized as the first-line agents in the treatment of both CHF and hypertension. Some of the distinguishing characteristics of the various agents that make up this large class of antihypertensives are summarized in Table 23-3.

Mechanism of Action

As is often the case with pharmaceutical discoveries, the development of the ACE inhibitors was spurred by the discovery of an animal substance found to have beneficial effects in human beings. This particular animal substance was the venom of the South American viper, which was found to inhibit kininase activity. Kininase is an enzyme that normally breaks down bradykinin, a potent vasodilator in the human body.

The ACE inhibitors have several beneficial cardiovascular effects. As their name implies, they inhibit the angiotensin-converting enzyme, which is responsible for converting angiotensin I to angiotensin II, the latter a potent vasoconstrictor and stimulator of aldosterone. Aldosterone stimulates sodium and water resorption. This whole system is referred to as the *renin angiotensin–aldosterone system.*

Drug Effects

The primary effects of the ACE inhibitors are cardiovascular and renal. Their cardiovascular effects are due to their ability to reduce blood pressure by decreasing SVR. They do this by preventing the breakdown of the vasodilating substance bradykinin and the formation of angiotensin II. These combined effects decrease afterload, or the resistance against which the left ventricle must eject its volume of blood during contraction. The ACE inhibitors are beneficial in the treatment of CHF because they prevent sodium and water resorption by inhibiting aldosterone secretion. This causes diuresis, which decreases blood volume and return to the heart. This in turn decreases preload, or the left ventricular end-diastolic volume, and the work on the heart.

Although the ACE inhibitors prevent sodium and water resorption in the kidney, potassium is resorbed. Therefore its levels may need to be monitored, especially in patients taking potassium-sparing diuretics, because hyperkalemia could develop in them and with it severe cardiac effects such as dysrhythmias.

Therapeutic Uses

The therapeutic effects of the ACE inhibitors are related to their potent cardiovascular effects. They are excellent antihypertensives and adjunctive agents for the treatment of CHF. They may be used alone or in combination with other agents such as diuretics in the treatment of hypertension or CHF.

The beneficial hemodynamic effects of the ACE inhibitors have been studied extensively. Because of their ability to decrease SVR as well as preload and afterload, ACE inhibitors can stop the progression of left ventricular hypertrophy. The various therapeutic effects of the ACE inhibitors are listed in Table 23-4, which shows the body substances the ACE inhibitors act on and the resulting beneficial hemodynamic effect.

Side Effects and Adverse Effects

Major CNS effects of the ACE inhibitors include dizziness, mood changes, and headaches. A characteristic dry, nonproductive cough is reversible upon discontinuation of the therapy. A first-dose hypotensive

Table 23-3 ACE Inhibitors: Distinguishing Characteristics

Generic Name	Trade Name	Combination with Hydrochlorothiazide	Interval	Route	Prodrug
Benazepril	Lotensin	Lotensin HCT			Yes
Fosinopril	Monopril	None			Yes
Lisinopril	Prinivil / Zestril	Prinizide 12.5 and 25 / Zestoretic 12.5 and 25	Once a day	PO	No
Quinapril	Accupril	None			No
Ramipril	Altace	None			Yes
↓Captopril	Capoten	Capozide 25/15 and 25/25, Capozide 50/15 and 50/25	Multiple	PO	Yes / No
Enalapril	Vasotec	Vaseretic		PO & IV	Yes

Table 23-4 ACE Inhibitors: Therapeutic Effects

Body Substance	Effect in Body	ACE Inhibitor Action	Resulting Hemodynamic Effect
Bradykinin	Potent vasodilator	Prevents its breakdown	↓ SVR = ↓ afterload
Angiotensin II	Potent vasoconstrictor	Prevents its formation	↓ SVR = ↓ afterload
Aldosterone	Causes sodium and water retention	Prevents its formation	Diuresis = ↓ plasma volume = ↓ filling pressures or ↓ preload

SVR, systemic vascular resistance; ↓ = decreased.

Table 23-5	**ACE Inhibitors: Drug Interactions**	
Drug	**Mechanism**	**Result**
Antacids	Decrease absorption	Reduced therapeutic effect
Antihypertensives/diuretics	Additive effect	Increased therapeutic effect
Aspirin, indomethacin, other NSAIAs	Antagonism	Reduced therapeutic effect
Lithium	Decreases excretion	Increased lithium toxicity
Potassium-sparing diuretics	Decrease lithium excretion	Hyperkalemia

NSAIAs, nonsteroidal antiinflammatory agents.

effect can cause a significant decline in blood pressure. Other side effects include loss of taste, proteinuria, hyperkalemia, rash, pruritus, anemia, neutropenia, thrombocytosis, and agranulocytosis.

Toxicity and Management of Overdose

The most pronounced symptom of an overdose of an ACE inhibitor is hypotension. Treatment is symptomatic and supportive, and includes the administration of IV fluids to expand the blood volume. Hemodialysis is effective for the removal of captopril and lisinopril.

Interactions

The ACE inhibitors can interact with nonsteroidal antiinflammatory agents and potassium-sparing diuretics. The drugs that interact with these agents, the mechanism responsible, and the result of the interaction are summarized in Table 23-5.

Acetone may be falsely detected in the urine of patients taking captopril.

Dosages

For information on the dosages for selected ACE inhibitors, see the dosages table on p. 329.

Drug Profiles

The ACE inhibitors are a large category of very effective antihypertensive agents. The currently available agents and some characteristics of the different agents are given in Table 23-3. The ACE inhibitors as a class are very similar and only differ in a few of their chem-

ical properties, but there are some significant differences between them in terms of their clinical properties. Knowing these differences can be helpful in selecting the proper agent for a particular patient.

Captopril has the shortest half-life and therefore must be dosed more frequently than any of the other ACE inhibitors. This may be an important drawback to its use in a patient who has a history of being noncompliant with his or her medication therapy. On the other hand, it may be best to start with a drug that has a short half-life in a patient who is still very critically ill and may not tolerate medications well, so if problems arise, they will be short-lived. Both captopril and enalapril can be dosed multiple times a day.

Captopril and lisinopril are the only two ACE inhibitors that are not prodrugs. A **prodrug** is a drug that is inactive in its present form and must be biotransformed in the liver to its active form to be effective. This is an important advantage in a patient with liver dysfunction, as all the other ACE inhibitors are prodrugs and their transformation to active forms in such patients would be hindered.

Enalapril is the only ACE inhibitor that is available in a parenteral preparation. All other agents are only available in oral formulations. All the newer ACE inhibitors, such as benazepril, fosinopril, lisinopril, quinapril, and ramipril, have long half-lives and durations of action allowing them to be given once a day. This is particularly beneficial in a patient who is taking many other medications and may have difficulty keeping track of the various dosing schedules for each. A once-a-day medication regimen promotes excellent patient compliance.

All ACE inhibitors have detrimental effects on the unborn fetus and neonate. They are classified as pregnancy category C agents for women in their first trimester and as pregnancy category D agents for women in their second or third trimester. ACE inhibitors should be used in pregnant women only if there are no safer alternatives. Fetal and neonatal morbidity and mortality have been reported to have occurred in at least 50 women who were receiving ACE inhibitors during their pregnancies. All ACE inhibitors are

DOSAGES

SELECTED ANTIHYPERTENSIVE AGENTS: ACE INHIBITORS

AGENT	PHARMACOLOGIC CLASS	DOSAGE RANGE	PURPOSE
⚓Captopril (Capoten) (Capozide)*		*Adult* PO: 25-150 mg 2-3 times/day	Hypertension and heart failure
		PO: Usual dose, 1-2 tablet/day or higher based on the ratio of the two drugs*	Hypertension
Enalapril (Vasotec)	ACE inhibitor	*Adult* PO: 10-40 mg/day as a single dose or in 2 equal doses	Hypertension
		PO: 50-20 mg/day as a single dose with dig. and diuretic	Congestive heart failure
(Vaseretic)*		IV: 1.25 mg q6h over a 5-min period PO: Usual dose, 1-2 tablet/day	Hypertension

*Fixed-combination tablet with hydrochlorothiazide.

contraindicated in patients with a known hypersensitivity to them, lactating women, children, and patients with heart block or bilateral renal artery stenosis.

⚓ CAPTOPRIL

Captopril (Capoten, Capozide) was the first ACE inhibitor to become available and is considered the prototypical agent for the class. Several large multicenter studies have shown its clinical efficacy in minimizing or preventing the left ventricular dilation and dysfunction (also called *ventricular remodeling*) that can arise in the acute period after a myocardial infarction, thereby improving the patient's chances of survival. It can also reduce the risk of heart failure in these patients, and thus the need for subsequent hospitalizations for the treatment of CHF. Because it has the shortest half-life of all the currently available ACE inhibitors, captopril is an excellent agent to give to hospitalized patients who are in a fragile condition but need afterload and preload reduction. Such a reduction will decrease the work load of a failing heart such as that which exists in the setting of CHF. A very long acting agent may reduce these hemodynamic variables too much and have lingering effects that may be difficult to compensate for acutely. Captopril is only available orally as 12.5-, 25-, 50-, and 100-mg tablets and as a combination product that includes hydrochlorothiazide. Recommended dosages are given in the dosages table above.

⬢⬢ PHARMACOKINETICS

HALF-LIFE	ONSET	PEAK	DURATION
<2 hr	15 min	1-2 hr	2-6 hr

ENALAPRIL

Enalapril (Vasotec, Vaseretic) is the only currently available ACE inhibitor that is available in both oral and parenteral preparations. The parenteral formulation offers the hemodynamic benefit of inhibiting ACE activity in an acutely ill patient who cannot tolerate oral medications. Although its half-life is slightly longer than that of captopril, it may in some instances still have to be given twice a day. Enalapril differs from captopril in that it is a prodrug and relies on a functioning liver to be converted to its active form. Like captopril it too has been shown in many large studies to improve a patient's chances of survival after a myocardial infarction and to reduce the incidence of heart failure and the need for subsequent hospitalizations for the treatment of CHF in these patients. The oral formulation comes as 2.5-, 5-, 10-, and 20-mg tablets. The parenteral form comes as a 1.25-mg/ml injection. Recommended dosages are given in the dosages table above.

⬢⬢ PHARMACOKINETICS

HALF-LIFE	ONSET	PEAK	DURATION
<2 hr	1 hr	4-6 hr	12-24 hr

CALCIUM CHANNEL BLOCKERS

The calcium channel blockers have been discussed in some detail in the two previous chapters on antidysrhythmic agents (Chapter 21) and antianginal agents (Chapter 22). As a class of medications they are used for many indications and have many beneficial effects and few side effects. They are primarily used for the treatment of hypertension and angina. Their effectiveness in treating hypertension is related to their ability to cause smooth muscle relaxation by blocking the binding of calcium to its receptors, thereby preventing contraction. Because of their effectiveness and safety they have been added to the list of first-line agents for the treatment of hypertension. The calcium channel blockers are used for many other indications as well. They are effective antidysrhythmics and migraine medications. They can prevent the cerebral artery spasms that can occur after a subarachnoid hemorrhage, and they are effective in the treatment of Raynaud's disease.

DIURETICS

The diuretics are a highly effective class of antihypertensive agents. Their primary therapeutic effects are decreasing the plasma and extracellular fluid volumes. This leads to a decrease in cardiac output and total peripheral resistance, all of which decrease the work load of the heart. This large group of antihypertensive are discussed in detail in Chapter 26 on diuretics.

VASODILATORS

Vasodilators act directly on arteriolar smooth muscle to cause relaxation. Some vasodilators (diazoxide IV and sodium nitroprusside) are particularly useful in the management of hypertensive emergencies when the blood pressure is severely, or even only moderately, elevated, but there is a threat of impending end-organ damage, particularly of the brain, heart, or eyes.

Mechanism of Action

The particular mechanism of action of the direct-acting vasodilators that makes them useful as antihypertensive agents is their ability to directly elicit peripheral vasodilation. This results in a reduction in peripheral vascular resistance.

Drug Effects

In general the most notable effect of the vasodilators is their hypotensive effect. However, in recent years minoxidil (in its topical form) has received increasing attention because of its effectiveness in restoring hair growth. Oral diazoxide has also proved to have significant antihypoglycemic effects.

Therapeutic Uses

All the vasodilators can be used to treat hypertension, either alone or in combination with other antihypertensives. Diazoxide is also an antihypoglycemic when administered orally. Sodium nitroprusside and diazoxide (IV) are reserved for the management of hypertensive emergencies. Minoxidil in its topical form is used to restore hair growth.

Side Effects and Adverse Effects

Undesirable effects of diazoxide include dizziness, headache, orthostatic hypotension, dysrhythmias, water retention, nausea, vomiting, rarely acute pancreatitis, and hyperglycemia in diabetic patients.

The adverse effects of hydralazine include dizziness, headache, anxiety, tachycardia, edema, nasal congestion, dyspnea, anorexia, nausea, vomiting, diarrhea, anemia, agranulocytosis, hepatitis, and rash.

Minoxidil effects include T-wave ECG change, pericardial effusion or tamponade, angina, breast tenderness, rash, and thrombocytopenia.

Sodium nitroprusside effects include bradycardia, decreased platelet aggregation, rash, hypothyroidism, hypotension, and possible cyanide toxicity.

Toxicity and Management of Overdose

The main symptom of diazoxide overdose or toxicity is hypotension, which can usually be controlled by having the patient assume the Trendelenburg position. Sympathomimetics such as dopamine or norepinephrine may also be required.

Hydralazine toxicity or overdose produces hypotension, tachycardia, headache, and generalized skin flushing. Treatment is supportive and symptomatic and includes the administration of IV fluids, digitalization, if needed, and the administration of beta-blockers for the control of tachycardia.

Minoxidil overdose or toxicity can precipitate excessive hypotension. Treatment is supportive and symptomatic and includes the administration of IV fluids. Norepinephrine and epinephrine should not be used to reverse the hypotension because of the possibility of this causing excessive cardiac stimulation.

The main symptoms of sodium nitroprusside overdose or toxicity are excessive hypotension and cyanide toxicity. Treatment for the hypotension is supportive and symptomatic, and cyanide toxicity can be treated using a standard antidote kit.

Interactions

Although the incidence of drug interactions with the direct-acting vasodilators, especially sodium nitroprusside, is low, as a class of agents they are associated with a variety of drug interactions. These are summarized in Table 23-6.

Dosages

For dosage information for selected vasodilator agents, see the dosages table on the following page.

DRUG PROFILES

DIAZOXIDE

Diazoxide (Hyperstat) is contraindicated in patients who have shown a hypersensitivity to it and in those with functional hypoglycemia or the compensatory hypertension associated with coarction or arteriovenous shunt. Its use as an antihypertensive agent is limited to the management of hypertensive emergencies. Oral agents can control hypoglycemia. See the dosages table on p. 332 for dosage information. Pregnancy category C.

✿ PHARMACOKINETICS

HALF-LIFE	ONSET	PEAK	DURATION
30-36 hr	<1 min	2-5 min	3-12 hr

HYDRALAZINE HYDROCHLORIDE

Hydralazine hydrochloride (Alazine, Apresoline) is contraindicated in patients with a known hypersensitivity to it as well as in those with coronary artery disease or mitral valvular or rheumatic heart disease. See the dosages table on p. 332 for dosage information. Pregnancy category C.

✿ PHARMACOKINETICS

HALF-LIFE	ONSET	PEAK	DURATION
3-7 hr	20-30 min	1-2 hr	2-4 hr

MINOXIDIL

Minoxidil (Loniten, Rogaine) is contraindicated in patients with a known hypersensitivity to it and in those with pheochromocytoma. A topical 2% minoxidil solution is used to treat hair loss. See the dosages table on p. 332 for dosage information. Pregnancy category C.

✿ PHARMACOKINETICS

HALF-LIFE	ONSET	PEAK	DURATION
4.2 hr	30 min	2-8 hr	2-5 days

Table 23-6	Direct-Acting Vasodilators: Drug Interactions	
DRUG	**MECHANISM**	**RESULT**
Diazoxide		
Antihypertensives/thiazides	Additive effects	Increased hypotensive/hyperglycemic effect
Hydralazine	Additive effects	Increased hypotensive effect
PO anticoagulants	Protein storage displacement	Increased anticoagulant effect
Hydralazine		
Adrenergics	Antagonism	Decreased hypotensive effect
Antihypertensives	Additive effects	Increased hypotensive effect
Monoamine oxidase inhibitors	Alters biotransformation	Increased hypotensive effect
Minoxidil		
Antihypertensives/thiazides	Additive effects	Increased hypotensive effect
Guanethidine	Additive effects	Significant hypotensive effect
Sodium nitroprusside		
Ganglionic-blocking agents	Additive effects	Increased hypotensive effect

DOSAGES

SELECTED ANTIHYPERTENSIVE AGENTS: VASODILATORS

AGENT	PHARMACOLOGIC CLASS	DOSAGE RANGE	PURPOSE
Diazoxide (Hyperstat)		*Pediatric/Adult* IV: 1-3 mg/kg repeated at 5-15 min intervals; maintenance doses can be given at 4-24 hr intervals if required.	Acute hypertension
Hydralazine hydrochloride (Alazine, Apresoline)	Direct-acting peripheral vasodilator	*Pediatric* PO: 0.75-7.5 mg/kg/day to a maximum of 200 mg/day *Adult* PO: 10 mg qid for 2-4 days followed by 25 mg qid for balance of week. Second and subsequent weeks, 50 mg qid, then adjust to lowest effective dose for maintenance. IV: 20-40 mg prn	Hypertension
Minoxidil (Loniten, Rogaine)		*Pediatric <12 y/o* PO: 0.25-1 mg/kg/day usually as a single dose; do not exceed 50 mg/day. *Pediatric >12 y/o/Adult* PO: 10-40 mg/day as a single dose or divided; do not exceed 100 mg/day	Hypertension
Sodium nitroprusside (Nipride, Nitropress)		*Pediatric/Adult* IV: 0.3-10 mg/kg/min	

SODIUM NITROPRUSSIDE

Sodium nitroprusside (Nipride, Nitropress) is contraindicated in patients with a known hypersensitivity to it, as well as in those with the compensatory hypertension associated with coarction or arteriovenous shunt, congenital Leber's optic atrophy, tobacco amblyopia, or inadequate cerebral circulation. This drug's use is limited to the management of hypertensive emergencies. See the dosages table above for dosage information. Pregnancy category C.

NURSING PROCESS

As just discussed, there are a variety of agents used to treat hypertension. Although much of the nursing process related to their use is similar for the agents as a whole, there are some considerations very specific to the use of the particular classes of agents. Therefore the overall nursing process called for in patients receiving any of the antihypertensive agents is described

☣ PHARMACOKINETICS

HALF-LIFE	ONSET	PEAK	DURATION
2 min	Immediate	Immediate	Short

here, with the patient teaching tips giving details on the nursing process called for for the individual classes of antihypertensives.

ASSESSMENT

Before administering any antihypertensive agent to a patient, the nurse should obtain a thorough health history and perform a head-to-toe physical examination, as this is crucial to ensuring safe drug therapy. During the nursing assessment, it is important to look for underlying causes of the hypertension such as renal or liver dysfunction, a stressful life-style, Cushing's disease, Addison's disease, renal artery stenosis, coarctation of the aorta, peripheral vascular disease, or pheochromocytoma because many of these diseases demand cautious administration of the antihypertensive agent or may even constitute a contraindication to its use. In addition, if it is primary (idiopathic) hypertension that is being treated, the identification of an underlying cause of what would then be secondary hypertension means that eradication of the primary disease could alleviate the high blood pressure, ruling

out the need for antihypertensive therapy. Cautious use of antihypertensives is called for in elderly patients and patients who have chronic illnesses. Specifically, diuretics should be used cautiously in elderly patients and patients with hypotension suffering from fluid and electrolyte disturbances. Beta-blockers should be used cautiously in patients with chronic obstructive pulmonary disease (COPD), diabetes mellitus, or hyperlipidemia. The adrenergic inhibitor clonidine should be used cautiously in patients suffering from coronary insufficiency, those with Raynaud's disease or a history of mental depression, and recent victims of MI. In addition to cautions listed for clonidine therapy, methyldopa, another adrenergic inhibitor, should not be used in patients with active liver disease and should be used cautiously in patients with hemolytic anemia.

Contraindications to the use of the peripherally acting adrenergic inhibitors include COPD, peptic ulcer disease or colitis, hypersensitivity to them, and frank CHF not related to hypertension. Cautious use of these agents is called for in the settings of severe

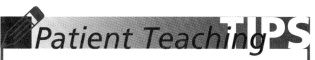

Patient Teaching TIPS

Diuretics

✔ If patients are diabetic or have gout, they must monitor their condition carefully because diuretics may cause an increase in uric acid levels as well as hyperglycemia.

✔ Encourage patients to always be cautious about their potassium levels and report any leg cramping, weakness, and muscle cramps.

✔ Encourage patients to increase their intake of potassium-rich foods such as bananas, apricots, and citrus fruits.

✔ Patients should take their diuretics ("fluid pill") early in the day so that they won't be up all night voiding.

✔ Patients should be encouraged to take their blood pressure at least three times a week, unless otherwise specified by the physician, and to keep a record of the readings.

✔ If patients are also taking digitalis products, they must be careful to report any of the following symptoms to their physician immediately: very slow pulse (<50 beats/min), nausea, vomiting, loss of appetite, or visual disorders.

✔ Alcohol, barbiturates, and narcotics will react with any of these medications and cause the patients' blood pressure to decrease further, which may cause dizziness or fainting.

Patient Teaching TIPS

Peripherally Acting Agents

✔ Dizziness, light-headedness, and fainting occur frequently in patients taking these medications, especially when patients change positions suddenly.

✔ Hot tubs, showers, or baths; hot weather; prolonged sitting or standing; physical exercise; and alcohol ingestion are all conditions that can aggravate low blood pressure, and this may lead to fainting and possible injury. If patients experience dizziness, they should sit or lie down until the symptoms subside.

✔ Patients should inform any other health care personnel who may be treating them (e.g., dentist, surgeons) that they are taking antihypertensives.

✔ Taking medications as prescribed is very important to controlling hypertension and preventing complications.

✔ Patients should be warned not to take any other medications or OTC drugs that might contain a sympathomimetic that can precipitate high blood pressure.

✔ Follow-up care with the physician is very important to the patient's health and overall well-being.

✔ Encourage patients to always carry a Medic-Alert card naming their condition and the medications they are taking.

NURSING ▪ CARE ▪ PLAN

Hypertension

Mr. J.C., a 58-year-old black male, reports to the doctor's office today and is newly diagnosed as hypertensive. He has never taken any medications for any disorder and has been extremely healthy until this recent bout with headaches and chest pain. His blood pressure at the office today is 172/98, P92, R22, and he is somewhat anxious about his blood pressure and taking any medication. His wife of 25 years is very supportive and has attended each visit with him to the doctor's office. He is an executive vice-president for a local computer company and is a hard-driving, hard-working individual. He denies smoking and drinking, and his weight and height are within normal limits. Nursing assessment is negative for any edema, chest pain, distress, dyspnea, palpitations, or other problems. He exercises regularly and will be instructed on a low-fat diet and be supervised at a local cardiac rehab center for appropriate exercising and stress management. The main concern today is education about his medication, enalapril maleate.

Assessment with nursing diagnoses	Planning with goals and outcome criteria	Implementation with patient education	Evaluation
Subjective "I really am not sure about how to take this new blood pressure medicine or anything about its side effects" "Are there any medications I can't take when I'm taking this blood pressure medicine?" **Objective** New diagnosis of hypertension Addition of enalapril maleate to regimen BP 168/106 P88 RR 22 SMA6 within normal limits Renal and liver function studies within normal limits **Nursing diagnoses** Knowledge deficit, need for patient teaching, related to the use of enalapril maleate	**Goals** Patient will remain compliant and with minimal side effects to enalapril maleate therapy within 1 mo **Outcome criteria** Patient will repeat the following instructions: How to take the medication How not to skip or double up on doses missed or forgotten How to measure and record BPs with pulse Side effects associated with therapy Ways to maximize the effects of the medication Side effects to report to the physician immediately; Importance of compliance to therapy Drug interactions and importance of a holistic approach to therapy such as with exercise, diet, etc.	Patient education focused on the following instructions: Take medication at least 1 hr before meals as ordered Avoid OTC preparations that are used for colds due to their vasoconstricting properties, which in turn elevate blood pressure It is important that you take this medication exactly as prescribed and without missing any doses or doubling up on doses; if stopped abruptly it may lead to a "rebound" hypertensive problem in which your blood pressure could elevate at high and dangerous levels Light-headedness occurs for the first few days of therapy and usually subsides after this time; however, you should always rise slowly to sitting or standing position to avoid postural hypotension and fainting	Patient will display therapeutic response to medication as a result of compliance to drug therapy as evidenced by: Taking meds as prescribed Blood pressures within normal limits with systolic consistently <90 mmHg Avoiding interacting medications Contacting physician appropriately with problems or concerns Positioning self slowly from sitting or standing without fainting or falls Taking meds before meals Reporting improved health and sense of well being Normal appetite Without weight gain, edema, dyspnea, wet rales, and signs and symptoms of CHF Wearing sunscreen when outdoors Suffering minimal side effects and without mouth sores, edema, or irregular heartbeats or chest pain

NURSING ▪ CARE ▪ PLAN—cont'd

Assessment with nursing diagnoses	Planning with goals and outcome criteria	Implementation with patient education	Evaluation
		Make sure you always comply with dosage schedule even if you are feeling better	Contacting physician when ill and possibly dehydrated
		Photosensitivity may occur, so avoid sunlight or wear sunscreen if outdoors	Patient monitored for side effects but experiences minimal problems
		Contact your physician if you have problems with mouth sores, fever, swelling of hands or feet, palpitations, or irregular heartbeats and chest pain	Recording blood pressures in a journal and sharing them with the physician at appointments; gradual decline in elevated blood pressure to within normal limits
		If you perspire heavily or suffer from dehydration, vomiting, diarrhea, you could have a fall in blood pressure with resulting fainting, dizziness or falling; contact physician should this occur	
		Take and record in a journal your blood pressures at least 3 times/wk or have a local rescue/fire squad member take it for you. They often will provide this service for you if you go by their station	

renal disease, recent MI, cerebrovascular disease, CHF, sinus bradycardia, diabetes mellitus, impaired liver function, and fever. Rauwolfia alkaloids such as reserpine should be used cautiously in patients with a history of mental depression, gallstones, renal insufficiency, cerebral hemorrhage, epilepsy, cardiac damage, COPD, or parkinsonism. Contraindications to their use include mental depression, ulcerative colitis, and acute peptic ulcers.

Cautious use of the alpha$_1$-blockers is warranted in patients with angina or severe cardiac disease and in the elderly. Vasodilators should be used cautiously in patients with impaired cerebral or cardiac circulation. Arterial and venous dilator drugs should not be used in patients with inadequate cerebral circulation and should be used cautiously in patients suffering from impaired renal or hepatic function or vitamin B$_{12}$ deficiency. ACE inhibitors should not be used as first-line agents because of their potentially serious side ef-

fects, and they should be used cautiously in patients with hyperkalemia or reduced renal function.

Calcium channel blockers should be used cautiously in patients suffering from severe aortic stenosis, bradycardia, heart failure, or cardiogenic shock. Their cautious use is recommended in elderly patients as well as in those with impaired renal or liver function.

NURSING DIAGNOSES

Nursing diagnoses appropriate to patients receiving antihypertensive agents include, but are not limited to:

- Knowledge deficit related to the new treatment program, its rationale, the side effects of the agent, and those symptoms of either their side effects or toxicity or of the hypertension to report to the physician immediately.
- Noncompliance with the therapy related to lack of

familiarity with or acceptance of the disease process.

■ Risk for sexual dysfunction related to the effects of the antihypertensive medication.

■ Risk for injury related to side effects of the antihypertensive agent such as dizziness, orthostatic hypotension, and syncope.

■ Risk for pain (headache and dry mouth) related to side effects of the medication.

■ Risk for altered tissue perfusion (decreased cardiopulmonary) related to the disease process.

■ Risk for excess fluid volume related to side effects of medications.

■ Altered nutritional status (less than body requirements) related to side effects of the agent.

■ Altered bowel elimination (constipation) related to side effects of the medication.

Patient Teaching TIPS

Adrenergic Agents

✔ Follow-up visits to the physician are very important so that patients' blood pressure and medication levels can be monitored closely.

✔ Patients should not miss doses or stop taking their medication abruptly without a physician's order, as this could precipitate a considerable increase in their blood pressure (rebound hypertension), which could lead to life-threatening problems. These serious problems could occur within 8 to 24 hours after the drug is stopped.

✔ If patients are experiencing serious side effects or believe that they should stop taking their medication or have the dose changed, they should contact their physician immediately.

✔ The symptoms of a hypertensive crisis or of blood pressure that is elevated such that stroke or other life-threatening problems may ensue are anxiety, sweating, increased pulse, salivation, muscle pain, and stomach pain.

✔ Patients should always keep an adequate supply of these medications on hand, especially while traveling.

✔ As with any antihypertensive agent, patients should always wear a Medic-Alert tag or bracelet and have periodic (every 6 months) eye examinations.

✔ The use of clonidine with other CNS depressants can cause severe drowsiness.

Patient Teaching TIPS

Alpha₁-Adrenergic Blockers

✔ There is a first-dose effect with prazosin. This means that patients will experience a considerable drop in their blood pressure after they take their first dose, so they should take it while lying down or before bedtime and arise slowly. This first-dose effect decreases with time or with a reduction in the dose, as ordered by the physician.

✔ It often takes 4 to 6 weeks for this drug to be working at its full potential.

✔ Patients should weigh themselves daily and report any increase to their physician.

✔ Patients should know the importance of taking this medication exactly as instructed by their physician.

✔ Patients should not take other medications, including OTC drugs, without first getting the okay of their physician.

✔ Patients should take their blood pressure frequently and keep a record of the readings.

Patient Teaching TIPS

All Antihypertensives

✔ Patients should be encouraged to take their medication exactly as prescribed by the physician.

✔ If a dose is missed, patients should check with their physician for instructions on what to do. They should never double up on doses.

✔ Medication should be taken with a full glass of fluid, preferably orange juice (unless this is not allowed) because it is high in potassium. Other foods high in potassium are citrus fruits, dried fruits, apricots, bananas, nuts, cantaloupe, watermelon, beef, and fowl.

✔ Remember that medication is only part of a treatment program. Patients need to watch their diet, stress level, weight, and alcohol intake. They should avoid smoking and eating foods high in sodium such as lunch meats, processed cheese, snack foods, and Chinese food, and they should engage only in supervised exercise.

✔ Keep all medications out of the reach of children.

✔ Patients should wear a Medic-Alert tag or bracelet and a medical ID card specifying their condition and the medications they are taking.

Patient Teaching TIPS

Rauwolfia Alkaloids

✔ Patients should change positions slowly to prevent possible dizziness and fainting.

✔ These medications have a sedating effect, so patients should be careful about operating hazardous machinery.

✔ Patients should not take other CNS depressants.

✔ Patients should report any awareness of mental depression to their physician.

✔ Sugarless hard candy or gum and/or saliva substitutes may help to relieve the dry mouth that is a side effect of these agents.

✔ Patients should not stop taking this drug without their physician's approval.

✔ Patients should understand the importance of follow-up care with their physician.

✔ Patients should always carry a Medic-Alert card naming their condition and the medication they are taking.

Patient Teaching TIPS

Vasodilators (Arteriolar)

✔ Patients should be encouraged to take their pulse and blood pressure frequently and report any changes to the physician.

✔ Patients should weigh themselves daily and report any increase to their physician.

✔ Patients should report any shortness of breath, chest pain, cough, or fatigue to their physician.

✔ Systemic lupus may occur in patients taking more than 200 mg of oral hydralazine per day, so they should report any fever, sore throat, joint pain, chest pain, or fatigue to their physician.

✔ Patients should know they must never stop taking their medications on their own without their physician's okay because this may lead to a very dangerous increase in their blood pressure and life-threatening problems.

✔ Hypertrichosis occurs in about 80% of patients taking minoxidil and involves thickening and increased pigmentation of the fine body hair over the face, shoulders, back, legs, and forearms. It is reversible within 2 to 6 months after the drug is discontinued. Patients should report any problems with hair overgrowth to their physician.

Patient Teaching TIPS

Calcium Channel Blockers

✔ Patients should always keep a record of their medications. Patients should be encouraged to always keep a record of any chest pain that occurs and note its pattern, duration, and severity. Blood pressure readings should also be recorded.

✔ Encourage patients to change positions slowly.

✔ It is important for patients to see their physician regularly.

✔ Patients should monitor their blood pressure and pulse regularly and keep a record of the values. They should report a pulse of less than 50 beats/min, headaches, nausea, rashes, vomiting, edema, or a weight gain to their physician.

✔ Patients are encouraged to wear a Medic-Alert tag at all times that names their condition and the medication they are taking.

✔ Patients should never omit or double up on a dose, and they should notify their physician if this should occur. Patients should be encouraged to never stop taking their medication abruptly because this may precipitate a life-threatening increase in their blood pressure.

✔ Patients should continue to take this medication, even if they are feeling much better.

✔ Patients should get the okay of their physician before taking any OTC or other medication.

Patent Teaching TIPS

ACE Inhibitors

✔ It may take several weeks before patients experience the benefits of this medication.

✔ Patients should report any signs of infection and easy bruising or bleeding.

✔ Patients should report any weight gain or loss.

✔ The impaired taste associated with these medications usually goes away in 2 to 3 months.

✔ Patients should be encouraged to not take potassium supplements or increase potassium intake because this may be harmful.

✔ Patients need to wear a Medic-Alert tag specifying their condition and the medication they are taking.

PLANNING

Nursing goals of antihypertensive therapy should focus on educating the patient and his or her family to the need for adequate management to prevent end-organ damage. These goals include making sure the patient understands the nature of the disease, its symptoms and treatment, and the importance of complying with the treatment regimen. The patient must also come to terms with the diagnosis as well as with the fact that there is no cure for the disease and treatment will be lifelong. The impact of chronic illness as well as the importance of nonpharmacologic therapy and stress reduction, and of follow-up care must also be underscored. The nurse needs to plan for ongoing assessment of blood pressure, weight, diet, exercise, smoking habits, alcohol intake, compliance with therapy, and sexual function in such patients.

Specific patient goals include:
- Patient will state the rationale and importance of medication therapy.
- Patient maintains record of medication administration and of any associated side effects that occur.
- Patient reports any change in sexual patterns and function, bowel pattern changes, or activity intolerance.
- Patient implements measures to take to decrease the occurrence of side effects.
- Patient remains compliant to therapy.

Outcome Criteria

Outcome criteria related to the use of antihypertensive agents are as follows:
- Patient will state importance of lifelong compliance to the pharmacologic treatment of hypertension to decrease end-organ damage and complications to every organ system.
- Patient follows instructions to change position slowly, monitor blood pressure, and keep a journal, to help decrease injury from side effects of drugs.
- Patient will communicate openly with nurses and other members of the health care team regarding the disease and the treatment prescribed and any concerns related to changes in body image or function.

TAKE HOME POINTS

Blood Pressure
- BP is the product of cardiac output (CO) times the systemic vascular resistance (SVR).
- All antihypertensives in some way affect CO and/or SVR.
- CO = amount of blood ejected from left ventricle measured in liters per minute.
- SVR = force the left ventricle must overcome to eject its end-diastolic volume.
- Four main categories of antihypertensives: diuretics, beta-blockers, ACE inhibitors, and calcium channel blockers.

Angiotensin-Converting Enzyme Inhibitors
- Work by blocking a critical enzyme system responsible for the production of angiotensin II (a potent vasoconstrictor).
- By blocking angiotensin converting enzyme, ACE inhibitors prevent vasoconstriction caused by angiotensin II.
- They also prevent aldosterone secretion and therefore sodium and water resorption.
- They also prevent bradykinin (a potent vasodilator) from being broken down by angiotensin II.

Calcium Channel Blockers
- May be used to treat angina, dysryhthmias, and hypertension.
- Relieve high blood pressure by causing smooth muscle relaxation and dilation of blood vessels.
- If calcium not present smooth muscle cannot contract.
- Three chemical categories of calcium channel blockers; the dihydropyridines have the greatest affinity for the peripheral blood vessels.

Nursing Considerations
- A thorough nursing assessment should include finding out whether the patient has any underlying causes of hypertension, such as renal or liver dysfunction, a stressful life-style, Cushing's disease, Addison's disease, renal artery stenosis, peripheral vascular disease, or pheochromocytoma.
- Always check for the existence of contraindications, cautions, and drug interactions before administering any of the antihypertensive agents.
- Patients should be managed not only by pharmacologic means but should also be encouraged to consume a diet low in fat, to make any other modifications in their diet, to engage in regular, supervised exercise, and to reduce stress in their life.

- Patient will report to the physician immediately any edema or weight gain of more than 2 lbs in 1 week.
- Patient will maintain normal nutritional status through adherence to a prescribed diet high in fiber and fluids and avoidance of alcohol.

IMPLEMENTATION

Generally speaking, nursing interventions can help the patient achieve stable blood pressures and can minimize adverse effects. Many patients have problems complying with treatment because the disease itself is silent whereas the medications often have very altering effects on one's self-concept and sexual function. Any

RESEARCH

There is much controversy about the need for salt restriction in patients who are hypertensive. Read any recent research article on hypertension and its treatment, as well as the article by Rodman (Hypertension: step-care management, *RN* 54 [2]: 24, 1991) and answer the following question based on your research: Should sodium be restricted in a 33-year-old patient with moderate hypertension? Why or why not?

Tips for Nurses Caring for Antihypertensive Patients

- Nurses need to be proactive in screening patients for hypertension and take every opportunity to provide patients with both verbal and written information about the disease and the lifestyle changes needed. Information about medications is also important!
- Home health care nurses should take every opportunity to participate in blood pressure screenings in their community and seek occasions to answer patients' questions about hypertension—its causes, risks, complications, and treatment.
- Whenever a nurse identifies a patient with a diastolic blood pressure that exceeds 120 mm Hg, because this is a hypertensive crisis, he or she should make sure the patient gets immediate medical attention.

symptoms patients experience may well be side effects of the medication.

Besides monitoring vital signs and educating patients (see the boxes for patient teaching tips), the nurse should encourage patients to lose weight; avoid stress; engage in supervised exercise; pay attention to their skin condition, note any skin turgor, leg cramps, or general muscle weakness (hypokalemia); watch for interactions with OTC or other drugs; monitor for signs of depression such as nightmares, poor appetite, and insomnia; change positions slowly; avoid straining, smoking, and consuming alcohol; watch their blood glucose levels if they are diabetic; inform all health care personnel of medications they are currently taking; and protect their extremities from the cold and from possible injury from falls as the result of side effects such as orthostatic hypotension. Although the restriction of sodium intake has always been a standard aspect of the nonpharmacologic therapy for hypertension, the actual need for it is now being debated (see research box at left). Treatment of their hypertension should be managed holistically, and it should be emphasized that the medication therapy is only part of the overall treatment. Tips for nurses caring for patients with hypertension are presented below left.

EVALUATION

Because patients with hypertension are at high risk for incurring cardiovascular injury, it is critical for them to be compliant with both their pharmacologic and nonpharmacologic treatment. Monitoring patients for the adverse and toxic effects of the various types of antihypertensive agents is important to the identification of potentially life-threatening complications. The most important aspect of the evaluation process, though, is collecting data and monitoring patients for evidence of controlled blood pressure. Blood pressure should be maintained at less than 140/90 mm Hg. The physician also needs to examine the fundus of patients' eyes, because this is a more reliable indicator of the long-term effectiveness of treatment than blood pressure readings. The patient must constantly be monitored for the development of end-organ damage as well as for specific problems that the medication can cause. Men receiving an antihypertensive agent should be questioned about impotence because they often are not aware that this is an expected side effect of most antihypertensive agents. Follow-up visits to the physician are important for monitoring patient compliance, the effectiveness of or problems with treatment, and complications of the hypertension.

Critical Thinking **A C T I V I T I E S**

1. Primary hypertension has been diagnosed in J.M., a 53-year-old woman, and reserpine (0.1 mg PO qd) has been prescribed. Before initiating reserpine therapy, what past medical conditions should the nurse inquire about during the nursing assessment?

2. B.T. is a 78-year-old woman who has been admitted to the emergency room for the treatment of a possible acute myocardial infarction. One of your standing orders is to start a nitroglycerin infusion at a rate of 33 μg/min. The concentration of nitroglycerin in a standard, premixed nitroglycerin infusion bag is 200 μg/ml. What rate in milliliters per hour should you set the infusion pump at to deliver the prescribed dose?

Case Study

Hypertension was diagnosed in G.S. when she was 33 years old. Both her mother and sister suffer from hypertension, and both were also in their 30s when it was diagnosed. G.S.'s most current blood pressure is 150/96 mm Hg, and for this reason, the nurse practitioner has recommended she see her primary care provider. After examining her, the physician prescribes hydrochlorothiazide and puts her on a diet low in table salt. After 14 days of this therapy; G.S.'s blood pressure is found to be 145/86 mm Hg. Stress reduction has been the biggest obstacle in her treatment. She is a lawyer in a prominent law firm and has found that her blood pressure is consistently elevated (diastolic readings >100 but <110 mm Hg) whenever she measures it at work.

Questions

1. What should Ms. Smith know about her antihypertensive medication therapy?

2. What life-style changes would you, as her nurse, recommend she make, and even more importantly, what information would you give her to help her change her life-style and more effectively reduce the stress in her life?

3. What questions would you ask G.S. to find out more about her stress level and the life-style changes she should make?

BIBLIOGRAPHY

Abdou-Awdi N et al: New support for the failing heart, *Am J Nurs* 9 (1):38, 1991.

Albanese J, Nutz P: *Mosby's 1995 nursing drug cards,* St Louis, 1995, Mosby.

Bennet NE: Hypertension in the elderly, *Lancet* 344:447, 1994.

Cerrato PL: Hypertension: the role of diet and lifestyle, *RN* 53 (12):46, 1990.

Gover MP: Top 25 discharge drugs, *Nursing* June 1991, p 53.

Hockenberry B: Multiple drug therapy in the treatment of essential hypertension, *Nurs Clin North Am* 26:417, 1991.

Johnson KB: *Harriet Lane handbook,* ed 13, St Louis, 1993, Mosby.

The Joint National Committee on Detection, Evaluation, and Treatment of High Blood Pressure: The Fifth Report of the Joint National Committee on Detection, Evaluation, and Treatment of High Blood Pressure (JNC V), *Arch Intern Med.* 153:154, 1993.

Keen JH: *Critical care and emergency drug reference,* St Louis, 1994, Mosby.

Knoben JE, Anderson PO: *Handbook of critical drug data,* ed 6, Hamilton, Ill, 1988, Drug Intelligence Publications.

Levy RA: *Ethnic and racial differences in response to medicines: preserving individualized therapy in managed pharmaceutical programs,* Reston, Va, 1993, National Pharmaceutical Council.

McEvoy GK: *AHFS drug information,* Bethesda, Md, 1994, American Society of Hospital Pharmacists.

Rodman MJ: Hypertension: first line therapy, *RN,* 54(1):32, 1991.

Rodman MJ: Hypertension: step-care management, *RN* 54(2):24, 1991.

Skidmore-Roth L: *Mosby's 1995 nursing drug reference,* St Louis, 1995, Mosby.

Swales JD: Pharmacological treatment of hypertension, *Lancet* 344:380, 1994.

Teplitz L: Hypertensive crisis: review and update, *Crit Care Nurse* 13(6):20, 30, 35, 1993.

Winer N: Hypertensive crises, *Crit Care Nurs Q* 13(4):23, 1990.

Objectives

When you reach the end of this chapter, you will be able to:

1 Discuss the mechanism of action of coagulation modifiers such as anticoagulants, antiplatelet agents, antifibrinolytics, and the thrombolytics.

2 Identify the indications for and contraindications to the use of coagulation modifiers.

3 Discuss the administration procedures for these medications.

4 Identify the drug interactions associated with the use of coagulation modifiers, specific observations related to their use, and the antidotes for an overdose.

5 Develop a nursing care plan for patients receiving anticoagulants, antiplatelet agents, antifibrinolytics, and the thrombolytics.

CHAPTER OUTLINE

Hemostasis

Coagulation Modifiers

Anticoagulants
 Mechanism of action
 Drug effects
 Therapeutic uses
 Side effects and adverse effects
  Toxicity and management of overdose
 Interactions
 Dosages

Drug Profiles
  Anisindione and Warfarin Sodium
  ⚓ Heparin

Antiplatelet Agents
 Mechanism of action
 Drug effects
 Therapeutic uses
 Side effects and adverse effects
 Interactions
 Dosages

Drug Profiles
  ⚓ Aspirin
  Dipyridamole
  Ticlopidine
  Pentoxifylline

Antifibrinolytics
 Mechanism of action
 Drug effects
 Therapeutic uses

Side effects and adverse effects
Interactions
Dosages

Drug Profiles
  Aminocaproic Acid
  Desmopressin

Thrombolytics
 Mechanism of action
 Drug effects
 Therapeutic uses
 Side effects and adverse effects
  Toxicity and management of overdose
 Interactions
 Dosages

Drug Profiles
  ⚓ Streptokinase
  Alteplase
  Anistreplase
  Urokinase

Nursing Process

Anticoagulants

Assessment
Nursing Diagnoses
Planning
 Outcome criteria
Implementation
Evaluation

Antiplatelet Agents

Assessment

continued

Nursing Diagnoses
Planning
  Outcome criteria
Implementation
Evaluation

Antifibrinolytics

Assessment
Nursing Diagnoses
Planning
  Outcome criteria
Implementation
Evaluation

Thrombolytics

Assessment
Nursing Diagnoses
Planning
Evaluation

Glossary

Anisolated plasminogen streptokinase activator complex A plasminogen-streptokinase complex that has been chemically modified by acylation, allowing a prolonged half-life. (p. 356)

Anticoagulants (an' tĭ ko ag' u lənt) A substance that prevents or delays coagulation of the blood. (p. 342)

Antifibrinolytic (an' tĭ fi' brĭ no lit ik) Drug that prevents the lysis of fibrin and in doing so promotes clot formation. (p. 353)

Antiplatelet drug (an' tĭ plāt' lət) Substance that prevents platelet plugs from forming, which can be beneficial in defending the body against heart attacks and strokes. (p. 342)

Antithrombin III (an' tĭ throm' bin) Substance that turns off the three main activating factors: activated II (thrombin), activated X, and activated IX. (p. 343)

Beta-hemolytic streptococci (group A) The pyogenic streptococci of group A that cause hemolysis of red blood cells in blood agar in laboratory setting. These organisms cause most of the acute streptococcal infections seen in human beings. (p. 356)

Clot specific Causing blood to clot. (p. 356)

Deep vein thrombosis (throm bo' sis) The formation of a thrombus in one of the deep veins of the body. The deep veins most commonly affected are the iliac and femoral veins. (p. 345)

Embolus (em' bo ləs) A blood clot that has been dislodged from the wall of a blood vessel and is traveling throughout the bloodstream. (p. 345)

Fibrin (fi' brin) A stringy, insoluble protein produced by the action of thrombin on fibrinogen during the clotting process. (p. 343)

Fibrinolysis (fi' brĭ nol' ə sis) The continual process of fibrin decomposition produced by the actions of fibrinolysin. It is the normal mechanism for removing small fibrin clots. It is stimulated by anoxia, inflammatory reactions, and other kinds of stress. (p. 343)

Fibrinolytic system A system undergoing fibrinolysis. (p. 343)

Hemorrheologic drugs (he' mo re' ol aj ik) Drug that alters platelet function without preventing them from working. (p. 343)

Hemostasis (he' mo sta' sis) The termination of bleeding by mechanical or chemical means or by the complex coagulation process of the body, consisting of vasoconstriction, platelet aggregation, and thrombin and fibrin synthesis. (p. 342)

Hemostatic agent A procedure, device, or substance that arrests the flow of blood. (p. 343)

Plasmin (plaz' min) The enzyme that breaks down fibrin into fibrin degradation products. (p. 343)

Plasminogen (plaz min' ə jən) A plasma protein that is converted into fibrin by thrombin in the presence of calcium ions. (p. 343)

Pulmonary emboli (pool' mo nar e) The blockage of a pulmonary artery by foreign matter such as fat, air, tumor, or a thrombus that usually arises from a peripheral vein. (p. 345)

Streptokinase (strep' to ki' nāse) A fibrinolytic activator that enhances the conversion of plasminogen to the fibrinolytic enzyme plasmin. It is used in the treatment of certain cases of pulmonary and coronary embolism. (p. 357)

Stroke Occlusion of the blood vessels of the brain by an embolus, thrombus, or cerebrovascular hemorrhage, resulting in ischemia of the brain tissue normally perfused by the damaged blood vessels. (p. 345)

Thromboembolic event An event in which a blood vessel is blocked by an embolus carried in the bloodstream from the site of its formation. The area supplied by an obstructed artery may tingle and become cold, numb, and cyanotic. (p. 345)

Thrombolytic drug (throm bo' lit ik) A drug or other agent that dissolves thrombi. (p. 343)

Thrombus (throm' bəs) An aggregation of platelets, fibrin, clotting factors, and the cellular elements of the blood that is attached to the interior wall of a vein or artery, sometimes occluding the lumen of the vessel. (p. 345)

Tissue plasminogen activator A naturally occurring plasminogen activator secreted by vascular endothelial cells (the walls of the blood vessels). (p. 343)

The process that halts bleeding after injury to a blood vessel is called **hemostasis**. Normal hemostasis involves the complex interaction of substances that promote clot formation and substances that either inhibit coagulation or dissolve the formed clot. The drugs discussed in this chapter aid the body in achieving hemostasis, and they can be broken down into several main categories based on their actions. The **anticoagulants** inhibit the action or formation of clotting factors and therefore prevent clots from forming. The **antiplatelet drugs** prevent platelet plugs from forming by inhibiting platelet aggregation, which can be beneficial in preventing heart attacks and strokes. Other agents alter platelet function without preventing them

Table 24-1	Coagulation Modifiers: Categories and Agents

TYPE OF COAGULATION MODIFIER	DRUG CLASS	INDIVIDUAL AGENTS
Prevent clot formation:		
Inhibit certain clotting factors	Anticoagulants	Anisindione, enoxaparin, heparin, warfarin
Prevent platelets from working	Antiplatelet drugs	Aspirin, dipyridamole, ticlopidine, pentoxifylline
Promote clot formation:		
Prevent lysis of fibrin	Antifibrinolytics	Aminocaproic acid, tranexamic acid, aprotinin
Lyse a preformed clot:		
Directly lyse the clot	Thrombolytics	Alteplase, anistreplase, streptokinase, urokinase
Reversal agents	Heparin antagonist	Protamine
	Warfarin sodium antagonist	Vitamin K

from working. These are sometimes referred to as **hemorrheologic drugs**. Sometimes clots may form and totally block a blood vessel. When this happens in one of the coronary arteries, a heart attack occurs, and the clot blocking the blood vessel must be lysed for the patient to survive. The **thrombolytic drugs** lyse or break down such preformed clots. This is a unique difference between them and the anticoagulants, which can only prevent the formation of a clot. **Hemostatic agents** have just the opposite effect of these other classes of agents; they promote blood coagulation and are helpful in the management of conditions in which excessive bleeding would be harmful. The various agents in each category of coagulation modifiers are listed in Table 24-1. Understanding the individual coagulation modifiers and their mechanism of action requires a basic working knowledge of the coagulation pathway and coagulation factors, and this is provided in the next section.

Hemostasis

As just mentioned, normal hemostasis involves a complex relationship between substances that promote clot formation (platelets, von Willebrand factor, activated clotting factors, and tissue thromboplastin) and substances that either inhibit coagulation (prostacyclin, **antithrombin III**, protein C) or dissolve a formed clot **(tissue plasminogen activator)**. Each of these systems is discussed along with the description of the actions of the various classes of coagulation modifiers.

The coagulation system is called a *cascade* because each activated factor serves as a catalyst that amplifies the next reaction. The end result is a very large concentration of a clot-forming substance called **fibrin**.

The coagulation cascade is typically divided into the intrinsic and the extrinsic pathways, and these pathways are activated by different types of injury. When blood vessels are damaged, thromboplastin, a substance contained in the walls of blood vessels, is released. This activates the extrinsic pathway by activating factors VII and X. All the components of this intrinsic pathway are present in the blood in their inactive forms. This pathway is activated when factor XII comes in contact with exposed collagen in damaged blood vessels. Figures 24-1 and 24-2 illustrate the steps that occur in the extrinsic and intrinsic pathways, respectively, and the factors involved. They also show where in these pathways the various coagulation modifiers work.

Once a clot is formed and fibrin is present, the **fibrinolytic system** is activated. This is the system that regulates the breakdown of clots and keeps the coagulation system from going out of control. **Fibrinolysis** is the mechanism by which formed thrombi are lysed to prevent excessive clot formation and blood vessel blockage. **Plasmin** is the enzyme that eventually breaks fibrin down into the fibrin degradation products, though it must first be activated by **plasminogen**. It is the fibrin in the clot that binds to circulating plasminogen, which in turn activates plasmin and keeps the clot localized. Figure 24-3 illustrates the fibrinolytic system.

Coagulation Modifiers

ANTICOAGULANTS

Drugs that prevent the formation of a clot by inhibiting certain clotting factors are called *anticoagulants*. These

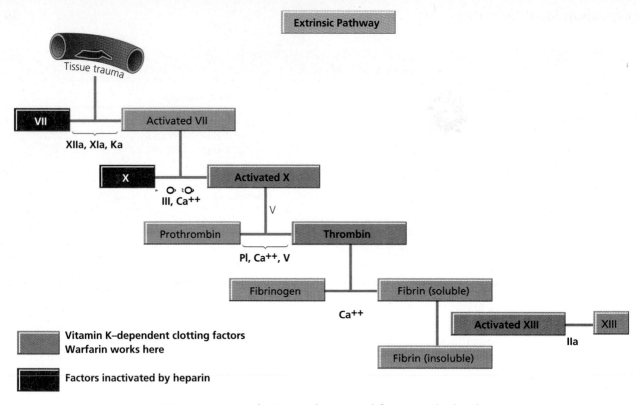

▼ **FIG. 24-1** Coagulation pathway and factors. *Pl*, platelets.

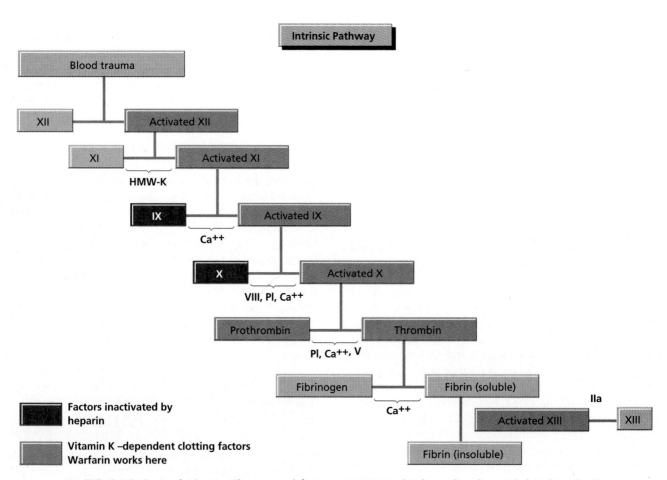

▼ **FIG. 24-2** Coagulation pathway and factors. *HMW-K,* high-molecular weight vitamin K; *Pl,* platelets.

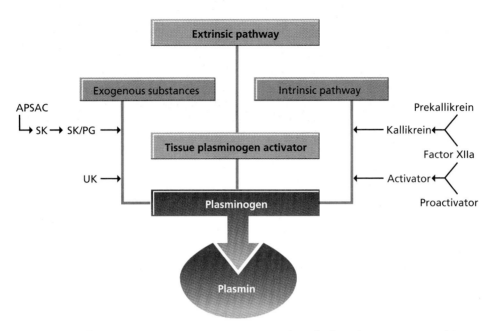

▼ **FIG. 24-3** The fibrinolytic system. *APSAC,* anisoylated plasminogen streptokinase activator complex; *PG,* plasminogen; *SK,* streptokinase; *UK,* urokinase.

agents are only given prophylactically because they have no direct effect on a blood clot that has already formed or on ischemic tissue injured as the result of an inadequate blood supply caused by the clot. By decreasing blood coagulability, anticoagulants prevent intravascular thrombosis. Their uses vary from preventing clot formation to preventing the extension of a preformed clot, or a **thrombus**.

Once a clot forms on the wall of a blood vessel, it may dislodge and travel through the bloodstream. This is referred to as an **embolus**. If it goes to the brain, it causes a **stroke**; if it goes to the lungs, it is a **pulmonary emboli**; and if it goes to the veins in the legs, it is a **deep vein thrombosis**. Collectively these complications are called **thromboembolic events** because they involve a thrombus becoming an embolus and causing an "event." Anticoagulants can prevent all of these from occurring if used in the correct manner. There are both orally and parenterally administered anticoagulants, and each agent has slightly different mechanisms of action and indications. All of them have their own risks, mainly that of causing bleeding.

Mechanism of Action

The mechanisms of action of the anticoagulants vary depending on the agent. Although other antico-

agulants exist such as anisindione and enoxaparin, by far the most frequently used anticoagulants are heparin and warfarin, and these are the anticoagulants focused on in this chapter. All anticoagulants work in the clotting cascade but do so at different points. As shown in Figs. 24-1 and 24-2, heparin works by binding to a substance called antithrombin III, which turns off three main activating factors: activated II (also called *thrombin*), activated X, and activated IX. Of these, the thrombin is the most sensitive to the actions of heparin. The overall effect of heparin is that it turns off the coagulation pathway and prevents clots from forming. As already noted, however, it cannot lyse or break down a clot.

Warfarin also works by inhibiting certain clotting factors, in particular clotting factors II, VII, IX, and X. These factors rely heavily on vitamin K for their synthesis, a process that takes place in the liver. Warfarin and the indanedione derivatives (anisindione and dicumarol) specifically work by interfering with the proper production of vitamin K. The end result is that the vitamin K needed for the production of clotting factors II, VII, IX, and X is dysfunctional, and this causes the clotting factors to be dysfunctional. As with heparin, the final effect is the prevention of clot formation. Figures 24-1 and 24-2 show where in the clotting cascade this occurs.

Drug Effects

The primary drug effects of the anticoagulants are confined to the coagulation system and bleeding. Besides preventing the formation of clots, heparin can also reduce the plasma lipid levels, and once the heparin therapy is stopped, a rebound increase in the lipid levels may occur.

Therapeutic Uses

The ability of anticoagulants to prevent clot formation is of benefit in certain settings in which there is a high likelihood of clot formation. These include a myocardial infarction, indwelling devices such as mechanical heart valves, and conditions in which blood flow may be slowed and blood may pool. As already mentioned, the ultimate consequence of a clot can be a stroke or a heart attack, so the prevention of these serious events is the ultimate benefit of these agents.

Side Effects and Adverse Effects

Bleeding is the main complication of anticoagulation therapy, and the risk increases with increasing dosages. It also depends on the nature of the patient's underlying clinical disorder and is increased in patients also taking high doses of aspirin or other drugs that impair platelet function. Some of the possible side effects of anticoagulant therapy are listed in Table 24-2.

Toxicity and Management of Overdose

Treatment of the toxic effects of anticoagulants is aimed at reversing the underlying cause. Although the toxic effects of heparin and warfarin are both hemorrhagic in nature, the management of each is different. Symptoms that may be attributed to toxicity or an overdose of anticoagulants are hematuria, melena, petechiae, ecchymoses, and gum or mucous membrane

Table 24-2	Anticoagulants: Adverse Effects
BODY SYSTEM	**SIDE/ADVERSE EFFECTS**
Blood	Bleeding, thrombocytopenia, thrombosis
Gastrointestinal	Nausea, vomiting, abdominal cramps, ulcerations, bleeding
Other	Osteoporosis, skin necrosis, hypoaldosteronism, anaphylactic reactions

bleeding. In the event of either heparin or warfarin toxicity, the anticoagulant should be discontinued. In the case of heparin, this may be enough to reverse the toxic effects because of the short half-life of the drug (1-2 hours). In severe cases or when large doses have been given intentionally (i.e., during cardiopulmonary bypass for heart surgery), a reversal agent may need to be given. If large amounts of blood have been lost, replacement with packed red blood cells may be necessary. The anticoagulant effects of heparin can be reversed with protamine sulfate. The protamine does this by forming a complex with heparin, and this has the effect of completely reversing the heparin's anticoagulant properties. This takes place in as fast as 5 minutes. As a rule of thumb, 1 mg of protamine can reverse the effects of 100 units of heparin. Because heparin comes from three different sources and each source has a different anticoagulant potency, in theory, however, the protamine dosing should vary depending on the type of heparin given (1 mg of protamine for 90 units of heparin-sodium from bovine lung tissue, 100 units of heparin calcium from porcine intestinal mucosa, and 115 units of heparin sodium from porcine intestinal mucosa).

In the event of warfarin sodium toxicity or overdose, as already mentioned, the first step is to discontinue the anticoagulant, but the reversal agent and the therapy after discontinuation differs from heparin's. As with heparin, the toxicity associated with sodium warfarin use is an extension of its therapeutic effects on the clotting cascade. However, because sodium warfarin functionally inactivates the vitamin K–dependent clotting factors and because these clotting factors are synthesized in the liver, it may take 36 to 42 hours before the liver can resynthesize enough clotting factors to reverse the warfarin effects. Treatment with warfarin's reversal agent, vitamin K (phytonadione), can hasten the return to normal coagulation. The dose of the vitamin K depends on the clinical situation and its acuity, that is, how quickly the sodium warfarin–induced effects must be reversed. High doses of vitamin K (10 to 15 mg) given intravenously should reverse the anticoagulation within 6 hours. If the warfarin therapy must be reinstated, resistance to its effect will be encountered because the large dose of vitamin K will maintain its reversal effects for up to a week. In acute situations in which bleeding is severe and the time it would take for the vitamin K to take effect is not rapid enough, it may be necessary to administer plasma or factor concentrates.

Interactions

The drug interactions involving the oral anticoagulants are profound and complicated, and the drugs and the result of an interaction are given in Table

24-3. The main interaction mechanisms responsible for increasing anticoagulant activity include:

■ Enzyme inhibition of biotransformation
■ Displacement of the agent from inactive protein-binding sites
■ A decrease in vitamin K absorption or synthesis by the bacterial flora of the large intestines
■ An alteration in the platelet count or activity

Drugs that can increase the activity of heparin include aspirin, IV ethacrynic acid, and the oral anticoagulants. Antihistamines, digitalis, and the tetracyclines may partially antagonize the anticoagulant effects of heparin.

The main interaction mechanism responsible for decreasing anticoagulant activity is an increase in the biotransformation of the oral agents (enzyme inducers). The drugs that cause this are listed in Table 24-3.

Heparin can alter the serum levels of lipids, glucose, thyroxine, SGOT, SGPT, and also affect T_3 uptake.

Dosages

For the dosages of anticoagulants, see the dosages table on the following page.

DRUG PROFILES

All three anticoagulants discussed here (anisindione, heparin sodium, and warfarin sodium) are prescription medications. Anisindione and warfarin are available in tablets; heparin can be given only by SC or IV injection.

ANISINDIONE AND WARFARIN SODIUM

Anisindione (Miradon) is an indanedione derivative, whereas warfarin sodium (Coumadin) is a coumarin derivative. Both drugs are contraindicated in patients who have shown a hypersensitivity to them and in those with subacute bacterial endocarditis or any type of potential or actual bleeding condition. Because both drugs can also pass the placental barrier, they are also

Table 24-3	Anticoagulants: Drug Interactions	
DRUG	**MECHANISM**	**RESULT**
Anisindione/Warfarin		
Acetaminophen (high doses)		
Bumetanide	Displaces from inactive protein-binding sites	Increased anticoagulant effect
Ethacrynic acid		
Furosemide		
↓Aspirin/other NSAIDs		
Cephalosporin	Decreases platelet activity	Increased anticoagulant effect
Broad-spectrum antibiotics		
Mineral oil	Interferes with vitamin K	Increased anticoagulant effect
Vitamin E		
Aminoglutethimide		
Barbiturates		
Carbamazepine	Enzyme inducer	Decreased anticoagulant effect
Glutethimide		
Rifampin		
↓Heparin		
Aspirin/other NSAIDs	Decrease platelet activity	
Ethacrynic acid	Additive	Increased anticoagulant effect
Oral anticoagulants	Additive	

DOSAGES

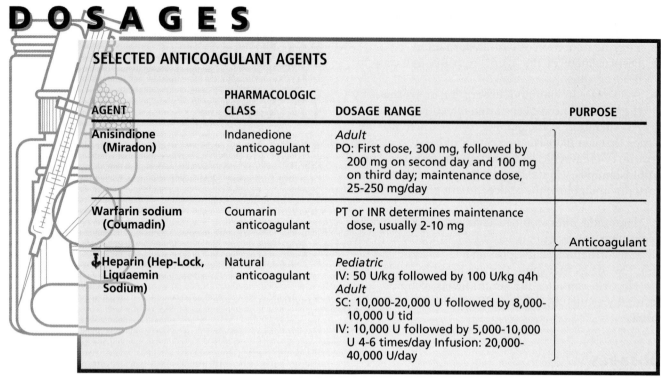

SELECTED ANTICOAGULANT AGENTS

AGENT	PHARMACOLOGIC CLASS	DOSAGE RANGE	PURPOSE
Anisindione (Miradon)	Indanedione anticoagulant	*Adult* PO: First dose, 300 mg, followed by 200 mg on second day and 100 mg on third day; maintenance dose, 25-250 mg/day	
Warfarin sodium (Coumadin)	Coumarin anticoagulant	PT or INR determines maintenance dose, usually 2-10 mg	Anticoagulant
⚓ **Heparin (Hep-Lock, Liquaemin Sodium)**	Natural anticoagulant	*Pediatric* IV: 50 U/kg followed by 100 U/kg q4h *Adult* SC: 10,000-20,000 U followed by 8,000-10,000 U tid IV: 10,000 U followed by 5,000-10,000 U 4-6 times/day Infusion: 20,000-40,000 U/day	

PT, prothrombin time; *INR,* International Normalization Ratio.

contraindicated in pregnant women. Both are noted as pregnancy category X agents. Anisindione is available as 50-mg tablets. Warfarin sodium (Coumadin) is available as an injection (50 mg per vial) and as 1-, 2-, 2.5-, 5-, 7, 7.5-, and 10-mg tablets. See the dosages table above for dosage information on both agents.

❖ PHARMACOKINETICS

HALF-LIFE	ONSET	PEAK	DURATION
Anisindione: 3-5 days	Unknown	1-3 days	1-6 days
Warfarin: 0.5-3 days	12-24 hr	0.5-3 days	2-5 days

⚓ HEPARIN

Heparin (Hep-Lock, Liquaemin Sodium) is a natural mucopolysaccharide anticoagulant obtained from the lungs, intestinal mucosa, or other suitable tissues of domestic mammals used for food. It is contraindicated in the settings of hypersensitivity and any potential or actual bleeding condition. Both forms of heparin are rated as pregnancy category C agents. Hep-Lock is available only as 10- to 100-U/ml IV or SC injections. Liquaemin Sodium is only available as a 1,000- to 40,000-U/ml infusion. See the dosages table above for dosage recommendations.

❖ PHARMACOKINETICS

HALF-LIFE	ONSET	PEAK	DURATION
1-2 hr	SC: 20-60 min IV: Immediate	SC: 2-4 hr	Dose-dependent

ANTIPLATELET AGENTS

Another class of coagulation modifiers that prevent clot formation are the antiplatelet drugs, but they accomplish this in an entirely different manner. Whereas the anticoagulants work in the clotting cascade, the antiplatelet drugs work at the initial step of the coagulation process, preventing platelet formation. As with the anticoagulants, an understanding of the role of platelets in the clotting process is essential to understanding how the antiplatelet drugs work.

Platelets normally flow through blood vessels without adhering to their surfaces. When blood vessels are injured by a disruption to blood flow, trauma, or the rupture of plaque from the vessel wall, substances such as collagen and fibronectin are present in the walls of blood vessels and are exposed. Collagen is a potent stimulator of platelet adhesion. Once platelet adhesion occurs, stimulators (adenosine diphosphate [ADP], thrombin, thromboxane A_2[TXA_2], and prostaglandin H_2) are released from the damaged blood vessels. These cause the platelets to aggregate at the

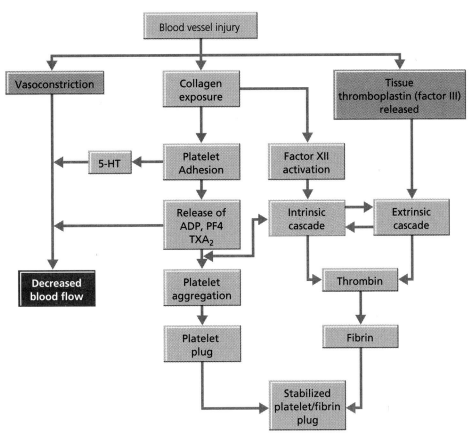

▼ **FIG. 24-4** Relationship between platelets and clotting cascade. *ADP*, adenosine diphosphate; *5-HT*, serotonin; *PF4*, platelet factor 4; *TXA₂*, thromboxane A₂.

site of injury. Once there, they change shape and release their contents, which include ADP, serotonin, and platelet factor 4 (PF4). The hemostatic function of these substances is twofold. First, they attract platelets to the site of injury (platelet recruiters); second, they are potent vasoconstrictors. Vasoconstriction limits blood flow to the damaged blood vessel, thus also decreasing blood loss.

A platelet plug that has formed at a site of injury to plug the damaged blood vessel is not stable and can be dislodged. The clotting system is therefore stimulated to form a more permanent fibrin plug. The role of the platelet and the relationship between platelets and the clotting cascade in the generation of a stabilized fibrin clot are illustrated in Fig. 24-4.

Mechanism of Action

The mechanisms of action of the antiplatelet drugs vary depending on the agent. Aspirin, dipyridamole, pentoxifylline, and ticlopidine all affect the normal function of platelets. Many of the antiplatelet drugs affect the cyclooxygenase pathway, which is one of the common final enzymatic pathways in the complex ar-

achidonic acid pathway that operates in platelets and on blood vessel walls. This pathway as it functions in both platelets and blood vessel walls is illustrated in Fig. 24-5.

Aspirin (acetylsalicylic acid) acetylates and inhibits cyclooxygenase in the platelet irreversibly such that the platelet cannot regenerate this enzyme. Therefore the effects of aspirin last the life span of a platelet, or 7 days. This irreversible inhibition of cyclooxygenase in the platelet prevents the formation of thromboxane (TX), a substance that causes blood vessels to constrict and platelets to aggregate. Thus by preventing TX formation, aspirin prevents these actions, with the result that blood vessels dilate and the platelets are prevented from aggregating or forming a clot. This system also exists in the blood vessel. However, much higher doses of aspirin (>80 mg per day) are needed to inhibit the cyclooxygenase pathway in the blood vessels, and this has the drawback of not only inhibiting the cyclooxygenase but also preventing the formation of prostacyclin, a beneficial substance that causes blood vessel dilation and inhibits platelet aggregation. If prostacylin is prevented from forming, vasoconstriction and platelet aggregation occur. By interfering with the

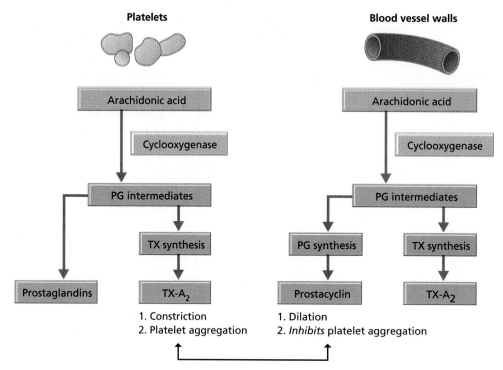

▼ **FIG. 24-5** Cyclooxygenase pathway. *PG*, prostaglandin; *TX-A₂*, thromboxane A₂.

function of the coagulation pathway, aspirin may also have a hematologic action. This is believed to consist in altering the hepatic synthesis of blood coagulation factors VII, IX, and X. Aspirin accomplishes this in much the same way that warfarin does, by interfering with the action of vitamin K.

Dipyridamole, another antiplatelet agent, also works by inhibiting platelet aggregation, which it does by preventing the release of ADP, PF4, and TX-A₂, substances that stimulate platelets to aggregate or form a clot. Figure 24-4 shows how these substances accomplish this. Dipyridamole may also directly stimulate the release of prostacyclin and inhibit the formation of TX-A₂ (see Fig. 24-5).

Ticlopidine is one of the newest antiplatelet drugs. Its mechanism of action is entirely different from aspirin's, in that it inhibits platelet aggregation by altering the platelet membrane so that it can no longer receive the signal to aggregate and form a clot. This signal is usually sent by fibrinogen, which attaches to a glycoprotein receptor (GP IIb-IIIa) on the surface of the platelet. Ticlopidine blocks this receptor. It may take 24 to 48 hours for this action to take effect, which suggests that these therapeutic effects may be produced by ticlopidine metabolites rather than by the ticlopidine itself.

Pentoxifylline, another antiplatelet agent, is a methylxanthine derivative with properties similar to those of theobromine, caffeine, and theophylline and other methylxanthines, but in contrast to other methylxanthines, it has little cardiac effects. It has many effects on blood. It can both increase the flexibility of red blood cells (RBCs) and reduce the aggregation of platelets. It is sometimes referred to as a hemorrheologic agent, or a drug that alters the normal function of the blood. It affects the RBCs by increasing the flexibility (deformability) of the cells and reducing the viscosity of whole blood, which it appears to do by facilitating the ability of the RBCs to maintain their integrity. The antiplatelet effects of pentoxifylline are that it inhibits platelet aggregation, which it does by inhibiting ADP, serotonin, and platelet factor 3 (see Fig. 24-4). Pentoxifylline also stimulates the synthesis and release of prostacyclin from blood vessels (see Fig. 24-5). In addition, it may have effects on the system that is responsible for lysing or breaking down clots, the fibrinolytic system. This may involve its increasing the breakdown of fibrin by raising the plasma concentrations of the tissue plasminogen activator (see Fig. 24-3).

Drug Effects

The drug effects of the antiplatelet drugs are multiple, but their primary ones are on the blood and the various mechanisms that maintain hemostasis. Although they have multiple effects on various components of the blood, they primarily inhibit the actions of platelets.

Table 24-4	Antiplatelet Drugs: Adverse Effects
BODY SYSTEM	**SIDE/ADVERSE EFFECT**
Aspirin	
Hematologic	Thrombocytopenia, agranulocytosis, leukopenia, neutropenia, hemolytic anemia, bleeding
Central nervous system	Stimulation, drowsiness, dizziness, confusion, flushing
Gastrointestinal	Nausea, vomiting, GI bleeding, diarrhea, heartburn
Dipyridamole	
Central nervous system	Headache, dizziness, weakness, fainting, syncope
Gastrointestinal	Nausea, vomiting, diarrhea
Ticlopidine	
Gastrointestinal	Nausea, vomiting, diarrhea, cholestatic jaundice, hepatitis, increased cholesterol level
Hematologic	Bleeding, agranulocytosis, neutropenia, thrombocytopenia
Pentoxifylline	
Central nervous system	Headache, anxiety, tremors, confusion, dizziness
Gastrointestinal	Nausea, vomiting, bloating, constipation, dry mouth, thirst, bad taste
Cardiovascular	Angina, dysrhythmias, palpitation, hypotension, chest pain, dyspnea

Table 24-5	Adrenergics: Interactions with Selected Agents		
DRUG	**INTERACTS WITH**	**MECHANISM**	**RESULT**
Dipyridamole	Anticoagulants	Inhibits PLT aggregation	Increased chance for bleeding
Ticlopidine			
Pentoxifylline			

Therapeutic Uses

The therapeutic effects of the antiplatelet drugs depend on the particular agent. Aspirin has multiple therapeutic effects, but many of them vary depending on the dose. Aspirin has analgesic, antiinflammatory, and antipyretic properties. It also has potent antithrombotic and hematologic effects. Dipyridamole is used as an adjunct to warfarin in the prevention of postoperative thromboembolic complications. It is also used to decrease platelet aggregation in the setting of a number of other thromboembolic disorders. Ticlopidine's therapeutic effects are similar to a few of the therapeutic effects of aspirin. It has antithrombotic effects and is useful for reducing the risk of fatal and nonfatal thrombotic stroke.

Side Effects and Adverse Effects

The potential adverse effects of the various antiplatelet drugs can be serious. The most common ones are listed in Table 24-4.

Interactions

There are some potentially very dangerous drug interactions that can occur with the antiplatelet agents. The most common of these are listed in Table 24-5, and more details on the drug interactions of aspirin are provided in Table 24-6. When ticlopidine is coadministered with antacids, this results in its decreased absorption. Its use with digoxin causes the plasma levels of the digoxin to be decreased. Concurrent use with aspirin is not recommended. The concurrent use of both dipyridamole and aspirin produces additive antiplatelet activity.

Ticlopidine can produce elevations in the alkaline phosphatase activity, the bilirubin level, and the transaminase activity.

Dosages

For information on the dosages of selected antiplatelet agents, see the dosages table on the following page.

DRUG PROFILES

The antiplatelet drugs are extremely useful in the management of thromboembolic disorders. Each has unique pharmacologic properties that make them all somewhat different from the other.

Table 24-6	Aspirin: Drug Interactions
INTERACTS WITH	**RESULT**
Steroids	Increase ulcerogenic effects and bleeding tendencies
Anticoagulants	Increased bleeding
Oral antidiabetic agents	Loss of diabetic control
NSAIDs	If allergic to aspirin, may also be allergic to these agents; potentiates bleeding because of salicylate components; increases ulcerogenic effects
Furosemide	Increased toxicity

ASPIRIN

Aspirin is available in many combinations with other prescription and nonprescription drugs and goes by many product names. It is classified as a pregnancy category D agent. Aspirin is contraindicated in patients with a known hypersensitivity to salicylates, in those with GI bleeding or bleeding disorders, in children under 12 years of age or with flulike symptoms, in lactating women, and in patients with vitamin K deficiency or peptic ulcer disease. It is available orally and rectally. Orally it comes in many doses and dosage forms. It is available as chewing gum containing 227 mg per stick; as tablets of numerous strengths: 324, 325, 500, and 650 mg; as 75- and 81-mg chewable tablets; as 165-, 324-, 325-, 500-, 650-, and 975-mg delayed-release tablets; as 650- and 800-mg extended-release tablets; and as 325- and 500-mg film-coated tablets. For commonly recommended dosages, see the dosages table below.

PHARMACOKINETICS

HALF-LIFE	ONSET	PEAK	DURATION
2-3 hr	15-30 min	0.25-2 hr	4-6 hr

DIPYRIDAMOLE

Dipyridamole (Persantine) works by inhibiting platelet aggregation and is used as an adjunct to warfarin in the prevention of postoperative thromboembolic complications. It also has been used to decrease plate-

DOSAGES

SELECTED ANTIPLATELET AGENTS

AGENT	PHARMACOLOGIC CLASS	DOSAGE RANGE	PURPOSE
Aspirin	Salicylate antiplatelet	*Adult* PO: 325-650 mg 2-4 times/day	Antithrombotic for MI prophylaxis and TIA
Dipyridamole (Persantine)	Antiplatelet	*Adult* PO: 75-100 mg qid	Antithrombotic for prosthetic heart valve replacement
Ticlopidine (Ticlid)	Antiplatelet	*Adult* PO: 250 mg bid with food	Reduce risk of thrombotic stroke in high-risk patients
Pentoxifylline (Trental)	Antiplatelet/ hemorrheologic	*Adult* PO: 400 mg tid with meals	Claudication associated with peripheral arterial disease

MI, myocardial infarction; *TIA*, transient ischemic attack.

let aggregation in the setting of a number of other thromboembolic disorders. Dipyridamole is a prescription-only drug and is classified as a pregnancy category C agent. It is contraindicated in patients with a known hypersensitivity to it and in those suffering from hypotension. Dipyridamole is available in oral preparations as 25-, 50-, and 75-mg tablets. For commonly recommended dosages, see the dosages table on p. 352.

❖❖ P H A R M A C O K I N E T I C S

HALF-LIFE	ONSET	PEAK	DURATION
10-12 hr	20-30 min	75 min	3 hr

TICLOPIDINE

Ticlopidine (Ticlid) is used to reduce the risk of fatal and nonfatal thrombotic stroke in patients who have suffered either a completed thrombotic stroke or stroke precursors (e.g., transient ischemic attacks, reversible ischemic neurologic deficit, or minor stroke). Its use should be reserved for patients unable to tolerate aspirin therapy because of the life-threatening neutropenia and agranulocytosis it can precipitate. It is classified as a pregnancy category B agent and is contraindicated in patients with a known hypersensitivity to it, as well as in those with active liver disease or a blood dyscrasia. It is only available orally as 250-mg film-coated tablets. For commonly recommended dosages, see the dosages table on p. 352.

❖❖ P H A R M A C O K I N E T I C S

HALF-LIFE	ONSET	PEAK	DURATION
12.6 hr then 4-5 days	<4 days	2 hr	2 wks after discontinuation

PENTOXIFYLLINE

As already noted, pentoxifylline (Trental) has many effects on the blood. It can both increase the flexibility of RBCs and reduce the aggregation of platelets. It is a prescription-only drug with many uses other than its antiplatelet one. It is contraindicated in patients with a known hypersensitivity to it or any methylxanthine. It is classified as a pregnancy category C agent and is only available orally as a 400-mg film-coated, extended-release tablet. For commonly recommended dosages, see the dosages table on p. 352.

❖❖ P H A R M A C O K I N E T I C S

HALF-LIFE	ONSET	PEAK	DURATION
0.4-8 hr	Unknown	0.8-2.6 hr	Unknown

ANTIFIBRINOLYTICS

The individual antifibrinolytic agents have varying mechanisms of action, but all prevent the lysis of fibrin, the substance that helps make the platelet plug insoluble and anchors the clot to the damaged blood vessel (see Figs. 24-1 and 24-2). The term **antifibrinolytic** refers to what these drugs do, which is to prevent the lysis of fibrin; in doing so, they promote clot formation. They have the opposite effects of the anticoagulant and antiplatelet agents, which prevent clot formation. There are two synthetic antifibrinolytics, aminocaproic acid and tranexamic acid; one natural antifibrinolytic agent, aprotinin; and another antifibrinolytic with a different mechanism of action, desmopressin. Other drugs used to stop excessive bleeding are referred to as hemostatic agents, and these comprise thrombin, microfibrillar collagen, absorbable gelatin, and oxidized cellulose. These agents are not discussed here.

Mechanism of Action

The antifibrinolytics vary in several ways, depending on the particular agent. The various antifibrinolytic agents and their proposed mechanisms of action are described in Table 24-7.

Drug Effects

The drug effects of the antifibrinolytics are very specific and limited. They do not have many effects outside of their hematologic ones. Aminocaproic acid, tranexamic acid, and aprotinin prevent the breakdown of fibrin, which prevents the destruction of the formed platelet clot. Desmopressin increases the resorption of water by the collecting ducts in the kidneys, resulting in increased urine osmolality and a decreased urinary flow rate. It also causes a dose-dependent increase in the concentration of plasma factor VIII (von Willebrand factor) along with an increase in the plasma concentration of tissue plasminogen activator. The overall effect of this is increased platelet aggregation and clot formation.

Therapeutic Uses

The antifibrinolytics are useful in both the prevention and treatment of excessive bleeding resulting from systemic hyperfibrinolysis or surgical complications. They have also proved successful in arresting excessive oozing from surgical sites such as chest tubes as well as in reducing the total blood loss and the duration of bleeding in the postoperative period.

Desmopressin's therapeutic effects exceed those of the antifibrinolytics. It can be given either intranasally or parenterally to prevent or control polydipsia, poly-

Table 24-7	Antifibrinolytics: Mechanism of Action
ANTIFIBRINOLYTIC AGENT	**MECHANISM OF ACTION**
Synthetic agents: aminocaproic acid and tranexamic acid	Forms a reversible complex with plasminogen and plasmin. By binding to the lysine-binding site of plasminogen, it displaces plasminogen from the surface of fibrin. This prevents plasmin from lysing the fibrin clot. Therefore these drugs can only work if a clot has formed.
Natural agent: aprotinin	Inhibits the proteolytic enzymes trypsin, plasmin, and kallikrein, which lyse proteins that destroy fibrin clots. By inhibiting these enzymes, aprotinin prevents the degradation of the fibrin clot. It is also thought to inhibit the action of the complement system.
Other: desmopressin (DDAVP)	Works by increasing factor VIII (von Willebrand factor), which anchors platelets to damaged vessels via the glycoprotein Ib platelet receptor. It appears that desmopressin acts as a general endothelial stimulant, stimulating factor VIII, prostaglandin I_2, and plasminogen-activated release.

Table 24-8	Antifibrinolytics: Adverse Effects
BODY SYSTEM	**SIDE/ADVERSE EFFECT**
Gastrointestinal	Nausea, vomiting, abdominal cramps, diarrhea
Central nervous system	Headache, dizziness, fatigue, hallucinations, psychosis, convulsions
Cardiovascular	Dysrhythmias, orthostatic hypotension, bradycardia

uria, and dehydration in patients with diabetes insipidus caused by a deficiency of endogenous posterior pituitary vasopressin and in patients with polyuria and polydipsia stemming from trauma or surgery in the pituitary region. It may also be used in patients who have hemophilia A or type I von Willebrand's disease. Desmopressin increases the levels of clotting factors these patients are deficient in.

Side Effects and Adverse Effects

The adverse effects of the antifibrinolytic drugs are infrequent and mild. There have been rare reports of these agents causing thrombotic events such as acute cerebrovascular thrombosis and acute myocardial infarction. The common side effects of antifibrinolytics are listed in Table 24-8.

Interactions

The drug interactions associated with the antifibrinolytics are few, and these are listed in Table 24-9. The concurrent use of drugs such as estrogens or oral contraceptives with aminocaproic acid, tranexamic acid, and aprotinin may have an additive effect, re-

sulting in increased coagulation. Few specific interactions have been reported for desmopressin, though it should be given cautiously in patients receiving lithium, large doses of epinephrine, demeclocycline, heparin, or alcohol because this may lead to a reduced antidiuretic response to the desmopressin. Drugs such as chlorpropamide and fludrocortisone may potentiate the antidiuretic response. The concurrent administration of clofibrate and desmopressin may prolong the antidiuretic effect of desmopressin.

Dosages

For information on the dosages for aminocaproic acid and desmopressin, see the dosages table on the next page.

DRUG PROFILES

The antifibrinolytics have a very limited use in preventing the lysis of fibrin, which promotes clot formation. The prototypical antifibrinolytic is aminocaproic acid. The effects of tranexamic acid and aprotinin are similar to those of aminocaproic acid, but desmopressin's effects are totally different from those of the other three agents.

AMINOCAPROIC ACID

Aminocaproic acid (Amicar) is a synthetic antifibrinolytic agent used to prevent and control the excessive bleeding that can result from surgery or overactivity

Table 24-9	Antifibrinolytics: Interactions	
DRUG	**INTERACTS WITH**	**RESULT**
Estrogens Oral contraceptives	Additive	Increased coagulation

DOSAGES

AMINOCAPROIC ACID AND DESMOPRESSIN

AGENT	PHARMACOLOGIC CLASS	DOSAGE RANGE	PURPOSE
Aminocaproic acid (Amicar)	Hemostatic	*Adult* IV infusion: 4-5 gm during first hour then 1-1.25 g at 1-hr intervals up to a daily maximum of 30 g	Excessive bleeding due to systemic hyperfibrin-olysis or urinary fibri-nolysis
Desmopressin (DDAVP)	Synthetic posterior pituitary hormone	*Adult* IV: 0.3 μg/kg infused over 15-30 min. Preop use: agent is administered 30 min before surgery	Surgical and postop he-mostasis and manage-ment of bleeding in patients with hemo-philia A or type I von Willebrand's disease

of the fibrinolytic system. Its use is contraindicated in patients who have had a hypersensitivity to it, as well as in the settings of postpartum bleeding, disseminated intravascular coagulation, upper urinary tract bleeding, and new burns. It is considered a pregnancy category C drug. It is available in both oral and parenteral preparations. Orally it comes as a 1.25-mg/ml solution and a 500-mg tablet. Parenterally it comes as a 250-mg/ml injection for intravenous infusion. For commonly recommended dosages, see the dosages table above.

PHARMACOKINETICS

HALF-LIFE	ONSET	PEAK	DURATION
2 hr	Unknown	1.2 hr	Unknown

DESMOPRESSIN

Desmopressin (DDAVP) is a synthetic polypeptide. It is structurally very similar to vasopressin, which is antidiuretic hormone, the natural human posterior pituitary hormone. Because of these physical characteris-

tics, it is often used to increase the resorption of water by the collecting ducts in the kidneys to prevent or control polydipsia, polyuria, and dehydration in patients with diabetes insipidus caused by a deficiency of endogenous posterior pituitary vasopressin or in patients with polyuria and polydipsia resulting from trauma or surgery in the pituitary region.

Desmopressin also causes a dose-dependent increase in plasma factor VIII (von Willebrand factor) along with an increase in tissue plasminogen activator, with the overall effect increased platelet aggregation and clot formation. Desmopressin is classified as a pregnancy B agent and is contraindicated in patients with a known hypersensitivity to it and in those with nephrogenic diabetes insipidus. It is available as a 10–μg/0.1 ml intranasal solution and a 4-μg/ml parenteral injection. For commonly recommended dosages, see the dosages table above.

PHARMACOKINETICS

HALF-LIFE	ONSET	PEAK	DURATION
<2 hr	15-30 min	1.1-2 hr	Unknown

THROMBOLYTICS

Thrombolytics are coagulation modifiers that break down, or lyse, performed clots (thrombi) in the blood vessels that supply the heart with blood, the coronary arteries. This reestablishes blood flow to the blood-starved heart muscle. If the blood flow is reestablished soon, the heart muscle and left ventricular function can be saved. If blood flow is not reestablished early, the heart muscle becomes ischemic, then necrotic, and eventually nonfunctional.

Thrombolytic therapy made its debut in 1933 when a substance that would break down fibrin clots was isolated from a patient's blood. This substance was observed to be produced by a bacteria growing in the patient. The bacteria was found to be group A **beta-hemolytic streptococci**, and the substance was eventually called streptokinase (SK). SK was first used in a patient in 1947 to dissolve a clotted hemothorax, but it was not until 1958 when the first patient with an acute myocardial infarction (AMI) received it. In 1960 a naturally occurring human plasminogen activator called urokinase came available that was found to exert fibrinolytic effects on pulmonary emboli (clots in the lungs). However, the results of the early thrombolytic trials conducted during the 1960s and 1970s and made up of patients who had had an AMI were not taken seriously by the medical community. It was not until the 1980s when DeWood and colleagues demonstrated that the underlying cause of AMIs was a coronary artery occlusion that the use of thrombolytics for the early treatment of AMIs took off.

During the past decade, new thrombolytics have been developed and launched. Tissue plasminogen activator and **anisylated plasminogen streptokinase activator complex** are two of these agents. With the advent of these new thrombolytics came the performance of several large landmark thrombolytic research studies, which showed that early thrombolytic therapy could bring about a 50% reduction in mortality, a reduction in the infarct size, an improvement in left ventricular function, and a reduction in the incidence and severity of congestive heart failure. These findings and developments along with a better understanding of the pathogenesis of AMIs have led the way in the advancements made in the treatment of AMIs.

Mechanism of Action

There is a fine balance between the formation and dissolution of a clot. The coagulation system is responsible for clot formation while the fibrinolytic system is responsible for dissolving the clot. The natural fibrinolytic system within blood takes days to break down a clot, and this is of little value in the case of a clotted blood vessel supplying blood to the heart muscle. Necrosis of the myocardium would not be prevented by these natural means, but thrombolytic therapy can activate the fibrinolytic system to break down the clot (thrombus) in the blood vessel quickly so that the delivery of blood to the heart muscle via the coronary arteries is quickly reestablished. This prevents myocardial tissue (heart muscle) and heart function from being destroyed. The thrombolytics accomplish this by activating the conversion of plasminogen to plasmin, which breaks down, or lyses, the thrombus (see Fig. 24-3). Plasmin is a proteolytic enzyme, which means that it breaks down proteins. It is a relatively nonspecific serine protease that is capable of degrading such proteins as fibrin, fibrinogen, and other procoagulant proteins such as factors V, VIII, and XII. In other words, the substances that form clots are destroyed by plasmin. Essentially, these drugs work by mimicking the body's own process of clot destruction. Although the individual thrombolytic agents are somewhat diverse in their actions, they all have this common end result.

SK binds with plasminogen to form an SK-plasminogen complex, which then acts on other plasminogen molecules to form plasmin. The plasmin formed then lyses the clots. SK is not **clot specific**, in that not only does it break down the thrombus in the coronary artery but it also breaks down clots anywhere in the body. It activates fibrinolysis throughout the body. Tissue plasminogen activator (t-PA) is a naturally occurring plasminogen activator secreted by vascular endothelial cells (the walls of blood vessels). However, the amount secreted naturally is not sufficient to dissolve a coronary thrombus quickly enough to restore circulation to the heart and save the heart muscle. t-PA is now made through recombinant DNA techniques and can thus be administered in quantities sufficient enough to dissolve a coronary thrombus quickly. It is fibrin specific and also clot specific, meaning that only the fibrin clot stimulates t-PA to convert plasminogen to plasmin. Therefore it does not induce a systemic lytic state. The anisoylated plasminogen-streptokinase activator complex (APSAC) is an SK-plasminogen complex that has been chemically modified by acylation, allowing a prolonged half-life. It, like SK, is not clot specific, so systemic fibrinolysis is induced with its use.

Drug Effects

The drug effects of the thrombolytics are primarily related to their action on the fibrinolytic system. They stimulate the fibrinolytic system to lyse preformed clots, and their action is limited solely to the fibrinolytic system.

Therapeutic Uses

The purpose of all the thrombolytic agents is to activate the conversion of plasminogen to plasmin, the enzyme that breaks down a thrombus. The presence of a thrombus that interferes significantly with normal blood flow on either the venous or the arterial side of the circulation is an indication for the use of thrombolytic therapy. Until further information is available, an exception to this may be a thrombus that has formed in blood vessels that directly connect with the central nervous system. The indications for thrombolytic therapy include AMI, arterial thrombosis, deep vein thrombosis, occlusion of shunts or catheters, and pulmonary embolism. Its use for other thrombotic disorders is currently being evaluated.

Side Effects and Adverse Effects

The most frequent undesirable effect of thrombolytic therapy is internal and superficial bleeding. Other problems include hypersensitivity, anaphylactoid reactions, nausea, vomiting, and hypotension. These drugs can also induce dysrhythmias, and urokinase therapy has been associated with the development of a Guillain-Barré–type syndrome.

Toxicity and Management of Overdose

Acute toxicity primarily causes an extension of the side effects of the thrombolytic agent, and treatment is symptomatic and supportive.

Interactions

The most common effect of drug interactions is an increased bleeding tendency resulting from the concurrent use of anticoagulants and antiplatelets or drugs that affect platelet function.

A laboratory test interaction that can occur with thrombolytic agents is a reduction in the plasminogen and fibrinogen levels.

Dosages

For information on the dosages for SK, alteplase, and urokinase, see the dosages table on the next page.

DRUG PROFILES

All thrombolytic agents exert their effects by activating plasminogen and converting it to plasmin, which is capable of digesting fibrinogen, a major component of clots. The three thrombolytic agents currently approved for intravenous use in the management of AMIs are SK, APSAC, and t-PA. The fourth thrombolytic agent available is urokinase. However, it is administered to lyse peripheral vascular thrombi and is seldom used to treat AMIs.

⚓ STREPTOKINASE

SK (Streptase, Kabikinase) is the oldest thrombolytic agent, the one produced from beta-hemolytic streptococci. It binds with plasminogen, and this SK-plasminogen complex then acts on other plasminogen molecules to form plasmin. As pointed out earlier, SK is not clot specific. Because it is made from a nonhuman source, it is antigenic and may provoke allergic reactions. This happens because the body's immune system recognizes it as a foreign substance (an antigen) and launches an antibody against it, with an antigen-antibody reaction the result. These antibodies develop approximately 5 days after SK therapy and persist for 6 months to 1 year afterwards. It is therefore recommended that patients not be retreated with SK or APSAC during that time. Hypotension secondary to vasodilation occurs in approximately 10% to 15% of patients given SK.

SK is a pregnancy category C agent and is contraindicated in patients with a known hypersensitivity to it, as well as in the settings of active internal bleeding, an aneurysm, uncontrolled hypotension, an intracranial or intraspinal neoplasm, surgery, and trauma. It is only available parenterally in doses of 250,000, 750,000, and 1,500,000 IU per vial. For the commonly recommended dosages, see the dosages table on the next page.

⬡ PHARMACOKINETICS

HALF-LIFE	ONSET	PEAK	DURATION
18 min then 83 min	1 hr	Varies with dose	24-36 hr

ALTEPLASE

Alteplase (Activase) is a naturally occurring t-PA secreted by vascular endothelial cells. The pharmaceutically available t-PA is made through recombinant DNA techniques, and modified mammalian hamster ovary cells produce the substance. It is clot (fibrin) specific, and thus it does not produce a systemic lytic state. In addition, because it is present in our bodies in a natural state, its administration for therapeutic use does not induce an antigen-antibody reaction. It can therefore be readministered immediately in the event of reinfarction. t-PA has a very short half-life of 5 minutes. It is believed to open the clogged artery faster, but its action is short-lived. Therefore, it is given con-

DOSAGES

SELECTED THROMBOLYTIC AGENTS

AGENT	PHARMACOLOGIC CLASS	DOSAGE RANGE	PURPOSE
Streptokinase (Streptase, Kabikinase)	Thrombolytic enzyme	*Adult* IV: initial bolus of 200,000 IU followed by a maintenance infusion of 2000 IU/min for 1 hr or intracoronary infusion initiated with a bolus of 20,000 IU followed by 2000 IU/min for 1 hr	Acute evolving MI
		IV: loading dose of 250,000 IU over 30 min followed by a maintenance infusion of 100,000 IU/hr for 24-72 hr	Deep vein thrombosis, arterial thrombosis and embolism, pulmonary embolism
		IV: 250,000 IU into each occluded limb of the cannula over 25-35 min and clamped for 2 hr followed by aspiration of the infused cannula with saline and reconnection of the cannula	Arteriovenous cannula occlusion
Urokinase (Abbokinase)	Thrombolytic enzyme	*Adult* IV: initial dose of 2000 IU/1b given over 10 min followed by a continuous infusion of 2000 IU/1b/hr for up to 12 hr	Pulmonary embolism
		Infuse into occluded artery at 6000 IU/min for up to 12 hr following an initial bolus dose of 2,500-10,000 U of heparin	Coronary artery thrombi
		1 ml or 5000 IU for each catheter clearance	Occluded IV catheters
Alteplase (Activase; tissue plasminogen activator)	Thrombolytic enzyme	*Adult* IV: 100 mg administered over 3 hr. First hour: 60 mg (34.8 million IU), of which 6-10 mg is given as a bolus dose, followed by 20 mg/hr given during the second and third hour.	Acute MI
		100 mg over 2 hr or 30 or 50 mg over 1.5-2 hr via pulmonary artery with concurrent heparin	Pulmonary embolism

comitantly with heparin to prevent reocclusion of the infarcted blood vessel.

The contraindications to alteplase use and its pregnancy rating are the same as SK's. Alteplase is also only available parenterally as 20-, 50-, and 100-mg injections for intravenous infusion. For the commonly recommended dosages, see the dosages table above. Pregnancy category C.

PHARMACOKINETICS

HALF-LIFE	ONSET	PEAK	DURATION
30-35 min	Unknown	Varies with dose	Unknown

ANISTREPLASE

Anistreplase (APSAC) is a new second-generation thrombolytic agent that has been developed for the purpose of overcoming some of the limitations of SK. APSAC is an SK-plasminogen complex that has been chemically modified by acylation, allowing a prolonged half-life. It is a sustained-release form of SK. It has a greater affinity for fibrin and a longer duration of action than SK and alteplase. These properties simplify intravenous administration, potentially improve coronary reperfusion, and reduce the reocclusion rates. It is similar to SK in that it is not clot specific and it has the same potential for causing allergic reactions as SK.

APSAC has the same contraindications and pregnancy rating as SK and is also only available parenterally. It comes as a 30-U/vial injection for intravenous infusion. Pregnancy category C.

✿ PHARMACOKINETICS

HALF-LIFE	ONSET	PEAK	DURATION
1.75-2 hr	Unknown	Unknown	Unknown

UROKINASE

Human urokinase (Abbokinase) was the first t-PA. It was initially purified from human urine but in North America is currently prepared from transformed fetal renal parenchymal cells in tissue culture. Urokinase is occasionally used as a thrombolytic agent in the treatment of AMIs, but clinical experience with this use is considerably more limited than that with the other thrombolytics. It is primarily used for the treatment of pulmonary embolism and occluded intravenous catheters. Its contraindications are the same as those of the other thrombolytics, but it is a pregnancy category B agent. Urokinase is only available in a parenteral preparation and comes in doses of 250,000, 5000, and 9000 per vial for intravenous injection. For commonly recommended dosages, see the dosages table on p. 358.

✿ PHARMACOKINETICS

HALF-LIFE	ONSET	PEAK	DURATION
10-20 min	Unknown	Unknown	<3 hr

NURSING PROCESS

There are a variety of conditions that warrant the use of coagulation modifiers. These conditions range from venous or arterial thromboembolism to vessel injury, and any of the coagulation modifiers such as heparin, warfarin, aspirin, dipyridamole, SK, and urokinase may be required for treatment. These agents with their different mechanisms of action and indications require some very specific nursing processes, and each is discussed under each category of coagulation modifier.

Anticoagulants

ASSESSMENT

The nursing assessment of patients receiving the anticoagulants heparin or warfarin sodium is very important to the safe care of these patients with some very life-threatening conditions. It is important to obtain a medical and medication history on the patient as well as information on any hypersensitivity reactions to medications before initiating treatment with an anticoagulant. Contraindications to the use of these agents include any condition in which there is a risk of hemorrhage, conditions such as severe hypertension, ulcer disease, ulcerative colitis, aneurysms, malignant hypertension, alcoholism, and head injuries. Women who are pregnant or breast feeding should also not be given warfarin sodium or indanedione derivatives. Extreme caution is necessary when heparin is used in patients undergoing major surgery or in patients receiving any other agents that may precipitate bleeding, agents such as those listed in Table 24-1. Patients with a history of congestive heart failure may also show an increased sensitivity to warfarin sodium and the indanedione derivatives.

NURSING DIAGNOSES

Nursing diagnoses that pertain to patients receiving anticoagulants include:
- Pain related to symptoms of underlying disorder or ischemia.
- Knowledge deficit related to new medication regimen and need for altered life-style.
- Risk for altered mobility related to underlying tissue disorder or ischemia.
- Risk for injury to self related to side effects of medications.
- Altered tissue perfusion (decreased) related to underlying disorder or ischemia.

PLANNING

Goals for the patient receiving anticoagulants include:
- Patient experiences increased comfort and relief of pain.
- Patient exhibits improved blood flow as the result of the therapeutic effects of the anticoagulants.
- Patient remains free from injury stemming from either the disease or the medication being taken.
- Patient will be compliant with the life-style changes required and with the medication therapy.
- Patient demonstrates adequate knowledge regard-

ing medication therapy and its potential side effects.

Outcome Criteria

Outcome criteria pertaining to the use of anticoagulants include:

- Patient will experience relief of symptoms such as decreased pain, swelling, and edema once tissue perfusion is regained as the result of medication therapy.
- Patient will show improved circulation with warm extremities, strong pedal pulses or experience a return to his or her predisease state of tissue perfusion.
- Patient will be free of bruising, bleeding problems, or any other adverse reaction to the medication.
- Patient states the rationale for the use of the medication regimen such as decreased clotting or clot formation.
- Patient states the nature of and rationale for the life-style changes needed, such as improved diet, exercise, and no smoking.
- Patient states side effects, how to monitor for complications of the anticoagulants, the importance of coming in for follow-up appointments with the physician and of frequent laboratory studies, and when to contact the physician so as to prevent complications such as hemorrhage.

IMPLEMENTATION

Vital signs are routinely monitored in all patients initially taking an anticoagulant as well as during therapy. Various laboratory values should also be monitored in patients receiving an anticoagulant. Any change in pulse rate or rhythm, blood pressure, or level of consciousness, and the occurrence of unexplained restlessness are significant because they are possible indications of bleeding problems related to the anticoagulant. The physician should be notified immediately of the occurrence of any of these problems.

Safe and effective treatment with anticoagulants requires that the nurse have an adequate knowledge about the similarities of and differences between the various anticoagulants. Knowledge of the proper techniques of administration is also crucial to their safe use. For example, it is important to remember that heparin should only be given subcutaneously or intravenously, not intramuscularly. To prevent inadvertent IM injection during subcutaneous injection, a ⅝-inch (1.5 cm) needle should be used. Sites of injection include areas of deep subcutaneous fat such as the fatty layer of the abdomen 2 inches (5 cm) away from the umbilicus or the area near the iliac crest. Incisional areas or wounds should be avoided by at least 2 inches. See the box

---

Subcutaneous ⬇Heparin Administration

- After thoroughly checking the physician's order, assess the patient for the existence of any allergies, contraindications, or cautions.

- Wash your hands thoroughly. Check the heparin bottle for the proper dilution of the agent, the expiration date, and the clarity of the solution. Using a tuberculin syringe, especially for small doses, draw up the exact dose of heparin. Always double-check with another registered nurse to make sure of the right dose. Replace the needle with a new sterile ⅝-in (1.5-cm), 26- to 28-gauge needle so that there is no residual on the needle and to ensure adequate sharpness of the needle for injection.

- Check the patient's identification band to make sure you have the correct patient.

- Put on disposable gloves and select the injection site outside a 2-in (5-cm) area around the umbilicus. Although the abdominal area or the area around the iliac crest is the preferred site of injection, any of the subcutaneous sites may be used. Always check where previous injections have been administered so that you can rotate the sites appropriately.

- Cleanse the site thoroughly with antiseptic but be careful not to massage or rub the site before or after the injection. Let the antiseptic dry before giving the injection.

- Grasp the subcutaneous tissue firmly so as to form a fat pad, then quickly insert the needle at a 90-degree angle. *Do not aspirate*, and be careful not to pinch the skin. Release the skin gently, and slowly inject the heparin. Count for 10 seconds, then withdraw the needle without changing its angle. Press a sterile 2 × 2–in (5 × 5–cm) gauze pad or sponge over the area and maintain gentle but firm pressure for 10 sec. *Be careful not to massage, rub, or traumatize the skin.*

- Check the site for bleeding or bruising and document the site, time, dose, and any other pertinent information in the appropriate places in the patient's chart and/or medication record. Make sure your patient is comfortable, then remove your gloves and wash your hands.

---

above for the procedure to follow subcutaneous for heparin administration.

When rapid anticoagulation is needed, the physician will generally order heparin to be given IV, either by continuous or intermittent infusion. During continuous IV heparin infusion, blood levels can be maintained and the effects can be easily reversed with the IV administration of protamine sulfate. The effects of SC heparin can also be reversed with protamine sulfate, but it often takes several doses to produce this effect because of the variable rates of absorption of the SC forms. See the box on the following page for the

---

Intravenous ⚓Heparin Administration

- For the continuous IV administration of heparin, an IV pump must be used to ensure a steady and precise rate of infusion.
- Always double-check the physician's order for the dose, rate, time, and route before initiating therapy. Generally, about a 6- to 12-hr supply is ordered.
- No other medication should be administered with the heparin or through the heparin line.
- For intermittent infusions, a heparin lock was used in years past. Nowadays in most institutions, heparin locks are called *intermittent infusion locks* and they are generally flushed with normal saline. Some institutions still use heparin locks and administer 10 to 100 USP units of heparin per milliliter of a flushing solution.
- Intermittent infusions of heparin are usually ordered to be given every 4 to 6 hr because of heparin's short half-life. The drug should be infused slowly and given either undiluted or diluted with 50 to 100 ml of isotonic saline solution, though the latter practice is preferred.
- Guidelines for intermittent infusions include injection through the lock after cleansing the diaphragm with 70% alcohol and using a 25- to 27-gauge needle, which helps the diaphragm to reseal after repeated injections.
- Regardless of whether the injection is given through an IV pump or by intermittent or continuous IV infusion, it is crucial to always check the site to determine whether infiltration has occurred, so as to prevent a hematoma from forming there. Should this occur, the lock should be removed and replaced in a new site before the next scheduled infusion. Document your actions appropriately in the nurse's notes.

Oral Anticoagulant Administration

- It is important to recheck the physician's orders and the patient's medication and medical history before administering the agent. Always check to make sure the patient has no known hypersensitivity to the agent.
- There are many more drugs that can interact with oral anticoagulants than with heparin, especially those that are highly protein bound such as the ones listed in Table 24-3. Always check the patient's medication list before initiating therapy with warfarin sodium or indanedione.
- The dose of the medication is calculated on the basis of the patient's clotting values.
- Oral anticoagulants should be administered at the same time every day to maintain steady blood levels.
- Document the dose, time of administration, and any other pertinent facts.

---

procedure for the intermittent or continuous IV administration of heparin.

When oral anticoagulants such as warfarin sodium and the indanedione derivatives are prescribed, therapy is often initiated with heparin until the prothrombin times indicate an adequate therapeutic response. This is necessary because the action of oral anticoagulants does not appear until about 12 to 24 hours after the first dose, by which time the normal removal of circulating clotting factors has occurred. The administration procedures for the oral anticoagulants are outlined in the box above right.

Patient education is a vital part of the nursing care plan for patients receiving anticoagulants. Not only do patients need to understand the reason why they are receiving anticoagulants, but they also need to understand the importance of laboratory testing to monitor

the therapeutic, side, and toxic effects of these drugs. Patient teaching tips for all the anticoagulants are listed in the box on the next page.

Should uncontrolled bleeding occur, the nurse must institute emergency measures to stabilize the patient's condition. Laboratory values should be reported to the physician. The antidote to hemorrhage or uncontrolled bleeding resulting from heparin therapy is protamine sulfate and that to oral anticoagulant therapy is vitamin K, which can be administered IV, IM, or orally. However, this may precipate resistance to future use of the oral anticoagulant which may last for some time.

EVALUATION

Monitoring for the therapeutic and adverse effects of anticoagulants is crucial to their safe use. Adverse effects of heparin therapy include elevated blood pressure, headache, hematoma formation, irritation and pain at the injection site, hemorrhage, thrombocytopenia, shortness of breath, chills, and fever. Early signs of an overdose of anticoagulants include bleeding of the gums while brushing teeth, unexplained nosebleeds or bruising, and heavier-than-usual menstrual bleeding. Abdominal pain, back pain, bloody or tarry stools, bloody urine, constipation, blood in the sputum, severe or continuous headaches, and the vomiting of frank red blood or a "coffee ground" substance (old blood) are all indications of internal bleeding. Warfarin sodium and the indanedione derivatives can also cause hair loss, rash, abdominal pain, diarrhea, nausea, vomiting, and leukopenia.

Therapeutic levels of anticoagulants can be monitored by laboratory tests. The standard tests for determining the effects of heparin therapy are the clotting times, and these consist of the Lee-White whole blood clotting time, the whole blood activated partial thromboplastin time (WBAPTT), and the activated partial thromboplastin time (APTT), the latter being the test most commonly used. A whole blood clotting time of 2½ to 3 times the control value indicates therapeutic levels have been reached. With IV heparin administrations, especially continuous IV infusions, coagulation studies should be performed every 4 hours. Prothrombin times are used to determine the dose of warfarin

sodium. Prothrombin times are determined daily in patients just starting warfarin sodium therapy until a time of 1½ to 2½ times the normal control value is reached, which indicates a therapeutic effect. Once the level of the particular agent stabilizes, the times may be determined at 1- to 4-week intervals depending on the patient's response and physical condition.

Should a heparin overdose occur, the antidote is protamine sulfate, given IV over 1 to 3 minutes. Vitamin K, or phytonadione, is the antidote to oral anticoagulant overdose and can be given IM, SC, IV, or orally, depending on the patient's condition.

Because of the complexity and life-threatening nature of the conditions anticoagulants are used for, the nurse must continually reassess and monitor the patient's response to the treatment and document the response accordingly. The continuous monitoring of the patient for the signs and symptoms of internal or external bleeding is crucial during both the initiation and maintenance of therapy.

Antiplatelet Agents

Another group of agents used to alter coagulation are the antiplatelet agents. Aspirin, dipyridamole, and ticlopidine are the most commonly used drugs in this category.

ASSESSMENT

The nursing assessment of patients receiving any of these agents should begin with the taking of a medication and medical history. Specific contraindications to the use of these agents include hypersensitivity, hypotension, and pregnancy. Aspirin is contraindicated in patients with any bleeding disorder, in children younger than 16 years old, in children with flulike symptoms, in pregnant or lactating women, and in patients with a vitamin K deficiency or peptic ulcer disease. Ticlopidine is contraindicated in the settings of hypersensitivity, sever liver impairment, or active bleeding, and when the results of clotting studies show an alteration. Additive antiplatelet effects occur when these agents are coadministered with other aspirin products or with any of the nonsteroidal antiinflammatory agents. Increased bleeding would occur in conjunction with the use of warfarin sodium. There are several drugs that interact with aspirin, and these are listed in Table 24-6.

Baseline vital signs also need to be determined in all patients. Lying and standing blood pressures are important to monitor because of the orthostatic hypotension these agents can precipitate. Before aspirin therapy is initiated, the patient's renal function, the complete blood count, hematocrit, hemoglobin level, and prothrombin time should all be assessed.

NURSING DIAGNOSES

Nursing diagnoses relevant to the patient receiving antiplatelet agents include:
- Altered tissue perfusion (decreased) as the result of the clotting disorder or thrombus formation.
- Altered mobility related to tissue injury or decreased tissue perfusion.
- Risk for injury related to possible adverse reactions to antiplatelet therapy.
- Knowledge deficit related to lack of information about the medication therapy.

PLANNING

Goals for patients receiving antiplatelet agents include:
- Patient will regain normal or near-normal tissue perfusion.
- Patient resumes normal daily activities.
- Patient remains free from injury related to medication therapy.
- Patient remains compliant with therapy.

Outcome Criteria

Outcome criteria pertaining to the patient receiving antiplatelet agents include:
- Patient will show signs of improved blood flow and tissue perfusion once therapy is initiated, signs such as improved distal pulses and color and temperature of distal areas.
- Patient will increase mobility gradually every day, as ordered, such as from walking to doorway to walking down hallway.
- Patient will protect self from skin injuries such as abrasions or bruising and avoid contact sports.
- Patient will take medication as prescribed and report any unusual side effects or adverse reactions such as bleeding, easy bruising, or palpitations to the physician immediately.

IMPLEMENTATION

Safe and effective treatment with antiplatelet agents requires that the nurse have an adequate knowledge about these agents, including knowledge of the drug interactions that can occur and the life-style changes the patient must make. Dipyridamole should be taken on an empty stomach or either 1 hour before or 2 hours after meals so that maximal absorption can take place, whereas aspirin should be taken 30 minutes before or 2 hours after meals to minimize GI upset. Patients taking either of these agents should quit smoking because

---

Patient Teaching TIPS

- ✔ Patients taking aspirin or aspirin products should know to report any of the following symptoms to their physician: decrease in urine output; constant ringing of the ears; swelling of the feet, ankles, or legs; dark urine; clay-colored stools; abdominal pain; rash (discontinue use if rash occurs); and blurred vision or the perception of halos around objects.

- ✔ Make sure patients know to keep these products out of the reach of children.

- ✔ Patients should be told about not consuming alcohol or smoking.

- ✔ Patients should understand that these medications are not cures and often need to be taken long term.

- ✔ Patients should be told to avoid hazardous activities until they are stabilized on dipyridamole therapy because of the dizziness the drug can cause.

- ✔ Patients should report any unusual symptoms to their physician immediately.

- ✔ Patients should avoid taking ticlopidine with aspirin or dipyridamole, unless ordered to do so by the physician, because this can precipitate bleeding.

- ✔ Patients should avoid taking antacids with these medications or space the dosing of the two at least 2 hours apart. The concurrent use of digoxin and ticlopidine will result in decreased digitalis levels.

---

of the vasoconstriction induced by the nicotine. It is important to remember that aspirin will interfere with the results of certain laboratory tests, such as coagulation studies, liver function tests, serum uric acid levels, and serum potassium and cholesterol levels. Ticlopidine can alter the serum alkaline phosphatase, bilirubin, and transaminase levels. Patient teaching tips are given in the box above.

EVALUATION

Monitoring for both the therapeutic and adverse effects of antiplatelet agents is crucial to their safe use. The therapeutic effects include decreased chest pain, dizziness and other neurologic symptoms, and platelet adhesion. Adverse effects of aspirin use include GI upset, GI bleeding, heartburn, headache, hepatitis, thrombocytopenia, agranulocytosis, leukopenia, neutropenia, hemolytic anemia, prolonged prothrombin time, tinnitus, hearing loss, rapid pulse, wheezing, hypoglycemia, hyponatremia, and hypokalemia. Adverse effects of dipyridamole use include postural hypotension, headache, weakness, syncope, GI upset, rash, flushing of the face, and dizziness. It is necessary to continually monitor liver, renal, and clotting function with laboratory studies in patients on long-term aspirin therapy. It is also critical to the safe care of patients receiving these medications that the nurse reassess and monitor the patient's response to the treatment and document the response accordingly. Continuous monitoring of the patient for signs of internal or external bleeding is of utmost importance both during the initiation of therapy and during ongoing therapy.

Antifibrinolytics

ASSESSMENT

Nursing assessment of patients receiving these agents should begin with the taking of medication and medical history. Baseline vital signs should also be obtained and recorded as well as blood clotting studies performed. Drug interactions to assess for include concurrent use of oral contraceptives. Cautious use of desmopressin is recommended in patients receiving lithium, large doses of epinephrine, heparin, or alcohol. Amino caproic acid is contraindicated in hypersensitivity, postpartum bleeding, disseminated intravascular coagulation, new burns, and upper–urinary tract bleeding. Desmopressin is contraindicated in patients with hypersensitivity and nephrogenic diabetes insipidus.

NURSING DIAGNOSES

Nursing diagnoses pertaining to the patient receiving antifibrinolytics include:
- Altered tissue perfusion (decreased) related to excessive bleeding.
- Risk for injury or shock related to excessive bleeding.
- Risk for injury related to side effects of antifibrinolytics.

PLANNING

Goals pertaining to patients receiving antifibrinolytics include:
- Patient maintains/regains normal to near normal tissue perfussion.
- Patient will have improved hemostasis with drug therapy and supportive treatment.
- Patient experiences minimal adverse or toxic effects of antifibrinolytic agents.

Outcome Criteria

Outcome criteria pertaining to patients receiving antifibrinolytics include the following:
- Patient experiences increased strength of pulses and increased to normal skin temperature and color.
- Patient exhibits a return to normal vital signs with improved blood pressure (BP), pulse (P), and respiration (R) (BP: 120/80 mm Hg; P: more than 60 but less than 100 beats per min; and R: more than 16 but fewer than 20 respirations per min).
- Patient will be free of signs and symptoms of acute cerebrovascular thrombosis (cerebrovascular accident, i.e., stroke) or acute myocardial infarction.

IMPLEMENTATION

Before administering IV, check the rate of infusion and dilutional factor for amino caproic acid because infusion that is too rapid may result in bradycardia or hypotension. Desmopressin should be infused IV over 15-30 minutes for doses of 0.3 μg/kg. Intranasal dosage form should be administered exactly as ordered.

EVALUATION

Therapeutic effects of antifibrinolytics include arrest of oozing of blood from surgical site or decrease in blood loss. In addition, desmopressin may result in control or prevention of polyuria, polydypsia, and dehydration in patients with diabetes insipidus.

Thrombolytics

Another group of agents used to alter clotting mechanisms are the enzymes used as thrombolytics. These agents are used in patients who are in very acute situations, such as those suffering acute myocardial infarctions.

ASSESSMENT

A nursing assessment should be performed prior to initiation of therapy. Possible drug interactions include concurrent use with anticoagulants and antiplatelet agents or any agent altering platelet function. Contraindications and cautions for the use of these drugs are similar to those in previous discussions on coagulation modifiers. Baseline vital signs as well as related laboratory studies are also important to obtain and monitor.

NURSING DIAGNOSES

Nursing diagnoses appropriate to the use of these agents are similar to the ones discussed in the previous sections on anticoagulants and antiplatelets.

PLANNING

Goals and outcome criteria are also similar to the two previously discussed groups of coagulation modifiers.

EVALUATION

The therapeutic effects of thrombolytics include improved tissue perfusion, decreased chest pain, decreased leg pain, improved shunt performance, and prevention of further myocardial damage. Adverse effects to monitor for include hypersensitivity, nausea, vomiting, and hypotension. Dysrhythmias may also occur.

TAKE HOME POINTS

Coagulation Modifiers
- Work by (1) preventing clot formation, (2) promoting clot formation, (3) lysing a preformed clot, or (4) reversing the action of anticoagulants.
- Anticoagulants, antiplatelet agents, antifibrinolytics, thrombolytics, and reversal agents are all examples.

Coagulation System
- Clot formation going on at same time as clot destruction.
- Clot destruction is governed by the fibrinolytic system.
- Clot formation is accomplished by the coagulation pathway, of which there is an extrinsic and an intrinsic pathway.
- The extrinsic pathway is initiated by blood vessels.
- The intrinsic pathway is initiated by blood cells.

Warfarin (Coumadin)
- Prevents clot formation by inhibiting vitamin K–dependent clotting factors (II, VII, IX, and X).
- Used prophylactically to prevent clots from forming.
- Cannot lyse preformed clots.
- The degree of anticoagulation or "thinning of the blood" is monitored by the prothrombin time.

Heparin
- Prevents clot formation by binding to antithrombin III and by doing so turns off certain activating factors.
- Overall effect is to turn off the coagulation pathway and prevent clots from forming.
- Cannot lyse or break down a clot.

Antiplatelet Agents
- Prevent clot formation by preventing platelet involvement in clot formation.
- Aspirin, dipyridamole, pentoxifylline, and ticlopidine all affect normal platelet function.

- Aspirin is the primary antiplatelet agent.
- At high doses works by inhibiting cyclooxygenase in platelets as well as blood vessels.

Antifibrinolytics
- Prevent lysis of fibrin, thus promoting clot formation.
- Have opposite effects of anticoagulants.
- Examples of agents include aminocaproic acid, tranexamic acid, aprotinin, and desmopressin.
- Work in opposition to anticoagulants, antiplatelets, and thrombolytics.
- Used to arrest oozing of blood from surgical sites such as chest tubes and to reduce total blood loss volume postoperatively.

Thrombolytics
- Anticoagulants that break down or lyse *preformed* clots in blood vessels that supply the heart with blood.
- Examples of agents include streptokinase (SK), urokinase, +−PA, and APSAC.
- SK derived from group A beta-hemolytic streptococci.
- Converts plasminogen to plasmin, which breaks down thrombi.
- Therapeutic effects include improved tissue perfusion, decreased chest pain, and prevention of further myocardial damage.
- Adverse effects include nausea, vomiting, and hypotension.

Nursing Considerations
- Therapeutic effects of most coagulation modifier agents include improved circulation, tissue perfusion, decreased pain, and prevention of further tissue damage.
- Before using any of these agents, it is important to perform a thorough physical assessment and record findings as well as monitor any pertinent laboratory values.

Critical Thinking **A C T I V I T I E S**

1. L.P. is a 69-year-old woman who has just had hip replacement surgery. Her orthopedic surgeon has prescribed 5000 U of subcutaneous heparin to be given twice a day for 7 days because she is at high risk for the development of a pulmonary embolism. The concentration of heparin for subcutaneous injections is 2500 U/ml, and it comes in a 10-ml vial. How many vials of subcutaneous heparin will be needed to complete L.P.'s 7-day course of therapy?

2. There are many side effects of the anticoagulant heparin. One of your patients has been on IV heparin for 72 hours. She is complaining of numbness and tingling of the extremities and fell when you got her out of bed, an activity she tolerated 6 hours before. What would your first action be and why? What would be some other data to collect on this patient at this time?

Case Study

3. In the past 2 years, L. L., a 56-year-old attorney, has suffered three episodes of deep vein thrombosis, but all occurred without complications and all were treated successfully with anticoagulant therapy and bed rest. He now presents to the urgent care center because of increased pain and swelling in the left calf that has lasted for the past 3 days. Initially he is given 5000 units of heparin. At admission to the hospital for anticoagulant therapy he is started on a continuous infusion of 25,000 units of heparin in 1000 ml of 0.9% sodium chloride.
   a. What nursing actions should be implemented to ensure the accuracy and safety of the continuous heparin infusion?
   b. What patient findings would indicate a therapeutic response to the heparin therapy?
   c. If L.L. suddenly complains of numbness and tingling in his lower extremities with accompanying changes in muscle strength and sensation 12 hours after the initiation and continuation of heparin therapy, what would be the most appropriate nursing action(s) to implement?

BIBLIOGRAPHY

Albanese J, Nutz P: *Mosby's 1995 nursing drug cards*, St Louis, 1995, Mosby.

Aragon D, Martin M: What you should know about thrombolytic therapy for acute MI, *Am J Nurs* 93(9):24, 1993.

Bell WR: Thrombolytic therapy: agents, indications, and laboratory monitoring, *Med Clin North Am* 78(3):745, 1994.

Campbell RK: Clinical update on pentoxifylline therapy for diabetes-induced peripheral vascular disease, *Ann Pharmacother* 27:1099, 1993.

Dalen JE, Hirsh J: Antithrombotic therapy: introduction, *Chest* 102(4 suppl):303S, 1992.

Fong LN: Balancing anticoagulant therapy, *Geriatr Nurs* 12(1):15, 1991.

Grines CL: Thrombolytic, antiplatelet, and antithrombotic agents, *Am J Cardiol* 70(12):181, 1992.

Herrera CR, Grasela TH, Walawander CA: A nationwide investigation of a possible protamine drug-product defect, *Ann Pharmacother* 26:643, 1992.

Hirsh J et al: Oral anticoagulants, mechanism of action, clinical effectiveness, and optimal therapeutic range, *Chest* 102(4 suppl):312S, 1992.

Johnson KB: *Harriet Lane handbook,* ed 13, St Louis, 1993, Mosby.

Keen JH: *Critical care and emergency drug reference,* St Louis, 1994, Mosby.

Knoben JE, Anderson PO: Handbook of critical drug data, ed 6, Hamilton, Ill, 1988, Drug Intelligence Publications.

McConnell EA: Administering SC heparin, *Nursing* 21(12):24, 1990.

McEvoy GK: *AHFS drug information,* Bethesda, Md, 1994, American Society of Hospital Pharmacists.

Ostrow CL: Thrombolytics, *AACN Clin Issues Crit Care Nurs* 3(2):423, 1992.

Rapaport E: Thrombolysis, anticoagulation, and reocclusion, *Am J Cardiol* 68(16):17E, 1991.

Samlaska CP, Winfield EA: Pentoxifylline, *J Am Acad Dermatol* 30:603, 1994.

Skidmore-Roth L: *Mosby's 1995 nursing drug reference,* St Louis, 1995, Mosby.

Chapter 25

Antilipemic Agents

Objectives

When you reach the end of this chapter, you will be able to:

1 Explain the nature of hyperlipidemia.
2 Discuss the different types of lipoproteins.
3 List the various antilipemic agents commonly used to treat hyperlipidemia.
4 Explain the rationale for antilipemic treatment and cite the dosages, side effects, cautions, contra-indications, and drug interactions associated with the use of the various antilipemics.
5 Develop a comprehensive nursing care plan for patients receiving antilipemics that includes patient outcomes and education.
6 Cite the therapeutic responses produced by antilipemic agents.

CHAPTER OUTLINE

Lipids and Lipid Abnormalities

Primary Forms of Lipids
Cholesterol Homeostasis
Atherosclerotic Plaque Formation
Link between Cholesterol and Coronary Artery
  Disease
Hyperlipidemias and Treatment Guidelines

Antilipemic Agents

Bile Acid Sequestrants
  Mechanism of action
  Drug effects
  Therapeutic uses
  Side effects and adverse effects
    Toxicity and management of overdose
  Interactions
  Dosages
Drug Profiles
  Cholestyramine
  Colestipol hydrochloride
HMG–CoA Reductase Inhibitors
  Mechanism of action
  Therapeutic uses
  Side effects and adverse effects
    Toxicity and management of overdose
  Interactions
  Dosages

Drug Profile
  ⚓ Lovastatin
Fibric Acid Derivatives
  Mechanism of action
  Drug effects
  Therapeutic uses
  Side effects and adverse effects
    Toxicity and management of overdose
  Interactions
  Dosages
Drug Profiles
  Clofibrate
  Gemfibrozil
Nicotinic Acid
  Mechanism of action
  Drug effects
  Therapeutic uses
  Side effects and adverse effects
  Interactions
  Dosages
Drug Profile
  Nicotinic acid
Probucol
  Mechanism of action
  Drug effects
  Therapeutic uses
  Side effects and adverse effects
  Interactions
  Dosages

continued

Drug Profile
  Probucol
Nursing Process
Assessment
Nursing Diagnoses
Planning
  Outcome criteria
Implementation
Evaluation

Glossary

Antilipemic (an′ tĭ li pe′ mik) Drug that reduces lipid levels. (p. 368)

Apoproteins (ap′ o pro tēn) A polypeptide chain not yet complexed to its specific prosthetic group. (p. 368)

Cholesterol (kə les′ tər ol) A fat-soluble crystalline steroid alcohol found in animal fats and oils and egg yolk and widely distributed in the body, especially in the bile, blood, brain tissue, liver, kidneys, adrenal glands, and myelin sheaths of nerve fibers. (p. 368)

Chylomicrons (ki′ lo mi′ kron) Minute droplets of lipoproteins. Chylomicrons consist of about 90% triglycerides and small amounts of cholesterol, phospholipids, and proteins. (p. 368)

Exogenous lipids (ek soj′ ə nəs \lip′ idz) Lipids originating outside the body or an organ or produced as the result of external causes, such as a disease caused by a bacterial or viral agent foreign to the body. (p. 368)

Foam cells The characteristic initial lesion of atherosclerosis, also known as the *fatty streak*. (p. 370)

Hypercholesterolemia (hi′ pər kə les tər ol e me ə) A condition in which greater-than-normal amounts of cholesterol are present in the blood. High levels of cholesterol and other lipids may lead to the development of atherosclerosis. (p. 369)

Lipoproteins (lip′ o pro tēnz) Conjugated proteins in which lipids form an integral part of the molecule. They are synthesized primarily in the liver; contain varying amounts of triglycerides, cholesterol, phospholipids, and protein; and are classified according to their composition and density. (p. 368)

Triglycerides (tri glis′ ər īd) A compound consisting of a fatty acid (oleic, palmitic, or stearic) and glycerol. Triglycerides make up most animal and vegetable fats and are the principal lipids in the blood, where they circulate bound to a protein, forming high- and low-density lipoproteins. (p. 368)

An understanding of **antilipemic** drugs begins with an understanding of how **cholesterol** and **triglycerides** are transported and used in the human body and how **lipoproteins**, apolipoproteins, receptors, and enzyme systems are involved in these processes. Also essential is an understanding of the basic mechanisms underlying lipid abnormalities and the link between hyperlipidemia and coronary heart dis-

ease (CHD). Armed with this knowledge, the clinician can develop and implement a rational approach to treatment using both nonpharmacologic and pharmacologic interventions.

Lipids and Lipid Abnormalities

PRIMARY FORMS OF LIPIDS

Triglycerides and cholesterol are the two primary forms of lipids in the blood. Triglycerides function as an energy source and are stored in adipose (fat) tissue. Cholesterol is primarily used to make steroid hormones, cell membranes, and bile acids. Triglycerides and cholesterol are both water-insoluble fats that must be bound to specialized lipid-carrying proteins called **apoproteins**. This combination of triglycerides and cholesterol with an apoprotein is referred to as a lipoprotein. Lipoproteins transport lipids via the blood. They are made up of a lipid core of triglycerides or cholesterol esters, or both, which is surrounded by a thin layer of phospholipids, apoproteins, and cholesterol. There are various types of lipoproteins, and they are classified according to their density and the type of apoproteins they contain. These various types of lipoproteins and their classification are listed in Table 25-1.

CHOLESTEROL HOMEOSTASIS

Fats are taken into the body through our diet, and these dietary fats are broken down in the small intestine to form triglycerides. These triglycerides are in turn incorporated into **chylomicrons**, which are taken up into the lymphatic system. The primary purpose of chylomicrons is to transport lipids obtained from dietary sources (**exogenous lipids**) from the intestines to the liver to be used to make steroid hormones, peripheral cells, and bile acids.

The liver is the major organ where lipid metabolism occurs. The liver produces very-low-density lipoprotein (VLDL) from both endogenous and exogenous sources. The major role of VLDL is the transport of endogenous lipids to peripheral cells. Once VLDL is circulating, it is enzymatically cleaved by lipoprotein lipase and loses triglycerides. This creates intermediate-density lipoprotein (IDL), which is soon also cleaved by lipoprotein lipase, creating low-density lipoprotein (LDL). Cholesterol is almost all that is left in LDL after this process. Any tissues that require LDL, such as endocrine cells, possess LDL receptors. LDL

Table 25-1	Lipoprotein Classification	
LIPID CONTENT	**LIPOPROTEIN CLASSIFICATION**	**PROTEIN CONTENT**
Most ↑ Least	Chylomicron Very-low-density lipoprotein Low-density lipoprotein Intermediate-density lipoprotein High-density lipoprotein	Least ↓ **Most**

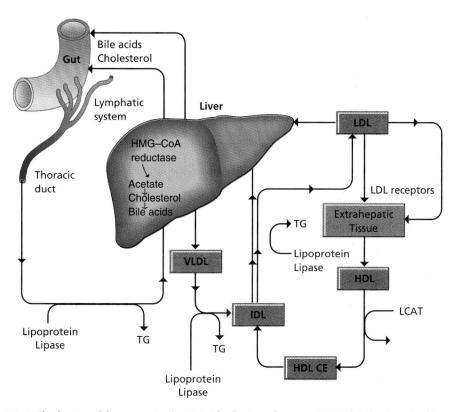

▼ **FIG. 25-1** Cholesterol homeostasis. *CE,* Cholesterol ester; *HDL,* high-density lipoprotein; *HMG–CoA,* hydroxymethylglutaryl–coenzyme A; *IDL,* intermediate-density lipoprotein; *LCAT,* lecithin cholesterol acetyltransferase; *LDL,* low-density lipoprotein; *TG,* triglyceride; *VLDL,* very-low-density lipoprotein.

and about half of the IDL are returned to the liver by means of LDL receptors on the liver.

High-density lipoprotein (HDL) is produced in the liver and intestines and is also formed when chylomicrons are broken down. Lipids that are not used by peripheral cells are transferred as cholesterol esters to HDL. HDL then transfers the cholesterol esters to IDL to be returned to the liver. HDL is responsible for the "recycling" of cholesterol. HDL is sometimes referred to as the "good" lipid because it is believed to be cardioprotective.

If the liver has an excess amount of cholesterol, the number of LDL receptors on the liver decreases, resulting in an accumulation of LDL in the blood. One explanation for **hypercholesterolemia** (cholesterol in the blood) therefore is this down-regulation of hepatic LDL receptors. A major function of the liver is to manufacture cholesterol, a process that requires acetyl coenzyme A (CoA) reductase. Inhibition of this enzyme thus results in decreased cholesterol production by the liver. The entire process of cholesterol homeostasis is illustrated in Fig. 25-1.

ATHEROSCLEROTIC PLAQUE FORMATION

Fundamental to the study of hyperlipidemia is an understanding of the processes by which lipids and lipoproteins participate in the formation of atherosclerotic plaque and subsequently the development of CHD. When the serum cholesterol levels are elevated, circulating monocytes adhere to the smooth endothelial surface of the coronary vasculature. These monocytes burrow into the next layer of the blood vessel, the subendothelial tissue, and change into macrophage cells, which then take up cholesterol from circulating lipoproteins until they become filled with fat. At this point, they become **foam cells**, the characteristic precursor lesion of atherosclerosis, also known as the *fatty streak*. Once this process is established, it is usually present throughout the coronary and systemic circulation.

LINK BETWEEN CHOLESTEROL AND CORONARY ARTERY DISEASE

Numerous epidemiologic trials have shown that as blood cholesterol levels increase in the members of a population, the incidence of death and disability related to CHD also increases. The risk of CHD in patients with cholesterol levels of 300 mg/dl is three to four times greater than that in patients with levels less than 200 mg/dl. The absolute incidence of CHD in women is approximately 25% less than that of men. This is thought to be secondary to the effects of estrogen, because the risk of CHD climbs considerably in ostmenopausal women.

Statistics show that half of all Americans, both male and female, will die of a heart attack. Thus, the thrust of treatment is two pronged: one aimed at treating the disease in patients who have it, and one aimed at preventing it in those who don't.

Measures taken early in a person's life to reduce and maintain cholesterol levels in a desirable range should have a dramatic effect in terms of preventing CHD and the death and disability it causes.

HYPERLIPIDEMIAS AND TREATMENT GUIDELINES

The decision to prescribe hyperlipemic drugs as an adjunct to diet therapy in patients with an elevated cholesterol level should be based on the patient's clinical profile. This includes the patient's age, sex, menopausal status (if the patient is a woman), family history, and response to dietary treatment, as well as the presence of risk factors (other than hyperlipidemia) for premature coronary artery disease and the cause, du-

---

High Blood Cholesterol: Risk Factors

Positive Risk Factors
Age
  Male: ≥45 years
  Female: ≥55 years or women with premature menopause not on estrogen replacement therapy
Family history
  History of premature CHD (e.g., myocardial infarction or sudden death before 55 years of age in father or other male first-degree relative, or before 65 years of age in mother or other female first-degree relative.)
Current cigarette smoker
Hypertension: ≥140/90 mm Hg, or on antihypertensive medication
Low HDL cholesterol level: <35 mg/dl
Diabetes mellitus

Negative Risk Factors
High HDL cholesterol: ≥60 mg/dl—if the HDL cholesterol is ≥60 mg/dl, subtract one risk factor.

---

ration, and the phenotypic pattern of the patient's hyperlipidemia.

A major source of guidance for antilipemic treatment at the disposal of health care professionals in the United States has been the National Cholesterol Education Program (NCEP), which has been developed in close cooperation with other major professional organizations such as the American Heart Association. This program has two main thrusts, both aimed at reducing the total risk of CHD in the population of the United States. One is focused on the entire population and consists of general guidelines for the prevention of CHD. It emphasizes the appropriate dietary intake of total cholesterol and saturated fat, weight control, physical activity, and the control of other life-style risk factors. The other aspect is focused on the management of individual patients who are at increased risk for CHD. The original guidelines for the detection, evaluation, and treatment of high serum cholesterol levels in adults were published in 1988, and revised guidelines were made available in June 1993. In these guidelines, the selection of diet and drug therapy options is determined by whether certain risk factors are present. These risk factors are listed in the box above.

When the decision to institute drug therapy has been made, the choice of drug should then be determined by the specific lipid profile of the patient. There are four patterns of hyperlipidemia, and possibly a fifth, and these are determined by the nature of the plasma (serum) concentrations of total cholesterol and triglycerides. These various types of hyperlipidemias are listed in Table 25-2. The process of determining a patient's specific cholesterol profile is referred to as *phenotyping*.

Table 25-2	Types of Hyperlipidemias	
	LIPID COMPOSITION	
PHENOTYPE	**CHOLESTEROL**	**TRIGLYCERIDE**
IIa	Elevated	Normal
IIb and III	Elevated	Elevated (1-3 × higher than cholesterol)
IV	Normal or mildly elevated	Elevated
I and V	Elevated (>300 mg/dl)	Elevated (>1000 mg/dl)

One of the basic tenets of the NCEP guidelines is that all reasonable nonpharmaceutical means of controlling the blood cholesterol level (diet, exercise, and so on) should be tried and found to fail before drug therapy is considered. However, generally this means that diet modifications have been tried for at least 6 months and failed. Because the drug therapy for hyperlipidemias entails a long-term commitment to the therapy, factors that should be considered before the initiation of therapy should be the magnitude of hypercholesterolemia, the age and life-style of the patient, the relative contraindications to the first-choice drug, potential drug interactions, and the overall cost of therapy. The NCEP guidelines recommend that all patients with LDL cholesterol levels exceeding 190 mg/dl and those with LDL cholesterol levels between 160 and 190 mg/dl who have CHD or two or more risk factors be considered for drug therapy after an adequate trial of dietary and other nondrug therapies has proved ineffective.

The major classes of drugs are the bile acid sequestrants (cholestyramine, colestipol), nicotinic acid, and the hepatic hydroxymethylglutaryl (HMG)–CoA reductase inhibitors (lovastatin, pravastatin, simvastatin, fluvastatin). Other classes of drugs include fibric acid derivatives (gemfibrozil, clofibrate) and probucol. Estrogen replacement therapy may also be considered.

Antilipemic Agents

BILE ACID SEQUESTRANTS

The bile acid sequestrants, also called *bile acid–binding resins* and *ion-exchange resins,* are cholestyramine and colestipol. Both these agents have been used widely for more than 20 years and have been evaluated extensively in well-controlled clinical trials. Generally these drugs lower the plasma concentrations of LDL cholesterol by 15% to 30%. They also increase the HDL cholesterol level by 3% to 8% and increase hepatic triglyceride and VLDL production, which may result in a 10% to 50% increase in the triglyceride level.

Mechanism of Action

The bile acid resins bind bile, and this prevents the resorption of the bile acids from the small intestine. Bile acids are necessary for the absorption and enterohepatic resorption of cholesterol. The hepatic synthesis of bile acids from cholesterol is stimulated by the depletion of the bile acid pool, and this results in a decreased pool of cholesterol in the liver. To compensate for this, both cholesterol biosynthesis and the number of high-affinity LDL receptors expressed on the liver's surface are increased, and this results in an increased rate of LDL catabolism (increased removal of LDL from the bloodstream). In this way, the bile acid sequestrants lower the plasma LDL levels by enhancing the efficiency of the receptor-mediated removal of LDL from plasma. The result of the ion-exchange resin binding to the bile acids is an insoluble resin–bile acid complex that is excreted by means of the feces.

Drug Effects

The fecal excretion of bile acids leads to a proportional breakdown of cholesterol into bile acids, which in turn lowers the serum cholesterol and LDL (beta) levels.

These drugs may also cause mild increases in the triglyceride levels and lower the absorption of fat-soluble vitamins.

Therapeutic Uses

The bile acid sequestrants are used as adjuncts in the management of type II hyperlipoproteinemia. In addition, cholestyramine is used to relieve the pruritus associated with partial biliary obstruction.

Side Effects and Adverse Effects

The adverse effects of colestipol and cholestyramine are similar; constipation is a frequent problem and may be accompanied by heartburn, nausea, belching, and bloating. These adverse effects tend to disappear over time, however. Many patients require extra education and support to help them deal with the gastrointestinal effects and comply with the medication regimen. It is important to initiate therapy with low doses and instruct patients to take the drugs with meals to reduce the side effects. Increasing the dietary fiber intake or taking a fiber supplement such as psyllium (Metamucil and others) may relieve constipation and bloating. The most common side effects and adverse effects of the bile acid sequestrants are listed in Table 25-3.

Toxicity and Management of Overdose

Because the bile acid sequestrants are not absorbed, an overdose could cause obstruction of the GI tract. Therefore treatment of an overdose involves restoring gut motility.

Table 25-3	Bile Acid Sequestrants: Adverse Effects
BODY SYSTEM	**SIDE/ADVERSE EFFECT**
Gastrointestinal	Constipation, heartburn, nausea, belching, bloating
Other	Bleeding, headache, tinnitus, burnt odor to urine

Interactions

The significant drug interactions associated with the use of bile acid sequestrants are limited to the absorption of concurrently administered drugs. All drugs should be taken at least 1 hour before or 4 to 6 hours after the administration of the ion-exchange resins. In addition, high doses of a bile acid sequestrant will decrease the absorption of fat-soluble vitamins (A, D, E, and K), resulting in their malabsorption.

Dosages

For dosage information on cholestyramine and colestipol hydrochloride, see the dosages table below.

DRUG PROFILES

The bile acid sequestrants cholestyramine and colestipol are indicated for the treatment of type IIa and IIb hyperlipidemia. They lower the cholesterol level, in particular the LDL cholesterol level, by increasing the destruction of LDL. However, their use may result in increases in the VLDL cholesterol level. Because of the high incidence of gastrointestinal side effects in patients taking these agents, compliance with the prescribed dosage schedules is often poor. Therefore ed-

DOSAGES

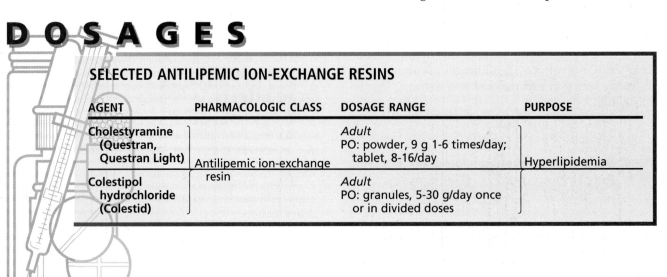

SELECTED ANTILIPEMIC ION-EXCHANGE RESINS

AGENT	PHARMACOLOGIC CLASS	DOSAGE RANGE	PURPOSE
Cholestyramine (Questran, Questran Light)	Antilipemic ion-exchange resin	*Adult* PO: powder, 9 g 1-6 times/day; tablet, 8-16/day	Hyperlipidemia
Colestipol hydrochloride (Colestid)		*Adult* PO: granules, 5-30 g/day once or in divided doses	

ucating the patient to the purpose of therapy and to the expected side effects of the therapy and their treatment can foster improved compliance. Because of the pronounced drug interactions that can result from the concurrent administration of other drugs with the bile acid sequestrants, patients must also be warned about this and the need to take these other drugs at other times of the day. The importance of patient education in the recipients of bile acid sequestrants cannot be overemphasized.

CHOLESTYRAMINE

Cholestyramine (Questran, Questran Light) is a prescription-only drug that is contraindicated in patients with a known hypersensitivity to it and in those suffering from complete biliary obstruction. It may interfere with the distribution of the proper amounts of fat-soluble vitamins to the fetus or nursing infant of pregnant or nursing women taking the agent. It is therefore classified as a pregnancy category C agent. The drug is only available orally as 4- and 9-gm packets of powder to be taken as an oral suspension. The recommended dosages are given in the dosages table on the preceding page.

COLESTIPOL HYDROCHLORIDE

Colestipol hydrochloride (Colestid) is a prescription-only drug. It is contraindicated in patients who have shown a hypersensitivity reaction to it. It may interfere with the distribution of the proper amounts of fat-soluble vitamins to the fetus or nursing infant of pregnant or nursing women taking the agent. This drug is available in 5-gm packets or bottles of 300 and 500. The recommended dosages of colestipol are given in the dosages table on the preceding page. Pregnancy category B.

HMG–CoA REDUCTASE INHIBITORS

The specific competitive inhibitors of the rate-limiting enzyme in cholesterol synthesis, HMG–CoA reductase, are the most potent of the drugs available for reducing plasma concentrations of LDL cholesterol. Lovastatin was the first agent in this drug class to be approved for use, and this occurred in 1987. More recently three other HMG-CoA reductase inhibitors have come available: pravastatin, simvastatin, and fluvastatin. The HMGs, or "statins" as they are sometimes called, are more effective than other types of antilipemic drugs in lowering the plasma concentrations of LDL and total cholesterol. The maximum extent to which these lipid levels are lowered does not occur until 6 to 8 weeks after the start of therapy. The findings from few direct comparisons of the HMGs have been published.

However, the authors of the published account of one such study concluded that the following doses of agents would yield the same reduction in the LDL cholesterol level: simvastatin, 10 mg; pravastatin, 20 mg; and lovastatin, 20 mg. This particular study did not assess fluvastatin. The HMGs are primarily used in the treatment of type IIa and IIb hyperlipidemias.

Mechanism of Action

The HMGs lower the blood cholesterol level by decreasing the rate of cholesterol production. The liver requires HMG–CoA reductase to produce cholesterol. It is the rate-limiting enzyme in the reactions needed to make cholesterol. The "statins" inhibit HMG–CoA reductase, thereby decreasing cholesterol production. When less cholesterol is produced, the liver increases the number of LDL receptors in order to augment the recycling of LDL from the circulation back into the liver, where it is needed for the synthesis of other needed substances such as steroids, bile acids, and cell membranes. Lovastatin and simvastatin are administered as inactive drugs or prodrugs that must be biotransformed into their active metabolites in the liver. In contrast, pravastatin is administered in its active form.

Therapeutic Uses

The HMG-CoA reductase inhibitors appear to be equally effective in their ability to reduce LDL cholesterol concentrations. They are primarily indicated for the treatment of type IIa and IIb hyperlipidemias and have been shown to reduce the plasma concentrations of LDL cholesterol by 30% to 40%. Their cholesterol-lowering properties are dose dependent, in that the larger the dose, the greater the cholesterol-lowering effects. A 10% to 30% decrease in the concentrations of plasma triglycerides has been observed in patients receiving any of these drugs. Another very important therapeutic effect of the HMGs is an overall tendency for the HDL cholesterol level to increase by 2% to 15%.

RESEARCH

It has been reported that maximal therapeutic effects associated with the use of fluvastatin (Lescol) usually occur in approximately 1 month. The adult dose is 20 mg taken in the evening. Because of drug interactions, especially with cimetidine (Tagamet), ranitidine (Zantac), and omeprazole (Prilosec), it is recommended that other medications be taken 2 hours after fluvastatin.

Side Effects and Adverse Effects

The HMG–CoA reductase inhibitors available for clinical use have proved to be well tolerated, with significant side effects being fairly uncommon. Mild, transient gastrointestinal disturbances, rash, and headache have been the most common problems. The common undesirable effects of the HMGs are listed in Table 25-4. Less common but still clinically important side effects include myopathy (muscle pain) and elevations in liver enzyme activity. The myopathy is uncommon (less than 0.1%) during monotherapy but appears to be dose dependent and is more common in patients receiving an HMG–CoA reductase inhibitor in combination with cyclosporin, nicotinic acid, gemfibrozil, or erythromycin. The serum creatine phosphokinase concentrations may be increased by more than ten times the normal level in patients receiving these agents. Dose-dependent elevations in liver enzyme activity to values greater than three times the upper limit of normal have been noted in 0.4% to 1.9% of patients taking HMG–CoA reductase inhibitors. Most of these patients have remained asymptomatic, however.

Toxicity and Management of Overdose

Very limited data are available on the nature of toxicity and overdose in patients taking HMG–CoA reductase inhibitors. Treatment, if needed, is supportive.

Interactions

As far as the drug interactions that can occur with the HMG–CoA reductase inhibitors, they should be used cautiously in patients taking oral anticoagulants. In addition, the coadministration of these drugs with erythromycin, gemfibrozil, or niacin has been observed to rarely lead to the development of rhabdomyolysis.

As far as the laboratory interactions that can occur, increases in the SGOT levels and activated clotting

time, thrombocytopenia, and transient eosinophilia have all been observed.

Dosages

For dosage information on lovastatin, see the drug profile for this agent.

*D*RUG PROFILE

The HMG–CoA reductase inhibitors (lovastatin, pravastatin, simvastatin, and fluvastatin) are all potent inhibitors of the enzyme that catalyzes the rate-limiting step in the synthesis of cholesterol. All four agents are prescription-only drugs and are contraindicated in pregnant or lactating women and in those suffering from active liver dysfunction or with elevated serum transaminase levels of unknown cause. They are pregnancy category X agents. There is little evidence to recommend one agent over another.

⚓ LOVASTATIN

Lovastatin (Mevacor) was the first HMG–CoA reductase inhibitors to come available for clinical use, and for this reason it is considered the prototype. It is indicated primarily for the treatment of type IIa and IIb hyperlipidemias. It is effective in lowering the LDL cholesterol level and to some degree the triglyceride levels. It may also beneficially increase the HDL cholesterol level. There are very little significant differences in the clinical effects of the four currently available HMG–CoA reductase inhibitors. The recommended dosage for lovastatin is 20 to 80 mg/day by mouth. Pregnancy category X.

� P H A R M A C O K I N E T I C S

HALF-LIFE	ONSET	PEAK	DURATION
1.1-1.7 hr	2 wk	4-6 hr	Unknown

FIBRIC ACID DERIVATIVES

Currently clofibrate and gemfibrozil are the only two fibric acid antilipemics approved for clinical use in the United States. These agents primarily affect the triglyceride levels but may also lower the total cholesterol and LDL cholesterol levels and raise the HDL cholesterol level.

Table 25-4	HMG–CoA Reductase Inhibitors: Common Adverse Effects

BODY SYSTEM	SIDE/ADVERSE EFFECT
Gastrointestinal	Constipation, cramps, diarrhea, nausea, changes in bowel function
Central nervous system	Headache, dizziness, blurred vision, ophthalmoplegia, fatigue, insomnia
Other	Myalgias, skin rashes

Mechanism of Action

The fibric acid agents are believed to work by activating lipoprotein lipase, an enzyme responsible for the breakdown of cholesterol. This enzyme usually cleaves off a triglyceride molecule from VLDL or LDL, leaving behind lipoproteins. Fibric acid derivatives can also suppress the release of free fatty acid from adipose tissue, inhibit the synthesis of triglycerides in the liver, and increase the secretion of cholesterol into bile.

Drug Effects

The fibric acid derivatives decrease the serum VLDL and LDL concentrations. They have also been shown to reduce the triglyceride levels. Independent of their lipid-lowering actions, the fibric acid derivatives can also induce changes in blood coagulation. This involves a tendency for them to decrease platelet adhesiveness. They can also increase plasma fibrinolysis, the process that causes fibrin and therefore clots to be broken down. Clofibrate has also been reported to increase the release of antidiuretic hormone from the posterior pituitary, to block arginine-induced insulin and glucagon secretion by the pancreas, and to lower fasting blood glucose concentrations and serum insulin concentrations in patients with diabetes mellitus.

Therapeutic Uses

The fibric acid derivatives, gemfibrozil and clofibrate, both decrease the triglyceride levels and increase the HDL cholesterol level by as much as 25%. Both decrease the LDL concentrations in patients with type IIa and IIb hyperlipidemias but increase the LDL levels in patients with type IV and V hyperlipemias. They are indicated for the treatment of type III, IV, and V hyperlipidemias, and in some cases the type IIb form.

Side Effects and Adverse Effects

As a class, the most common adverse effects of the fibric acid derivatives are abdominal discomfort, diarrhea, nausea, headache, blurred vision, increased risk of gallstones, and prolonged prothrombin time. Liver function tests may also show increased function. The more common side effects and adverse effects are listed in Table 25-5.

Toxicity and Management of Overdose

Supportive therapy is called for in the management of an overdose of clofibrate. The pharmacokinetic data for clofibrate are very limited. The oral absorption of the drug is good, and its ability to bind to protein is high (>95%). It is excreted in the urine, primarily as metabolites.

Table 25-5	Fibric Acid Derivatives: Common Adverse Effects
BODY SYSTEM	**SIDE/ADVERSE EFFECT**
Gastrointestinal	Nausea, vomiting diarrhea, gallstones, acute appendicitis
Genitourinary	Impotence, decreased urine output, hematuria, increased risk of urinary tract infections and viral infections
Other	Drowsiness, dizziness, rash, pruritus, alopecia, eczema, vertigo, headache

The management of gemfibrozil overdose is also supportive. The drug is well absorbed, and the levels peak in 1 to 2 hours.

Interactions

Careful dosage adjustment of oral anticoagulants is necessary in patients also receiving clofibrate because clofibrate enhances their action. Furosemide can also displace clofibrate from inactive storage sites.

Gemfibrozil can also enhance the action of oral anticoagulants, thus also necessitating careful dose adjustments of these latter agents. When it is given in conjunction with an HMA-CoA reductase inhibitor, the risk of myositis, myalgias, and rhabdomyolysis is increased.

Laboratory test interactions that can occur in patients taking gemfibrozil include a decrease in the hemoglobin level, hematocrit value, and white blood cell count. In addition, the SGOT, activated clotting time (ACT), lactate dehydrogenase, and bilirubin levels can be increased.

Dosages

For dosage information on clofibrate and gemfibrozil, see the dosages table on p. 376.

DRUG PROFILES

The fibric acid derivatives, clofibrate and gemfibrozil, are prescription-only drugs. They are both pregnancy category C agents and are contraindicated in the set-

DOSAGES

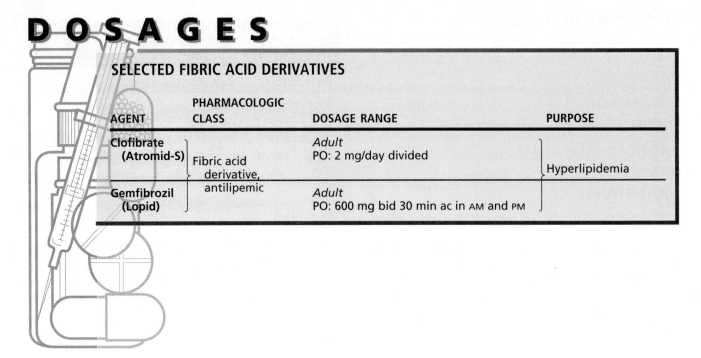

SELECTED FIBRIC ACID DERIVATIVES

AGENT	PHARMACOLOGIC CLASS	DOSAGE RANGE	PURPOSE
Clofibrate (Atromid-S)	Fibric acid derivative, antilipemic	*Adult* PO: 2 mg/day divided	Hyperlipidemia
Gemfibrozil (Lopid)		*Adult* PO: 600 mg bid 30 min ac in AM and PM	

tings of hypersensitivity, preexisting gallbladder disease, significant hepatic or renal dysfunction, and primary biliary cirrhosis. Both agents decrease the triglyceride and increase the HDL levels by as much as 25%. They are good agents for the treatment of mixed hyperlipidemias.

CLOFIBRATE

Clofibrate (Atromid-S) was the first fibric acid antilipemic drug approved by the FDA. It is seldom used now because large multicenter studies failed to show that it prevented atherosclerosis. Clofibrate has also been found to be associated with an increased incidence of gallstones and gastrointestinal tract malignant tumors, as shown by a recent study of 5000 men with hypercholesterolemia who were treated with the agent. This study showed not only an increased mortality rate stemming from malignant and gastrointestinal disease in these men but also a higher rate of cholecystectomy necessitated by gallstone disease. Its use should now probably be limited to patients with severe hypertriglyceridemia unresponsive to gemfibrozil.

Clofibrate is indicated for the management of type III, IV, and V hyperlipidemias. It is only available orally as 500-mg liquid-filled capsules. Specific dosage recommendations for clofibrate are given in the dosage table above. Pregnancy category C.

♥ PHARMACOKINETICS

HALF-LIFE	ONSET	PEAK	DURATION
12-22 hr	Unknown	4-6 hr	Unknown

GEMFIBROZIL

Gemfibrozil (Lopid) is a fibric acid derivative that decreases the synthesis of apolipoprotein B and lowers the VLDL level. It can also increase the HDL level. In addition, it is highly effective for lowering the plasma triglyceride levels. In a very large trial, the Helsinki study, the triglyceride levels of the group receiving gemfibrozil were reduced by as much as 43% compared with the control group. The total cholesterol and LDL levels were reduced by 11% and 10%, respectively, and the high-density lipoprotein level was increased by 10%.

Gemfibrozil is indicated for the treatment of type IV and V hyperlipidemias and in some cases of the type IIb form. Gemfibrozil is only available orally as a 600-mg film-coated tablet. The specific dosing recommendations are given in the dosage table above. Pregnancy category B.

♥ PHARMACOKINETICS

HALF-LIFE	ONSET	PEAK	DURATION
1.3–1.5 hr	Unknown	1-2 hr	Unknown

NICOTINIC ACID

Nicotinic acid, or niacin, is not only a very unique lipid-lowering agent it is also a vitamin. For its unique lipid-lowering properties to be realized, much larger doses of the agent are required than are commonly given when it is used as a vitamin. Nicotinic acid, or niacin, is a B vitamin, specifically vitamin B_3. It is an effective and inexpensive medication that exerts favorable effects on the plasma concentrations of all lipoproteins. Niacin is often given in combination with other antilipemic drugs to enhance the lipid-lowering effects.

Mechanism of Action

Although the exact mechanism of action of nicotinic acid is unknown, the beneficial effects are believed to be related to its ability to reduce the breakdown of lipids by increasing the activity of lipoprotein lipase, the enzyme that breaks down lipids; directly inhibiting the synthesis of certain lipids (VLDL and LDL) in the liver; and changing the metabolism of HDL, resulting in increased HDL levels. Niacin also inhibits the release of free fatty acids from adipose tissue (fat tissue).

Drug Effects

The drug effects of nicotinic acid are primarily limited to its ability to reduce the metabolism or catabolism of cholesterol and triglycerides. Niacin decreases the LDL levels moderately, decreases the triglyceride levels, and increases the HDL levels moderately. Niacin is also a vitamin needed for many bodily processes. In large doses it may produce vasodilation that is limited to the cutaneous vessels. This effect seems to be induced by prostaglandins. Niacin also causes the release of histamine, resulting in an increase in gastric motility and acid secretion. Niacin may also stimulate the fibrinolytic system to break down fibrin clots.

Therapeutic Uses

Nicotinic acid has been shown to be effective in lowering lipid levels. This includes the triglyceride, total serum cholesterol, and LDL cholesterol levels. It also brings about an increase in the HDL cholesterol levels. Niacin may also lower the lipoprotein (a) level, except in patients with severe hypertriglyceridemia. It has been shown to be effective in the treatment of types IIa, IIb, III, IV, and V hyperlipidemias.

Nicotinic acid's effects on the triglyceride levels begin to be noticed after 1 to 4 days of therapy, with the decrease in the levels ranging from 20% to 80%. The decline in the LDL levels is less, with the maximum decrease ranging from 10% to 15%. The maximum effects of niacin are seen after 3 to 5 weeks of continuous therapy.

Side Effects and Adverse Effects

Niacin can cause flushing, pruritus, and gastrointestinal distress. Sometimes small doses of aspirin or nonsteroidal antiinflammatory drugs may be taken with the agent to minimize the cutaneous flushing. These undesirable effects can also be minimized by

Table 25-6	Nicotinic Acid: Common Adverse Effects
BODY SYSTEM	**SIDE/ADVERSE EFFECT**
Skin	Cutaneous flushing, pruritus, hyperpigmentation
Gastrointestinal	Abdominal discomfort, gastrointestinal distress
Other	Blurred vision, glucose intolerance, hyperuricemia, rarely dry eyes, hepatotoxicity

starting patients off on a low initial dosage and increasing it gradually and having patients take the drug with meals. The most common side effects and adverse effects associated with nicotinic acid therapy are listed in Table 25-6.

Interactions

The major drug interactions associated with nicotinic acid are minimal. Niacin reportedly potentiates the hypotensive effects of ganglionic blockers (discussed in Chapter 19). In addition, when niacin is taken concomitantly with an HMG–CoA reductase inhibitor, the likelihood of myopathy developing is greatly increased.

Dosages

For dosage information on nicotinic acid, see the drug profile for this agent.

DRUG PROFILE

NICOTINIC ACID

Used alone or in combination with other lipid-lowering drugs, nicotinic acid (niacin; Nicor, Nicolar) is a very effective, inexpensive medication that, as already mentioned, has beneficial effects on the LDL cholesterol, triglyceride, and HDL cholesterol levels. Drug therapy with nicotinic acid is usually initiated at a small daily dose taken with or after meals to minimize the side effects previously discussed.

Nicotinic acid is a pregnancy category A agent that is contraindicated in patients who have shown a hypersensitivity to it, in those with peptic ulcer, hepatic disease, hemorrhage, or severe hypotension, and in lactating women. Niacin is available over the counter as well as by prescription. Nicotinic acid is only available orally as 25-, 50-, 100-, 250-, 500-, and 750-mg tablets and is commonly given in 2 to 4 divided doses of 1.5 to 6 g/day.

⬡ PHARMACOKINETICS

HALF-LIFE	ONSET	PEAK	DURATION
45 min	Unknown	30-70 min	Unknown

PROBUCOL

Three other drugs that can be considered in the treatment of selected patients with hypercholesterolemia are probucol, neomycin, and D-thyroxine, but of these, only probucol is discussed here. Probucol (Lorelco) does not fit into any of the general categories of cholesterol-lowering agents. It is a synthetic lipophilic antioxidant that has been used as an antilipemic agent for almost 20 years. It is not frequently prescribed because it actually lowers the HDL level even more than it does the LDL level. The HDL level is lowered by as much as 30%, and the LDL level is often lowered by less than 10%; the total cholesterol level is lowered by 10% to 15%.

Mechanism of Action

The mechanism of action of probucol is uncertain, but it does not affect the production or degradation of LDL as many of the other antilipemic agents do. Instead it prevents unoxidized LDL from being oxidized and taken up by macrophages. By doing so, probucol prevents the formation of foam cells, which, as already discussed, are the precursors of atheromas and atherosclerosis.

Drug Effects

The drug effects of probucol are limited to its ability to lower the cholesterol level, primarily the HDL and LDL levels. It has antioxidant properties as well. It may also affect the cardiac conduction system and cause prolongation of the QT interval, which is an occasional effect of membrane-stabilizing drugs such as the class I antidysrhythmics.

Therapeutic Uses

The therapeutic effects of probucol are cholesterol lowering. Probucol can decrease the LDL cholesterol level by approximately 8% to 15%, but unfortunately it also decreases the HDL cholesterol level by as much as 25%. The role of probucol in the manage-

ment of hyperlipidemia remains controversial. It may be best considered a second-line drug in the treatment of primary types IIa and IIb hypercholesterolemias.

Side Effects and Adverse Effects

Probucol is generally well tolerated. The most common undesirable effects include abdominal pain, changes in bowel function, and nausea, but these occur in less than 8% of the patients taking it. The drug should not be used in patients with an initially prolonged QT interval or in those with a history of ventricular dysrhythmias.

Interactions

Specific drug interaction information is unavailable. However, because antilipemic agents in general reduce or delay the absorption of other oral medications, probucol should be taken either 1 hour before or 4 to 6 hours after these agents.

Patients taking probucol have been found to have low hemoglobin and hematocrit values.

Dosages

For dosage information on probucol, see the drug profile of this agent.

*D*RUG *P*ROFILE

PROBUCOL

As of 1995, the antilipemic agent known as Probucol (Lorelco) will no longer be distributed in the United States. The product will still be available in other countries.

Probucol (Lorelco) is indicated for the treatment of type IIa and IIb hyperlipidemias and should probably be reserved for those patients who have failed to respond to other more effective antilipemic agents. Probucol has little if any effect on the triglyceride levels. Probucol is a pregnancy category B agent that is contraindicated in patients with a known hypersensitivity to it. It should be used cautiously in patients with a history of dysrhythmias. It is available orally as 250- and 500-mg film-coated tablets. A common dosage is a 500-mg tablet given twice a day, once in the morning and once in the evening with meals.

PHARMACOKINETICS

HALF-LIFE	ONSET	PEAK	DURATION
2-3 mo*	5-11 days†	Unknown	25 days*

*Until serum cholesterol levels are back to baseline values.
†Until therapeutic effect.

NURSING PROCESS

Assessment

Before initiating antilipemic therapy in a patient, the nurse should obtain a thorough health and medication history, including the nature of any hypersensitivity reactions. The patient's dietary patterns; the exercise programs he or she is involved in; his or her weight, height, and vital signs; the nature of tobacco and alcohol use; and the patient's family history are important data to be used for developing a nursing care plan in patients receiving these medications.

Contraindications to the use of antilipemics include hypersensitivity to them, biliary obstruction, liver dysfunction, and active liver disease. Cautious use is indicated in children and in lactating or pregnant women. Some of the major drug interactions that can occur involve other antilipemics, insulin, oral antidiabetic agents, and oral anticoagulants.

RESEARCH

Is the Rate of Procedures Linked to Outcomes?
According to a study conducted by Noraloo Roos and colleagues at the University of Manitoba, in some instances at least as many deaths could be prevented by decreasing an area's surgical rates to the US average as by improving the quality of technology and associated care with which procedures are performed. In a study of adverse outcomes associated with CABG surgery experienced by elderly residents of US cities in 1986, it was found that death rates were strongly associated with both the technical quality of the surgery and the surgical rate of the specific geographic area. The death rate per 1,000 Medicare enrollees was 0.09 for the 30 cities (43.7 deaths or less per 1000 procedures) with the best technical quality as compared with a death rate of 0.23 per 1000 population in an area where the procedure was performed most frequently. The communities with the lowest surgical rates had about half the rates of adverse outcomes.

From Roos NP et al: A population-based approach to monitoring adverse outcomes of medical care, *Med Care* 33(2): 127, 1995.

Patient Teaching TIPS

✔ Patients should take these medications as ordered, and the dosing should not be changed without the physician's approval.

✔ Patients should not stop taking the medication without the physician's approval.

✔ Patients must be counseled concerning diet and nutrition. This is an important part of antilipemic therapy.

✔ Patients should be told they must take powder forms with a liquid. These should be mixed thoroughly but not stirred!

✔ Other medications should be taken 1 hour before or 4 to 6 hours after antilipemics because they can interfere with the absorption of antilipemics.

✔ The patient should notify the physician of the occurrence of any new or troublesome symptoms or of persistent GI upset, constipation, gas, bloating, heartburn, nausea, vomiting, abnormal or unusual bleeding, and yellow discoloration of the skin. Other symptoms to report include decreased sex drive, impotence, and difficulty urinating.

✔ These medications, as with all medications, should be kept out of the reach of children.

✔ Patients should eat lots of raw vegetables, fruit, and bran and drink at least 2 quarts (2 liters) of fluids a day to prevent the constipation associated with antilipemic use.

✔ It has been observed that high-fiber foods also bring about a decrease in cholesterol levels, so this is an added benefit of the high-fiber foods consumed to prevent constipation.

✔ Women receiving these agents should check with their physician about the possible interaction with oral birth control pills, should they be taking them.

✔ Taking these medications with meals will help decrease any associated GI upset.

✔ Patients should eat less animal fat and red meat while taking these medications if their cholesterol levels are high.

✔ Patients should engage in moderate daily exercise, but only with their physician's approval.

✔ If a once-a-day dosage scheme is chosen, the medications should be taken at night with the evening meal.

NURSING DIAGNOSES

Nursing diagnoses in the patient receiving an antilipemic agent include:

- Altered nutrition (greater than body requirements) related to poor dietary habits of high fat intake.
- Knowledge deficit related to an understanding of hyperlipidemia, the risks of CHD, and the need for life-style changes.
- Knowledge deficit related to an understanding of drug therapy and the therapeutic as opposed to the toxic effects.
- Risk for noncompliance related to lack of knowledge about the new drug therapy and to the need for life-style changes.

PLANNING

Goals for the patient receiving antilipemics include:

- Patient remains compliant with both nonpharmacologic and pharmacologic therapy.
- Patient remains free of the complications associated with antilipemics because of appropriate use of the drug.
- Patient will see physician regularly and as indicated for the treatment of hyperlipidemia and to repeat laboratory studies.

Outcome Criteria

Outcome criteria related to the administration of antilipemics include:

- Patient states importance of pharmacologic and nonpharmacologic therapy to their overall health and safety such as decreasing the risk of CHD.
- Patient states the rationale of therapy as well as its side effects and expected therapeutic effects (i.e., decreasing lipid levels; GI side effects; and therapeutic response of improved lipid profile).
- Patient states those conditions that may arise which the physician should be notified of such as jaundice and abdominal pain.
- Patient states importance of follow-up care with physician so as to monitor for changes in liver function studies as well as lipid levels.

IMPLEMENTATION

Patients receiving any of these agents long term may require supplemental fat-soluble vitamins A, D, and K. Clofibrate often causes constipation so patients need to increase fiber and fluid intake to offset this effect. Probucol, however, causes diarrhea. If either of these problems occurs and cannot be managed at home, the physician should be consulted. Nicotinic acid may result in pruritus and flushing, but these may be minimized by starting patients off on decreased doses, with gradual increases in the dose as ordered by the physician.

The powder or granule forms of cholestyramine and colestipol hydrochloride (ion-exchange resins) must be mixed with either a noncarbonated liquid or pureed fruit and not given in dry forms. When mixing them with liquids, the powders need to be dissolved slowly, without stirring, for at least 1 minute because stirring causes the powder to clump. These medications must also be taken 1 hour before or 4 to 6 hours after other medications because of their ability to interact with other medications and food. Patient teaching tips are on p. 379.

EVALUATION

Patients receiving an antilipemic agent need to be monitored for therapeutic and side effects during their therapy. The therapeutic effects of both nonpharmacologic and pharmacologic measures would be evidenced by a decrease to normal cholesterol and triglyceride levels. The nonpharmacologic measures include a low-fat, low-cholesterol diet; supervised, moderate exercise; weight loss; cessation of smoking or drinking; and relaxation therapy. If there is no response to pharmacologic therapy after about 3 months, then the medication is generally withdrawn. Adverse effects to monitor for include GI upset, dyspepsia, increased liver enzyme levels, hepatomegaly, flatulence, weight gain, cholelithiasis, rash, fatigue, leukopenia, anemia, bleeding, dizziness, decreased libido, impotence, hematuria, myalgias, angina, and pulmonary emboli. Patients should also be closely monitored for the development of liver or renal dysfunction.

BIBLIOGRAPHY

Albanese J, Nutz P: *Mosby's 1995 nursing drug cards*, St Louis, 1995, Mosby.

Choice of cholesterol-lowering drugs, *Med Lett Drugs Ther* 35(891):19, 1993.

Hunninghake DB: Diagnosis and treatment of lipid disorders, *Med Clin North Am* 78(1):247, 1994.

Johnson KB: *Harriet Lane handbook*, ed 13, St Louis, 1993, Mosby.

Keen JH: *Critical care and emergency drug reference*, St Louis, 1994, Mosby.

Knoben JE, Anderson PO: *Handbook of critical drug data*, ed 6, Hamilton, Ill, 1988, Drug Intelligence Publications.

Larsen ML, Illingworth DR: Drug treatment of dyslipoproteinemia, *Med Clin North Am* 78(1):225, 1994.

McEvoy GK: *AHFS drug information*, Bethesda, Md, 1994, American Society of Hospital Pharmacists.

Milander MM, Kuhn M: Lipid-lowering drugs, *AACN* 3:494, 1992.

Skidmore-Roth L: *Mosby's 1995 nursing drug reference*, St Louis, 1995, Mosby.

United States Pharmacopeial Convention: *USPDI: drug information for the health care professional*, ed 14, Rockville, Md, 1994, The US Pharmacopeial Convention.

TAKE HOME POINTS

Lipids
- Two primary forms of lipids are triglycerides and cholesterol.
- Triglycerides function as an energy source and are stored in adipose (fat) tissue.
- Cholesterol is primarily used to make steroid hormones, cell membranes, and bile acids.
- Lipoproteins transport lipids via the blood.

Link between Cholesterol and CHD
- Lipids and lipoproteins participate in the formation of atherosclerotic plaques, which leads to CHD.
- Lipids or plaque form in the blood vessels that supply the heart with needed oxygen and nutrients.
- They eventually decrease the lumen size of these blood vessels, and this reduces the amounts of these substances that can reach the heart

Antilipemics
- Drugs used to lower high levels of lipid (triglycerides and cholesterol).
- Major classes of antilipemics: (1) bile acid sequestrants, (2) nicotinic acids, and (3) HMG–CoA reductase inhibitors.
- The mechanism of action differs for each agent.

HMG–CoA Reductase Inhibitors
- Lower blood cholesterol level by decreasing the rate of cholesterol production.
- Inhibit the enzyme necessary for the liver to produce cholesterol.
- Have very few side effects.
- Four agents: lovastatin, pravastatin, simvastatin, and fluvastatin.

Nursing Considerations
- Contraindications to the use of antilipemics include hypersensitivity, biliary obstruction, liver dysfunction, and active liver disease.
- While taking a nursing history it is important to find out whether the patient is taking drugs that interact with antilipemics, such as insulin, oral antidiabetic agents, or oral anticoagulants.
- Fat-soluble vitamins may need to be prescribed for patients taking these medications long term.
- Powder or granules must be mixed with noncarbonated liquid and *never* taken dry.
- Monitoring for side effects as well as liver and renal function is important.

Critical Thinking ACTIVITIES

1. Ms. Lane has been on cholestyramine therapy 6 months for the treatment of primary hyperlipidemia. She is complaining of frequent nosebleeds. What would you give to her as the reasons for this, and what would you recommend she do?

2. Which of the following vitamins or minerals would it be potentially important to add to the long-term antilipemic therapy in a patient taking cholestyramine?
   a. Zinc
   b. Vitamin C
   c. Tyramine
   d. Vitamin K

3. In evaluating a patient for the therapeutic effects of antilipemic medication for the treatment of primary hyperlipidemia, it is very important to monitor the cholesterol levels. Which of the following cholesterol levels is the most desirable and thus the one most reflecting a therapeutic response to antilipemic treatment?
   a. 500 mg/dl
   b. 400 mg/dl
   c. 300 mg/dl
   d. 200 mg/dl

PART 5

RENAL AND GENITOURINARY SYSTEM: STUDY SKILLS BRIEF

TEXT NOTATION

Highlighting or underlining text materials is a tool that can be very helpful when rehearsing and reviewing materials after the study reading. The problem as discussed in the study skills manual is that it is often difficult to limit the quantity of material that is marked. Although a good general guideline is to try to limit yourself to marking no more than 20% to 25% of the total, this guideline applies to large blocks of material. However, some paragraphs contain essential information and must be marked extensively, while other paragraphs may need only one or two sentences marked. In this Part study model, the object is to look at how the author's structure and language can help you to select what should be marked.

Text Notation Application

Reproduced below are two paragraphs from Chapter 27 with my model underlining completed, followed by a discussion of the reasons for which I made the choices. You should not view the model underlining as a "perfect" example. The decision as to what to mark is very much an individual choice based on a number of factors, including prior experience with the subject matter and awareness of personal learning objectives and needs. These model paragraphs with the accompanying discussion are intended to provide you with a basic model to adapt to your own learning style and needs.

Chapter 27, Paragraph One

"Fluid and electrolyte management is one of the cornerstones of patient care. Most disease processes, tissue injuries, and operative procedures greatly influence the physiologic status of fluids and electrolytes in the body. A prerequisite to the understanding of fluid and electrolyte management is knowledge of the extent and composition of the various body fluid compartments.

Sixty percent of the adult human body is water. This is referred to as the *total body water* (TBW), and it is distributed to the three main compartments in the following proportions: intracellular fluid (ICF) 67%, interstitial fluid (ISF) 25%, and plasma volume (PV) 8%.''

DISCUSSION

The first thing you should notice is that the underlining I have done exceeds the 20% to 25% guideline. This is the first paragraph in the chapter. First paragraphs are usually introductions to the topic and may vary a great deal in the quantity of important information. This chapter, in my view, contains a number of key points that must be considered. Because the content seems important, I have chosen to underline more.

Sentence one was chosen because of the word "cornerstones." This word suggests that fluid management is extremely important in patient care and I must be sure to keep that focus throughout the chapter. Paying careful attention to the author's word choices plays a major role in selecting materials for text notation.

Paying attention to language led me to the third sentence, which begins: "A prerequisite to the understanding . . ." That phrase should immediately capture your attention. The phrase says that there is something that must be understood before anything else that follows will make complete sense. The phrase should also serve as an instant cue to generate a question for reading. "What is the prerequisite to understanding fluid and electrolyte management?" This question is answered directly by the sentence containing the phrase. The phrase serves as a language cue that there is something important. This in turn suggests that you probably will want to underline or highlight some information. The question helps you to select what should be marked. Everything you do at this point serves as a guide to help you establish clear learning objectives and makes the process of selecting the best information for marking easier to accomplish.

The next segment was chosen because it stands out from the body of the paragraph. *"Total body water (TBW)"* is italicized. This is a print convention used as a means of putting emphasis on something that the author believes to be of special importance. The decision to underline words and phrases that are already emphasized is a personal one. You may feel that, since the author has already marked it, you have no need to add your own marks. I find that my own marking, even of italicized or bold print material, serves as a double reminder of the importance of the information. This is an excellent example of what I mean when I say that text notation is highly personal. Whether you choose to add your own marking or not there is one aspect of this phrase that is essential. "Total body water" is part of the vocabulary of fluids and electrolytes. That means it is time to add to your vocabulary cards.

VOCABULARY CARD FRONT

total body water

Standard Abbreviation – TBW

VOCABULARY CARD BACK

Chapter 27

Page __404__

Definition – 60% of the human body is water.

This is referred to as total body water.

Total body water may be abbreviated as TBW.

This term served as a lead-in to the next key point that I have marked. The next sentence is "TBW is distributed to the three main compartments . . ." Whenever you see a phrase with a number and a word such as "main," you should be aware that this is potentially important material. This phrase should generate a new question that will aid in your selection of material to mark. "What are the three main compartments?" You see immediately that the rest of this sentence answers that question, and therefore identifies what needs to be

marked. This marking also identifies three additional vocabulary items to be added to your cards for this chapter. As you set up your cards be careful. One fluid is "intra-," and the second is "inter-." It would be easy to confuse the two, but they have very different meanings. If you are not sure what the difference is between intra- and inter-, make use of a dictionary.

Chapter 27, Paragraph Three

"The TBW can be described as being in or out of the blood vessels, or vasculature. If this terminology is used, then the term intravascular fluid (IVF) describes fluid inside the blood vessels, and the term extravascular fluid (EVF) describes the fluid outside the blood vessels. The term plasma is used to describe the fluid that flows through the blood vessels that is intravascular. Interstitial fluid is the fluid that is in the spaces between cells, tissues, and organs. Both plasma and interstitial fluid make up extracellular volume. Both interstitial fluid and intracellular fluid make up extravascular volume. These terms are often confused and misused. Table 27-1 lists these definitions for further clarity and understanding."

DISCUSSION

The language conventions and the print conventions, ***bold italics***, are the same that I used to help in the previous paragraph. This paragraph also makes a point about the possibility of confusing and/or misusing the terms introduced. Being told that there is confusing material suggests that it is crucial that you be able to identify, define, and explain each of the terms used, and that it will take some careful thought to do so. There is one additional point in this para-

graph that is important. The last sentence points you to a table, Table 27-1. There are many tables in this text. Always remember that tables are often used in an effort to simplify complex material and to clarify the relationships between the items presented in the table. In these opening paragraphs, with the repeated reference to the confusing nature of the descriptions, Table 27-1 will almost certainly be important to your learning.

Objectives

When you reach the end of this chapter, you will be able to:

1 Discuss the disorders diuretics are used to treat.

2 Discuss the different types of diuretics and their mechanisms of action as they relate to the various disorders they are used to treat.

3 List the commonly used diuretics and the different classes of agents.

4 Describe the rationale for diuretic treatment, the dosages of the agents, their side effects, and the cautions, contraindications, and drug interactions associated with their use.

5 Develop a comprehensive nursing care plan that includes patient outcomes and patient education for the patient receiving diuretics.

6 Summarize the therapeutic effects anticipated in patients receiving diuretics.

CHAPTER OUTLINE

Kidney Function

Diuretic Agents

Carbonic Anhydrase Inhibitors
  Mechanism of action
  Drug effects
  Therapeutic uses
  Side effects and adverse effects
  Interactions
  Dosages
Drug Profile
  Acetazolamide
Loop Diuretics
  Mechanism of action
  Drug effects
  Therapeutic uses
  Side effects and adverse effects
    Toxicity and management of overdose
  Interactions
  Dosages
Drug Profile
  ⚓ Furosemide
Osmotic Diuretics
  Mechanism of action
  Drug effects
  Therapeutic uses
  Side effects and adverse effects

Interactions
Dosages
Drug Profile
  Mannitol
Potassium-sparing Diuretics
  Mechanism of action
  Drug effects
  Therapeutic uses
  Side effects and adverse effects
  Interactions
  Dosages
Drug Profiles
  Amiloride
  Spironolactone
  Triamterene
Thiazides and Thiazide-like Diuretics
  Mechanism of action
  Drug effects
  Therapeutic uses
  Side effects and adverse effects
    Toxicity and management of overdose
  Interactions
  Dosages
Drug Profiles
  Hydrochlorothiazide
  Metolazone

Nursing Process
Assessment

continued

```
Nursing Diagnoses
Planning
  Outcome criteria
Implementation
Evaluation
```

Glossary

Afferent arterioles The small blood vessels leading to the glomerulus. (p. 386)

Aldosterone (al' dos tər ōn) A mineralocorticoid steroid hormone produced by the adrenal cortex that mediates the actions of the renal tubule in the regulation of sodium and potassium balance in the blood. (p. 386)

Ascites (ə si' tēz) An abnormal intraperitoneal accumulation of fluid containing large amounts of protein and electrolytes. Ascites may be detected when more than 500 ml of fluid has accumulated. (p. 390)

Collecting duct The final common pathway for filtered fluid that starts in the glomerulus. (p. 386)

Distal tubule The structure that anatomically follows the ascending loop of Henle. (p. 386)

Diuretics (di' u ret' ik) Drug or other substance that tends to promote the formation and excretion of urine. (p. 385)

Diuretic ceiling effect Daily doses of more than 50 mg of diuretic drugs in a 1-day period rarely produce additional clinical results but do increase drug toxicity. (p. 397)

Efferent arterioles The small blood vessels leaving the glomerulus. (p. 386)

Glomerular filtration rate (glo mer' u lər) The amount of ultrafiltrate formed per unit of time by the plasma flowing through the glomeruli of the kidney. (p. 385)

Glomerulus (glo mer' u ləs) Cluster of capillaries that surround each nephron. (p. 385)

Kaliuretic diuretics (ka le u ret' ik) Agents that induce potassium loss in the urine. (p. 392)

Nephron (nef' ron) A microscopic structural and functional unit of the kidney that resembles a funnel and consists of a long stem and two convoluted sections. (p. 385)

Open-angle glaucoma (glaw' ko mə) Elevated pressure in an eye because of obstruction of the outflow of aqueous humor. (p. 387)

Proximal tubule Structure that anatomically follows the glomerulus. (p. 386)

The drugs that accelerate the rate of urine formation are termed **diuretics,** and they accomplish this through a variety of mechanisms. The end result is that they remove sodium and water from the body.

The diuretics were discovered by accident when it was noticed that a mercury-based antibiotic had a very potent diuretic effect. Thus began the early developmental stages of diuretics. All the major classes of diuretic drugs in use today were developed between 1950 and 1970, and they remain among the most commonly prescribed drugs in the world. The fifth Joint National Committee on the Detection, Evaluation, and Treatment of Hypertension recently reaffirmed the role of diuretics as the first-line agents in the treatment of hypertension. Diuretics hypotensive activity may be due to many different mechanisms. They cause direct arteriolar dilation, decreasing peripheral vascular resistance. They also decrease extracellular fluid volume, plasma volume, and cardiac output, which may account for the decrease in blood pressure. They have long been the mainstay of therapy not only for this disease but also for congestive heart failure (CHF). In fact, the diuretics are so potent, so safe, and so inexpensive that they are almost universally the drug of choice in the treatment of many clinical conditions. The one main problem with their use is their metabolic side effects, which are dose related.

This chapter reviews the essential properties and actions of the following important classes of diuretic agents: carbonic anhydrase inhibitors (CAIs), loop diuretics, osmotic diuretics, potassium-sparing diuretics, and thiazide and thiazide-like diuretics. However, before these are discussed in detail, it is first important to quickly review kidney function, because this is the key to understanding the therapeutic effects of these agents.

Kidney Function

The kidney serves a very important role in the day-to-day functioning of our bodies. It filters out toxic waste products from the blood while simultaneously saving essential ones. This delicate balance between toxins and essential chemicals is maintained by the **nephron.** This is the main structural element in the kidney, and each kidney contains approximately one million of them. It is in them where diuretic agents exert their effect. The actual filtering takes place in the **glomerulus,** a cluster of capillaries surrounded by the glomerular capsule. The rate at which this occurs is referred to as the **glomerular filtration rate** (GFR), and it is used as a gauge of how well the kidneys are functioning as filters. Normally about 180 liters of blood is filtered through them per day. The GFR, which can also be thought of as the rate at which blood flows into and out of the glomerulus, is regulated by the small blood vessels leading to the glomerulus, the **afferent arterioles,** and the small blood vessels leaving the glomerulus, the **efferent arterioles.** Alterations in blood flow such as occurs in a patient in shock would therefore have a dramatic effect on kidney (renal) function. In low blood flow situations the kidney receives less blood, and therefore less diuretic gets to its site of action. For this reason diuretics may have diminished effects.

The **proximal tubule,** which anatomically follows the glomerulus, resorbs 60% to 70% of the sodium from the filtered fluid (filtrate) back into the bloodstream. Blood vessels surround the nephrons and allow substances to be directly absorbed from or secreted into the bloodstream. This process is an active one that requires energy. As sodium is actively transported back into the blood, this causes the passive resorption of chloride and water. The chloride and water simply follow the sodium. Another 20% to 25% of sodium is resorbed back into the bloodstream in the ascending loop of Henle. This is a passive process that does not require energy because here it is the chloride that is actively resorbed and the sodium that passively follows it.

The remaining 5% to 10% of sodium resorption takes place in the **distal tubule,** which anatomically follows the ascending loop of Henle. Here sodium is actively filtered in exchange for potassium or hydrogen ions, a process regulated by the hormone **aldosterone.** The **collecting duct** is the final common pathway for the filtrate that started in the glomerulus. It is here that antidiuretic hormone acts to increase the absorption of water back into the bloodstream, thereby preventing it from being lost in the urine. This entire process, along with the sites of action of the different classes of diuretics are shown in Fig. 26-1.

Diuretic Agents

The various diuretics are classified according to their sites of action, their chemical structure, and their diuretic potency, and the sites of action of the various diuretics are determined by the way in which in-

1. **Mannitol**
2. **Acetazolamide**
3. **Loop diuretics**
4. **Thiazide diuretics**
5. **Potassium-sparing diuretics**

▼ **FIG. 26-1** The nephron and diuretic sites of action. *ADH,* antidiuretic hormone.

hibit the sodium and other electrolyte transport systems located along the nephron (see Fig. 26-1). The commonly used classes of agents and the individual drugs in these classes are listed in Table 26-1. The most potent diuretics are the loop diuretics, followed by metolazone, a thiazide-like diuretic, the thiazides, and then the potassium-sparing diuretics. Their potency is a function of where they work in the nephron to inhibit sodium and water resorption. The more sodium and water they inhibit from resorption the greater the amount of diuresis and therefore the greater the potency.

CARBONIC ANHYDRASE INHIBITORS

The CAIs are chemical derivatives of sulfonamide antibiotics. As their name implies, the CAIs inhibit the enzyme carbonic anhydrase, which exists in the kidneys, eyes, and other parts of the body. The site of action of the CAIs depends on the distribution of carbonic anhydrase along the nephron. For instance, acetazolamide acts principally in the proximal tubule, which as just described is directly behind the glomerulus. Today CAIs are mainly used for the adjunct treatment of chronic simple glaucoma, sometimes referred to as **open-angle glaucoma.** The CAIs, and particularly acetazolamide, can also be extremely helpful in the management of patients with CHF who have become resistant to their present diuretic regimens.

Mechanism of Action

As just noted, the carbonic anhydrase system in the kidney is located just behind the glomerulus in the proximal tubules, where almost two thirds of all sodium and water is resorbed back into the blood. Here a specific transport system operates that exchanges sodium for hydrogen ions. For sodium and thus water to be resorbed back into the blood, hydrogen must be exchanged for it. Without the hydrogen, this cannot

occur, and the sodium and water are eliminated with the urine. The carbonic anhydrase helps make the hydrogen ions available for this exchange. When its actions are inhibited with a CAI such as acetazolamide, little sodium and water can be resorbed into the blood and they are eliminated with the urine. The clinical benefit from this is limited, however, because as early as 2 to 3 days after the start of therapy the diuretic action of acetazolamide is sharply reduced. Put another way, the CAIs reduce the formation of hydrogen (H^+) and bicarbonate (H_2CO_3) ions from carbon dioxide and water by the noncompetitive, reversible inhibition of carbonic anhydrase. This results in a reduction in the availability of these ions, mainly hydrogen, for active transport systems.

Drug Effects

As just mentioned, the inhibition of carbonic anhydrase causes the hydrogen ion concentration in the renal tubules to be reduced, resulting in an increased excretion of bicarbonate, sodium, water, and potassium. Because the resorption of water is decreased, the urine volume is increased and the urine becomes alkaline. This accounts for the diuretic effects of CAIs. Orally or parenterally administered CAIs can also decrease the formation of aqueous humor in the eye. This has the benefit of lowering intraocular pressure in patients who suffer from glaucoma. However, this effect of CAIs seems to be independent of its diuretic action.

The inhibited formation of bicarbonate and hydrogen ions the CAIs bring about has many effects on other parts of the body. The metabolic acidosis induced by CAIs is also beneficial in the prevention of seizures. In addition, the CAIs may induce respiratory and metabolic acidosis, which may in turn increase oxygenation during hypoxia by increasing ventilation, cerebral blood flow, and the dissociation of oxygen from oxyhemoglobin. An undesirable effect of the CAIs is that they elevate the blood glucose level and cause glycosuria in diabetic patients. This may be due

Table 26-1	**Classification of Diuretics**
CLASS	DRUGS
Carbonic anhydrase inhibitors	Dichlorphenamide, acetazolamide, methzolamide
Thiazide and thiazide-like diuretics	Chlorothiazide, hydrochlorothiazide, bendroflumethiazide, methyclothiazide, quinethazone, metolazone, chlorthalidone, indapamide
Loop diuretics	Furosemide, ethacrynic acid, bumetanide, torsemide
Osmotic diuretics	Mannitol
Potassium-sparing diuretics	Amiloride, spironolactone, triamterene

to the decline in the potassium level that the CAIs may induce.

Therapeutic Uses

The therapeutic applications of CAIs are wide and varied. They are commonly used in the treatment of glaucoma, edema, epilepsy, and high-altitude sickness.

The CAIs are used principally as adjunct agents in the long-term management of open-angle glaucoma that cannot be controlled by topical miotic agents or epinephrine derivatives alone. These agents together can increase the outflow of aqueous humor, the obstruction of which is responsible for the glaucoma. They are also used short term in conjunction with miotics to lower intraocular pressure in preparation for ocular surgery in patients with acute ocular disorders or narrow-angle glaucoma and as an adjunct in the treatment of secondary glaucoma.

The CAIs, particularly acetazolamide, are used to manage the edema secondary to CHF that has become resistant to other diuretics. However, as a class, the CAIs are much less potent diuretics than the loop diuretics or the thiazides, and the metabolic acidosis they induce diminishes their diuretic effect in 2 to 4 days.

Acetazolamide may be a useful adjunct to other anticonvulsants in the prophylactic management of various forms of epilepsy. However, tolerance to the anticonvulsant effects of CAIs develops quickly, and they may be ineffective for prolonged therapy. Acetazolamide is also effective in both the prevention and treatment of the symptoms of high-altitude sickness. These symptoms include headache, nausea, shortness of breath, dizziness, drowsiness, and fatigue.

Side Effects and Adverse Effects

The more common undesirable effects of the CAIs are metabolic abnormalities such as acidosis. They may also cause drowsiness, anorexia, paresthesias, hematuria, urticaria, photosensitivity, and melena.

Interactions

Significant drug interactions that occur with the CAIs include an increase in digitalis toxicity stemming from the hypokalemia CAIs may induce. Their concomitant use with corticosteroids may cause hypokalemia, and their use with oral hypoglycemic agents and quinidine will induce greater activity or toxicity of the latter agents.

Dosages

For information on the dosages of acetazolamide, see its drug profile.

DRUG PROFILE

Although there are three CAIs (see Table 26-1), by far the most widely prescribed one is acetazolamide, and it is thus the only one profiled here.

ACETAZOLAMIDE

Acetazolamide (Diamox, Diamox Sequels) is classified as a pregnancy category C agent and is contraindicated in patients who have shown a hypersensitivity to it, as well as in those with significant liver or kidney dysfunction, low serum potassium or sodium levels, acidosis, and adrenal gland failure. Acetazolamide is available both orally and parenterally. Orally it comes as 500-mg extended-release capsules and 125- and 250-mg tablets. Parenterally acetazolamide comes as a 500-mg injection. A recommended dosages for pediatric patients is oral administration of 5 mg/kg/day. A common oral dosage for adults is 250 to 375 mg/day given on alternate days.

☣ PHARMACOKINETICS

HALF-LIFE	ONSET	PEAK	DURATION
10-15 hr	1 hr	2-4 hr	8-12 hr

LOOP DIURETICS

The loop diuretics (bumetanide, ethacrynic acid, furosemide, and torsemide) are very potent diuretics that act primarily along the thick ascending limb of the loop of Henle, blocking chloride and secondarily sodium resorption. They are also believed to activate the renal prostaglandins, resulting in dilation of the blood vessels of the kidneys, the lungs, and the rest of the body (systemic and pulmonary vascular resistance). The beneficial hemodynamic effects of the loop diuretics are a reduction in both the preload and central venous pressures, which are the filling pressures of the ventricles. These actions make them very useful in the treatment of the edema associated with CHF, hepatic cirrhosis, and renal disease.

This class of drugs is particularly useful when rapid diuresis is desired because their onset of action is rapid. In addition, the diuretic effect lasts at least 2 hours. A distinct advantage they have over the thiazide diuretics is that their diuretic action continues even when the creatinine clearance decreases below 25 ml/min. Their combined use with a thiazide (especially metolazone) increases their effectiveness because this results in the blockade of sodium and water resorption at multiple sites in the nephron, a property referred to as *sequential nephron blockade*. Because of their potent diuretic effect and the duration of this effect they are effective as single-dose therapy. This allows the renal tubule time to partially compensate for the potassium depletion and other electrolyte derangements that often accompany around-the-clock diuretic therapy. Despite this, the major side effect of the loop diuretics is electrolyte disturbances. Though rare, prolonged high doses can also result in hearing loss stemming from ototoxicity. Bumetanide and furosemide are chemically related to the sulfonamides.

Mechanism of Action

The loop diuretics act directly on the ascending limb of the loop of Henle to inhibit sodium and chloride resorption. They have also been shown to inhibit electrolyte resorption in the proximal renal tubule and to increase the concentrations of renal prostaglandins, resulting in the dilation of blood vessels in the kidney, lungs, and possibly the entire body. This reduction in peripheral vascular resistance may account for their antihypertensive effects. However, this effect is reversed when nonsteroidal antiinflammatory drugs are given in conjunction with them.

Drug Effects

The loop diuretics have renal, cardiovascular, and metabolic effects. The renal effects just discussed constitute the loop diuretics' major mechanism of action.

As already noted, the loop diuretics produce a potent diuresis and subsequent loss of fluid, and the resulting decreased fluid volume leads to a decreased return of blood to the heart, or decreased filling pressures. This has the following cardiovascular effects: it reduces blood pressure, pulmonary vascular resistance, systemic vascular resistance, central venous pressure, and left ventricular end-diastolic pressure.

The metabolic effects of the loop diuretics are secondary to the electrolyte losses, specifically potassium depletion, produced by the potent diuresis. Changes in the plasma insulin, glucagon, and growth hormone levels have been seen as a result in patients taking loop diuretics.

Therapeutic Uses

The loop diuretics are used to manage the edema associated with CHF and hepatic or renal disease, to

Table 26-2	Loop Diuretics: Common Adverse Effects	
BODY SYSTEM	**SIDE/ADVERSE EFFECT**
Central nervous system	Dizziness, headache, tinnitus, blurred vision
Gastrointestinal	Nausea, vomiting, diarrhea
Hematologic	Agranulocytosis, thrombocytopenia, neutropenia

control hypertension, and to increase the renal excretion of calcium in patients with hypercalcemia.

Side Effects and Adverse Effects

Common undesirable effects of the loop diuretics are listed in Table 26-2. Those commonly associated with bumetanide therapy are muscle cramps, dry mouth, arthritic pain, and encephalopathy, and these are especially common in patients with preexisting liver disease. Ethacrynic acid may cause neutropenia and rare episodes of Henoch-Schönlein purpura. Furosemide can produce erythema multiforme, exfoliative dermatitis, photosensitivity, and rare cases of aplastic anemia. Torsemide may rarely cause thrombocytopenia, agranulocytosis, leukopenia, and neutropenia. It may also cause a severe skin disorder called *Stevens-Johnson syndrome*.

Toxicity and Management of Overdose

Electrolyte loss and dehydration, which can result in circulatory failure, are the main toxic effects of loop diuretics that require attention. Treatment involves electrolyte and fluid replacement.

Interactions

The loop diuretics exhibit both neurotoxic and nephrotoxic properties, and they produce additive effects when given in combination with drugs that have similar toxicities. The drug interactions are summarized in Table 26-3.

Loop diuretics also affect certain laboratory results. They cause increases in the serum levels of uric acid, glucose, SGPT, and SGOT.

Dosages

For the recommended dosages of loop diuretics, see the dosages table on p. 391.

Table 26-3	Loop Diuretics: Drug Interactions	
DRUG	**MECHANISM**	**RESULT**
Aminoglycosides Capreomycin Chloroquine Oxyphenbutazone Phenylbutazone Vancomycin Viomycin	Additive effect	Increased neurotoxicity, especially ototoxicity
Corticosteroids Digitalis	Hypokalemia	Additive hypokalemia Increased digitalis toxicity
Lithium	Decreases renal excretion	Increased lithium toxicity
Indomethacin	Not determined	Decreased diuretic activity

DRUG PROFILE

The currently available loop diuretics are bumetanide, ethacrynic acid, furosemide, and torsemide. As a class they are very potent diuretics, but this potency varies between the various agents. The equipotent doses for these various agents are as follows:

Bumetanide	Torsemide	Furosemide	Ethacrynic Acid
1 mg	10 mg	40 mg	50 mg

⚓ FUROSEMIDE

Furosemide (Lasix) is by far the loop diuretic most commonly used in clinical practice and the prototype agent in this class. Structurally it is related to the sulfonamides. It has all the therapeutic and adverse characteristics of the loop diuretics mentioned earlier. It is primarily used in the management of pulmonary edema and the edema associated with CHF, liver disease, nephrotic syndrome, and **ascites** (the accumulation of fluid in the peritoneal area). It has also been used in the treatment of hypertension, usually that caused by CHF.

Furosemide is classified as a pregnancy category C agent and is contraindicated in patients who have shown a hypersensitivity to sulfonamides, in infants and lactating women, and in patients suffering from anuria, hypovolemia, and electrolyte depletion. It is

available orally as a 40-mg/5 ml and a 10-mg/ml oral solution. It is also available as 20-, 40-, and 80-mg tablets. Parenterally it is available as a 10-mg/ml injection. Recommended dosages are given in the dosages table on the following page.

✿ PHARMACOKINETICS

HALF-LIFE	ONSET	PEAK	DURATION
1-2 hr	1 hr	1-2 hr	6-8 hr

OSMOTIC DIURETICS

The osmotic diuretics are mannitol, urea, organic acids, and glucose. Mannitol, a nonabsorbable, solute that works along the entire nephron, is the most commonly used of these agents. Its major site of action, however, is the proximal tubule. Because it is nonabsorbable, it produces an osmotic effect, that is, it pulls fluid, or water, into the blood vessels and nephrons from the surrounding tissues. Ultimately this increases urine production and causes diuresis. However, it produces only a slight loss of electrolytes, especially sodium. Because of this, mannitol is not indicated for patients in an edematous state because it does not promote sufficient sodium excretion.

Mannitol may induce vasodilation and in doing so increase both glomerular filtration and renal plasma flow. This makes it an excellent agent for preventing kidney damage during acute renal failure (ARF). It has also been shown to reduce intracranial pressure and cerebral edema resulting from head trauma. In addition, mannitol treatment may be tried when elevated intraocular pressure is unresponsive to other drug therapies.

Mannitol may crystallize when exposed to low

DOSAGES

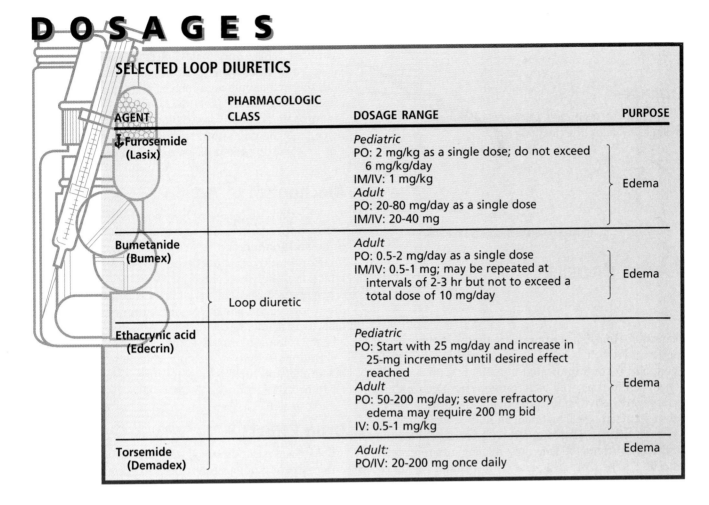

SELECTED LOOP DIURETICS

AGENT	PHARMACOLOGIC CLASS	DOSAGE RANGE	PURPOSE
↓Furosemide (Lasix)		*Pediatric* PO: 2 mg/kg as a single dose; do not exceed 6 mg/kg/day IM/IV: 1 mg/kg *Adult* PO: 20-80 mg/day as a single dose IM/IV: 20-40 mg	Edema
Bumetanide (Bumex)		*Adult* PO: 0.5-2 mg/day as a single dose IM/IV: 0.5-1 mg; may be repeated at intervals of 2-3 hr but not to exceed a total dose of 10 mg/day	Edema
Ethacrynic acid (Edecrin)	Loop diuretic	*Pediatric* PO: Start with 25 mg/day and increase in 25-mg increments until desired effect reached *Adult* PO: 50-200 mg/day; severe refractory edema may require 200 mg bid IV: 0.5-1 mg/kg	Edema
Torsemide (Demadex)		*Adult:* PO/IV: 20-200 mg once daily	Edema

temperatures, and this is more likely to occur when concentrations exceed 15%. Because of this, mannitol should always be administered intravenously through a filter.

Mechanism of Action

Mannitol and the other osmotic diuretics induce diuresis mainly by increasing the osmotic pressure of the glomerular filtrate, which in turn inhibits the tubular resorption of water and solutes, producing a rapid diuresis. The resulting osmotic effect pulls fluid from the extravascular spaces intravascularly into the tubules or into the blood vessels from the surrounding tissue.

Drug Effects

Besides increasing the osmotic pressure of the glomerular filtrate, mannitol can also induce the rapid excretion of water, sodium, and other electrolytes as well as the rapid excretion of toxic substances from the kidney. This drug also reduces excessive intraocular pressure.

Therapeutic Uses

Mannitol is the osmotic diuretic of choice. It is commonly used in the treatment of patients in the early, oliguric phase of ARF. However, for it to be effective in this setting, enough renal blood flow and glomerular filtration must exist to enable the drug to reach the tubules. Increased renal blood flow resulting from the dilation of blood vessels supplying blood to the kidneys is another therapeutic benefit of mannitol therapy in such patients. It can also be used to promote the excretion of toxic substances, reduce intracranial pressure, and treat cerebral edema. In addition, it can be used as a genitourinary irrigant in the preparation of patients for transurethral surgical procedures and as supportive treatment in patients with edema induced by other conditions.

Side Effects and Adverse Effects

Significant undesirable effects of mannitol include convulsions, thrombophlebitis, and pulmonary congestion. Other less significant effects are headaches, chest pains, tachycardia, blurred vision, chills, and fever.

Interactions

There are no drugs that interact significantly with mannitol.

Dosages

For the recommended dosages of mannitol, see the dosages table on the next page.

DRUG PROFILE

MANNITOL

Mannitol (Resectial, Osmitrol) is the prototypical osmotic diuretic. It is rated as a pregnancy category C agent and is contraindicated in patients with a hypersensitivity to it as well as in those suffering from anuria, severe dehydration, pulmonary congestion, or cerebral hemorrhage. Treatment should be terminated if severe cardiac or renal impairment develops after the initiation of therapy. It is only available parenterally as a 5%, 10%, 15%, 20%, and 25% solution for intravenous injection. Recommended dosages are given in the dosages table on the next page.

♥♥ PHARMACOKINETICS

HALF-LIFE	ONSET	PEAK	DURATION
1.5 hr	30-60 min	Dose and time dependent	6-8 hr

POTASSIUM-SPARING DIURETICS

The most commonly prescribed potassium-sparing diuretics are amiloride, spironolactone, and triamterene. These diuretics are also referred to as the *aldosterone-inhibiting diuretics* because they block the aldosterone receptors. These agents work in the collecting ducts and the distal convoluted tubules, where they interfere with sodium-potassium exchange. They also competitively bind to aldosterone receptors and therefore block the resorption of sodium and water that is induced by aldosterone secretion. They are often prescribed in children with CHF because the cardiac disorder in this setting is often accompanied by an excess secretion of aldosterone and the loop and thiazide diuretics are frequently ineffective in its management.

Because little more than 3% of the total filtered load reaches the collecting ducts, the potassium-sparing diuretics are weak as diuretics. When diuresis is needed, they are generally used as adjuncts to thiazide treatment. This combination is beneficial in two aspects. First, it has synergistic diuretic effects, and second, the two agents counteract the adverse metabolic effects of each other: The thiazide diuretics cause potassium, magnesium, and chloride to be lost in the urine, and the potassium-sparing diuretics counteract this by elevating the potassium and chloride levels.

Mechanism of Action

The diuretic action of the potassium-sparing diuretics varies for the different drugs in the class. Amiloride and triamterene, which have similar pharmacologic properties, act directly on the distal renal tubule, which is under the control of the mineralocorticoids, especially aldosterone, to inhibit the resorption of sodium ions in exchange for potassium and hydrogen ions. This results in the diuresis of water and sodium and the retention of potassium.

Spironolactone is a competitive antagonist of aldosterone, and for this reason causes sodium and water to be excreted and potassium to be retained.

Drug Effects

As their name implies, the potassium-sparing diuretics prevent potassium from being pumped into the tubule, so it is not secreted. They do this by competitively blocking the aldosterone receptors and inhibiting the action of this mineralocorticoid. The excretion of sodium and water is promoted, however. In addition, with the exception of triamterene, these drugs have an antihypertensive effect.

Therapeutic Uses

The therapeutic applications of the potassium-sparing diuretics vary depending on the particular agent. Spironolactone and triamterene are used in the treatment of hyperaldosteronism and hypertension and for reversing the potassium loss caused by the **kaliuretic diuretics** or other potassium-losing drugs. The uses for amiloride are similar to those of spironolactone and triamterene, but it is less effective in the long term. It may be more effective than spironolactone or triamterene in the treatment of metabolic alkalosis, however. It is typically used in the treatment of CHF.

Side Effects and Adverse Effects

The potassium-sparing diuretics have several common undesirable effects. These are listed in Table 26-4. There are also some significant adverse effects that are specific to the individual agents. Spironolactone can

DOSAGES

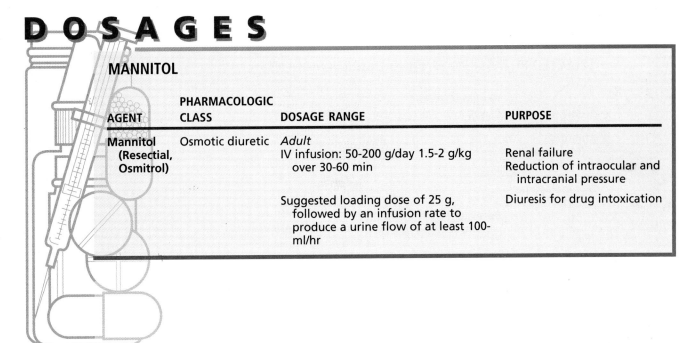

MANNITOL

AGENT	PHARMACOLOGIC CLASS	DOSAGE RANGE	PURPOSE
Mannitol (Resectial, Osmitrol)	Osmotic diuretic	*Adult* IV infusion: 50-200 g/day 1.5-2 g/kg over 30-60 min	Renal failure Reduction of intraocular and intracranial pressure
		Suggested loading dose of 25 g, followed by an infusion rate to produce a urine flow of at least 100-ml/hr	Diuresis for drug intoxication

Table 26-4	Potassium-Sparing Diuretics: Common Adverse Effects

BODY SYSTEM	SIDE/ADVERSE EFFECT
Central nervous system	Dizziness, headache
Gastrointestinal	Cramps, nausea, vomiting, diarrhea
Other	Urinary frequency, weakness

Table 26-5	Potassium-Sparing Diuretics: Drug Interactions

DRUG	MECHANISM	RESULTS
ACE inhibitors	Additive effect	Hyperkalemia
Lithium	Reduce excretion	Increased lithium toxicity
Potassium supplements	Additive effects	Hyperkalemia

cause gynecomastia, amenorrhea, irregular menses, and postmenopausal bleeding. Triamterene may reduce folic acid levels and cause the formation of kidney stones and urinary casts. It may also precipitate megaloblastic anemia. Hyperkalemia also may occur when triamterene is used alone or in combination with other diuretics. Side effects from triamterene use are rare.

Interactions

The concomitant use of these potassium-sparing diuretics with lithium, ACE inhibitors, or potassium supplements can result in significant drug interactions. These are summarized in Table 26-5.

Dosages

For recommended dosages of potassium-sparing diuretics, see the dosages table on p. 394.

DRUG PROFILES

AMILORIDE

Amiloride (Midamor) is generally used in combination with a thiazide or loop diuretic in the therapy for CHF. Hyperkalemia may occur in as much as 10% of the patients who are taking amiloride alone. It should be used with caution in patients suffering from renal impairment or diabetes mellitus and in elderly patients. Amiloride is contraindicated in the settings of hypersensitivity, hyperkalemia, and impaired renal function. It has only weak antihypertensive properties. It is

DOSAGES

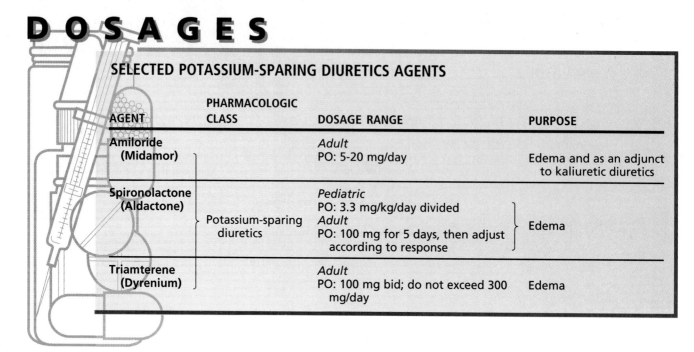

SELECTED POTASSIUM-SPARING DIURETICS AGENTS

AGENT	PHARMACOLOGIC CLASS	DOSAGE RANGE	PURPOSE
Amiloride (Midamor)		*Adult* PO: 5-20 mg/day	Edema and as an adjunct to kaliuretic diuretics
Spironolactone (Aldactone)	Potassium-sparing diuretics	*Pediatric* PO: 3.3 mg/kg/day divided *Adult* PO: 100 mg for 5 days, then adjust according to response	Edema
Triamterene (Dyrenium)		*Adult* PO: 100 mg bid; do not exceed 300 mg/day	Edema

a pregnancy category B agent and is only available orally as a 5-mg tablet. It also comes in combination with hydrochlorothiazide in a product called Moduretic. Recommended dosages are given in the dosages table above.

❖ PHARMACOKINETICS

HALF-LIFE	ONSET	PEAK	DURATION
6-9 hr	2 hr	6-10 hr	24 hr

SPIRONOLACTONE

Structurally spironolactone (Aldactone) is a synthetic steroid that blocks aldosterone receptors. It is used in high doses for the treatment of ascites. This condition is commonly associated with cirrhosis of the liver. The serum potassium level should be monitored frequently in patients taking it who have impaired renal function or who are currently taking potassium supplements because hyperkalemia is a frequent complication of spironolactone therapy. It is the potassium-sparing diuretic most frequently prescribed for children who have CHF because this form of CHF frequently causes excess aldosterone to be secreted, which in turn causes increased sodium and water resorption. It is contraindicated in patients who have a hypersensitivity to it and those suffering from anuria, significant renal impairment, or hyperkalemia. Of the three commonly used potassium-sparing diuretics, spironolactone has the greatest antihypertensive activity. It is a pregnancy category D agent and is only available orally as 25-mg tablets and as 25-, 50-, and 100-mg film-coated tablets. It also comes in combination with hydrochlorothiazide

in a product called Spironazide or Aldactazide. Recommended dosages are given in the dosages table above.

❖ PHARMACOKINETICS

HALF-LIFE	ONSET	PEAK	DURATION
13-24 hr	1-3 days	2-3 days	2-3 days

TRIAMTERENE

As previously mentioned, the pharmacologic properties of triamterene (Dyrenium) are similar to those of amiloride. Therefore, like amiloride, triamterene acts directly on the distal renal tubule of the nephron to depress the resorption of sodium and the excretion of potassium and hydrogen, processes otherwise stimulated at that site by aldosterone. However, unlike spironolactone, which induces diuresis by directly inhibiting aldosterone, triamterene does so independent of aldosterone. Triamterene is contraindicated in the settings of hypersensitivity, anuria, significant renal or hepatic insufficiency, and hyperkalemia. It has little or no antihypertensive effect. It is a pregnancy category D agent and is only available orally as 50- and 100-mg capsules. It also comes in combination with hydrochlorothiazide in a product called Dyazide or Maxzide. Recommended dosages are given in the dosages table above.

❖ PHARMACOKINETICS

HALF-LIFE	ONSET	PEAK	DURATION
2-3 hr	2-4 hr	6-8 hr	7-9 hr

THIAZIDES AND THIAZIDE-LIKE DIURETICS

Thiazide and thiazide-like diuretics are all generally considered equivalent in their effects, though chlorthalidone is somewhat different because of its long duration of action and metolazone, which is also frequently prescribed, and quinethazone may be more effective than other agents in the class in the treatment of patients with renal dysfunction. Hydrochlorothiazide is one of the most commonly used and the least expensive of the generic preparations. The thiazide diuretics consist of bendroflumethiazide, benzthiazide, chlorothiazide, polythiazide, and trichlormethiazide. The thiazide-like diuretics are very similar in action to the thiazides and include chlorthalidone, indapamide, metolazone, and quinethazone.

Thiazides are used as adjunct agents in the management of CHF, hepatic cirrhosis, and edema of various origins. The primary site of action of thiazides and the thiazide-like diuretics is the distal convoluted tubule, where they inhibit sodium and chloride resorption. The thiazides also cause direct relaxation of the arterioles (small blood vessels), with decreased preload (filling pressures) and decreased afterload (the force the ventricles must overcome to eject the volume of blood they contain) the beneficial hemodynamic effects. This makes them very effective for the treatment of both CHF and hypertension.

As renal function decreases, the efficacy of thiazides diminishes, probably because delivery of the drug to the active site is impaired. Thiazides generally should not be used if the creatinine clearance is less than 30 to 50 ml/min. The only exception is metolazone, which remains effective to a creatinine clearance of 10 ml/min. Major side effects of the agents stem from the electrolyte disturbances they produce, as they are noted for precipitating hypokalemia and hypercalcemia as well as metabolic disturbances such as hyperlipidemia, hyperglycemia, and hyperuricemia.

Mechanism of Action

The thiazide diuretics are chemical derivatives (benzothiadiazines) of the sulfonamides. Their diuretic effect stems from their ability to inhibit the tubular resorption of sodium and chloride ions, primarily in the ascending loop of Henle and in the early distal tubule of the nephron. As a result, water, sodium, and chloride, and to a lesser extent potassium, are excreted.

Drug Effects

The thiazides and related diuretics cause water, sodium, chloride, and potassium ions to be excreted without altering the pH of the urine. By dilating the arterioles these drugs also lower peripheral vascular resistance.

Table 26-6	Thiazide and Thiazide-Like Diuretics: Common Adverse Effects
Body System/Process	**Side/Adverse Effect**
Central nervous system	Dizziness, headache, blurred vision, paresthesia
Gastrointestinal	Anorexia, nausea, vomiting, diarrhea, pancreatitis, cholecystitis
Hematologic	Jaundice, leukopenia, purpura, agranulocytosis, aplastic anemia, thrombocytopenia
Dermatologic	Urticaria, photosensitivity
Metabolic	Hypokalemia, glycosuria, hyperglycemia, hyperuricemia, hypochloremic alkalosis

The antihypertensive effect of the thiazides is the result of sodium depletion and lowered peripheral vascular resistance. They are one of the most prescribed group of agents for the treatment of hypertension.

Therapeutic Uses

In addition to hypertension, the thiazide and thiazide-like diuretics are used in the treatment of edematous states, idiopathic hypercalciuria, and diabetes insipidus. Any of these drugs can be used either as a sole agent or in combination with other agents. This group of diuretics may also be useful as adjunct agents in the treatment of edema related to CHF, hepatic cirrhosis, and corticosteroid or estrogen therapy.

Side Effects and Adverse Effects

As already mentioned, major side effects of the thiazide and thiazide-like diuretics relate to the electrolyte disturbances they cause; these mainly comprise reduced potassium levels and elevated levels of calcium, lipids, glucose, and uric acid. Other effects, such as gastrointestinal disturbances, skin rashes, photosensitivity, thrombocytopenia, pancreatitis, and cholecystitis, are less common. Dizziness and vertigo are common side effects of metolazone therapy and are attributed to sudden shifts in the plasma volume brought about by the agent. Headache, impotence, and decreased libido are other important side effects of these agents. The more common side effects of the thiazide and thiazide-like diuretics are listed in Table 26-6.

Toxicity and Management of Overdose

An overdose of these drugs can lead to an electrolyte imbalance resulting from hypokalemia. Symptoms include anorexia, nausea, lethargy, muscle weakness, mental confusion, and hypertension. Treatment involves electrolyte replacement.

Interactions

The thiazides and related agents interact with corticosteroids, diazoxide, digitalis, and oral hypoglycemics. The mechanisms and results of these interactions are summarized in Table 26-7.

Besides the drug interactions, these agents can increase the serum levels of SGOT and SGPT and alter the glucose levels in urine. In addition, the excessive consumption of licorice can lead to an additive hypokalemia in patients taking them.

Dosages

For information on the dosages for thiazide and thiazide-like diuretics, see the dosages table below.

DRUG PROFILES

The thiazide diuretics and thiazide-like diuretics are listed in the box below. These drugs fall into several

Table 26-7	Thiazide and Thiazide-like Diuretics: Drug Interactions	
DRUG	**MECHANISM**	**RESULT**
Corticosteroids	Additive effect	Hypokalemia
Diazoxide	Additive effect	Hyperkalemia
Digitalis	Hypokalemia	Increased digitalis toxicity
Oral hypo-glycemics	Antagonism	Reduced therapeutic effect

Thiazide and Thiazide-like Diuretics

Thiazide Diuretics
Bendroflumethiazide (Naturetin)
Benzthiazide (ExNa)
Chlorothiazide (Diuril)
Cyclothiazide (Anhydron)
Hydrochlorothiazide (Esidrex, Hydro-Diuril)
Hydroflumethiazide (Saluron, Diucardin)
Methyclothiazide (Enduron, Aquatensen)
Polythiazide (Renese)
Trichloromethiazide (Metahydrin, Naqua)

Thiazide-Like Diuretics
Chlorthalidone (Hygroton)
Indapamide (Lozol)
Metolazone (Mykrox, zaroxolyn)
Quinethazone (Hydromox)

DOSAGES

THIAZIDE AND SELECTED THIAZIDE-LIKE DIURETICS AGENTS

AGENT	PHARMACOLOGIC CLASS	DOSAGE RANGE	PURPOSE
Hydrochlorothiazide (Esidrex, Hydro-Diuril)	Thiazide diuretic	*Pediatric* PO: <6 mo, 3.3 mg/kg/day; <2 y/o, 12.5-37.5 mg/day in 2 doses; 2-12 y/o, 37.5-100 mg/day in 2 doses *Adult* PO: 25-200 mg/day, usually divided	Edema
Metolazone (Mykrox, Diulo, Zaroxolyn)	Thiazide-like diuretic	*Adult* PO: 2.5-20 mg/day	Edema

pregnancy categories. Chlorothiazide, hydrochlorothiazide, indapamide, methyclothiazide, and metolazone are category B agents. Benzthiazide, polythiazide, and trichloromethiazide are category C agents, and hydro-

flumethiazide is the only category D agent in this class. Bendroflumethiazide, chlorthalidone, and quinethazone are not classified in any pregnancy category.

Patient Teaching TIPS

Diuretic Therapy

✔ The patient should be told to always maintain proper nutritional and fluid volume status and to eat more potassium-rich foods when taking *any but the potassium-sparing diuretics.* Foods high in potassium include bananas, oranges, dates, raisins, plums, fresh vegetables, potatoes (especially potato skins), meat, and fish.

✔ If patients are taking a diuretic along with a digitalis preparation, they and/or their family members should be shown how to monitor the pulse rate and know to call the physician at the first signs of toxicity. The symptoms of this consist of anorexia, nausea, vomiting, and bradycardia, or a pulse of less than 60 beats/min.

✔ Diabetic patients who are taking thiazide diuretics should be told to closely monitor their blood sugar levels because these drugs can raise them.

✔ Patients taking diuretics should be told to change positions slowly and rise slowly after sitting or lying to prevent dizziness and possible fainting (syncope) related to the orthostatic hypotension resulting from the diuretic therapy.

✔ Encourage patients to return to their physician for follow-up visits and especially for laboratory workups.

✔ Patients taking diuretics should keep a journal or log of their daily weights.

✔ Patients who have been ill and experienced nausea, vomiting, and/or diarrhea should notify their physician of this because of the electrolyte and fluid loss this may have precipitated. Patients should ask whether to institute fluid volume replacement to prevent any excess fluid or electrolyte loss.

✔ Signs and symptoms of hypokalemia include muscle weakness, constipation, irregular pulse rate, and an overall feeling of lethargy.

✔ Patients should be encouraged to notify the physician immediately should they experience rapid heart rates or syncope, as this may be a result of hypotension or fluid volume loss.

✔ Any weight gain of 2 or more pounds (1 kg) a day or 5 or more pounds (2.25 kg) in a week should be reported to the physician immediately.

HYDROCHLOROTHIAZIDE

Hydrochlorothiazide (Esidrix, Hydro-Diuril), which is considered the prototypical thiazide diuretic, is a very commonly prescribed and inexpensive thiazide diuretic. It is also a very safe and effective diuretic. There are many combination-drug products that contain hydrochlorothiazide, the other agent being methyldopa, propranolol, spironolactone, triamterene, hydralazine, the angiotensin-converting enzyme inhibitors, the beta-blockers, or labetalol. Daily doses exceeding 50 mg a day rarely produce additional clinical results and may only increase drug toxicity. This property is known as the **diuretic ceiling effect.**

Hydrochlorothiazide is a pregnancy category D agent and is contraindicated in patients with a known hypersensitivity to thiazides or sulfonamides, and in those suffering from anuria, renal decompensation, or hypomagnesemia. It is only available orally as a 50-mg/5 ml solution and as 25-, 50-, and 100-mg tablets. Recommended dosages are given in the dosages table on the previous page.

⬡ PHARMACOKINETICS

HALF-LIFE	ONSET	PEAK	DURATION
5.6-14.8 hr	2 hr	4 hr	6-12 hr

METOLAZONE

Metolazone (Mykrox, Diulo, Zaroxolyn) is a thiazide-like diuretic that appears to be more potent than the thiazide diuretics. This is most visible in patients with renal dysfunction. One striking advantage of metolazone is that it remains effective to a creatinine clearance as low as 10 ml/min. It may also be given in combination with loop diuretics to obtain a potent diuresis in patients with severe symptoms of CHF.

Metolazone is classified as a pregnancy D agent and is contraindicated in patients with a known hypersensitivity to thiazides or sulfonamides, in those with anuria, and in pregnant or lactating women. It is only available orally as 0.5-, 2.5-, 5-, and 10-mg tablets. Recommended dosages are given in the dosages table on the previous page.

⬡ PHARMACOKINETICS

HALF-LIFE	ONSET	PEAK	DURATION
8 hr	1 hr	1-2 hr	up to 24 hr

NURSING PROCESS

ASSESSMENT

Before administering any type of diuretic, the nurse should obtain a thorough history in the patient. A physical examination must also be completed and the findings documented. Because fluid volume levels and electrolyte concentrations are affected by diuretics, the patient's baseline fluid volume status, intake and output measurements, serum electrolyte values, weight, and vital signs should be documented. Skin turgor, the

serum creatinine level, arterial blood gas values, blood pH, and the uric acid level should also be documented before the start of diuretic therapy. Often it is necessary to measure postural blood pressures (lying and standing) in patients who are to receive these agents because they cause fluid to be lost from the intravascular spaces first, and this may precipitate blood pressure changes (both a decrease and postural changes).

Cautious use of diuretics, with close monitoring, is recommended in patients with the following disorders or conditions: hypokalemia, hypovolemia, renal disease, liver disease, lupus, diabetes, chronic obstructive pulmonary disease, and gout. Potassium-sparing diuretics should be used cautiously in patients who are dehydrated, those with renal disease, and lactating women. Cautious use of osmotic diuretics is recommended in patients with severe renal disease or CHF, those who are dehydrated, and pregnant or lactating women.

Contraindications to the use of diuretics include allergies to the specific medication, or to sulfonamides in the case of furosemide treatment; anuria; dehydration; hypovolemia; hypotension; and electrolyte disturbances. Their use is also contraindicated in infants and in breast-feeding women. Thiazide diuretics are also contraindicated in patients suffering from altered

NEONATAL CONSIDERATIONS
Diuretics Therapy

■ Thiazide diuretics can cross the placenta and pass through to the fetus. They are also secreted in breast milk. Therefore they can produce exaggerated and even toxic or lethal effects in the fetus or neonate of women taking them.

■ CAI diuretics are only for adult use.

■ Potassium-sparing diuretics are contraindicated in pregnant women.

GERIATRIC CONSIDERATIONS
Diuretic Therapy

■ Always obtain baseline measurements of the patient's height, weight, intake and output amounts, and serum sodium, potassium, and chloride levels.

■ Diuretics should be taken early in the day to prevent nocturia, or voiding at night, which could lead to lack of sleep and possible injury because of the need to get out of bed during the night.

■ If the elderly patient is living alone and has no assistance or minimal assistance with his or her medication regimen, visits from a home health or public health professional may help ensure the safety of the therapy and compliance with therapy and diet.

PEDIATRIC CONSIDERATIONS
Thiazide Diuretics

■ Pediatric dosages of these medications should be calculated carefully. Admission and daily weights should be measured and recorded so that a possible overdose can be identified. Fluid volume and electrolyte loss, hypotension, shock, and possibly death are the consequences of overdose.

■ Weights, intake and output amounts, and vital signs, including the rate, depth, and rhythm of respirations, should be checked daily to make sure the child is responding appropriately and to help identify possible adverse reactions to or complications of the therapy.

■ The oral forms may be taken with food or milk and should be taken early in the day.

■ Sunscreen containing PABA should be avoided, and clothing worn to protect the child from the sun during even brief exposure. Lengthy exposure to either heat or sun should be avoided because of the heat stroke, exhaustion, and fluid volume loss this may precipitate.

renal function or hypomagnesemia. Potassium-sparing diuretics are contraindicated in patients suffering from hyperkalemia and in pregnant women. The osmotic diuretics are contraindicated in patients with severe pulmonary edema, severe edema, active intracranial bleeding, and severe dehydration.

NURSING DIAGNOSES

Nursing diagnoses associated with the use of diuretics include:

- Decreased cardiac output related to adverse effects of diuretics.
- Electrolyte imbalances related to adverse effects of diuretics.
- Risk for injury (falls) stemming from postural hypotension and dizziness.
- Knowledge deficit related to new use of diuretic therapy.
- Pain (headache, nausea, fatigue) related to adverse effects of diuretics.
- Noncompliance related to side effects of diuretics.

PLANNING

Goals related to the administration of diuretics include:

- Patient regains fluid and electrolyte balance.
- Patient remains free of the complications associated with diuretic use.
- Patient will remain free of injury to self while on diuretics.
- Patient will remain compliant with therapy.

Outcome Criteria

The outcome criteria in patients receiving diuretics are as follows:

- Patient will maintain normal electrolyte values (sodium, potassium, and chloride values) while on diuretics.
- Patient will continue to show or regain normal cardiac output while on diuretic therapy as evidenced by vital signs, adequate intake and output within normal limits (P <100, >60), (BP 120/80); (urine output ≥30 cc/hr).
- Patient's skin turgor will be pliable and without edema or dryness.
- Patient will rise slowly and change positions slowly and cautiously while receiving diuretics.
- Patient will state importance and rationale for follow-up visits with the physician such as monitoring for adverse effects, dehydration, fluid and electrolyte imbalances.
- Patient will report dizziness, fainting, palpitations, tingling, confusion, or disorientation to physician immediately.

IMPLEMENTATION

The diuretics, including patient education guidelines, were discussed in Chapter 23 on antihypertensive agents. Additional guidelines are given in the box on p. 397. As a reminder, however, diuretics should be taken in the morning as much as possible to avoid their interference with sleep patterns. Potassium supplements are generally not recommended when potassium levels exceed 3.0 mEq/L. For other nursing interventions please also refer to Chapter 23 and the boxes on p. 398 on neonatal and geriatric considerations. For the considerations in pediatric patients receiving thiazide diuretics, see the box on p. 398.

EVALUATION

The therapeutic effects of diuretics include the resolution of or a reduction in the edema, fluid volume overload, CHF, or hypertension or a return to normal intraocular pressures. The patient must also be monitored for the occurrence of adverse reactions such as metabolic alkalosis (monitor arterial blood gas values), drowsiness, lethargy, hypokalemia, tachycardia, hypotension, leg cramps, restlessness, and a decrease in mental alertness.

TAKE HOME POINTS

Types of Diuretics

■ Five main types of diuretics: carbonic anhydrase inhibitors and loop, osmotic, potassium-sparing, and thiazide and thiazide-like diuretics.

■ The loop, potassium-sparing, and thiazide and thiazide-like diuretics are the most commonly used.

■ All increase the rate of urine formation.

■ Their purpose is to cause a net loss of water from the body and to increase urine output.

Nephron

■ The main structural element in the kidney.

■ The site where diuretics work.

■ Composed of the glomerulus, afferent and efferent arterioles, proximal and distal tubules, and collecting ducts.

Loop Diuretics

■ Very potent diuretics that work in the loop of Henle, where the most of the sodium is resorbed.

■ Three main ones currently used: furosemide, bumetanide, and torsemide.

■ Ethacrynic acid seldomly used.

■ Potency differences: 1 mg of bumetanide = 10 mg of torsemide = 40 mg of furosemide = 50 mg of ethacrynic acid.

Thiazide and Thiazide-Like Diuretics

■ Frequently used and least expensive because several generic preparations are available.

■ Hydrochlorothiazide is considered the prototypical thiazide diuretic.

■ Used as adjunctive therapy to manage hepatic cirrhosis, edema, and CHF.

■ May cause adverse metabolic effects: hypokalemia, hypercalcemia, hyperlipidemia, hyperglycemia, hyperuricemia.

Nursing Considerations

■ Fluid volume status should be monitored in patients receiving diuretics because of the serious excess and deficit states they can cause.

■ Skin and mucous membrane status and sodium, potassium, and chloride levels are ways of monitoring for excess and deficit states.

■ Intake and output amounts should be monitored in patients receiving diuretics.

■ Elderly patients are very susceptible to the effects of diuretics.

■ Adverse reactions to diuretics include metabolic alkalosis, drowsiness, lethargy, hypokalemia, tachycardia, hypotension, leg cramps, restlessness, and decreased mental alertness.

NURSING ■ CARE ■ PLAN

Diuretic Therapy

Mr. L.P. is a 59-year-old attorney who is a partner in a local prestigious law firm. His typical work day begins at 7:30 AM and lasts till about 8 PM at night. He exercises 2 to 3 times a week, but not regularly. However, he is in good health and cholesterol and lipid profiles are within normal limits. He has been diagnosed with hypertension and needs to lose about 22 pounds per physician's or-ders. He is to begin taking chlorothiazide (Diuril) at a dosage of 500 mg twice daily and is to follow up in 1 week with the physician and dietician (for further consultation). He has been asked to have his blood pressure taken 3 times a week and to keep a daily journal of any symptoms as well as record blood-pressure readings.

Assessment with nursing diagnoses	Planning with goals and outcome criteria	Implementation with patient education	Evaluation

Subjective
 	
Complaint of severe headaches
 	
Objective
 	
Attorney × 24 yr
History of stress ulcers
Family history of hypertension
Blood pressure at physician's office was 180/98
 	
Nursing diagnoses
 	
Knowledge deficit related to new drug therapy with a diuretic
	Goals
	
	Patient will remain compliant to diuretic therapy within 1 mo
	
	Outcome criteria
	
	Patient will verbalize safe and accurate means of taking diuretic medication as evidenced by:
	  < side effects and
	  < therapeutic effects within 1 mo of therapy
		Chlorothiazide, a diuretic that will help eliminate water to help decrease your blood pressure. It also eliminates, through urine, sodium, chloride, potassium, and magnesium, which means we monitor electrolytes frequently, along with BPs
		
		Weigh yourself weekly and report a gain in weight of 2 lb or more in 1 wk
		
		Take plenty of fluids, up to 2-3 L/day
		
		Change positions slowly when you rise from sitting or standing to avoid fainting and dizziness
		
		Take your medication with food
		
		Take this medication early in the morning to prevent urination at nighttime
		
		Eat a diet high in potassium with foods such as strawberries, orange juice, apricots, and bananas to help counter the potassium lost in the urine
		
		Contact physician should you experience muscle cramps, dizziness, nausea, and muscle weakness
		
		Record and monitor your BPs at least 3x/wk for now
		
		Follow up with the physician in 1 wk
			Patient shows a therapeutic response to diuretic therapy as evidenced by:
			  Improved blood pressure
			  Less edema in feet and hands
			  Improved energy levels
			
			Patient is monitored for side effects such as:
			  Dizziness
			  Drowsiness
			  Postural hypotension
			  nausea, vomiting, anorexia
			  Muscle cramps
			  Fatigue
			  Headache
			  Hyperglycemia
			  Polyuria
			  Blurred vision

Critical Thinking **A C T I V I T I E S**

1. G.G. is a 64-year-old man who has been admitted to the coronary care unit because he is suffering from heart failure. He has been given 80 mg of furosemide every 6 hours, but with no relief of his pulmonary and peripheral edema. The physician would like to change him to bumetanide. What would be the equivalent daily dose of bumetanide?

2. What type of caution would you give a patient who is beginning treatment with a potassium-sparing diuretic?

Case Study

3. Primary hypertension has been diagnosed in S.G., a 47-year-old woman. Her blood pressures have been ranging between 158 and 172 mm Hg systolic and 94 and 110 mm Hg diastolic. Her average blood pressure over the past month has been 156/98 mm Hg. She has a strong family history of hypertension and is a single parent of two adolescents. She is also trying to keep up with her responsibilities as a full-time assistant professor of education at a local urban university. There is no evidence of renal insufficiency or cardiac damage at this time nor is there evidence of retinopathy or other signs and symptoms of end-organ disease. No other problems are reported, and S.G. is begun on 50 mg of hydrochlorothiazide daily.

a. Discuss the antihypertensive effects of hydrochlorothiazide.
b. What sort of guidelines must you give this patient so that she does not have adverse reactions to the diuretic therapy?
c. What nonpharmacologic measures should the nurse tell the patient about that can help control her blood pressure?

BIBLIOGRAPHY

Albanese J, Nutz P: *Mosby's 1995 nursing drug cards,* St Louis, 1995, Mosby.

Aranda P, Lopez de Novales E: Diuretics and the treatment of systemic hypertension, *Am J Cardiol* 65(17):72H–76H, 1990.

Baker LK, Alyn IB: Pharmacologic manipulation of preload, afterload, and contractility in the young, *J Cardiovasc Nurs* 6(3):12, 1992.

Ellison DH: Diuretic drugs and the treatment of edema: from clinic to bench and back again, *Am J Kidney Dis* 23:623, 1994.

Hockenberry B: Multiple drug therapy in the treatment of essential hypertension, *Nurs Clin North Am* 26(2):417, 1991.

Johnson KB: *Harriet Lane handbook,* ed 13, St Louis, 1993, Mosby.

Keen JH: *Critical care and emergency drug reference,* St Louis, 1994, Mosby.

Kellick KA: Diuretics, *AACN* 3:472, 1992.

Knoben JE, Anderson PO: *Handbook of critical drug data,* ed 6, Hamilton, Ill, 1988, Drug Intelligence Publications.

McEvoy GK: *AHFS drug information,* Bethesda, Md, 1994, American Society of Hospital Pharmacists.

Mende CW: Pharmacologic treatment of heart failure, *Nurs Clin North Am* 26:401, 1991.

Mujais SK: Nora NA, Levin ML: Principles and clinical uses of diuretic therapy, *Prog Cardiovasc Dis* 35:221, 1992.

Purcell JA, Holder CK: Cardiomyopathy: understanding the problem, *Am J Nurs* 89(1):58, 1989.

Skidmore-Roth L: *Mosby's 1995 nursing drug reference,* St Louis, 1995, Mosby.

Chapter 27

Fluids and Electrolytes

Objectives

When you reach the end of this chapter, you will be able to:

1. Identify the various fluid and electrolyte solutions commonly used in the management of fluid and electrolyte disorders.
2. Discuss the mechanism of action of the various fluid and electrolyte solutions, the indications for their use, the dosages, the contraindications and cautions to their use, and their side effects.
3. Develop a comprehensive nursing care plan appropriate for the patient receiving any of the fluid and electrolyte solutions.
4. Discuss the patient education guidelines related to fluid and electrolyte management.

CHAPTER OUTLINE

Physiology of Fluid Balance

Crystalloids
  Mechanism of action
  Drug effects
  Therapeutic uses
  Side effects and adverse effects
  Interactions
  Dosages

Drug Profile
  Sodium Chloride

Colloids
  Mechanism of action
  Drug effects
  Therapeutic uses
  Side effects and adverse effects
  Interactions
  Dosages

Drug Profiles
  Albumin
  Dextran
  Hetastarch

Blood Products
  Mechanism of action
  Drug effects
  Therapeutic uses
  Side effects and adverse effects
  Interactions
  Dosages

Drug Profiles
  Plasma Protein Fractions
  Fresh Frozen Plasma

  Packed Red Blood Cells
  Whole Blood

Physiology of Electrolyte Balance

Potassium
  Mechanism of action
  Drug effects
  Therapeutic uses
  Side effects and adverse effects
    Toxicity and management of overdose
  Interactions
  Dosages

Drug Profile
  Potassium Supplements

Sodium
  Mechanism of action
  Drug effects
  Therapeutic uses
  Side effects and adverse effects
    Toxicity and management of overdose
    Interactions
  Dosages

Drug Profile
  Sodium chloride

Nursing Process
Assessment
Nursing Diagnoses
Planning
  Outcome criteria
Implementation
Evaluation

Glossary

Colloid (kol′ oid) A state of matter in which large molecules or aggregates of molecules that do not precipitate and that measure between 1 and 100 nm are dispersed in another medium. (p. 405)

Colloid oncotic pressure (ong kot′ ik) The osmotic pressure exerted by a colloid in solution, such as that produced when the concentration of protein in the plasma on one side of a cell membrane is higher than that in the neighboring interstitial fluid. (p. 405)

Crystalloids (kris′ tə loid) A substance in a solution that diffuses through a semipermeable membrane. (p. 406)

Dehydration (de′ hi dra′ shən) Excessive loss of water from the body tissues. It is accompanied by an imbalance in the essential electrolyte concentrations, particularly sodium, potassium, and chloride. (p. 406)

Edema (ə de mə) The abnormal accumulation of fluid in interstitial spaces, such as in the pericardial sac, intrapleural space, peritoneal cavity, and joint capsules. (p. 405)

Extracellular fluid (eks′ trə sel′ u lər) That portion of the body fluid comprising the interstitial fluid and blood plasma. The adult body contains about 11.2 liters of interstitial fluid, constituting about 16% of the body weight, and about 2.8 liters of plasma, constituting about 4% of the body weight. (p. 405)

Extravascular fluid (eks′ trə vas′ ku lər) Fluids in the body that are outside the blood vessels. Examples include lymph and cerebrospinal fluid. (p. 405)

Hydrostatic pressure (hi′ dro stat′ ik) The pressure exerted by a liquid. (p. 405)

Hypokalemia (hi′ po kə le′ me ə) A condition in which there is an inadequate amount of potassium, the major intracellular cation, in the bloodstream. (p. 413)

Hyponatremia (hi′ po nə tre′ me ə) A condition in which there is an inadequate amount of sodium in the blood, caused either by inadequate excretion of water or by excessive water in the bloodstream. (p. 415)

Interstitial fluid (in′ tər stish′ əl) Extracellular fluid that fills in the spaces between most of the cells of the body and provides a substantial portion of the liquid environment of the body. (p. 405)

Intracellular fluid Fluid located within cell membranes throughout most of the body. It contains dissolved solutes that are essential to maintaining electrolytic balance and healthy metabolism. (p. 405)

Intravascular fluid The fluid inside blood vessels. (p. 405)

Isotonic (i′ so ton′ ik) Having the same concentration of a solute as another solution, hence exerting the same osmotic pressure as that solution, such as an isotonic saline solution that contains an amount of salt equal to that found in the intracellular and extracellular fluid. (p. 405)

Osmotic pressure The pressure exerted on a semipermeable membrane separating a solution from a solvent; the membrane being impermeable to the solutes in the solution and permeable only to the solvent. (p. 405)

Plasma (plaz′ mə) The watery, straw-colored fluid component of lymph and blood in which the leukocytes, erythrocytes, and platelets are suspended. (p. 405)

Fluid and electrolyte management is one of the cornerstones of patient care. Most disease processes, tissue injuries, and surgical procedures greatly influence the physiologic status of fluids and electrolytes in the body. A prerequisite to the understanding of fluid and electrolyte management is knowledge of the extent and composition of the various body fluid compartments.

Physiology of Fluid Balance

Sixty percent of the adult human body is water. This is referred to as the *total body water* (TBW), and it is distributed to the three main compartments in the following proportions: intracellular fluid (ICF), 67%; interstitial fluid (ISF), 25%; and plasma volume (PV), 8%. This distribution is illustrated in Fig. 27-1, and the actual volume of fluid that would normally be in each compartment in an average 70-kg man with a TBW content of 60% of his total body weight is diagrammed in Fig. 27-2.

The terms used to identify the various spaces within which the TBW is distributed can be quite confusing, and in addition, there are two basic approaches

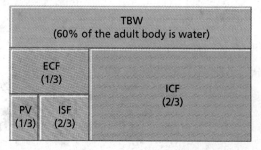

▼ **FIG. 27-1** Distribution of total body water (TBW). *ECF*, extracellular fluid; *ICF*, intracellular fluid; *ISF*, interstitial fluid; *PV*, plasma volume.

to distinguishing among the locations of the fluid. The TBW can be described as being in or out of the blood vessels, or vasculature. If this terminology is used, then the term **intravascular fluid** (IVF) describes fluid inside the blood vessels, and the term **extravascular fluid** (EVF) describes the fluid outside the blood vessels. The term **plasma** is used to describe the fluid that flows through the blood vessels that is intravascular. **Interstitial fluid** is the fluid that is in the space between cells, tissues, and organs. Both plasma and interstitial fluid make up extracellular volume. Both interstitial fluid and intracellular fluid make up extravascular volume. These terms are often confused and misused. Table 27-1 lists these definitions for further clarity and understanding.

▼ **FIG. 27-2** Actual volume of fluid in each compartment in a 70-kg man with a total body water content of 60% of his total body weight.

What then keeps fluid inside the blood vessels? All the fluid outside the cells, the ECF, which consists of both the plasma and the ISF, has about the same concentration of electrolytes. However, there is one big difference between the plasma and the ISF; the plasma has a protein concentration, primarily consisting of albumin but also including globulin and fibrinogen, four times greater than that of the ISF, and it is this difference that explains how fluid is kept inside the blood vessels. The reason for this higher concentration of protein is that these solutes (proteins) have a molecular weight that exceeds 69,000 daltons, and this makes them too large to pass through the walls of the blood vessels. Because of the difference in this concentration of plasma proteins (also known as **colloids**), fluid flows from the area of low protein concentration in the interstitial compartment to the area of high concentration inside the blood vessel in order to try and create an isotonic environment. (**Isotonic** means an equal concentration of solutes.) The protein in the blood vessels therefore exerts a constant **osmotic pressure** that prevents the leakage of too much plasma through the capillaries into the tissues. This pressure is called the **colloid oncotic pressure** (COP), and normally it is 24 mm Hg. The opposing pressure, that exerted by the ISF, is called the **hydrostatic pressure** (HP), and normally it is 17 mm Hg, which, of course, is less than the COP. The phenomenon of COP is illustrated in Fig. 27-3.

The regulation of the volume and composition of body water is essential for life because it is the medium in which all metabolic reactions occur. The body maintains the volume and composition remarkably constant by maintaining a balance between intake and excretion: The amount of water gained each day is kept equal to the amount of water lost. When for some reason the body cannot maintain this equilibrium, therapy with various agents becomes necessary. If the amount of water gained exceeds the amount of water lost, a water excess or overhydration occurs. This is referred to as **edema**. If the quantity of water lost ex-

Table 27-1	Fluid Location: Descriptive Terms	
LOCATION OF FLUID	**NAME**	**DEFINITION/LOCATION**
Cells (in or out)	Intracellular fluid Extracellular fluid	Inside cells Outside cells
Blood vessels (in or out)	Intravascular fluid (plasma) Extravascular fluid	Inside blood vessels Outside blood vessels
Tissues (in between)	Interstitial fluid	In the spaces between cells, tissues, and organs

ceeds that gained, a water deficit, or **dehydration**, occurs. It has been estimated that death usually occurs when 20% to 25% of the body water is lost.

Dehydration leads to a disturbance in the balance between the amount of fluid in the extracellular compartment and that in the intracellular compartment. In the initial stages of dehydration, water is lost first from the extracellular compartments. The nature of further fluid losses or COP changes, or both, depends on the type of clinical dehydration, and these various types are listed in the box below. Clinical conditions that can result in dehydration and fluid loss as well as the symptoms of dehydration and fluid loss are listed in the box below right.

When fluid that has been lost must be replaced, there are three categories of agents that can be used to accomplish this: crystalloids, colloids, and blood products. The clinical situation dictates which category of agents is most appropriate.

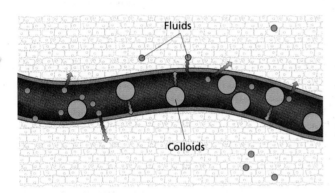

▼ **FIG. 27-3** Colloid oncotic pressure. As can be seen, the colloids inside the blood vessel are too large to pass through the vessel wall. The resulting oncotic pressure exerted by the colloids draws fluid from the surrounding tissues and other extravascular spaces into the blood vessels and also keeps fluid inside the blood vessel.

CRYSTALLOIDS

Crystalloids are fluids that supply water and sodium to maintain the osmotic gradient between the extravascular and intravascular compartments. Their PV-expanding capacity is related to the sodium concentration. They are generally used as maintenance fluids to compensate for insensible fluid losses, as replacement fluids to correct body fluid deficits, and for special purposes (i.e., the treatment of specific fluid and electrolyte disturbances). The different crystalloids are listed in Table 27-2.

Mechanism of Action

As just mentioned, the crystalloids supply sodium and water to maintain the osmotic gradient between the fluid outside the blood vessels (the EVF) and the fluid inside the blood vessels (the IVF). This capacity to expand the PV is related to the sodium content. Therefore hypertonic saline (3% sodium chloride) is more efficient than normal saline (0.9% sodium chloride) for expanding the PV.

Dehydration and Fluid Loss: Conditions and Symptoms

CONDITIONS	SYMPTOMS
Fever	Dry skin and mucous membranes
Bowel obstruction	Decreased perspiration and mucous secretions
Diarrhea	Decreased urine output
Vomiting	Decreased tears and saliva
Bleeding	Increased bleeding and pulse rate

Types of Dehydration

TYPE OF DEHYDRATION	CHARACTERISTICS
Isotonic	Caused by a loss of sodium and water from the body, resulting in a decrease in the volume of extracellular fluid. *Examples*: diarrhea and vomiting.
Hypotonic	Caused when sodium loss is greater than water loss, resulting in higher concentrations of solute inside the cells, thus pulling fluid from outside the cells (plasma and interstitial spaces) into the cells. *Examples*: renal insufficiency and inadequate aldosterone secretion.
Hypertonic	Caused when water loss is greater than sodium loss, resulting in a concentration of solutes outside the cells and causing the fluid inside the cells to move to the extracellular space, thus dehydrating the cells. *Example*: elevated temperature resulting in perspiration.

Drug Effects

Crystalloid solutions contain fluids and electrolytes that are normally found in the body. They do not contain proteins (colloids), which are necessary to maintain the COP and prevent water from leaving the plasma compartment. In fact, the administration of large quantities of crystalloid solutions for fluid resuscitation decreases the COP. Compared with the distribution of colloids, crystalloids are also distributed faster into the interstitial and intracellular compartments, which makes them better for treating dehydration than for expanding the PV, such as in the setting of hypovolemic shock. That is to say, crystalloids cannot expand the PV as well as colloids, and besides this, much larger quantities are initially required to accomplish this.

Therapeutic Uses

The crystalloid solutions are most commonly used as maintenance fluids. They are used to compensate for insensible fluid losses, to replace fluids when there are body fluid deficits, and to manage specific fluid and electrolyte disturbances. Crystalloids also promote urinary flow. They are much less expensive than colloids and blood products. In addition, there is no risk of viral transmission or anaphylaxis and no alteration in the coagulation profile associated with their use. The choice whether to use a crystalloid or colloid in these situations depends on the severity of the condition. Following are the common indications for either crystalloid or colloid replacement therapy.

- Shock
- Adult respiratory distress syndrome
- Acute nephrosis
- Burns
- Cardiopulmonary bypass
- Renal dialysis
- Hypoproteinemia
- Acute liver failure
- To reduce the risk of deep vein thrombosis

Side Effects and Adverse Effects

The crystalloids are a very safe and effective means of replacing needed fluid. They do, however, have some unwanted effects. Because they contain no large particles such as proteins, they do not stay within the blood vessels but can leak out of the plasma into the tissues and cells. This may result in edema anywhere in the body. Peripheral edema and pulmonary edema are two common examples. Crystalloids also dilute the proteins that are in the plasma, further reducing the COP. Because the crystalloids cannot carry oxygen as the blood products do, their use may result in decreased oxygen tension. Typically, large volumes are required for them to be effective (liters of fluid). As a result, large or prolonged infusions may worsen tissue acidosis or adversely affect CNS function in patients suffering from hepatic insufficiency, renal failure, or hypovolemic shock. Another disadvantage of the crystalloids is that their effects are short-lived (transient).

Interactions

Interactions with the crystalloid solutions are rare because they are very similar if not identical to normal physiologic substances. Certain electrolytes contained in lactated Ringer's solution may interact with other electrolytes, forming a complex that results in the formation of a precipitate. However, this would be an incompatibility rather than a true interaction.

Dosages

For the recommended dosages of crystalloids, see Table 27-3.

Table 27-2	Crystalloids							
	COMPOSITION (MEQ/L)							
PRODUCT	**NA**	**CL**	**K**	**CA**	**MG**	**LACTATE**	**VOLUME (ML)**	**COST***
Normal saline	154	154	0	0	0	0	1000	2×
Hypertonic saline	513	513	0	0	0	0	500	1
Lactated ringer's	130	109	4	3	0	28	1000	2.5×
5% Dextrose (D5W)	0	0	0	0	0	0	1000	2×
Plasmalyte	140	103	10	5	3	8	1000	5×

Na, sodium; *Cl*, chloride; *K*, potassium; *Ca*, calcium; *Mg*, magnesium.
*Relative cost; example: normal saline is two times the cost of hypertonic saline.

Table 27-3	Crystalloids and Colloids: Dosing Guidelines

	CRYSTALLOIDS AND COLLOIDS			
	0.9% NS	3% NS	5% COLLOID*	25% COLLOID†
To raise plasma volume by 1 liter administer:				
	5-6 liters	1.5-2 liters	1 liter	0.5 liter
Fluid compartment distributed to:				
Plasma	25%	25%	100%	200%-300%
Interstitial space	75%	75%	0	Decreased fluid levels
Intracellular space	0	0	0	Decreased fluid levels

NS, normal saline.
*Isooncotic solutions such as 5% albumin, dextran 70, and hetastarch.
†Hyperoncotic solutions such as 25% albumin.

DRUG PROFILE

The most commonly used crystalloid solutions are normal saline (0.9% sodium chloride) and lactated Ringer's solution. The available crystalloid solutions and their compositions are summarized in Table 27-2.

SODIUM CHLORIDE

Sodium chloride (salt, NaCl) comes in many different concentrations, the most common being 0.9%. This is the normal concentration of sodium chloride, and for this reason, it is referred to as *normal saline*. Other commonly used concentrations are 0.45% or half-normal saline, and 3%, or hypertonic saline. These solutions have different indications, and they are used in different situations depending on how urgently fluid volume restoration is needed and/or the extent of the sodium loss.

Sodium chloride is a physiologic fluid that is present throughout our body. For this reason there are no hypersensitivity reactions to it. It is safe to administer it during any stage of pregnancy, but it is contraindicated in patients with conditions in which the administration of sodium and chloride would be detrimental. Hypertonic saline injections (3% and 5%) are contraindicated in the presence of increased, normal, or only slightly decreased serum electrolyte concentrations. Sodium chloride comes as a 650-mg tablet and as 0.45%, 0.9%, 3%, and 5% solutions.

♆ PHARMACODYNAMICS

PLASMA VOLUME EXPANSION	COLLOID ONCOTIC PRESSURE	DURATION OF EXPANSION
60-70 ml*	−30 mm Hg	Few hours

*500 ml of normal saline will expand the plasma volume by 60 to 70 ml.

The dose of sodium chloride administered depends on the clinical situation. As a general rule, 20% or less of blood is lost more slowly then sodium chloride is required. The amounts of crystalloid or colloid needed to expand the PV by 1 liter, or 1000 milliliters, are given in Table 27-3, and this can be used as a general guide to dosing.

COLLOIDS

Colloids are substances that increase the COP and effectively move fluid from the interstitial compartment to the plasma compartment by pulling the fluid into the blood vessels. Normally this task is performed by the three blood proteins, albumin, globulin, and fibrinogen. However, for them to be effective, the total protein level must be in the range of 7.4 gm/dl. If this level drops below 5.3 gm/dl, the COP then becomes less than the HP (hydrostatic pressure) and fluid shifts into the tissues. When this happens, colloid replacement therapy is required to reverse this process by increasing the COP. The COP decreases with age and also in the settings of hypotension and malnutrition. The commonly used colloids are listed in Table 27-4.

Mechanism of Action

The mechanism of action of colloids is related to their ability to increase the COP. As already explained, because the colloids cannot pass into the extravascular

	COMPOSITION (MEQ/L)			
PRODUCT	**NA**	**CL**	**VOLUME (ML)**	**COST***
⚓Dextran 70†	154	154	500	1
⚓Dextran 40†	154	154	500	2×
Hetastarch	154	154	500	5×
5% Albumin	145	145	500	10
25% Albumin	145	145	100	10

Table 27-4 Commonly Used Colloids

*Using the cost of dextran 70 as the means of comparison.
†Dextran is available in NaCl, which has 154 mEq/L of both Na and Cl. It is also available in D5W, which contains no Na or Cl.

space, there is ordinarily a higher concentration of solutes (solid particles) inside the blood vessels (intravascular space) than outside the blood vessels. Fluid thus moves toward this hypertonic area in an attempt to make it isotonic. The end result is that fluid is pulled from the extravascular space to the intravascular space, thereby increasing the blood volume. Because colloids increase the blood volume, they are sometimes called *plasma expanders*. They also make up part of the total PV.

Drug Effects

Colloids increase the COP and move fluid from outside the blood vessels to inside the blood vessels. They can maintain the COP for several hours. They are naturally occurring products and consist of proteins (albumin), carbohydrates (dextrans or starches), and animal collagen (gelatin). Usually they contain a combination of both small and large particles. The small particles are eliminated quickly and promote diuresis and perfusion of the kidneys; the larger particles maintain the PV. Albumin is the one exception in that it contains particles that are all the same size.

Therapeutic Uses

The colloids are used to treat a wide variety of conditions (see list on page 407). Clinically the colloids are superior to the crystalloids in their ability to expand the PV. However, crystalloids are less expensive and are less likely to promote bleeding. On the other hand, they are more likely to cause edema because of the larger volumes needed to achieve the desired clinical effect.

Side Effects and Adverse Effects

The colloids are relatively safe agents, though there are some disadvantages to their use. They can alter the coagulation system, resulting in impaired coagulation and possibly bleeding. They have no oxygen-carrying ability and contain no clotting factors. They may also dilute the plasma protein concentration, and this may impair the function of platelets. Rarely dextran therapy precipitates anaphylaxis or renal failure. All these undesirable effects should be closely monitored for.

Interactions

Because colloid solutions are so compatible with drugs, they are sometimes used as the medium for delivering them. The drug propofol (Diprivan) is such an example. It is delivered in a 10% lipid emulsion. There are no drugs that interact with colloid solutions.

Dosages

For the recommended dosages of colloids, see Table 27-3.

*D*RUG PROFILES

The specific colloid used for replacement therapy at a particular institution varies from institution to institution. The three most commonly used ones are dextran 40, hetastarch, and 5% albumin. They are all very quick in onset and have a long duration of action. They are metabolized in the liver and excreted by the kidneys, with albumin the one exception. It is metabolized by the reticuloendothelial system and excreted by the kidneys and the intestines.

ALBUMIN

Albumin (Albuminar, Albutein, Buminate, Plasbumin) is a natural protein that is normally produced by the liver. It is responsible for generating about 70% of the COP. Albumin human is a sterile solution of serum albumin prepared from pooled blood, plasma serum, or placentas obtained from healthy human donors. It is pasteurized (heated at 60° C for 10 hours) to destroy any contaminants.

Albumin is classified as a pregnancy category C agent and is contraindicated in patients with a known hypersensitivity to it and in those with congestive heart failure, severe anemia, or renal insufficiency. Albumin is only available in a parenteral form and comes in concentrations of 5% and 25%. See Table 27-3 for the dosing guidelines. Pregnancy category C.

⚗ P H A R M A C O K I N E T I C S

HALF-LIFE	ONSET	PEAK	DURATION
21 days	<1 min	Unknown	<24 hr

⚓ DEXTRAN

Dextran (Gentran, LMD, Rheomacrodex) is a solution of glucose. It is available in two concentrations, dextran 40 and the more concentrated dextran 70, and it has a molecular weight similar to that of albumin. Dextran 40 is the more commonly utilized of the two and is a low-molecular-weight polymer of glucose. It is a derivative of sugar that has actions similar to those of human albumin in that it expands the PV by drawing fluid from the interstitial space to the intravascular space.

Dextran is classified as a pregnancy category C agent and is contraindicated in the settings of hypersensitivity, congestive heart failure, renal insufficiency, and extreme dehydration. It is only available in a parenteral form and comes in either a 5% dextrose solution or a 0.9% sodium chloride solution. See Table 27-3 for the dosing guidelines.

⚗ P H A R M A C O K I N E T I C S

HALF-LIFE	ONSET	PEAK	DURATION
2-6 hr (D-40)	<5 min	Unknown	4-6 hr
12 hr (D-70)	1 hr	Unknown	12 hr

HETASTARCH

Hetastarch (Hespan) is a synthetic colloid derived from cornstarch. Its molecular weight is similar to that of albumin, and the colloidal properties of the 6% hetastarch solution resemble those of human albumin and dextran. It is similar to dextran in that it is a synthetic colloid and has no protein-binding properties.

Hetastarch is classified as a pregnancy category C agent and is contraindicated in patients who have shown a hypersensitivity to it and in those with severe bleeding disorders, congestive heart failure, or renal insufficiency. Hetastarch is only available in a parenteral form and comes as a 6% concentration in a 0.9% sodium chloride solution. See Table 27-3.

⚗ P H A R M A C O K I N E T I C S

HALF-LIFE	ONSET	PEAK	DURATION
17-48 days	<1 min	Unknown	24-36 hr

BLOOD PRODUCTS

Blood products are also known as *oxygen-carrying resuscitation fluids*. They are the only class of fluids that are able to carry oxygen because they are the only fluid that contains hemoglobin. They not only can increase the PV but also can improve tissue oxygenation. They are also the most expensive and least available of the three types of fluids (crystalloids, colloids, and blood products) because they are natural products and require human donors. The available blood products are listed in Table 27-5. Their use is called for when a patient has lost more than 25% of his or her blood volume.

Mechanism of Action

The mechanism of action of blood products is related to their ability to increase the COP, and hence the PV. They do so in the same manner as the colloids and crystalloids, by pulling fluid from the extravascular space to the intravascular space. Because of this they are also considered plasma expanders. Some also have the ability to carry oxygen. These are the oxygen-carrying resuscitation fluids, and they consist of packed red blood cells (PRBCs) and whole blood.

Table 27-5	Blood Products	
PRODUCT	**DOSAGE**	**COST***
Cryoprecipitate		1
Fresh frozen plasma (FFP)		1.7×
Packed RBCs	1 unit	2.2×
Plasma protein fractions (PPF)		1
Whole blood		3.3×

*Using the cost of cryoprecipitate as the means of comparison.

Drug Effects

Blood products increase COP and move fluid from outside the blood vessels to inside the blood vessels. They can maintain the COP for several hours to days, and because they come from human donors, they have all the effects that our own blood products have. They are administered when our own body is deficient in these products.

Therapeutic Uses

The blood products are used to treat a wide variety of clinical conditions, and the blood product used depends on the specific indication. The available blood products and the specific conditions they are used to treat are listed in the box below.

Side Effects and Adverse Effects

The undesirable effects of the blood products are many, with some being potentially serious. Because these products come from other human beings, they can be incompatible with the recipient's immune system. These incompatibilities are tested for before the administration of the particular blood product by determining the respective blood types of the donor and recipient and by doing cross-matching tests. This helps reduce the likelihood of the recipient rejecting the blood products, which would in turn precipitate transfusion reactions and anaphylaxis. These products can also transmit pathogens from the donor to the recipient. Examples of such pathogens are hepatitis and AIDS. Various preparation techniques are now utilized to reduce this risk of pathogen transmission, with the result that there has been a drastic reduction in the incidence of such problems.

Interactions

As with crystalloids and colloids, blood products are very similar if not identical to normal physiologic substances, so they interact with very few substances. Calcium and drugs such as aspirin, which normally affect coagulation, may interact with these substances when infused in the body in much the same way they interact with the body's own blood products.

Dosages

For the dosage guidelines pertaining to blood products, see Table 27-6.

DRUG PROFILES

Whole blood and PRBCs are currently the most commonly used oxygen-carrying resuscitation fluids. They should be used in patients who have lost more than 25% of their total blood volume. All the blood products are derived from pooled human blood donors. For this reason they can do all of the following: carry oxygen, increase the PV, and improve tissue oxygenation.

PLASMA PROTEIN FRACTIONS

PPF is obtained using a process very similar to the one used to obtain albumin. It involves the fractionation of human plasma with ethanol and its pasteurization at 60° C for 10 hours. More than 83% of PPF is albumin and more than 1% is gamma-globulin. It and albumin are similar in that both have similar colloidal properties. The primary advantages to the use of PPF are that it is simpler to manufacture and greater amounts of protein per unit of plasma are yielded. The disadvantage to its use is that it is more antigenic than albumin. The suggested guidelines are given in Table 27-6.

Blood Products: Indications

BLOOD PRODUCT	INDICATION
Cryoprecipitate and PPF	To manage acute bleeding (>50% blood loss slowly or 20% acutely)
FFP	To increase clotting factor levels in patients with a demonstrated deficiency
PRBCs	To increase oxygen-carrying capacity in patients with anemia, in patients with substantial hemoglobin deficits, and in patients who have lost >25% of their total blood volume
Whole blood	Same as for PRBCs

Table 27-6	Suggested Guidelines for Blood Products: Management of Bleeding
AMOUNT OF BLOOD LOSS	**FLUID OF CHOICE**
20% or less (slow loss)	Crystalloids
20%-50% (slow loss)	Nonprotein plasma expanders (dextran and hetastarch)
>50% (slow loss) or 20% (acutely)	Whole blood or PPF and FFP
80% or more lost	As above, but for every 5 units of blood given, administer 1-2 units of FFP and 1-2 units of platelets to prevent the hemodilution of clotting factors and bleeding

FRESH FROZEN PLASMA

FFP is obtained by centrifuging whole blood and thereby removing the cellular elements. The resulting plasma is then frozen at −18° C. FFP is not recommended for routine fluid resuscitation but may be used as an adjunct to massive blood transfusion in the treatment of patients with underlying coagulation disorders. The plasma-expanding capability of FFP is similar to that of dextran but slightly less than that of hetastarch. The disadvantage to FFP use is that it can transmit pathogens. The suggested guidelines are given in Table 27-6.

PACKED RED BLOOD CELLS

PRBCs are obtained by the centrifugation of whole blood, and their separation from plasma and the other cellular elements. The advantage to PRBC use is that their oxygen-carrying capacity is better than that of the other blood products and they are less likely to cause cardiac fluid overload. They are small, compact oxygen carriers. The disadvantages are that they have a poor shelf life, their availability fluctuates, they can transmit viruses, they can cause allergic reactions, they can precipitate bleeding abnormalities, and they are expensive. The suggested guidelines are given in Table 27-6.

WHOLE BLOOD

Whole blood is a complete and physiologic volume expander. One unit provides hemoglobin, protein, and water that not only restores lost oxygen-carrying ca-

pacity but also expands the PV. The advantages and disadvantages of whole blood transfusion are the same as those associated with PRBC use. The suggested guidelines are given in Table 27-6.

Physiology of Electrolyte Balance

The chemical composition of the fluid compartments varies from compartment to compartment. The principal electrolytes in the ECF are sodium cations (Na^+) and chloride anions (Cl^-), and the major electrolyte of the ICF is the potassium cation (K^+). Other important electrolytes are calcium, magnesium, and phosphorus. These different chemical compositions are vital to the normal function of all systems in the body, and they are controlled by the renin-angiotensin-aldosterone system, antidiuretic hormone system, and sympathetic nervous system. When these compositions are imbalanced, adverse consequences occur.

POTASSIUM

Potassium is the most abundant cationic (positively charged) electrolyte inside cells (the intracellular space), where the normal concentration is approximately 150 mEq/L. Approximately 95% of the potassium in the body is intracellular. In contrast, the potassium content outside the cells in the plasma ranges from 3.5 to 5.0 mEq/L. These plasma levels are critical to normal body function and are maintained by the adrenal gland hormone aldosterone.

We obtain potassium from a variety of foods, the most common sources being fruit and juices, fish, vegetables, poultry, meats, and dairy products. It has been estimated that for normal body functions to be maintained, a person must consume 5 to 10 mEq of potassium in their diet per day. Fortunately the average daily diet usually provides 35 to 100 mEq of potassium, which is well above the required daily amount. Excess dietary potassium is usually excreted by the kidneys in the urine. However, if the kidneys lose their ability to filter and secrete waste products, potassium can accumulate, leading to toxic levels, and these in turn can precipitate ventricular fibriliation and cardiac arrest. *Hyperkalemia* is the term for an excessive serum potassium level, and it is defined as a serum potassium level exceeding 5 mEq/L. There are several causes of hyperkalemia. One, renal failure, was just mentioned. Others are:

- Renal failure
- Burns

- Trauma
- Infections
- Metabolic acidosis
- Excessive loss from cells
- Potassium supplements
- Potassium-sparing diuretics

The opposite of hyperkalemia is **hypokalemia,** or a deficiency of potassium. This condition is more a result of excessive potassium loss than of poor dietary intake, however. As with hyperkalemia, there are a multitude of clinical conditions that can cause it. These include:

- Malabsorption
- Diarrhea
- Burns*
- Thiazide-like diuretics
- Corticosteroids
- Alkalosis
- Vomiting
- Crash diets
- Loop diuretics
- Ketoacidosis
- An increased secretion of mineralocorticoids (hormones of the adrenal cortex)
- Large amounts of licorice
- Thiazide diuretics
- Prolonged laxative misuse

Too little serum potassium can also greatly increase the toxicity associated with digitalis preparations, and this can precipitate serious ventricular dysrhythmias.

The early detection of hypokalemia is important to the prevention of the serious, life-threatening consequences of this metabolic disturbance if it goes undetected. The key to early detection is knowing its early symptoms, which are generally mild and can easily go undetected. Both the early (mild) symptoms and late (severe) symptoms of hypokalemia are listed in the box above right. The treatment of hypokalemia involves both identifying and treating the cause and restoring the serum potassium levels to normal (>3.5 mEq/L). The consumption of potassium-rich foods can usually correct mild hypokalemia, but clinically significant hypokalemia requires the oral or parenteral administration of a potassium supplement, which usually contains potassium chloride.

Mechanism of Action

Potassium's importance as the primarily intracellular electrolyte is highlighted by the enormous number of life-sustaining reactions and everyday physiologic functions that require it, functions that we take

---

*Burn patients can exhibit either hyperkalemia or hypokalemia.

Symptoms of Hypokalemia
Early
Anorexia
Lethargy
Mental confusion
Nausea
Muscle weakness
Hypotension
Late
Neuropathy
Paralytic ileus
Secondary alkalosis
Cardiac dysrhythmias

for granted and that would not be possible without it. Muscle contraction, the transmission of nerve impulses, and the regulation of heartbeats (the pacemaker function of the heart) are just a few of these functions.

Potassium is also essential for the maintenance of acid-base balance, isotonicity, and the electrodynamic characteristics of the cell. It plays a role in many enzymatic reactions, and it is an essential component of gastric secretion, renal function, tissue synthesis, and carbohydrate metabolism.

Drug Effects

The drug effects of potassium are numerous, as evidenced by the enormous number of physiologic functions and reactions throughout the body it is involved in. As mentioned earlier, it is the major cation inside cells.

Therapeutic Uses

Potassium replacement therapy is called for in the treatment or prevention of potassium depletion in patients whenever dietary measures prove inadequate. The potassium salt used for this purpose is potassium chloride. The chloride is required to correct the hypochloremia (low chloride) that frequently accompanies potassium deficiency.

Other therapeutic effects of potassium are related to its role in the contraction of muscles and the maintenance of the electrical characteristics of cells. Potassium salts may be used to stop irregular heartbeats (dysrhythmias) and to manage the tachyarrhythmias that can occur after cardiac surgery. Potassium may also be used to treat thallium poisoning and to help increase muscular strength in some patients with myasthenia gravis.

Side Effects and Adverse Effects

The adverse effects of potassium therapy are primarily limited to the GI tract and occur with the oral administration of potassium preparations. These GI effects include diarrhea, nausea, and vomiting. More significant ones include GI bleeding and ulceration. The parenteral administration of potassium usually produces pain at the injection site. Rare cases of phlebitis have been associated with IV administration, and the excessive administration of potassium salts can lead to hyperkalemia and toxic effects.

Toxicity and Management of Overdose

The toxic effects of potassium are the result of hyperkalemia. Symptoms include muscle weakness, paresthesia, paralysis, cardiac rhythm irregularities that can result in ventricular fibrillation, and cardiac arrest. The treatment instituted depends on the degree of the hyperkalemia and ranges from regimens for reversing life-threatening problems to simple dietary restrictions. In the event of severe hyperkalemia, the IV administration of sodium bicarbonate, calcium gluconate or other calcium salt, and dextrose solution is required. Less critical levels can be reduced with ion-exchange resins and by means of dietary restrictions.

Interactions

The use of potassium-sparing diuretics can produce a hyperkalemic state. The use of diuretics, amphotericin B, and mineralosteroids can produce a hypokalemic state.

Dosages

Fluid and electrolyte therapy involves replacing any deficit losses and/or providing maintenance levels for specific patient requirements. Accordingly, specific dosage amounts of fluids or electrolytes depend on several clinical factors that include the following:

- Specific patient losses
- Efficacy of patient physiologic systems involved in fluid and electrolyte metabolism, especially adrenal, cardiovascular, and kidney functions
- Current drug therapy for pathologic conditions that complicate the amount and duration of replacement
- Selection of oral or parenteral replacement formulations

Suggested dosage guidelines with subsequent adjustments for potassium are 10 to 20 mEq administered orally several times a day or parenteral administration of 30 to 60 mEq every 24 hours.

DRUG **P**ROFILE

POTASSIUM SUPPLEMENTS

Potassium supplements are administered to either prevent or treat potassium depletion. The acetate, bicarbonate, chloride, citrate, and gluconate salts of potassium are available for oral administration. The parenteral salt forms of potassium for intravenous administration are acetate, chloride, and phosphate.

The dosage of potassium supplements is usually expressed in milliequivalents of potassium and depends on the requirements of the individual patient. The different salt forms of potassium deliver varying milliequivalent amounts of potassium. These various salt forms and how many grams of each are needed to yield 40 mEq are given in the box below.

Potassium is classified as a pregnancy category A agent and is contraindicated in patients with severe renal disease, severe hemolytic disease, or Addison's disease, and in those suffering from hyperkalemia, acute dehydration, or extensive tissue breakdown stemming from multiple trauma. Potassium is available in many different oral and intravenous formulations. It comes as a tablet and powder for solution, an extended-release capsule and tablet, and an elixir and oral solution. It is also comes as an injection for intravenous use.

⬡ P H A R M A C O K I N E T I C S

HALF-LIFE	ONSET	PEAK	DURATION
IV: Variable	IV: Immediate	IV: Rapid	IV: Variable
PO: Variable	PO: <30 min	PO: 30 min	PO: Variable

Potassium: Various Salt Forms

SALT FORM	AMOUNT (IN GRAMS) NEEDED TO YIELD 40 mEq OF POTASSIUM
Acetate	3.9
Bicarbonate	4.0
Chloride	3.0
Citrate	4.3
Gluconate	9.4
Monobasic phosphate	5.4
Dibasic phosphate	3.5

SODIUM

Sodium is the counterpart to potassium in that potassium is the principal cation (positively charged substance) inside cells and sodium is the principal cation outside cells. The normal concentration of sodium outside cells is 135 to 145 mEq/L, and it is maintained through the dietary intake of sodium in the form of sodium chloride, which is obtained from salt, fish, meats, and other foods flavored, seasoned, or preserved with salt.

Hyponatremia is the condition of sodium loss or deficiency and occurs when the serum levels decrease below 135 mEq/L. It is manifested by lethargy, hypotension, stomach cramps, vomiting, diarrhea, and seizures. Some of the same conditions that cause hypokalemia can also cause hyponatremia, and these are listed on p. 413. Other causes of hyponatremia are excessive perspiration, occurring during hot weather or physical work; prolonged diarrhea or vomiting, especially in young children; renal disorders; and adrenocortical impairment.

Hypernatremia is the condition of sodium excess and occurs when the serum levels of sodium exceed 145 mEq/L. Some of the causes are water retention (edema) and hypertension. The most common cause, however, is poor renal excretion stemming from kidney malfunction. Inadequate water consumption and dehydration are other causes. Symptoms of hypernatremia include red, flushed skin; dry, sticky mucous membranes; increased thirst; temperature elevation; and decreased or absent urination.

Mechanism of Action

As one of the body's electrolytes, sodium performs many physiologic roles necessary for the normal functioning of the body. It is the major cation in ECF and is principally involved in the control of water distribution, fluid and electrolyte balance, and osmotic pressure of body fluids. Sodium also participates along with both chloride and bicarbonate in the regulation of acid-base balance. Chloride, the major extracellular anion (negatively charged substance), closely complements the physiologic action of sodium. Sodium is also capable of causing diuresis.

Drug Effects

The drug effects of sodium are numerous. Because it is the major cation, it is involved in an enormous number of physiologic functions and reactions throughout the body.

Therapeutic Uses

Sodium is primarily administered in the treatment or prevention of sodium depletion when dietary measures have proved inadequate. Sodium chloride is the primary salt used for this purpose. Mild hyponatremia is usually treated with the oral administration of sodium chloride tablets. Pronounced sodium depletion is treated with normal saline or lactated Ringer's solution administered intravenously. These agents have been discussed earlier in this chapter.

Side Effects and Adverse Effects

The oral administration of sodium chloride can cause gastric upset consisting of nausea, vomiting, and cramps. Venous phlebitis can be a consequence of its parenteral administration.

Toxicity and Management of Overdose

Hypernatremia leads to hypertension, edema, thirst, tachycardia, weakness, convulsions, and possibly coma. Treatment consists of increased fluid intake and dietary restrictions. The intravenous administration of dextrose solution may be required in more serious cases to help promote renal excretion.

Interactions

Sodium is not known to interact significantly with any drugs.

Dosages

Fluid and electrolyte therapy involves replacing any deficit losses and/or providing maintenance levels for specific patient requirements. Accordingly, specific dosage amounts of fluids or electrolytes depend on several clinical factors that include the following:

- Specific patient losses
- Efficacy of patient physiologic systems involved in fluid and electrolyte metabolism, especially adrenal, cardiovascular, and kidney functions
- Current drug therapy for pathologic conditions that complicate the amount and duration of replacement
- Selection of oral or parenteral replacement formulations

Suggested dosage guidelines with subsequent adjustments for sodium chloride are 1 to 2 g administered orally several times a day or parenteral administration of 1 liter of sodium chloride injection (normal saline).

DRUG PROFILE

SODIUM CHLORIDE

Sodium chloride is primarily used as a replacement electrolyte for either the prevention or treatment of sodium loss. It is also used as a diluent for the infusion of compatible drugs and in the assessment of kidney function after a fluid challenge. Sodium chloride is classified as a pregnancy category C agent and is contraindicated in patients who are hypersensitive to it. It is available in many intravenous preparations and orally as a 650-mg tablet.

☙ PHARMACOKINETICS

HALF-LIFE	ONSET	PEAK	DURATION
Unknown	Immediate	Rapid	Variable

NURSING PROCESS

ASSESSMENT

Parenterally administered hydrating solutions such as 5% dextrose are used mainly for the prevention of dehydration. Isotonic solutions such as normal saline are customarily used to augment extracellular volumes diminished as the result of blood loss, severe vomiting, or any condition that leads to a chloride loss equal to or greater than the sodium loss. Normal saline is also used as the medium for blood transfusions because 5% dextrose in water results in the hemolysis of red blood cells. Hypertonic solutions such as 3.5% sodium chloride are used to treat hypotonic expansion, such as that resulting from water intoxication. Plasmalyte 56 or Plasmalyte 148 are maintenance solutions used to replace electrolytes and water lost as the result of severe diarrhea or vomiting.

Although the physician selects which solution is to be administered, it is the nurse who by monitoring and assessing the patient diagnoses the problem and the complications of the therapy and determines the effectiveness or ineffectiveness of the therapy. Today many patients needing replacement therapy are in home care settings, making the nurse now even more responsible for ensuring their adequate and proper assessment.

The assessment of a patient who is to receive any of the parenteral replacement solutions should focus on the patient's past and present medical history, including diseases and GI, renal, cardiac, or hepatic dysfunction or disorders. The nurse should question patients about prescription and OTC medications they are taking and their dietary habits. Patients' fluid volume and electrolyte status and baseline vital signs should be determined and laboratory studies performed. The skin, mucous membranes, daily weights, and intake and output measurement should also be assessed and any skin turgor noted in patients being treated for a fluid or electrolyte disorder.

Before administering potassium to patients, it is important to assess the ECG for the presence of peaking T waves, depressed R waves, a prolonged Q-R interval, or a widening QRS complex, as well as the potassium levels and intake and output amounts. Contraindications to the use of potassium include renal disease, severe hemolytic disease, hyperkalemia, Addison's disease, acute dehydration, and multiple trauma that involves severe tissue breakdown. Potassium supplementation should be avoided or used with extreme caution in patients taking angiotensin-converting enzyme inhibitors. Cautious use is recommended in patients suffering from cardiac disease or systemic acidosis and those taking potassium-sparing diuretics. Patients' pulse rate, blood pressure, and evidence of edema also need to be reported and documented.

Albumin and other colloids are contraindicated in patients with congestive heart failure or severe anemia and in those who have shown a hypersensitivity to it. Cautious use is called for in the settings of decreased salt intake, decreased cardiac reserve, hepatic disease, and pregnancy, as well as in the absence of an albumin-deficient state. The hematocrit, hemoglobin levels, and serum protein levels should also be noted and documented. Baseline assessment of patients' blood pressure, pulse rate, respiratory status, and intake and output amounts should also be performed and documented and any dyspnea or hypoxia noted.

Before administering blood or blood components, the nurse should obtain a thorough history regarding transfusions patients have received and their response to them. If the patient has any history of adverse reactions, this should be reported to the physician and blood bank or laboratory and the nature of them documented. It is also important to assess venous access as well as to check the patient's laboratory values (e.g., Hct, Hgb, WBC, RBC, clotting factors) and baseline vital signs before infusing the blood or blood product. Even the general appearance of the patient and his or her affect can be a source of early evidence of adverse reactions to a transfusion or infusion of blood components.

NURSING DIAGNOSES

Nursing diagnoses relevant to the patient who is to receive blood products, blood components, or related agents include:

■ Risk for injury related to adverse reaction to transfusion or infusion or allergic reaction.

■ Altered mobility because of fatigue resulting from anemia.

■ Risk for injury (skin trauma or abnormal clotting) related to altered blood component levels.

■ Knowledge deficit regarding treatment with replacmenet products or other parenteral replacement solutions.

■ Risk for self-injury related to complications of the transfusion or infusion of blood products, blood components, or related agents.

PLANNING

Following are the goals related to the administration of fluids and electrolytes and blood components:

■ Patient has minimal problems with volume overload related to the transfusion or infusion.

■ Patient begins minimal exercise and show increased tolerance daily.

■ Patient participates in activities as he or she can tolerate them.

■ Patient states measures to implement to minimize self-injury related to altered blood component levels or altered fluid and electrolytes.

■ Patient states rationale for treatment and the side effects of replacement agents.

■ Patient states symptoms and problems to report to physician.

Outcome Criteria

Following are the outcome criteria for patients receiving fluid, electrolytes, or blood components:

■ Patient remains free of injury to self as the result of adverse reactions (dizziness, volume overload, hypersensitivity) to the transfusion or infusion or of an allergic reaction.

■ Patient regains ability to engage in normal or near-normal exercise showing increased tolerance daily as evidenced by walking small distances and increasing to regular supervised exercise.

■ Patient participates in activities according to his or her ability to tolerate them without dyspnea or chest pain.

■ Patient demonstrates return to normal or near-

normal values of blood components or fluid and electrolyte levels.

■ Patient sees physician for follow-up as ordered to monitor laboratory values pertinent to treatment.

IMPLEMENTATION

Continued reassessment of the patient during therapy is crucial in ensuring safe and effective treatment and also important in preventing the complications of overtreatment and undertreatment, which may be life-threatening. Serum electrolyte levels should not exceed normal ranges (sodium, 135-145 mEq/L; chloride, 95-108 mEq/L; potassium, 3.5-5.0 mEq/L; calcium, 4.5-5.8 mEq/L; magnesium, 1.5-2.5 mEq/L) and should be watched carefully after the conclusion of treatment as well. It is important to document all changes in the patient and any changes in assessment findings. Besides monitoring the infusion rate, the appearance of the fluid or solution, and the infusion site, the nurse must also constantly watch for infiltration of the solution, thrombosis, thrombophlebitis, pain at the IV site, pulmonary edema, fever, and air emboli.

With the administration of any of the fluid and electrolyte solutions, a steady and even flow rate must be maintained to prevent complications. If for some reason the nurse cannot administer the solution ordered or in the amount or at the rate specified, this must be dealt with immediately, the situation resolved, the physician notified, an incident report filed, and the matter documented. The nurse must always perform in an especially prudent, safe, and thorough manner when administering fluids to elderly or pediatric patients because they are more sensitive to changes in fluid and electrolyte levels.

When administering potassium replacements parenterally, the nurse should carefully monitor the dosage during infusion. When given intravenously, potassium *must always be given in diluted form* and administered slowly and only to persons with a documented urine output. It is generally recommended that IV solutions should not contain more than 40 mEq/L of potassium and the rate should not exceed 20 mEq/hr. Oral preparations of potassium should be prescribed whenever possible and in conjunction with a high potassium diet so as to avoid the need for intravenous administration. Potassium chloride is the salt customarily used for IV infusions.

Oral forms of potassium are usually prepared in doses of 10, 20, or 40 mEq/15 ml and must be diluted in water or fruit juice to minimize GI distress or irritation. Powder or effervescent forms should be prepared according to the package guidelines. Both enteric-coated and uncoated forms can cause GI ulcers with bleeding, so their use should always be closely monitored. Any complaints of nausea, vomiting, GI pain, or GI bleeding should be assessed, noted, and reported to the physician immediately and all doses withheld until further orders are received.

Symptoms of hyponatremia include lethargy, hypotension, stomach cramps, vomiting, diarrhea, and seizures. Treatment with Ringer's solution or normal saline is usually helpful in alleviating them, but sodium can also be taken in by consuming a diet high in salt, obtained from such sources as catsup, mustard, cured meats, cheeses, potato chips, peanut butter, popcorn, and table salt. Careful administration with constant monitoring of the IV solution and the rate and site of administration is recommended in any patient undergoing electrolyte replacement therapy.

The intravenous infusion of albumin and other colloids should always be done slowly and cautiously, with careful monitoring, to prevent fluid overload and possible congestive heart failure, especially in those patients at particular risk for this. The hematocrit and hemoglobin values should also be determined in advance so that any anemia can be detected and care taken not to overload the heart pump with an increased volume. Albumin and any blood products should be infused at room temperature.

The patients should be carefully assessed and all findings documented at the start of the administration of a blood product or component (e.g., PPF, platelets, and FFP) and then assessed and the findings documented every 15 minutes, or more frequently if needed, thereafter. At this point the product should be infused at a rate of about 20 drops per minute. Vital signs should be checked and recorded every 15 minutes, or more frequently if possible. Should a reaction occur, the transfusion should be stopped immediately, appropriate nursing measures implemented, the physician notified, and the nature of the event, the corresponding measures taken, and the patient's response documented. Apprehension, restlessness, flushed skin, increased pulse and respirations, dyspnea, rash, swelling, fever and chills (a febrile reaction beginning 1 hour after the start of administration and lasting up to 10 hours), nausea, weakness, and jaundice need to be reported to the physician immediately. The expiration date of blood components should be checked to make sure they are fresh. No outdated blood or blood components should be used. See the box above right for patient teaching tips.

EVALUATION

The therapeutic response to fluid, electrolyte, and blood or blood component therapy includes the normalization of the following laboratory values: RBCs, WBCs, Hgb, Hct, sodium, potassium, and calcium. In

---

Patient Teaching TIPS

✔ Patients should consume foods high in potassium in order to take in the recommended daily allowance, which is between 40 and 50 mEq for adults and 2 to 3 mEq/kg of body weight for infants. Two medium-sized bananas or an 8-oz. glass of orange juice contains 45 mEq; 20 large dried apricots contain 40 mEq; and a level teaspoon of salt substitute (KCl) contains 60 mEq of potassium. Oral doses are usually increased gradually over about 1 week to prevent hyperkalemia.

✔ Sodium may be lost as the result of major tissue or body trauma, vomiting, the syndrome of inadequate antidiuretic hormone secretion, diuretic use, tap water enemas, wound drainage, loss of GI fluids, and excessive perspiration. Patients should follow replacement instructions carefully and as the physician prescribed.

✔ Encourage patients taking any type of fluid or electrolyte substance, colloid, or blood component to report any unusual side effects immediately to their physician. Such complaints include chest pain, dizziness, weakness, shortness of breath, or any unusual symptom.

✔ Water intake is important in all patients, especially the elderly and anyone in a hot, humid environment or losing fluids as the result of perspiration, drainage, and the like. Patients should understand that water is important because it is the medium in which all metabolic reactions occur and it is needed for the precise regulation of the volume and composition of body fluid, both of which are essential for life.

---

addition, the fluid levels, volume status, and cardiac function should return to normal and the patient should be able to resume his or her normal or near-normal activities. The patient should also show an increased tolerance to activity, improved skin color, and minimal to no dyspnea, chest pain, weakness, or fatigue. The therapeutic response to albumin therapy includes increased blood pressure, decreased edema, and increased serum albumin levels. Monitoring for the side effects of any of these products as well as for conditions stemming from either an excess or deficit of the particular product is also part of the evaluation process, and any such findings should be reported to the physician, if necessary, and documented. Adverse reactions to albumin include distended neck veins, shortness of breath, anxiety, insomnia, expiratory rales, frothy blood-tinged sputum, and cyanosis.

TAKE HOME POINTS

Total Body Water
- Broken down into intracellular (inside the cell) and extracellular (outside the cell) volume.
- The fluid that is outside the cells is either in the plasma (intravascular volume) or between the tissues, cells, or organs (interstitial fluid).

Colloid Oncotic Pressure
- The concentration of colloids such as albumin is four times greater inside blood vessels than outside them.
- Colloids are large protein particles that cannot leak out of the blood vessels.
- Because of their greater concentration inside blood vessels, fluid is pulled into the blood vessels.
- Albumin, hetastarch, and dextran are examples of colloids.

Crystalloids
- Fluids that supply water and sodium to maintain the osmotic gradient between extravascular and intravascular compartments.
- Their PV-expanding capacity is related to the sodium concentration.
- They contain fluids and electrolytes that are normally found in the body.

Blood Products
- Also known as *oxygen-carrying resuscitation fluids.*
- Only class of fluids able to carry oxygen because they are the only fluids that contain hemoglobin.
- They not only increase the oxygen-carrying capabilities but also the COP.

Nursing Considerations—Hydration
- Hydrating solutions include 0.45%, 0.9%, or higher saline in water (hypertonic solutions = 3% and 5%); these are used to hydrate patients and prevent dehydration. Hypertonic solutions should be given slowly (<100 cc/hr).
- Dehydration may be hypotonic, resulting from the loss of salt; hypertonic, resulting from fever with perspiration; or isotonic, resulting from diarrhea or vomiting.
- Each form of dehydration is treated differently.

Nursing Considerations—Potassium Therapy
- Symptoms of hypokalemia include lethargy, weakness, fatigue, respiratory difficulty, paralysis, and ileus.
- IV potassium should always be given slowly and only in appropriate concentrations.
- Hyperkalemia may lead to ventricular fibrillation and cardiac arrest.

Nursing Considerations—Sodium Therapy
- Hyponatremia is manifested by lethargy, hypotension, stomach cramps, vomiting, diarrhea, and possibly seizures.
- Hypernatremia is manifested by red, flushed skin; dry, sticky mucous membranes; increased thirst; temperature elevation; and a decrease in or absence of urination.

Nursing Considerations—Blood Products
- Blood products may cause hemolysis of RBCs, and so adverse reactions such as fever, chills, back pain, to name just a few, should be watched for. If noted, the physician should be notified immediately, the IV infusion discontinued, and the nature of the reactions and all actions taken documented.

Albumin
- During the infusion of albumin and like products, the patient should be constantly monitored for the development of increased central venous pressure, as manifested by the occurrence of distended neck veins, shortness of breath, expiratory rales, anxiety, and frothy, blood-tinged sputum.

Critical Thinking **A C T I V I T I E S**

1. The normal serum levels of potassium are:
   a. 185-190 mg/L
   b. 3.5-5.0 mEq/L
   c. 13-18 mg/L
   d. 120-135 mEq/L

2. Ms. Wall takes 2500 mg of calcium carbonate daily in the form of an OTC calcium supplement. How much elemental calcium is she actually taking?

▲▲

BIBLIOGRAPHY

Albanese J, Nutz P: *Mosby's 1995 nursing drug cards,* St Louis, 1995, Mosby.

Johnson KB: *Harriet Lane handbook,* ed 13, St Louis, 1993, Mosby.

Keen JH: *Critical care and emergency drug reference,* St Louis, 1994, Mosby.

Knoben JE, Anderson PO: *Handbook of critical drug data,* ed 6, Hamilton, Ill, 1988, Drug Intelligence Publications.

McEvoy GK: *AHFS drug information,* Bethesda, Md, 1994, American Society of Hospital Pharmacists.

McKenry L, Salerno E: *Mosby's pharmacology in nursing,* ed 19, St Louis, 1995, Mosby.

Skidmore-Roth L: *Mosby's 1995 nursing drug reference,* St. Louis, 1995, Mosby.

Wagner B, D'Aemio L: Pharmacologic and clinical considerations in selecting crystalloid, colloidal, and oxygen-carrying resuscitation fluids, part 1, *Clin Pharmacol* 12:335, 1993.

Wagner B, D'Aemio L: Pharmacologic and clinical considerations in selecting crystalloid, colloidal, and oxygen-carrying resuscitation fluids, part 2, *Clin Pharmacol* 12:415, 1993.

Chapter 28

Female Reproductive Agents

Objectives

When you reach the end of this chapter, you will be able to:

1 List the disorders estrogens and progestins are used in the treatment of.

2 Discuss the normal hormonally mediated feedback system and how it regulates the female reproductive system.

3 List the various estrogen and progestin drugs commonly used in the treatment of disorders of the female reproductive system.

4 Describe the rationale for treatment and cite the dosages, side effects, cautions, contraindications, and drug interactions associated with estrogen and progestin therapy.

5 Develop a comprehensive nursing care plan that includes patient outcomes and patient education for the patient receiving estrogens, progestins, oral contraceptives, and the drugs used in labor and delivery.

6 List the expected therapeutic responses to estrogen and progestin therapy.

7 Discuss the use of oral contraceptives as it relates to therapeutic and adverse effects.

8 List the therapeutic responses to uterine stimulants and relaxants.

CHAPTER OUTLINE

The Female Reproductive System

Female Sex Hormones

Estrogens
  Mechanism of action
  Drug effects
  Therapeutic uses
  Side effects and adverse effects
  Interactions
  Dosages
Drug Profiles
    Estrogen
Progestins
  Mechanism of action
  Drug effects
  Therapeutic uses
  Side effects and adverse effects
  Interactions
  Dosages
Drug Profiles
    Medroxyprogesterone
    ⚓ Megestrol
Oral Contraceptives
  Mechanism of action
  Drug effects

Therapeutic uses
Side effects and adverse effects
Interactions
Dosages
Drug Profiles
Labor and Delivery Drugs

Uterine Stimulants
  Mechanism of action
  Drug effects
  Therapeutic uses
  Side effects and adverse effects
  Interactions
  Dosages
Drug Profiles
    Dinoprostone
    Ergonovine and Methylergonovine
    Oxytocin
Uterine Relaxants
  Mechanism of action
  Drug effects
  Therapeutic uses
  Side effects and adverse effects
    Toxicity and management of overdose
  Interactions
  Dosages

continued

Drug Profiles
  Ritodrine
  Terbutaline

Fertility Agents
  Mechanism of action
  Drug effects
  Therapeutic uses
  Side effects and adverse effects
  Interactions
  Dosages
  Drug Profiles
  ⚓ Clomiphene
    Chorionic Gonadotropin
    Menotropins

Nursing Process
  Assessment
  Nursing Diagnoses
  Planning
    Outcome criteria
  Implementation
  Evaluation

Glossary

Corpus luteum (kor′ pəs loo′ te əm) Structure that forms on the surface of the ovary after every ovulation and acts as a short-lived endocrine organ that secretes progesterone. (p. 437)

Endocrine gland (en′ do krin) Part of a system of glands that secrete hormones into the blood. (p. 422)

Endometrium (en′ do me′ tre əm) Mucous membrane lining the uterus. (p. 422)

Fallopian tube (fə lo′ pe ən) Passage through which an ovum is carried to the uterus. (p. 422)

Gonadotropin (gon′ə do tro′ pin) Hormone that stimulates the testes and ovaries. (p. 422)

Implantation The attachment, penetration, and embedding of the blastocyst in the lining of the uterine wall. (p. 422)

Menarche (mə nahr′ ke) The first menstruation and the beginning of cyclic menstrual function. (p. 422)

Menopause (men′ o pawz) The cessation of menses. (p. 422)

Menses (men′ sēz) The normal flow of blood that occurs during menstruation. (p. 424)

Menstrual cycle (men′ stroo əl) The recurring cycle of changes in the endometrium when the decidual layer is shed, regrows, proliferates, is maintained for several days, and is shed again at menstruation. (p. 422)

Nucleic acid (noo kle′ ik) Compound involved in energy storage and release and in the determination and transmission of genetic characteristics. (p. 424)

Ova (o′ və) Female reproductive or germ cells. (p. 422)

Ovaries (o′ və rez) Pair of female gonads located on each side of the lower abdomen beside the uterus. (p. 422)

Puberty (pu′ bər te) Period of life when the ability to reproduce begins. (p. 424)

Uterus (u′ tər əs) Hollow, pear-shaped female organ in which the fertilized ovum is implanted and the fetus develops. (p. 422)

Vagina (və ji′ nə) Part of the female genitalia that forms a canal from the orifice through the vestibule to the uterine cervix. (p. 422)

The Female Reproductive System

The female reproductive system consists of the ovaries, fallopian tubes, uterus, vagina, and an external structure (the vulva). The development of these primary sex characteristics, their subsequent reproductive functions (starting at puberty), and their maintenance are controlled by pituitary **gonadotropins** and the female steroid sex hormones, estrogens. Estrogens are also responsible for stimulating the development of secondary female sex characteristics.

The **ovaries** (female gonads) are paired glands located on each side of the uterus and function both as an **endocrine gland** and as a reproductive gland. As a reproductive gland they produce mature **ova** from ovarian follicles, which are then ovulated and transported down the **fallopian tube** to the uterus. As an endocrine gland the ovaries are responsible for producing estrogens and progesterone.

The **uterus** consists primarily of smooth muscle and an inner layer called the **endometrium.** It is a mucous membrane and the site of:

- **Implantation** of a fertilized ovum and the subsequent development of the fetus
- The initiation of labor and the birthing of the infant
- Menstruation

The **vagina** serves as a common passageway for birthing and menstrual flow. In addition, it is a receptacle for the penis during sexual intercourse and the sperm after male ejaculation.

The **menstrual cycle** usually takes 1 month to complete. It commences during puberty with the first menses **(menarche)** and ceases with **menopause**, which in most women occurs between 45 and 55 years of age. The hormonally controlled menstrual cycle consists of three distinct but interrelated phases:

Phase 1 The **menstrual phase,** which initiates the cycle and lasts from 5 to 7 days.

Phase 2 The follicular phase, during which a mature ovum develops from an ovarian follicle. This phase is also called the proliferative or preovulatory phase. It terminates on or about day 14 of the cycle.

Phase 3 The final phase of the cycle is called the luteal or postovulatory phase, and it is when the corpus luteum forms from the ruptured graafian follicle and progesterone is produced. The endometrium is developed to receive the fertilized ovum, and it is here that it is implanted. If fertilization does not occur, the corpus luteum degenerates and the cycle begins again on or about day 28.

Figure 28-1 illustrates the sequence of hormone secretions and related events that take place during the menstrual cycle.

Female Sex Hormones

ESTROGENS

There are three major endogenous estrogens: estradiol, estrone, and estriol. All are synthesized from cholesterol in the ovarian follicles and have the basic structure of a steroid. For this reason they are sometimes

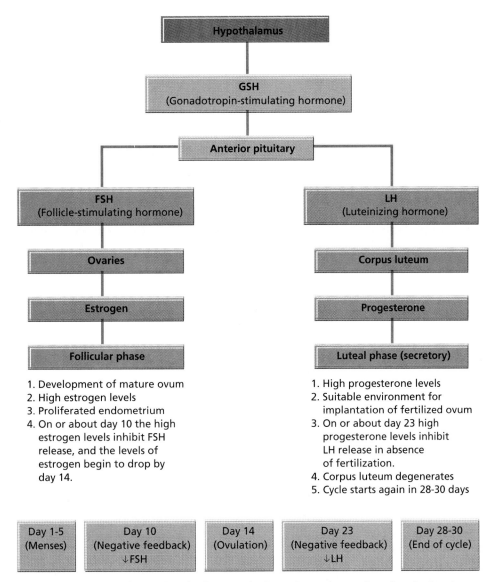

▼ **FIG. 28-1** Hormonal activity during ovulation. Gonadotropin-stimulating hormone (GSH) from the hypothalamus stimulates the pituitary, causing a surge in the production of follicle-stimulating hormone (FSH). The maturing follicle secretes estrogen, which inhibits the production of FSH. When the level of estrogen reaches an appropriately high level, it stimulates the hypothalamus and pituitary to secrete luteinizing hormone (LH). The LH brings the follicle to full maturation, causing it to release an ovum. In the absence of a fertilized ovum, estrogen and progesterone are then secreted by the ovary, which inhibit the production of LH and end the cycle.

referred to as *steroid hormones*. Estradiol is the principal and most active of the three and represents the end-product of estrogen synthesis.

The exogenous estrogenic agents, those used for therapeutic reasons, were developed because most of the endogenous estrogens are inactive orally. These synthetic agents fall into two categories: steroidal and nonsteroidal, and the agents in the two categories are as follows:

Steroidal
- Conjugated estrogens (Premarin)
- Esterified estrogens (Estratab, Menest)
- Estradiol transdermal (Estraderm, Estrace)
- Estradiol cypionate (Depoestradiol, Depogen)
- Estradiol valerate (Delestrogen, Duragen)
- Ethinyl estradiol (Estinyl, Feminone)
- Estrone (Gynogen, Theelin aqueous)
- Estropipate (Ogen)
- Quinestrol (Estrovis)

Nonsteroidal
- Chlorotrianisene (TACE)
- Dienestrol (DV)
- Diethylstilbestrol
- Diethylstilbestrol diphosphate (Stilphostrol)

The natural (steroidal) estrogenic agents are all obtained from the urine of pregnant mares, thus the agent Premarin (*pregnant mare urine*). Ethinyl estradiol is one of the most potent of these estrogens. The nonsteroidal agents do not have the basic steroid structure but can still act on estrogenic tissues throughout the body.

Mechanism of Action

The binding of estrogen to estrogen receptors stimulates the synthesis of **nucleic acid** (DNA and RNA) and proteins, which are the building blocks for all living tissue. Estrogens are also required at **puberty** for the development and maintenance of the female reproductive system and the development of secondary sex characteristics (feminization).

Drug Effects

The estrogens produce their effects in estrogen-responsive tissues, which have a high content of estrogen receptors. These tissues comprise the female genital organs, the breasts, the pituitary, and the hypothalamus.

At the time of puberty the production of estrogen increases greatly. This causes **menses** to be initiated, the breasts to develop, body fat to be redistributed, soft skin to form, and other feminizing changes to occur. Estrogens play a role in the shaping of body contours and the skeleton. For instance, long bones are usually inhibited from growing, with the result that females are usually considerably shorter than males.

Therapeutic Uses

Estrogens are utilized in the treatment or prevention of an assortment of disorders that primarily result from estrogen deficiency. These conditions are listed in the box below.

Side Effects and Adverse Effects

The most serious side and adverse effects of the estrogens are thromboembolic events. Rarely they can cause erythema multiforme, a rare skin disorder in which acute eruptions of macules, papules, or subdermal vesicles that exhibit a multiforme appearance appear on the hands and forearms. It can be recurrent or may run a severe course and fatally terminate in the Stevens-Johnson syndrome. The most common undesirable effects of estrogens are listed in Table 28-1.

Interactions

The estrogens can decrease the activity of the oral anticoagulants, and their concurrent use with rifampin can decrease the estrogenic effect. Their use with tricyclic antidepressants may result in a toxic response. Smoking during estrogen therapy is best avoided because this too can diminish the estrogenic effect.

Dosages

Please see the dosages table on p. 425 for the recommended dosages of estrogens.

Indications for Estrogen Therapy

- Atrophic vaginitis (shrinkage of the vagina and/or urethra)
- Hypogonadism
- Oral contraception (in combination with a progestin)
- Ovarian failure or castration
- Uterine bleeding
- Breast/prostate cancer (palliative treatment of advanced inoperable cases)
- Kraurosis vulvae (atrophy and shrinkage of the skin of the vagina and vulva)
- Osteoporosis
- Postpartum lactation (prevention of)
- Dysmenorrhea (painful or difficult menstruation)

Table 28-1	Estrogens: Common Adverse Effects
BODY SYSTEM	**SIDE/ADVERSE EFFECTS**
Gastrointestinal	Nausea, vomiting, diarrhea, constipation, cramps, weight gain
Genitourinary	Amenorrhea, breakthrough uterine bleeding, enlarged uterine fibromyomas
Cardiovascular	Hypertension, thrombophlebitis, edema
Other	Tender breasts, fluid retention, decreased carbohydrate tolerance, headaches

DRUG PROFILES

ESTROGEN

Estrogen replacement is indicated for the treatment of many clinical conditions, but primarily those resulting from estrogen deficiency. (See box on p. 424.) Therefore it follows that many of these conditions occur around the time of menopause when the endogenous estradiol level is declining. Any estrogen capable of binding to the estrogen receptors in target organs can alleviate

DOSAGES

SELECTED ESTROGENIC AGENTS

AGENT	PHARMACOLOGIC CLASS	DOSAGE RANGE	PURPOSE
STEROIDAL Conjugated estrogens (Premarin) and Esterified estrogens (Estratab, Menest)	Estrogenic hormone mixture	*Adult* PO: 0.3-1.25 mg/day cyclically	Atropic vaginitis, kraurosis vulvae, vasomotor symptoms of menopause
		PO: 10 mg tid for at least 3 mo	Breast cancer
		PO: 1.25 mg/day cyclically	Castration, ovarian failure
		PO: 2.5-7.5 mg/day divided for 20 days, followed by a 10-day rest period	Female hypogonadism
		PO: 3.75 mg q4h for 5 doses or 1.25 mg q4h for 5 days	Pospartum breast engorgement
		PO: 1.25-2.5 mg tid	Prostate cancer
		IM/IV: 25 mg repeat in 6-12 hr prn	Abnormal uterine bleeding
Estradiol (Estrace)	Estrogenic hormone	*Adult* PO: 1-2 mg/day cyclically	Atropic vaginitis, kraurosis vulvae, vasomotor symptoms of menopause
		PO: 10 mg tid for at least 3 mo	Breast cancer
		PO: 1-2 mg/day tid	Prostate cancer
		PO: 0.5 mg/day cyclically	Osteoporosis prophylaxis
Estradiol transdermal (Estraderm)	Estrogenic hormone	*Adult* Apply 0.05 mg system to abdominal skin twice weekly, either cyclically (intact uterus) or continuously (nonintact uterus). Dosage must be adjusted.	Symptoms of menopause

continued

SELECTED ESTROGENIC AGENTS—cont'd

AGENT	PHARMACOLOGIC CLASS	DOSAGE RANGE	PURPOSE
Estradiol cypionate (Dep Gynogen, Depolen)	Estrogenic hormone	*Adult* IM: 1-5 mg every 3-4 wk IM: 1.5-2 mg every mo	Symptoms of menopause Female hypogonadism
Estradiol valerate (Delestrogen, Duragen, Valergen)	Estrogenic hormone	*Adult* IM: 10-20 mg every 4 wk IM: 10-25 mg administered at first stage of labor IM: 30 mg or more every 1-2 wk	Symptoms of menopause Postpartum breast engorgement Prostate cancer
Ethinyl estradiol (Estinyl)	Estrogenic hormone	*Adult* PO: 0.02-1.5 mg/day cyclically PO: 0.05 mg 1-3 times/day for 2 wk, followed by progesterone for 2 wk. Continue this regimen for 3-6 mo. PO: 1 mg tid PO: 0.15-2 mg/day	Symptoms of menopause Female hypogonadism Breast cancer Prostate cancer
Estropipate (Ogen)	Estrogenic hormone (solubilized estrone)	*Adult* PO: 0.625-5 mg/day cyclically PO: 1-25-7.5 mg/day cyclically PO: 0.625 mg/day for 25 days of a 31-day cycle	Atrophic vaginitis, kraurosis vulvae, symptoms of menopause Female castration, hypogonadism, primary ovarian failure Osteoporosis prophylaxis
Quinestrol (Estrovis)	Synthetic estrogenic hormone	*Adult* PO: 100 μg/day for 7 days, followed by 100-200 μg once weekly	Atrophic vaginitis, kraurosis vulvae, female castration/hypogonadism, primary ovarian failure, symptoms of menopause
NONSTEROIDAL **Chlorotrianisene (TACE)**	Synthetic nonsteroidal estrogenic agent	*Adult* PO: 12-25 mg/day cyclically PO: 12 mg qid for 7 days or 50 mg q6h for 6 doses PO: 12-25 mg/day	Atrophic vaginitis, kraurosis vulvae, symptoms of menopause Postpartum breast engorgement Prostate cancer
Dienestrol (DV)	Synthetic nonsteroidal estrogenic agent	*Adult* Intravaginal: apply 1-2 applicators full/day for 1-2 wk. Reduce dosage as indicated. Usual maintenance dose is 1 applicator full 1-3 times/day	Atrophic vaginitis, kraurosis vulvae
Diethylstilbestrol	Synthetic nonsteroidal estrogenic agent	*Adult* PO: 15 mg/day PO: 1-3 mg/day	Breast cancer Prostate cancer

continued

SELECTED ESTROGENIC AGENTS—cont'd

AGENT	PHARMACOLOGIC CLASS	DOSAGE RANGE	PURPOSE
Diethylstilbestrol diphosphate (Stilphostrol)	Synthetic nonsteroidal estrogenic agent	*Adult* PO: 50 mg tid and adjusted; do not exceed 1 g/day IV: 0.5 g/day and increased to 1 g on next ≥5 days, followed by 0.25-0.5 g maintenance dose 1-2 times/wk	Prostate cancer

these menopausal symptoms. As a general rule, however, the smallest dose of estrogen that alleviates the symptoms or prevents the condition is used for the shortest possible time.

Estrogenic agents are contraindicated in the following clinical settings: hypersensitivity, active or past history of estrogen-associated thromboembolic disorders (except for cancer palliation), abnormal genital bleeding, estrogen-dependent neoplasms, and breast cancer. These agents are also classified as pregnancy category X agents by the FDA.

The principal pharmacologic effects of all the estrogens are similar because there are only slight differences in their chemical structure. These differences make for different potencies, which in turn make them useful for a variety of indications. They also allow the agents to be given by different routes of administration.

PROGESTINS

Progestational agents consist of both natural and synthetic agents. *Progesterone* is the principal natural progestational hormone. It is produced by the corpus luteum and during pregnancy by the placenta. Because orally administered progesterone is relatively inactive and parenterally administered progesterone causes local reactions and pain, chemical derivatives were developed that are effective orally and also more potent. Their actions are also more specific and of longer duration. These are the progestins, and the commonly used ones are:

■ Hydroxyprogesterone (Duralutin, Gesterol LA)
■ Medroxyprogesterone (Amen, Cycrin, Provera, Depo-Provera)
■ Norethindrone (Norlutin, Micronor)
■ Norethindrone acetate (Aygestin, Norlutate)
■ Norgestrel (Ovrette, Ovral)
■ Megestrol (Megace)
■ Progesterone (Gesterol 50)

The progestins produce all the same responses as those produced by progesterone. These include inducing secretory changes in the endometrium, increasing the basal body temperature, producing changes in the vaginal epithelium, relaxing uterine smooth muscle, stimulating mammary alveolar tissue growth, inhibiting the pituitary, and producing withdrawal bleeding in the presence of estrogen.

Mechanism of Action

When exogenous progestins are given, the body senses that it does not need to produce and release more progestins. These progestins in the blood signal the pituitary gland to inhibit gonadotropin. This mechanism is called feedback inhibition.

Drug Effects

Progestins affect the pituitary gland, the uterus (especially during the menstrual cycle), the vaginal mucosa, and the mammary glands. Because gonadotropin normally stimulates the ovaries, its suppressed release as the result of feedback inhibition causes the function of the ovaries to be suppressed. The subsequent effects on the uterus include an increase in the secretory (luteal) phase of endometrial development during the menstrual cycle and relaxation of uterine smooth muscle during pregnancy. In addition, the vaginal mucosa increases in thickness and mammary tissue growth is stimulated during therapy with progestins.

Therapeutic Uses

The progestins are useful in the treatment of functional uterine bleeding caused by a hormonal imbalance, fibroids, or uterine cancer; the treatment of primary and secondary amenorrhea; the adjunctive and palliative treatment of some cancers and endometriosis; and alone or in combination with estrogens for the prevention of conception. They may also be useful to prevent a threatened miscarriage and alleviate the symptoms of the premenstrual syndrome. Specifically, medroxyprogesterone, hydroxyprogesterone, norethindrone, and progesterone have all been used to treat hormone imbalance, primary or secondary amenorrhea, and functional bleeding of the uterus, though medroxyprogesterone is the one most commonly used for this. Norethindrone and norgestrel may be used to treat female hormone imbalance and endometriosis but are more commonly used alone or in combination with estrogens as contraceptives to prevent pregnancy. Megestrol is commonly used to treat breast and endometrial cancers.

Side Effects and Adverse Effects

The most serious undesirable effects of progestins include liver dysfunction, commonly manifested as cholestatic jaundice; thrombophlebitis; and thromboembolic disorders such as pulmonary embolism. The more common of these effects are listed in Table 28-2.

Interactions

Reports of possible decreases in glucose tolerance when progestins are taken with antidiabetic agents may require that the dose of the antidiabetic agent be adjusted. The concurrent use of medroxyprogesterone or norethindrone with aminoglutethimide or rifampin induces increased metabolism of the progestin.

Dosages

For recommended dosages of the progestins, see the dosages table on p. 429.

*D*RUG *P*ROFILES

MEDROXYPROGESTERONE

Medroxyprogesterone (Amen, Cycrin, Provera, Depo-Provera) inhibits the secretion of pituitary gonadotropins, which prevents follicular maturation and ovulation; stimulates the growth of mammary tissue; and has an antineoplastic action against endometrial cancer. It is used to treat uterine bleeding, secondary amenorrhea, endometrial cancer, and renal cancer, and is also used as a contraceptive. It is classified as a pregnancy category X agent and is contraindicated in patients with a history of thrombophlebitis, thrombo-

Table 28-2	Progestins: Common Adverse Effects
BODY SYSTEM	**SIDE/ADVERSE EFFECTS**
Gastrointestinal	Nausea, vomiting
Genitourinary	Amenorrhea, breakthrough uterine bleeding, spotting, changes in menstrual flow, changes in cervical erosion and secretions
Other	Edema, weight gain or loss, allergic rash, pyrexia, somnolence or insomnia, mental depression

embolic disorders, cerebral apoplexy, liver disease, undiagnosed vaginal bleeding, suspected breast cancer, or drug hypersensitivity.

Medroxyprogesterone is available in both oral and parenteral preparations. Orally it comes as 2.5-, 5-, and 10-mg tablets. Parenterally it comes as a 100-, 150-, and 400-mg/ml sterile suspension for intramuscular injection. Recommended dosages are given in the following dosages table.

❧ P H A R M A C O K I N E T I C S

HALF-LIFE	ONSET	PEAK	DURATION
14.5 hr	Unknown	IM: 2-7 hr	IM: 3 mo

⚓ MEGESTROL

Megestrol (Megace) is a synthetic progestin that differs structurally from progesterone only in the addition of a methyl group on the steroid nucleus and a double bond. Although megestrol shares the actions of the progestins, it is primarily used in the palliative management of recurrent, inoperable, or metastatic endometrial or breast cancer. It has also been used in the management of anorexia, cachexia, or an unexplained, substantial weight loss in patients with the acquired immunodeficiency syndrome. In addition, it may be used to stimulate appetite and promote weight gain in patients with cancer. It is also classified as a pregnancy category X agent, and the contraindications to its use are the same as those of the other progestins. It is only available orally as a 200-mg/5 ml oral suspension and as 20- and 40-mg tablets. Recommended dosages are given in the following dosages table.

❧ P H A R M A C O K I N E T I C S

HALF-LIFE	ONSET	PEAK	DURATION
x̄ = 34 hr	6-8 wk	Unknown	4-10 mo

D O S A G E S

SELECTED PROGESTATIONAL AGENTS

AGENT	PHARMACOLOGIC CLASS	DOSAGE RANGE	PURPOSE
Hydroxyprogesterone caproate (Duralutin, Gesterol LA 250, Pro-Depo)	Progestin	*Adult* IM: 375 mg	Amenorrhea, uterine bleeding
Medroxyprogesterone acetate (Amen, Cycrin, Provera, Depo-Provera)	Progestin	*Adult* PO: 5-10 mg/day for 5-10 days. Withdrawal bleeding usually starts 3-7 days after ending therapy.	Amenorrhea
		PO: 5-10 mg each day for 5-10 days beginning on calculated day 16 or 21 of cycle.	Uterine bleeding
		IM: 400-1000 mg/wk	Metastatic endometrial or renal cancer
Norethindrone (Norlutin)	Progestin	*Adult* PO: 5-20 mg starting on day 5 and ending on day 25 of the cycle	Amenorrhea, uterine bleeding
		PO: 10 mg/day for 2 wk and increase by 5 mg every 2 wk until 30 mg/day is reached, then continue for 6-9 mo; if breakthrough bleeding occurs, therapy should be stopped temporarily	Endometriosis
Norethindrone acetate (Aygestin, Norlutate)	Progestin	*Adult* PO: 2.5-10 mg starting on day 5 and ending on day 25 of cycle	Amenorrhea, uterine bleeding
		PO: 5 mg/day for 2 wk and increase by 2.5 mg every 2 wk until 15 mg/day is reached, then continue for 6-9 mo; if breakthrough bleeding occurs, therapy should be stopped temporarily	Endometriosis
Progesterone	Progestin	*Adult* IM: 5-10 mg/day for 6-8 days	Amenorrhea
		IM: 5-10 mg/day for 6 days	Uterine bleeding
⤓Megestrol Acetate (Megace)	Progestin	*Adult* PO: 400-800 mg/day	Weight loss in AIDS patients
		PO: 40 mg qid	Breast cancer
		PO: 40-320 mg/day	Endometrial cancer

ORAL CONTRACEPTIVES

The oral contraceptives are the most effective form of birth control currently available. Estrogen-progestin combinations, sometimes referred to as "the pill," are oral contraceptives that contain both estrogenic and progestinic steroids. The estrogenic component is either ethinyl estradiol or mestranol. Ethinyl estradiol is a semisynthetic steroidal estrogen, and as previously noted, it is the most orally active estrogenic drug currently available. It is about twenty times more potent than diethylstilbestrol. Mestranol is slightly less active. The progestinic component is ethynodiol diacetate, levonorgestrel, norethindrone, norethindrone acetate, norethynodrel, or norgestrel.

The currently available oral contraceptives may be biphasic or triphasic in terms of the doses taken at different times in the menstrual cycle. The biphasic agents contain a fixed estrogen dose but a low progestin dose for the first 10 days and a higher dose for the rest of the cycle in 21- or 28-day dosage packages. The triphasic oral contraceptives contain three different estrogen-progestin dose ratios that are administered sequentially during the cycle in 21- or 28-day dosage packs. The triphasic products closely duplicate the normal hormonal levels of the female cycle. These contraceptives also come in a monophasic form, in which the estrogen and progestin doses are the same throughout the cycle.

Mechanism of Action

The oral contraceptives prevent ovulation by inhibiting the release of gonadotropins and by increasing uterine mucous viscosity resulting in (1) decreased sperm movement and fertilization of ovum; and (2) possible inhibition of implantation of fertilized egg (zygote).

Drug Effects

The oral contraceptives have many of the same effects as those normally produced by the endogenous estrogens and progesterone. The contraceptive effect mainly results from the suppression of the hypothalamic-pituitary system they induce, which in turn prevents ovulation. Other incidental benefits to their use are that they improve menstrual cycle regularity and decrease blood loss during menstruation. A decreased incidence of functional ovarian cysts and ectopic pregnancies has also been associated with their use. Drawbacks to their use include alterations in carbohydrate and lipid metabolism, increases in serum hormone concentrations, and alterations in serum metal and plasma protein levels. It is the estrogen component that appears to be the source of most of these metabolic effects.

Therapeutic Uses

The oral contraceptives are primarily utilized to prevent pregnancy. In addition, they are used to treat endometriosis and hypermenorrhea and to produce cyclic withdrawal bleeding.

Side Effects and Adverse Effects

Common side effects and adverse effects associated with the use of oral contraceptives are listed in Table 28-3.

Interactions

Drugs that decrease the effectiveness of the oral contraceptives when taken in conjunction with them include:

- Ampicillin
- Analgesics
- Antihistamines
- Barbiturates
- Chloramphenicol
- Griseofulvin
- Isoniazid
- Migraine preparations
- Neomycin
- Nitrofurantoin
- Penicillin V
- Phenytoin
- Primidone
- Rifampin
- Sulfonamides
- Tetracycline
- Tranquilizers

Table 28-3	Oral Contraceptives: Common Adverse Effects
BODY SYSTEM	SIDE/ADVERSE EFFECTS
Central nervous system	Dizziness, headache, migraines, depression, stroke
Cardiovascular	Hypotension, thrombophlebitis, edema, thromboembolism, pulmonary embolism, myocardial infarction
Gastrointestinal	Nausea, vomiting, diarrhea, anorexia, pancreatitis, cramps, constipation, increased appetite, increased weight, cholestatic jaundice
Genitourinary	Amenorrhea, cervical erosion, breakthrough bleeding, dysmenorrhea, breast changes

Drugs that have reduced effectiveness when taken with the oral contraceptives include:
- Anticonvulsants
- Beta-blockers
- Guanethidine
- Hypnotics
- Hypoglycemic agents
- Oral anticoagulants
- Theophylline
- Tricyclic antidepressants
- Vitamins

Dosages

For the recommended dosages of oral contraceptives, see the dosages table below.

*D*RUG *P*ROFILES

The oral contraceptives are contraindicated in the following settings: known or suspected breast cancer, estrogen neoplasia, pregnancy, present or past thrombophlebotic disorders, undiagnosed abnormal genital bleeding, cerebrovascular and coronary disease, and benign or malignant liver tumors associated with estrogen use. The oral contraceptives are classified as pregnancy category X agents.

Labor and Delivery Drugs

There are many drugs that can be used during labor and delivery. There are agents that stimulate uterine contraction, those that relax the uterus, those that stimulate ovulation, those that inhibit lactation, and those that suppress the immune response. Many of these drugs have other uses and may be discussed in greater detail in other chapters, but all will be discussed briefly here.

UTERINE STIMULANTS

There are three types of drugs that are used to stimulate uterine contractions: the ergot derivatives, the prostaglandins, and oxytocin. All work on the uterus,

DOSAGES

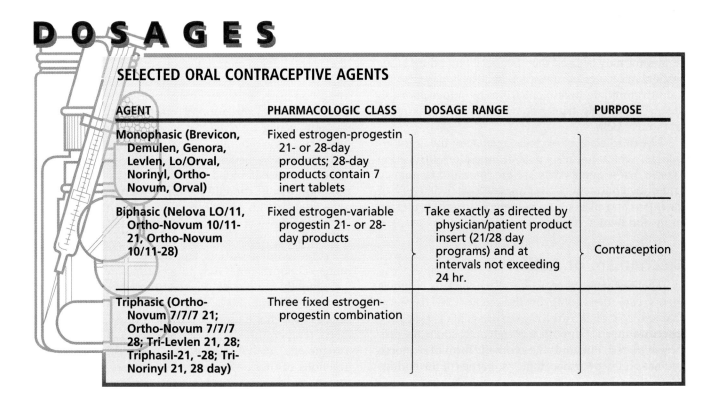

SELECTED ORAL CONTRACEPTIVE AGENTS

AGENT	PHARMACOLOGIC CLASS	DOSAGE RANGE	PURPOSE
Monophasic (Brevicon, Demulen, Genora, Levlen, Lo/Orval, Norinyl, Ortho-Novum, Orval)	Fixed estrogen-progestin 21- or 28-day products; 28-day products contain 7 inert tablets		
Biphasic (Nelova LO/11, Ortho-Novum 10/11-21, Ortho-Novum 10/11-28)	Fixed estrogen-variable progestin 21- or 28-day products	Take exactly as directed by physician/patient product insert (21/28 day programs) and at intervals not exceeding 24 hr.	Contraception
Triphasic (Ortho-Novum 7/7/7 21; Ortho-Novum 7/7/7 28; Tri-Levlen 21, 28; Triphasil-21, -28; Tri-Norinyl 21, 28 day)	Three fixed estrogen-progestin combination		

a highly muscular organ that has a complex network of smooth muscle fibers and a large blood supply. The uterus undergoes several changes during normal gestation and child birth that at different times make it either resistant or susceptible to various hormones and drugs. These agents are sometimes referred to as oxytocic agents, named after the naturally occurring hormone oxytocin whose action they mimic. It is one of the two hormones secreted by the posterior pituitary. The other is vasopressin, or antidiuretic hormone. The uterus of a woman who is not pregnant is relatively insensitive to oxytocin, but during pregnancy the uterus becomes more sensitive to oxytocin, being most sensitive at term (the end of gestation).

During childbirth, oxytocin stimulates uterine contraction, and during lactation it promotes the movement of milk from the mammary glands to the nipples. Oxytocin is available in a synthetic form called *Pitocin,* and this agent is used to induce labor at or near full-term gestation and to stimulate labor when uterine contractions are weak and ineffective. Oxytocic agents are also used to prevent or control uterine bleeding after delivery, to complete an incomplete abortion, and to promote milk ejection during lactation.

Another class of oxytocic agents are the prostaglandins, natural hormones involved in regulating the muscles of the uterus, referred to as the myometrium. These hormones cause very potent contractions of the myometrium and may be responsible for the natural induction of labor. When the prostaglandin concentrations increase during the final few weeks of pregnancy, this stimulates mild myometrial contractions, commonly known as *Braxton Hicks contractions.* The prostaglandins may be used therapeutically to induce labor and enhance uterine muscle tone. They may also be used to stimulate the myometrium to induce abortion during the second trimester when the uterus is resistant to oxytocin.

The third class of oxytocic agents are the ergot alkaloids, which are also potent simulators of uterine muscle. These agents increase the force and frequency of uterine contractions and are used after delivery of the infant and placenta to prevent postpartum uterine atony and hemorrhage.

Mechanism of Action

The mechanisms of action of the various oxytocic agents vary depending on the agent. One common characteristic of all three classes of agents is that they stimulate uterine smooth muscle contraction. As previously noted, Pitocin is the synthetic form of oxytocin and has all the pharmacologic properties of the endog-

enously produced hormone. It indirectly stimulates contraction of uterine smooth muscle by increasing the sodium permeability of uterine myobrils. In the term uterus, oxytocin increases the amplitude and frequency of uterine contractions; decreases cervical activity, producing dilation; and impedes uterine blood flow. During lactation, oxytocin causes the cells surrounding the alveoli of the breast to contract, forcing milk from the alveoli into the larger ducts and thus facilitating milk ejection. Prostaglandins such as dinoprostone directly stimulate uterine and gastrointestinal smooth muscle. Like Pitocin, dinoprostone increases the frequency and amplitude of uterine contractions but the uterus is more responsive to it than to Pitocin in early pregnancy. This is why it may be used to induce abortion. Dinoprostone-induced uterine contractions are usually sufficient to cause evacuation of both the fetus and the placenta. It also produces cervical dilation and softening. The ergot alkaloids, such as ergonovine and methylergonovine are pharmacologically similar; both directly stimulate contractions of uterine and vascular smooth muscle. In large doses they elicit sustained, forceful contractions of the uterus. Like the other two classes of oxytocic drugs the ergot alkaloids also increase the amplitude and frequency of uterine contractions and uterine tone, which together impedes uterine blood flow. Ergonovine and methylergonovine also increase contractions of the cervix.

Drug Effects

The drug effects of the oxytocic agents are primarily limited to the uterine smooth muscle. The drug effects other than those on the uterus vary depending on the agent. Pitocin stimulates the smooth muscle of the uterus, causing uterine contraction and decreased uterine blood flow. It also facilitates milk ejection and may also produce vasodilation of vascular smooth muscle, thereby increasing renal, coronary, and cerebral blood flow. However, an initial decrease in blood pressure it may produce is usually followed by a small but sustained increase in blood pressure. Prostaglandins such as dinoprostone directly stimulate uterine and gastrointestinal smooth muscle. Its effects on the uterus are similar to those of oxytocin, but it has the unique feature of being able to stimulate the uterine smooth muscle prior to full gestation. This makes it useful in abortions. Dinoprostone may also stimulate the circular smooth muscle of the gastrointestinal tract and increase GI motility. When inhaled, dinoprostone causes bronchodilation. It may also cause increases in body temperature. The ergot alkaloids such as ergonovine and methylergonovine directly stimulate contractions of uterine and vascular smooth muscle and produce vasoconstriction. This vasoconstriction causes increases in the central venous pressure, blood pressure, and rarely peripheral ischemia, resulting in gangrene.

Therapeutic Uses

The therapeutic uses of the oxytocic agents vary depending on the particular agent. Pitocin is commonly used to induce labor in near-term or term pregnancies, to augment labor and promote contractions if labor is prolonged, to promote expulsion of the placenta and control uterine bleeding postpartum, to facilitate the completion of incomplete abortions after prostaglandin induction of the abortion, to promote milk ejection when the milk supply is inadequate, and to reduce postpartum breast engorgement. Prostaglandins such as dinoprostone are administered intravaginally to induce abortion during the second trimester (beyond the twelfth week of gestation). Dinoprostone cervical gel may also be used to improve cervical inducibility (cervical "ripening") near or at term in women with a medical or obstetric need for labor induction. This agent prepares the cervix for the induction of labor and makes the process easier. Intranasally administered dinoprostone may also be used to dilate the bronchi in patients with bronchial asthma, but its effects in this setting have been inconsistent, thus limiting its use for this purpose. Ergot alkaloids such as ergonovine and methylergonovine are primarily used for the prevention and treatment of postpartum and postabortion hemorrhage caused by uterine atony or subinvolution.

Side Effects and Adverse Effects

The most common undesirable effects of dinoprostone, ergonovine, methylergonovine, and oxytocin are listed in Table 28-4.

Interactions

There are few clinically significant drug interactions that occur with the oxytocic agents. The most common and important of these involve sympathomimetic drugs. The combination of drugs that produce vasoconstriction, such as sympathomimetics, with the oxytocic agents can result in severe hypertension.

Dosages

For the recommended dosages of selected oxytocic agents, see the dosages table on p. 434.

Table 28-4	Oxytocic Agents: Most Common Adverse Effects	
BODY SYSTEM	**SIDE/ADVERSE EFFECTS**
Central nervous system	Headache, dizziness, fainting
Cardiovascular	Hypotension or hypertension, chest pain
Gastrointestinal	Nausea, vomiting, diarrhea
Genitourinary	Vaginitis, vaginal pain, cramping
Other	Leg cramps, joint swelling, chills, fever, weakness, blurred vision

DRUG PROFILES

DINOPROSTONE

Dinoprostone (Prostin E2) is a synthetic derivative of the naturally occurring hormone prostaglandin E_2. The use of dinoprostone is contraindicated in the following settings: hypersensitivity, uterine fibrosis, cervical stenosis, pelvic inflammatory disease, and respiratory disease. It is also contraindicated in patients who have undergone pelvic operations. It is available only as a 20-mg vaginal suppository. Commonly recommended dosages are given in the dosages table on p. 434. Pregnancy category C.

PHARMACOKINETICS

HALF-LIFE	ONSET	PEAK	DURATION
Gel			
N/A	Rapid	30-45 min	Unavailable
Suppository (vaginal)			
N/A	10 min	Unavailable	2-3 hr

ERGONOVINE AND METHYLERGONOVINE

The ergot alkaloids ergonovine (Ergotrate) and methylergonovine (Methergine) are pharmacologically similar. Their use is contraindicated in patients with a known hypersensitivity to ergot medications and in those with pelvic inflammatory disease. They also should not be used to augment labor, before delivery of the placenta, or during a spontaneous abortion. Methylergonovine is available orally as 0.2-mg tablets and is a pregnancy category C agent. It is also available parenterally as a 0.2-mg/ml injection. Ergonovine is no longer being produced by the manufacturer and is a pregnancy category X agent. Commonly recommended dosages are given in the dosages table below.

☙ P H A R M A C O K I N E T I C S

HALF-LIFE	ONSET	PEAK	DURATION
<2 hr	PO: 5-15 min	30 min	3 hr
	IM: <5min		

OXYTOCIN

Pitocin (Syntocinon) is the synthetic form of the endogenous hormone oxytocin and has all of its pharmacologic properties. Oxytocin is contraindicated in patients with a history of hypersensitivity to the drug. Use of the nasal spray is contraindicated during pregnancy. Commonly recommended dosages are given in the dosages table below.

☙ P H A R M A C O K I N E T I C S

HALF-LIFE	ONSET	PEAK	DURATION
3-5 min	IV: Immediate	IV: Immediate	IV: <1 hr
	IM: <5 min	IM: Immediate	IM: 2-3 hr

UTERINE RELAXANTS

When contractions of the uterus begin before term, it may be desirable to stop labor, because premature birth, or labor before term, can have many detrimental effects, death of the neonate being the most serious consequence. Postponing delivery by relaxating the uterine smooth muscles and helping prevent contractions and the induction of labor increases the likelihood of the infant's survival. However, this measure is generally only employed after the twentieth week of gestation because spontaneous labor occurring before the twentieth week is frequently associated with a defective fetus and thus is usually not interrupted. Only uterine contractions occurring between about 20 and 37 weeks of gestation are considered premature labor.

The nonpharmacologic treatment of premature la-

D O S A G E S

SELECTED UTERINE STIMULANTS

AGENT	PHARMACOLOGIC CLASS	DOSAGE RANGE	PURPOSE
Dinoprostone (Prostin E2)	Prostaglandin E$_2$ oxytoxic (abortifacient)	*Adult* Vaginal: Insert one suppository (20 mg) q3-5h until abortion occurs	Abortion induction
Methylergonovine (Methergine)	Oxytoxic ergot alkaloid	*Adult* PO: 0.2-0.4 mg q6-12h for 2-7 days IM: 0.2 mg after delivery of placenta and repeated q2-4h prn for a total of 5 doses IV: Reserved for excessive bleeding; dosage the same as for IM route	Postpartum uterine atony and hemorrhage
Oxytocin (Pitocin, Syntocinon)	Oxytoxic hypothalamic hormone	*Adult* IV: Infusion rate 1-2 mU/min; can be increased slowly until contractions reach desired rate/intensity	Labor induction
		IV: 10-40 U in 1000 ml infused at a rate sufficient to control uterine atony IM: 3-10 U after delivery of placenta	Postpartum uterine atony and hemorrhage
		Intranasal spray: 1 spray in one/both nostrils 2-3 min before nursing/pumping breast	Assist postpartum milk ejection

bor includes bed rest, sedation, and hydration. Drugs given to inhibit labor and maintain the pregnancy are called tocolytics, the three most commonly used ones being ritodrine, terbutaline, and magnesium sulfate. Terbutaline and ritodrine are classified as beta-adrenergic agents (see Chapter 15) and work by directly relaxing uterine smooth muscle. Magnesium sulfate is most commonly used as an anticonvulsant in the treatment of pregnancy-induced hypertension (preeclampsia), but it is also an effective tocolytic agent.

Mechanism of Action

One common characteristic of all three tocolytics is that they relax uterine smooth muscle and stop the uterus from contracting. As just mentioned terbutaline and ritodrine work by directly relaxing uterine smooth muscle and they do so by stimulating beta-adrenergic receptors located on the bronchial tree, peripheral vasculature, and uterine smooth muscles. These are believed to be primarily beta$_2$-adrenergic receptors. (The beta$_1$-adrenergic receptors are located on the heart and are not stimulated by terbutaline or ritodrine except at high doses.)

Drug Effects

The drug effects of terbutaline and ritodrine are related to their beta-adrenergic effects. When the bronchial beta-adrenergic receptors are stimulated by these beta agonists, the bronchi dilate and airway resistance decreases. When the beta-adrenergic receptors of the peripheral vasculature are stimulated by these beta agonists, these blood vessels dilate and blood pressure decreases. Finally, when the beta-adrenergic receptors located on the uterine smooth muscle are stimulated by the beta agonists terbutaline and ritodrine, the uterine smooth muscle relaxes, thus stopping premature contractions.

Therapeutic Uses

Both terbutaline and ritodrine are used to inhibit uterine contractions in preterm labor, but this is generally done only after the twentieth week of gestation, because, as previously noted, spontaneous labor before the twentieth week is frequently associated with a defective fetus and therefore is usually not interrupted. Terbutaline may also be used as a bronchodilator in the symptomatic treatment of bronchial asthma and reversible bronchospasm.

Side Effects and Adverse Effects

The most common adverse effects of terbutaline and ritodrine are listed in Table 28-5.

Toxicity and Management of Overdose

The toxicity stemming from an overdose of oxolytics and its management are similar to those of the other adrenergic agents and are discussed in Chapter 15.

Interactions

For information on the drugs that interact with the tocolytic agents, see Table 28-6.

Dosages

For the recommended dosages of ritodrine and terbutaline, see the dosages table on the following page.

Table 28-5	Tocolytic Agents: Most Common Adverse Effects
BODY SYSTEM	**SIDE/ADVERSE EFFECTS**
Central nervous system	Tremors, anxiety, insomnia, headache, dizziness, nervousness
Cardiovascular	Palpitations, tachycardia, hypertension, dysrhythmias, altered maternal and fetal heart rate and blood pressure, chest pain
Gastrointestinal	Nausea, vomiting, anorexia, bloating, constipation, diarrhea
Metabolic	Hyperglycemia, hypokalemia
Other	Rash, dyspnea, hyperventilation, glycosuria, lactic acidosis

Table 28-6	Drug Interactions: Uterine Relaxants	
DRUG	**MECHANISM**	**RESULT**
Sympathomimetic agents	Additive	Additive cardiovascular effects
Beta-blockers	Antagonism	Increased effects of uterine relaxants

DOSAGES

SELECTED UTERINE RELAXANTS

AGENT	PHARMACOLOGIC CLASS	DOSAGE RANGE	PURPOSE
Ritodrine (Yutopar)	Beta adrenergic	*Adult* Starting IV infusion dose, 50-100 μg/min; usual effective dose, 150-350 μg/min	Management of preterm labor
Terbutaline sulfate (Brethine, Bricanyl)	Beta adrenergic	*Adult* 10 μg/min to a maximum of 80 μg/min IV if needed; 2.5 mg po q4-6h for maintenance	Unlabeled management of preterm labor

DRUG PROFILES

Ritodrine and terbutaline are contraindicated in the following settings: hypersensitivity, eclampsia, hypertension, dysrhythmias, thyrotoxicosis, before the twentieth week of pregnancy, antepartum hemorrhage, intrauterine fetal death, maternal cardiac disease, pulmonary hypertension, and uncontrolled diabetes.

RITODRINE

Ritodrine (Yutopar) is indicated for the prevention of preterm labor. Parenterally it comes as a 10- and 15-mg/ml injection for intravenous infusion, and orally it comes as a 10-mg tablet. Commonly recommended dosages are given in the dosages table above. Pregnancy category B.

▼ PHARMACOKINETICS

HALF-LIFE	ONSET	PEAK	DURATION
IM/IV: 2-3 hr	IM: <15 min	IM: 20-40 min	IM: Unknown
PO: 2 hr	PO: <1 hr	PO: 30-60 min	PO: Unknown

TERBUTALINE

Terbutaline (Brethine, Bricanyl) is indicated for the prevention of preterm labor and may also be used as a bronchodilator in the symptomatic treatment of bronchial asthma and occasionally in the treatment of hyperkalemia. It is available parenterally as a 1-mg/ml injection for subcutaneous administration and orally as a 2.5- and 5-mg tablet. It is also available as a 200-μg/metered spray for oral inhalation. Commonly recommended dosages are given in the dosages table above. Pregnancy category B.

▼ PHARMACOKINETICS

HALF-LIFE	ONSET	PEAK	DURATION
PO: 20 hr	PO: 30-45 min	PO: 1-2 hr	PO: 6-8 hr
IV: 20 hr	IV: 5 min	IV: 30-60 min	IV: 1.5-4 hr

Fertility Agents

Loss of fertility in women occurs for various reasons, and some of these disorders are amenable to treatment with fertility agents. These agents are bromocriptine, clomiphene, gonadorelin, chorionic gonadotropin, menotropins, and urofollitrophin.

In cases of infertility in which the hypophysis (pituitary gland) and the ovaries are normal but the stimulus that activates follicular development is absent, clomiphene can stimulate the hypothalamus and thus the ovaries to develop ovarian follicles. In women who are infertile because they cannot supply sufficient gonadotropins to properly stimulate the ovary, the hypophysis or pituitary is usually dysfunctional. Menotropins, gonadorelin, chorionic gonadotropin, and urofollitrophin may be useful in treating this form of infertility because they stimulate the release of follicle-stimulating hormone (FSH) and luteinizing hormone (LH). Chorionic gonadotropin and gonadorelin are used when primarily LH release must be stimulated.

Mechanism of Action

The mechanism of action of the various fertility agents varies depending on the agent.

Chorionic gonadotropin and gonadorelin have the principal pharmacologic effects of human chorionic gonadotropin (hCG). In fact, gonadorelin has the same amino acid sequence as hCG. The pharmacologic effects and mechanisms of action of the two agents are identical to those of LH. They may also have a minimal effect on FSH. During the normal menstrual cycle, LH and FSH are responsible for stimulating the development and maturation of the normal ovarian follicle. The abrupt midcycle increase in the LH concentration triggers ovulation. Because gonadotropin and gonadorelin can substitute for LH in this function, they can cause ovulation as well.

Menotropins and urofollitrophins have pharmacologic effects similar to those of FSH, which stimulates the development and maturation of the ovarian follicle. They also have properties similar to those of LH, which causes ovulation and stimulates the development of the **corpus luteum**. The administration of menotropins for 9 to 12 consecutive days stimulates ovarian follicular growth and maturation in women whose infertility is not due to primary ovarian failure. To induce ovulation, a single, large dose of gonadotropin, which has LH activity, is then given when the clinical assessment shows that sufficient follicular maturation has occurred.

Clomiphene appears to stimulate the release of FSH and LH, which results in the development and maturation of the ovarian follicle, induces ovulation, and causes the subsequent development and function of the corpus luteum. Gonadotropin release may result either from direct stimulation of the hypothalamic-pituitary axis or from a decreased inhibitory influence of estrogens on the hypothalamic-pituitary axis, the latter occurring because of the competing influence of the endogenous estrogens from the uterus, pituitary, or hypothalamus. Clomiphene may also directly affect the biosynthesis of ovarian hormones.

Drug Effects

The drug effects of the ovulation stimulants, or fertility agents, are primarily the same as the effects of FSH and LH. By manipulating these drugs in various ways, they can be made to mimic these hormones' natural effects. They may also stimulate spermatogenesis in men.

Therapeutic Uses

The ovulation stimulants are primarily used in the treatment of female infertility. Clomiphene is used chiefly to induce ovulation in women who do not ovulate but want to get pregnant. It is also used in the treatment of other disorders, ranging from menstrual abnormalities to gynecomastia to fibrocystic disease of the breast. Gonadotropin and gonadorelin are customarily used in conjunction with menotropins in the treatment of infertility. Their action is almost identical to that of pituitary LH and they may also have slight FSH activity. In addition, they may be used in men for the treatment of various conditions such as prepubertal cryptorchidism and hypogonadotropic hypogonadism. Menotropins is used to induce ovulation in women who do not ovulate. It also stimulates spermatogenesis in men. Urofollitrophin is pharmacologically similar to menotropins and therefore has similar therapeutic effects.

Side Effects and Adverse Effects

The most common adverse effects of the ovulation stimulants are listed in Table 28-7. Some of the agents may cause more and some fewer undesirable effects.

Table 28-7	Fertility Agents: Most Common Adverse Effects
BODY SYSTEM	**SIDE/ADVERSE EFFECTS**
Central nervous system	Dizziness, headache, flushing, depression, restlessness, anxiety, nervousness, fatigue, fever
Cardiovascular	Tachycardia, phlebitis, deep vein thrombosis, hypovolemia
Gastrointestinal	Nausea, bloating, constipation, abdominal pain, vomiting, anorexia
Other	Urticaria, ovarian hyperstimulation, multiple pregnancies, blurred vision, diplopia, photophobia, breast pain

Interactions

For information about drugs that interact with the fertility agents, see Table 28-8.

Dosages

For recommended dosages of the fertility agents, see the dosages table below.

Table 28-8	Drug Interactions: Fertility Agents	
DRUG	**MECHANISM**	**RESULT**
Tricyclic antidepressants, butyrophenones, methyldopa, phenothiazines, and reserpine	Antagonism	Increase prolactin concentrations while bromocriptine is trying to reduce them
Antihypertensives	Additive	Additive hypotensive effects when taken with bromocriptine

DOSAGES

SELECTED FERTILITY AGENTS

AGENT	PHARMACOLOGIC CLASS	DOSAGE RANGE	PURPOSE
⬇Clomiphene (Clomid, Serophene)	Ovulation stimulant	*Women* PO: 50 mg/day for 5 days. If ovulation does not occur, a second course of 100 mg/day for 5 days and a third and final course of 100 mg/day for 5 days can be administered.	Female infertility in selected patients
Chorionic gonadotropin (A.P.L., Follutein, Chorex-5, Gonic, Pregryl, Profasi HP)	Gonotropin (placental) ovulation stimulant	*Adult* IM: 4000 USP units 3 times/wk for 3 wk	Prepubertal cryptorchidism
		IM: 500-1000 USP units 3 times/wk for 3 wk followed by same dose 2/wk for 3 wk	Hypogonadotropic hypogonadism
		IM: 5000-10,000 USP units given 1 day after the last dose of menotropins	Female infertility
Menotropins (Pergonal)	Gonadotropins (FSH/LH) ovulation stimulant	*Women* IM: 1 ampule (75 IU of FSH/LH) for 9-12 days followed by 5000-10,000 U of hCG 1 day after the last dose of menotropins. Repeat course if required with 1 ampule of 150 IU of FSH/LH for 9-12 days followed by 10,000 U of hCG. A third and final course may be required.	Female infertility
		Men IM: after pretreatment with hCG, administer 1 ampule (75 IU of FSH/LH) 3 times/wk with 2000 U of hCG 2 times/wk for at least 6 mo.	Male infertility

DRUG PROFILES

⚓ CLOMIPHENE

Clomiphene (Clomid, Serophene) is primarily used to stimulate the production of pituitary gonadotropins, which in turn induces the maturation of the ovarian follicle and eventually ovulation. It is contraindicated in women with a known hypersensitivity to it and in those with hepatic disease or undiagnosed vaginal bleeding. It is classified as a pregnancy category X agent and is available as a 50-mg oral tablet. Commonly recommended dosages are given in the dosages table on page 438.

⬡ PHARMACOKINETICS

HALF-LIFE	ONSET	PEAK	DURATION
5 days	4-12 days	Unknown	1 mo

CHORIONIC GONADOTROPIN

Chorionic Gonadotropin (A.P.L., Chorex-5, Follutein, Gonic, Pregnyl, Profasi HP) is a hormone that is normally secreted by the placenta, and its principal pharmacologic effects are the same as hCG's. It is classified as a pregnancy category B agent and is contraindicated in patients with a known hypersensitivity to it, in patients with ovarian cysts or hormonally dependent tumors, and in those with anovulation stemming from causes other than those of hypothalamic origin. It only comes parenterally as 5,000-, 10,000-, and 20,000-unit injections. Commonly recommended dosages are given in the preceding dosages table.

⬡ PHARMACOKINETICS

HALF-LIFE	ONSET	PEAK	DURATION
5.6 hr	2 hr	6 hr	36 hr

MENOTROPINS

Menotropins (Pergonal) is a purified preparation of gonadotropins extracted from the urine of postmenopausal women. It is classified as a pregnancy category C agent and is contraindicated in the settings of primary ovarian failure, abnormal bleeding, thyroid or adrenal dysfunction, an organic intracranial lesion, ovarian cysts, and primary testicular failure. It only

comes as a parenteral injection in the following potencies: 75 IU of FSH activity with 75 IU of LH activity or 150 IU of FSH activity with 150 IU of LH activity. Commonly recommended dosages are given in the preceding dosages table.

⬡ PHARMACOKINETICS

HALF-LIFE	ONSET	PEAK	DURATION
Unknown	Unknown	Unknown	Unknown

NURSING PROCESS

ASSESSMENT

Before administering estrogen or progesterone agents, the nurse should determine whether the patient has any contraindications to its use. These include a history of breast cancer, thromboembolic disorders, malignancies of the reproductive tract, or abnormal vaginal bleeding. They also should not be used in breast-feeding or pregnant women. Cautious use of the estrogens and progestins is called for in patients with hypertension, asthma, blood dyscrasias, diabetes, headaches, congestive heart failure, depressive disorders, seizure

CULTURAL IMPLICATIONS
Premature Birth

Because the childbearing experience is influenced by one's culture, it is important to understand and appreciate other cultures' views of the birthing experience. Many Haitian people are Catholic, but also participate in the practices of voodoo, a religion of African origin. In voodoo, the spirits are believed to be angels who have rebelled against God and are thought to have great powers and to provide favors related to protection, health, and wealth. Those persons practicing voodoo also believe their illnesses are a result of an evil spirit, which may result in their bypassing western health services. In the case of pregnancy, a premature birth may be seen as evil and health services therefore not be obtained.

From Corrine L et al: The unheard voices of women: spiritual interventions in maternal child health, *MCN* 17(3): 141, 1992.

CULTURAL IMPLICATIONS

Is Racial-Ethnic Status, Socioeconomic Status, or Geographic Access a Consideration in Choice of Obstetrician?

Pregnant women with obstetric risks who live in rural areas are far more likely to initiate care with family practitioners than with obstetricians. As stated by the research of Sharon Dobie of the University of Washington, this choice probably has more to do with socioeconomics, insurance coverage, and geographic access than with rational planning. On average, she found that rural pregnant women are poorer and younger than their urban counterparts, and are more likely to be covered by Medicaid, have limited mobility, and be reluctant to travel long distances for prenatal care, even if referred to an obstetrician. It was also found in this study that women seeking care from rural family physicians were most likely to be uninsured (12.5% of 14,281 patients) and more likely than their urban women counterparts to begin prenatal care late in pregnancy, and have a documented history of alcohol or substance abuse, both of which are pregnancy risk factors.

From Dobie SA et al: Do women choose their obstetric providers based on risks at entry into prenatal care? *Obstet Gynecol* 84(4): 557, 1994.

disorders, liver disease, renal disease, or a family history of breast or reproductive tract cancer.

The patient's baseline blood pressure, weight, blood glucose levels, liver function, and urinary output should also be determined and documented. Drug allergies and any prescription and nonprescription drugs being used should also be recorded. Drugs that interact with estrogens include anticoagulants, oral antidiabetic agents, tricyclic antidepressants, anticonvulsants, barbiturates, and steroids. Drugs that interact with progestins include anticoagulants, oral antidiabetic agents, tricyclic antidepressants, anticonvulsants, barbiturates, and steroids.

Before administering uterine stimulants such as oxytocin and prostaglandins, the nurse should determine and document the patient's blood pressure, pulse, and respiration. The fetal heart rate and contraction fetal heart rate should also be determined and recorded. The same considerations apply to the ergot alkaloids, with assessment of the patient being particularly critical because these agents are most often used for the prevention and control of postpartum and postabortion hemorrhage. The most notable drug interaction that occurs is that resulting from their concurrent use with sympathomimetic drugs, which can precipitate severe hypertension.

As previously mentioned, uterine relaxants such as ritodrine, terbutaline, and magnesium sulfate should only be used in women presenting in premature labor who are in their twentieth to thirty-seventh week of gestation. Cautious administration is recommended in any patient receiving them, but especially in women who have other complications of pregnancy or any condition such as seizures, hypertension, diabetes, a cardiac dysrhythmia, angina, or hypokalemia. Contraindications to their use include allergies, eclampsia, hypertension, thyrotoxicosis, antepartum hemorrhage, intrauterine fetal death, and other conditions listed earlier in this chapter. Testing of reflexes and a head-to-toe neurologic assessment are also necessary before magnesium sulfate therapy is initiated.

Before any of the fertility agents are administered, it is important to determine whether there are any contraindications to their use and to identify any cautions. Contraindications include allergies, pregnancy, liver disease, and undiagnosed vaginal bleeding. Cautious use is recommended in patients with hypertension, seizure disorders, or diabetes mellitus. The drug interactions are presented in Table 28-8.

NURSING DIAGNOSES

Nursing diagnoses in patients receiving estrogens or progestins include:
- Altered body image related to physiologic or pathologic effects stemming from changes in the female hormone levels.
- Knowledge deficit related to first-time therapy.

Nursing diagnoses in patients receiving drugs to promote labor and delivery include:
- Pain related to pain and delivery and associated abnormalities.
- Altered body image related to abnormal pregnancy or associated complications.
- Anxiety concerning possible fetal death or the complications of labor and pregnancy.
- Knowledge deficit related to unknown events and outcome of pregnancy.

Nursing diagnoses related to the use of fertility drugs include:
- Altered self-image related to inability to conceive.
- Anxiety related to unknown effects of treatment.
- Knowledge deficit related to the new treatment.

PLANNING

Goals in patients receiving drugs for the treatment of various disorders and conditions of the female reproductive tract include:

- Patient will be free of body image disturbances.
- Patient will state the rationale for hormonal replacement, uterine relaxants, or fertility drugs.
- Patient will state the side effects of specific medications.
- Patient will state the importance of compliance with hormonal therapy and other recommended pharmacologic and nonpharmacologic measures for the treatment of premature labor, preeclampsia, or fertility disorders.

Outcome Criteria

Outcome criteria in patients receiving agents used to treat various disorders and conditions of the female reproductive tract include:

- Patient will openly verbalize her concerns, fears, and anxieties with staff about body image changes.
- Patient will be compliant with pharmacologic and nonpharmacologic therapy with successful management of infertility, preeclampsia, premature labor, or experience effective birth control.
- Patient will be free of complications and disturbing side effects associated with each group of drugs, such as chest pain, leg pain, blurred vision.
- Patient returns for regular follow-up visits with physician to monitor therapeutic and adverse effects of treatment.

IMPLEMENTATION

Both estrogens and progestins should be administered in the lowest doses possible and then the doses titrated as needed. Intramuscular doses should be given deep in large muscle masses and the injection sites rotated. Oral forms should be taken with food or milk to minimize GI upset. Patient teaching tips are given in the box above right.

Ritodrine should be administered using an IV infusion pump or orally, as ordered. Only clear parenteral solutions should be used and administered only after accurate dilutions have been mixed in such solutions as 5% dextrose in water or normal saline. Generally they should only be infused at a rate of 0.3 mg/min, with a dilution of 150 mg/500 ml given at a rate of 0.1 mg/min, or as ordered. The patient should be positioned in the left lateral recumbent position to minimize hypotension and increase renal blood flow.

Oxytocin should only be administered using an IV infusion pump and only after dilution in 5% dextrose in water or 0.9% normal saline and given at a rate of 20 to 40 mU/min, or as ordered, for completing an incomplete abortion; at no greater than 20 mU/min for stimulating labor; and at 20 to 40 mU/min for controlling postpartum bleeding. A crash cart should be

Patient Teaching TIPS

Estrogens and Progestins

✔ Patients should take oral forms of hormones with food or milk to minimize GI upset.

✔ Patients should perform regular breast exams and report any unusual lumps or bumps.

✔ Patients should report chest pain, leg pain, blurred vision, headache, neck stiffness and pain, edema, yellow discoloration of the skin or sclera, clay-colored stools, and vaginal bleeding.

✔ Breast-feeding is not recommended in patients on estrogen therapy.

✔ Patients should report any weight gain of more than 5 pounds (2.25 kg) in a week.

✔ While on estrogen therapy, patients should avoid sunlight or wear sunscreen because these agents make the skin more susceptible to sunburn.

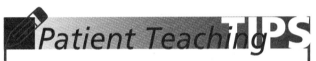

Patient Teaching TIPS

Uterine Stimulants

✔ Specific instructions for the use of oxytocin should be reviewed for patients administering it intranasally. They should be told to blow their nose, sit upright, hold the container upright, insert it into the nostril, and squeeze it during inspiration.

✔ The physician should be notified immediately by the patient if she begins to experience excessively strong contractions, edema or other symptoms of water intoxication, palpitations, chest pain, or changes in fetal movement.

✔ Patients should receive explicit instructions regarding the self-administration of these drugs.

kept on the unit and magnesium sulfate should be kept at the patient's bedside.

Fertility agents such as clomiphene are often self-administered. Specific instructions regarding their administration at home and the way to monitor drug effectiveness is very important to enhancing the success of treatment.

Teaching tips for patients receiving uterine stimulants, uterine relaxants, and fertility agents are presented in the boxes above and on the next page.

Patient Teaching TIPS

Uterine Relaxants

✔ Patients should understand the rationale for treatment with a uterine relaxant.

✔ Patients should understand the need for complying with other aspects of treatment such as bed rest while experiencing premature onset of labor (POL).

✔ Tell the patient that the oral preparation of ritodrine is often used as a form of maintenance treatment, if needed.

✔ It is important for patients on maintenance ritodrine therapy to understand the importance of regular monitoring of the blood glucose and electrolyte levels.

✔ Patients should report any increase in the intensity, duration, or frequency of their contractions as well as palpitations, anxiety, shortness of breath, vomiting, dizziness, or tachycardia to the nurse or physician.

✔ Any loss of fetal movement should be immediately reported to the physician or nurse.

Patient Teaching TIPS

Fertility Agents

✔ Patients should keep a journal of all medications, body changes and any other changes, their emotional and physical status, and any related signs and symptoms.

✔ It is important to emphasize the importance of regular follow-up visits to the physician in patients undergoing treatment for infertility.

✔ Make sure patients understand all instructions regarding the treatment regimen and the medication (use, dose, route, timing, side effects, drug interactions, and so on), because this is critical to ensuring compliance and safe self-administration.

✔ Teach patients how to monitor for the therapeutic effects and side effects.

EVALUATION

Therapeutic responses to estrogens include the disappearance of menopausal symptoms, absence of breast engorgement, and a decrease in the size of prostatic tumors. The side effects of estrogens include thromboembolism, edema, jaundice, abnormal vaginal bleeding, hyperglycemia, nausea, vomiting, increased appetite, and weight gain.

Therapeutic responses to progestins include a decrease in abnormal uterine bleeding and disappearance of menstrual disorders such as amenorrhea. The side effects of progestins include edema, hypertension, cardiac symptoms, depression, changes in mood and affect, and jaundice.

Therapeutic effects of oxytocin and other uterine stimulants include stimulation of labor and control of postpartum bleeding. Adverse reactions include changes in vital signs with bradycardia, dysrhythmias and premature ventricular contractions, severe abdominal pain and shocklike symptoms with a decrease in blood pressure, and increased pulse. All of these indicate possible uterine rupture and fetal distress. The

patient should also be closely monitored for the occurrence of acceleration or deceleration as well as for the signs and symptoms of water intoxication. In addition, the physician should be notified if contractions last longer than 1 minute or do not occur.

The primary therapeutic effect of the uterine relaxants is the absence of preterm labor. Adverse maternal effects to monitor for include palpitations, nausea, vomiting, headache, jitteriness, tremors, chest pain, cardiac dysrhythmias, and anxiety. Adverse neonatal effects include hypoglycemia, ileus, hypotension, and hypocalcemia. Both maternal and fetal heart rates as well as the maternal blood pressure should be closely monitored either as set out in the institutional policy and procedure manual or as ordered by the physician, or as the needs of the patient dictate. Nursing actions in the latter instance should be documented in the nurses' notes on the patient. The IV fluid rate and volume must also be closely monitored so that fluid volume overload is not allowed to occur.

The therapeutic effect of fertility agents would be the successful fertilization of an ovum and resultant pregnancy. Adverse reactions to monitor for in patients receiving these agents include hot flashes, abdominal discomfort, blurred vision, GI upset, nervousness, depression, weight gain, and hair loss. Multiple births and birth defects are other possible consequences of therapy.

TAKE HOME POINTS

Menstrual Cycle

- First menses or menstrual cycle is called *menarche,* which then occurs once a month until it ceases with menopause.
- Consists of three phases: menstrual phase (1st), follicular phase (2nd), and luteal phase (3rd).
- Follicular phase associated with high levels of estrogen.
- Luteal phase associated with high levels of progesterone.

Estrogens

- Three major estrogens are synthesized in the ovaries: estradiol (principal estrogen), estrone, and estriol.
- Exogenous estrogens can be broken down into two main groups: steroidal estrogens (e.g., conjugated estrogens, esterified estrogens, estradiol) and nonsteroidal estrogens (e.g., chlorotrianisene, dienestrol, diethylstilbestrol).
- Work by binding to and interacting with the estrogen receptors, increasing the synthesis of DNA and RNA.
- Ethinyl estradiol is a semisynthetic steroidal estrogen and the most orally active estrogenic drug.

Progestins

- Progesterone is a hormone secreted by the corpus luteum.
- Progesterone is the principal natural progestational hormone.
- Chemical derivatives of progesterone are called *progestins.*
- Have a variety of uses: uterine bleeding, amenorrhea, adjunctive and palliative treatment of some cancers, and others.

Oral Contraceptives

- Most effective form of birth control currently available.
- Combinations of both estrogenic and progestinic steroids.

Labor and Delivery Drugs

- Uterine stimulants = ergot derivatives, prostaglandins, and oxytocin.
- Uterine stimulants are sometimes called *oxytocic agents.*
- Uterine relaxants = used to stop preterm labor and maintain pregnancy by stopping uterine contractions.
- Uterine relaxants are sometimes called *tocolytics.*

Nursing Considerations

- A thorough nursing assessment is necessary to ensure the safe and effective use of female reproductive agents, including information on the patient's past medical problems, history of menses and problems with menstrual cycle, medications taken (prescribed and over-the-counter), the number of pregnancies and miscarriages, the last menstrual period, and any related surgical or medical treatments.
- Patient education should focus on the medication therapy and its importance to the management of the specific disease or disorder and also on means to ensure a positive self-image and open communication.

Critical Thinking A C T I V I T I E S

1. K.T. has spent 14 hours in labor with her first pregnancy and has made little progress. She is becoming exhausted and the uterine contractions have decreased in strength. Oxytocin is ordered to be given at a rate of 1 mU/min. The normal concentration of oxytocin is 10 mU/ml. What rate (in milliliters per hour) should the infusion be run at to deliver 1 mU/min?

2. Why are oxytocics such as Pitocin and Ergotrate used to treat postpartum and postabortion bleeding caused by uterine relaxation and enlargement?

3. What is the primary mechanism by which oral contraceptives prevent pregnancy?

BIBLIOGRAPHY

Albanese J, Nutz P: *Mosby's 1995 nursing drug cards,* St Louis, 1995, Mosby.

Corrine L et al: The unheard voices of women: spiritual interventions in maternal child health, *MCN* 17(3): 141, 1992.

Johnson KB: *Harriet Lane handbook,* ed 13, St Louis, 1993, Mosby.

Keen JH: *Critical care and emergency drug reference,* St Louis, 1994, Mosby.

Knoben JE, Anderson PO: *Handbook of critical drug data,* ed 6, Hamilton, Ill, 1988, Drug Intelligence Publications.

Knowlden HA: The pill and cancer: a review of the literature, *J Adv Nurs* 15:1016, 1990.

McEvoy GK: *AHFS drug information,* Bethesda, Md, 1994, American Society of Hospital Pharmacists.

McKenry L, Salerno E: *Mosby's pharmacology in nursing,* ed 19, St Louis, 1995, Mosby.

McKeon VA: Estrogen replacement therapy: current guidelines for education and counseling, *J Gerontol Nurs* 16(10):6, 1990.

Skidmore-Roth L: *Mosby's 1995 nursing drug reference,* St Louis, 1995, Mosby.

Chapter 29

Male Reproductive Agents

Objectives

When you reach the end of this chapter, you will be able to:

1 List the disorders for which androgen treatment is indicated.

2 Discuss the normal anatomy and physiology of the male reproductive system.

3 List the various androgenic agents.

4 Explain the rationale for androgen treatment, give the dosages and side effects of the agents as well as the cautions and contraindications to their use, and name the drugs that interact with them.

5 Develop a comprehensive nursing care plan that includes outcomes and education for the patient receiving androgens.

6 Describe the therapeutic responses anticipated in patients receiving androgens.

CHAPTER OUTLINE

Male Reproductive System
Male Reproductive Agents
  Mechanism of action
  Drug effects
  Therapeutic uses
  Side effects and adverse effects
  Interactions
  Dosages
Drug Profiles
  ⚓ Danazol
  Finasteride
  Methyltestosterone
  Fluoxymesterone

Nursing Process
Assessment
Nursing Diagnoses
Planning
  Outcome criteria
Implementation
Evaluation

Glossary

Anabolic activity (ə nab′ ə lik) The activity produced by testosterone that causes the development of bone and muscle tissue. (p. 446)

Androgenic activity (an dro jen′ ik) The activity pro-duced by testosterone that causes the development and maintenance of the male reproductive system. (p. 446)

Androgens Male sex hormones responsible for me-diating the development and maintenance of male sex characteristics. (p. 446)

Benign prostatic hypertrophy Enlargement of the prostate gland. (p. 446)

Erythropoietic effect (ə rith′ ro poi et′ ik) Effect that stimulates the production of red blood cells. (p. 446)

Testosterone (təs tos′ tə rōn) The main androgenic hormone. (p. 446)

MALE REPRODUCTIVE SYSTEM

The male reproductive system consists of several struc-tures, the testes and seminiferous tubules being the im-portant ones from the standpoint of the discussion here. The testes are the male gonads, and they are a pair of oval glands that are located in the scrotal sac. They are the site of both reproductive (androgenic) and endocrine activity. The seminiferous tubules, which are channels in the testes, are the site of spermatogen-esis, which is the process by which mature sperm cells are produced.

The normal development and maintenance of the primary male sex characteristics (the normal male anatomy) as well as the secondary ones (the growth and maturation of the prostate, seminal vesicles, penis, and scrotum; the male hair distribution, such as the beard and pubic, chest, and axillary hair; laryngeal en-largement and the thickening of the vocal cords; and the alterations in body musculature and fat distribution) are mediated by the male sex hormones—the **androgens**—which must be secreted in adequate amounts for these characteristics to appear. One of the primary androgens is **testosterone.** It is produced from clusters of interstitial cells located between the seminiferous tubules. Besides its **androgenic activity,** testosterone is also involved in the development of bone and muscle tissue, the inhibition of protein catabolism (its breakdown), and the retention of nitrogen, phosphorus, potassium, and sodium. These constitute its **anabolic activity.** The hormone initiates the synthesis of specific proteins needed for androgenic and anabolic activity by binding to chromatin in the nucleus of interstitial cells. In addition, testosterone appears to have an **erythropoietic effect,** in that it stimulates the production of red blood cells.

MALE REPRODUCTIVE AGENTS

There are several synthetic derivatives of testosterone, and these were developed with the intention of improving on the pharmacokinetic and pharmacodynamic characteristics of the naturally occurring hormone. One way in which this was accomplished was by combining various esters with testosterone, with the result that the hormone's duration of action has been prolonged. For example, testosterone propionate is formulated in an oily solution and its hormonal effects last for 2 to 3 days; the effects of testosterone cypionate and testosterone enanthate in oil last even longer. They can be administered once every 2 to 4 weeks. Orally administered testosterone has very poor pharmacokinetic and pharmacodynamic characteristics because most of a dose of it is metabolized and destroyed by the liver before it can reach the circulation. To circumvent this problem, researchers developed methyltestosterone. Both the serum levels and effectiveness of buccally administered methyltestosterone are increased. Fluoxymesterone, another testosterone derivative, is effective when administered orally.

There are other chemical derivatives of the naturally occurring testosterone known as anabolic steroids. These are synthetic agents that closely resemble the natural hormone, but they possess high anabolic and low androgenic activity, unlike the androgens whose activity is more balanced. Anabolic steroids have a great potential for being misused by such people as athletes, especially body builders and weight lifters, because of their muscle-building properties. Improper use of these substances can have many serious consequences, and for this reason, the anabolic steroids are currently classified as controlled (schedule III) substances by the U.S. Drug Enforcement Administration. (This classification implies that misuse of the agent can lead to psychologic or physical dependence, or both.)

Androgen inhibitors are agents that block the effects of the naturally occurring (endogenous) androgens. The specific enzyme they inhibit is 5-alpha-reductase, and for this reason, they are called 5-alpha-reductase inhibitors. As previously mentioned, the androgens maintain secondary sex characteristics, one of which is the growth and maintenance of the prostate. When androgens are secreted in excessive amounts, the prostate enlarges, a condition known as **benign prostatic hypertrophy** (BPH) and one amenable to treatment with a 5-alpha-reductase inhibitor. Currently, however, the only such agent available is finasteride.

The currently available natural and synthetic androgens, synthetic anabolic steroids, and androgen inhibitors are listed in the box below.

Mechanism of Action

Androgens such as testosterone stimulate the synthesis and activity of the building blocks of protein—RNA. The increased synthesis of protein aids in the formation and maintenance of muscular and skeletal proteins. Another potent anabolic, or building, effect of androgens is the retention of nitrogen, a substance essential for the manufacture of protein. They also promote the storage of inorganic phosphorus, sulfate, sodium, and potassium.

Finasteride works by inhibiting the enzymatic process responsible for converting testosterone to 5-alpha-dihydrotestosterone (DHT), which is the principal androgen responsible for stimulating prostatic growth. It can dramatically lower the prostatic DHT concentrations, thereby reducing the testosterone concentrations and causing the hypertrophied prostate to decrease in size.

Androgens, Anabolic Steroids, and Androgen Inhibitors: Available Agents

Androgens
⚓Danazol
Fluoxymesterone
Methyltestosterone
Testosterone

Anabolic Steroids
Nandrolone
Oxymetholone
Stanozolol

Androgen Inhibitors
Finasteride

Drug Effects

The natural and synthetic androgens as well as the synthetic anabolic steroids have effects similar to those of the endogenous androgens. These are the stimulation of the normal growth and development of the male sex organs (the primary sex characteristics) and the maintenance of the secondary sex characteristics. They also cause the retention of the substances (nitrogen, potassium, and phosphorus) needed for the building of proteins and retard the breakdown of amino acids. This may result in weight gain and an increase in musculature and strength. The administration of exogenous androgens causes the release of endogenous testosterone to be inhibited as the result of the feedback inhibition of pituitary luteinizing hormone. Large doses of exogenous androgens may also suppress sperm production as the result of the feedback inhibition of pituitary follicle-stimulating hormone. Androgens also stimulate the production of erythrocytes by promoting the production of erythropoietic stimulating factor.

The drug effects of finasteride are limited primarily to the prostate, but this agent may also affect 5-alpha-reductase processes elsewhere in the body, such as in the skin and liver. As just noted, inhibition of this enzyme system leads to a dramatic reduction in prostate size in men with BPH.

Therapeutic Uses

The therapeutic uses for the androgenic agents vary depending on the particular agent, and these uses are listed in the box below.

Side Effects and Adverse Effects

Although rare, some of the most devastating effects of the steroids occur in the liver, where they cause the formation of blood-filled cavities, a condition known as *peliosis of the liver*. This is a potential consequence of the long-term administration of androgenic anabolic steroids and can be life-threatening. Other serious hepatic effects are hepatic neoplasms, cholestatic hepatitis, jaundice, and abnormal liver function. Fluid retention is another undesirable effect of androgens and may account for some of the weight gain seen in persons taking them. All in all, the serious adverse effects that can be caused by the androgens far outweigh the advantages to be gained from their use in those seeking improved athletic ability.

Other less serious adverse effects of androgens are listed in Table 29-1.

Table 29-1	Androgens: Common Adverse Effects
BODY SYSTEM	**SIDE/ADVERSE EFFECT**
Endocrine	Acne, gynecomastia, amenorrhea, menstrual irregularities, and virilization (deepening of voice, hirsutism, and clitoral enlargement)
Hematologic	Polycythemia; suppression of clotting factors II, V, VII, X; increased serum cholesterol level
Central nervous system	Headache, anxiety, mental depression, generalized paresthesias
Other	Priapism or excessive sexual stimulation in males; male-pattern baldness; water retention, along with retention of sodium, chloride, potassium, and inorganic phosphates; stomatitis; hypercalcemia from osteolysis

---

Androgens and Androgen Inhibitors: Therapeutic Uses

ANDROGEN OR ANDROGEN INHIBITOR	THERAPEUTIC USE
↓Danazol	Endometriosis
↓Danazol	Fibrocystic breast disease
Fluoxymesterone and methyltestosterone	Inoperable breast cancer
Nandrolone	Metastatic breast cancer
Fluoxymesterone and methyltestosterone	Postpartum breast engorgement
Danazol and stanozolol	Hereditary angioedema
Oxymetholone	Various anemias
Fluoxymesterone and methyltestosterone	Male hypogonadism
Methyltestosterone	Postpubertal cryptorchidism
Finasteride	Benign prostatic hypertrophy

Interactions

Methyltestosterone when used with oral anticoagulants can significantly increase anticoagulant activity.

Dosages

For recommended dosages of the male reproductive agents, see the dosages table on the next page.

DRUG PROFILES

⚓ DANAZOL

Danazol (Danocrine) is a synthetic derivative of ethisterone that possesses weak androgenic activity. It is classified as a pregnancy category C agent, and its use is contraindicated in patients with significant cardiac, hepatic, or renal dysfunction and those with porphyria; in men with undiagnosed abnormal genital bleeding; and in pregnant or lactating women. Refer to the dosages table for the dosage information.

FINASTERIDE

Finasteride (Proscar) is contraindicated in patients who have shown a hypersensitivity to it and in pregnant women. It is classified as a pregnancy category X agent. Refer to the dosages table for dosage information.

⬡ PHARMACOKINETICS

HALF-LIFE	ONSET	PEAK	DURATION
4-15 hr*	Unknown	8 hr† 3-12 mo‡	Unknown

*Varies with age.
†To lower DHT concentrations.
‡To reduce prostate size.

METHYLTESTOSTERONE

Methyltestosterone (Android, Oreton-M) is contraindicated in patients with significant cardiac, hepatic, or renal dysfunction; pregnant or breast-feeding women; and men with breast carcinoma or known or suspected prostate cancer. It is a pregnancy category X agent.

Refer to the dosages table for the recommended dosages.

⬡ PHARMACOKINETICS

HALF-LIFE	ONSET	PEAK	DURATION
10-100 min	Unknown	1-2 hr (serum)	Unknown

FLUOXYMESTERONE

Fluoxymesterone (Halotestin) is a synthetic androgen hormone that is contraindicated in patients with significant cardiac, hepatic, or renal dysfunction; pregnant or breast-feeding women (pregnancy category X); and men with breast carcinoma or known or suspected prostate cancer. For recommended dosages, see the dosages table.

⬡ PHARMACOKINETICS

HALF-LIFE	ONSET	PEAK	DURATION
9.2 hr	Unknown	Unknown	Unknown

NURSING PROCESS

ASSESSMENT

Androgenic agents are used for the treatment of a variety of disorders and diseases, including malignancies. Before administering an androgenic agent to a patient, however, the nurse should first find out the purpose for its use in the patient. Contraindications to the use of testosterone and related products include an allergy to the medication; renal, cardiac, or liver disease; and pregnancy. Cautious use is recommended in patients with diabetes and those with a history of cardiovascular disease or myocardial infarction. Because androgenic anabolic steroids such as testosterone and nandrolone increase weight and raise the potassium, chloride, nitrogen and phosphorus levels, it is important to determine and record the patient's baseline weight, height, vital signs, and serum electrolyte levels. It is also important to look at the results of laboratory tests that assess renal, cardiac and liver functions, such as the BUN, creatinine, SGOT, lactate dehydrogenase, creatine phosphokinase, and bilirubin levels.

Danazol is contraindicated in patients with signif-

DOSAGES

SELECTED MALE REPRODUCTIVE AGENTS

AGENT	PHARMACOLOGIC CLASS	DOSAGE RANGE	PURPOSE
Danazol (Danocrine)	Synthetic androgenic hormone	*Adult* PO: 200-800 mg/day in 2 divided doses and reduced to a dose that maintains amenorrhea. Therapy requires 3-9 mo.	Endometriosis
		100-400 mg/day in 2 divided doses for 4-6 mo	Fibrocystic breast disease
		200 mg 2-3 times/day and reduced by 50% after a favorable response at 1- to 3-mo intervals	Hereditary angioedema
Finasteride (Proscar)	Androgen inhibitor, antiprostatitis agent	*Adult* PO: 5 mg once/day	Benign prostatic hypertrophy
Methyltestosterone (Android, Oreton-M)	Synthetic androgenic hormone	*Adult* PO: 10-50 mg/day or 5-25 mg/day—buccal tablets	Male hypogonadism
		50-200 mg/day or 25-50 mg/day—buccal tablets	Breast cancer
		80 mg/day for 3-5 days after delivery	Postpartum breast pain/engorgement
Testosterone cypionate (Dep-Android, Depo-Testosterone)	Natural androgenic hormone	*Adult* IM: 50-400 mg every 2-4 wk	Male hypogonadism
		200-400 mg every 2-4 wk	Breast cancer
Testosterone transdermal (Testoderm)	Natural androgenic hormone	*Adult* Skin: 4- or 6-mg system applied daily	Male hypogonadism
Fluoxymesterone (Halotestin)	Synthetic androgenic hormore	*Adult* PO: 10-40 mg/day divided	Breast cancer
		2.5 mg after delivery followed by 5-10 mg/day divided for 4-5 day	Postpartum breast pain/engorgement
		5-20 mg/day divided	Male hypogonadism

icant cardiac, hepatic, or renal dysfunction; in pregnant or lactating women; and in women with abnormal genital bleeding. Finasteride is contraindicated in patients with known allergies to the medication. Nandrolone is contraindicated in patients with severe cardiac, liver, or renal disease; pregnant women and those with abnormal genital bleeding; and men with breast or prostate cancer. The androgenic agents interact with oral anticoagulants, steroids, insulin, and oral antidiabetic agents.

NURSING DIAGNOSES

Nursing diagnoses relevant to patients receiving androgenic agents include:

■ Altered body image related to disease process or side effects of androgenic agents.

■ Fatigue related to side effects of androgenic agents.

■ Electrolyte imbalance (excess sodium) related to sodium retention caused by large dosages of androgenic agent.

Patient Teaching TIPS

Androgenic Treatment

✔ Patients taking an androgenic or any type of hormone-related agent should be told to *never* abruptly stop taking the medication. Discontinuing the medication should only be done with a physician's order and the patient monitored over the several weeks during which the dose is tapered.

✔ Patients taking danazol should report any abnormal vaginal discharge or bleeding and should perform routine breast examinations.

✔ Patients taking finasteride should understand the rationale for therapy and know its side effects.

✔ Patients taking any of the androgenic medications should always be careful about taking other prescription or over-the-counter medications or eating foods that interact with these agents.

✔ A woman taking nandrolone should notify her physician of any menstrual irregularities or of any decrease in the therapeutic effects.

✔ Patients being given testosterone IM should be aware of the indicated route of administration and the proper technique of administration.

■ Altered sexual integrity or function stemming from side effects of androgenic agents.
■ Knowledge deficit related to androgenic agents.

PLANNING

Goals for patients receiving androgenic agents include:
■ Patient maintains positive body image.
■ Patient maintains normal activity levels during androgenic therapy.
■ Patient maintains normal sodium and fluid volume levels.
■ Patient experiences minimal alterations in sexual integrity and function during androgenic therapy.
■ Patient remains compliant with androgenic therapy.

Outcome Criteria

Outcome criteria related to the administration of androgenic agents include:
■ Patient verbalizes feelings, fears, and anxieties concerning potential for alteration in body image related to disease process or the side effects of androgenic therapy.

TAKE HOME POINTS

Androgens
■ Male sex hormones.
■ Responsible for normal development and maintenance of male sex characteristics.
■ Primary androgen is testosterone.
■ Danazol, fluoxymesterone, methyltestosterone, and testosterone are exogenous agents.

Testosterone
■ Responsible for development and maintenance of male reproductive system and secondary sex characteristics.
■ Oral testosterone has very poor pharmacokinetic and pharmacodynamic characteristics.
■ Primarily administered by parenteral route.
■ Methyltestosterone was developed to circumvent the problems associated with oral administration.

Anabolic Steroids
■ Nandrolone, oxymetholone, and stanozolol.
■ Chemical derivatives of testosterone.
■ Responsible for bone and muscle development and decreased protein breakdown.
■ Classified as controlled substances by the U.S. Drug Enforcement Administration (schedule III).

Androgen Inhibitors
■ Used to block the effects of naturally occurring androgens.
■ Also called *5-alpha-reductase inhibitors* because of the enzyme they block, the enzyme needed to form testosterone.
■ Currently the only agent is finasteride (Proscar).
■ Used to stop growth of the prostate in men with BPH.

Nursing Considerations
■ Testosterone and related products, if administered IM, should be given deep in the upper outer quadrant of the gluteus muscle injection site.
■ Therapeutic effects of androgenic agents often take 3 to 4 months to appear.
■ These agents should never be withdrawn abruptly.

- Patient maintains healthy activity level during androgenic therapy and suffer minimal fatigue with increased ADLs.
- Patient states measures to be taken to minimize edema related to sodium retention stemming from use of large dosages of androgens such as dietary cautions.
- Patient verbalizes feelings, anxieties, and fears of alteration in their sexual integrity or function during androgenic therapy and seeks counseling if needed.
- Patient takes medications as prescribed.

IMPLEMENTATION

When administered intramuscularly, testosterone and related products should be injected deep into the upper outer quadrant of the gluteus muscle injection site. Generally the lowest dose possible is prescribed to prevent as many of the side effects as possible. Other dosage forms, such as sublingual or oral ones, need to be given exactly as instructed. The manufacturer's guidelines for the administration of some of the sublingual or buccal forms of androgenic agents recommend that the patient not swallow, chew, eat, or drink the buccal tablet but must let it be completely absorbed.

Danazole should be taken with food or milk to minimize the gastric upset often associated with its use. Finasteride is an antiprostatitis agent that is used in the management of BPH. It is administered orally for 6 to 12 months and then the condition is reevaluated.

Nandrolone, an anabolic steroid, should be taken exactly as ordered and at the lowest possible dose. If edema occurs, a low sodium diet may be recommended. Teaching tips for patients receiving androgenic medications are presented in the box on p. 450.

EVALUATION

The therapeutic effect of androgenic agents is essentially the amelioration of whatever condition they are being used to treat. Some of the therapeutic effects may not be seen for 3 or 4 months, such as in the case of osteoporosis. It may also take up to 4 weeks for some of these medications, such as testosterone, to take effect. It is important to observe and monitor the patient for the side effects of these medications, effects such as hypercalcemia, hypoglycemia, hypertension, edema, changes in sexual functioning, and mood changes.

Critical Thinking **A C T I V I T I E S**

1. How do finasteride and methyltestosterone differ in their mechanisms of action?

2. Why might an androgen be prescribed in a patient suffering from anemia?

3. Which one of the following side effects is most commonly associated with the use of androgenic agents?
   a. Sodium depletion
   b. Dysphagia
   c. Virilization in women
   d. Hyperglycemia

BIBLIOGRAPHY

Albanese J, Nutz P: *Mosby's 1995 nursing drug cards,* St Louis, 1995, Mosby.

Johnson KB: *Harriet Lane handbook,* ed 13, St Louis, 1993, Mosby.

Keen JH: *Critical care and emergency drug reference,* St Louis, 1994, Mosby.

Knoben JE, Anderson PO: *Handbook of critical drug data,* ed 6, Hamilton, Ill, 1988, Drug Intelligence Publications.

McEvoy GK: *AHFS drug information,* Bethesda, Md, 1994, American Society of Hospital Pharmacists.

Skidmore-Roth L: *Mosby's 1995 nursing drug reference,* St Louis, 1995, Mosby.

Yelverton GA: Anabolic steroids, *Pediatr Nurs* 15(11):63, 1989.

PART 6

ENDOCRINE SYSTEM: STUDY SKILLS BASICS

QUESTIONING STRATEGY

One of the most important activities for learning is to become actively involved with the text. The best way to achieve this involvement is to develop the habit of asking questions. These questions can be generated using a number of different cues and structures which are part of the part and chapter structure. Some of what you anticipate as related material will not be correct. You will adjust your expectations as you read the material. For now focus on asking a lot of questions and making use of everything you know, which can help to start the process of answering your questions.

Part Title

As you begin each new part, ask a question to focus your attention. What do all the chapters in this part have in common? In Part 6 this question is: "What is the endocrine system?" This same question could be asked of Parts 2 through 8 by simply replacing "endocrine" with the appropriate system for the specific part. Looking at the chapter titles in the part tells us that the endocrine system has to do with the pituitary agents, thyroid agents, antidiabetic agents, and adrenal and corticosteroid agents. While this answer is far too general to demonstrate any real understanding of the endocrine system, it is a beginning and helps keep you aware of what you need to learn from each chapter.

Chapter Titles

Chapter titles provide the first mechanism that can be used to generate questions. The first question to ask about each chapter is a very basic one. What is this chapter about? That question is also answered immediately. "What is Chapter 30 about?" It is about pituitary agents.

The next question is equally obvious but also extremely important. The question to ask next is: "To what do pituitary (Chapter 30), thyroid (Chapter 31), antidiabetic (Chapter 32), and adrenal (Chapter 33) refer?" Take the chapter title and state it as a question. What do you know about these subjects?

Chapter Objectives

To enhance your study turn each chapter objective into one or more questions. Here are some possible questions using the objectives from Chapter 32.

Objective 1: Discuss the normal actions and functions of the pancreas and the feedback system that regulates it.

- What are the normal actions and functions of the pancreas?
- What is the feedback system for the pancreas?

Objective 2: Describe the differences in the hyposecretion and hypersecretion of insulin and the difference between non–insulin-dependent (NIDDM) and insulin-dependent diabetes mellitus (IDDM).

- What does hypo- mean?
- What does hyper- mean?
- What is hypersecretion of insulin?

- What is hyposecretion of insulin?
- What are the differences between hyposecretion and hypersecretion?
- What is NIDDM?
- What is IDDM?

Since the objectives tell you what the authors expected you to know at the end of the chapter, starting out with questions based on the objectives will improve your learning and probably save you time.

Chapter Outline

The same principle can be applied to each of the topic headings set out in the chapter outline. Continuing to use Chapter 32 as a model, here are some samples of questions that might be useful as preparation for reading.

Insulin-Dependent Diabetes Mellitus (IDDM)
- What is insulin-dependent diabetes?
- What is mellitus?

As you start to process the chapter outline, you should also notice that it serves to begin to answer some of the questions from the chapter objectives. And another reminder, this is a good time to begin setting up vocabulary cards.

Mechanism of Action
- What is the mechanism of action in IDDM?
- Is there more than one mechanism?

Drug Effects
- What are the most important drug effects in IDDM?
- Where do these effects take place?
- What is the evidence of these effects?

The idea is to focus on the major content of the chapter, and establish a guide for learning as you read.

Print Conventions Within the Body of the Chapter

Print conventions are useful in this study skills strategy. The use of *italics*, **bold**, <u>underlining</u>, and multiple colors of ink are examples of print conventions. They are designed to catch your attention. Use them as a basis for questions.

Print Conventions, Chapter 32

In paragraph one of this chapter the first obvious print convention is the word **glucose**. It is printed in bold. If you let your eyes float down the page and do not read anything, this word stands out. It must be important.
- What is glucose?
- What is the relationship between glucose and IDDM?

There are more words on the first page of the chapter text that are in the same print style. Apply the same procedure to these terms. Also, notice that two of the terms, **glycogen** and **glycogenolysis**, must have some direct relationship, since the second term contains the first word. The basic question in each case is, what does the term mean? But there should be more to your questions than just the basics. Glycogenolysis seems to mean that there is some operation or activity taking place. Ask yourself:
- What happens in glycogenolysis?
- Where does glycogenolysis occur?
- When?
- How does it relate to IDDM?

Chapter Tables

Tables serve as a summary of information discussed in the chapter. You can learn a great deal from tables if you take the time.

Look at Table 32-1. The table summarizes characteristics of Type I and Type II diabetes. There are two obvious questions for each type.
- What is Type I (Type II) diabetes?
- What are its characteristics?

Use these questions to study Table 32-1 and you will find that all the information you need to respond to these questions is found here. It may be useful to make a first pass through the chapter focusing only on the tables before you begin to read. You will learn a great deal about some of the topics, and you will have established background information that will help you to ask better questions and read with better understanding.

The time you spend asking questions makes the reading and learning go more quickly. Another benefit is that some of the questions you ask appear on tests. These questions will be easy for you to answer. This promotes test-taking confidence, and better scores result in better grades. If you have not been using questioning strategy up to this point in your text, begin now. After you use the strategy for two or three chapters, you will find that the benefits far outweigh the time it takes.

Chapter 30

Pituitary Agents

Objectives

When you reach the end of this chapter, you will be able to:

1 Describe the normal function of the anterior and posterior aspects of the pituitary gland.

2 Identify the various pituitary agents.

3 Discuss the mechanism of action of, indications for, side effects of, and contraindications to, pituitary agents, as well as the nursing care called for in patients receiving them.

4 Develop a comprehensive nursing care plan, including education, for patients receiving pituitary agents.

CHAPTER OUTLINE

The Endocrine System
Pituitary Agents
  Mechanism of action
  Drug effects
  Therapeutic uses
  Side effects and adverse effects
  Interactions
  Dosages
Drug Profiles
  Corticotropin
  Somatropin and Somatrem
  ♵ Octreotide
  ♵ Desmopressin
  Lypressin
  ♵ Vasopressin
Nursing Process
Assessment
Nursing Diagnoses
Planning
  Outcome criteria
Implementation
Evaluation

Glossary

Negative feedback A way in which hormone secretion is regulated that involves a decrease in function in response to a stimulus. (p. 455)

Neuroendocrine system (nùr ō en′ də krən) The system that regulates the reactions of the organism to both internal and external stimuli and that involves the integrated activities of the endocrine glands and nervous system. (p. 455)

Pituitary gland (pǐ too′ ǐ tar′ e) An endocrine gland suspended beneath the brain that supplies numerous hormones that control many vital processes (p. 455)

THE ENDOCRINE SYSTEM

The maintenance of physiologic stability is the main goal of the endocrine system, and it must accomplish this task despite constant changes in the internal and external environments. Every cell, and hence organ, in the body comes under its influence. The endocrine system communicates with the nearly fifty million target cells in the body using a chemical "language" called hormones. These are natural substances that are secreted into the bloodstream in response to the body's needs, which then conveys them to their site of action—the target cell.

For decades the pituitary gland was believed to be the master gland that regulated and controlled the other endocrine glands in this very diverse system. However, the discovery of strong evidence that the central nervous system, specifically the hypothalamus, controls the pituitary has caused this old belief to be discarded, and the hypothalamus and pituitary are now viewed as functioning together as an integrated unit, with the primary direction coming from the hypothalamus. For this reason, the system is now frequently referred to as the **neuroendocrine system.** In fact, the endocrine system can be considered in much the same way as the nervous system. Each is basically a system for signaling, and each operates in a stimulus-and-response manner. Together these two systems essentially govern all bodily functions.

The **pituitary gland** is made up of two distinct glands—the anterior (adenohypophysis) and posterior (neurohypophysis) pituitary. They are individually linked to and communicate with the hypothalamus, and each gland secretes its own set of hormones. These various hormones are listed in the box above.

Hormones are either water or lipid soluble. The water-soluble hormones are protein-based substances such as the catecholamines norepinephrine and epinephrine. The receptors for these hormones are usually located on cell membranes, and these hormones bind to their receptors on the cell surface, whereupon they either directly activate the cell to perform a function or cause a signal to be sent by means of a "second messenger" to generate an appropriate cellular response. The lipid-soluble hormones consist of the steroid and thyroid hormones. They are capable of crossing the plasma membrane through the process of simple diffusion and of binding with receptors within the cell nucleus, where they stimulate a specific cellular response.

The activity of the endocrine system is regulated by a system of surveillance and signaling usually dictated by the body's needs. Hormone secretion is commonly regulated by the process of **negative feedback**. This is best explained using a fictional example: When gland X releases hormone X, this stimulates target cells to release hormone Y. When there is an excess of hormone Y, gland X "senses" this and inhibits the release of hormone X.

PITUITARY AGENTS

There are a variety of drugs that affect the pituitary gland. They are generally used for the following purposes: as replacement therapy to make up for a hormone deficiency, as drug therapy to produce a particular hormone response, in a patient with a specific disorder, and as diagnostic aids to determine whether there is hypofunction or hyperfunction of hormones. Many of the anterior and posterior pituitary hormones listed in the box at left have been synthesized, and some of these have already been discussed in other chapters. The currently identified anterior and posterior pituitary hormones and the drugs that mimic or antagonize their actions are listed in the box on the next page.

The anterior pituitary drugs discussed in this chapter include corticotropin, somatotropin, somatrem, and octreotide; the posterior pituitary drugs discussed in this chapter consist of vasopressin, lypressin, and desmopressin. The many other drugs that have effects on the pituitary are covered in depth in other chapters.

Mechanism of Action

The mechanisms of action of the various pituitary agents differ depending on the agent, but overall they either augment or antagonize the natural effects of the pituitary hormones. Exogenously administered corticotropin elicits all the same pharmacologic responses as those elicited by the endogenous corticotropin, or ACTH. Regardless of whether it is exogenous or endogenous in origin, corticotropin travels to the adrenal cortex located just above the kidneys and stimulates the secretion of the mineralocorticoid cortisol (hydrocortisone), corticosterone, several weakly androgenic substances, and, to a very limited extent, aldosterone.

The drugs that mimic GH are somatropin and somatrem. These agents promote growth by stimulating the anabolic processes that cause growth. A drug that antagonizes the effects of the natural GH is octreotide, and it does so by inhibiting GH release. It is a synthetic polypeptide that is structurally and pharmacologically similar to GH release–inhibiting factor.

The drugs that affect the posterior pituitary such as vasopressin, lypressin, and desmopressin mimic the actions of the naturally occurring ADH. Exogenous vasopressin elicits all the same pharmacologic responses as those elicited by endogenous vasopressin (ADH). It increases water resorption in the distal tubules and collecting ducts of the nephrons, concentrates urine, and is a potent vasoconstrictor. It does all these by increasing the resorption of sodium and water in the distal tubules and collecting ducts.

Drug Effects

The drug effects of the various pituitary drugs also differ depending on the agent, and many of the effects are the same as those of the pituitary hormones. By stimulating the cortex of the adrenal gland to secrete cortisol, corticotropin causes sodium to be retained, with edema and hypertension the result. Cortisol can also decrease inflammation by preventing the release of destructive substances from leukocytes. It also inhibits macrophage accumulation in inflamed areas, reduces leukocyte adhesion to capillary walls, and reduces capillary wall permeability and edema formation. Other effects of corticotropin are a decrease in the level of complement components, the antagonism of histamine activity, a reduction in fibroblast prolif-

---

Anterior and Posterior Pituitary Hormones and Drugs

HORMONE	FUNCTION/MIMICKING DRUG
Anterior Pituitary	
Adrenocorticotropic hormone	Targets adrenal gland; mediates adaptation to physical and emotional stress and starvation; redistributes body nutrients; promotes synthesis of adrenocortical hormone (glucocorticoids, mineralocorticoids, androgens); involved in skin pigmentation. Corticotropin: diagnosis of adrenocortical insufficiency.
Follicle-stimulating hormone	Stimulates oogenesis and follicular growth in females and spermatogenesis in males. Menotropins: same pharmacologic effects as FSH; many of the other gonadotropins also stimulate FSH (Chapter 28).
Growth hormone	Regulates anabolic processes related to growth and adaptation to stressors; promotes skeletal and muscle growth; increases protein synthesis; increases liver glycogenolysis; increases fat mobilization. Somatotropin: human GH for hypopituitary dwarfism. Octreotide: a synthetic polypeptide structurally and pharmacologically similar to growth hormone release–inhibiting factor; it inhibits GH.
Luteinizing hormone	Stimulates ovulation and estrogen release by ovaries in females; stimulates interstitial cells in males to promote spermatogenesis and testosterone secretion. Gonadotropins: many of the agents discussed in Chapter 28 stimulate LH.
Prolactin	Targets mammary glands; stimulates lactogenesis and breast growth. Bromocriptine: inhibits action of PH and therefore inhibits lactogenesis (Chapter 12).
Thyroid-stimulating hormone	Stimulates secretion of thyroid hormones (triiodothyronine [T3] and thyroxine [T4]) by the thyroid. Thyrotropin: increases the production and secretion of thyroid hormones (Chapter 31).
Posterior Pituitary	
Antidiuretic hormone	Increases water resorption in distal tubules and collecting duct of nephron; concentrates urine; causes potent vasoconstriction. Vasopressin: ADH; performs all the physiologic functions of ADH. Lypressin: a synthetic vasopressin; has uses similar to those of vasopressin. Desmopressin: a synthetic vasopressin.
Oxytocin	Targets mammary glands; stimulates ejection of milk and contraction of uterine smooth muscle. Pitocin: has all the physiologic actions of oxytocin (Chapter 28)

eration, the deposition of collagen, and the subsequent formation of scar tissue.

Somatropin and somatrem have pharmacologic effects equivalent to those of human GH. They both promote linear growth in children who lack normal amounts of the endogenous hormone. In addition, they cause increased cellular protein synthesis, nitrogen retention, liver glycogenolysis, impaired glucose tolerance, lipid mobilization, a reduction in body fat stores, and increased plasma levels of fatty acids. GH derivatives also cause the retention of sodium, potassium, and phosphorus.

Octreotide is a synthetic polypeptide that is structurally and pharmacologically related to somatostatin (GH release–inhibiting factor). It can eliminate or alleviate certain symptoms (e.g., severe diarrhea, flushing) of carcinoid tumors. It is also effective in the management of the potentially life-threatening hypotension associated with a carcinoid crisis. Octreotide decreases the stool volume, electrolyte loss, and plasma concentrations of vasoactive intestinal polypeptide (VIP), a substance secreted by VIPomas that causes profuse watery diarrhea.

The synthetically made hormones that are structurally identical or similar to ADH are vasopressin, lypressin, and desmopressin. By increasing the resorption of sodium and water in the distal tubules and collecting duct of the nephron, they decrease the urinary flow rate, thereby causing as much as 90% of the water that might otherwise be excreted in the urine to be conserved. In large doses, vasopressin directly stimulates the contraction of smooth muscle, particularly of the capillaries and small arterioles, causing vasoconstriction. Desmopressin causes a dose-dependent increase in the plasma levels of factor VIII (antihemophilic factor, or von Willebrand's factor) and tissue plasminogen activator.

Therapeutic Uses

Corticotropin's primary therapeutic effect is the stimulation of the release of cortisol from the adrenal cortex, making it an excellent agent in the diagnosis of adrenocortical insufficiency. It is also used for the treatment of multiple sclerosis and corticotropin insufficiency caused by long-term corticosteroid use. Its antiinflammatory and immunosuppressant properties may be therapeutic in patients with normal adrenocortical function. Somatropin and somatrem are recombinantly made human GH. They are effective in stimulating skeletal growth in patients suffering from an inadequate secretion of normal endogenous GH, such as those with hypopituitary dwarfism. Octreotide is a synthetic polypeptide that is structurally and pharmacologically related to somatostatin (GH release–inhibiting factor). It is of benefit in alleviating or elim-

inating certain symptoms of carcinoid tumors stemming from the secretion of VIP. (These symptoms have been described in the previous section.) Vasopressin, lypressin, and desmopressin are used to prevent or control polydipsia, polyuria, and dehydration in patients with diabetes insipidus caused by a deficiency of endogenous ADH. Because of their vasoconstrictor properties they are useful in the treatment of various types of bleeding, in particular GI hemorrhage. Because of its unique ability to increase the plasma level of factor VIII (von Willebrand's factor) and tissue plasminogen activator, desmopressin is especially useful in the treatment of hemophilia A and type I von Willebrand's disease.

Side Effects and Adverse Effects

Many of the adverse effects of the pituitary drugs are specific to the individual agents. Those agents possessing similar hormonal effects generally have similar adverse effects. The most common adverse effects of the pituitary drugs described here are listed in Tables 30-1 to 30-3.

Table 30-1	**Corticotropin: Common Adverse Effects**
Body System	**Side/Adverse Effect**
Central nervous system	Convulsions, dizziness, euphoria, insomnia, headache, depression, psychosis
Gastrointestinal	Nausea, vomiting, peptic ulcer perforation, pancreatitis
Genitourinary	Water and sodium retention, hypokalemia
Other	Sweating, acne, hyperpigmentation, weakness, muscle atrophy, myalgia, arthralgia

Table 30-2	**Desmopressin, Lypressin, and Vasopressin: Common Adverse Effects**
Body System	**Side/Adverse Effect**
Central nervous system	Drowsiness, headache, lethargy, flushing
Gastrointestinal	Nausea, heartburn, cramps,
Genitourinary	Uterine cramping
Cardiovascular	Increased BP
Other	Nasal irritation and congestion, tremor, sweating, vertigo

Interactions

For information on the drugs that interact with pituitary agents, see Table 30-4.

Dosages

For the recommended dosages of pituitary agents, see the dosages table on the following page.

DRUG PROFILES

CORTICOTROPIN

Corticotropin (Acthar, H.P. Acthar Gel) is classified as a pregnancy category C agent. It is contraindicated in patients who have shown a hypersensitivity to it, in those with scleroderma, osteoporosis, CHF, peptic ulcer disease, hypertension, or primary adrenocortical insufficiency or hyperfunction, and in those who have undergone recent surgery. It is available in two parenteral forms, a regular form that may be given by intravenous, intramuscular, or subcutaneous injection, and a repository form, which may be given intramuscularly or subcutaneously, that has more prolonged effects. The parenteral form is available in 25- and 40-U strengths and the repository form in 40 and 80-U/ml strengths. Common dosages are listed in the following dosages table.

PHARMACOKINETICS

HALF-LIFE	ONSET	PEAK	DURATION
Unknown	Rapid	1 hr	3 days*

*For repository form.

SOMATROPIN AND SOMATREM

Somatropin (Humatrope, Nutropin) and somatrem (Protropin) are both made by recombinant DNA techniques. They are contraindicated in anyone whose bones have stopped growing, that is, those with closed epiphyses. They should also not be used in any patient showing evidence of an active tumor. These GHs are available only for injection and come as 5-mg/5 ml vials for this purpose. Common dosages are listed in the following dosages table. Both are pregnancy category C agents.

PHARMACOKINETICS

HALF-LIFE	ONSET	PEAK	DURATION
<30 min	SC: 3-6 hr	SC: 3-5 hr	Variable

OCTREOTIDE

Octreotide (Sandostatin) is contraindicated only in patients who have shown a hypersensitivity to it. It is only available parenterally as 50-, 100-, 200-, 500-, and 1000-μg/ml injections. Common dosages are listed in the following dosages table. Pregnancy category B.

PHARMACOKINETICS

HALF-LIFE	ONSET	PEAK	DURATION
1.7 hr	Unknown	15-30 min	12 hr

Table 30-3	Drugs That Affect Growth Hormone: Common Adverse Effects

BODY SYSTEM	SIDE/ADVERSE EFFECT
Central nervous system	Headache
Genitourinary	Hypercalciuria
Endocrine	Hyperglycemia, ketosis, hypothyroidism
Other	Rash, urticaria, antibodies to GH, inflammation at injection site

Table 30-4	Pituitary Drug Interactions	
DRUG	**MECHANISM**	**RESULT**
ACTH with diuretics and amphotericin B	Additive	Additive effect on lowering potassium levels
Desmopressin with carbamazepine, chlorpropamide, and clofibrate	Additive	Increased response to desmopressin
Desmopressin with lithium, alcohol, demeclocycline, and heparin	Antagonism	Decreased response to desmopressin

DOSAGES

SELECTED PITUITARY DRUGS

AGENT	PHARMACOLOGIC CLASS	DOSAGE RANGE	PURPOSE
Corticotropin (Acthar)		*Pediatric* Suggested dose, 1.6 μg/kg/day or 50 μg/m^2/day in 3-4 divided doses	Replacement or therapeutic
		Adult IM/SC: 20 μg qid	Antiinflammatory immunosuppressant
	Adrenal cortex stimulating hormone	IM: 80-120 μg/day in divided doses for 2-3 wk	Exacerbation of multiple sclerosis
		IV: 10-25 μg in 500 ml of a suitable IV fluid (usually 5% dextrose) infused over 8 hr	Diagnosis of adrenocortical insufficiency
		IV: up to 100 μg over 8 hr for 10 days	Myasthenia gravis
Repository injection (H.P. Acthar Gel)		*Adult* IM: 40-80 μg q24-72 hr	Antiinflammatory, immunosuppressant
		IM: 80-120 μg/day for 14-21 days	Exacerbation of multiple sclerosis
Desmopressin acetate (DDAVP, Stimate)	Antidiuretic antihemophilic hormone	*Pediatric* ≥6 y/o: 0.2 ml (20 μg) of the nasal spray hs, with ½ dose administered to each nostril	Primary nocturnal enuresis
		3 mo-12 y/o: 0.05-0.3 ml (5-30 μg) of the nasal spray/day hs	Diabetes insipidus
		Adult/Pediatric ≥3 mo: IV: 0.3 μg/kg over 30 min	Hemophilia A, type I von Willebrand's disease
		Adult 0.1-0.4 ml (10-40 μg) of the spray hs or divided	Diabetes insipidus
Lypressin (Diapid)	Synthetic antidiuretic hormone	*Pediatric/Adult* 1-2 sprays (7-14 μg) of the nasal spray administered 1-2 times in each nostril qid	Diabetes insipidus
⚓Octreotide (Sandostatin)	Growth hormone inhibitor	*Adult* IV/SC: 50 μg tid and adjust	Treatment of acromegaly
		IV/SC: 100-600 μg/day in 2-4 divided doses	Carcinoid tumors
		IV/SC: 200-300 μg/day in 2-4 divided doses	VIPoma
Somatrem (Protropin)	Growth hormone	*Pediatric* IM/SC: Up to 0.1 mg/kg (0.26 μI/kg) 3 times/wk	Growth failure due to inadequate levels of natural GH
Somatropin (Humatrope, Nutropin)	Growth hormone	*Pediatric* IM/SC: up to 0.06 mg/kg (0.16 μI/kg) 2 times/wk	

continued

SELECTED PITUITARY DRUGS—cont'd

AGENT	PHARMACOLOGIC CLASS	DOSAGE RANGE	PURPOSE
Vasopressin (Pitressin)	Antidiuretic hormone	*Pediatric* IM/SC: 2.5-10 μg 3-4 times/day	Diabetes insipidus
		Adult IM/SC: 5 μg to start and up to 10 U prn	Postop abdominal distention
		IM/SC: 10 μg given 2 hr and ½ hr before procedure	Abdominal roentgenography
		5-10 μg repeated 2-3 times/day prn	Diabetes insipidus
Vasopressin tannate in oil		*Adult* IM: 1.6-5 μg (0.3-1 ml) repeated prn	Diabetes insipidus

⚓ DESMOPRESSIN

Desmopressin (DDAVP) is a synthetically made hormone that is structurally related to the endogenous hormone arginine vasopressin (ADH), but its effects differ slightly from those of the natural vasopressin (see the sections Drug Effects, Therapeutic Uses). It is classified as a pregnancy category B agent and is contraindicated in patients who have shown a hypersensitivity to it and in those with nephrogenic diabetes insipidus. It is available as a 10-μg/0.1 ml and a 100-μg/ml metered-dose nasal spray and a 4-μg/ml parenteral injection. Common dosages are listed in the dosages table.

✸ PHARMACOKINETICS

HALF-LIFE	ONSET	PEAK	DURATION
IV: 1.5-2.5 hr	IV: 30 min	IV: 1.5-2 hr	IN:* 12 hr

*Intranasal.

LYPRESSIN

Lypressin (Diapid) is lysine vasopressin, and it is identical to the vasopressin produced naturally in swine (pig) pituitaries. However, this synthetic vasopressin differs from that produced in humans in that it contains lysine instead of arginine in its structure, though the principal pharmacologic action of the two is similar. They both increase the resorption of sodium and water in the distal tubules and collecting duct of the nephron and in so doing block diuresis.

Lypressin is classified as a pregnancy B agent and is contraindicated in patients who have shown a hypersensitivity to it and in those with nephrogenic diabetes insipidus. It is available as a 185-μg/ml nasal spray. Common dosages are listed in the dosages table.

✸ PHARMACOKINETICS

HALF-LIFE	ONSET	PEAK	DURATION
15 min	Rapid	0.5-2 hr	3-8 hr

⚓ VASOPRESSIN

Vasopressin (Pitressin) is a synthetic arginine vasopressin that structurally is identical to endogenous vasopressin (ADH) and produces all the same effects as the endogenous hormone. It is classified as a pregnancy C agent and is contraindicated in patients who have shown a hypersensitivity to it and in those with chronic nephritis. It is available as a 20-U/ml parenteral injection. Common dosages are listed in the dosages table.

✸ PHARMACOKINETICS

HALF-LIFE	ONSET	PEAK	DURATION
10-35 min	Unknown	Unknown	2-8 hr

NURSING PROCESS

ASSESSMENT

Before administering any of the pituitary agents in a patient, the nurse should perform a thorough nursing assessment and obtain a complete medication history,

Pituitary Agents: Assessment Data

ASSESSMENT PARAMETERS	CAUTIONS AND DRUG INTERACTIONS	CONTRAINDICATIONS
Corticotropin		
Baseline vital signs	*Cautions:*	Allergy
Electrolyte values	Pregnancy	Osteoporosis
Blood glucose levels	Lactation	CHF
Chest x-ray study	Liver disease	Ulcer disease
CBC, I&O, weight	Mental illness	Scleroderma
Cortisol levels	Myasthenia gravis	Fungal infections
Allergy to pork, because of	Gout	Recent surgery
cross-sensitivity	Hypothyroidism	Adrenocortical hypo/hyper
	Latent TB	function (primary)
	Drug interactions: Alcohol	
	Aspirin	
	Steroids	
	Diuretics	
	Amphotericin B	
Somatropin and Somatrem		
Thyroid function studies	*Cautions:*	Drug allergy
GH antibodies	Diabetes mellitus	Intracerebral lesions
	Hypothyroidism	Closed epiphyseal plates
	Pregnancy	
	Drug interactions:	
	Glucocorticoids	
	Androgens	
	Thyroid hormones	
⚓Desmopressin		
Vital signs with BP lying and	*Cautions:*	Allergy to drug or to tricyclic
standing q4h	Depression or suicidal ten-	antidepressants
CBC: leukocytes	dencies	Glaucoma
Cardiac enzymes	Narrow-angle glaucoma	MI (recovery phase)
Liver enzymes	Increased intraocular pres-	BPH
Weight every week	sure	Seizure disorder
ECG	Seizure disorder	Children under 12 y/o
	Children under 12 y/o	
⚓Vasopressin and Lypressin		
Pulse-vital signs, especially	*Cautions:*	Allergy
with IM/IV dosage forms	Coronary artery disease	Chronic renal disease
I&O	Pregnancy	
Weights		
Edema		

and then document the findings. There are many contraindications and cautions to the use of these agents and many drugs that interact with them, and all of this should be checked for before their administration. A hypersensitivity reaction to any of these medications is also a contraindication to their use. Further assessment data are provided in the box on the next page.

NURSING DIAGNOSES

Nursing diagnoses related to the administration of pituitary agents include:

■ Altered body image related either to the specific disease process or to side effects of the medications.

■ Fluid volume overload related to side effects of the medications.

■ Electrolyte imbalances related to side effects of the medications.

■ Fatigue related to the disease and its treatment.

■ Altered tissue perfusion (decreased) related to drug-induced hypertension.

■ Pain (epigastric discomfort) related to ulcerogenic side effects of the medications.

■ Knowledge deficit related to new treatment.

PLANNING

Goals pertaining to patients receiving pituitary medications include:

- Patient maintains positive body image.
- Patient maintains normal fluid volume status.
- Patient maintains normal serum electrolyte levels while on medication.
- Patient returns to normal or pretherapy levels of activity.
- Patient maintains adequate tissue perfusion.
- Patient experiences little to no pain related to medication-induced GI upset or epigastric distress.
- Patient remains compliant with medication therapy.
- Patient is without self-injury related to adverse effects of medications.

Outcome Criteria

The outcome criteria for patients receiving pituitary agents include:

- Patient will openly verbalize fears, anxieties, and concerns with healthcare professionals regarding body image changes related to disease process and medication therapy.
- Patient's sodium level will be within normal limits while on medication therapy.
- Patient will state ways to decrease edema caused by medication such as dietary precautions.
- Patient will experience minimal GI upset and gastric distress by taking medication with food or at mealtimes.
- Patient will state measures to employ to diminish the risk of falls related to the musculoskeletal and neurologic (seizures) side effects of medication.
- Patient will perform ADLs and other normal activity without difficulty.
- Patient will state importance of follow-up visits to the physician such as monitoring compliance, therapeutic effects, and adverse reactions.

Patient Teaching TIPS

Pituitary Agents

Corticotropin
- ✔ Patients receiving corticotropin and corticotropin-like drugs should be encouraged to maintain adequate hydration of up to 2000 ml per day, unless this is contraindicated.
- ✔ Patients receiving corticotropin should avoid vaccinations during drug therapy.
- ✔ Patients should not take any over-the-counter medications during therapy.
- ✔ Patients should avoid consuming alcohol.
- ✔ Patients should be told not to discontinue the medication abruptly.
- ✔ Patients should wear a Medic-Alert tag at all times, naming the medication they are taking.
- ✔ Patients should be informed that the medication does not lead to a cure but does help alleviate the symptoms of the disease.
- ✔ Patients should notify their physician should they experience infection, fever, sore throat, joint pain, or muscular pain.
- ✔ Patients should tell all other health care professionals, such as dentists, that they are taking corticotropin.

Somatropin
- ✔ Patients should be given instructions regarding the dosage form and amount and the importance of compliance with therapy.

- ✔ Discolored or cloudy solutions should not be used.
- ✔ Show the parents of children receiving the agent how to keep a journal of the growth measurements.

Desmopressin
- ✔ The technique for nasal instillation should be demonstrated to the child and caregiver and reevaluated at later visits, with repeat demonstrations if necessary. Written instructions should also be provided.
- ✔ The patient should not take any over-the-counter medications for colds, cough, allergies, or hay fever because of the epinephrine in these preparations that can interact with the desmopressin.
- ✔ Patients should avoid consuming alcohol.
- ✔ A Medic-Alert bracelet or necklace should be worn at all times, naming the medication being taken.

Lypressin
- ✔ Patients should be encouraged to carry the medication with them at all times.
- ✔ The nasal spray should be used according to instructions and only after patients have cleared their nasal passages. The spray should not be INHALED!

Octreotide
- ✔ Inform patients with carcinoid tumors who are taking this drug that symptoms of flushing and severe diarrhea will improve or be eliminated.

IMPLEMENTATION

Corticotropin is available in IM, SC, and IV forms as well as in gel and repository forms. Gel forms should be at room temperature when administered, and IM injections should be administered using a 21-gauge needle. IV injections should be given over 2 minutes, or as designated in the packaging insert, and should be diluted with the recommended amounts of normal saline solution. The patient's protein intake should be increased because of the protein loss and the potential negative nitrogen balance that can occur. Patients are usually encouraged to decrease their sodium intake and increase their potassium intake to counteract the side effects of the medication. Teaching tips for patients receiving pituitary agents are presented in the box below.

EVALUATION

Following are the therapeutic responses expected in patients receiving pituitary agents: corticotropin should eliminate the pain associated with inflammation, and produce increased comfort and muscle strength in patients with myasthenia gravis; somatropin should increase growth in children; and desmopressin, lypressin, and vasopressin should eliminate severe thirst and decrease urinary output. Side effects to monitor for in patients receiving corticotropin include dependent edema, moon face, pulmonary edema, infection, and mental status changes that include increased aggressive behavior and irritability. Allergic reactions to corticotropin include rash, urticaria, fever, and dyspnea. If these occur, the drug should be discontinued and the physician notified. The side effects of somatropin include hypercalciuria. Desmopressin, lypressin, and vasopressin cause similar side effects, and these include hypertension, nausea, GI upset, tremors, respiratory distress, and drowsiness.

TAKE HOME POINTS

Pituitary Gland
- Composed of two distinct glands: anterior and posterior.
- Each has its own set of hormones: anterior = TSH, GH, ACTH, PH, FSH, LH; posterior = ADH, oxytocin.

Pituitary Drugs
- Either mimic or antagonize the action of endogenous pituitary hormones.
- Those that mimic are corticotropin, somatropin, somatrem, vasopressin, lypressin, and desmopressin.
- Octreotide antagonizes.

Somatropin
- Human GH that is made by recombinant DNA techniques.
- Mimics the effects of GH.
- So does somatrem (also made by recombinant DNA techniques).

Octreotide
- Antagonizes the effects of natural GH.
- Suppresses or inhibits certain symptoms of carcinoid tumors.
- Decreases plasma concentrations of vasoactive intestinal polypeptide (VIP).

Desmopressin
- Synthetically made hormone that is structurally related to endogenous arginine vasopressin, also known as *antidiuretic hormone* (ADH).
- Increases plasma levels of factor VIII (von Willebrand's factor) and tissue plasminogen activator.
- Used in the treatment of hemophilia A and type I von Willebrand's disease.

Nursing Considerations
- Assessment in patients receiving corticotropin should include baseline vital signs, electrolyte values, blood glucose levels, chest x-ray studies, weight, cortisol levels, and allergy to pork because of cross-sensitivity.
- Assessment in patients receiving somatropin should include thyroid function and GH levels.
- Assessment in patients receiving desmopressin should include vital signs with lying and standing blood pressures, CBCs, cardiac and liver enzyme activity, ECG, and weight.
- Assessment in patients receiving vasopressin or lypressin should include vital signs, intake and output amounts, weight, and presence and status of edema.

Critical Thinking **A C T I V I T I E S**

1. Vasopressin, lypressin, and desmopressin are structurally identical or similar to what endogenous hormone?

2. What are the two recombinantly made human GH products?

3. A therapeutic response to lypressin therapy includes which of the following:
   a. Excitability
   b. Edema
   c. Oliguria
   d. Dysphagia

BIBLIOGRAPHY

Albanese J, Nutz P: *Mosby's 1995 nursing drug cards,* St Louis, 1995, Mosby.

Johnson KB: *Harriet Lane handbook,* ed 13, St Louis, 1993, Mosby.

Keen JH: *Critical care and emergency drug reference,* St Louis, 1994, Mosby.

Knoben JE, Anderson PO: *Handbook of critical drug data,* ed 6, Hamilton, Ill, 1988, Drug Intelligence Publications.

McEvoy GK: *AHFS drug information,* Bethesda, Md, 1994, American Society of Hospital Pharmacists.

Skidmore-Roth L: *Mosby's 1995 nursing drug reference,* St Louis, 1995, Mosby.

Objectives

When you reach the end of this chapter, you will be able to:

1 Discuss the normal actions and functions of the thyroid hormones.

2 Describe the differences in the diseases resulting from the hyposecretion and hypersecretion of the thyroid hormones.

3 Identify the various agents that are used to manage the hyposecretion and hypersecretion states.

4 Discuss the mechanism of action of, indications for, contraindications and cautions to, and side effects of thyroid agents.

5 Develop a nursing care plan as it relates to the nursing process in patients receiving thyroid or antithyroid agents.

6 Identify the teaching guidelines for patients receiving thyroid or antithyroid agents.

CHAPTER OUTLINE

Thyroid Function
Hypothyroidism
Hyperthyroidism
Thyroid Agents
  Mechanism of action
  Drug effects
  Therapeutic uses
  Side effects and adverse effects
  Interactions
  Dosages
Drug Profiles
  Thyroid
  Thyroglobulin
 ⚓ Levothyroxine
  Liothyronine
  Liotrix
Antithyroid Agents
  Mechanism of action
  Drug effects
  Therapeutic uses
  Side effects and adverse effects
  Interactions
  Dosages
Drug Profiles
  Methimazole
 ⚓ Propylthiouracil

Nursing Process
Assessment
Nursing Diagnoses
Planning
  Outcome criteria
Implementation
Evaluation

Glossary

Hyperthyroidism (hi′ pər thi′ roid iz əm) Condition characterized by excessive production of the thyroid hormones. (p. 466)

Hypothyroidism Condition characterized by decreased activity of the thyroid gland. (p. 466)

Thyroid-stimulating hormone *Endogenous* substance secreted by the pituitary gland that controls the release of thyroid hormone and is necessary for the growth and function of the thyroid gland. (p. 466)

Thyrotropin (thi ro′ tro pin) *Exogenous* preparation that increases the uptake of radioactive iodine in the thyroid and the secretion of thyroxine by the thyroid. (p. 466)

Thyroxine (thi rok′ sen) Thyroid hormone that influences the metabolic rate. (p. 466)

Triiodothyronine (tri i′ o do thi′ ro nēn) Hormone that helps regulate growth, development, metabolism, and body temperature and inhibits the secretion of thyrotropin by the pituitary. (p. 466)

Thyroid Function

The thyroid gland lies on either side of the neck and is responsible for the secretion of three hormones essential for the proper regulation of metabolism: **thyroxine** (T_4), **triiodothyronine** (T_3), and calcitonin. It is in close to and communicates with the parathyroid gland, which lies just above and behind it. The parathyroid gland is a bean-shaped gland and consists of two pairs. These glands are made up of encapsulated cells, which are responsible for maintaining adequate levels of calcium in the extracellular fluid, primarily by mobilizing calcium from bone.

T_4 and T_3 are produced in the thyroid gland through the iodination and coupling of the amino acid tyrosine. The iodide needed for this process is acquired from our diet, and for normal function to be maintained, we need about 1 mg of iodide per week. This iodide is sequestered by the thyroid gland, where it is trapped and concentrated to twenty times its concentration in blood. It is here that it is also converted to iodine, which is combined with the tyrosine to make diiodotyrosine. The combination of two molecules of diiodotyrosine causes the formation of thyronine, which therefore has four iodine molecules in its structure (T_4). Triiodothyronine is formed by the coupling of one molecule of diiodotyrosine with one molecule of monoiodotyrosine, thus it has three iodine molecules in its structure (T_3). The biologic potency of T_3 is about four times greater than that of T_4, but T_4 is present in much greater quantities. After the synthesis of these two thyroid hormones, they are stored in a complex with thyroglobulin (a protein that contains tyrosine and an amino acid) in the follicles in the thyroid gland called the colloid. When the thyroid gland is signaled to do so, the thyroglobulin–thyroid hormone complex is then enzymatically broken down to release either T_3 or T_4 into the circulation. This entire process is triggered by **thyroid-stimulating hormone** (TSH), also called **thyrotropin**. Its release from the anterior pituitary is stimulated when the blood levels of T_3 and T_4 levels are low.

The thyroid hormones are involved in a wide variety of bodily processes. They regulate lipid and carbohydrate metabolism, they are essential for normal growth and development, they control the heat-regulating system (thermoregulatory center), and they have multiple effects on the cardiovascular, endocrine, and neuromuscular systems. Therefore hyperfunction or hypofunction of the thyroid gland can lead to a wide range of serious consequences.

HYPOTHYROIDISM

A deficiency in thyroid hormones can be caused by a number of different diseases, and these diseases affect the thyroid in different ways, such that there are three types of **hypothyroidism**. Primary hypothyroidism stems from an abnormality in the thyroid gland itself and occurs when the thyroid gland is not able to perform one of its many functions, such as releasing the thyroid hormones from their storage sites, coupling iodine with tyrosine, trapping iodide, or converting iodide to iodine, or any combination of these defects. It is the most common of the three. Secondary hypothyroidism results when the pituitary gland is dysfunctional and does not secrete the TSH needed to trigger the release of the T3 and T4 stored there. Tertiary hypothyroidism is similar to the secondary form in that the stimulus needed to trigger the secretion of the next hormone is absent. However, the source of the problem is that the level of the thyrotropin-releasing hormone (TRH) secreted from the hypothalamus is reduced, which in turn results in decreased TSH levels and hence decreased thyroid hormone levels. Knowledge of the underlying cause of the hypothyroidism allows one to treat the cause and by so doing eliminate the deficiency.

Some forms of hypothyroidism may result in the formation of a goiter, which is an enlargement of the thyroid gland resulting from its overstimulation by elevated levels of TSH. The TSH level is elevated because of little or no thyroid hormone in the circulation. Common symptoms of hypothyroidism are thickened skin, hair loss, lethargy, constipation, anorexia, and many others.

HYPERTHYROIDISM

The excessive secretion of thyroid hormones, or **hyperthyroidism**, may be caused by several different diseases and drugs. Some of the more common diseases are Graves' disease, which is the most common cause; Plummer's disease, which is also known as *toxic nodular disease* and is the least common cause; multinodular disease; and thyroid storm, which is usually induced by stress or infection.

Hyperthyroidism can affect multiple body systems, resulting in an overall increase in metabolism. Frequently reported symptoms are diarrhea, flushing, increased appetite, muscle weakness, fatigue, palpitations, irritability, nervousness, sleep disorders, heat intolerance, and altered menstrual flow.

THYROID AGENTS

All three types of hypothyroidism are amenable to thyroid hormone replacement using various thyroid preparations. These agents can be either natural or synthetic in origin. The natural thyroid preparations are derived from the thyroids of animals such as cattle and hogs and include thyroid and thyroglobulin. All the natural preparations used to be standardized according to their iodine content, an indirect indicator of the true hormonal biologic activity, but now the measurable amounts of levothyroxine (T4) and liothyronine (T3) in each 65 mg of thyroid or thyroglobulin is used for this purpose. The synthetic thyroid preparations include levothyroxine, liothyronine, and liotrix, the latter agent containing a combination of T4 and T3 in a 4:1 ratio. The approximate clinically equivalent doses of the agents are given in the box below, and this information is useful for guiding dosage adjustments when switching a patient from one thyroid hormone to another.

Mechanism of Action

The thyroid preparations are given to replace what the thyroid gland cannot itself produce in order to achieve normal thyroid levels (euthyroid). The thyroid drugs work in the same manner as the endogenous thyroid hormone. At the cellular level they work to induce changes in the metabolic rates, stimulate the cardiovascular system, and increase oxygen consumption, body temperature, blood volume, growth, and overall cellular growth.

Drug Effects

The drugs that are used to treat hypothyroid conditions affect many body systems, and they do this in the same way the endogenous thyroid hormones do. The principal pharmacologic effect of the drugs is an increase in the rate of protein, carbohydrate, and lipid metabolism. Thyroid hormones are also involved in the regulation of cell growth and differentiation and have a cardiostimulatory effect, which involves increasing the sensitivity of the heart to catecholamines or increasing the number of myocardial beta-adrener-

gic receptors, or both. In addition, thyroid hormones increase cardiac output, renal blood flow, and the glomerular filtration rate, which results in a diuretic effect.

Therapeutic Uses

The various thyroid preparations are used in the treatment of all three forms of hypothyroidism, though levothyroxine is generally the preferred agent because its hormonal content is standardized and its effect is therefore predictable. The thyroid drugs can also be used for the diagnosis of suspected hyperthyroidism and in the prevention or treatment of various types of goiters.

Side Effects and Adverse Effects

The adverse effects of thyroid medications are usually the result of overdose. The most significant adverse effect is cardiac dysrhythmia. Other more common undesirable effects are listed in Table 31-1.

Interactions

When thyroid preparations are taken in conjunction with oral anticoagulants, the activity of the oral anticoagulants is increased, thus necessitating reduced anticoagulant doses. Their concurrent use with cholestyramine results in reduced oral absorption of the antilipemic, and diabetic patients taking a thyroid agent may require increased doses of their hypoglycemic agents. In addition, their use with epinephrine in patients with coronary disease may induce coronary insufficiency.

Dosages

For the recommended dosages of the thyroid agents, see the dosages table on p. 468.

Thyroid Drugs: Clinically Equivalent Doses

THYROID DRUG	APPROXIMATE EQUIVALENT DOSE
Natural thyroid preparations	
Thyroid	60-65 mg (1 grain)
Synthetic thyroid preparations	
Levothyroxine	100 μg or less
Liothyronine	25 μg
Liotrix	50 μg/12.5 μg

Table 31-1	Thyroid Drugs: Common Adverse Effects
BODY SYSTEM	**SIDE/ADVERSE EFFECT**
Central nervous system	Insomnia, tremors, headache
Cardiovascular	Tachycardia, palpitations, angina, dysrhythmias, hypertension, cardiac arrest
Gastrointestinal	Nausea, diarrhea, increased or decreased appetite, cramps
Other	Menstrual irregularities, weight loss, sweating, heat intolerance, fever, thyroid storm

DOSAGES

SELECTED THYROID AGENTS

AGENT	PHARMACOLOGIC CLASS	DOSAGE RANGE	PURPOSE
Thyroid (S-P-T, Armour Thyroid, Thyrar, Thyroid Strong, Westhroid)	Desiccated thyroid gland	*Adult* PO: 65-195 mg/day	Hypothyroidism
↓**Levothyroxine (Levoxine, Levothroid, Synthyroid)**	Synthetic levothyroxine (T4) thyroid hormone	*Pediatric* PO: 0-6 mo, 8-10 μg/kg/day PO: 6-12 mo, 6-8 μg/kg/day PO: 1-5 y/o, 5-6 μg/kg/day PO: 6/12 y/o, 4-5 μg/kg/day *Adult* PO: 50-200 μg/day	Hypothyroidism
Liothyronine (Cytomel, Triostat)	Synthetic liothyronine (T3) thyroid hormone	*Pediatric* PO: Infants: usually require 20 μg/day PO: 1-3 y/o: usually require 50 μg/day PO: >3 y/o: may require full adult dose *Adult* PO: 25-75 μg/day PO: 50-100 μg/day	Hypothyroidism Myxedema
Liotrix (Thyrolar, Euthroid)	Synthetic T3/T4 thyroid hormone combination	*Adult* PO: start with a single daily dose of Thyrolar ¼ or ½ or of Euthroid ½ and adjust as needed at 2-wk intervals	Hypothyroidism

DRUG PROFILES

As already mentioned, there are a variety of agents that may be used for the treatment of hypothyroidism. The selection of a natural as opposed to a synthetic agent is based on many factors. These include the proportion of T3 to T4 desired, the cost, and the desired duration of effect. The thyroid drugs are classified as pregnancy category A agents. They are all contraindicated in patients who have had a hypersensitivity reaction to them in the past and in those suffering from adrenal insufficiency, myocardial infarction, or thyrotoxicosis.

Thyroid

Thyroid (S-P-T, Armour Thyroid, Thyrar, Thyroid Strong, Westhroid) is the cleaned, dried, and powdered thyroid gland of domesticated animals, usually hogs, and it is a combination of both T3 and T4 in a normal physiologic ratio. Each 60 to 65 mg of thyroid is approximately equivalent to 100 μg or less of T4 or 25 μg of T3. There is also a Thyroid Strong preparation that is 50% more potent than regular thyroid. Thyroid is only available orally as 60-, 120-, 180-, and 300-mg capsules; 15-, 30-, 60-, 65-, 90-, 120-, 130-, 180-, 240-, and 300-mg tablets; 30-, 60-, and 120-mg bovine (cattle-derived) tablets; 15-, 30-, 60-, 120-, 200-, 250-, and 300-mg pork (hog-derived) tablets; 60- and 120-mg enteric-coated tablets; and 32.5-, 65-, 130-, and 200-mg Thyroid Strong tablets. Common dosages are given in the dosages table above. Pregnancy category A.

PHARMACOKINETICS

HALF-LIFE	ONSET	PEAK	DURATION
6-7 days	2 days	8-10 days	3-5 days

THYROGLOBULIN

Thyroglobulin (Proloid) is a purified extract obtained from the thyroid of hogs. To ensure certain biologic activity, it has been standardized to contain a ratio of T4 to T3 of 2.5:1. It only comes as an oral preparation in the form of 32-, 65-, 100-, 130-, and 200-mg tablets. Common dosages are given in the preceding dosages table. Pregnancy category A.

PHARMACOKINETICS

HALF-LIFE	ONSET	PEAK	DURATION
6-7 days	2 days	8-10 days	3-5 days

LEVOTHYROXINE

Levothyroxine (Levoxine, Levothroid, Synthyroid), or T4, is the most commonly prescribed synthetic thyroid hormone. One advantage it has over the natural thyroid preparations is that it is chemically pure, being 100% T4. Its half-life is also long enough that it only needs to be administered once a day. It comes in both an oral and a parenteral form. As an oral preparation it comes as 12.5-, 25-, 50-, 75-, 88-, 100-, 112-, 125-, 150-, 175-, 200-, and 300-μg tablets. Parenterally it comes as a 200- and 500-μg injection. Common dosages are given in the preceding dosages table. Pregnancy category A.

PHARMACOKINETICS

HALF-LIFE	ONSET	PEAK	DURATION
6-7 days	2 days	8-10 days	3-5 days

LIOTHYRONINE

Liothyronine (Cytomel, Triostat) is also a chemically pure synthetic thyroid hormone preparation, but it is 100% T3. Another way in which it differs from levothyroxine is that it has a rapid onset and a short duration of action. These pharmacokinetic differences are important because they make liothyronine the preferred agent when either a rapid effect or a rapidly reversible effect is desired, such as for diagnostic procedures requiring short-term thyrotropin suppression or for the treatment of myxedema coma. On the other hand, its more pronounced adverse cardiovascular effects along with its short duration of action make it unsatisfactory for long-term use. It is only available

orally as 5-, 25-, and 50-μg tablets. Common dosages are given in the preceding dosages table. Pregnancy category A.

PHARMACOKINETICS

HALF-LIFE	ONSET	PEAK	DURATION
6-7 days	2 days	8-10 days	3-5 days

LIOTRIX

Liotrix (Thyrolar, Euthroid) is another synthetic thyroid hormone that is essentially a combination of the other two synthetic thyroid hormones, levothyroxine (T4) and liothyronine (T3). In the standard dose of liotrix, which is equivalent to 60 mg of thyroid, the respective amounts of T3 and T4 in the two commercial preparations differ slightly. Thyrolar contains 50 μg of T4 and 12.5 μg of T3. Euthyroid contains 60 μg of T4 and 15 μg of T3. The clinical significance of this is questionable. Liotrix is only available orally as tablets that contain T4 and T3 in the following amounts:

Levothyroxine (μg)	Liothyronine (μg)	Trade name
12.5	3.1	Thyrolar ¼
25	6.25	Thyrolar ½
30	7.5	Euthyroid ½
50	12.5	Thyrolar-1
60	15	Euthyroid-1
100	25	Thyrolar-2
120	30	Euthyroid-2
150	37.5	Thyrolar-3
180	45	Euthyroid-3

Common dosages are given in the preceding dosages table. Pregnancy category A.

PHARMACOKINETICS

HALF-LIFE	ONSET	PEAK	DURATION
6-7 days	2-3 days	8-10 days	3-5 days

ANTITHYROID AGENTS

The treatment of hyperthyroidism may be aimed at treating either the primary cause or the symptoms of the disease. Antithyroid drugs, iodides, ionic inhibitors, and radioactive isotopes of iodine are used to treat the underlying cause, and drugs such as beta-blockers are used to treat the symptoms. The focus of the discussion here is on the antithyroid drugs called the *thioamide derivatives,* which mainly consist of methimazole and propylthiouracil. Surgery is a nonpharmacologic means of treating hyperthyroidism and involves removal of part of the thyroid gland. It is usually a very effective way to treat hyperthyroidism.

Mechanism of Action

Methimazole and propylthiouracil act by inhibiting the incorporation of iodine molecules into the amino acid tyrosine, a process required to make both monoiodotyrosine and diiodotyrosine, the precursors of T3 and T4. By doing this, the formation of thyroid hormone is impeded. Propylthiouracil has the added ability to inhibit the conversion of T4 to T3 in the peripheral circulation. Neither drug can inactivate already existing thyroid hormone, however.

Drug Effects

The drug effects of methimazole and propylthiouracil are primarily limited to the thyroid gland, their overall effect being a decrease in the thyroid hormone level. The administration of these medications to patients suffering from hyperthyroidism lowers the high levels of thyroid hormone, thereby normalizing the overall metabolic rate.

Therapeutic Uses

The antithyroid agents are used to palliate hyperthyroidism and to prevent the surge in thyroid hormones that occurs after the surgical treatment of or during the radioactive iodine therapy for hyperthyroidism. In some types of hyperthyroidism such as that seen in the Graves' disease, the long-term administration of these agents (several years) may induce a spontaneous remission. However, most patients eventually require surgery or radioactive iodine therapy to ablate the condition.

Side Effects and Adverse Effects

The most damaging or serious adverse effects of the two antithyroid medications are liver and bone marrow toxicity. These and the more common adverse effects of methimazole and propylthiouracil are listed in Table 31-2.

Interactions

Drug interactions that occur with the antithyroid agents include an additive agranulocytosis when they are taken in conjunction with other bone marrow depressants and an increase in the activity of oral anticoagulants.

Dosages

See the dosages table on the next page for the recommended dosages of methimazole and propylthiouracil.

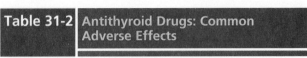

Table 31-2	Antithyroid Drugs: Common Adverse Effects
BODY SYSTEM	**SIDE/ADVERSE EFFECT**
Central nervous system	Drowsiness, headache, vertigo, fever, paresthesia
Skin	Rash, pruritus, hyperpigmentation
Gastrointestinal	Nausea, vomiting, diarrhea, jaundice, hepatitis, loss of taste
Musculoskeletal	Myalgia, arthralgia, nocturnal muscle cramps
Hematologic	Agranulocytosis, leukopenia, thrombocytopenia, hypothrombinemia, lymphadenopathy, bleeding
Other	Enlarged thyroid, nephritis

DRUG PROFILES

METHIMAZOLE

Methimazole (Tapazole) is one of the two thioamide antithyroid agents and is rated as a pregnancy category D agent. It is contraindicated in patients who have shown a hypersensitivity to it and in pregnant women during the third trimester. It is only available orally as a 5- and 10-mg tablet. Common dosages are given in the following dosages table.

PHARMACOKINETICS

HALF-LIFE	ONSET	PEAK	DURATION
5-13 hr	30-40 min	1 hr	2-4 hr

PROPYLTHIOURACIL

Propylthiouracil (PTU) is the other thioamide antithyroid agents and is also rated as a pregnancy category D agent. The contraindications to its use are the same as those for methimazole. It is only available orally and comes as a 50-mg tablet. Common dosages are given in the following dosages table.

PHARMACOKINETICS

HALF-LIFE	ONSET	PEAK	DURATION
1-2 hr	30-40 min	1-1.5 hr	2-4 hr

DOSAGES

SELECTED ANTITHYROID AGENTS

AGENT	PHARMACOLOGIC CLASS	DOSAGE RANGE	PURPOSE
Methimazole (Tapazole)		*Pediatric* PO: 0.4 mg/kg/day in 3 divided doses q8h; usual maintenance dose is half initial dose. *Adult* PO: 15-60 mg in 3 divided doses q8h; maintenance dose is 5-10 mg/day.	Hyperthyroidism
Propylthiouracil (PTU)	Antithyroid	*Pediatric* PO: 6-10 y/o: 50-150 mg/day in 3 divided doses at 8-hr intervals; maintenance dose depends on response. >12 y/o: 150-300 mg in 3 divided doses at 8-hr intervals *Adult* PO: 300-900 mg/day in 3 divided doses at 8-hr intervals; usual maintenance dose is 100-150 mg/day.	Hyperthyroidism

NURSING PROCESS

ASSESSMENT

Before administering any of the thyroid agents, the nurse should assess the patient to make sure he or she has none of the conditions that would contraindicate their use. These include adrenal insufficiency, myocardial infarction, and hyperthyroidism. Their cautious use is recommended in patients with coronary heart disease, hypertension, angina, or cardiac disease, and in pregnant women. See also the box at right, which summarizes some of the special considerations that apply to geriatric patients receiving these agents.

The antithyroid hormones methimazole and propylthiouracil are contraindicated in patients who have shown a hypersensitivity to the medication and in pregnant women during the third trimester. Cautious use is recommended in patients with liver disease, infections, or bone marrow disease (because of the agranulocytosis and other blood dyscrasias they can cause)

GERIATRIC CONSIDERATIONS
Thyroid Hormones

- The elderly patient is much more sensitive to thyroid hormone replacement therapy and also more liable to suffer more adverse reactions to thyroid hormones than patients in any other age group.

- Make sure that the medication regimen in an elderly patient is highly individualized. Often the dose in elderly patients must be 25% less than that given to patients of other age groups.

- Because the symptoms of hypothyroidism may be confused with the symptoms of other diseases, nonspecific symptoms such as stumbling, falling, depression, incontinence, cold intolerance, and weight gain should be thoroughly evaluated and documented before a diagnosis of hypothyroidism is rendered.

and during the first and second trimesters of pregnancy.

Baseline weights and vital signs should be obtained and recorded in any patients receiving either a thyroid or antithyroid preparation.

NURSING DIAGNOSES

Nursing diagnoses appropriate to patients receiving a thyroid or antithyroid preparation include:

- Risk for injury to self as the result of the side effects of the medications.
- Risk for infection as the result of the bone marrow depression caused by antithyroid medications.
- Pain (acute) related to the side effects of the medications.
- Altered cardiac output (decreased) related to side effects of the thyroid agents.
- Knowledge deficit regarding the medication therapy.

PLANNING

Goals pertaining to patients receiving a thyroid or antithyroid prreparation include:

- Patient remains free from injury as the result of the side effects of the medications.
- Patient will be monitored closely, such as the blood cell counts, while taking the medication.
- Patient remains free of infection while receiving antithyroid medication.
- Patient maintains normal energy levels while on thyroid agents.
- Patient experiences minimal side effects resulting from the medications.
- Patient demonstrates an understanding of the use of the thyroid agent and its side effects and need for compliance by stating such information.

Outcome Criteria

Outcome criteria that pertain to patients receiving a thyroid or antithyroid preparation include:

- Patient will state measures to implement to decrease the likelihood of self-injury related to the drug's side effects such as frequent laboratory checks and monitoring vital signs.
- Patient states the importance of follow-up appointments with the physician for frequent blood studies and monitoring of therapeutic effects.
- Patient states ways to decrease the risk of infection while receiving an antithyroid medication such as avoiding persons with infections and eating a proper diet and getting adequate rest.
- Patient uses relaxation techniques to deal with the nervousness and irritability caused by the agents or the diseases.

IMPLEMENTATION

When administering thyroid agents, it is important to give the medication at the same time each day in order to maintain consistent blood levels of the agent. If pos-

Patient Teaching TIPS

Thyroid and Antithyroid Agents

✔ Patients should never discontinue their medication without the physician's approval or order.

✔ It is important for patients taking thyroid agents to take the medication exactly as prescribed, at the same time everyday, and not to switch brands, unless approved by the physician.

✔ A too high dose of a thyroid agent will result in nervousness, irritability, and insomnia.

✔ Patients taking thyroid agents should report any unusual symptoms, chest pain, or heart palpitations.

✔ Patients taking either thyroid or antithyroid drugs should not take any over-the-counter medications.

✔ Patients taking antithyroid medications may be advised to avoid eating foods high in iodine, such as soy, tofu, turnip, seafood, and some breads, as well as to avoid using iodized salt.

✔ Patients should understand that the therapeutic effects of thyroid agents may take several months to occur.

✔ Patients taking thyroid and antithyroid agents should keep a log or journal of their responses to the therapy and a graph of their pulse, weight, and mood status.

sible, it is also best to administer thyroid agents given once a day in the morning to decrease the likelihood of insomnia that may result from evening dosing. If administering levothyroxine intravenously, the nurse should follow the manufacturer's guidelines regarding the dilutional substances and the rate of administration. If the patient is scheduled to undergo any radioactive isotope studies, the thyroid medication is usually discontinued about 4 weeks before the test, but only with a physician's order.

Antithyroid medications are better tolerated orally when taken with meals. These agents should also be given at the same time every day to maintain consistent blood levels of the agent. In addition, these medications should never be withdrawn abruptly.

Teaching tips for patients receiving thyroid or antithyroid agents are presented in the box above.

EVALUATION

A therapeutic response to thyroid agents is reflected by the disappearance of the symptoms of hypothy-

TAKE HOME POINTS

Thyroid Hormone

- Thyroxine (T4) and tyrosine (T3) are the two hormones produced by the thyroid gland.
- Made by iodination and coupling with the amino acid tyrosine.
- T4 is made by combining two molecules of diiodotyrosine (it has four iodine molecules).
- T3 is formed by coupling one molecule of diiodotyrosine with one molecule of monoiodotyrosine (it has three iodine molecules).
- T3 is about four times more biologically potent than thyroxine.

Hypothyroidism

- Primary hypothyroidism caused by an abnormality in the thyroid gland itself.
- Secondary hypothyroidism may result from a dysfunctional pituitary gland (lowered TSH level).
- Tertiary hypothyroidism similar to secondary in that the stimulus needed for secretion of thyroid hormone is absent.
- Tertiary hypothyroidism is due to hypothalamic rather than pituitary dysfunction (lowered TRH level).

Thyroid Replacement

- Natural and synthetic thyroid hormone.
- Natural preparations are derived from animal thyroid and include thyroid and thyroglobulin.
- Synthetic preparations include levothyroxine, liothyronine, and liotrix.

Hyperthyroidism

- Caused by excessive secretion of thyroid hormone from the thyroid gland.
- Due to different diseases or drugs.
- Diseases = Graves' disease, Plummer's disease, and multinodular disease.

Antithyroid Drugs

- Called *thioamide derivatives* and consist of mainly methimazole and propylthiouracil.
- Surgery is a nondrug therapy for hyperthyroidism.
- Drugs act by inhibiting the incorporation of iodine molecules into the amino acid tyrosine.
- By inhibiting the formation of the precursors of thyroid hormone they prevent its formation.

Nursing Considerations

- Children taking thyroid replacement hormones will show almost immediate behavior and personality changes reflecting their improved thyroid state.
- Patients on thyroid hormone replacement therapy should avoid iodine food containing iodized salt, soybeans, tofu, turnips, some types of seafood, and some breads. A nutritional consult is recommended as part of the therapy protocol.
- Patients should report the occurrence of excitability, irritability, or anxiety to their physician or health care provider, as these may indicate toxicity.
- Hair loss in children taking thyroid replacements is temporary.

RESEARCH ACTIVITY

Read and prepare a written review of one research article published within the past 5 years that deals with the use of thyroid hormones in patients with hypothyroidism. Discuss the research's impact on nursing care.

roidism; these include depression, constipation, loss of appetite, weight gain, cold intolerance, syncope, and dry and brittle hair. Increased nervousness, irritability, mood changes, angina, and palpitations are side effects that need to be reported to the physician immediately. Clues to the fact that a patient is receiving inadequate doses include tachycardia, irritability, nervousness, and fever.

A therapeutic response to antithyroid medications would be characterized by weight gain, decreased pulse, a return to a normal blood pressure, and decreased serum levels of T4. Symptoms of overdose include cold intolerance, depression, and edema. The patient should be encouraged to report the development of any swelling, sore throat, lesions, or other signs of inflammation. Clues to the fact that a patient is not receiving adequate doses include tachycardia, insomnia, irritability, fever, and diarrhea.

Critical Thinking **A C T I V I T I E S**

1. Your patient has been taking thyroid agents for about 16 months and has recently noted palpitations and some heat intolerance. Should you be concerned about this? Explain your answer.

2. D.W. is a 63-year-old woman who has just had her thyroid gland removed and is being started on thyroid hormone replacement with levothyroxine (Synthroid) at a dose of 200 μg once a day.
   a. How much is 200 μg of levothyroxine in milligrams?
   b. How many grains of thyroid would this be equivalent to?

3. You are caring for a patient who has just been transferred to your floor from the intensive care unit. The patient underwent a thyroidectomy 2 days ago, and the transfer orders instruct that he should be started on his home medications. The written orders specify that 25 μg of levothyroxine should be given once daily. However, the pharmacy has sent 25 μg of liothyronine, another thyroid replacement product. Because the dose of each is the same, is it okay to administer the liothyronine?

4. In an attempt to control the insomnia associated with thyroid hormone replacement therapy, the patient may be encouraged to do which of the following:
   a. Take one half of the dose in the morning and the other half at dinner or at bedtime.
   b. Try to switch the dosing to every other day, and if this is unsuccessful in relieving the insomnia, to notify the physician of the problem.
   c. Take the medication in the morning, if possible.
   d. Try lowering the dose every day by one fourth until the insomnia is gone.

▲▲▲

BIBLIOGRAPHY

Albanese J, Nutz P: *Mosby's 1995 nursing drug cards,* St Louis, 1995, Mosby.

Johnson KB: *Harriet Lane handbook,* ed 13, St Louis, 1993, Mosby.

Keen JH: *Critical care and emergency drug reference,* St Louis, 1994, Mosby.

Knoben JE, Anderson PO: *Handbook of critical drug data,* ed 6, Hamilton, Ill, 1988, Drug Intelligence Publications.

McEvoy GK: *AHFS drug information,* Bethesda, Md, 1994, American Society of Hospital Pharmacists.

Roberts A: The thyroid gland and its disorders in later life, *Nursing Times,* 86(28):663, 1990.

Skidmore-Roth L: *Mosby's 1995 nursing drug reference,* St Louis, 1995, Mosby.

Chapter 32

Antidiabetic and Hypoglycemic Agents

Objectives

When you reach the end of this chapter, you will be able to:

1. Discuss the normal actions and functions of the pancreas and the feedback system that regulates it.
2. Describe the differences in the hyposecretion and hypersecretion of insulin and the difference between non–insulin-dependent and insulin-dependent diabetes mellitus.
3. Describe the various factors influencing the blood glucose levels in the presence or absence of diabetes mellitus.
4. Identify the various agents used to manage non–insulin-dependent and insulin-dependent diabetes mellitus.
5. Identify the signs and symptoms of hypoglycemia and hyperglycemia.
6. Discuss the mechanism of action of indications for, contraindications and cautions to, and side effects of the insulin, oral antidiabetic, and hypoglycemic agents
7. Develop a nursing care plan as it relates to the nursing process in patients receiving insulin, oral antidiabetic agents, or hypoglycemic agents.
8. Identify the teaching guidelines for patients receiving insulin, oral antidiabetic agents, or hypoglycemic agents.

CHAPTER OUTLINE

The Pancreas

Diabetes Mellitus
  Insulin-dependent diabetes mellitus
  Non–insulin-dependent diabetes mellitus
Hypoglycemia

Antidiabetic Agents

Insulins
  Mechanism of action
  Drug effects
  Therapeutic uses
  Side effects and adverse effects
  Interactions
  Dosages

Drug Profiles
  Rapid-acting Insulin
  Intermediate-acting Insulin
  Long-acting Insulin
  Fixed-combination Insulins
Oral Antidiabetic Agents
  Mechanism of action
  Drug effects
  Therapeutic uses
  Side effects and adverse effects

Interactions
Dosages
Drug Profiles
  Chlorpropamide
  Glipizide
  Glyburide
Investigational Drugs
Glucose-Elevating Drugs

Nursing Process
Assessment
Nursing Diagnoses
Planning
  Outcome criteria
Implementation
Evaluation

Glossary

Diabetes mellitus (di ə be′ tēz me′ lə təs) Complex disorder of carbohydrate, fat, and protein metabolism primarily resulting from the lack of insulin secretion by the beta cells of the pancreas or from defects of the insulin receptors. (p. 477)

Diabetic ketoacidosis (ke′ to as ĭ do′ sis) Diabetic coma. (p. 477)

Glucagon (gloo′ kə gon) Hormone produced by the alpha cells in the islets of Langerhans that stimulates the conversion of glycogen to glucose in the liver. (p. 476)

Glucose (gloo′ kōs) Simple sugar found in fruits that serves as a major source of energy. (p. 476)

Glycogen (gli′ co jən) A polysaccharide that is the major carbohydrate stored in animal cells. (p. 476)

Glycogenolysis (gli′ co jə nol′ ə sis) Breakdown of glycogen to glucose. (p. 476)

Hyperglycemia (hi′ pər gli se′ me ə) A greater than normal amount of glucose in the blood. (p. 476)

Hypoglycemia A less than normal amount of glucose in the blood. (p. 478)

Insulin (in′ sə lin) Naturally occurring hormone secreted by the beta cells of the islands of Langerhans in response to increased levels of glucose in the blood. (p. 476)

Insulin-dependent diabetes mellitus An inability to metabolize carbohydrate caused by an overt insulin deficiency that occurs in children and adults. (p. 477)

Ketones (ke′ tōnz) Organic chemical compound produced through the oxidation of secondary alcohols. (p. 477)

Nephropathy (nə frop′ ə the) Disorder of the kidney that includes inflammatory, degenerative, and sclerotic conditions. (p. 477)

Neuropathy (noŏ rop′ ə the) Inflammation or degeneration of the peripheral nerves. (p. 477)

Non–insulin-dependent diabetes mellitus Type of diabetes mellitus in which patients are not insulin dependent but they may take insulin to correct the hyperglycemia. (p. 477)

Polydipsia (pol ĭ-dip′ se-ə) Chronic excessive intake of water. (p. 476)

Polyphagia (pol e-fa′ jə) Excessive eating. (p. 476)

Polyuria (pol e-u′ re-ə) The passage of a large volume of urine in a given period, a characteristic of diabetes. (p. 476)

Retinopathy (ret ĭ nop′ ə the) Noninflammatory eye disorder resulting from changes in the retinal blood vessels. (p. 477)

The Pancreas

The pancreas is a large, elongated organ that is located behind the stomach. It is both an exocrine (secreting digestive enzymes) and endocrine organ, but it is its endocrine function that is relevant to the discussion here. There are two main hormones produced by the pancreas—insulin and glucagon, and both play an important role in the regulation of the endocrine system, specifically the utilization, mobilization, and storage of **glucose,** which is one of the primary sources of energy for the cells of our body. There is a normal amount of

glucose that circulates in the blood to meet quick energy requirements. However, not all the glucose we consume is needed. When the quantity of glucose in the blood is sufficient, the excess is stored as **glycogen** in the liver, where it remains until the body needs it.

When blood glucose is needed, the glycogen in the storage sites in the liver is converted back to glucose through a process called **glycogenolysis**. The hormone responsible for initiating this process is **glucagon**.

At the same time that the glucagon is released from the alpha cells of the islets of Langerhans in the pancreas, the beta cells of these same islets secrete insulin, a protein hormone composed of two chains, the A chain, which is acidic, and the B chain, which is basic, with the two chains joined by a disulfide linkage. The actions of **insulin** oppose those of glucagon. Essentially insulin takes the excess glucose from the blood and places it in the liver for storage. It also inhibits further glucagon release. These opposing actions of insulin and glucagon serve as a check and balance for each other, and both are needed to maintain normal glucose levels in the blood.

Two other substances that function as glucose regulators are cortisol and epinephrine, and these work synergistically with glucagon to counter the effects of insulin and cause increases in the blood glucose level. Insulin actually serves many important functions in the body, all of them related to metabolism. It stimulates carbohydrate metabolism in skeletal and cardiac muscle and adipose tissue by facilitating the transport of glucose into these cells. In the liver, insulin facilitates the phosphorylation of glucose to glucose-6-phosphate, which is then converted to glycogen for storage. By causing glucose to be stored in the liver as glycogen, insulin keeps the kidney free of glucose, which without it would cause the kidney to contain spillage substances such as glucose, ketones, and other substances that would otherwise draw water into the nephron, causing **polydipsia**, **polyuria**, and **polyphagia**.

Insulin also has a direct effect on fat metabolism. It stimulates lipogenesis and inhibits lipolysis and the release of fatty acids from adipose cells. In addition, insulin stimulates protein synthesis and promotes the intracellular shift of potassium and magnesium, thereby decreasing elevated blood concentrations of these electrolytes. The actions of insulin are antagonized by the following body substances: somatropin (growth hormone), epinephrine, adrenocortical hormones, thyroid hormones, and estrogens.

DIABETES MELLITUS

Hyperglycemia is the state in which there is too much glucose in the blood and results when the counterbalancing actions of glucagon and insulin go away. One of the most common causes is a syndrome known as diabetes mellitus. **Diabetes mellitus** is primarily a disorder of carbohydrate metabolism that involves either a deficiency of insulin or a resistance to insulin, or both. Whatever the cause of the diabetes, the result is hyperglycemia.

Diabetes mellitus has been recognized since 1550 B.C. when Egyptians wrote of a malady they called "honeyed urine." The first step toward discerning the cause of it occurred in 1788 when Thomas Cawley, an English physician, voiced his suspicion that the source of the illness lay in the pancreas. However, it took over a century to prove this, and it took even longer to discover the substance, insulin, that is secreted from the pancreas, the lack of which is responsible for causing the disease. It was known that the substance, whatever it was, was needed by those afflicted with the illness, but the substance could not be isolated. It was not until the early 1920s that insulin was finally discovered. Its discovery is now considered one of the greatest triumphs of twentieth-century medicine, and its use in the therapy for diabetes mellitus has proved to be a life-saving remedy for millions.

Diabetes mellitus is not actually a single disease, however, but a group of diseases, and this is why it is often regarded as a syndrome rather than a disease. The relative or absolute lack of insulin is believed to result from the destruction of beta cells in the pancreas such that insulin can neither be produced nor secreted. Hyperglycemia can also be caused by insulin receptor-defects. When the receptors that normally function in coordination with insulin in removing glucose from the blood are defective, they no longer recognize insulin and therefore the glucose remains in the blood. In addition, other cells throughout the body that are supposed to recognize insulin may become insulin resistant and refuse to use circulating insulin. These differences in the source of the hyperglycemia account for

the two types of diabetes mellitus that have been recognized: type I, or **insulin-dependent diabetes mellitus** (IDDM), and type II, or **non–insulin-dependent diabetes mellitus** (NIDDM). There are also three categories of diabetes mellitus; these are secondary diabetes, gestational diabetes, and impaired glucose tolerance. The differences between IDDM and NIDDM are listed in Table 32-1.

Insulin-Dependent Diabetes Mellitus

Type I diabetes mellitus, or IDDM, is characterized by a lack of insulin production or by the production of a defective insulin, and affected patients require exogenous insulin to treat and prevent its many complications. Common complications of the disorder are the destruction of the retina of the eye, **retinopathy**; the destruction of nerves, **neuropathy**; and the destruction of the nephrons of the kidney, **nephropathy**. These occur because rather than the glucose being broken down into the normal carbohydrates, lipids, and proteins for use in maintaining the body's vital functions, they are broken down into other nutrients that are harmful to the body. For instance, fatty acids are converted to **ketones**, and these in turn cause the development of **diabetic ketoacidosis** (DKA), a complex multisystem disorder and a common complication of uncontrolled IDDM that results in coma. The person experiencing DKA is suffering from extreme hyperglycemia, positive serum ketone levels, acidosis, dehydration, and electrolyte imbalances. Approximately 25% to 30% of the patients with IDDM present with DKA, the most common precipitator of DKA being physical or emotional stress. The stress triggers it by causing the release of the counterregulatory hormones cortisol and epinephrine, which then mobilize glucagon and release glucose from the storage sites in the liver, further

Table 32-1	Type I and II Diabetes: Characteristics	
CHARACTERISTIC	**TYPE I (IDDM)**	**TYPE II (NIDDM)**
Onset	Juvenile-onset diabetes, <20 yr old	Maturity-onset diabetes, >40 yr old
Endogenous insulin	Little or none	Normal
Treatment	Insulin	Weight loss, diet and exercise, oral hypoglycemics; only a third of patients need insulin
Incidence	10%	90%
Receptors	Normal	Decreased or defective
Body weight	Usually nonobese	Obese (80%)
Etiology	Autoimmune destruction of beta cells in the pancreas	Multifactorial genetic defects; strong association with obesity and insulin resistance resulting from a reduction in insulin receptors

adding to the already elevated levels of glucose in the blood.

Non–Insulin-Dependent Diabetes Mellitus

NIDDM, which was once thought to be a mild form of IDDM, is an important but poorly treated disorder. Of all the forms of diabetes mellitus, it is by far the most common, accounting for about 85% of all the cases of diabetes mellitus and affecting as much as 10% of the population over 70. There are many common and dangerous misconceptions regarding NIDDM: that it is a mild diabetes, that it is easy to treat, and that tight metabolic control is unnecessary because these patients, being mostly old, will die before diabetic complications develop. None of these are true, however.

NIDDM is due to both insulin resistance and insulin deficiency. As already noted, one of insulin's normal roles is to take circulating glucose and transport it to tissues to be used as energy. In the setting of NIDDM all the main target tissues of insulin (muscle, liver, and adipose tissue) are hyporesponsive (resistant) to the effects of the hormone. Not only is the absolute number of insulin receptors on these tissues reduced but their sensitivity and responsiveness to insulin are reduced as well. Therefore it is possible for a patient with NIDDM to have normal or even elevated levels of insulin yet have high blood glucose levels as well. The reason for this paradoxical situation is that the altered insulin-sensing mechanism causes the liver to overproduce glucose, adding to the already present hyperglycemic condition.

The reduction in insulin secretion that can occur in patients with NIDDM is the result of a loss of the response of the beta cells in the pancreas to the elevated blood glucose levels and other stimuli. If these beta cells do not recognize glucose, they do not secrete insulin, and glucose is not transported into cells or tissues nor is it stored in the liver. There also seems to be an alteration in the response to meals in patients with NIDDM. Either insulin resistance or insulin deficiency may lead to or induce the other.

Although NIDDM is a multifaceted disorder, lipid abnormalities, obesity, and hypertension are the primary findings in most persons afflicted with it. The dyslipidemias of NIDDM typically involve hypertriglyceridemia and the atherogenic combination of decreased high-density (HDL) and elevated low-density (LDL) lipoprotein cholesterol.

HYPOGLYCEMIA

Hypoglycemia is the condition in which the blood glucose level is abnormally low. When the cause is organic and the effects mild, treatment usually consists of dietary modifications, primarily a high intake of protein and low intake of carbohydrates. The condition can also be caused by the antidiabetic agents and occurs when the effect of these agents is greater than that expected. There are also other drugs that can cause it. Common symptoms of the disorder when it is more severe are confusion, sweating, hypothermia, tremor, headache, irritability, hallucinations, convulsions, and ultimately coma and death if it is not treated. Because the brain needs a constant amount of glucose to function, often some of the first symptoms of hypoglycemia are the central nervous system manifestations—the confusion, irritability, hallucinations, and so on.

Antidiabetic Agents

The two largest classes of drugs used to treat diabetes mellitus are the insulins and the oral hypoglycemics. These drugs may broadly be referred to as *antidiabetic agents* because they are aimed at preventing the hyperglycemia induced by diabetes mellitus.

⬇INSULINS

The primary treatment for IDDM is insulin therapy. Today there are two main sources of insulin. It can be extracted from domesticated animals or synthesized in laboratories using recombinant DNA technology. The two insulins that come from animal sources are cattle (bovine) insulin, which differs from the human form by only two amino acids, and pig (porcine) insulin, which differs from human insulin by only one amino acid. Recombinantly made insulin is made by feeding bacteria or yeast the genetic information necessary for them to reproduce an insulin that is exactly like human insulin. The pharmacokinetic properties of exogenous insulin (the onset of action, peak effect, and duration of action) have been manipulated so that there are now five different insulin preparations. Several combination preparations are also available. This manipulation of insulin activity was required to help meet the various time-oriented metabolic demands for insulin in diabetic patients. Further modifications can be accomplished by mixing compatible insulin preparations before administration. Regular insulin can be mixed with any insulin preparation. Semilente is compatible with lente and ultralente insulin.

Mechanism of Action

Exogenous insulin elicits all the same physiologic responses as those usually elicited by the endogenous

Table 32-2 ⚓ Insulin: Common Adverse Effects

Body System	Side/Adverse Effect
Central nervous system	Headache, lethargy, tremors, weakness, fatigue, delirium, sweating
Cardiovascular	Tachycardia, palpitations
Metabolic	Hypoglycemia
Other	Blurred vision, dry mouth, hunger, nausea, flushing, rash, urticaria, anaphylaxis

hormone and is administered to replace either what is not made or is made defectively.

Drug Effects

The drug effects of exogenously administered insulin are many and affect many body systems. They are the same as those of normal endogenous insulin. That is, exogenously administered insulin restores the diabetic's ability to metabolize carbohydrates, fats, and proteins; to store glucose in the liver; and to convert glycogen to fat.

Therapeutic Uses

As already discussed, endogenous insulin has many positive effects on several body systems. Its primary therapeutic effect, however, is maintaining normal blood levels of glucose. By causing the appropriate utilization, mobilization, and storage of glucose, exogenous insulin can serve as a replacement for the defective or insufficient natural hormone.

Side Effects and Adverse Effects

Hypoglycemia resulting from an insulin overdose can result in shock and possibly death. This is the most immediate and serious adverse effect of insulin. Other more common adverse effects of insulin therapy are listed in Table 32-2.

Interactions

Drug interactions that can occur with the insulins are significant. Chlorthalidone, corticosteroids, diazoxide, epinephrine, ethacrynic acid, furosemide, phenytoin, thiazides, and thyroid hormones can all antagonize the hypoglycemic effects of insulin. Alcohol, anabolic steroids, guanethidine, MAO-inhibitors, propranolol, and the salicylates can all increase insulin's hypoglycemic effects.

Dosages

See the dosages table on the next page for the recommended dosages of the various insulin agents.

DRUG PROFILES

The primary treatment for IDDM is insulin therapy, and there are three basic types of insulin, as determined by their pharmacokinetic properties—rapid, intermediate, and long acting. They are classified as pregnancy category B agents and are contraindicated in patients who have shown hypersensitivity reactions to them.

RAPID-ACTING INSULIN

There are many rapid-acting insulin products, Humulin, Iletin, and Velosulin being just a few of these. There is both a regular and a semilente insulin that comes from each of the three main sources: beef, pork, and human. Both the regular and semilente forms are considered rapid acting because of their rapid onset of action. Regular insulin is also the only insulin that is clear. All other insulins are cloudy. Their effects are most like those of the endogenous insulin produced from the pancreas in response to a meal. After a meal, the glucose that is ingested stimulates the pancreas to secrete insulin. This insulin then takes the excess glucose and stores it in the liver as glycogen. In persons with diabetes mellitus, the insulin response to meals is deficient, so a rapid-acting insulin product such as regular or semilente is used.

All the currently available beef, pork, and human regular and semilente insulins come in a strength of 100 U/ml. Iletin II, from purified pork, also comes in a 500-U/ml strength. The usually recommended doses are given in the dosages table on the next page. Pregnancy category B.

❇ PHARMACOKINETICS

	ONSET	PEAK	DURATION
Regular:	0.5-1 hr	2-3 hr	8 hr
Semilente:	0.5-1.5 hr	5-10 hr	12-16 hr

INTERMEDIATE-ACTING INSULIN

There are two main types of intermediate-acting insulin products—lente and NPH insulin—and there is an intermediate-acting agent from each of the three

D O S A G E S

INSULINS

AGENT	PHARMACOLOGIC CLASS	DOSAGE RANGE	PURPOSE
Insulin injection (regular) (Humulin BR, Iletin, Velosulin)	Rapid-acting insulin (unmodified)	SC: Must be individualized to patient's needs	Diabetes and diabetic coma
Prompt insulin zinc (Semilente)	Rapid-acting insulin zinc suspension	SC: Usual starting dose, 10-20 U bid and adjusted	Diabetes
Isophane insulin (NPH) (Humulin N, Iletin NPH, Novolin-N)	Intermediate-acting insulin zinc suspension	SC: Usual starting dose, 7-26 U 30-60 min before breakfast and adjusted	Diabetes
Insulin zinc (Lente)	Intermediate-acting insulin zinc suspension	SC: Usual starting dose, 7-26 U 30-60 min before breakfast and adjusted	Diabetes
Extended insulin zinc (Ultralente, Iletin)	Long-acting insulin zinc suspension	SC: Usual starting dose, 7-26 U 30-60 min before breakfast and adjusted	Diabetes
Combination insulins (NPH/regular) (Humulin 70/30, Humulin 50/50, Mextard 70/30, Novolin 70/30)	Rapid/intermediate-acting insulin mixture	SC: Must be individualized to patient's needs	Diabetes

main sources: beef, pork, and human. As the experience with the regular insulins grew, a search was mounted for a longer-acting insulin that would eliminate the need for relatively frequent dosing. It was found that the duration of the effects of insulin could be prolonged through the addition of a basic protein such as protamine or a substance such as zinc. This led to the development in the late 1930s and 1940s of protamine-zinc insulin (PZI) and neutral protamine hagedorn (NPH) insulin.

Lente insulin is an intermediate-acting insulin that contains zinc, 70% of which is long-acting insulin zinc (ultralente) and 30% of which is rapid-acting insulin zinc (semilente). The result is a cloudy insulin solution with a usual onset of action of about 1 to 2.5 hours. Neutral Protamine Hagedorn (NPH) insulin, also known as isophane insulin, is a sterile suspension of zinc insulin crystals and protamine sulfate in buffered water for injection. The resulting suspension is a cloudy or milky suspension.

Because of their intermediate onset of action, the effects of these insulins are slower in onset and more prolonged than those of endogenous insulin. Both of

these intermediate-acting insulins come in a strength of 100 U/ml. The usually recommended dosages are given in the dosages table above. Pregnancy category B.

☙ P H A R M A C O K I N E T I C S

ONSET	PEAK	DURATION
Lente: 1-2.5 hr	7-15 hr	18-24 hr
Isophane: 1-2 hr	4-12 hr	18-24 hr

LONG-ACTING INSULIN

There is only one type of long-acting insulin product—ultralente insulin. It is available as both a human and beef insulin and comes in a 100 U/ml strength. Its duration of action was prolonged through the addition of even more zinc, specifically zinc chloride, than that added to create the intermediate-acting insulins.

Ultralente insulin, or extended insulin zinc, is a sterile suspension of insulin in buffered water that is given by injection. The resulting suspension is cloudy or milky. The ultralente insulins have an onset of ac-

Table 32-3	Available Insulin Products		
TYPE	**BEEF**	**PORK**	**HUMAN**
Rapid-acting			
Regular	Iletin I*	Iletin II	Humulin R
PZI	Iletin II	Regular Pork	Novolin R
	Semilente	Iletin I Semilente*	—
Intermediate-acting			
Lente	Iletin I Lente*	Iletin II Lente	Humulin L
NPH	Lente Beef	Lente Pork	Novolin L
	Iletin I NPH*	Ilentin II NPH	Humulin N
	NPH Beef	NPH Pork	Novolin N
		Insulatard NPH	
Long-acting EZI	Iletin I Ultralente*	—	Humulin U
	Ultralente Beef		

PZI, prompt zinc insulin; *EZI*, extended zinc insulin.
*Iletin I is a combination of beef and pork regular insulin.

tion that exceeds 4 hours. Besides being slower in onset, their effects are also more prolonged than those of endogenous insulin. The usually recommended dosages are given in the preceding dosages table. Pregnancy category B.

❇ P H A R M A C O K I N E T I C S

ONSET	PEAK	DURATION
4 hr	10-30 hr	36 hr

FIXED-COMBINATION INSULINS

Fixed-combination insulins (Humulin 50/50 and 70/30, Mextard 70/30, Novolin 70/30) were developed to more closely simulate the varying levels of endogenous insulin that occur normally in nondiabetic persons. To maintain constant blood glucose levels both after and in between meals, insulin must be present. In some insulin regimens, patients take a combination of a rapid-acting insulin to deal with the surges in glucose that occur after meals and an intermediate or long-acting insulin for in between meals when the glucose levels are less. However, this requires the mixing of insulins and the use of different types of insulins. Fixed-combination products were developed in an attempt to simplify matters. These agents can more closely simulate the body's own varying levels of insulin.

The fixed-combination insulin products from a human source are available in the following combinations: 50 U of isophane insulin (intermediate-acting) with 50 U of regular (short-acting) insulin and 70 U of isophane insulin with 30 U of regular insulin. The fixed-combination insulin product from a pork source contains 70 U of pork isophane insulin and 30 U of regular pork insulin.

The available insulin products are classified by their source and pharmacokinetic characteristics in Table 32-3. Pregnancy category B.

ORAL ANTIDIABETIC AGENTS

The treatment of NIDDM is a multipronged one. Because of the dyslipidemia of NIDDM, most (75%) of the patients with it are obese at the time of its initial diagnosis, and the obesity only worsens the insulin resistance. Therefore the initial treatment of NIDDM should consist of weight loss and life-style changes. The benefits of weight loss are that it lowers not only the blood glucose and lipid levels in these patients, but it also reduces the high blood pressure common in them. The life-style changes include stopping smoking, decreasing alcohol consumption, and exercising regularly. The reason why smoking should be stopped is that it doubles the risk of cardiovascular disease in these patients. In fact, stopping smoking would probably save far more lives than antihypertensive or antilipemic drug treatment together!

If normal blood glucose levels are not achieved after 2 to 3 months of these dietary and life-style modifications, treatment with a sulfonylurea is indicated, but these agents should never be used in lieu of dietary regulation—only as a supplement.

The sulfonylureas are a group of oral antidiabetic agents that are able to stimulate insulin secretion from the beta cells of the pancreas. This increased insulin then helps transport the glucose out of the blood and into the tissues, cells, and organs where it is needed. Because of these actions, the sulfonylureas may also be broadly considered oral hypoglycemic agents. These agents have many other beneficial effects besides their ability to stimulate insulin release from the pancreas.

They may also enhance the actions of insulin in muscle, liver, and adipose tissue, allowing these tissues to take up and store glucose more easily as a later source of energy. They may also increase the availability of insulin by preventing the liver from breaking it down as fast as it ordinarily would (reduced hepatic clearance). In summary, the overall effect of the sulfonylureas is that they improve both insulin secretion and the sensitivity to insulin in tissues.

The sulfonylureas have been the backbone of the oral pharmacologic therapy for NIDDM for more than 30 years. Because their primary beneficial effect in patients with NIDDM is that they stimulate insulin secretion from beta cells in the pancreas, for them to work, there must be functioning beta cells to stimulate. Thus these drugs work best during the early stages of the disease when there is preserved beta cell function. The commonly used sulfonylurea drugs are listed in Table 32-4.

Other drugs or drug categories that may be used in the treatment of NIDDM are the biguanides (metformin and phenformin) and insulin. Insulin has already been extensively discussed in this chapter, and the biguanides will be briefly described later in the chapter. By far most of the oral therapy makes use of the sulfonylurea compounds, and these are the focus of the following discussion.

Mechanism of Action

As already noted, the sulfonylurea compounds exert their antidiabetic activity by stimulating the beta cells of the pancreas to secrete insulin. In patients with NIDDM this forces the extra glucose out of the blood, where it does all its harm, and into cells, tissues, and organs, where it can be used as energy or stored as fuel. The sulfonylurea compounds also increase the sensitivity of the cells of the muscles, liver, and fat to the effects of insulin.

Drug Effects

The primary drug effects of the oral hypoglycemic agents are on the pancreas, where, as already mentioned, they stimulate the secretion of insulin from the beta cells. In addition, by enhancing the actions of insulin on muscle, liver, and adipose tissue, they cause these tissues to take up and store glucose more easily. This is of benefit in those cases of NIDDM in which there is plenty of insulin to transport the glucose out of the blood and into the tissues but the tissues are not sensitive to the effects of insulin and therefore do not accept the glucose. By preventing the liver from breaking insulin down, they also cause more insulin to be available.

Therapeutic Uses

The oral hypoglycemic agents such as the sulfonylurea drugs are used to lower the blood glucose levels in patients when diet and life-style changes have failed to do so, though beta cell function must be preserved for this to happen.

Side Effects and Adverse Effects

The most serious adverse effects involve the hematologic system and include agranulocytosis, hemolytic anemia, thrombocytopenia, and cholestatic jaundice. Effects on the GI system include nausea, epigastric fullness, and heartburn. Erythrema, photosensitivity, hypoglycemia, and morbilliform and maculopapular eruptions are other undesirable effects.

Interactions

The potential drug interactions that can occur with the sulfonylureas are significant. Their hypoglycemic effect is increased when they are taken concurrently with alcohol, anabolic steroids, beta-blockers, chlor-

Table 32-4	Sulfonylurea Agents				
Agent	**Potency**	**Onset of Action**	**Duration of Action**	**Active Metabolite**
First generation				
Chlorpropamide	Low	Slow	Very long	Yes
Tolazamide	Low	Slow	Short	Yes
Tolbutamide	Low	Fast	Short	Yes
Second generation				
⇓Glipizide	High	Very fast	Short	No
⇓Glyburide	High	Intermediate	Long	Yes

amphenicol, guanethidine, MAO inhibitors, oral anticogulants, phenylbutazone, and sulfonamides.

Drugs that are capable of reducing their hypoglycemic effect include adrenergics, corticosteroids, thiazides, and thyroid preparations.

Dosages

For the recommended dosages of oral antidiabetic agents, see the dosages table below.

DRUG PROFILES

There are two classes, or generations, of sulfonylurea drugs. The first-generation sulfonylureas are the older, low-potency drugs acetohexamide, tolbutamide, chlorpropamide, and tolazamide. The second-generation sulfonylureas are the newer, high-potency drugs glyburide and glipizide.

CHLORPROPAMIDE

Chlorpropamide (Diabinese) is a first-generation sulfonylurea agent that is structurally similar to the other first-generation agents acetohexamide, tolazamide, and tolbutamide and is the most commonly used of the first-generation agents. It differs from the other first-generation agents in that it has a very long duration of action. The chlorpropamide-induced decrease in the blood glucose may be prolonged in patients with decreased renal function because the drug is dependent on the kidneys for elimination. Like the other first-generation agents, it has active metabolites that can accumulate if they are not eliminated by the kidneys, with a prolongation of their effects and possible toxicity the consequences. This would be manifested by hypoglycemia.

Chlorpropamide is classified as a pregnancy category D drug and is contraindicated in patients with a known hypersensitivity to sulfonylureas and those with juvenile or brittle diabetes or in renal failure. Profound flushing of the skin and in particular the face occurs if it is taken with alcohol. Although this can occur with any of the sulfonylurea compounds, it is most prominent with chlorpropamide use and is called the *chlorpropamide-alcohol flush*. The facial temperature can also increase. Chlorpropamide is available orally as a 100- and 250-mg tablet. Common dosages are listed in the dosages table below.

PHARMACOKINETICS

HALF-LIFE	ONSET	PEAK	DURATION
24-48 hr	1 hr	3-6 hr	60 hr

DOSAGES

SELECTED ORAL ANTIDIABETIC AGENTS

AGENT	PHARMACOLOGIC CLASS	DOSAGE RANGE	PURPOSE
Chlorpropamide (Diabinese)	1st-generation sulfonylurea (oral hypoglycemic)	*Adult* PO: 100-500 mg/day as a single dose	NIDDM
⬇Glipizide (Glucotrol, Glucotrol XL)	2nd-generation sulfonylurea (oral hypoglycemic)	*Adult* PO: 2.5-40 mg/day as a single dose	NIDDM
⬇Glyburide (DiaBeta, Micronase, Glynase Prestab)	2nd-generation sulfonylurea (oral hypoglycemic)	*Adult* PO: 1.25-20 mg/day as a single dose	NIDDM

⚓ GLIPIZIDE

Glipizide (Glucotrol, Glucotrol XL) is a second-generation sulfonylurea agent with a potency much greater than that of the first-generation agents. This explains why the common doses of glipizide are 5 and 10 mg compared with the 100- to 500-mg doses of the first-generation agents. In contrast to the other second-generation agent glyburide, glipizide has a very rapid onset and short duration of action with no active metabolites. This confers many benefits. The rapid onset of action allows it to function much like the body's normal response to meals when greater levels of insulin are rapidly required to deal with the increased glucose in the blood. When a patient with NIDDM takes glipizide, it rapidly stimulates the pancreas to release insulin and transport the extra glucose in the blood to the muscles, liver, and adipose tissues.

Its short duration of action compared with that of glyburide prevents the long-term stimulation of the beta cells in the pancreas, which may otherwise cause the beta cells to become resistant to the effects of the sulfonylurea agents. It may also cause them to make too much insulin, thereby inducing hyperinsulinemia, which can cause the muscle, liver, and fat tissues to become resistant to the effects of insulin. Glipizide also does not have any active metabolites.

Glipizide is a pregnancy category C drug that has the same contraindications as chlorpropamide, except that it is not contraindicated in patients with renal failure. It works best if given 30 minutes before meals. This allows the timing of the insulin secretion induced by the glipizide to correspond to the elevation in the blood glucose level induced by the meal in much the same way as the endogenous levels are raised in a normal person. It is only available orally as 5- and 10-mg regular-release and extended-release (XL) tablets. Common dosages are listed in the dosages table on the previous page.

⬡⬡ P H A R M A C O K I N E T I C S

HALF-LIFE	ONSET	PEAK	DURATION
2-4 hr	1-1.5 hr	1-3 hr	10-24 hr

⚓ GLYBURIDE

Glyburide (DiaBeta, Micronase, Glynase Prestab) is the other second-generation sulfonylurea drug. It differs from the first-generation oral hypoglycemic agents in its greater potency and from glipizide in its slower onset and longer duration of action and the fact that it has active metabolites. These differences can have significant consequences. Because of its relatively slow onset of action, glyburide is less desirable for the treatment of the short-term elevations in the blood glucose

levels that occur after meals. However, its longer duration of action make it better for the long-term, constant stimulation of the pancreas, causing it to release a constant amount of insulin. This may be beneficial in controlling blood glucose levels during the night or throughout the day. Because of the varying glucose levels, it is possible and therefore rationale to use glipizide and glyburide together, with glyburide dosed either in the morning or in the morning and the evening to control the blood glucose levels throughout the day or evening, and with glipizide dosed 30 minutes before meals to deal with the elevations in the blood glucose levels after meals.

Glyburide is a pregnancy category B drug, and the contraindications to its use are the same as glipizide's. It is only available orally as 1.25-, 2.5-, and 5-mg tablets. Common dosages are listed in the preceding dosages table.

⬡⬡ P H A R M A C O K I N E T I C S

HALF-LIFE	ONSET	PEAK	DURATION
2-4 hr	1-1.5 hr	4 hr	20-24 hr

*When assays have been performed to measure the metabolite levels, the terminal elimination half-life has been found to average 10 hours.

INVESTIGATIONAL DRUGS

Many of the long-term complications associated with diabetes mellitus stem from the effects of a breakdown product of glucose called sorbitol, and it is an enzyme called aldose reductase that converts or breaks down the glucose to sorbitol. The accumulation of this substance in various sites such as the eyes, nerves, and kidneys causes damage resulting in the complications of diabetic retinopathy, neuropathy, and nephropathy. The incidence of these can be reduced through the use of a group of investigational drugs called aldose reductase inhibitors. As their name suggests, these agents inhibit the aldose reductase and thereby the breakdown of glucose to sorbitol, thus eliminating the agent responsible for causing the complications of hyperglycemia. The agents that are currently being investigated for this purpose are sorbinil, statil, and tolrestat (Alredase).

GLUCOSE-ELEVATING DRUGS

There are two drugs used for the treatment of hypoglycemia. Glucagon, a natural hormone secreted by the pancreas, has also been synthesized in the laboratory and is now available as a tablet to be given when a quick response to hypoglycemia is needed. Diazoxide is another agent that may be given to correct abnormally low blood glucose levels. It works by inhibiting the release of insulin from the pancreas and is most commonly given to patients with long-term illnesses that are causing hypoglycemia. An example of such an illness is pancreatic cancers that cause the pancreas to oversecrete insulin, resulting in too much insulin in the blood, or hyperinsulinemia. The oral form of diazoxide is used for the treatment of hypoglycemia and the intravenous form is used for the treatment of hypertensive emergencies (very high blood pressures).

NURSING PROCESS

ASSESSMENT

Before administering any type of insulin, it is important to question patients about allergies they may have to insulin, beef, or pork and whether they are taking drugs that interact with insulin. Those that produce a greater hypoglycemic effect include alcohol, steroids, oral hypoglycemic agents, and MAO inhibitors. The use of insulin with thyroid hormones, oral contraceptives and steroids results in a decreased hypoglycemic effect.

Oral antidiabetic agents are contraindicated in patients with allergies to the medication proper or to the sulfonylureas in general. The oral agents are also contraindicated in the treatment of juvenile-onset diabetes because these patients have no functioning beta cells in the pancreas, which is where the oral agents work. The oral agents should be administered with caution to elderly patients or to anyone with cardiac, renal, hepatic, or thyroid disease. Drugs that interact with them include warfarin sodium, aspirin, digoxin, insulin, diuretics, beta-blockers, calcium channel blockers, corticosteroids, phenobarbital, and phenytoin, to name just a few. Because of the many drugs oral antidiabetic agents interact with, it is crucial for the nurse to check what other medications a patient who is to receive an oral antidiabetic is also taking.

Questions about the patient's past medical history are important in determining whether the patient's diabetes is well controlled or whether there are problems with polyuria, polydipsia, polyphagia, weight loss, visual changes, and fatigue. The nurse should ask about problems with hypoglycemia such as the acute onset of nervousness, sweating, lethargy, weakness, cold and clammy skin, and a change in sensorium. Symp-

toms of hyperglycemia would include tachycardia, blood glucose levels that exceed 150 mg/dl, and a change in respiration (Kussmaul's).

Before administering any glucose elevating drug,

Antidiabetic Agent

✔ Patients need to have a thorough understanding of their type of diabetes and its specific management, including special diets and exercise, as ordered by the physician. Provide the patient with any available literature, pamphlets, and videos on diabetes. The American Diabetic Association can also provide the patient with information on diabetes and other resources available.

✔ Patients should always carry an identification card and wear a Medic-Alert bracelet or necklace that identifies them as diabetics, and also carry a supply of readily available sugar.

✔ Patients should know the signs and symptoms of hyperglycemia, such as an increased pulse rate, abnormal breathing, and a fruity, acetone odor to their breath. Patients should also know the signs and symptoms of hypoglycemia, such as weakness, nervousness, cold and clammy skin, sweating, paleness of the skin, and shallow, rapid breathing. The physician or health care provider should be notified if any of these symptoms occur!

✔ Patients taking oral antidiabetic agents should know how to measure their blood glucose level with a glucometer and perform this as ordered by their physician. Patients should notify their physician should they note yellow discoloration of the skin, dark urine, fever, sore throat, weakness or any unusual bleeding, or easy bruising.

✔ Patients taking insulin should always carry an extra supply of medication, syringes, needles, and alcohol or antiseptic swabs when traveling.

✔ Diabetics are very sensitive to changes in blood glucose levels when they are ill, have an infection, are vomiting or not able to eat, or under stress. If any of these conditions occur, patients may require a change in their diabetic treatment. They should therefore notify their physician should any of these illnesses or stressors occur.

✔ Diabetic patients should avoid consuming alcohol because it will make their blood glucose level drop, causing them to become very ill.

✔ Patients taking insulin injections should know the importance of rotating the injection sites.

a thorough history should be obtained and documented. Baseline vital signs and blood glucose levels as well as the patient's sensorium should also be documented.

NURSING DIAGNOSES

Nursing diagnoses in patients receiving antidiabetic agents include:

- Risk for self-injury stemming from changes in sensorium and the pathophysiologic impact of diabetes.
- Risk for infection related to the diabetes.
- Altered nutrition (more than body requirements) related to the disease process.
- Knowledge deficit regarding diabetes mellitus, its management, and the prevention of its complications.

PLANNING

Goals in patients receiving antidiabetic agents include:

- Patient remains free of self-injury and complications of diabetes.
- Patient remains free from infection.
- Patient maintains adequate weight control and dietary habits in the overall management of diabetes.
- Patient states the effects of diabetes on body function.
- Patient remains compliant with the medical regimen.

TAKE HOME POINTS

Antidiabetic Agents

- Drugs that affect the pancreas (insulin and oral hypoglycemics).
- Insulin takes glucose from the blood and puts it in the liver to be stored.
- Oral hypoglycemics stimulate insulin secretion from the beta cells of the pancreas as well as enhance insulin's effectiveness.

Glucagon

- The second hormone secreted by the pancreas.
- Responsible for initiating glycogenolysis.
- Glycogenolysis opposes the action of insulin; it increases the blood glucose level.

Glycogen

- The storage form of glucose.
- Most is stored in the liver.
- Broken down by the synergistic actions of glucagon, cortisol, and epinephrine.

Types of Diabetes

- Insulin-dependent diabetes mellitus (IDDM):
  Also known as *type I diabetes* or *juvenile-onset diabetes.*
  Little or no endogenous insulin produced.
  Much less common—about 10% of all diabetics.
  Patients are usually nonobese.
- Non–insulin-dependent diabetes mellitus (NIDDM):
  Also known as *type II diabetes* or *adult-onset diabetes.*
  Insulin secretion is usually normal.
  Much more common—about 90% of all diabetics.
  80% of patients are obese.

Complications Associated with Diabetes

- Retinopathy, neuropathy, nephropathy.
- Severe complication of uncontrolled diabetes is diabetic ketoacidosis (DKA).
- DKA is due to the body utilizing other sources of energy besides glucose, such as fatty acids.
- Fatty acids are broken down into ketones, which leads to acidosis.

Nursing Considerations

- Always check for allergies to specific medications and to beef and pork insulins before initiating therapy.
- Correct diet is an important component of the entire medical treatment regimen for a diabetic.
- Patients need to learn about their disease and the type of insulin they are taking—its onset of action, peak effect, and duration of action, as well as the importance of always having a rapidly active form of sugar available.
- Patients also need to learn the signs and symptoms of hypoglycemia and hyperglycemia and the methods of treating it at home, as well as when to contact their physician.
- Foot care and the prevention of infection should be part of the patient education given to diabetics.

- Patient will state the action and side effects of insulin or the oral hypoglycemic agents.

Outcome Criteria

Outcome criteria in patients receiving antidiabetic agents include:

- Patient will perform self-assessment and foot care as directed and as needed to maintain healthy skin.
- Patient will immediately report elevated temperature, difficult-to-heal lesions or sores, and any unusual redness of an area to their healthcare provider.
- Patient will observe the diet recommended by the American Diabetic Association or other dietary consultant per the physician's orders or nutritional consult.
- Patient will eat a healthy diet, get sufficient rest and relaxation, and notify the physician should any unusual problems occur with changes in usual activity (problems such as nausea and vomiting).
- Patient will keep all scheduled appointments with health care providers to monitor therapeutic effectiveness or for complications of therapy.
- Patient will take medication as scheduled, monitor blood glucose levels, and watch for any signs and symptoms of hyperglycemia or hypoglycemia.

IMPLEMENTATION

In any patient who is to receive insulin or the oral antidiabetic agents, it is critical to always check the blood glucose levels before administering the agent so that there is an accurate baseline reading. Always check the order at least three times before administering the medication and always have another registered nurse check the injection you prepare to make sure it is in accordance with the physician's order. Roll the vial, do not shake it, before withdrawing the medication. Insulin may be stored at room temperature if it is to be used within 1 month, otherwise it needs to be refrigerated. Never use insulin that is discolored or past its expiration date. Administer the insulin subcutaneously and at a 90-degree angle, unless the patient is emaciated. Only regular insulin can be administered intravenously. A 25- to 28-gauge needle should be used and always use an insulin syringe, which is calibrated in units. If mixing insulins, always withdraw the regular or rapid-acting (unmodified) insulin first and then the intermediate or NPH (modified) insulin. Always rotate the injection sites as follows: upper back, buttocks, thighs, and upper arm, and document the site in the patient's nursing record.

Insulin is usually given about 15 to 30 minutes before meals, so be sure that the meal trays are either on their way to the unit or are there. The oral antidiabetic agents should be administered at least 30 minutes before meals.

Patient education is crucial to ensuring the safe and effective use of the antidiabetic agents, and these teaching tips are on p. 485.

EVALUATION

A therapeutic response to any of the antidiabetic agents includes a decrease in the blood glucose levels to the level prescribed by the physician, one at which the patient is free of the symptoms of hyperglycemia and hypoglycemia. Patients with diabetes need to be monitored to make sure they are complying with therapy, and the nurse also needs to watch for the manifestations of hypoglycemia or hyperglycemia. An insulin allergy is manifested by local swelling, itching, and redness at the injection site.

A therapeutic response to glucose elevating drugs would include elevation of blood glucose levels to within normal limits (fasting blood sugar >60, <120, or level as designated by physician).

Critical Thinking A C T I V I T I E S

1. IDDM has recently been diagnosed in a 240-pound, 45-year-old woman. When she is admitted to your unit for additional testing and control of her diabetes, she is placed on a 1500-calorie diabetic diet and on 30 U of NPH insulin to be given every day at 7:30 AM. At 4 PM on the first day of therapy she becomes diaphoretic, weak, and pale. How would you explain these symptoms to this patient?

2. Which of the following substances would eliminate the polydipsia, polyuria, and a low specific gravity of urine in a diabetic: insulin, glucagon, ADH, or aldosterone? Explain your answer.

BIBLIOGRAPHY

Albanese J, Nutz P: *Mosby's 1995 nursing drug cards,* St Louis, 1995, Mosby.

Bliss M: The history of insulin, *Diabetes Care* 16[suppl 3]:4, 1993.

Genuth S: Insulin use in NIDDM, *Diabetes Care* 13(2):1240, 1990.

Groop LC: Sulfonylureas in NIDDM, *Diabetes Care* 15(6):737, 1992.

Heinemann L: Clinical pharmacology of human insulin, *Diabetes Care* 16[suppl 3]:90, 1993.

Johnson KB: *Harriet Lane handbook,* ed 13, St Louis, 1993, Mosby.

Keen JH: *Critical care and emergency drug reference,* St Louis, 1994, Mosby.

Knoben JE, Anderson PO: *Handbook of critical drug data,* ed 6, Hamilton, Ill, 1988, Drug Intelligence Publications.

McEvoy GK: *AHFS drug information,* Bethesda, Md, 1994, American Society of Hospital Pharmacists.

Melander A: Sulfonylureas: why, which, and how?, *Diabetes Care* 13[suppl 3]:18, 1990.

Mulcahy K: Hypoglycemic emergencies, *AACN Clin Issues* 3(2):361, 1992.

Sauve DO: Hyperglycemic emergencies, *AACN Clin Issues* 3(2):350, 1992.

Skidmore-Roth L: *Mosby's 1995 nursing drug reference,* St Louis, 1995, Mosby.

Tsai SC, Burnakis TG: Aldose reductase inhibitors: an update, *Ann Pharmacother* 27:751, 1993.

White JR: Drug interactions in diabetic patients: the risk of losing glycemic control, *Postgrad Med* 93(3):131, 1993.

Williams G: Management of non-insulin-dependent diabetes mellitus, *Lancet* 343:95, 1994.

Chapter 33

Adrenal Agents

Objectives

When you reach the end of this chapter, you will be able to:

1 Discuss the normal actions and functions of the adrenal system and its feedback mechanism.

2 Describe the differences in the hyposecretion and hypersecretion of the adrenal hormones.

3 Describe the various diseases that are attributed to the hyposecretion and hypersecretion of adrenal hormones.

4 Identify the various agents used to manage the hyposecretion and hypersecretion of adrenal hormones as well as other indications for the use of adrenal agents.

5 Discuss the mechanism of action of, indications for, contraindications and cautions to, and side effects of adrenal medications.

6 Develop a nursing care plan as it relates to the nursing process for patients receiving adrenal medications.

7 Identify the teaching guidelines for patients receiving adrenal medications.

CHAPTER OUTLINE

The Adrenal System

Adrenal Agents
 Mechanism of action
 Drug effects
 Therapeutic uses
 Side effects and adverse effects
 Interactions
 Dosages

Drug Profiles

Corticosteroids
 ⚕ Hydrocortisone
 ⚕ Prednisone
 Dexamethasone
 Fludrocortisone

Antiadrenals
 Aminoglutethimide

Nursing Process

Assessment

Nursing Diagnoses

Planning
 Outcome criteria

Implementation

Evaluation

Glossary

Addison's disease Life-threatening condition caused by failure of adrenocortical function. (p. 491)

Adrenal cortex (ə dre′ nəl kor′ teks) Outer portion of the adrenal gland. (p. 490)

Adrenal medulla (ə dre′ nəl mə dul′ə) Inner portion of the adrenal gland. (p. 490)

Aldosterone (al dos′ tər ōn) Mineralocorticoid hormone produced by the adrenal cortex that acts on the renal tubule to regulate sodium and potassium balance in the blood. (p. 490)

Cortex Outer layer of a body organ or other structure. (p. 490)

Corticosteroid (kor tǐ ko ster′ oid) Any one of the natural or synthetic adrenocortical hormones (p. 490)

Cushing's syndrome Metabolic disorder characterized by abnormally increased secretion of the adrenocortical steroids caused by increased secretion of adrenocorticotropic hormone from the pituitary. (p. 491)

Epinephrine (ep′ ǐ nef′ rin) An endogenous adrenal hormone and synthetic adrenergic vasoconstrictor. (p. 490)

Norepinephrine (nor′ ep ǐ nef′ rin) Adrenergic hormone that increases blood pressure by causing vasoconstriction but does not affect cardiac output. (p. 490)

The Adrenal System

The adrenal gland is an endocrine organ that sits on top of the kidneys like a cap. It is composed of two distinct parts called the **adrenal cortex** and the **adrenal medulla** that both structurally and functionally are very different. The adrenal cortex is made up of regular endocrine tissue, and the adrenal medulla is made up of neurosecretory tissue. Therefore the adrenal gland actually functions as two different endocrine glands, with each secreting different hormones.

The adrenal medulla secretes two important hormones, both of which are catecholamines. These are **epinephrine**, or adrenaline, which accounts for about 80% of the secretion, and **norepinephrine**, or noradrenaline, which accounts for the other 20%. (Both of these hormones are discussed in Chapter 15 and will not be discussed further here in any detail.) The differences between the adrenal cortex and the adrenal medulla and the various hormones secreted by each are listed in Table 33-1.

The hormones secreted from the adrenal cortex, which are the focus of this chapter, are broadly referred to as **corticosteroids** because they arise from the **cortex** and they are made from the crystalline *steroid* alcohol cholesterol. There are two types of corticosteroids—the glucocorticoids and the mineralocorticoids—and these are secreted by two different layers, or zones, of the cortex. The zona glomerulosa, which is the outer layer, secretes the mineralocorticoids, and the zona fasciculata, which lies under the zona glomerulosa, secretes the glucocorticoids. A third, inner layer, the zona reticularis, secretes small amounts of sex hormones. All the hormones secreted by the adrenal cortex are steroid hormones.

The mineralocorticoids get their name from the fact that they play an important role in regulating the way in which mineral salts (electrolytes) are processed in the body. In humans the only physiologically important mineralocorticoid is **aldosterone.** Its primary role is to maintain normal levels of sodium in the blood (sodium homeostasis), and it does this by causing sodium to be resorbed from the urine back into the blood in exchange for potassium and hydrogen ions. In this way aldosterone not only regulates the blood sodium levels but also influences the potassium levels of the blood and its pH.

Overall, the corticosteroids are necessary for many vital bodily functions, and some of the important ones are listed in the box below. Without these hormones, life-threatening consequences may arise.

The adrenal corticosteroids are synthesized as needed; the body does not store them as it does other hormones. The body levels of these hormones are regulated by the hypothalamus-pituitary-adrenal (HPA) axis in much the same way as the levels of hormones secreted by the already discussed endocrine glands (the pancreas, thyroid, and pituitary) are regulated. As the name implies, this axis consists of a very organized system of communication between the adrenal gland, the pituitary, and the hypothalamus and, as is the case for the other endocrine glands, uses hormones as the messengers and a negative feedback mechanism as the controller and maintainer of the process. This feedback process operates as follows: When the level of a particular corticosteroid is low, corticotropin-releasing

---

Adrenal Cortex Hormones: Biologic Functions

Glucocorticoids
Antiinflammatory actions
Maintenance of normal blood pressure
Carbohydrate and protein metabolism
Fat metabolism
Stress effects

Mineralocorticoids
Sodium and water resorption
Blood pressure control
Potassium levels and pH of blood

Table 33-1 | Adrenal Gland: Characteristics

TYPE OF TISSUE	TYPE OF HORMONE	SPECIFIC HORMONES
Adrenal cortex		
Endocrine	Glucocorticoids	Betamethasone, corticotropin (ACTH), cortisone, dexamethasone, hydrocortisone, methylprednisolone, paramethasone, prednisolone, triamcinolone
	Mineralocorticoids	Aldosterone, fludrocortisone, desoxycorticosterone
Adrenal medulla		
Neuroendocrine	Catecholamines	Epinephrine, norepinephrine

hormone is released from the hypothalamus into the bloodstream and travels to the anterior pituitary, where it triggers the release of corticotropin (ACTH). The corticotropin is then transported in the blood to the adrenal cortex, where it stimulates the production of the corticosteroid. The corticosteroid is then released into the bloodstream, and when it reaches a peak level, this sends a signal (negative feedback) to the hypothalamus, and the HPA axis is inhibited until the level of the corticosteriod is depleted, whereupon the axis is stimulated once again.

The oversecretion (hypersecretion) of the adrenocortical hormones can lead to a collection of symptoms called **Cushing's syndrome**. The hypersecretion of glucocorticoids results in the redistribution of body fat from the arms and legs to the face, shoulders, trunk, and abdomen, resulting in the "moon face" characteristic of patients with Cushing's syndrome. The hypersecretion of aldosterone, or primary aldosteronism, leads to increased water retention and muscle weakness resulting from the potassium loss.

The undersecretion (hyposecretion) of adrenocortical hormones causes a condition referred to as **Addison's disease**. It is associated with increased blood sodium levels, decreased blood glucose and potassium levels, dehydration, and weight loss. The combination of a mineralocorticoid (fludrocortisone) and a glucocorticoid (prednisone or some other suitable agent) are used for treatment.

ADRENAL AGENTS

All the naturally occurring corticosteroids are available as exogenous agents, and there are also higher-potency synthetic analogues. The adrenal glucocorticoids are an extremely large group of steroids, and they are classified in various ways. They can be classified by whether they are a natural or synthetic corticosteroid; by the method of administration (e.g., systemic, topical); by their salt and water retention potential; by their duration of action (i.e., short, intermediate, or long acting), or by some combination of these schemes. The only synthetic mineralocorticoid on the market is fludrocortisone. The currently available synthetic adrenal hormones and adrenal steroid inhibitors are listed in Table 33-2.

Mechanism of Action

The action of the corticosteroids is related to their involvement in the synthesis of specific proteins. There are several steps to this process. Initially the steroid hormones bind to a receptor on the surface of a target cell to form a steroid-receptor complex, which is then transported to the nucleus of that target cell. Once inside the nucleus of the target cell, the complex stimulates the cell's DNA to produce messenger-RNA, which is then used as a template for the synthesis of a specific protein. It is these proteins that exert specific drug effects.

Drug Effects

Most of the corticosteroids exert their effects by modifying enzyme activity, so their role is more intermediary than direct.

As already mentioned, the naturally occurring mineralocorticoid aldosterone affects electrolyte and

Table 33-2	Available Synthetic Corticosteroids	
HORMONE TYPE	**METHOD OF ADMINISTRATION**	**INDIVIDUAL DRUGS**
Glucocorticoid	Topical	Alclometasone dipropionate, amcinonide, betamethasone benzoate, betamethasone dipropionate, betamethasone valerate, clobestasol propionate, clocortolone pivalate desonide, desoximethasone, dexamethasone sodium phosphate, diflorasone diacetate, fluocinolone acetonide, fluocinonide, flurandrenolide, fluticasone propionate, halobitasol propionate, halcinonide, hydrocortisone acetate, hydrocortisone valerate, methylprednisolone acetate, mometasone furoate, triamcinolone
	Systemic	Betamethasone, cortisone, dexamethasone, hydrocortisone, methylprednisolone, prednisolone, prednisone, triamcinolone
	Inhaled	Beclomethasone, dexamethasone, flunisolide, triamcinolone acetonide
	Nasal	Beclomethasone dipropionate, dexamethasone sodium phosphate, flunisolide, triamcinolone acetonide
Mineralocorticoid	Systemic	Fludrocortisone acetate
Adrenal steroid inhibitor	Systemic	Aminoglutethimide, trilostane

Table 33-3 Systemic Glucocorticoids: A Comparison

DRUG	ORIGIN	DURATION OF ACTION	EQUIVALENT DOSE (MG)	SALT AND WATER RETENTION POTENTIAL
Betametasone	Synthetic	Long	0.6	Very low
Cortisone	Natural	Short	25.0	High
Dexamethasone	Synthetic	Long	0.75	Very low
⚓Hydrocortisone	Natural	Short	20.0	High
Methylprednisolone	Synthetic	Intermediate	4.0	Very low
⚓Prednisone	Synthetic	Intermediate	5.0	Low
Prednisolone	Synthetic	Intermediate	5.0	Low
Triamcinolone	Synthetic	Intermediate	4.0	Very low

fluid balance by working on the distal renal tubule to promote sodium resorption from the nephron into the blood, which pulls water and fluid along with it. In doing so it causes fluid and water retention, which leads to edema and hypertension. It may also promote potassium and hydrogen excretion.

The naturally occurring glucocorticoids hydrocortisone (cortisol) and cortisone have some mineralocorticoid activity and therefore have some of the same effects as aldosterone (i.e., fluid and water retention). Their other main effect is the inhibition of inflammatory and immune responses. They do this by stimulating the cells that eventually become red blood cells called erythroid cells. The stimulation of these cells in the bone marrow prolongs the survival of erythrocytes (RBCs and platelets). The glucocorticoids also promote the breakdown (catabolism) of protein, the production of glycogen (gluconeogenesis), and the redistribution of fat from peripheral to central areas of the body.

Therapeutic Uses

All the systemically administered glucocorticoids have a similar clinical efficacy but differ in their potency and duration of action and in the extent to which they cause salt and fluid retention. (Refer to Table 33-3 for details.) They are indicated in the treatment of the following conditions:

- Adrenocortical deficiency
- Adrenogenital syndrome
- Bacterial meningitis
- Cerebral edema
- Collagen diseases (e.g., systemic lupus erythematosus)
- Dermatologic diseases (e.g., exfoliative dermatitis, pemphigus)
- Endocrine disorders (thyroiditis)
- GI diseases (ulcerative colitis, regional enteritis)

- Hematologic disorders (reduce bleeding tendencies)
- Ophthalmic disorders (nonpyogenic inflammations)
- Organ transplant recipients
- Palliative management of leukemias and lymphomas
- Remission of proteinurea in nephrotic syndrome
- Spinal cord injury

The glucocorticoids are administered by inhalation for the control of steroid-responsive bronchospastic states. Nasally administered glucocorticoids are used in the management of rhinitis and to prevent the recurrence of polyps after surgical removal. The topical steroids are the largest group and are used in the management of inflammations in the eye, ear, and skin.

Side Effects and Adverse Effects

The potent metabolic, physiologic, and pharmacologic effects of the corticosteroids can influence every body system, with the result that they can produce a wide variety of significant undesirable effects. The more common of these are summarized in Table 33-4.

Interactions

The systematically administered corticosteroids can interact with many agents:

- Their use with non–potassium-sparing diuretics (e.g., thiazides, loop diuretics) can lead to severe hypocalcemia.
- Their use with aspirin, other NSAIDs, and other ulcerogenic drugs produces additive effects.
- Their use with anticholinesterase drugs produces weakness in patients with myasthenia gravis.

Table 33-4	Corticosteroids: Common Adverse Effects	
BODY SYSTEM	**SIDE/ADVERSE EFFECT**
Central nervous system	Convulsions, headache, vertigo, mood swings, psychic impairment
Cardiovascular	Congestive heart failure, cardiac edema, hypertension—all due to electrolyte imbalances
Endocrine	Growth suppression, Cushing's syndrome, menstrual irregularities, carbohydrate intolerance, hyperglycemia, HPA axis suppression
Gastrointestinal	Peptic ulcers with possible perforation, pancreatitis, ulcerative esophagitis, abdominal distention
Skin	Fragile skin, petechiae, ecchymoses, facial erythema, poor wound healing, hirsutism, urticaria
Musculoskeletal	Muscle weakness, loss of muscle mass
Ocular	Increased intraocular pressure, glaucoma, exophthalmos, cataracts

- Their use with immunizing biologicals inhibits the immune response to the biological.
- Their use with antidiabetic agents may reduce the hypoglycemic affect.

Dosages

For information on the recommended dosages of adrenal agents, see the dosages table on the next page.

DRUG PROFILES

CORTICOSTEROIDS

The systemic corticosteroids consist of 13 chemically different but pharmacologically similar hormones. They all exert varying degrees of glucocorticoid and mineralocorticoid effects. Their differences arise out of slight changes in their chemical structures.

Corticosteroids can cross the placenta and produce fetal abnormalities. For this reason, they are classified as pregnancy category C agents. They may also be secreted in breast milk and cause abnormalities in the nursing infant. They are contraindicated in patients who have exhibited hypersensitivity reactions to them in the past as well as in patients with fungal infections. Long-term use can lead to a condition known as *steroid psychosis*. In addition, the cessation of long-term treatment with these agents requires a tapering of the daily dose because the administration of the exogenous hormones causes the endogenous production of the hormones to stop. Tapering daily doses allows the HPA axis the time it needs to recover and start to stimulate the normal production of the endogenous hormones.

⚕ HYDROCORTISONE

Hydrocortisone (Cortef, Hydrocortone, Solu-Cortef) is a short-acting adrenocortical steroid. Both it and cortisone are the only two short-acting agents. Compared with other glucocorticoids they have the strongest mineralocorticoid actions (potassium excretion and sodium and water retention) and weakest glucocorticoid actions (antiinflammatory, immunosuppressant, and metabolic-type effects). They have relatively short half-lives (0.5-2 hours) and therefore short durations of action. Because they have both glucocorticoid and mineralocorticoid properties, either hydrocortisone or cortisone is usually the corticosteroid of choice for replacement therapy in patients with adrenocortical insufficiency.

Hydrocortisone is available in oral, injectable, and topical preparations. Orally it comes as 5-, 10-, and 20-mg tablets and as a 10–mg/5 mg oral suspension; parenterally it comes as a 25-, 50-, 100-, 250-, 500-, and 1000-mg injection; topically it comes as a cream, lotion, ointment, and spray preparation. Recommended dosages are given in the dosages table. Pregnancy category C.

⬡ PHARMACOKINETICS

HALF-LIFE	ONSET	PEAK	DURATION
0.5-2 hr	Unknown	1 hr	30-36 hr

⚕ PREDNISONE

Prednisone (Orasone, Meticorten, Deltasone, Cortan, Sterapred) is one of the four intermediate-acting glucocorticoids, the others being methylprednisolone, prednisolone, and triamcinolone. These agents have half-lives that are over more than double those of the short-acting steroids (2-5 hours), and therefore they have much longer durations of action. Prednisone is the preferred oral glucocorticoid for antiinflammatory

D O S A G E S

SELECTED CORTICOSTEROID AND ANTIADRENAL AGENTS

AGENT	PHARMACOLOGIC CLASS	DOSAGE RANGE	PURPOSE
⚓Hydrocortisone (Cortef, Hydrocortone)	Natural short-acting glucocorticoid	*Pediatric* PO: 0.56-8 mg/day in 3-4 divided doses *Adult* PO: 10-320 mg/day in 3-4 divided doses	Adrenocortical insufficiency
Hydrocortisone sodium succinate (Solu-Cortef)	Natural water-soluble, short-acting glucocorticoid	*Pediatric* IM/IV: 0.16-1 mg/kg administered 1-2 times/day *Adult* IM/IV: 100 mg-8 g/day	Adrenocortical insufficiency
⚓Prednisone (Orasone, Meticorten, Deltasone, Cortan, Sterapred)	Synthetic intermediate-acting glucocorticoid	*Pediatric* PO: 0.14-2 mg/kg/day divided *Adult* PO: 5-60 mg/day divided	Allergic, autoimmune, collagen, inflammatory conditions; cerebral edema; immunosuppression; palliation of selected neoplasms
Dexamethasone (Decadron, Hexadrol, Dexone, Solurex, Dexeject-LA)	Synthetic long-acting glucocorticoid	*Pediatric* PO: 0.025-0.35 mg/day divided *Adult* PO: 0.75-9 mg/day divided	Allergic, autoimmune, collagen, inflammatory conditions; cerebral edema; immunosuppression; palliation of selected neoplasms
Dexamethasone acetate (Decadron-LA, Dexaject-LA, Solurex LA)	Synthetic long-acting repository glucocorticoid	*Adult* IM: 8-16 mg every 1-3 wk prn for systemic effects	Same as dexamethasone
		Intraarticular: 4-16 mg every 1-3 wk prn	Antiinflammatory
		Intralesional: 0.8-1.6 mg/injection site	Antiinflammatory
Fludrocortisone (Florinef)	Synthetic gluco/mineralocorticoid	*Adult* PO 0.1 mg 3 times/wk to 0.2 mg/day PO: 0.1-0.2 mg/day	Addison's disease Salt-losing adrenogenital syndrome
Aminoglutethimide (Cytadren)	Adrenal steroid inhibitor	*Adult* PO: Start with 250 mg qid and adjust according to response	Selected cases of Cushing's syndrome

or immunosuppressant purposes. These agents have only minimal mineralocorticoid properties and therefore alone are inadequate for the management of adrenocortical insufficiency.

Prednisone is available orally as a 5-mg/5 ml oral solution; as a 5-mg/5 ml syrup; as 1-, 2.5-, 5-, 10-, 20-, 25-, and 50-mg tablets; and as a 5-mg film-coated tablet. Recommended dosages are given in the dosages table. Pregnancy category C.

PHARMACOKINETICS

HALF-LIFE	ONSET	PEAK	DURATION
18-36 hr	Unknown	1-2 hr	36 hr

DEXAMETHASONE

Dexamethasone (Decadron, Hexadrol, Dexone, Solurex, and Dexaject-LA) is one of the three long-acting glucocorticoids, the other two being betamethasone and paramethasone. These agents have half-lives that range from 3 to 5 hours and durations of action of 36 to 54 hours. Usually dexamethasone and the other long-acting steroids are used for antiinflammatory or immunosuppressant purposes. They have only minimal mineralocorticoid properties and therefore alone are inadequate for the management of adrenocortical insufficiency. Dexamethasone may be administered by inhalation for the treatment of bronchial asthma. A dexamethasone suppression test may be performed to establish the diagnosis of Cushing's syndrome or an adrenal adenoma. Dexamethasone inhibits the release of corticotropin (ACTH) from the pituitary and decreases the output of endogenous corticosteroids. Dexamethasone has also been shown to be very effective in preventing the nausea and vomiting associated with emetogenic cancer chemotherapy.

Dexamethasone is available orally as a 0.5-mg/5 ml oral elixir; as a 0.5–mg/5 ml solution; and as 0.25-, 0.5-, 0.75-, 1-, 1.5-, 2-, 4-, and 6-mg tablets. Dexamethasone as an acetate salt is given intramuscularly and is available as a 8- and 16-mg injection. Dexamethasone sodium phosphate is given either intramuscularly or intravenously and comes as a 4-, 10-, 20-, and 24 mg/ml injection. Recommended dosages are given in the dosages table. Pregnancy category C.

PHARMACOKINETICS

HALF-LIFE	ONSET	PEAK	DURATION
36-54 hr	Unknown	1-2 hr	66 hr

FLUDROCORTISONE

Fludrocortisone (Florinef) is a synthetic mineralocorticoid with very weak glucocorticoid but very potent mineralocorticoid activity. It is used for oral replacement therapy in patients suffering from an adrenocortical insufficiency such as Addison's disease. It has also been used to increase systolic and diastolic blood pressure in patients suffering from chronic severe postural hypotension. It is only available as a 0.1-mg oral tablet. Recommended dosages are given in the dosages table.

PHARMACOKINETICS

HALF-LIFE	ONSET	PEAK	DURATION
18-36 hr	10-20 min	1.7 hr (PO)	Unknown

ANTIADRENALS

Aminoglutethimide, metyrapone, and trilostane are antiadrenals, or adrenal steroid inhibitors. They inhibit the normal actions or function of the adrenal cortex by inhibiting the conversion of cholesterol into adrenal corticosteroids. They are indicated for the treatment of Cushing's syndrome, which results from an overproduction of corticosteroids by the adrenal gland. They are contraindicated in patients who have shown a previous hypersensitivity reaction to them and many are classified as pregnancy category X agents. Their most common adverse effects are nausea, anorexia, dizziness, and skin rash.

AMINOGLUTETHIMIDE

Aminoglutethimide (Cytadren) is the most commonly used of the three antiadrenal drugs in the treatment of Cushing's syndrome, metastatic breast cancer, and adrenal cancer. It is only available orally as a 250-mg tablet. Recommended dosages are given in the dosages table. Pregnancy category D.

PHARMACOKINETICS

HALF-LIFE	ONSET	PEAK	DURATION
9 hr	Unknown	Unknown	Unknown

NURSING PROCESS

ASSESSMENT

Before administering any of the adrenal agents, the nurse should perform a thorough physical assessment to determine the patient's baseline weight, intake and

Patient Teaching TIPS

Adrenal Agent

✔ Because of their suppressed immune system, patients taking corticosteroids should avoid persons with infections and report any fever, increased weakness and lethargy, or sore throat.

✔ Encourage patients to tell the nurse and other members of the health care team about unpleasant side effects and changes in appearance.

✔ Encourage patients to get adequate rest, exercise, and nutrition.

✔ Evaluate and monitor patients' nutritional status, weight, fluid volume, electrolyte status, and skin turgor during therapy.

✔ Encourage patients to keep a daily log of their general feelings of well-being and any response to the medication, along with any questions for the physician.

✔ Emphasize the importance of not discontinuing any of the corticosteroids and of keeping all medications out of the reach of children.

✔ Patients should take all adrenal medications exactly as prescribed and at the same time every day.

✔ Topical corticosteroids should be applied as recommended by the manufacturer as well as according to the physician's orders.

✔ Hydrocortisone and prednisone should be taken exactly as ordered, and one daily AM dose is recommended, if ordered by the physician, to minimize adrenal suppression. Sudden discontinuation of these agents can precipitate an adrenal crisis caused by a sudden drop in the serum levels of cortisone. Cushingoid symptoms include moon face, weight gain, muscle wasting, and increased deposition of fat in the trunk area, leading to

truncal obesity. Patients should notify the physician of any weakness, joint pain, dyspnea, fever, dysrhythmias, depression, edema, or any other unusual symptom.

✔ Topical agents should be applied as ordered, and often the site should be covered with an occlusive dressing; the method for doing this should be demonstrated to the patient. The skin should be clean and dry before topical administrations.

✔ Nasal sprays should be administered per the manufacturer's guidelines and the physician's orders. (See Chapter 4 for more information on the administration of nasal agents.)

✔ Aminoglutethimide should be administered as ordered and careful attention paid to the overall nutritional status and well-being of the patient. In addition, the patient should report the development of jaundice, rash, fever, or skin lesions. If masculinization occurs, this will disappear once the therapy is stopped.

Nursing Considerations

✔ Patients should be monitored frequently for weight gain, changes in nutritional status, electrolyte imbalances, and fluid volume excess.

✔ Patients should not be taken off these agents abruptly.

✔ Once-a-day dosing corticosteroids should be administered between 6 and 9 AM to minimize adrenal suppression, and this needs to be explained to the patient.

✔ Patients taking antiadrenal agents should be monitored carefully for development of jaundice, rash, fever, or skin lesions.

---

output status, vital signs (especially blood pressure), hydration status, skin condition, and immune status. Important baseline laboratory values include the serum Na, K, BUN, and Hgb levels, as well as the Hct. All this is crucial for ensuring the safe and most effective use of these adrenal agents and for identifying any specific cautions or contraindications in advance of treatment, as well as for monitoring the patient's response to the treatment. Any edema or electrolyte imbalances need to be documented and brought to the attention of the physician. Because glucocorticoids can elevate a patient's blood glucose level, a baseline level must be determined. Because corticosteroids often aggravate peptic ulcer disease, the nurse should find out

whether the patient has a history of ulcer disease, gastritis, or heartburn.

There are many drugs that interact with corticosteroids (see previous discussion), so the nurse should always find out what prescription and over-the-counter medications the patient is currently taking to prevent these interactions from occurring.

The antiadrenal agents are contraindicated in patients with a known hypersensitivity to them.

NURSING DIAGNOSES

Nursing diagnoses appropriate to the patient receiving adrenal agents include:

- Altered nutrition more than body requirements related to changes in appetite resulting from corticosteroid therapy or antiadrenal agents.
- Body image disturbance related to side effects of long-term corticosteroid therapy or from antiadrenal agents.
- Increased cardiac output related to increased volume or fluid retention associated with mineralocorticoid therapy.
- Risk for infection related to side effects of glucocorticoid therapy.
- Impaired skin and oral mucosa integrity related to the side effects of corticosteroid therapy.
- Risk for injury stemming from changes in sensorium and possible confusion related to side effects of corticosteroid therapy or from adverse reactions of antiadrenal agents.

PLANNING

The goals in patients receiving corticosteroids or antiadrenals include:
- Patient describes the healthy diet to observe during treatment.
- Patient experiences minimal body image disturbances.
- Patient exhibits minimal complications resulting from the fluid retention caused by mineralocorticoid therapy.
- Patient will be free of infection during corticosteroid therapy.
- Patient's skin and mucous membranes will remain intact during treatment.
- Patient will maintain normal electrolyte levels.
- Patient will remain free of changes in sensorium and possible confusion or dizziness from adrenal or antiadrenal therapy.
- Patient states symptoms to report immediately to the physician should they occur.

Outcome Criteria

Outcome criteria for patients receiving adrenal agents include:
- Patient will eat adequate foods from the four major food groups and maintain weight within normal range with adequate menu planning.
- Patient will openly verbalize fears about body image disturbances to health care providers.
- Patient will experience minimal problems with fluid volume excess and not gain more than 2 lb/week.
- Patient will notify the physician if fever (>100.0° F or 38° C) occurs.
- Patient performs frequent mouth and skin care to prevent infections and maintain intactness.

TAKE HOME POINTS

Adrenal Gland
- An endocrine organ that sits on top of the kidneys.
- Composed of two distinct tissues: the adrenal cortex and the adrenal medulla.
- Adrenal medulla secretes two important hormones: epinephrine (80%) and norepinephrine (20%).
- Adrenal cortex secretes hormones known as *corticosteroids:* glucocorticoids and mineralocorticoids.

Corticosteroids
- Glucocorticoid biologic functions: antiinflammatory actions, maintenance of normal blood pressure, carbohydrate and protein metabolism, fat metabolism, and stress effects.
- Mineralocorticoid biologic functions: sodium and water resorption, blood pressure control, and potassium levels in and pH of blood.

Nursing Considerations
- Adrenal agents may be administered orally, IM, or IV; some are also administered by means of a rectal enema.
- Parenteral forms should be diluted and administered according to the manufacturer's guidelines.
- IM forms of adrenal agents should be administered deep into a large muscle such as in the gluteal area.
- Steroid inhalers should be used as ordered and only after adequate patient education.
- Adverse effects to monitor for include weight gain (if more than 5 pounds [2.25 kg] in a week), increase in blood pressure, pulse irregularities, mental status changes such as aggression or depression, electrolyte disturbances, elevated glucose levels, decreased healing, GI tract upset, and ulcer-related symptoms.

- Patient implements measures to minimize major electrolyte imbalances during corticosteroid or mineralocorticoid therapy such as forcing fluids and possible salt restrictions or additives as ordered.
- Patient will change positions slowly and walk carefully to prevent injuries from dizziness or syncope.
- Patient will identify symptoms to report to the physician such as a weight gain of more than 2 lb/

week, shortness of breath, edema, dizziness, or syncope.

■ Patient must be weaned off corticosteroids to prevent Addison's crisis.

IMPLEMENTATION

Systemic adrenal agents, such as hydrocortisone and prednisone, may be given by the oral, IM, IV, and rectal (enema) (hydrocortisone) routes. Parenteral forms of these agents should be diluted according to the manufacturer's guidelines and administered over the recommended time span; for example, hydrocortisone should be given at a rate of 25 mg or less per minute. All liquid and parenteral forms should be mixed thoroughly before administration. IM forms should always be administered in a large-muscle (e.g., gluteal) site as opposed to the deltoid muscle, and the sites rotated to prevent tissue trauma and damage. Oral forms should be given with food or milk so as to minimize GI upset. Injections should not be given subcutaneously because this may lead to tissue damage.

Topical agents should be applied as ordered and only according to the instructions in the package insert, which, for example, may specify the use of an occlusive dressing. The skin should be clean and dry before application, and the nurse should wear gloves and apply the medication with either a sterile tongue depressor or cotton-tipped applicator, if the skin is intact. A sterile technique should be used if the skin is not intact!

Beclomethasone is a nasally administered synthetic corticosteroid that should be used as ordered. Any written instructions that come with the product should be read and followed carefully. Before administering a nasal corticosteroid, the patient should clear the nasal passages, and this may require a decongestant, which the physician may need to prescribe. See Chapter 4 for more instructions on nasal sprays.

Steroid inhalers should be used as ordered and the patient adequately taught the technique for administration (also covered in Chapter 4). It is important to emphasize to patients receiving them that, once the inhaler has been used, they should clean out the oral cavity with mouthwash to prevent possible oral fungal infections from developing.

Patients receiving fludrocortisone should take it with food or milk to minimize GI upset. Any weight gain of more than 5 pounds (2.25 kg) a week during mineralocorticoid therapy should be reported to the physician. Abrupt withdrawal is not recommended because this may precipitate an adrenal crisis.

Aminogluthethimide should be taken with an antacid (before the steroid) to minimize GI upset. Because this drug is often used in patients with malignant tumors, it is also important to enhance the patient's nutritional and general well-being during therapy, such as by giving him or her nutritional supplements or vitamins.

See the box on p. 496 for more teaching tips for patients receiving adrenal agents.

EVALUATION

A therapeutic response to corticosteroids includes a resolution of the underlying manifestations of the disease, such as a decrease in inflammation. Adverse effects to monitor for include weight gain, increased blood pressure, pulse irregularities, mental status changes such as aggression or depression, electrolyte disturbances, elevated glucose levels, decreased healing, GI upset, and ulcer-related symptoms. The systemic agents may cause potassium depletion, and this is manifested by fatigue, nausea, vomiting, muscle weakness, and dysrythymias.

A therapeutic response to aminoglutethimide includes a decrease in the size of the tumor or a decrease in the Cushing's syndrome. Side effects to watch for include jaundice, skin lesions, hypotension, headache, lethargy, weakness, GI upset, and hepatotoxicity.

Critical Thinking **A C T I V I T I E S**

1. A 19-year-old man is admitted through the emergency room after a motorcycle accident. He is conscious upon admission, has stable vital signs, and minimal cuts and abrasions on the left side of his body. You perform a thorough neurologic examination and find absence of sensation to light touch and pinprick and lower extremity paralysis. Reflexes are absent below the groin area. The physician orders a high dose IV methylprednisolone. What is the purpose of this medication and what should you, as the nurse, watch for while the patient is receiving this medication?

2. You are caring for a patient who is taking 100 mg of hydrocortisone orally. The physician decides that he is more familiar with prednisone and wants to change the patient over to the equivalent oral dose of prednisone. What should you recommend?

3. One of the most important points to emphasize to a patient taking corticosteroids is which one of the following:
   a. Report a weight gain of 1 to 2 pounds (0.5 to 1 kg) that occurs within 10 days.
   b. Immunosuppression is not an expected side effect of these drugs.
   c. Corticosteroids should *never* be discontinued abruptly.
   d. All doses of corticosteroids should be taken before 9:00 AM.

▲▲

BIBLIOGRAPHY

Albanese J, Nutz P: *Mosby's 1995 nursing drug cards,* St Louis, 1995, Mosby.

Cutie AJ, Sciarra JJ: Therapeutic inhalation of aerosols in the treatment of asthma, *J Pract Nurs*, 40(12):41, 1990.

Gift AG: Dyspnea, *Nurs Clin North Am* 25:955, 1990.

Johnson KB: *Harriet Lane handbook,* ed 13, St Louis, 1993, Mosby.

Keen JH: *Critical care and emergency drug reference,* St Louis, 1994, Mosby.

Knoben JE, Anderson PO: *Handbook of critical drug data,* ed 6, Hamilton, Ill, 1988, Drug Intelligence Publications.

Levin RH: Advances in pediatric therapy of asthma, *Nurs Clin North Am.* 26:263, 1991.

McEvoy GK: *AHFS drug information,* Bethesda, Md. 1994, American Society of Hospital Pharmacists.

Skidmore-Roth L: *Mosby's 1995 nursing drug reference,* St Louis, 1995, Mosby.

Thibodeau GA, Patton KT: *Anatomy and physiology,* ed 2, St Louis, 1993, Mosby.

Wingard L, et al: *Human pharmacology: molecular to clinical,* St Louis, 1991, Mosby.

PART 7

RESPIRATORY SYSTEM: STUDY SKILLS BRIEF

STUDY ON THE RUN, PURR

The basic approach in applying Study on the Run (SOTR) is to make use of small blocks of time that are otherwise nonproductive. Plan, Rehearse, and Review (PURR) do not require that the entire chapter be covered in one study session. These steps produce their benefits by promoting repetition of learning.

Where Is the Time

SOTR time is everywhere. In the course of a single day you might have an hour or more that can be used for SOTR actions. It is just a matter of becoming aware of little bits and pieces of your day that can ordinarily slip away without being productive. Small blocks of time are everywhere in your day; it just takes a little creativity on your part to become aware of them. Finishing an exam early, standing in the checkout line, waiting for the teakettle to boil, or even waiting for the washing machine to finish the last spin before you change loads can be time used for SOTR. Get creative and be flexible. Remember, every minute of time you use this way is a minute of time you will not have to find later.

SOTR and Plan

I have repeatedly stressed the importance of questioning as an essential component in Plan. Look at the chapter objectives for Chapter 35. There are seven objectives presented for this chapter. You got out of class a little early today, and have 10 minutes before you must fulfill your next obligation. Work on the questions for as many of these objectives as can be accomplished in the time you have. If you complete questions for only two objectives, do not look upon it as failure to complete something. Instead learn to view what you have done as that much less to do later. The time you spend now frees up that much more time during your large blocks of study time for intense study reading.

Will you forget the questions you generated in this session before you have the opportunity to read the chapter? If you make it a habit to ask questions as a continuing part of all study, you will find that you remember the focus questions very well. If you have trouble remembering your own questions, use a pencil. Write questions in the margins of the text. Gradually you will find questioning becomes such an automatic procedure that you will be able to dispense with writing questions. You will remember them.

SOTR and Vocabulary

One of the most challenging aspects of a course like this is the almost overwhelming vocabulary load. If the new vocabulary load is not enough, there is also the need to keep reviewing previous parts and chapters because some term that was introduced three chapters ago has reappeared and you do not remember it clearly. Creating your own vocabulary cards is a perfect SOTR activity.

The basic card model is simple. The word, common form, prefix, or suffix appears on the card front. The back of the card may have just a little information, the minimum being a definition of what is on the front, or the back of the card may contain considerable information. I recommend that you include part, chapter, and page number on the back so that you can locate the term quickly if the need arises. In addition, you may want to add a specific example from the text or of your own creation to help clarify the term. Put as much information on the back as you find useful.

Creating Vocabulary Cards with SOTR

Use the time between classes to create several personal vocabulary cards. Grab your text and your blank note cards. Open to the next chapter you will be studying. Flip over to the glossary pages. Write the first word from the glossary on the front of a blank note card. Flip the card over. Write the part and chapter numbers and the page number for the glossary on the card. Pick a standard location for this. Put these numbers in a top corner or a bottom corner, but make sure you put them in the same corner every time. Eventually this becomes a habit and makes the preparation process faster. It also helps when you are making use of the cards because you will know exactly what information you put on the card and where you put it. Put this card aside and repeat the process with the next term in the glossary. In those few minutes before you go to class you can have completed the basic preparation for a full set of cards covering the 21 terms in the Chapter 35 glossary.

Notice that all I proposed was that you copy the term and the locating information. I did not tell you to copy the definition in the glossary at this time. The term, used in the context of a sentence and a paragraph, may be much easier to understand. If, as you read the chapter, you feel that the glossary definition is also useful to have on this card you can always flip back using the locating information you put on the card.

SOTR and Vocabulary Review

Your vocabulary cards are ideal for SOTR action. Carry a deck of cards with you at all times. Whenever you have even a minute or two, you can pull out a stack of cards—cards from previous chapters or the current chapter. Use the oral ask and answer method discussed in the *Study Skills Manual*. For instance, the first term in the glossary for Chapter 35 is *allergen*. Ask yourself aloud, "What is an allergen?" Then try to answer the question aloud. Answer: "An allergen is a substance that produces an allergic reaction." It is not necessary to recall the exact answer presented in the glossary and/or the chapter. What is important is that you respond with a clear and meaningful answer. The answer given above is not exactly the same as that stated in the glossary, but the general concept is the same. Once you have stated your answer turn the card over and check to make sure that you were correct. Each time you do this with a term, you are strengthening your long-term memory and will find that it takes less and less time to recall the terms you need.

SOTR and Chapter Review

It can be overwhelming if you think that review means rereading the material, and therefore you need large blocks of uninterrupted time. There is a much more efficient way to review, and it works well in short time blocks, which makes it a perfect technique for SOTR.

Look at the first page of Chapter 34. You should instantly see a number of visible structures that make it easy to review key terms and concepts without rereading the entire block of material. First, there is the chapter title: *Antihistamines, Decongestants, Antitussives, and Expectorants*. What are antihistamines? This is a question you would have generated when you were engaged in the Plan step of PURR. Now that you have read the chapter repeat the question and answer it aloud. Answer aloud because you will hear what you say, and will either know the material or need to mark it to come back and reread. Now ask a more complex question, "What is the role of antihistamines? What do they do?" Now try to answer these questions. If you can, then you do not need to reread to find out what antihistamines are. Next, looking at p. 503, you will notice some things in **bold print**. Apply the same process. Using the bold face words and phrases as stimulus, ask questions and try to answer them to your own satisfaction. If you cannot develop a satisfactory answer, then you know that some rereading is needed. But it is very focused. You are not trying to reread everything on the page, only the material right there associated with the term.

Looking further down the page you will see a list. Look at the previous sentence, "This explains why, when excessive amounts of histamine are released, this can lead to anaphylaxis and severe allergic symptoms and result in any or all of the following physiologic changes." Ask questions. If you can answer, no reading is necessary. If you cannot answer, you know that the answers are found immediately after this sentence in the indented list. Use the structures in the chapter to accomplish focused review. Comprehension is improved, long-term memory is strengthened, and your test grades will reflect this.

The benefits of SOTR are enormous. There is no drawback. You are using time that otherwise would be "wasted." This time now becomes productive study time. The more active you become in looking for SOTR opportunities, the more you will find. The more SOTR time you spend the better student you will become.

Chapter 34

Antihistamines, Decongestants, Antitussives, and Expectorants

Objectives

When you reach the end of this chapter, you will be able to:

1 Discuss the actions of and indications for the antihistamines, decongestants, antitussives, and expectorants.

2 Identify the various agents representative of antihistamines, decongestants, antitussives, and expectorants.

3 Discuss the contraindications to and adverse effects related to the antihistamines, decongestants, antitussives, and expectorants.

4 Develop a nursing care plan as it relates to the nursing process in patients taking antihistamines, decongestants, and expectorants.

CHAPTER OUTLINE

Histamine and the Antihistamines

Mechanism of action
Drug effects
  Therapeutic uses
  Side effects and adverse effects
  Interactions
  Dosages
Drug Profiles
Nonsedating Antihistamines
    Astemizole
    Loratadine
  ⚓ Terfenadine
Traditional Antihistamines
    Diphenhydramine
Other Antihistamines

Cold Medications

Decongestants
  Mechanism of action
  Drug effects
  Therapeutic uses
  Side effects and adverse effects
  Interactions
  Dosages
Drug Profiles
    Naphazoline

Antitussives
  Mechanism of action
  Drug effects
  Therapeutic uses
  Side effects and adverse effects
  Interactions
  Dosages
Drug Profiles
  ⚓ Dextromethorphan
    Benzonatate
  Codeine
Expectorants
  Mechanism of action
  Drug effects
  Therapeutic uses
  Side effects and adverse effects
  Interactions
  Dosages
Drug Profiles
  ⚓ Guaifenesin

Nursing Process

Assessment
Nursing Diagnoses
Planning
  Outcome criteria
Implementation
Evaluation

Glossary

Adrenergics (sympathomimetics) (a drə nər' jiks) Of or pertaining to sympathetic nerve fibers of the autonomic nervous system that use epinephrine or epinephrine-like substances as neurotransmitters. (p. 510)

Ammonium chloride (ə mo' ne əm klor' īd) Works by initially irritating the gastrointestinal tract, which causes a reflex stimulation or irritation of the respiratory tract. (p. 514)

Antagonist (an tag' ə nist) Any agent that exerts an action opposite to that of another or competes for the same receptor sites. (p. 503)

Anticholinergics (parasympatholytics) (an tǐ co lin'ər jikz) Of or pertaining to the blockade of acetylcholine receptors that results in the inhibition of the transmission of parasympathetic nerve impulses. (p. 510)

Antihistamines (an' tǐ his' tə mīn) Any substance capable of reducing the physiologic and pharmacologic effects of histamine, including a wide variety of drugs that block histamine receptors. (p. 503)

Benzonatate (ben zo' nə tāt) A nonopiate antitussive. (p. 512)

Corticosteroids Any one of the natural or synthetic hormones produced by the adrenal cortex. They influence or control key processes of the body, such as carbohydrate and protein metabolism, the maintenance of serum glucose levels, electrolyte and water balance, and the functions of the cardiovascular system, skeletal muscle, the kidneys, and other organs. (p. 510)

Dextromethorphan (deks' tro məth or' fan) An antitussive derived from morphine, but lacking narcotic effects. (p. 512)

Empiric therapy (em pir' ik) A method of treating disease based on observations and experience without an understanding of the cause of or mechanism responsible for the disorder or the way in which the therapeutic agent or procedure effects improvement or cure. (p. 510)

Expectorant (ek spek' tə rənt) An agent that increases the flow of fluid in the respiratory tract, reducing the viscosity of bronchial and tracheal secretions and facilitating their removal by the cough reflex and ciliary action. (p. 514)

Guaifenesin (gwi' fen' əsin) Glyceryl guaiacolate, a white to slightly gray powder with a bitter taste and faint odor. It is widely used as an expectorant. (p. 514)

Histamine antagonist (his' tə mēn) Drug that competes with histamine for histamine receptors. (p. 503)

Influenza Highly contagious infection of the respiratory tract caused by a myxovirus and transmitted by airborne droplets. (p. 509)

Iodinated glycerol (i o' dǐ nā ted glis' ər ol) One of the substances that makes up iodine. (p. 514)

Ipecac syrup (ip' ə kak) An emetic prescribed for the treatment of certain types of poisoning and drug overdose. (p. 514)

Nonsedating antihistamines Substances that work peripherally to block the actions of histamine and therefore do not have the central nervous system effects that many of the older antihistamines have. (p. 506)

Peripherally acting antihistamines Another name for nonsedating antihistamines. (p. 506)

Potassium iodide One of the products that makes up iodine. (p. 514)

Reflex stimulation An irritation of the respiratory tract occurring in response to an irritation of the gastrointestinal tract. (p. 514)

Rhinovirus (ri' no vi' rəs) Any of about 100 serologically distinct, small RNA viruses that cause about 40% of acute respiratory illnesses. (p. 509)

Sympathomimetic A pharmacologic agent that causes effects that mimick those resulting from stimulation of organs and structures by the sympathetic nervous system. They do this by occupying adrenergic receptor sites and acting as an agonist or by increasing the release of norepinephrine at postganglionic nerve endings. (p. 510)

Terpin hydrate (tər' pin hi' drāt) Diminishes secretions and promotes healing of the mucous membrane. (p. 514)

Upper respiratory tract infection Any infectious disease of the upper respiratory tract, including the common cold, laryngitis, pharyngitis, rhinitis, sinusitis, and tonsillitis. (p. 509)

Histamine and the Antihistamines

Histamine is a bodily substance that performs many functions. It is involved in CNS transmission, the dilation of capillaries, the contraction of smooth muscles, the stimulation of gastric secretion, and the acceleration of the heart rate. There are two types of cellular receptors for histamine. The histamine-1 (H-1) receptors, which mediate smooth muscle contraction and the dilation of capillaries, and the histamine-2 (H-2) receptors, which mediate the acceleration of the heart rate and gastric acid secretion. This explains why, when excessive amounts of histamine are released, this can lead to anaphylaxis and severe allergic symptoms and result in any or all of the following physiologic changes:

- Constriction of smooth muscle, especially in the stomach and lungs
- Increase in body secretions
- Vasodilation and increased capillary permiability resulting in fluid movement out of the blood vessels and into the tissues, causing a drop in blood pressure and edema
- Dramatic decrease in blood pressure

Antihistamines are drugs that directly compete with histamine for specific receptor sites. For this reason they are also called antagonists. Those antihistamines that compete with histamine for the H-2 receptors are called **histamine-2 antagonists** (also *H-2 blockers*) and include such agents as cimetidine, ranitidine, famotidine, and nizatidine. Because they act on the gastrointestinal system, they are discussed in detail in Unit XI, which focuses on the agents that affect this system. The focus of this chapter is on the **histamine-1 antagonists;** these are the agents more commonly known as antihistamines. They are especially useful agents because approximately 10% to 20% of the general population is sensitive to various environmental allergies, and it is histamine that mediates the resulting disorders, ones such as allergic rhinitis (e.g., hay fever, mold and dust allergies), anaphylaxis, angioneurotic edema, drug fevers, insect bite reactions, and urticaria (itching).

The H-1 antagonists (also called *H-1 blockers*) include such drugs as diphenhydramine, chlorpheniramine, terfenadine, and astemizole. They are of greatest value in the treatment of nasal allergies, particularly seasonal hay fever. They are also given to relieve the symptoms of the common cold such as sneezing and running nose. In this regard they are palliative, not curative; that is, they can help alleviate the symptoms of a cold but can do nothing to destroy the virus causing it.

The clinical efficacy of the more than a dozen different antihistamines is extremely similar, though they all have varying degrees of antihistaminic, anticholinergic, and sedating properties. The particular actions of, and hence indications for, a particular antihistamine are determined by its specific chemical make-up. All antihistamines compete with histamine for the H-1 receptors in areas such as the smooth muscle surrounding blood vessels and bronchioles. They also affect the secretions of the lacrimal, salivary, and respiratory mucosal glands. Because of their antihistamic properties, they are indicated for the treatment of allergies. These agents also differ from each other in their potency and their adverse effects, especially in the degree of drowsiness they produce. The antihistaminic, anticholinergic, and sedative properties of some of the commonly used antihistamines are summarized in Fig. 34-1. Some of the commonly used antihistamines are listed in Table 34-1, which also summarizes their various anticholinergic and sedative effects. These effects make them useful for the treatment of such problems as vertigo, motion sickness, insomnia, and cough.

Mechanism of Action

The H-1 blockers (antihistamines) work by blocking or inhibiting the action of histamine throughout the body. They do not push off histamine that is already bound to its receptor but compete with the substance for unoccupied receptors. Therefore these agents are most beneficial when given early in a reaction before all the histamine binds to receptors. This binding of H-1 blockers to these receptors prevents the adverse consequences of histamine stimulation—vasodilation, increased GI and respiratory secretions, and increased capillary permeability.

▼ **FIG. 34-1** Comparison of efficacy and side effects of selected antihistamines. (Modified from McKenry L, Salerno E: *Mosby's pharmacology in nursing,* ed 19, St Louis, 1995, Mosby.)

| Table 34-1 | Effects of Various Antihistamines | | |

CHEMICAL CLASS	ANTICHOLINERGIC EFFECTS	SEDATIVE EFFECTS	COMMENTS
Alkylamines			
Brompheniramine	Moderate	Low	Cause less drowsiness and more CNS stimulation; suitable
Chlorpheniramine	Moderate	Low	for daytime use.
Dexchlorpheniramine	Moderate	Low	
Ethanolamines			
Clemastine	High	Moderate	Substantial anticholinergic effects; commonly cause se-
Diphenhydramine	High	Low	dation; with usual doses drowsiness occurs in about
Dimenhydrinate	High	Low	50% of patients; diphenhydramine and dimenhydri-
			nate also used as antiemetics.
Ethylenediamines			
Pyrilamine	Low to none	Low	Weak sedative effects, but adverse GI effects are
Tripelennamine	Low to none	Moderate	common.
Phenothiazines			
Promethazine	High	High	Principally used as antipsychotics; some are useful as
Trimeprazine	High	Moderate	antihistamines, antipruritics, and antiemetics.
Piperadines			
Azatadine	Moderate	Moderate	Commonly used in the treatment of motion sickness;
Cyproheptadine	Moderate	Low	hydroxyzine is used as a tranquilizer, sedative,
Hydroxyzine	Moderate	Moderate	antipruritic, and antiemetic.
Phenindamine	Moderate	Low to none	
Miscellaneous			
Astemizole	Low to none	Low to none	Very few adverse effects from anticholinergic or sedative
↓Terfenadine	Low to none	Low to none	effects; almost exclusively antihistaminic effects; can
Loratadine	Low to none	Low to none	take during day because no sedative effects. In
			general they are longer acting and have fewer side
			effects.

Drug Effects

By blocking the H-1 receptors, and thereby preventing histamine from acting on the cell, antihistamines have the opposite effects of histamine. Whereas histamine causes extravascular smooth muscle (e.g., in the bronchial tree) to contract, antihistamines cause it to relax. They also prevent or reduce salivary, gastric, lacrimal, and bronchial secretions. By stimulating nerve endings, histamine causes pruritus. Antihistamines can prevent or alleviate the itching. Histamine causes microvascular dilation (involves both H-1 and H-2 receptors) and increased vascular permeability (involves only H-1 receptors). Antihistamines have the opposite effect. During allergic reactions, histamine and other substances are released from mast cells, basophils, and other cells in response to antigens (foreign substances) circulating in the blood. It then binds to and activates specific receptors in the nose, eyes, respiratory tract, and skin, producing the characteristic allergic signs and symptoms. Antihistamines can prevent or alleviate these reactions. The various drug effects of antihistamines are listed in Table 34-2.

Therapeutic Uses

The antihistamines are more effective in preventing the actions of histamine than in reversing them once they have taken place. Because of their anticholinergic actions, they have a drying effect and reduce nasal, salivary, and lacrimal gland hypersecretion (runny nose and tearing and itching eyes). In the skin they block capillary permeability, wheal-and-flare formation, and itching. The antihistamines are most beneficial in the management of nasal allergies, seasonal allergic rhinitis (e.g., hay fever), and some of the typical symptoms of the common cold. They are also very useful in the treatment of various allergic reactions, motion sickness, Parkinson's disease, and vertigo. In addition, they have proved to be safe and effective as sleep aids.

Side Effects and Adverse Effects

Drowsiness is usually the chief complaint of people who take antihistamines, but these sedative effects vary from class to class (see Table 34-1). The anticholinergic (drying) effects of antihistamines can cause

Table 34-2	Antihistamines: Drug Effects	
BODY SYSTEM	**HISTAMINE EFFECT**	**ANTIHISTAMINE EFFECT**
Cardiovascular system (small blood vessels)	Dilation of blood vessels, increased blood vessel permeability (allows substances to leak into tissues).	Prevents dilation of blood vessels and increased permeability.
Smooth muscle (on exocrine glands)	Stimulates salivary, gastric, lacrimal, and bronchial secretions.	Prevents salivary, gastric, lacrimal, and bronchial secretions.
Immune system (release of various substances commonly associated with allergic reactions)	Mast cells release histamine and several other substances, resulting in allergic reactions.	Do not stabilize mast cells nor do they prevent the release of the substances such as histamine, but they bind to histamine receptors and prevent the actions of histamine.

Table 34-3	Antihistamines: Common Adverse Effects
BODY SYSTEM	**SIDE/ADVERSE EFFECT**
Central nervous system	Sedation (mild drowsiness to deep sleep), dizziness, muscular weakness, paradoxical excitement, restlessness, insomnia, nervousness, seizures
Cardiovascular	Local anesthetic (quinidine-like) effect on the cardiac conduction system resulting in dysrhythmias, arrest, hypotension, palpitations, syncope, dizziness, death (see Interactions section)
Gastrointestinal	Anorexia, nausea, vomiting, diarrhea or constipation, hepatitis, jaundice
Other	Dryness of mouth, nose, and throat; urinary retention; impotence; vertigo; visual disturbances; blurred vision; tinnitus; headache; rarely agranulocytosis, hemolytic anemia, leukopenia, thrombocytopenia, pancytopenia

such side effects as dry mouth, difficulty urinating, constipation, and cardiovascular system problems. The most frequent side effects and adverse effects of the antihistamines are listed in Table 34-3.

Interactions

The nonsedating histamines should not be used concurrently with erythromycin, ketoconazole, or itraconazole because of the life-threatening cardiovascular

disorders that can result. These include cardiac arrest, torsades de pointes, and other ventricular dysrhythmias.

Dosages

For the recommended dosages for selected antihistamines, see the dosages table on the next page.

DRUG PROFILES

Although most of the antihistamines are prescription drugs, many are also available over the counter (OTC). The antihistamines come in many dosage forms to be administered orally, intramuscularly, intravenously, or topically.

NONSEDATING ANTIHISTAMINES

A major advance in antihistamine therapy occurred with the development of the **nonsedating antihistamines,** terfenadine, astemizole, and loratadine. These agents were developed in part to eliminate many of the unwanted side effects of the older antihistamines, mainly sedation. These agents work peripherally to block the actions of histamine and therefore do not have the central nervous system effects that many of the older antihistamines have. For this reason these agents are also called **peripherally acting antihistamines.** Another advantage these agents have over the older antihistamines is that they have longer durations

DOSAGES

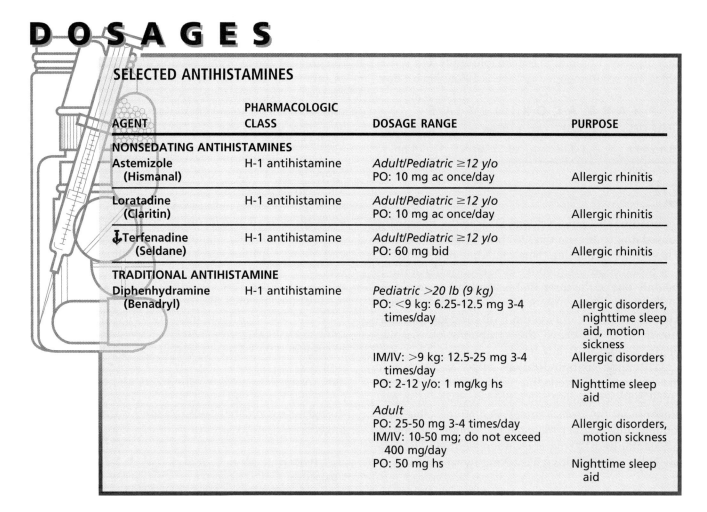

SELECTED ANTIHISTAMINES

AGENT	PHARMACOLOGIC CLASS	DOSAGE RANGE	PURPOSE
NONSEDATING ANTIHISTAMINES			
Astemizole (Hismanal)	H-1 antihistamine	*Adult/Pediatric ≥12 y/o* PO: 10 mg ac once/day	Allergic rhinitis
Loratadine (Claritin)	H-1 antihistamine	*Adult/Pediatric ≥12 y/o* PO: 10 mg ac once/day	Allergic rhinitis
⇩Terfenadine (Seldane)	H-1 antihistamine	*Adult/Pediatric ≥12 y/o* PO: 60 mg bid	Allergic rhinitis
TRADITIONAL ANTIHISTAMINE			
Diphenhydramine (Benadryl)	H-1 antihistamine	*Pediatric >20 lb (9 kg)* PO: <9 kg: 6.25-12.5 mg 3-4 times/day	Allergic disorders, nighttime sleep aid, motion sickness
		IM/IV: >9 kg: 12.5-25 mg 3-4 times/day	Allergic disorders
		PO: 2-12 y/o: 1 mg/kg hs	Nighttime sleep aid
		Adult PO: 25-50 mg 3-4 times/day	Allergic disorders, motion sickness
		IM/IV: 10-50 mg; do not exceed 400 mg/day	
		PO: 50 mg hs	Nighttime sleep aid

of action, which allows some of them to be taken only once a day. This further increases compliance. Unlike many of the older antihistamines, the nonsedating antihistamines are only available by prescription, in part because of some of the life-threatening drug interactions associated with these agents.

ASTEMIZOLE

Astemizole (Hismanal) has many pharmacologic characteristics that distinguish it from the other antihistamines. It has the longest half-life of the three nonsedating antihistamines (20-60 hours), allowing it to be dosed only once a day. It also has very poor anticholinergic effects, which means it does not cause some of the unwanted effects of the older antihistamines, effects such as dry mouth, difficulty urinating, constipation, and cardiovascular effects.

Astemizole is indicated for the treatment of seasonal allergic rhinitis and chronic idiopathic urticaria, but as with all antihistamines, it merely provides palliative therapy. Because seasonal allergic rhinitis may be a chronic, recurrent condition, affected patients often may require long term intermittent therapy with the drug.

Contraindications to astemizole use include hy-

persensitivity. It should be used with caution in patients with impaired liver function, because this may allow astemizole to accumulate and would lead to life-threatening reactions similar to the cardiovascular problems that occur if the agent is taken with erthromycin, ketoconazole, or itraconazole. Astemizole is classified as a pregnancy category C agent and is available in 10-mg tablets. The recommended dosage is 10 mg per day, given as a single dose.

PHARMACOKINETICS

HALF-LIFE	ONSET	PEAK	DURATION
11-20 hr	Slow	1 hr	≤24 hr

LORATADINE

Loratadine (Claritin) is the newest of the nonsedating antihistamines. It also only needs to be taken once a day. Structurally it is similar to cyproheptadine and azatadine, but unlike these other agents, it cannot distribute into the central nervous system. Loratadine is used to relieve the symptoms of seasonal allergic rhinitis (e.g., hay fever).

Loratadine is classified as a pregnancy category B agent and is contraindicated in patients who have shown a hypersensitivity to it, those suffering from an acute asthma attack, and those with lower respiratory tract diseases. Loratadine is available orally as a 10-mg tablet. The recommended dosage is 10 mg once a day.

⬡ PHARMACOKINETICS

HALF-LIFE	ONSET	PEAK	DURATION
8.4-24 hr	1-3 hr	8-12 hr	24 hr

⚓ TERFENADINE

Terfenadine (Seldane, Seldane-D) was the first of the nonsedating antihistamines to come available. Because it has a shorter half-life than loratadine or aztemizole, it is dosed more frequently. However, terfenadine is the only one of the three that is available in combination with the decongestant pseudoephedrine. Terfenadine alone or in combination with the pseudoephedrine is used to relieve the symptoms of seasonal allergic rhinitis (e.g., hay fever).

The same contraindications apply to astemizole and loratadine. Terfenadine is classified as a pregnancy category C agent and is only available as an oral preparation. By itself it comes as a 60-mg tablet; the combination product (Seldane-D) contains 60 mg of terfenadine and 120 mg of pseudoephedrine. The usually recommended dosage is 60 mg twice a day.

⬡ PHARMACOKINETICS

HALF-LIFE	ONSET	PEAK	DURATION
20 hr	1-2 hr	3-4 hr	>12 hr

TRADITIONAL ANTIHISTAMINES

The traditional antihistamines are the older agents that work both peripherally and centrally. They also have anticholinergic effects, which in some cases make them more effective than the nonsedating antihistamines. Some of these commonly used older agents are diphenhydramine, brompheniramine, chlorpheniramine, dimenhydrinate, doxylamine, meclinzine, and promethazine. These agents are used either alone or in combination with other drugs in the symptomatic relief of many disorders ranging from insomnia to motion sickness. Many patients respond to and tolerate the older agents quite well, and because many are generically available, they are much less expensive. These agents are available both OTC and by prescription.

DIPHENHYDRAMINE

Diphenhydramine (Benadryl) is an older, traditional antihistamine that works both peripherally and centrally. It also has potent anticholinergic effects. It is one of the most commonly used antihistamines, in part because of its excellent safety profile and efficacy. It has the greatest range of therapeutic indications of any of the antihistamines available. It is used for the relief or prevention of histamine-mediated allergies and motion sickness, the treatment of Parkinson's disease, and as a sleep-aid. It is also used in conjunction with epinephrine in the management of anaphylaxis.

Diphenhydramine is classified as a pregnancy category B agent and is contraindicated in patients with a known hypersensitivity to it, nursing mothers, neonates, and patients with lower respiratory tract symptoms. It is available in oral, parenteral, and topical preparations. Orally diphenhydramine comes as a 25- and 50-mg capsules and regular and film-coated tablets; as a 12.5–mg/5 ml elixir; and in several combination products that contain other cough and cold medications. Parenterally diphenhydramine comes as a 10- and 50-mg/ml injection. Topically diphenhydramine is available as a 1% and 2% cream. It also comes in combination with several other drugs that are commonly given topically, such as calamine, camphor, and zinc oxide. These combination preparations come as aerosols, creams, gels, and lotions. The recommended dosages are given in the dosages table on the preceding page.

⬡ PHARMACOKINETICS

HALF-LIFE	ONSET	PEAK	DURATION
2-7 hr	15-30 min	1-2 hr	4 hr

OTHER ANTIHISTAMINES

Brompheniramine and chlorpheniramine are other antihistamines commonly used alone or in combination with other drugs as OTC cough and cold preparations. Dimenhydrinate (Dramamine) is commonly used in the treatment of motion sickness. It is available as a chewable tablet that can be quickly absorbed, making its onset of action rapid. This is of use in patients suffering from vertigo or motion sickness of sudden onset. Because of its potent sedating effects, doxylamine (Unisom) is very frequently used in combination with cough and cold medications such as acetaminophen (Tylenol) to induce sleep in cold sufferers. Meclizine (Antivert or Bonine), which is used for the treatment of vertigo, is available both OTC and by prescription in higher doses. One of the most commonly used antiemetic agents is an antihistamine. This agent, promethazine (Phenergan), is commonly given for the treatment of various types of nausea and vomiting. It is available in oral and rectal preparations and as an injection. Following is a listing of all the antihistamines that includes the commonly recommended dosages and other pertinent information:

■ **Azatadine** (Optimine) is available by prescription

as 1-mg tablets. The recommended dosage is 1 to 2 mg twice daily, given with a full glass of water. It is rated as a pregnancy category B agent.

■ **Brompheniramine** (Dimetane) is available as a 2-mg/5 ml elixir and as 4-, 8-, and 12-mg tablets. These dosage forms may be either obtained by prescription or OTC, depending on the dose and dosage instructions. The recommended oral dosage is 4 to 8 mg three to four times daily, taken with a full glass of water. It is rated as a pregnancy category C agent.

■ **Buclizine** (Bucladin-S, Softabs) is available by prescription as 50-mg tablets. The usual adult dosage is 50 mg taken a half hour before travel and repeated after 4 to 6 hours, if needed. It has no pregnancy category designation.

■ **Chlorpheniramine** (Chlor-Trimeton) is available as 4-, 8-, and 12-mg tablets. These dosage forms are available either by prescription or OTC, depending on the dose and dosage instructions. The recommended oral dosage is 4 mg every 4 to 6 hours, given with a full glass of water. It is rated as a pregnancy category B agent.

■ **Clemastine** (Tavist) is a prescription drug available as a 0.67-mg/5 ml syrup and in 1.34- and 2.68-mg tablets. The recommended oral adult dosage is 1.34 to 2.68 mg one to three times daily, given with a full glass of water. It is rated as a pregnancy category B agent.

■ **Cyclizine** (Marezine) is available OTC as 50-mg tablets. The recommended adult dosage is 50 mg taken a half hour before travel and repeated after 4 to 6 hours, if needed. The total daily dose should not exceed 200 mg. The recommended dosage in 6 to 12-year-old children is 25 mg, given up to three times per day. It is rated as pregnancy category B agent.

■ **Cyproheptadine** (Periactin) is available as a 2-mg/5 ml syrup and as 4-mg tablets. The usual adult dosage is 4 mg three to four times per day, given with a full glass of water. It is rated as a pregnancy category B agent.

■ **Dexchlorpheniramine** (Polaramine) is a prescription drug available as a 2-mg/5 ml syrup and as 2-, 4-, and 6-mg tablets. The recommended adult dosage is 2 mg three to four times per day, given with a full glass of water. It is rated as a pregnancy category B drug.

■ **Dimenhydrinate** (Dramamine) is a prescription drug available as 50-mg tablets. The recommended oral adult dosage is 50 to 100 mg every 4 to 6 hours, taken a half hour before travel. The recommended dosage for 6 to 12-year-old children is 25 to 50 mg every 6 to 8 hours, taken a half hour before travel. It is rated as a pregnancy category B drug.

■ **Doxylamine** (Unisom) is an OTC drug available as

25-mg tablets. The recommended adult dosage is 25 mg at bedtime, taken with a full glass of water. It is rated as a pregnancy category B drug.

■ **Meclizine** (Antivert, Bonine) comes as 12.5-, 25-, and 50-mg tablets and as 25-mg chewable tablets, available either by prescription or OTC, depending on the dose and dosage instructions. The recommended adult oral dosage is 25 to 50 mg, repeated once daily and given with a full glass of water. It is rated as a pregnancy category B drug.

■ **Methdilazine** (Tacaryl) is available by prescription as a 4-mg/5 ml syrup and as 4- and 8-mg tablets. The recommended adult dosage is 8 mg, taken with a full glass of water two to four times per day. It is rated as a pregnancy category B drug.

■ **Promethazine** (Phenergan) is a prescription drug available as a 25- and 50-mg/ml injection, as a 6.25- and 25-mg/5 ml syrup, and as 12.5-, 25-, and 50-mg tablets. The recommended adult dosage is 12.5 to 25 mg three times daily, taken with a full glass of water. It is rated as a pregnancy category C drug.

■ **Trimeprazine** (Temaril) is a prescription drug available as 5-mg capsules, 2.5-mg tablets, and a 2.5-mg/5 ml syrup. The recommended adult dosage is 2.5 mg four times a day, given with a full glass of water. It has no pregnancy category designation.

■ **Tripelennamine** (PBZ) is a prescription drug available as 25-, 50-, and 100-mg tablets. The recommended adult dosage is 25 to 50 mg every 4 to 6 hours, given with a full glass of water. It has no pregnancy category designation.

■ **Triprolidine** (Actidil) is an OTC drug available as a 1.25-mg/5 ml syrup and 2.5-mg tablet. The recommended adult dosage is 2.5 mg every 4 to 6 hours, taken with a full glass of water. It is rated as a pregnancy category C drug.

Cold Medications

The agents used to treat the symptoms of the common cold are decongestants, antitussives (cough suppressants), and expectorants. Most common colds are due to a viral infection, most often a **rhinovirus** or an **influenza** virus such as myxovirus. These viruses normally invade the tissues (mucosa) of the upper respiratory tract (nose, pharynx, and larynx) to cause an **upper respiratory tract infection** (URI). The inflammatory response elicited by these invading viruses stimulates excessive mucus production. This fluid drips down the pharynx and into the esophagus and lower respiratory tract, which leads to symptoms typical of cold—sore throat, coughing, and upset stomach.

The irritation of the nasal mucosa often triggers the sneeze reflex and also causes the release of several inflammatory and vasoactive substances, which results in the dilation of the small blood vessels in the nasal sinuses and leads to nasal congestion. The treatment of the common symptoms of URIs involves the combined use of antihistamines, nasal decongestants, antitussives, and expectorants. However, they can only relieve the symptoms of URIs. They can do nothing to eliminate the causative pathogen. Antivirals and antibiotics are currently the only agents that can do this, but treatment with these is often hampered by the fact that the viral or bacterial cause cannot be readily identified. Because of this, the treatment rendered can only be determined on the basis of what is believed to be the most likely cause. This is called **empiric therapy.**

DECONGESTANTS

Nasal congestion is due to excessive nasal secretions and inflamed and swollen nasal mucosa, and the primary causes are allergies and URIs, especially the common cold. There are three separate groups of nasal decongestants: the **adrenergics (sympathomimetics),** which are the largest group; the **anticholinergics (parasympatholytics),** which are rarely used; and selected topical **corticosteroids** (intranasal steroids).

Nasal decongestants can be applied orally to produce a systemic effect, inhaled, or administered topically to the nose. Each method of administration has its advantages and disadvantages.

The decongestants administered by the oral route are exclusively adrenergic agents that possess alpha-adrenergic activity. They include:

- Phenylephrine
- Phenylpropanolamine
- Pseudoephedrine* (Afrin tablets, Sudafed)

The agents administered by the oral route produce prolonged decongestant effects, but the onset of activity is more delayed and the effect less potent than those of the decongestants applied topically. However, the clinical problem of rebound congestion associated with the topically administered agents is almost nonexistent.

Decongestants suitable for being inhaled must be aromatic, and include:

- Deoxyephedrine (Vicks inhaler)
- Propylhexedrine (Benzedrex inhaler)

The topical administration of adrenergics and intranasal steroids produces a potent decongestant effect with a prompt onset of action. However, sustained use of these agents for several days causes a rebound congestion, which only exacerbates the condition. These agents include:

Adrenergics
- Ephedrine (Vicks Vatronol)
- Naphazoline (Privine)
- Oxymetazoline (Afrin, Sinex Long-Acting)
- Phenylephrine (Neo-Synephrine)
- Tetrahydrozoline (Tyzine, Tyzine Pediatric)

Intranasal steroids
- Beclomethasone dipropionate (Beconase, Vancenase)
- Dexamethasone sodium phosphate (Decadron Phosphate Turbinase)
- Flunisolide (Nasalide)

Mechanism of Action

The nasal decongestants are most commonly used for their ability to shrink engorged nasal mucous membranes and relieve nasal stuffiness. The adrenergic agents (e.g., ephedrine, oxymetazoline) accomplish this by constricting the small blood vessels that supply the structures of the upper respiratory tract, the primary ones being the blood vessels surrounding the nasal sinuses. When these blood vessels are stimulated by alpha-adrenergic drugs, they constrict. Because sympathetic nervous system stimulation produces the same effect, these agents are sometimes referred to as **sympathomimetics.** Once these blood vessels shrink, the nasal secretions in the swollen mucous membranes are better able to drain.

The nasal steroids are aimed at the inflammatory response elicited by the invading organisms—the viruses and bacteria, which the body responds to by producing inflammation, walling off the area and attracting various cells of the immune system. The steroids exert their antiinflammatory effect by causing these cells to be turned off or rendered unresponsive.

Drug Effects

The drug effects of the topical alpha-adrenergic agents are predominantly limited to the mucosal surface on which they are administered. They constrict the arterioles in the mucous membranes, resulting in local vasoconstriction of the dilated blood vessels and a subsequent reduction in blood flow and nasal congestion. The drug effects of the intranasal steroids are discussed in Chapter 35.

Therapeutic Uses

Nasal decongestants relieve the nasal congestion associated with acute or chronic rhinitis, the common cold, sinusitis, and hay fever or other allergies. They may also be used to reduce swelling of the nasal pas-

---

*Pseudoephrine is an alpha-beta agent, but the alpha activity is the greater of the two.

sage and to facilitate visualization of the nasal and pharyngeal membranes before surgery or diagnostic procedures.

Side Effects and Adverse Effects

The adrenergic agents are usually well tolerated. Rare adverse effects of these agents include nervousness, insomnia, palpitations, and tremor.

Occasionally a topically applied adrenergic nasal decongestant is somewhat absorbed into the bloodstream, producing drug effects elsewhere in the body. These include cardiovascular effects such as hypertension and palpitations and central nervous system effects such as headache, nervousness, and dizziness. These systemic effects are the result of alpha-adrenergic stimulation of the heart, blood vessels, and central nervous system. The most common side effects of the intranasal steroids include local mucosal irritation and dryness.

Interactions

See Table 34-4.

Dosages

For the recommended dosages of naphazoline, the only nasal decongestant profiled, see the dosages table on p. 513.

DRUG PROFILES

Many of the decongestants are OTC agents, but the more potent agents that can cause serious side effects are available only by prescription. The adrenergic agents are usually contraindicated in patients with diabetes, hypertension, cardiac disease, thyroid dysfunction, prostatitis, or a known hypersensitivity to them. Although the nasal steroids are relatively safe, they too are contraindicated in some circumstances, specifically nasal mucosal infections and drug hypersensitivity.

Many of the adrenergic agents (phenylephrine, phenylpropanolamine, prophylhexedrine, and pseudoephedrine) and some of the steroids (beclomethasone, dexamethasone, and flunisolide) are discussed in greater detail in other chapters. The adrenergic agents such as naphazoline are discussed here. These are usually the first-line agents used in the treatment of nasal congestion because they are available OTC.

NAPHAZOLINE

Naphazoline (Privine) is chemically and pharmacologically very similar to the other sympathomimetic agents oxymetazoline, tetrahydrozoline, and xylometazoline. When these agents are administered intranasally, they cause dilated arterioles to constrict, thereby reducing nasal blood flow and congestion. During a cold the blood vessels that surround the nasal sinus are usually dilated or swollen and engorged with white blood cells, histamines, and many other cells that are involved in fighting infections of the respiratory tract. This swelling, or dilation, occludes the nasal passage, resulting in the nasal congestion. When agents such as naphazoline are applied to this area, they relieve this swelling and congestion by constricting these blood vessels.

Naphazoline and its chemically related cousins are classified as pregnancy category C agents and have the same contraindications as the other nasal decongestants. Nasally administered naphazoline is available as a 0.05% nasal solution and is meant to be instilled into each nostril. Common dosages for this agent are given in the following dosages table.

✿ P H A R M A C O K I N E T I C S

HALF-LIFE	ONSET	PEAK	DURATION
Unknown	5-10 min	Unknown	2-6 hr

ANTITUSSIVES

Coughing is a normal physiologic function and serves the purpose of removing potentially harmful foreign substances and excessive secretions from the respiratory tract. The cough reflex is stimulated when receptors in the bronchi, alveoli, and pleura (lining of the lungs) are stretched. This causes a signal to be sent to

Table 34-4	Drug Interactions: Nasal Decongestants		
DRUG	**MECHANISM**	**RESULT**	
Sympathomimetics	Additive	Increased toxicity	
MAOIs	Additive	Potentiate the pressor effect	

the cough center in the medulla of the brain, which in turn stimulates the cough. Although most of the time coughing is a beneficial response, there are times when it is nonproductive (dry) and may even be harmful. In these situations, this otherwise normal response must be stopped or inhibited through the use of an antitussive agent. There are two main categories of these agents—the narcotic and nonnarcotic antitussives.

Although all narcotic agents have antitussive effects, only codeine and its semisynthetic derivative hydrocodone are used as antitussives. Both agents are effective in suppressing the cough reflex and, if used in the prescribed manner, their use should not lead to dependency. The two drugs are usually incorporated into various dosage formulations and are rarely used as sole agents.

The nonnarcotic antitussive drugs are less effective than the narcotic ones and are available either alone or in combination with other agents in an array of OTC cold and cough preparations. Dextromethorphan is the most widely used of these antitussive agents and is a derivative of the synthetic narcotic levorphanol. Benzonatate is another nonnarcotic agent.

Mechanism of Action

The narcotic antitussives codeine and hydrocodone suppress the cough reflex through a direct action on this cough center. The nonnarcotic cough suppressant **dextromethorphan** works in the same way. However, because it is not an opioid narcotic, it does not have analgesic properties nor does it cause addiction or CNS depression. Another nonnarcotic antitussive is **benzonatate.** Its mechanism of action is entirely different from that of the other agents. Benzonatate suppresses the cough reflex by anesthetizing (numbing) the stretch receptors and thus keeping the cough reflex from being stimulated in the medulla.

Drug Effects

Codeine, hydrocodone, and dextromethorphan directly suppress the cough reflex while benzonatate anesthetizes, or numbs, the stretch receptors. The narcotic antitussives also provide analgesia as well as have a drying effect on the mucosa of the respiratory tract. They also tend to increase the viscosity of the bronchial secretions.

Therapeutic Uses

Although they have other properties, such as the analgesic effect of the narcotic agents, the antitussives are used primarily to stop the cough reflex when the cough is nonproductive and harmful.

Side Effects and Adverse Effects

Following are the side effects and adverse effects of selected antitussive agents:

- Benzonatate: dizziness, headache, sedation, nausea, constipation, pruritus, and nasal congestion
- Codeine: sedation, nausea, vomiting, lightheadedness, and constipation
- Dextromethorpan: dizziness, drowsiness, and nausea
- Diphenhydramine: sedation, dry mouth, and other anticholinergic effects
- Hydrocodone: sedation, nausea, vomiting, lightheadedness, and constipation

Interactions

There are very few drug interactions that occur with benzonatate, though there are some associated with the use of the narcotic antitussives and dextromethorphan. The narcotic antitussives (codeine and hydrocodone) may potentiate the effects of other opioid narcotics, general anesthetics, tranquilizers, sedatives and hypnotics, tricyclic antidepressants, monoamine oxidase inhibitors, alcohol, and other CNS depressants. Dextromethorphan should not be given in conjunction with the monoamine oxidase inhibitors.

Dosages

For the recommended dosages of selected antitussive agents, see the dosages table on the following page.

*D*RUG PROFILES

The antitussives come in many oral dosage forms and are available both with and without a prescription. Most of the narcotic antitussives are available only by prescription because of the associated abuse potential. Dextromethorphan is the most popular nonnarcotic antitussive available OTC.

⚓ DEXTROMETHORPHAN

Dextromethorphan (Vicks Formula 44, Robitussin-DM, and many others) is a nonnarcotic antitussive that is available alone or in combination with many other cough and cold preparations. It is very widely used because it is very safe and nonaddicting and does not cause respiratory and CNS depression. It is classified as a pregnancy category C agent and is contraindicated in the following settings: hypersensitivity, asthma and emphysema, and persistent headache. Dextromethrophan is available as lozenges, a solution, liquid-filled capsules, granules, tablets (oral, chewable, extended-release, and film-coated), and an extended-release suspension. Common dosages are listed in the dosages table below.

BENZONATATE

Benzonatate (Tessalon) is a nonnarcotic antitussive agent that works by anesthetizing or numbing the cough receptors. It is only available with a prescription and only as a 100-mg capsule, to be taken orally. It is classified as a pregnancy category C agent and is contraindicated in patients with a known hypersensitivity to it. Common dosages are listed in the dosages table below.

PHARMACOKINETICS

HALF-LIFE	ONSET	PEAK	DURATION
Unknown	15-30 min	Unknown	3-6 hr

PHARMACOKINETICS

HALF-LIFE	ONSET	PEAK	DURATION
Unknown	15-20 min	Unknown	3-8 hr

DOSAGES

SELECTED DECONGESTANT, EXPECTORANT, AND ANTITUSSIVE AGENTS

AGENT	PHARMACOLOGIC CLASS	DOSAGE RANGE	PURPOSE
Naphazoline (Privine)	Alpha-adrenergic vasoconstrictor	*Adult/Pediatric ≥12 y/o* 0.05% solution 1-2 drops or sprays in each nostril prn	Nasal decongestant
↓Dextromethorphan (Vicks Formula 44, Robitussin-DM, others)	Nonnarcotic antitussive	*Pediatric* PO: 2-6 y/o: 2.5-7.5 mg q4-8h; do not exceed 30 mg/day PO: 6-12 y/o: 5-10 mg q4h or 15 mg q6-8 h; do not exceed 60 mg/day *Adult/Pediatric >12 y/o* PO: 10-30 mg q4-8 h; do not exceed 120 mg/day	Cough suppression
Benzonatate (Tessalon)	Nonnarcotic antitussive	*Adult/Pediatric > 10 y/o* PO: 100 mg tid; do not exceed 600 mg/day	Cough suppression
Codeine (Dimetane-DC, Tussar SF, Novahistine DH, Robitussin A-C, others)	Narcotic antitussive	*Pediatric* PO: 2-6 y/o: 2.5-5 mg q4-6h; do not exceed 30 mg/day PO: 6-12 y/o: 5-10 mg q4-6h; do not exceed 60 mg/day *Adult* PO: 10-20 mg q4-6h; do not exceed 120 mg/day	Cough suppression
↓Guaifenesin (glyceryl guaiacolate) (Guiatuss, Humibid, Robitussin, others)	Expectorant	*Pediatric* PO: 2-6 y/o: 50-100 mg q4h; do not exceed 600 mg/day PO: 6-12 y/o: 100-200 mg q4h; do not exceed 1200 mg/day *Adult/Pediatric ≥12 y/o* PO: 100-400 mg q4h; do not exceed 2400 mg/day	Respiratory congestion

CODEINE

Codeine (Dimetane-DC, Tussar SF, Novahistine DH, Robitussin A-C, and many others) is a very popular narcotic antitussive agent. It is used in combination with many other common cough and cold medications in the treatment of coughs. Because it is a narcotic, it is potentially addictive and can depress respirations and the CNS. For this reason, codeine-containing cough suppressants are more tightly controlled substances. These cough suppressants are available in many oral dosage forms—solutions, tablets, capsules, and suspensions. They are classified as pregnancy category C agents and are contraindicated in patients with a known hypersensitivity to opiates, and those suffering from respiratory depression, increased intracranial pressure, seizure disorders, or severe respiratory disorders. Common dosages are listed in the preceding dosages table.

✷ P H A R M A C O K I N E T I C S

HALF-LIFE	ONSET	PEAK	DURATION
2.9 hr (plasma)	30-60 min	1-2 hr	4-6 hr

EXPECTORANTS

Expectorants aid in the expectoration (removal) of excessive mucus that has accumulated in the respiratory tract by disintegrating and thinning out the secretion. They are administered orally either as single agents or in combination with other drugs to facilitate the flow of respiratory secretions by reducing the viscosity of tenacious secretions. The actual clinical effectiveness of expectorants is highly questionable, however. Placebo-controlled clinical evaluations have failed to show that expectorants reduce the viscosity of sputum. Despite this, expectorants are popular drugs and are contained in most OTC cold and cough preparations. The most common expectorant in OTC products is guaifenesin (formerly known as glyceryl guaiacolate). The various expectorants include:

- Ammonium chloride
- Guaifenesin (Robitussin)
- Iodinated glycerol (Organidin)
- Ipecac syrup
- Potassium iodide (Pima syrup)
- Terpin hydrate elixir

Mechanism of Action

The expectorants work by means of one of two different mechanisms of action, depending on the agent. The first is **reflex stimulation**. In it, the loosening and thinning of the respiratory tract secretions occurs in response to an irritation of the gastrointestinal tract produced by the agent. **Guaifenesin** is one of the most commonly used of these agents. **Ipecac syrup** and **ammonium chloride** are others. The secretory glands can also be stimulated directly to increase their production of respiratory tract fluids. **Terpin hydrate** works in this way. The iodine-containing products (**iodinated glycerol** and **potassium iodide**) have been conjectured to work by both directly and indirectly stimulating the production of respiratory tract fluids.

Drug Effects

The expectorants primarily affect the gastrointestinal and respiratory tracts, either directly by stimulating the respiratory tract or indirectly by irritating the gastrointestinal tract.

Therapeutic Uses

The expectorants are used for the relief of the nonproductive coughs commonly associated with the common cold, bronchitis, laryngitis, pharyngitis, pertussis, influenza, and measles. They may also be used for the suppression of coughs caused by chronic paranasal sinusitis. By loosening and thinning sputum and the bronchial secretions, they may indirectly diminish the tendency to cough.

Side Effects and Adverse Effects

The side effects and adverse effects of expectorants are minimal. The most common side effects of the individual expectorants are listed in Table 34-5.

Table 34-5	Expectorants: Common Adverse Effects
EXPECTORANT	**SIDE/ADVERSE EFFECT**
Ammonium chloride	Nausea, vomiting, metabolic acidosis, acidification of urine
⚓Guaifenesin	Nausea, vomiting, gastric irritation
Iodinated iodine	Gastrointestinal irritation, rash, enlarged thyroid gland
Ipecac	Nausea, vomiting
Potassium iodide	Iodism, nausea, vomiting, taste perversion
Terpin hydrate	Gastric upset; elixir also has a high alcohol content

Interactions

The drug interactions most commonly seen in conjunction with expectorant use occur with the iodinated products. They may produce an additive or synergistic hypothyroid effect when used concurrently with lithium. Their use with antithyroid agents may result in an additive hypothyroid effect, and their use with potassium iodide, potassium-containing drugs, or potassium-sparing diuretics may lead to the development of hyperkalemia, which can result in cardiac dysrhythmias or cardiac arrest.

Dosages

The recommended dosages of guaifenesin, the only expectorant profiled, are given in the dosages table on p. 513.

DRUG PROFILES

⚓ GUAIFENESIN

Guaifenesin (Guiatuss, Humibid, Robitussin, and many others) is a very commonly used expectorant that is available in several different oral dosage forms—capsules, tablets, solutions, and granules. It is used in the symptomatic management of coughs of varying origin. It is beneficial in the treatment of productive coughs because it waters down thick, difficult-to-cough-up mucus in the respiratory tract. Pharmacokinetics for guaifenesin are not available. See the dosages table on p. 513 for the common dosages. Pregnancy category C.

NURSING PROCESS

ASSESSMENT

Before administering antihistamines, it is important for the nurse to make sure the patient has no allergies to this group of medications, even though these agents are actually used mostly for the treatment of drug allergies and other allergic symptoms. They are also contraindicated in patients suffering from an acute asthma attack and those with lower respiratory tract disease. Cautious use or very close monitoring is called for in patients with a history of increased intraocular pressure; those with cardiac or renal disease, hypertension, bronchial asthma, chronic obstructive pulmonary disease, peptic ulcer disease, convulsive disorders, or benign prostatic hypertrophy; and pregnant women.

The one contraindication to the use of nonsedating antihistamines such as astemizole is hypersensitivity. They should not be given concurrently with erythromycin, ketoconazole, or itraconazole because of the serious cardiovascular disorders this can precipitate. Cautious use is called for in patients with impaired liver function.

Before administering an antitussive agent, the patient should be assessed for hypersensitivity to the agent, and a respiratory and cough assessment should be performed and documented. Decongestants may result in hypertension, palpitations, and CNS stimulation, and their use may be contraindicated in patients with disorders of these systems. Expectorants should be used with caution in the elderly or debilitated patient or in those individuals with asthma or respiratory insufficiency.

NURSING DIAGNOSES

Nursing diagnoses appropriate to patients receiving any of the respiratory agents include the following:
- Ineffective airway clearance related to respiratory congestion.
- Knowledge deficit regarding the proper use of respiratory and cold products.
- Risk for injury related to side effects of the antihistamines, decongestants, antitussives, or expectorants.

PLANNING

Goals for patients receiving any of these respiratory-related agents include the following:
- Patient states rationale for the use of antihistamines, expectorants, antitussives, or decongestants.
- Patient states the side effects of medication.
- Patient states the importance of compliance with therapy.
- Patient identifies symptoms to report to the physician.
- Patient states the importance of follow-up appointments with the physician.

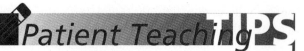

Patient Teaching TIPS

Antihistamine Agents

✔ Patients should be encouraged to contact the physician or other health care provider should excessive sedation, confusion, or hypotension occur.

✔ Patients taking any of the cold products or antihistamines should be told to avoid driving or operating heavy machinery.

✔ Patients taking antihistamines should not consume alcohol or take other CNS depressants.

✔ Patients should be thoroughly educated regarding the purpose of the medication, the expected side effects, and the drugs they interact with.

✔ Patients taking one of the nonsedating antihistamines should know to always inform any other physician or health care provider, including dentists, that they are taking this medication because they interact with erythromycin, ketoconazole, and itraconazole, with serious consequences.

✔ Patients should always check the package inserts that come with OTC cold preparations to find out the drugs they may interact with.

Patient Teaching TIPS

Decongestants and Expectorants

✔ Patients should report a fever (>100.0° F), cough, or other symptoms lasting longer than a week to their physician.

✔ Patients taking expectorants should force fluids, unless contraindicated, to increase expectoration of sputum.

✔ Some decongestants cause cardiac and CNS stimulating effects that may result in palpitations, insomnia, restlessness, and nervousness.

Patient Teaching TIPS

Antitussive Agents

✔ Because nonopiod antitussives may cause sedation, drowsiness, or dizziness, patients taking them should be told to avoid driving or operating heavy machinery.

✔ Patients should report any of the following symptoms to their physician: a cough that lasts longer than a week, a persistent headache, fever, and/or a rash.

✔ Patients taking antitussive lozenges or chewable tablets should not drink liquids for 30 to 35 minutes afterwards.

Outcome Criteria

Outcome criteria pertaining to patients receiving any of these respiratory-related agents include the following:

■ Patient will remain compliant with antihistamine therapy until symptoms are resolved or by physician's order.

■ Patient will take medications exactly as prescribed, no more and no less, to avoid complications of therapy and to experience maximal effectiveness.

■ Patient will report any of the following symptoms to the physician immediately: increase in cough, congestion, shortness of breath, chest pain fever (>100.0° F), or any change in sputum production or color (i.e., if not clear).

IMPLEMENTATION

Patients on antihistamines should take the medications as prescribed, and most of these medications are best tolerated when taken with meals. Even though this slightly minimizes absorption of the agent, it has the benefit of also minimizing the GI upset it can cause. If patients complain of dry mouth, they can suck on candy or chew gum, preferably sugarless, and perform frequent mouth care to ease the discomfort. OTC medications and other prescribed medications should not be taken with an antihistamine unless okayed by the physician because of the serious drug interactions that can occur. Education guidelines for patients receiving these agents are presented in the box above left.

Patients taking expectorants should receive more fluids, unless contraindicated, to help loosen and liquify secretions and to help with expectoration. Any cough or symptoms of fever (>100.0° F) should be reported to the physician.

Patients taking chewable or lozenge antitussive agents should avoid fluid for 30 to 35 minutes after their use to prevent "washing away" their effect. Drowsiness or dizziness may occur with the use of nonopiod antitussives, so patients should be cautioned against driving a car or operating heavy machinery.

TAKE HOME POINTS

Antihistamines

- Two types of histamine blockers: histamine$_1$ (H$_1$) blockers and histamine$_2$ (H$_2$) blockers.
- H$_2$-blockers are used in the treatment of gastric acid disorders such as ulcers.
- H$_1$-blockers are the agents most people are referring to when they use the term *antihistamine*.
- H$_1$-blockers prevent the harmful effects of histamine.
- Used for treatment of seasonal allergic rhinitis, anaphylaxis, insect reactions, etc.

Nonsedating Antihistamines

- Drugs such as astemizole (Hismanal), loratadine (Claritin), and terfenadine (Seldane).
- Devoid of the sedating effect that most antihistamines have.
- Nonsedating because they avoid the central nervous system and work peripherally.

Decongestants

- Consist of adrenergics and corticosteroids.
- Most are adrenergic drugs such as phenylpropanolamine, pseudoephedrine, and phenylephrine.
- The adrenergics work by stimulating engorged and swollen blood vessels in the sinuses to constrict, which decreases pressure and allows mucous membranes to drain.

Antitussives

- Antitussives are used to stop or reduce coughing.
- Are either narcotic or nonnarcotic.
- Narcotic agents = codeine and hydrocodone.
- Nonnarcotic antitussives = benzonatate and dextromethorphan.

Expectorants

- Drugs that aid in expectoration or removal of mucus.
- Work by reducing the viscosity of secretion by thinning or watering them down.
- Guaifenesin and terpin hydrate are two common expectorants.
- Their mechanism of action is related to their ability to irritate the GI tract and to cause reflex stimulation or irritation of the respiratory tract.

Nursing Considerations

- Contraindications to the use of antihistamines include hypersensitivity, acute asthma attack, and lower respiratory tract disease.
- Cautious use of antihistamines or use with very close monitoring of the patient is called for in patients with a history of increased intraocular pressure or those with cardiac or renal disease, hypertension, bronchial asthma, COPD, peptic ulcer disease, convulsive disorders, or BPH, as well as in pregnant women.
- Nonsedating antihistamines have important contraindications to their use, such as their concurrent use with erythromycin, ketoconazole, or itraconazole.
- If patients are taking any of the cold products or antihistamines, they should avoid driving and operating heavy machinery.
- Patients should avoid consuming alcohol and taking other CNS depressants while they are taking antihistamine agents.

EVALUATION

A therapeutic response to respiratory agents would include a decrease in the symptoms of the condition for which they were prescribed. These include cough; congestion; nasal, salivary, and lacrimal gland hypersecretion; motion sickness; allergic rhinitis; Parkinson's disease; and vertigo. Some of the antihistamines, such as diphenhydramine, are also helpful as sleep aids, and a therapeutic response would of course be successful induction of sleep. Adverse effects to monitor for in patients using an antitussive, antihistamine, expectorant, or decongestant include excessive dry mouth, drowsiness, oversedation, dizziness, paradoxical excitement, nervousness, dysrhythmias, palpitations, GI upset, urinary retention, fever, dyspnea, chest pain, palpitations, headache, or insomnia depending on the agent prescribed. (See Table 34-3 for other common side effects.)

Critical Thinking **A C T I V I T I E S**

1. Why should antihistamines be used with caution in asthmatic patients?

2. Decongestants that have beta-stimulating effects may also result in which of the following adverse effects?
   a. hypertension
   b. fever
   c. bradycardia
   d. CNS depression

3. Antihistamines have all of the following therapeutic effects, *except* that:
   a. they prevent the dilation of blood vessels.
   b. they stimulate salivary, gastric, lacrimal, and bronchial secretions.
   c. they bind to receptors and prevent histamine from being released from mast cells.
   d. they prevent increased vascular permeability.

4. Adrenergic decongestants work by stimulating blood vessels to _____ , thereby decreasing pressure and allowing nasal secretions to drain from swollen mucous membranes.
   a. dilate   b. constrict

5. Steroidal decongestants work by decreasing the _____ response caused by the cells of the _____ .
   1. first   2. inflammatory   3. bacterial
   4. immune system   5. blood vessels   6. bone marrow

6. Antitussives are drugs that are used to:
   a. aid in the removal of mucus by reducing the viscosity of secretions.
   b. block the effects of histamine on the blood vessels.
   c. constrict the blood vessels and relieve congestion.
   d. stop or reduce coughing.

7. Dextromethorphan is a _____ type of antitussive and works by _____ the cough reflex in the _____ .
   1. narcotic   2. nonnarcotic   3. decongestant   4. stimulating
   5. medulla   6. suppressing   7. cortex   6. numbing
   a. 1, 6, & 7   b. 2, 6, & 5   c. 1, 4, & 5   d. 2, 6, & 7

8. The expectorants have the common therapeutic effect of increasing the viscosity of secretions so that they are more easy to remove.
   a. True   b. False

▲▲

BIBLIOGRAPHY

Albanese J, Nutz P: *Mosby's 1995 nursing drug cards*, St Louis, 1995, Mosby.

Johnson KB: *Harriet Lane handbook*, ed 13, St Louis, 1993, Mosby.

Keen JH: *Critical care and emergency drug reference*, St Louis, 1994, Mosby.

Knoben JE, Anderson PO: *Handbook of critical drug data*, ed 6, Hamilton, Ill, 1988, Drug Intelligence Publications.

McEvoy GK: *AHFS drug information*, Bethesda, Md, 1994, American Society of Hospital Pharmacists.

Skidmore-Roth L: *Mosby's 1995 nursing drug reference*, St Louis, 1995, Mosby.

Chapter 35

Bronchodilators and Other Respiratory Agents

Objectives

When you reach the end of this chapter, you will be able to:

1 Describe the anatomy and physiology of the respiratory system.
2 Describe how lower respiratory tract diseases affect the respiratory system.
3 Discuss the manifestations of lower respiratory tract diseases.
4 Identify the factors that precipitate lower respiratory tract diseases.
5 Identify the various respiratory agents, both the classes and specific agents, used in the treatment of lower respiratory tract disease.
6 Discuss the mechanism of action of, indications for, contraindications to, dosage forms and amounts of, side effects and toxic effects of, and therapeutic and toxic effects of the agents used to treat lower respiratory tract diseases.
7 Explain the nursing process as it relates to patients with lower respiratory tract diseases.

CHAPTER OUTLINE

The Respiratory System
Diseases of the Respiratory System

Asthma
Chronic Bronchitis
Emphysema

Treatment of Diseases of the Lower Respiratory Tract

Bronchodilators
  Xanthine derivatives
    Mechanism of action
    Drug effects
    Therapeutic uses
    Side effects and adverse effects
    Interactions
    Dosages
Drug Profile
  Theophylline
Beta-Agonists
  Mechanism of action
  Drug effects
  Therapeutic uses
  Side effects and adverse effects
  Interactions
  Dosages
Drug Profiles
  ⚓ Albuterol
  Metaprotereneol

⚓ Epinephrine, Ephedrine, Ethylnorepinephrine
Other Respiratory Agents
  Anticholinergics
  Corticosteroids
    Mechanism of action
    Drug effects
    Therapeutic uses
    Side effects and adverse effects
    Interactions
    Dosages
Drug Profile
  Beclomethasone Dipropionate
  Indirect-acting antiasthmatic agents
    Mechanism of action
    Drug effects
    Therapeutic uses
    Side effects and adverse effects
    Dosages
Drug Profiles
  ⚓ Cromolyn
  Nedocromil
Nursing Process
Assessment
Nursing Diagnoses
Planning
  Outcome criteria
Implementation
Evaluation

519

Glossary

Allergen (al' ər jen) Any substance that evokes an allergic response. (p. 521)

Allergic asthma (as' mə) Asthma caused by hypersensitivity to an allergen or allergens. (p. 521)

Alveoli (al' ve o li) Microscopic sacs where oxygen is exchanged for carbon dioxide. (p. 520)

Antibody (an' tĭ bod' e) An immunoglobulin produced by lymphocytes in response to bacteria, viruses, or other antigenic substances. (p. 521)

Antigen (an' tĭ jən) Substance, usually a protein, that causes the formation of an antibody and reacts specifically with that antibody. (p. 521)

Asthma attack Onset of wheezing together with difficulty breathing. (p. 521)

Bronchial asthma (brong' ke əl) Recurrent and reversible shortness of breath resulting from narrowing of the bronchi and bronchioles. (p. 521)

Chronic bronchitis (brong ki' tis) Chronic inflammation of the bronchi. (p. 521)

Emphysema (em' fə se' mə) Condition of the lungs resulting from enlargement of the air spaces distal to the bronchioles. (p. 521)

Idiopathic asthma (id' e ə pa' thik): Asthmatic condition for which no specific cause has been truly identified; also called *intrinsic asthma*. (p. 521)

Immunoglobulin (im' u no glob' u lin) Any of five structurally and antigenically distinct antibodies present in the serum and external secretions of the body. (p. 521)

Intrinsic asthma (in trin' sik) Asthmatic condition for which no specific cause has been truly identified; also called *idiopathic asthma*. (p. 521)

Ipratropium bromide (ip' rə tro' pe əm bro' mīd) The only anticholinergic drug used in the treatment of asthma. (p. 528)

Lower respiratory tract Division of the respiratory system composed of organs located almost entirely within the chest. (p. 520)

Mast cell stabilizers Drugs such as cromolyn and nedocromil that stabilize the membranes of cells that normally release very harmful bronchoconstricting substances. (p. 531)

Nonseasonal allergic asthma Asthmatic condition caused by the continuous presence of an allergen such as animal dander, mold, or dust. (p. 521)

Seasonal asthma Asthmatic condition caused by the periodic appearance of a particular allergen. (p. 521)

Status asthmaticus (sta' təs az mat'ik əs): A prolonged asthma attack. (p. 521)

Sympathomimetic bronchodilators Group of drugs commonly used during the acute phase of an asthmatic attack to quickly reduce airway constriction and restore normal airflow; also called *beta-agonists*. (p. 524)

Upper respiratory tract Division of the respiratory system composed of organs located outside the chest cavity (thorax). (p. 520)

Xanthine bronchodilators (zan' thēn brong' ko di la' torz) Xanthine derivatives that produce bronchodilation by competitively inhibiting the enzyme phosphodiesterase and increasing the cyclic adenosine monophosphate level. (p. 522)

The Respiratory System

The main function of the respiratory system is to deliver oxygen to the cells that make up the body and then to remove carbon dioxide from these cells. To perform this deceptively simple task requires a very intricate system of tissues, muscles, and organs called the *respiratory system*. It consists of two divisions, or tracts—the upper and lower respiratory tracts. The **upper respiratory tract** (URT) is composed of the structures that are located outside the chest cavity (thorax). These are the nose, nasopharynx, oropharynx, laryngopharynx, and larynx. The **lower respiratory tract** (LRT) is located almost entirely within the chest, and it is composed of the trachea, all segments of the bronchial tree, and the lungs. The URT and LRT have four main accessory structures that aid in their overall function. These are the oral cavity (mouth), the rib cage, the muscle of the rib cage (intercostal muscles), and the diaphragm. The URT and LRT together with the accessory structures make up the respiratory system, and they are in constant communication with each other as they perform the vital function of respiration and the exchange of oxygen for carbon dioxide.

The air we breathe is a mixture of many gases, and the lung, by filtering, warming, and humidifying the air, is able to extract the oxygen needed for sustaining life. The oxygen is actually delivered to the cells by the blood vessels that make up the circulatory system, and the transfer of oxygen from the respiratory system to the circulatory system takes place in the microscopic sacs at the end of the bronchial tree called **alveoli**. It is here that the respiratory system "hands off" the oxygen it has extracted from inhaled air to the hemoglobin in red blood cells. It is also here that the unnecessary carbon dioxide that has been deposited in the blood by the cells and transported back to the lungs by the circulatory system is diffused back into the respiratory system and then exhaled into the air.

Besides performing this vital function of oxygen and carbon dioxide exchange, the respiratory system is also involved in speech, it has specialized cells that make smell possible, and it helps regulate pH (acid-base balance) in the body.

Diseases of the Respiratory System

There are several diseases or disorders that impair the function of the respiratory system. Those that affect the

URT include colds, rhinitis, and hay fever, and they and the agents used to treat them are discussed in Chapter 34. The diseases that impair the function of the LRT include asthma, **emphysema,** and **chronic bronchitis.** The one feature these diseases have in common is that they all involve the obstruction of airflow through the airways. *Chronic obstructive pulmonary disease* (COPD) is the name applied collectively to emphysema and chronic bronchitis because the obstruction is relatively constant. Asthma that is persistent and present most of the time despite treatment is also considered a COPD. Cystic fibrosis and infant respiratory distress syndrome are other disorders that affect the LRT, but because the treatment for them places more emphasis on nonpharmacologic than on pharmacologic measures, they are not a focus of the discussion in this chapter.

ASTHMA

Bronchial asthma is defined as a recurrent and reversible shortness of breath and occurs when the airways of the lung—the bronchi and bronchioles—become narrow as the result of bronchospasm, inflammation and edema of the bronchial mucosa, and the production of viscid mucus. The alveolar ducts and alveoli distal to the bronchioles remain open, but the obstruction to the airflow in the airways prevents carbon dioxide from getting out of the air spaces and oxygen from getting into them. Wheezing and difficulty breathing are the symptoms, and because of the sudden and dramatic onset of these episodes, they are commonly referred to as **asthma attacks.** Most of the attacks are short, and normal breathing is subsequently recovered. However, an asthma attack may be prolonged for days to weeks, a condition known as **status asthmaticus.** The onset of asthma occurs before 10 years of age in 50% of the patients and before 40 years of age in about 30%.

There are three categories of asthma: allergic, idiopathic, and mixed allergic/idiopathic asthma, and approximately 2% of the general population is affected by one of the three types. Allergic asthma accounts for approximately 30% to 35% of the cases of asthma and idiopathic asthma for about 35% to 50%, with the mixed form accounting for the remaining cases.

Allergic asthma is caused by a hypersensitivity to an allergen or allergens in the environment. An **allergen** is any substance that elicits on allergic reaction. In patients with **seasonal asthma** the allergen is a substance such as pollen, which is present only periodically (seasonally). The offending allergens in patients with **nonseasonal asthma** are substances such as dust, mold, and animal danders, which are present in the environment throughout the year. Exposure to the offending allergen in a patient with either type of allergic asthma causes an immediate allergic reaction—the asthma attack, and this is mediated by hypersensitive antibodies already present in the patient's body that sense the allergen to be a foreign substance, or **antigen.** The **antibody** in asthma sufferers is usually **immunoglobulin E** (IgE), which is one of the five types of antibodies in the body, the others being IgG, IgA, IgM, and IgD. Upon exposure to the allergen, the patient's body responds by mounting an immediate and potent antigen-antibody reaction. This reaction occurs on the surface of cells such as mast cells that are rich in histamines and other mediators and stimulates the release of histamine, which, as known from the previous chapter, triggers the allergic reaction, in this case the asthma attack. The sequence of events that occur in a patient with allergic asthma are listed in the box below.

The specific cause of **idiopathic, or intrinsic, asthma,** is unknown. It is not mediated by IgE, and there is no family history of allergies in affected patients. There are, however, certain factors that have been noted to precipitate asthma attacks in these patients, and these include respiratory infections, stress, cold weather, and strenuous work or exercise.

As the name implies, mixed allergic/idiopathic asthma results from a combination of allergic and idiopathic factors.

The three types of asthma and their most likely causes are summarized in the box below.

Steps Involved in an Attack of Allergic Asthma

- The offending allergen(s) provokes the production of hypersensitive antibodies (most commonly IgE) that are specific to the allergen. This immunologic response initiates patient sensitivity.

- The IgE antibodies are homocytotrophic and collect on the surface of most cells, thus sensitizing the patient to the allergen(s).

- Subsequent allergen contact provokes the antigen-antibody reaction on the surface of mast cells.

- Mast cell integrity is then violated, and these cells release chemical mediators. They also synthesize and then release other chemical mediators. These mediators include bradykinin, eosinophil chemotactic factor of anaphylaxis (ECF-A), histamine, prostaglandins, and slow-reacting substance of anaphylaxis (SRS-A).

- The released chemical mediators, especially histamine and SRS-A, trigger the bronchial constriction and the asthma attack.

CHRONIC BRONCHITIS

Chronic bronchitis is a continuous inflammation of the bronchi, though it is the inflammation of the bronchioles that occurs in the disorder that is responsible for the obstruction to airflow. The disease can arise as the result of repeated attacks of acute bronchitis or in the context of chronic generalized diseases. It is usually precipitated by prolonged exposure to bronchial irritants, primarily cigarette smoke, but patients who acquire the disease may be affected by other predisposing factors such as viral or bacterial pulmonary infections during childhood, mild impairment of the ability to inactivate proteolytic enzymes, or certain as yet unknown genetic characteristics. Pathologically it involves the excessive secretion of mucus and certain structural changes in the bronchi.

EMPHYSEMA

Emphysema is the condition that results when the air spaces enlarge as a result of the destruction of the alveolar walls. This appears to stem from the effect of proteolytic enzymes released from leukocytes in the setting of alveolar inflammation. Because the alveolar walls are then partially destroyed, the area where oxygen and carbon dioxide exchange takes place is reduced, thus impairing effective respiration. As with chronic bronchitis, smoking appears to be the primary irritant responsible for precipitating the underlying inflammation that leads to the development of emphysema.

Treatment of Diseases of the Lower Respiratory Tract

The treatment of asthma and the other COPDs makes use of different classes of drugs that in various ways cause the airways to dilate. These various classes of bronchodilating agents include the beta-agonists, selected anticholinergics, xanthine derivatives, corticosteroids, and the indirect-acting antiasthmatic drugs such as cromolyn sodium and nedocromil sodium. A synopsis of how these agents work is provided in the box below.

BRONCHODILATORS

The bronchodilator drugs are an important part of the pharmacotherapy for the COPDs such as asthma, chronic bronchitis, and emphysema. As their name implies, they are able to dilate the bronchi and bronchioles narrowed as the result of the disease process. There are two classes of such agents: the **xanthine derivatives** and the beta-agonists.

Xanthine Derivatives

The natural xanthines consist of the plant alkaloids caffeine, theobromine, and theophylline, but only theophylline and its chemical derivatives are used as bronchodilators. Caffeine is primarily utilized as a central nervous system stimulant (analeptic) and theobromine as a diuretic. Besides theophylline, the other xan-

---

Types of Asthma

TYPE OF ASTHMA	MOST LIKELY CAUSE
Allergic	Allergens (antigens) such as animal dander, dust, and molds.
Idiopathic	Poorly defined etiologic factors; may be induced by stress, respiratory infections, or strenuous exercise.
Mixed	Combination of allergens and some of the idiopathic factors.

Mechanism of Antiasthmatic Drugs

ANTIASTHMATIC	MECHANISM IN ASTHMA RELIEF
Beta-agonists and xanthine derivatives	Raise intracellular levels of cAMP, which in turn produces smooth muscle relaxation and dilates the constricted bronchi and bronchioles.
Anticholinergics	Block cholinergic receptors, thus preventing the binding of cholinergic substances that cause constriction.
Indirect-acting antiasthmatics (cromolyn and nedocromil)	Stabilize the cell membranes that the antigen-antibody reactions take place on (the mast cell), thereby preventing the release of substances such as histamine that cause constriction.
Corticosteroids	Prevent the inflammation commonly provoked by the substances released from mast cells.

thine bronchodilators used clinically for the treatment of bronchoconstriction are: aminophylline, Dyphylline, and oxtriphylline.

Because of their relatively slow onset of action, the xanthines are used more for the prevention of asthmatic symptoms than for the relief of acute asthma attacks. They are also used as bronchodilators in the symptomatic treatment of the asthma and reversible bronchospasm that may occur in patients with chronic bronchitis or emphysema. Intravenously administered theophylline (aminophylline) is used in patients with status asthmaticus who have not responded to fast-acting beta-agonists such as epinephrine.

Mechanism of Action

The mechanisms of action of theophylline and its chemical derivatives are similar. They all cause bronchodilation by increasing the levels of the energy-producing substance cAMP (cyclic adenosine monophosphate), and they do this by competitively inhibiting phosphodiesterase (PDE), the enzyme responsible for breaking down the cAMP. The cAMP plays an integral role in the maintenance of an open airway in patients with COPD because its intracellular concentration is what chiefly determines smooth muscle relaxation and the inhibition of the IgE-induced release of the chemical mediators (histamine, SRS-A, and others) that are responsible for causing an allergic reaction. An accumulation of cAMP therefore causes the constricted airways of the lung to dilate.

Drug Effects

Xanthines have many beneficial drug effects other than those beneficial to the respiratory system. In the respiratory system they mostly cause the airways of the lungs to dilate by relaxating the smooth muscle of the respiratory tract, thereby relieving bronchospasm and allowing greater airflow into and out of the lungs. The xanthines also stimulate all levels of the central nervous system, but to a lesser degree than caffeine, another xanthine. This stimulation of the CNS has the beneficial effect of directly stimulating the medullary respiratory center. In large doses, theophylline and its derivatives may stimulate the cardiovascular system, resulting in both an increased force of contraction (positive inotrope) and an increased heart rate (positive chronotrope). The increased force of contraction increases cardiac output and hence blood flow to the kidneys. This in combination with the xanthines' ability to dilate blood vessels in and around the kidney, thus increasing the glomerular filtration rate, results in a diuretic effect.

Therapeutic Uses

Theophylline and the other xanthine derivatives are used to dilate the airways in patients with asthma,

chronic bronchitis, or emphysema. They may be used in mild to moderate cases of acute asthma and as an adjunct agent in the management of a COPD. The combination of their ability to increase the force of contraction in a failing heart and to dilate the airways also make them useful as adjunctive therapy for the relief of the pulmonary edema and paroxysmal nocturnal dyspnea in patients with left-sided heart failure. Aminophylline may be used to increase urine output. Their ability to increase cardiac output and thus the blood flow to the kidneys causes diuresis.

Side Effects and Adverse Effects

The common side effects of the xanthine derivatives include nausea, vomiting, and anorexia. In addition, gastroesophageal reflux has been observed to occur during sleep in patients taking them. Cardiac side effects include sinus tachycardia, extrasystole, palpitations, and ventricular dysrhythmias. Transient increased urination and hyperglycemia are other side effects.

Interactions

The use of xanthine derivatives with any of the following agents causes the serum level of the xanthine derivative to be increased: allopurinol, cimetidine, erythromycin, flu vaccine, and the oral contraceptives. Their use with sympathomimetics can produce additive cardiac and CNS stimulation.

Dosages

For the recommended dosages of theophylline, the only xanthine derivative profiled, see the dosages table on the next page.

DRUG PROFILE

THEOPHYLLINE

Theophylline (Bronkodyl, Elixophyllin, Slo-bid, Theo-Dur, Theo-24, Quibron-T, Uniphyl) is one of the most commonly used of all the xanthine derivatives as well as of all the bronchodilators. It is used most frequently in the treatment of chronic respiratory disorders but may also be used for the relief of mild to moderate acute asthmatic attacks. Theophylline is available in oral, rectal, parenteral, and topical dosage forms, but only with a prescription. These various preparations are listed in the box on p. 524.

DOSAGES

THEOPHYLLINE

DRUG	PHARMACOLOGIC CLASS	DOSAGE RANGE	PURPOSE
Theophylline (Bronkodyl, Elixophyllin, Slo-bid, Theo-Dur, Theo-24, Quibron-T, Uniphyl)	Xanthine derivative	*Pediatric* PO: usual dose is 2.5 mg/kg q6h *Adult* PO: usual dose is ≥160 mg q6h*	Asthma

*Adjust dosage to achieve optimal patient response.

Available Theophylline Preparations

DOSAGE FORM	STRENGTHS
Oral	
Capsules	100 and 200 mg
Extended-release capsules	50, 60, 65, 75, 100, 125, 130, 200, 250, 260, and 300 mg
Solution	27 and 50 mg/5 ml
Tablets	100, 125, 200, 250, and 300 mg
Extended-release tablets	100, 200, 250, 300, 400, 450, and 500 mg
Parenteral	
Injection	25, 2500, and 5000 mg/ml
Injection for infusion	0.4, 0.8, 1.6, 2, 3.2, and 4 mg/ml
Rectal	
Suppository	250 and 500 mg

Theophylline is classified as a pregnancy category C agent and is contraindicated in patients with a known hypersensitivity to xanthines and in patients with tachyarrhythmias. Its beneficial effects can be maximized by maintaining levels in the blood within a certain target range. If these levels become too high, then many unwanted adverse effects can occur. If the levels become too low, then the patient receives little therapeutic benefit. Although the optimal level may vary from patient to patient, the common therapeutic range for theophylline in the blood is 10 to 20 mg/dl. The commonly recommended dosages are given in the dosages table above.

❧ PHARMACOKINETICS

HALF-LIFE	ONSET	PEAK	DURATION
7-9 hr	Unknown	1-2 hr	Varies with dosage form

BETA-AGONISTS

The beta-agonists are a large group of drugs that are commonly used during the acute phase of an asthmatic attack to quickly reduce airway constriction and restore airflow to normal. They are agonists or stimulators of the sympathetic nervous system receptors—the beta- and alpha-adrenergic receptors already discussed in depth in Unit III—and because they imitate the effects of norepinephrine on these receptors, they are also called **sympathomimetic bronchodilators.** For a beta-agonist to dilate the airways of the lungs, it must stimulate the beta$_2$-adrenergic receptors located throughout the lungs. When these receptors are stimulated, the constricted airways dilate; conversely, a nonspecific beta-blocker would cause the airways to constrict.

The beta-agonists, or sympathomimetic bronchodilators, are categorized according to the specific receptors they stimulate, and there are as a result three types of these bronchodilators:

1. Nonselective adrenergic drugs, which stimulate the alpha, beta$_1$ (cardiac), and beta$_2$ (respiratory) receptors. Example: epinephrine.
2. Nonselective beta-adrenergic drugs, which stimulate both beta$_1$ and beta$_2$ receptors. Example: isoproterenol.
3. Selective beta$_2$ drugs, which only stimulate the beta$_2$ receptors. Example: albuterol.

These drugs can also be categorized according to the route of administration as oral, parenteral, and inhalational agents. The various beta-agonist bronchodilators are listed in Table 35-1.

Mechanism of Action

The mechanism of action of the beta-agonist bronchodilators begins at the specific receptor stimulated and ends with the dilation of the airways, but many reactions must take place at the cellular level for this bronchodilation to occur. When a beta$_2$-adrenergic receptor is stimulated by a beta-agonist, adenylate cyclase, an enzyme needed to make cAMP, is activated. The bronchioles, which are the small airways that precede the alveoli, are surrounded by smooth muscle. If this smooth muscle contracts, the airways are narrowed and the amount of oxygen and carbon dioxide exchanged is reduced. The increased levels of cAMP made available by adenylate cyclase cause these smooth muscles to relax, which results in bronchial dilation and increased airflow into and out of the lungs.

Drugs such as epinephrine that also stimulate the alpha-adrenergic receptors produce vasoconstriction, which has the effect of reducing the amount of edema or swelling in the mucous membranes and limiting the quantity of secretions normally secreted from these membranes. However, beta$_1$-receptor stimulation also results in unwanted cardiac side effects such as an increased heart rate and force of contraction.

Drug Effects

Drugs such as albuterol that predominantly stimulate the beta$_2$-receptors have more specific drug effects. By predominantly stimulating the beta$_2$-adrenergic receptors of the bronchial, uterine, and vascular smooth muscles, they cause bronchodilation as one of the desirable effects. They may also have a dilating effect on the peripheral vasculature, resulting in a decrease in diastolic blood pressure. By stimulating intracellular shifts of potassium from the blood, the beta$_2$ stimulants are thought to stimulate Na$^+$/K$^+$-ATPase, resulting in a temporary decrease in potassium levels. This makes them useful in treating patients with hyperkalemia.

Some of the beta-agonist bronchodilators partially stimulate beta$_1$ receptors, and this causes central nervous system and cardiovascular system stimulation, which may result in nervousness, tremors, a fast heart rate, and elevated blood pressure.

Other beta-agonist bronchodilators may stimulate both alpha and beta receptors. This stimulation of the alpha-adrenergic receptors mostly results in constric-

Table 35-1	Beta-Agonist Bronchodilators		
DRUG	**TYPE**	**BRAND NAMES**	**ROUTE OF ADMINISTRATION**
⚓Albuterol	Beta$_2$	Proventil, Ventolin	PO, inhalation
Bitolterol	Beta$_2$	Tornalate	Inhalation
Ephedrine	Alpha-beta	None	PO, IM, IV, SC
⚓Epinephrine	Alpha-beta	Adrenalin, Primatene, Bronkaid, Bronitin, Medihaler-Epi	SC, IM, inhalation
Ethylnorepinephrine	Alpha-beta	Bronkephrine	IM, SC
Isoetharine	Beta$_1$-beta$_2$	Arm-a-Med Isoetharine	Inhalation
Isoproterenol	Beta$_1$-beta$_2$	Isuprel, Medihaler-Iso	IV, sublingual, inhalation
Metaproterenol	Beta$_1$-beta$_2$	Alupent, Metaprel	PO, inhalation
Pirbuterol	Beta$_2$	Maxair	Inhalation
Salmeterol	Beta$_2$	Serevent	Inhalation
Terbutaline	Beta$_2$	Brethine, Bricanyl	PO, SC, inhalation

tion, specifically of the arterioles in the skin, mucous membranes, and organs. However, it results in the dilation of the arterioles in skeletal muscles. Some of this vasoconstriction can be beneficial in the management of certain respiratory disorders. For instance, a beta-agonist such as ephedrine that also stimulates alpha receptors may also cause dilated blood vessels in the nasal mucosa to constrict, thereby producing nasal decongestion.

Therapeutic Uses

The therapeutic effects of the beta-agonists are mostly confined to the treatment of various pulmonary disorders. However, because they have effects outside the respiratory system, they may also be used for the management of other disorders. The primary respiratory system–related therapeutic effects are the relief of bronchospasm, bronchial asthma, bronchitis, and other pulmonary diseases.

Because some of these agents have the ability to stimulate both beta$_1$- and alpha-adrenergic receptors, they may be used to treat hypotension and shock. The agents that stimulate alpha receptors cause the blood vessels surrounding the nasal passages to constrict. This is a very useful property for the relief of the nasal congestion and stuffiness commonly affecting persons with colds, symptoms produced by dilated blood vessels in nasal passages.

Because terbutaline has the added ability to stimulate the beta$_1$-receptors on the uterus that control uterine contractions, it is used to produce uterine relaxation and prevent premature labor in pregnant women.

By stimulating a shift of potassium out of the blood and into cells, beta$_2$-agonists can be used to treat the hyperkalemia that often afflicts patients with renal failure.

Side Effects and Adverse Effects

The alpha-beta agonists produce the greatest array of undesirable effects. These include insomnia, restlessness, anorexia, cardiac stimulation, tremor, and vascular headache. The side effects of the nonselective beta-agonists are limited to beta-adrenergic effects, and these include cardiac stimulation, tremor, anginal pain, and vascular headache. The beta$_2$ agents can cause hypotension, vascular headaches, and tremor.

Interactions

The use of beta-agonist bronchodilators with a nonselective beta-adrenergic blocker antagonizes the bronchodilation. Their use with an MAO inhibitor and

other sympathomimetics is best avoided. Diabetics may require an adjustment in the dose of their hypoglycemic agent, especially patients taking epinephrine, because of the increased blood glucose levels that can occur.

Dosages

For recommended dosages of selected beta-agonists, see the dosages table on the next page.

DRUG PROFILES

Although the beta-agonists are commonly used in the treatment of an acute asthmatic attack, they are also used to treat hypotension and shock, as decongestants, to relax uterine muscles and prevent premature labor, and to lower serum potassium levels in patients with hyperkalemia.

⚓ ALBUTEROL

Albuterol (Proventil, Proventil Repetabs, Ventolin, Volmax) is one of five beta$_2$-specific bronchodilating beta-agonists, the others being bitolterol, pirbuterol, salmeterol, and terbutaline. It is most commonly used in the treatment of acute attacks of bronchial asthma but may also be used in the prevention of such attacks. If used too frequently, dose-related adverse effects may be seen, and these are the result of albuterol losing its beta$_2$-specific actions at larger doses. The consequence of this is that the beta$_1$ receptors are stimulated, and this causes nausea, increased anxiety, palpitations, tremors, and an increased heart rate.

Albuterol is classified as a pregnancy category C agent and is contraindicated in patients with a hypersensitivity to sympathomimetics, tachyarrhythmias, and severe cardiac disease. It is only available with a prescription and comes as an oral solution and tablet as well as an inhalational agent. Orally albuterol comes as a 2-mg/5 ml syrup, 2- and 4-mg tablets, 4- and 8-mg extended-release tablets, and 4-mg extended-release film-coated tablets. As an inhalational agent it comes in a metered-dose inhaler that releases 90-μg per spray, a 200-μg powder contained in a capsule, and a 0.083% solution and a 0.5% concentrated solution for nebulization. Commonly recommended dosages are given in the dosages table on the next page.

DOSAGES

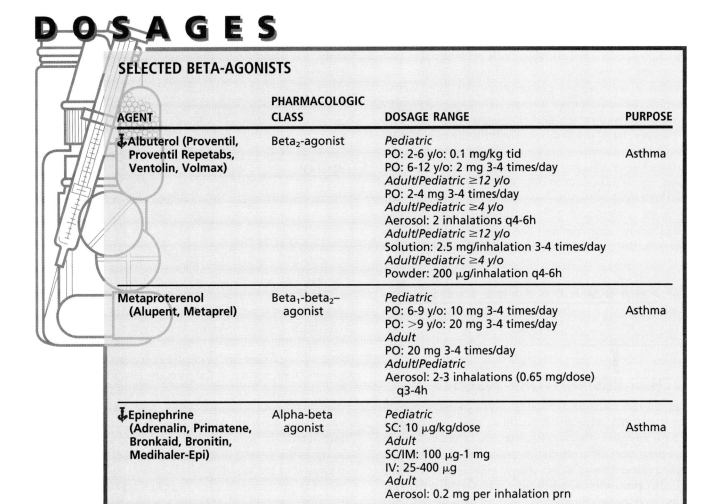

SELECTED BETA-AGONISTS

AGENT	PHARMACOLOGIC CLASS	DOSAGE RANGE	PURPOSE
⚓Albuterol (Proventil, Proventil Repetabs, Ventolin, Volmax)	Beta$_2$-agonist	*Pediatric* PO: 2-6 y/o: 0.1 mg/kg tid PO: 6-12 y/o: 2 mg 3-4 times/day *Adult/Pediatric ≥12 y/o* PO: 2-4 mg 3-4 times/day *Adult/Pediatric ≥4 y/o* Aerosol: 2 inhalations q4-6h *Adult/Pediatric ≥12 y/o* Solution: 2.5 mg/inhalation 3-4 times/day *Adult/Pediatric ≥4 y/o* Powder: 200 μg/inhalation q4-6h	Asthma
Metaproterenol (Alupent, Metaprel)	Beta$_1$-beta$_2$-agonist	*Pediatric* PO: 6-9 y/o: 10 mg 3-4 times/day PO: >9 y/o: 20 mg 3-4 times/day *Adult* PO: 20 mg 3-4 times/day *Adult/Pediatric* Aerosol: 2-3 inhalations (0.65 mg/dose) q3-4h	Asthma
⚓Epinephrine (Adrenalin, Primatene, Bronkaid, Bronitin, Medihaler-Epi)	Alpha-beta agonist	*Pediatric* SC: 10 μg/kg/dose *Adult* SC/IM: 100 μg-1 mg IV: 25-400 μg *Adult* Aerosol: 0.2 mg per inhalation prn	Asthma

✹ PHARMACOKINETICS

HALF-LIFE	ONSET	PEAK	DURATION
2.7-5 hr	PO: 5-15 min	2-3 hr	4-8 hr

METAPROTERENOL

Metaproterenol (Alupent, Metaprel) is a synthetic sympathomimetic bronchodilator that stimulates both beta$_1$ and beta$_2$ receptors. Other similar bronchodilating beta-agonists are isoetharine and isoproterenol. These agents produce dilation of the airways, but they also have beta$_1$-stimulating properties that are more pronounced at higher doses. CNS and cardiovascular system stimulation are the result.

Metaproterenol is only available with a prescription and is classified as a pregnancy category C agent. The contraindications to its use are the same as those for the beta$_2$-agonists such as albuterol, but it is also contraindicated in patients with narrow-angle glaucoma. Metaproterenol is available in both oral and inhalational preparations. Orally it comes as a 10-mg/5 ml solution and as 10- and 25-mg tablets. As an inhalational agent it comes in a metered-dose inhaler that releases 0.65 mg per spray. It also comes in a 0.4%, 0.6%, and 5% solution for nebulization. Common dosage recommendations are given in the dosages table above.

✹ PHARMACOKINETICS

HALF-LIFE	ONSET	PEAK	DURATION
Unknown	PO: 15-30 min	1 hr	4 hr

⚓ EPINEPHRINE, EPHEDRINE, ETHYLNOREPINEPHRINE

Epinephrine (Primatene, Bronkaid, Adrenalin, Medihaler-Epi, Bronitin), ephedrine, and ethylnorepinephrine are all beta-agonist bronchodilators that work by stimulating both beta and alpha receptors. Their beta$_2$-stimulating properties result in the bronchodilation, but by also stimulating alpha receptors, they have effects elsewhere in the body. One of these is arteriolar constriction in the mucous membranes, making them useful as nasal decongestants.

Epinephrine is available with or without a prescription. Ephedrine and ethylnorepinephrine are available only with a prescription. All three agents come in several dosage forms and are used to treat a variety of respiratory and nonrespiratory disorders. However, those preparations used for the treatment of respiratory disorders are generally given by the inhalational or oral route. Epinephrine given for this purpose comes in a metered-dose inhaler that releases 160, 200, 220, and 250 µg per spray for oral inhalation and as a 1%, 1.83%, and 2.25% solution for nebulization. Commonly recommended dosages of epinephrine are given in the preceding dosages table.

☙ P H A R M A C O K I N E T I C S

HALF-LIFE	ONSET	DURATION	PEAK
Unknown	Inhalation: 1-5 hr	1-3 hr	Rapid

OTHER RESPIRATORY AGENTS

The bronchodilators are just one type of agent used to treat asthma, chronic bronchitis, and emphysema. There are also other agents that are effective in suppressing various underlying causes of some of these respiratory illness. These drugs include anticholinergics (ipratroprium), corticosteroids (beclomethasone, dexamethasone, flunisolide, and triamcinolone), and indirect-acting agents (cromolyn and nedocromil).

Anticholinergics

Currently the only anticholinergic agent that is used in the treatment of asthma is **ipratropium bromide** (atrovent). Chemically it is very similar to atropine and produces local bronchodilation after inhalation. It works in the following way. On the surface of the bronchial tree are receptors for acetylcholine (ACh), the neurotransmitter for the parasympathetic nervous system (PNS). When the PNS releases ACh from its nerve endings, the neurotransmitter binds to the ACh receptors on the surface of the bronchial tree, resulting in bronchial constriction and narrowing of the airways. An anticholinergic drug such as ipratropium bromide prevents this bronchoconstriction, thereby causing the airways to dilate. Because its actions are slow and prolonged, ipratropium is used for prevention of the bronchospasm associated with the COPDs (chronic bronchitis or emphysema), not for the management of acute exacerbations.

The most commonly reported adverse effects of ipratropium therapy are dry mouth or throat, gastrointestinal distress, headache, coughing, and anxiety. It

is classified as a pregnancy category B agent and is contraindicated in patients with a known hypersensitivity to it, atropine, or any of its derivatives. There are currently no drugs that are known to interact with ipratropium. The usual adolescent or adult dose is one or two inhalations three to four times daily.

☙ P H A R M A C O K I N E T I C S

HALF-LIFE	ONSET	DURATION	PEAK
1.6 hr	15-30 min	4-5 hr	1-2 hr

Corticosteroids

Corticosteroids are used in the treatment of chronic asthma for their antiinflammatory effects, which lead to decreased airway obstruction. As with ipratroprium bromide, the corticosteroids also do not relieve the symptoms of acute asthmatic attacks but are used prophylactically to prevent an attack. The corticosteroids do this by preventing the release of substances that produce inflammation in the lungs. They can be given by inhalation or by the oral route in severe cases of asthma when the agent cannot get to the airways because of the obstruction. Corticosteroids administered by inhalation have an advantage over orally administered corticosteroids in that their action is limited to the topical site of action—the lungs. This prevents systemic effects. The chemical structures of the corticosteroids given by inhalation have also been slightly altered so as to limit their systemic absorption from the respiratory tract. The corticosteroids administered by inhalation include:

1. Beclomethasone dipropionate (Beclovent, Vanceril)
2. Dexamethasone sodium phosphate (Decadron Phosphate Respihaler)
3. Flunisolide (AeroBid, AeroBid-M)
4. Triamcinolone acetonide (Azmacort)

Mechanism of Action

Although the exact mechanism of action of the corticosteroids has not been determined, it is conjectured that they have the dual effect of both reducing inflammation and enhancing the activity of beta-agonists.

The corticosteroids just mentioned produce their antiinflammatory effects through a complex sequence of actions. They essentially work by stabilizing the membranes of cells that normally release very harmful bronchoconstricting substances (e.g., histamine, SRS-A). These cells are called *leukocytes,* which is another name for white blood cells (WBCs), and there are five different types of these cells, each with their own specific characteristics. The five types of WBCs, their role in the inflammatory process, and the way in which the corticosteroids inhibit their normal action, combat inflammation, and produce bronchodilation are summarized in Table 35-2.

The corticosteroids have also been shown to restore or increase the responsiveness of bronchial smooth muscle to beta-adrenergic receptor stimulation, which results in more pronounced stimulation of the beta$_2$ receptors by beta-agonist drugs such as albuterol.

Drug Effects

Most of the drug effects of the inhaled corticosteroids are limited to their topical site of action in the lungs. Because of the chemical structure of the corticosteroids, there is very little systemic absorption of the agents when they are administered by inhalation. When there is significant systemic absorption (absorption into the bloodstream), the corticosteroids can affect any of the organ systems in the body. Some of these systemic-drug effects include adrenocortical insufficiency, increased susceptibility to infection, fluid and electrolyte disturbances, endocrine effects, dermatologic effects, and nervous system effects.

Therapeutic Uses

The inhaled corticosteroids are used for the treatment of bronchospastic disorders that are not adequately controlled by the conventional bronchodilators—the beta-agonists and the xanthine derivatives. They are not considered first-line agents for the management of acute asthmatic attacks or status asthmaticus.

Side Effects and Adverse Effects

The main undesirable local effects of the corticosteroids on the respiratory system include pharyngeal irritation, coughing, dry mouth, and oral fungal infections. Systemic effects are rare (see Chapter 33) because of the low doses used for inhalation therapy.

Interactions

Inhaled corticosteroids are capable of causing few or no drug interactions. This is due in part to the fact that they are administered by nasal inhalation and so are delivered directly to the site of action in the respiratory tract. Because they are not administered systemically, they neither have systemic effects nor can they interact with other systemically administered drugs.

Dosages

For recommended dosages of selected corticosteroids, see the dosages table on the next page.

Table 35-2	White Blood Cells (Leukocytes)	
SPECIFIC WBC*	**ROLE IN INFLAMMATION**	**CORTICOSTEROID EFFECT**
Granulocytes		
Neutrophils (65%)	Contain powerful lysosomes, which are digestive-like enzymes; release chemicals that destroy invading organisms and also attack other WBCs.	Stabilize their cell membranes so that inflammation-causing substances not released.
Eosinophils (2%-5%)	Main function is in allergic reactions and in protecting against parasitic infections; ingest inflammatory chemicals and antigen-antibody complexes.	Little if any effect.
Basophils (0.5%-1%)	Contain histamine, an inflammation-causing substance, and heparin, an anticoagulant.	Stabilize their cell membranes so that histamine not released.
Agranulocytes		
Lymphocytes (25%)	Two types: T-lymphocytes and B-lymphocytes; T-cells attack infecting or cancerous cells; B-cells produce antibodies against specific antigens.	Decrease activity of the lymphocytes.
Monocytes (3%-5%)	Produce macrophages, which can migrate out of the bloodstream to such places as mucous membranes, where they are capable of engulfing large bacteria or virus-infected cells.	Inhibit macrophage accumulation in already inflamed areas, thus preventing more inflammation.

*Percentage in parentheses is the proportion of the total number of leukocytes they constitute.

DOSAGES

SELECTED CORTICOSTEROIDS

AGENT	PHARMACOLOGIC CLASS	DOSAGE RANGE	PURPOSE
Beclomethasone (Beclovent, Vanceril)	Synthetic glucocorticoid	*Adult/Pediatric 6-12 y/o* 1-2 inhalations 3-4 times/day. Each inhalation delivers 42 μg; do not exceed 840 μg/day	Asthma
Dexamethasone sodium phosphate (Decadron Phosphate Respihaler)	Synthetic glucocorticoid	*Pediatric* 2 inhalations 3-4 times/day. Each inhalation delivers 100 μg; do not exceed 800 μg/day. *Adult* 3 inhalations 3-4 times/day; do not exceed 1200 μg (1.2 mg)/day.	Asthma
Flunisolide (AeroBid, AeroBid-M)	Synthetic glucocorticoid	*Pediatric 6-12 y/o* 1-2 inhalations 3-4 times/day. Each inhalation delivers 250 μg; do not exceed 1200 μg (1.2 mg)/day. *Adult* 2 inhalations bid in AM and PM; do not exceed 2000 μg (2 mg)/day.	Asthma
Triamcinolone acetonide (Azmacort)	Synthetic glucocorticoid	*Pediatric 6-12 y/o* 1-2 inhalations 3-4 times/day. Each inhalation delivers 100 μg; do not exceed 1200 μg (1.2 mg)/day. *Adult* 2 inhalations 3-4 times/day; do not exceed 1600 μg (1.6 mg)/day.	Asthma

DRUG PROFILE

The inhaled corticosteroids are contraindicated in patients who are hypersensitive to glucocorticoids, patients whose sputum is positive for *Candida* organisms, and patients with systemic fungal infection. All four of the inhaled corticosteroids are classified as pregnancy category C agents and are only available with a prescription.

BECLOMETHASONE DIPROPIONATE

Beclomethasone dipropionate (Beclovent, Vanceril) is administered by oral inhalation for the treatment of bronchial asthma in patients who require corticosteroids on a long-term basis for the control of symptoms. It may also be used in patients who have not re-

sponded to an adequate trial of conventional therapy, usually xanthines and beta-agonists, as well as in the management of patients with a COPD such as chronic bronchitis whose disease has been stabilized with oral corticosteroid therapy. Beclomethasone in an oral solution or rectal suspension has also been used in the management of inflammatory diseases of the gastrointestinal tract.

When beclomethasone is administered by oral inhalation, the primary sites of action are the bronchi and the bronchioles. Very little drug reaches the bloodstream through the respiratory tract because it is metabolically inactivated. Compared with dexamethasone, another inhaled corticosteroid, beclomethasone appears to have greater topical antiinflammatory activity and to cause fewer adverse systemic effects. The use of an inhaled corticosteroid frequently allows for a reduction in the daily dose of the systemic corticosteroids often taken by patients with chronic bronchial asthma. Beclomethasone is available as an aerosolized mist in a metered-dose inhaler that releases 42 μg per spray and is given by oral inhalation. The available inhaled corticosteroids, their various dosage strengths, and their pharmacokinetic properties are summarized in the box below. Commonly recommended dosages are listed in the dosages table on the previous page. Pregnancy category C.

Indirect-Acting Antiasthmatic Agents

The indirect-acting antiasthmatic agents, cromolyn and nedocromil, are additional agents that can be used in the treatment of COPDs such as asthma, chronic bronchitis, and emphysema. Cromolyn and nedocromil are considered indirect acting because they prevent the release of the various chemical substances that cause bronchospasm. They have no direct bronchodilator activity and are used only prophylactically. They are most effective in preventing the asthma caused by extrinsic factors such as allergens and that caused by exercise.

Mechanism of Action

Both cromolyn and nedocromil are called **mast cell stabilizers.** The cells that these two indirect-acting antiasthmatic agents affect are those listed and described in Table 35-2. As already mentioned, these cells release the vasoconstrictive substances (e.g., histamine, SRS-A) responsible for causing the bronchoconstrictive disorders such as asthma. Cromolyn and nedocromil exert their actions by stabilizing the membranes of the cells that normally release these harmful substances in response to an antigen-antibody reaction, thereby suppressing the release of the substances.

Nedocromil and cromolyn share many of the pharmacologic effects just mentioned, but nedocromil is more potent on a weight basis in inhibiting mediator release and the bronchoconstriction induced by various stimuli. Nedocromil also appears to affect a broader range of inflammatory cells (eosinophils, neutrophils, macrophages, mast cells, monocytes, and platelets). Nedocromil can inhibit both an acute bronchoconstrictor response and a delayed inflammatory response to inhaled antigens and irritants. It may also suppress cough by inhibiting the neuronal reflexes in airways.

Drug Effects

The drug effects of cromolyn and nedocromil are primarily limited to the lungs, and when administered into the lungs, very little if any of the agents gets into the bloodstream to cause systemic effects. The primary drug effect of these agents is on the surface of cell membranes. Because these drugs can be administered by several different routes (orally, inhaled, and in the eye), they can get to all areas of the body where there are inflammatory cells (e.g., mast cells, monocytes, macrophages, neutrophils) and stabilize their cell membranes, thereby preventing the release of the harmful cellular contents that cause inflammation. Cromolyn and nedocromil may also inhibit the movement of some cells into and out of the tissues and blood vessels.

Therapeutic Uses

Cromolyn and nedocromil are used as adjuncts to the overall management of patients with COPDs such as asthma, chronic bronchitis, and emphysema and are used solely for prophylaxis. These agents are of no value in the treatment of acute asthma attacks, and the types of asthma they are used in the prevention of are exercise-induced bronchospasm and the bronchospasm induced by exposure to other known precipitating factors such as cold dry air, environmental pollutants, and allergens. They may also be used for the symptomatic prevention and treatment of seasonal or perennial allergic rhinitis. Cromolyn may be used to relieve allergic eye disorders that result in itching, tearing, redness, and discharge. It has also been administered orally for the prophylactic management of food allergies and for the treatment of chronic inflammatory bowel disease (Crohn's disease and ulcerative colitis).

Side Effects and Adverse Effects

Most of the side effects of cromolyn and nedocromil affect the respiratory system and include coughing, sore throat, rhinitis, and bronchospasm. Other effects include taste changes, dizziness, and headache.

Dosages

For the recommended dosages of cromolyn and nedocromil, see the dosages table on the following page.

✿ PHARMACOKINETICS

INHALED CORTICOSTEROIDS Beclomethasone Dipropionate (42 µg/metered spray)			
HALF-LIFE	**ONSET**	**PEAK**	**DURATION**
3-15 hr	10 min	15-30 hr	4-6 hr
Dexamethasone Sodium Phosphate (100 µg/metered spray)			
HALF-LIFE	**ONSET**	**PEAK**	**DURATION**
36-54 hr*	10-15 min	15-30 min	4-6 hr
Flunisolide (250 µg/metered spray)			
HALF-LIFE	**ONSET**	**PEAK**	**DURATION**
1-2 hr	Unknown	Unknown	1 hr
Triamcinolone (100 µg/metered spray)			
HALF-LIFE	**ONSET**	**PEAK**	**DURATION**
Unknown	Unknown	Unknown	Unknown

*Biologic half-life.

D O S A G E S

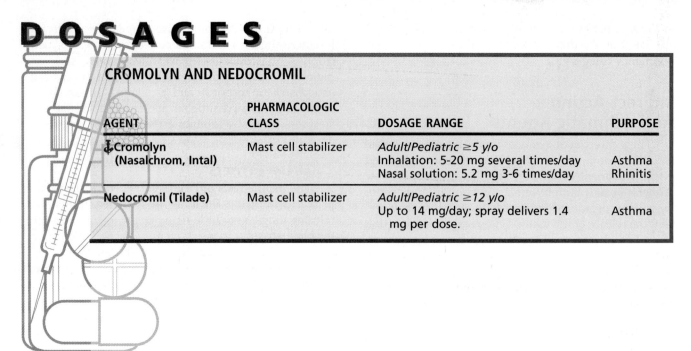

CROMOLYN AND NEDOCROMIL

AGENT	PHARMACOLOGIC CLASS	DOSAGE RANGE	PURPOSE
⚓Cromolyn (Nasalchrom, Intal)	Mast cell stabilizer	*Adult/Pediatric ≥5 y/o* Inhalation: 5-20 mg several times/day Nasal solution: 5.2 mg 3-6 times/day	Asthma Rhinitis
Nedocromil (Tilade)	Mast cell stabilizer	*Adult/Pediatric ≥12 y/o* Up to 14 mg/day; spray delivers 1.4 mg per dose.	Asthma

DRUG PROFILES

⚓ CROMOLYN

Cromolyn (Nasalcrom, Opticrom, Gastrocrom, Intal) is a mast cell stabilizer that is indicated for the prevention of bronchospasms and bronchial asthmatic attacks. It differs from nedocromil in that it seems to stabilize fewer cell types and is less potent. It was the first of the two agents in this drug class to be discovered and used in clinical practice.

Cromolyn is classified as a pregnancy category B drug and is contraindicated in patients who are hypersensitive to the drug or to its lactose filler. Patients who have lactose intolerance may exhibit symptoms of this disorder after the inhalation of cromolyn. Cromolyn is also contraindicated in patients who have status asthmaticus. It is available for both oral and ophthalmic administration as well as for nasal and oral inhalation, and because of its many dosage formulations, it may be used for the treatment of many disorders. The nasal solution delivers 5.2 mg per metered spray; the ophthalmic solution is a 4% solution; the oral capsules contain 100 mg of the agent; the aerosolized oral inhalation agent delivers 800 μg per metered spray; the

powder for oral inhalation comes as a 20-mg capsule; and the solution for nebulization has a concentration of 20 mg/2 ml. It is only available by prescription. Recommended dosages are given in the dosages table above.

⬡ PHARMACOKINETICS

HALF-LIFE	ONSET	PEAK	DURATION
1.5 hr	Unknown	15 min	4-6 hr

NEDOCROMIL

Nedocromil (Tilade) is indicated for the prevention of bronchospasms and bronchial asthma attacks. The contraindications to its use are the same as those for cromolyn and it is also a pregnancy category B agent. Its particular mechanism of action has already been described. Nedocromil is only available as an aerosolized inhaler, and it is only used as an adjunct agent in the overall management of patients with mild to moderate bronchial asthma. It too is only available with a prescription. It comes in a metered-dose inhaler that delivers 1.75 mg per spray for oral inhalation. Recommended dosages are given in the dosages table above.

⬡ PHARMACOKINETICS

HALF-LIFE	ONSET	PEAK	DURATION
1½ hr	Unknown	15 min	4-6 hr

NURSING PROCESS

ASSESSMENT

The net drug effect of all the bronchodilators—the beta-agonists, anticholinergics, xanthine derivatives, indirect-acting antiasthmatics, and corticosteroids—is relaxation of the bronchial smooth muscle. There are many indications for their use, but there are also many cautions and contraindications to their use, and these can be identified by means of thorough patient assessments. Beta-agonists are contraindicated in patients with a history of cardiac disease, dysrhythymias, angina, coronary artery disease, hypertension, diabetes, or convulsive disorders. The anticholinergic agents used as bronchodilators are contraindicated in patients with a history of benign prostatic hypertrophy or glaucoma. Xanthine derivatives such as aminophylline are contraindicated in patients with a history of peptic ulcer disease or GI disorders, and cautious use (with close monitoring) is recommended in patients with a history of a cardiac disorder. Corticosteroids are contraindicated in patients with an allergy to the drug, a psychosis, fungal infections, AIDS, TB, or idiopathic thrombocytopenia, as well as in children under 2 years of age. Cautious use is recommended in patients with diabetes mellitus, glaucoma, osteoporosis, ulcer disease, renal disease, congestive heart failure, edema, myasthenia gravis, seizure disorders, or esophagitis.

Cromolyn sodium is used in the management of asthma but only as preventive treatment, not for the control of acute exacerbations of asthma, so acute exacerbations represent a contraindication to its use. Use of this medication in children younger than 5 years of age and in pregnant or lactating women is not recommended.

In a thorough assessment of patients receiving any of the respiratory agents, the patient's skin color, temperature, and respirations (rate [<12 or >24 breaths/min] and rhythm) must be checked. The nurse should also find out whether the patient is having problems with cough, dyspnea, orthopnea, or respiratory distress; whether he or she has or is suffering from sternal retraction, cyanosis, restlessness, activity intolerance, or cardiac symptoms such as palpitations, hypertension, and tachycardia; and whether he or she is using accessory muscles to breathe. In addition, the nurse should ask patients whether they have a history of allergies and, if so, what they are, whether there is sputum production, and what other medications and non-

drug therapies they are using. Patients should also be asked to give a thorough history of their COPD.

NURSING DIAGNOSES

Nursing diagnoses related to the administration of respiratory agents include:
- Impaired gaseous exchange related to pathophysiologic changes caused by COPD.
- Fatigue related to disease process.
- Risk for injury related to side effects of medication.
- Anxiety related to disease process and medication therapy.
- Altered thought processes related to the CNS stimulation caused by bronchodilators.
- Knowledge deficit concerning disease process and its precipitating factors.
- Knowledge deficit related to the medication therapy.
- Noncompliance related to side effects of medication therapy.

PLANNING

Goals for the patient receiving respiratory agents include:
- Patient experiences minimal exacerbations of the disease while compliant with medication regimen.
- Patient states the importance of rest to recovery.
- Patient will be free of self-injury related to either the disease or the side effects of the medication.
- Patient remains compliant with the medication regimen as well as with nonpharmacologic therapies.
- Patient follows up with health care providers as instructed by the physician.
- Patient will not increase or decrease dose or stop taking the medication on their own.
- Patient's respiratory status will improve because of compliance with medication therapy.

Outcome Criteria

Outcome criteria for patients receiving respiratory agents include:
- Patient will briefly describe the disease process, its signs and symptoms, and the precipitating factors.
- Patient states measures to take to prevent self-injury resulting from the disease or the side effects of the medication such as taking medications as prescribed.
- Patient will be well rested, with plans to rest during periods of exacerbation.
- Patient will state the expected side effects of the drug such as palpitations, nervousness, mood changes, and insomnia.

(*Text continued on p. 536.*)

NURSING ▪ CARE ▪ PLAN

Asthma

Jennifer, a 13-year-old girl recently diagnosed with asthma, is to begin nebulizer treatments with cromolyn sodium (Intal) twice daily. She has been compliant with her steroid inhaler and with other treatments for her asthma, so the physician be-lieves that the cromolyn sodium will help prevent some of her asthmatic attacks. Since you are the nurse on the "well" side of the pediatrician's office today, you are to tell her about the medication and its use.

Assessment with nursing diagnoses	Planning with goals and outcome criteria	Implementation and patient education	Evaluation

Subjective
 	
"I'm not sure that this stuff is gonna work"
 	
Objective
 	
13-year-old newly diagnosed asthmatic
Success with other therapies
Listens and comprehends well
Anxious to get asthma under control
RR20
Lungs clear
BP 100/60
P66
 	
Nursing diagnoses
 	
Knowledge deficient (patient teaching) related to new diagnoses of asthma treatment
	Goals
	
	Patient will remain compliant to new asthma treatment within 1 mo
	
	Outcome criteria
	
	Patient will state the following about cromolyn sodium therapy:
	  Use
	  Side effects
	  Cautions
	  Side effects to report to the physician
		Remember that this medication is to be given by nebulizer for the time being and should be taken directly as ordered (bid)
		
		Make sure that after you do the treatment that you rinse your mouth out and gargle to prevent irritation to the mouth and throat
		
		You may not see its full effects for about 4 wk because it takes that long to get to its therapeutic effects of preventing some of your episodes of asthma
		
		Keep machinery clean as recommended by the manufacturer
		
		Once we have discussed the medication, you will be all set to go because you already know how to use the machine
		
		Side effects associated with cromolyn sodium include the following:
		  Throat irritation, cough, nasal stuffiness, burning of the eyes, headache, nausea, dry mouth, bitter taste
		
		Call the physician if you should experience severe headaches, dizziness, rash, or joint pain or swelling
			Patient will display a therapeutic response to cromolyn sodium as evidenced by:
			  Decrease in asthmatic symptoms
			  Decreased chest tightness and wheezing
			  Decrease in cough
			  Fewer asthma attacks
			  Regular respiratory rate and rhythm
			  No dyspnea
			
			Patient will experience minimal side effects and report those indicated

Patient Teaching TIPS

Respiratory Agents

✔ Patients should be encouraged to take measures that promote a generally good state of health and that can prevent, relieve, or decrease symptoms of the COPD. Such measures include avoiding exposure to conditions (e.g., allergens, stress, smoking, air pollutants) that can precipitate bronchoconstriction or that can worsen the symptoms; adequate fluid intake (at least 3000 ml/day, unless contraindicated, to thin the mucus); compliance with medical treatment, including frequent follow-up visits; and proper diet. They should also be told to avoid excessive fatigue, heat, and extremes in temperature and to avoid consuming caffeine-containing beverages, because these may increase bronchoconstriction.

✔ Patients should use the medications as ordered to prevent bronchoconstriction if they anticipate respiratory difficulty, such as using their inhaler before aerobic exercise.

✔ Patients should be encouraged to get prompt treatment for flu or other illnesses, especially respiratory illnesses, and to get vaccinated against pneumonia or flu, unless this is contraindicated.

✔ Encourage patients to always check with their physician before taking any other medication, even OTC medications.

✔ **Corticosteroid** treatment in patients with a COPD requires much patience on the part of the nurse as well as much patient education. Patients should first be made aware that abruptly *discontinuing* these medications can lead to serious consequences and that the agent should be weaned gradually over 1 to 2 weeks, and only under a physician's care and recommendation. They should wear an ID bracelet or necklace and carry a card at all times that identifies them as a steroid user. Patients should be told about the **cushingoid** symptoms that can be caused by steroids. These include moon face, acne, an increase in fat pads, and edema. Should they occur, the physician should be notified immediately. It is important to explain to the patient that these symptoms are the result of excess steroid levels. The signs and symptoms of **Addison's disease,** or adrenal insufficiency, resulting from inadequate steroid levels include nausea, dyspnea, joint pain, weakness, and fatigue and should also be reported to the physician. **Drugs** that can interact with corticosteroids, and that therefore should be avoided, include aspirin, alcohol, barbiturates, phenytoin, theophylline, anti-

coagulants, anticonvulsants, antidiabetic agents, antituberculin agents, antifungal agents, digitalis, diuretics, NSAIDs, oral contraceptives, estrogens, and macrolide antibiotics. *Patients should report any weight gain of more than 5 pounds (2.25 kg) a week or the occurrence of chest pain to their physician.*

✔ Patients taking a **beta-agonist** should be told to take the medication exactly as prescribed by the physician with no omissions or double dosing. Patients should notify the physician should they experience insomnia, jitteriness, restlessness, palpitations, chest pain, or any change in symptoms.

✔ Patients should be told to take **xanthine derivatives** exactly as ordered and to notify their physician should they experience palpitations, nausea, vomiting, weakness, dizziness, chest pain, or convulsions. The concurrent use of xanthine derivatives with other medications, such as cimetidine, allopurinol, oral contraceptives, and flu vaccine, or with large amounts of caffeine, which is also a xanthine, can have deleterious effects. Patients should never double up on doses if they have missed a dose; however, they may take it if only 1 hour has passed, but not if more than an hour has passed. They should never crush or chew sustained-released tablets, pills, or capsules.

✔ Patients should be told that **cromolyn sodium** needs to be administered consistently for the therapeutic effects to occur and that it may take up to 4 weeks before any of these effects are seen. Patients should be taught how to administer the medication and told to gargle and rinse the mouth with water afterward to minimize irritation to the throat and oral mucosa. Side effects include throat irritation, cough, headache, a bitter or bad taste in the mouth, and dry mouth.

✔ **Inhaled** forms of respiratory medications should be administered after patients have exhaled and then as they inhale deeply with the head tipped backward to produce maximal opening of the airway. Patients should then remove the inhaler and hold their breath for as much as 10 seconds, then exhale. Patients should be taught how to use a nebulizer and how to care for the equipment, such as changing the filters when they become discolored (grayish) and cleaning the tubing and mouthpieces frequently with soap, water, and white vinegar. Disposable tubing and mouthpieces are available.

- Patient will contact the physician with increased dyspnea, shortness of breath, increased cough, or fever.
- Patient will state the importance of taking the medication as prescribed, the reasons for not increasing or decreasing the dose of the agent, and the importance of not stopping the drug therapy to prevent complications and exacerbations related to disease or side effects of medications.

IMPLEMENTATION

Nursing interventions that apply to patients with a COPD in general include patient education and an emphasis on prevention, in addition to implementing the drug therapy prescribed. Measures to take to prevent, relieve, or decrease the manifestations of the disease should be emphasized to the patient at all times during treatment (see the box on p. 535 for patient teaching tips). Bronchodilators should be given exactly as prescribed and by the prescribed route (such as parenterally or orally or by intermittent positive pressure breathing). The proper method for administering the inhaled forms of these agents should be demonstrated to the patient, and the patient asked to demonstrate the method back. Patients should also be strongly discouraged from taking more than the prescribed dose of the beta-agonists because of the excessive cardiac demands (hypertension and tachycardia) this can cause. The nurse should always find out what other medications patients are taking to make sure that they are not taking one that can interact with any of the bronchodilators or antiasthmatic agents. Home health care implications applicable to patients receiving albuterol are given in the box at right.

Xanthine derivatives should be given exactly as prescribed. If they are to be given parenterally, the nurse should always determine the correct diluent to be used, the amount of the agent, and the time to infuse medication. Timed-release preparations should not be crushed or chewed because of the irritating effects they can have on the gastric mucosa. Suppository forms of the drug should be refrigerated, and patients should be told to notify their physician if rectal burning, itching, or irritation occurs in association with their use.

Corticosteroid inhalers should be used as prescribed, with cautions against overuse. All equipment, inhalers or nebulizers, should be kept clean and filters cleaned and changed (nebulizers) and in good working condition. Rinsing of the mouth after using the inhaler or nebulizer is recommended. Pediatric patients may need a physician's order to have these medications "on hand" at school and during athletic events or physical education. Peak flow meter use is also encouraged to help patients better regulate their disease.

HOME HEALTH POINTS
Patients Receiving Albuterol

- Instructions to patients regarding the proper use of inhaled forms of medications are crucial to ensuring their safe and effective use. Make sure to have patients demonstrate back the technique for using an inhaler or nebulizer.
- Instructions regarding the care of the inhaler or nebulizer and associated equipment are also important. This involves washing the inhaler in warm water every day and drying it before reuse or washing the tubing, and other apparatus used with the nebulizer. White vinegar can be used to rinse out the tubing of nebulizers. Always encourage patients to follow the manufacturer's recommendations regarding the use, storage, and cleaning of any equipment used.
- Patients must be warned not to let the inhaler spray get in their eyes.
- A therapeutic response to albuterol inhaler use includes absence of wheezing and dyspnea.
- Patients must be instructed and reminded during home health care visits to use these medications EXACTLY as prescribed and that an overdose may precipitate palpitations, angina, hypertension, or dysrhythmias.

Cromolyn sodium, although not a bronchodilator, does have a role to play in the *preventive* treatment of asthma. It comes as a powder contained in a capsule that is administered by a specific type of inhaler, but in both adults and children, it is most popularly administered by a nebulizer. During a treatment session using either delivery system, the patient may experience bronchospasms. If they continue, the patient's condition should be stabilized, the session discontinued, and the physician notified. The proper technique for inhalant administration is presented in the box on the pediatric implications pertaining to cromolyn sodium therapy (see p. 537). Other interventions such as forcing fluids and avoiding precipitating factors are also recommended!

Miscellaneous pediatric implications relevant to treatment with the various respiratory agents are presented in the box on p. 537. See the case study on p. 538 to test your understanding of the nursing process in a hospitalized patient with a COPD.

EVALUATION

The therapeutic effects of any of the agents used to treat or prevent respiratory diseases include decreased

PEDIATRIC IMPLICATIONS
Cromolyn Sodium

- Children over 6 years of age who are being treated with cromolyn sodium administered by nasal spray should be given only ONE spray in each nostril tid or qid BUT only as ordered by the physician and NOT to exceed six doses in 24 hours. This type of spray is usually indicated for the treatment of allergic rhinitis.

- Children over 5 years of age being treated for bronchospasms with inhaled forms are usually given 20 mg administered over less than 1 hour qid and nebulizer forms at a dose of 20 mg qid.

- Children over 5 years of age being treated for bronchial asthma are generally prescribed inhaler and nebulizer forms at a dose of 20 mg qid. Children are usually very willing and eager to learn about ways to prevent respiratory difficulty, so it is important to show them AND family members or caretakers the proper inhalation technique, which is as follows: Have the child exhale, then put the inhaler in place. Have the child inhale deeply with the head tipped back so as to maximize the opening of the air passages. The cromolyn sodium should be administered during this deep inhalation. After inhaling, instruct the child to remove the inhaler while holding the breath, than exhale when needed and repeat as instructed.

- Children should be told that capsules ARE NOT TO BE chewed.

- Be sure that the child, parents, or caretakers know that cromolyn sodium is preventive, not curative, treatment, that it must be used year-round, and that it may take up to 4 weeks before therapeutic effects are noticed.

- Nebulizer forms of cromolyn sodium should be administered as instructed and according to the physician's orders. All equipment, including the filter and tubing, should be kept clean. Filters need to be purchased or ordered well ahead of time, and manufacturer's guidelines suggest changing them when they begin to appear gray. The tubing and mouthpieces should be cleaned according to the manufacturer's guidelines using water and white vinegar. Specific instructions should be followed regarding the use of the machine and proper breathing during use of the machine. Once the nebulizer session is over, the mouthpiece should be rinsed. The child should also rinse out his or her mouth with water.

PEDIATRIC IMPLICATIONS
Respiratory Agents

- Bronchodilators are often used in children but should be used with *extreme caution* in these young patients. Monitor for adverse effects such as tremors, restlessness, GI tract upset, hallucinations, dizziness, palpitations, and tachycardia.

- Xanthine derivatives should be used very cautiously in children 6 months and older, with close monitoring of the blood levels and response to the medication. CNS-stimulating effects may be enhanced in children, and these effects should be watched for.

- Cromolyn sodium is generally used in children older than 6 years and should be used only if the child and parent or caregiver can accurately demonstrate the correct use of the nebulizer and how to care for the equipment. They should also show themselves capable of monitoring for the adverse effects.

- A daily journal or graph should be kept in which the date, time, drug used, signs and symptoms, and peak flowmeter results are documented. This will help chart the patient's compliance with the regimen and the therapeutic effects or lack there of.

dyspnea; decreased wheezing, restlessness, and anxiety; improved respiratory patterns with return to normal rate and quality; improved activity tolerance and arterial blood gas levels; increased quality of life; and decreased severity and incidence of respiratory symptoms. The therapeutic effects of bronchodilating agents such as xanthine derivatives or beta-agonists, include decreased symptoms and increased ease of breathing. The respiratory rate, rhythm, depth, and lung fields should also return to normal. Other antiasthmatic or bronchodilating agents should produce the same therapeutic effects.

Adverse effects to monitor for in patients receiving beta-agonists include tachyarrhythmias, chest pain, restlessness, agitation, nervousness, and insomnia. Adverse effects of anticholinergic agents consist of dry mouth, constipation, headache, nervousness, nausea, and blurred vision. The xanthine derivatives may cause palpitations, tachyarrhythmias, chest pain, GI upset, agitation, headache, insomnia, and restlessness. Besides watching for the side effects of xanthine derivatives, the therapeutic blood levels should also be checked. That for theophylline is 20 μg/ml. Any level above this is considered toxic and may cause fatal reactions. The adverse effects of cromolyn sodium include hypotension, bitter taste, dizziness, nausea, vomiting, dysrhythmias, and restlessness.

CASE STUDY

Chronic Obstructive Pulmonary Disorder

Ms. Brown is a 73-year-old woman who worked in the local traffic tunnel for about 25 years and has had a COPD for 10 years caused by her exposure to environmental pollutants while on the job. She is now retired and is frequently admitted to the hospital for treatment of her condition. She quit smoking about 8 years ago. She is now in the hospital for treatment of an acute exacerbation of her COPD and an upper respiratory tract infection. The physician has ordered the following: Aminophlline IV per respiratory therapy protocol, IV continuous infusion at a rate of 0.8 mg/kg/hr; chest physiotherapy bid and as needed; cephalothin antibiotic therapy, 1 gm IV in 30 ml NS q8h; I&O; daily weights; VS with breath sounds q2h and as needed until stable; and albuterol inhaler, two puffs q4h per respiratory therapy protocol.

- What nursing interventions would be most appropriate for helping this patient conserve energy while enhancing O_2 and CO_2 gas exchange?
- What is the rationale for using the continuous IV infusion of aminophylline?
- What are the reasons for prescribing the albuterol inhaler and the antibiotic? Be specific about the reasons for each.
- What would be the most important patient education guidelines to impart to Ms. Brown concerning the use of oral aminophylline and the albuterol inhaler at home?

TAKE HOME POINTS

Beta-Agonists

- Work by stimulating adenylate cyclase, which produces more cAMP and which in turn causes relaxation of the smooth muscle that surrounds the airways.
- Beta-agonists may stimulate alpha and beta receptors, beta$_1$ and beta$_2$ receptors, or just beta$_1$ receptors.
- Beta$_2$ stimulants are the most specific for the lungs and have the fewest side effects.

Xanthines

- Caffeine, theobromine, and theophylline are examples of xanthines.
- Work by inhibiting phosphodiesterase.
- Phosphodiesterase breaks down cAMP, which is needed to relax smooth muscles.
- Theophylline is the most common; aminophylline is the parenteral form of theophylline.

Anticholinergics

- Ipratropium bromide (Atrovent) is only agent used for treatment of asthma.
- Used for maintenance and not for relief of acute bronchospasms.
- Work by blocking the bronchoconstrictive effects of acetylcholine.

Corticosteroids

- Beclomethasone, dexamethasone, flunisolide, and triamcinolone are examples.
- Work by stabilizing the membranes of cells that release harmful bronchoconstricting substances.
- Not first-line agents; commonly used when conventional bronchodilators fail.

Indirect-Acting Agents

- Cromolyn (Nasalcrom) and nedocromil (Tilade).
- Only used prophylactically; used for management of chronic pulmonary disease.
- Work by stabilizing the mast cell wall, thereby preventing potentially harmful vasoconstrictive substances from being released.

Nursing Considerations

- Contraindications to beta-agonist use include history of cardiac disease, dysrhythmias, angina, coronary artery disease, hypertension, and seizure disorders.
- Anticholinergics are contraindicated in patients with BPH or glaucoma.
- Xanthine derivatives are contraindicated in patients with a history of GI tract disorders or peptic ulcer disease.
- Cromolyn sodium is used to prevent asthma, and treatment with this medication must be adhered to year-round.
- All respiratory agents should be given exactly as ordered and the diluent checked in terms of the proper amount and type of solution.

Critical Thinking A C T I V I T I E S

1. Your patient is taking a xanthine derivative and should not ingest xanthine-containing beverages. What are examples of these beverages, and why is it important to avoid consuming them while taking a xanthine derivative?

2. The physician prescribes cromolyn sodium (Intal) to be given by nebulizer at home for an 11-year-old girl with a 9-year history of asthma. The rationale for the use of this medication is that it:
   a. Inhibits histamine release.
   b. Stimulates the substances that release acetylcholine.
   c. Inhibits mast cell degeneration.
   d. Stimulates the release of bronchospastic agents.

3. Albuterol is a _____ type of beta-agonist that works by increasing the level of ____, which causes _____ of smooth muscle in the respiratory tract.

1. nonselective adrenergic	2. nonselective beta-adrenergic	3. selective beta$_2$	4. vasoconstriction
5. cAMP	6. relaxation	7. stimulation	8. potassium

   a. 1, 4, and 7   b. 2, 8, and 6   c. 3, 5, and 6   d. 3, 8, 6

4. Theophylline is a _____ type of bronchodilator that works by _____, which results in _____ the cAMP levels which _____ smooth muscle in the respiratory tract.

1. beta-agonist	2. xanthine	3. increasing	4. inhibiting PDE
5. stimulating beta receptors	6. relaxes	7. stimulates	8. decreasing

   a. 1, 4, 3, and 7   b. 2, 4, 3, and 6   c. 1, 5, 7, and 6   d. 2, 4, 8, 6

5. The indirect-acting agents (cromolyn and nedocromil), the corticosteroids (e.g., triamcinolone), and the anticholinergics (e.g., ipratroprium bromide) are all used _____ for patients with airway diseases such as asthma, chronic bronchitis, and emphysema.

   a. acutely   b. prophylactically   c. as needed   d. emergently

BIBLIOGRAPHY

Albanese J, Nutz P: *Mosby's 1995 nursing drug cards,* St Louis, 1995, Mosby.

Janson-Bjerklie S: Status asthmaticus, *Am J Nurs* 90(9):52, 1990.

Johnson KB: *Harriet Lane handbook,* ed 13, St Louis, 1993, Mosby.

Keen JH: *Critical care and emergency drug reference,* St Louis, 1994, Mosby.

Knoben JE, Anderson PO: *Handbook of critical drug data,* ed 6, Hamilton, Ill, 1988, Drug Intelligence Publications.

Lindell KO: Breaking bronchospasm's grip with MDIs, *Am J Nurs* 90(3):34, 1990.

McEvoy GK: *AHFS drug information,* Bethesda, Md, 1994, American Society of Hospital Pharmacists.

Skidmore-Roth L: *Mosby's 1995 nursing drug reference,* St Louis, 1995, Mosby.

PART 8

ANTIINFECTIVE AND ANTIINFLAMMATORY AGENTS: STUDY SKILLS BRIEF

This study model is focused on the "Nursing Process" section in Chapter 36. Since there is a "Nursing Process" section at the end of each chapter, the discussion of the example in Chapter 36 is applicable to all chapters.

NURSING PROCESS

Look at the opening paragraph of this section, which introduces the focus for the section and serves as your preliminary focus for learning.

"The discussion of the nursing process will <u>focus</u> on each <u>major classification of antibiotics</u> so that there is an <u>awareness of general and specific information</u> about the various antibiotics."

The underlining in this paragraph is intended to point out the important information found in this paragraph. The nursing process section focuses on major classifications. Another critical piece of this paragraph is the need to see both *General* and *Specific* information about the classifications. Although the paragraph is only one sentence in length, it clearly defines what you, as the student, need to keep in mind as you study this section.

ASSESSMENT

What is the purpose of this section? Each time you begin to read the nursing process section of a chapter you need to ask this question. What are you supposed to learn? What are you supposed to know? What are you supposed to be able to do? All these questions relate to your role as a nurse. Consider the following sentence from this section in Chapter 36:

"<u>Before the administration</u> of any antibiotic, it is <u>crucial to ensuring</u> the effectiveness and <u>appropriateness of treatment</u> for the nurse to <u>collect</u> data on the patient regarding his or her age; hypersensitivities to drugs; hepatic, renal, and cardiac function (i.e., pertinent laboratory test results); culture and sensitivity results; and CBC, Hgb, and Hct values."

Assessment clearly has to do with patient care. You are assessing the patient as he or she relates to the pharmacologic interventions that this chapter discusses. I have done some underlining in this section to bring into sharper focus some of the things that you must be very aware of as you study.

First, notice the use of the word *crucial* in the first line. Something is so important at this point that it cannot be ignored. Immediately the questioning process should be activated. What is crucial? The answer follows immediately in the sentence. You must have data collected on the patient. The sentence goes on to identify the kind of data that should be available, and the sentence makes it clear that it has to be done "before administration." Each of the data factors is important, and each relates to other parts and chapters in this text.

The patient's age should be known. There is a chapter in this text that deals with pediatric and geriatric concerns. Children and elderly patients respond to drugs differently than adults. This would directly affect dosage and possibly even the choice of antibiotics to be administered. This also ties directly to "effectiveness of treatment" referred to in this sentence.

The next data item is hypersensitivities. Some individuals are "allergic" to certain antibiotics. It would be dangerous and possibly fatal to administer an antibiotic to a patient if he or she is hypersensitive. This connects with the "appropriateness of treatment," which is the other crucial element specified in this sentence. As you consider each of the underlined elements in this sentence, you must keep in mind its relationship to effectiveness and appropriateness.

Another data item specifies hepatic-renal-cardiac functioning. As you read this you should instantly think to what hepatic, renal, and cardiac refer. Then you should try to recall information from this chapter that related the specific antibiotics to these functions. Learning is cumulative. The nursing process section assumes you have read and understood what was presented earlier in the chapter.

One more aspect of this sentence is the use of standard medical abbreviations. In earlier part introductions I have suggested that you prepare vocabulary cards for these abbreviations to help you in a situation such as this. You need to know what CBC, Hgb, and Hct mean, what they measure, and how they relate to appropriate and effective administration of antibiotics. If these letters are not meaningful to you, then you will not be able to link what you know about the antibiotics with what you must know about administering them as a nurse. Many test questions on nursing exams use the standard abbreviations, and you must know them instantly and be able to relate them to the situation covered. As you look at antibiotic administration and CBC, Hgb, and Hct, think what a test question might ask about these data elements in a real application in patient care? This is what nursing process is all about.

NURSING DIAGNOSES

The same first question applies here as in every other section. What am I supposed to learn? Since the focus is on administration of antibiotics, the expectation you should bring to this is an awareness of your role in diagnosis. What should you look for in working with patients that affects the administration of antibiotics?

This same procedure should be applied to the sections on Planning, Outcome Criteria, and Implementation. Consider what each of these headings suggests about the nursing process, and read and evaluate the information, relating it to what you have already learned. Also consider the implications of the information as possible test questions that may ask you to do more than recall specific facts. As an example, consider the following case:

Patient A, age 23, has a fever of 100.8° F. She was admitted yesterday and delivered a healthy infant 8 hours ago. She is breast feeding the newborn. What antibiotics might be administered for the fever? What specific antibiotics should be used with caution or eliminated from consideration?

This case demonstrates the need to read and think critically. You need to remember not only the specific facts from the chapter, but also be able to take a case study example and apply those facts to that specific situation.

EVALUATION

This is the final section under Nursing Process. What are you supposed to evaluate?

"The therapeutic effects of antibiotics in general include a decrease in the signs and symptoms of the infection; a return to normal vital signs, including temperature and negative results of culture and sensitivity tests; a decrease to a normal CBC; and improved appetite, energy level, and sense of well-being." This sentence makes it clear that you are evaluating the patient and his or her response to the antibiotics being administered. In evaluating the patient, what should you look for? Given the focus in nursing process on contraindications, cautions, hypersensitivity, and reactions related to the administration of antibiotics, you should be evaluating two aspects of the patient.

First you should look for the positive responses set forth in the above text sample that indicate the patient is responding favorably to the treatment. But when you read the next sentence in this section, you see: "Common adverse reactions to monitor for . . ." This says your role in evaluation is to monitor the patient for negative responses and be prepared to educate the patient as to the effects he or she is experiencing and possible steps to help alleviate the symptoms.

The Nursing Process section in each chapter should be read carefully and thoughtfully because it is in this section where you begin to see how the complex pharmacologic material presented earlier in the chapter fits into your role as a nurse. This material should be read with the same concern and care that you have given to the highly complex materials earlier in the chapter, as this is the section in which you must think about **application** of all you have learned. Apply the PURR model and be an active questioner and reader, and you will be successful in working with Nursing Process in each chapter.

Chapter 36

Antibiotics

Objectives

When you reach the end of this chapter, you will be able to:

1 Describe the general principles of antibiotic therapy.
2 Explain how antibiotics work to rid the body of infection.
3 Discuss the indications for, cautions and contraindications to, mechanism of action of, side effects of, and the toxicity associated with the various antibiotics.
4 Classify the various antibiotics with examples of specific drugs in each classification.
5 Develop a nursing care plan that includes education for the patient receiving antibiotics.

CHAPTER OUTLINE

Infection

General Principles of Antibiotic Therapy

Antibiotics

Sulfonamides
  Mechanism of action
  Drug effects
  Therapeutic uses
  Side effects and adverse effects
  Interactions
    Laboratory test interactions
  Dosages
Drug Profiles
  ⚓ Sulfamethoxazole
    Sulfisoxazole
Penicillins
  Mechanism of action
  Drug effects
  Therapeutic uses
  Side effects and adverse effects
  Interactions
  Dosages
Drug Profiles
  Natural penicillins
  ⚓ Penicillin G
    Penicillin V potassium
  Penicillinase-resistant penicillins
    Methicillin
Aminopenicillins
  ⚓ Ampicillin

Extended-Spectrum Penicillins
Cephalosporins
  Dosages
Drug Profiles
  First-generation cephalosporins
    ⚓ Cefazolin sodium
      Cephalexin
  Second-generation cephalosporins
    ⚓ Cefoxitin
      Cefuroxime
  Third-generation cephalosporins
      Cefixime
      Ceftriaxone
    ⚓ Ceftazidime
Tetracyclines
  Mechanism of action
  Drug effects
  Therapeutic uses
  Side effects and adverse effects
  Interactions
  Dosages
Drug Profiles
      Demeclocycline
    ⚓ Doxycycline
Aminoglycosides
  Mechanism of action
  Drug effects
  Therapeutic uses
  Side effects and adverse effects
  Interactions
  Dosages

continued

Drug Profiles
   Amikacin
  ⚓ Gentamicin
Quinolones
  Mechanism of action
  Drug effects
  Therapeutic uses
  Side effects and adverse effects
  Interactions
Drug Profiles
  ⚓ Ciprofloxacin
Macrolides
  Mechanism of action
  Drug effects
  Therapeutic uses
  Side effects and adverse effects
  Interactions
  Dosages
Drug Profiles
  ⚓ Erythromycin
  Azithromycin and Clarithromycin
Miscellaneous Antibiotics
  Aztreonam
  Clindamycin
  Imipenem-cilastatin
  ⚓ Vancomycin
Nursing Process
Assessment
  Penicillins
  Cephalosporins
  Sulfonamides
  Tetracyclines
  Aminoglycosides
  Clindamycin
  Quinolones
  Macrolides
  Vancomycin
Nursing Diagnoses
Planning
  Outcome criteria
Implementation
Evaluation

Glossary

Antibiotic Of or pertaining to the ability to destroy or interfere with the development of a living organism. (p. 544)

Bactericidal antibiotics Antibiotics that kill bacteria. (p. 559)

Bacteriostatic antibiotics Antibiotics that do not actually kill but rather inhibit the growth of bacteria. (p. 545)

Beta-lactams (lak′ təmz) The chemical structure of penicillins. (p. 547)

Empiric therapy A method of treating disease based on observations and experience without an understanding of the cause or mechanism of the disorder or the way in which the therapeutic agent or procedure employed effects improvement or cure. (p. 544)

Glucose-6-phosphate dehydrogenase deficiency An inherited disorder in which the red blood cells are partially or completely deficient in glucose-6-phosphate dehydrogenase, a critical enzyme in the aerobic glycolysis process. A sex-linked disorder, the defect is fully expressed in affected males despite a heterozygous pattern of inheritance. (p. 545)

Host factors Particular factors pertinent to patient with infection. (p. 544)

Prophylactic Preventing the spread of disease. (p. 544)

Slow acetylator (ə set′ ə la′ tor) A common genetic host factor. A peripheral neuropathy will develop in affected persons given isoniazid. (p. 545)

Subtherapeutic Referring to treatment that is considered ineffective. (p. 544)

Superinfection An infection occurring during antimicrobial treatment for another infection, resulting in overgrowth of nonsusceptible organism. (p. 544)

Teratogens (ter′ ə to jənz) Any substance, agent, or process that interferes with normal prenatal development and causes one or more developmental abnormalities in the fetus. (p. 545)

Therapeutic Of or relating to treatment that is considered beneficial. (p. 544)

Infection

A person is able to remain healthy and resistant to the microorganisms that cause infection because of the existence of certain host defenses. These defenses take various forms. They can be actual physical barriers such as intact skin and the ciliated respiratory mucosa. They can be physiologic defenses such as the gastric acid in the stomach and immune factors such as antibodies. They can also be the phagocytic cells—the macrophages and polymorphonuclear neutrophils—that are part of the reticuloendothelial system.

Microorganisms are everywhere in both the external environment as well as the internal environment of our bodies. They can be intrinsically harmful to humans, or they can be innocuous and even beneficial under normal circumstances but become harmful when these conditions are altered in some way. An example of an intrinsically harmful microorganism is *Rickettsia rickettsii*, which causes Rocky Mountain spotted fever. *Streptococcus viridans* is an example of a microorganism normally present in the body, but one that can cause endocarditis in patients whose heart valves have been damaged as the result of rheumatic fever.

When a person's normal host defenses are breached or somehow compromised, that person becomes susceptible to infection. The microorganisms invade and multiply in the body tissues, and if the infective process overwhelms the body's own defense system, the infection becomes clinically apparent. The patient then manifests the characteristic signs and symptoms of infection—fever, chills, sweats, redness, pain and swelling, fatigue, weight loss, increased white blood cell count, and the formation of pus.

To help the body combat an infection often requires antibiotic therapy, and these are the agents discussed in this chapter. However, before considering the specific agents and the therapy proper, there are certain general principles pertaining to antibiotic therapy that should be explained and understood first.

General Principles of Antibiotic Therapy

Therapy should begin with an initial assessment of the patient to determine whether he or she has the common signs and symptoms of infection just mentioned. The patient should also be assessed during and after antibiotic therapy to make certain the therapy is working, the infection is not recurring, and there are no untoward problems with the therapy.

Often the signs and symptoms of an infection appear long before an organism can be identified. When this happens and the risk of life-threatening or severe complications is high, an **antibiotic** is given to the patient immediately. The antibiotic selected is one that can best kill the microorganisms known to be the most common causes of infection. This is defined as **empiric therapy.** After the start of empiric antibiotic therapy, suspected areas of infection should be cultured in an attempt to identify a causative organism. If an organism is identified, it is then tested for various antibiotic susceptibilities, and the results of these tests can confirm whether the empiric therapy chosen is appropriate for eradicating the organism identified.

Antibiotics are also given for **prophylactic** reasons. This is done when patients are scheduled to have a procedure in which the likelihood of microorganisms being present is high. Prophylactic antibiotic therapy is used to prevent an infection. However, the risk of infection varies depending on the procedure being performed. For example, the risk of infection in a patient

undergoing coronary artery bypass surgery is relatively low compared with that in a person undergoing intraabdominal surgery for the treatment of injuries suffered in a motor vehicle accident. In the latter case, it is highly likely that the bacteria that normally live in the gastrointestinal tract will be present in the area of surgery. This would constitute a contaminated or dirty surgical field, and therefore the likelihood of infection would be high.

To optimize antibiotic therapy, the patient should be continuously monitored both to determine the effectiveness of therapy and whether the therapy is having any adverse effects. A **therapeutic** response to antibiotics is one in which there is a decrease in the specific signs and symptoms of infection compared with the baseline findings (e.g., fever, elevated WBC, redness, inflammation, drainage, pain). Antibiotic therapy is said to be **subtherapeutic** when it is ineffective, and this can result from using an incorrect route of administration, inadequate drainage of abscess, poor antibiotic penetration to the infected area, subtherapeutic serum levels of the agent, or bacterial resistance to the antibiotic. Antibiotic therapy is considered *toxic* when the serum levels of the antibiotic are too high, when the patient has an allergic reaction to the antibiotic, or when one of a host of patient-specific factors occurs; these include: rash, itching, hives, fever, chills, joint pain, difficulty breathing, or wheezing.

Superinfections and antibiotic interactions with food and other drugs are other problems to be watched for in patients taking antibiotics. Superinfections occur when antibiotics reduce or completely eliminate the normal bacterial flora. This consists of certain bacteria and fungi that are needed to maintain normal function in various organs. When these bacteria or fungi are killed by antibiotics, this permits other bacteria or fungi to take over and cause infection. An example of a superinfection is the diarrhea caused by vaginal yeast infections when the normal vaginal flora is reduced and yeast growth is no longer suppressed. The chemical makeup of antibiotics can also cause the body to react in many ways. Food-drug and drug-drug interactions are frequent problems in patients taking antibiotics. One of the more common food-drug interactions is that between milk or cheese and tetracycline. An example of an antibiotic-drug interaction is that between quinolone antibiotics and antacids.

Other important factors that are essential to the appropriate use of antibiotics are host-specific factors, or **host factors.** These are the particular factors that pertain to the infected patient and that can have an important bearing on the success or failure of antibiotic therapy. Some of these host factors are age, allergy history, organ function (kidneys and liver), pregnancy status, genetic characteristics, the site of infection, and host defenses.

Age-related host factors are those that apply to patients at either end of the age spectrum. For instance, infants and children may not be able to take certain antibiotics such as tetracyclines because of their effects on developing teeth or bones; quinolones may also affect bone development in children; and the sulfonamides may displace bilirubin from albumin and precipitate kernicterus in young patients. The aging process affects the function of various organ systems. As we age, there is a gradual decline in the function of such organs as the kidneys and liver, the organs responsible for eliminating and breaking down various antibiotics. Thus giving older patients antibiotics in doses appropriate only for younger patients could result in antibiotic toxicities.

If a patient has a history of an allergic reaction to an antibiotic, this plays an important role in the selection of the most appropriate antibiotic for that patient. Penicillins and sulfonamides are two broad categories of antibiotics that many persons have allergic or anaphylactic reactions to.

Pregnancy-related host factors are also important when it comes to selecting appropriate antibiotics, as several antibiotics can pass through the placenta to the fetus and cause harm to the developing fetus. Such drugs are called **teratogens,** and metronidazole, rifampin, and trimethoprim are examples of these agents. Their use in pregnant women can result in birth defects.

Many drugs, including certain antibiotics, depend on specific enzyme systems to break them down so that they can be eliminated. However, some patients have certain **genetic abnormalities** that may result in deficiencies of the enzymes needed by these systems, with the result that the antibiotic has abnormal effects. Two common examples of such genetic host factors are **glucose-6-phosphate dehydrogenase** (G6PD) **deficiency** and **slow acetylators** status. The administration of such antibiotics as sulfonamides, nitrofurantoin, pyrimethamine, and chloramphenicol to a person with G6PD deficiency will result in the hemolysis, or destruction, of red blood cells. A peripheral neuropathy will develop in a slow acetylator given isoniazid.

The **anatomic site of the infection** is another important host factor to consider when determining not only which antibiotic to use but also the dose, the route of administration, and the duration of therapy.

Consideration of these host factors helps ensure that the most appropriate antibiotic is selected for a particular patient. Appropriate assessment and routine monitoring of antibiotic therapy increase the likelihood that the antibiotic therapy is safe and effective.

Antibiotics

Antibiotics can be broken down into many broad categories based on their chemical structures. Some of the more common of these categories are the sulfonamides, penicillins, cephalosporins, macrolides, and quinolones. There are, however, many more such categories, ones such as the aminoglycosides, the tetracyclines, and other miscellaneous agents that do not easily fit into one of the broad categories. The characteristics that distinguish one class of agents from the next are the antibacterial spectrum, mechanism of action, potency, toxicity, and pharmacokinetic properties shared by the agents in that class.

SULFONAMIDES

Sulfonamides are a chemically related group of antibiotics that are all synthetic derivatives of sulfanilamide. They were one of the first group of drugs used as antibiotics, and some of the more commonly prescribed agents are sulfadiazine, sulfamethizole, sulfamethoxazole, and sulfisoxazole. Another sulfonamide, sulfasalazine, is used for other indications besides infections. Their antibiotic activity is the result of their ability to antagonize or inhibit an enzyme that is essential for the growth and proliferation of certain bacteria, and there are a wide range of organisms that the sulfonamide antibiotics are effective in combating. These antibiotics achieve very high concentrations in the kidneys, through which they are eliminated. Therefore they are primarily used in the treatment of urinary tract infections (UTIs). Sulfonamides are also used in the treatment of mild to moderate ulcerative colitis, active Crohn's disease, and rheumatoid arthritis. In addition, they may be combined with other antibiotics to increase their antibiotic potency.

Mechanism of Action

The sulfonamides do not actually destroy bacteria but inhibit their growth. For this reason they are considered **bacteriostatic antibiotics.** They inhibit the growth of susceptible bacteria by preventing the synthesis of a folic acid, a B-complex vitamin that is required for the proper synthesis of purines and nucleic acid. It is composed of a molecule of para-aminobenzoic acid (PABA), pteridine, and glutamic acid. Specifically, the sulfonamides compete (competitive inhibition) with the PABA for the enzyme that incorporates the PABA into the folic acid molecule during biosynthesis. Because the sulfonamides are capable of blocking a specific step in a biosynthetic pathway, they are also considered antimetabolites. However, those microorganisms that can utilize preformed folic acid are not affected by the sulfonamides.

As already mentioned, greater effectiveness of the sulfonamides' antibiotic potency is achieved by combining the sulfonamide agent sulfamethoxazole with trimethoprim (a nonsulfonamide). The resulting combination is called *co-trimoxazole*. Together the two antibiotics are capable of blocking two successive steps in the bacterial folic acid pathway. Unfortunately, however, many organisms once susceptible to the sulfonamides are now resistant to them.

Drug Effects

Only microorganisms that synthesize their own folic acid are inhibited by sulfonamides. Those animals and bacteria that are capable of utilizing folic acid precursors or preformed folic acid are not affected by them. Human cells can utilize preformed folic acid and are therefore not affected by sulfonamides.

Therapeutic Uses

The sulfonamides are used for the treatment of UTIs caused by susceptible strains *Enterobacter spp.*, *Escherichia coli*, *Klebsiella spp.*, *Proteus mirabilis*, *Proteus vulgaris*, and *Staphylococcus aureus*.

In addition, the sulfonamides are the drugs of choice for the treatment of nocardiosis; they are used as adjuncts in the treatment of malaria and toxoplasmosis and as alternative agents for the management of chlamydial infections and dermatitis herpetiformis. Following are the specific indications for the various sulfonamides: sulfapyridine is used for the treatment of dermatitis herpetiformis; sulfadiazine, sulfisoxazole, sulfamethoxazole, and triple sulfa are all used for the treatment of nocardiosis; and sulfasalazine is used to treat ulcerative colitis. Systemic antibacterial agents include sulfacytine, sulfadiazine, sulfamethiazole, sulfamethoxazole, sulfisoxazole, and triple sulfa.

Side Effects and Adverse Effects

The sulfonamides are capable of producing an array of significant side effects and adverse effects. The most common ones are listed in Table 36-1.

Interactions

The sulfonamides produce a fairly wide array of interactions when taken in conjunction with oral anticoagulants, PABA preparations, and urinary acidifiers.

Table 36-1	Sulfonamides: Common Adverse Effects
Body System	**Side/Adverse Effects**
Blood	Agranulocytosis, aplastic anemia, hemolytic anemia, thrombocytopenia
Skin	Epidermal necrolysis, exfoliative dermatitis, Stevens-Johnson syndrome, photosensitivity
Gastrointestinal	Nausea, vomiting, diarrhea, pancreatitis
Other	Convulsions, crystalluria, toxic nephrosis, headache, peripheral neuritis, urticaria

Laboratory Test Interactions

Sulfonamides can increase the serum levels of aspartate aminotransferase, acetyltransferase, and alkaline phosphatase.

Dosages

For recommended dosages of selected sulfonamides, see the dosages table on the following page.

DRUG PROFILES

The sulfonamides are classified as pregnancy category C agents and are contraindicated in patients with a known hypersensitivity to sulfonamides, in pregnant women at term, and in infants under 2 months of age.

⚓ SULFAMETHOXAZOLE

Sulfamethoxazole (Gantanol, Azo-Gantanol, Bactrim) is an intermediate-acting sulfonamide antibiotic. Because it is eliminated by means of the kidneys and reaches very high concentrations there, it is commonly used to treat UTIs caused by susceptible organisms. It is combined with phenazopyridine in a preparation known as Azo-Gantanol. The phenazopyridine is an analgesic-anesthetic that affects the mucosa of the urinary tract. Together the two agents not only inhibit susceptible bacteria in UTIs but also relieve any pain

DOSAGES

SELECTED SULFONAMIDE AGENTS

AGENT	PHARMACOLOGIC CLASS	DOSAGE RANGE	PURPOSE
⚓Sulfamethoxazole (Gantanol, Azo-Gantanol, Bactrim)	Sulfonamide	*Pediatric >2 mo* PO: 50-60 mg/kg loading dose, followed by 25-30 mg/kg q12h; do not exceed 75 mg/kg/day. *Adult* PO: 2 g loading dose, followed by 1-2 g 2-3 times/day The dose for Azo-Gantanol is the same. Do not exceed 2 days of treatment.	Nocardiosis, UTIs, adjunct for toxoplasmosis
Sulfisoxazole (Gantrisin, Azogantrisin, Pediazole)	Sulfonamide	*Pediatric >2 mo* PO: 75 mg/kg loading dose, followed by 150 mg/kg/day in 4-6 doses *Adult* PO: 2-4 g loading dose, followed by 4-8 g/day in 4-6 doses	Nocardosis, UTIs, adjunct for toxoplasmosis

associated with the infection. Sulfamethoxazole by itself comes as a 500-mg/5 ml oral suspension and a 500-mg tablet. In combination with phenazopyridine it comes as a film-coated tablet containing 500 mg of sulfamethoxazole and 100 mg of phenazopyridine.

Sulfamethoxazole is also combined with the antimetabolite trimethoprim in a fixed combination containing a 5:1 ratio of sulfamethoxazole to trimethoprim. As explained earlier, this combination of agents sequentially inhibits two steps in the folic acid pathway, giving it antibacterial synergism. It is commonly used in the treatment of UTIs caused by susceptible bacteria, *Pneumocystis carinii* pneumonia, ear infections (otitis media), bronchitis, gonorrhea, and many other infectious conditions. It is also used for prophylaxis in HIV-infected children. This fixed combination of sulfamethoxazole and trimethoprim is available as a 40-mg/5 ml oral suspension and in two strengths of oral tablets containing 80 and 400 mg and 180 and 800 mg of trimethoprim and sulfamethoxazole, respectively. It is also available in a fixed-combination agent containing 16 mg/ml of trimethoprim and 80 mg/ml of sulfamethoxazole to be given as an intravenous injection. Recommended dosages of the sulfamethoxazole products are listed in the dosages table above. Pregnancy category C.

✸ PHARMACOKINETICS

HALF-LIFE	ONSET	PEAK	DURATION
7-12 hr	Variable	2-4 hr (plasma)	Up to 12 hr

SULFISOXAZOLE

Sulfisoxazole (Gantrisin, Azogantrisin, Pediazole) is a short-acting sulfonamide antibiotic that is primarily used for its ability to effectively inhibit organisms in the urinary tract. It also is available as a fixed-combination product containing either phenazopyridine (azogantrisin) or erythromycin (Pediazole). It has good activity against those organisms that commonly cause ear infections (otitis media) in small children, so it is also available in an oral suspension for this purpose.

Unlike sulfamethoxazole, it is not available as a parenteral agent. It comes as a 500-mg tablet (Gantrisin); as a fixed-combination product containing 500 mg of sulfisoxazole and 50 mg of phenazopyridine (Azo-Gantrisin); as a 500-mg/5 ml oral solution and oral suspension; and as a fixed-combination product containing 600 mg of sulfisoxazole and 200 mg of erythromycin per 5 ml of the inert substance (Pediazole, E.S.P., or Eryzole). Pregnancy category C.

✸ PHARMACOKINETICS

HALF-LIFE	ONSET	PEAK	DURATION
4.6-7.8 hr	Variable	1-4 hr (plasma)	4-6 hr

PENICILLINS

The penicillins are a very large group of chemically related antibiotics that are derived from a fungus, or mold, often seen on bread or fruit. The penicillins may also be called **beta-lactams,** a term which refers to their chemical structure. The penicillins can be divided into four groups based on their structure and the bacteria they kill. These four groups comprise the natural penicillins, the penicillinase-resistant penicillins, the aminopenicillins, and the extended-spectrum penicillins. Examples of antibiotics in each group and a brief description of their characteristics are given in the box below.

The penicillins were first introduced onto the market in the early 1940s, and to this day they have remained very effective and safe antibiotics. They are bactericidal and can kill a wide variety of gram-positive and some gram-negative bacteria. The penicillins work by inhibiting bacterial cell wall synthesis, which they accomplish by interfering with the biosynthesis of structural substances needed in the cell walls of bacteria. However, bacteria have acquired the capacity to produce enzymes capable of destroying penicillins. These enzymes are called beta-lactamases, and they can destroy the structural component of the penicillin called the *beta-lactam ring*. This was a problem until chemicals were synthesized that inhibit these enzymes. Three of these beta-lactamase inhibitors are clavulanic acid, tazobactam, and sulbactam. By binding with the beta-lactamase they prevent the enzyme from breaking down the penicillin. Examples of currently available penicillin–beta-lactamase inhibitor combinations are:

- Ampicillin + sulbactam = Unasyn
- Amoxicillin + clavulanic acid = Augmentin
- Ticarcillin + clavulanic acid = Timentin
- Piperacillin + tazobactam = Zosyn

Mechanism of Action

The mechanism of action of the penicillins involves several steps that together result in the inhibition of bacterial cell wall synthesis. In the first step, the penicillins slide through the bacteria's cell walls to get to their site of action. However, some penicillins are too large to pass through these openings in the cell walls, and because they cannot get to their site of action, they cannot kill the bacteria. On the other hand, some bacteria can make the openings in their cell walls smaller so that the penicillin cannot get through to kill them. The penicillin that does gain entry into the bacteria must then find the appropriate binding site, in this case an enzyme called the penicillin-binding protein. By binding to this protein the penicillin interferes with the normal cell wall synthesis, causing the formation of defective cell walls that are unstable and easily break down. Bacteria death usually results from lysis.

Drug Effects

Penicillins only inhibit the cell wall synthesis of bacteria, not that of other cells in the body. Therefore the drug effects of penicillins are limited to the killing of bacteria. In humans this has the therapeutic effect of destroying invading bacteria that are responsible for infections.

Therapeutic Uses

The penicillins are indicated for the prevention and treatment of infections caused by susceptible bacteria. The microorganisms most commonly destroyed by penicillins are gram-positive bacteria, and this includes the *Streptococcus, Enterococcus*, and *Staphylococcus* species. Most penicillins have little if any ability to kill gram-negative bacteria, though some of the extended-spectrum penicillins can.

Penicillins: Classification

CLASS	ANTIBIOTICS	DESCRIPTION
Natural penicillins	penicillin G, penicillin V	Various natural penicillins have been produced by changing different side chains; penicillin exists as F, G, N, O, V, and X; only penicillin G and V are currently used clinically.
Penicillinase-resistant penicillins	Cloxacillin, dicloxacillin, methicillin, nafcillin, oxacillin	Stable against hydrolysis by most staphylococcal penicillinases (enzymes which normally break down the natural penicillins).
Aminopenicillins	Amoxicillin, ampicillin, bacampicillin	Have an amino group attached to their penicillin nucleus that enhances their activity against gram-negative bacteria compared with natural penicillins.
Extended-spectrum penicillins	Piperacillin, ticarcillin, carbenicillin, mezlocillin	Have wider spectra of activity than that of all the above types of penicillins.

Side Effects and Adverse Effects

The penicillins are generally well tolerated and associated with very few adverse effects. As with many drugs, the most common ones are gastrointestinal in nature. Their most common side effects and adverse effects are listed in Table 36-2.

Interactions

There are many drugs that interact with the penicillins; some have positive effects, and other have harmful effects. The most common and clinically significant drug interactions associated with penicillin use are listed in Table 36-3.

Dosages

For dosage information on selected penicillins, see the dosages table on the following page.

Table 36-2	Penicillins: Common Adverse Effects
BODY SYSTEM	**SIDE/ADVERSE EFFECTS**
Hematologic	Anemia, increased bleeding time, bone marrow depression, granulocytopenia
Gastrointestinal	Nausea, vomiting, diarrhea, increased liver function (SGOT and SGPT), abdominal pain, colitis
Central nervous system	Lethargy, hallucinations, anxiety, depression, twitching, coma, convulsions
Metabolic	Hyperkalemia, hypokalemia, alkalosis
Other	Taste alterations, sore mouth, dark, discolored, or sore tongue

DRUG PROFILES

The penicillins are classified as pregnancy category B agents. They are very safe antibiotics and are only contraindicated in patients with a hypersensitivity to them. Because of their relatively safe side effect profile, there are otherwise very few contraindications to their use.

Natural Penicillins

⚓ PENICILLIN G

Penicillin G (benzathine; potassium, sodium, and procaine salt forms) is one of the two currently available natural penicillins. Its four salt forms allow it to be given by several different routes. Penicillin G benzathine is the long-acting, depot, or repository, form of penicillin G. It is given by intramuscular injection and is expected to work over the course of several days. Penicillin G potassium and penicillin G sodium are commonly administered intravenously for the treatment of life-threatening illnesses such as septicemia, meningitis, pericarditis, or severe pneumonia. They are generally expressed in terms of units rather than weight. Like penicillin G benzathine, Penicillin G procaine is also a long-acting, depot, or repository, form of penicillin G. Unlike penicillin G benzathine, however, penicillin G procaine is generally not considered a suitable agent for the management of severe infections but should be used as a follow-up form of penicillin G benzathine in the treatment of less severe infections. All forms of penicillin G are given parenterally, either intravenously or intramuscularly.

Table 36-3	Penicillins: Drug Interactions	
DRUG	**MECHANISM**	**RESULT**
Aminoglycosides and clavulanic acid	Additive	More effective killing of bacteria
Rifampin	Inhibition	May inhibit the killing activity of penicillins
Probenecid	Competes for elimination	Prolongs the effects of penicillins
NSAIDs	Compete for protein binding	More free and active penicillin
Oral contraceptives	Decrease effectiveness	May decrease efficacy of the contraceptive
Warfarin	Increases metabolism	Penicillins may increase metabolism of warfarin, decreasing its effects

DOSAGES

SELECTED PENICILLINS

AGENT	PHARMACOLOGIC CLASS	DOSAGE RANGE	PURPOSE
⚓Penicillin G benzathine	Repository penicillin	*Neonates* IM: 50,000 U/kg once *Pediatric <27 kg* IM: 300,000-600,000 U once >27 kg: IM: 900,000-1.2 million U once *Adults* IM: 1.2 million U once	Antiinfective
⚓Penicillin G procaine	Repository penicillin	*Neonates* IM: 50,000 U/kg once daily *Adult/Pediatric* 600,000-1.2 million U 1-2 times/day do not exceed 4.8 million U/day.	Antiinfective
⚓Penicillin G potassium	Penicillin	*Infants* IM/IV: 300,000 U/kg bid *Pediatric* IM/IV: 300,000-1.2 million U/day; up to 10 million U may be required. *Adult* IM/IV: 300,000-8 million U/day; up to 60 million U may be given.	Antiinfective
Penicillin V potassium (Pen-Vee, Beepen-VK, V-Cillin, Ledercillin VK, and Veetids)	Acid-stable penicillin	*Pediatric <12 y/o* PO: 15-50 mg/kg/day in 3-6 doses *Adult* PO: 250-500 mg 3-4 times/day	Antiinfective
Methicillin (Staphcillin)	Penicillinase-resistant penicillin	*Pediatric* IM: 25 mg/kg q6h *Adult* IM: 1 g q4 or 6h IV: 1 g q6h	Penicillinase-producing staph infections
⚓Ampicillin (anhydrous, trihydrate, and sodium salt form)	Aminopenicillin	*Pediatric <20 kg* PO: 50-100 mg/kg divided q6-8h *Pediatric >20 kg* PO: 250-500 mg qid IM/IV: 25-50 mg/kg divided *Adult* PO: 250-500 mg qid IM/IV: 250-500 mg qid	Antiinfective
Ticarcillin disodium (Ticar)	Extended-spectrum penicillin	*Neonatal <2000 g* IM/IV: 75 mg/kg/12 hr for first 7 days; after 7 days of age, 75 mg/kg/8 hr. *Neonatal >2000 g* IM/IV: 75 mg/kg/8 hr for first 7 days; after 7 days of age, 100 mg/kg/8 hr. *Pediatric* *<40 kg* IM/IV: 50-100 mg/kg/day divided *Adult/Pediatric >40 kg* IM/IV: 150-300 mg/kg/day divided	Antiinfective

Penicillin G and its many salt forms are pregnancy category C agents and are contraindicated in patients who are hypersensitive to penicillins as well as in neonates. Penicillin G comes in many different dosages forms. Dosage recommendations are given in the dosages table on the previous page.

⬡ PHARMACOKINETICS

HALF-LIFE	ONSET	PEAK	DURATION
IM: 30-60 min	Variable	15-30 min	Variable

PENICILLIN V POTASSIUM

Penicillin V potassium (Pen-Vee K, Beepen-VK, V-Cillin K, Ledercillin VK, Veetids) is the other of the two currently available natural penicillins, and both are effective against a very similar spectrum of bacteria. Unlike penicillin G, however, it is only available in oral preparations. It is also contraindicated in patients hypersensitive to it and in newborns, and it is also a pregnancy category C agent. It comes as a 125- and 250-mg/5 ml oral solution; 250- and 500-mg tablets; and 125-, 250-, and 500-mg film-coated tablets. Commonly recommended dosages are given in the dosages table on the previous page.

⬡ PHARMACOKINETICS

HALF-LIFE	ONSET	PEAK	DURATION
30 min	Variable	30-60 min (plasma)	4-6 hr

Penicillinase-Resistant Penicillins
METHICILLIN

Methicillin (Staphcillin) is one of the five currently available penicillinase-resistant penicillins, the other four being cloxacillin, dicloxacillin, nafcillin, and oxacillin. The penicillinase-resistant penicillins are able to resist the breakdown of the penicillin-destroying enzyme (penicillinase) commonly produced by bacteria such as staphylococci. They accomplish this by attaching a large, bulky side chain around the beta-lactam ring that hinders the penicillinase and prevents it from attacking the beta-lactam ring, thus destroying the antibiotic. There are, however, certain strains of staphylococci, specifically *Staphylococcus aureus*, that are methicillin resistant. This bacteria can resist the actions of methicillin and therefore survive. Methicillin has the same contraindications and pregnancy rating as the natural penicillins. It is only available parenterally as a 1-, 4-, 6-, and 10-gm injection. Commonly recommended dosages are given in the dosages table on the previous page.

⬡ PHARMACOKINETICS

HALF-LIFE	ONSET	PEAK	DURATION
20-30 min	Variable	30-60 min	6 hr

Aminopenicillins

There are three aminopenicillins—amoxicillin, ampicillin, and bacampicillin. Because of the presence of a free amino group on the penicillin nucleus, the amino penicillins have enhanced activity against gram-negative bacteria, against which the natural and penicillinase-resistant penicillins are relatively ineffective. Amoxicillin is an analogue of ampicillin, and bacampicillin is a prodrug of ampicillin. Bacampicillin has no antibacterial activity until hydrolyzed to ampicillin in the body. The aminopenicillins have the same contraindications and pregnancy ratings (B) as the other penicillins.

⚓ AMPICILLIN

Ampicillin is the prototypical aminopenicillin, and it differs from penicillin G only in that it has the amino group on the penicillin nucleus. It is available in three different salt forms—anhydrous, trihydrate, and sodium. Like penicillin G, each salt form allows it to be administered by a different route. Ampicillin anhydrous and trihydrate are both administered orally, and ampicillin sodium is given parenterally. Anhydrous ampicillin (Omnipen) is available as 250- and 500-mg capsules and as a 250-mg/5 ml suspension. Trihydrate ampicillin (Polycillin, Principen, and Totacillin) is available as 250- and 500-mg capsules and 125-, 250-, and 500-mg/5 ml suspensions. Sodium ampicillin (Ampicillin sodium, Omnipen-N, and Totacillin-N) is available as 125-, 250-, 500-,1000-, 2000-, and 10,000-mg vials for injection. Commonly recommended dosages are given in the dosages table on the previous page.

⬡ PHARMACOKINETICS

HALF-LIFE	ONSET	PEAK	DURATION
PO: 0.7-1.4 hr	Variable	1-2 hr (serum)	4-6 hr

Extended-Spectrum Penicillins

By making a few changes in the basic penicillin structure, agents were produced with a wider spectra of activity than that possessed by either of the other two classes of semisynthetic penicillins—the penicillinase-resistant penicillins and the aminopenicillins—or by the natural penicillins. There are four of these extended-spectrum penicillins currently available—carbenicillin, piperacillin, ticarcillin, and mezlocillin, and these can be broken down into two main classes, as determined by their structure. These are:

- Carboxypenicillins = carbenicillin and ticarcillin
- Acylaminopenicillins = piperacillin and mezlocillin

The **carboxypenicillins** have a carboxylic acid group attached to the basic penicillin nucleus, which has endowed it with new activity against some bacteria that the other classes of penicillins cannot kill, bacteria such as the *Pseudomonas* spp., as well as with stability against the beta-lactams produced by *Proteus* organisms. The **acylaminopenicillins** have a basic group on one of the side chains off the main penicillin nucleus, giving them even greater activity against *Pseudomonas* spp. and Enterobacteriaceae than the carboxypenicillins. Carbenicillin differs structurally from ampicillin only in the substitution of a carboxy group for an amino group on the penicillin nucleus. Ticarcillin is an analogue of carbenicillin with a *B-thienyl* group, and mezlocillin is an ampicillin derivative that contains a ureido group on the penicillin nucleus. Piperacillin is a piperazine derivative of ampicillin. The end-result of all this is that small changes in the natural penicillin structure have translated into big changes in activity against new bacteria.

All the extended-spectrum penicillins are given parenterally (IV), except for carbenicillin, which is only given orally. The contraindications to their use are the same as those of the other penicillins, and they are also all pregnancy category C agents. Both ticarcillin and piperacillin come in fixed-combination products that include beta-lactamase inhibitors. The ticarcillin fixed-combination product (Timentin) includes clavulanate potassium. Piperacillin is combined with tazobactam in a product called Zosyn. Common dosage recommendations for ticarcillin (Ticar) are listed in the dosages table on p. 550.

CEPHALOSPORINS

The cephalosporins are semisynthetic antibiotic derivatives of cephalosporin C, a substance produced by a fungus but synthetically altered to produce an antibiotic. These chemically altered derivatives of this fungus are broadly referred to as cephalosporins, and they are structurally and pharmacologically related to the penicillins. Like the penicillins, the cephalosporins are also bactericidal and work by interfering with bacterial cell wall synthesis. They also bind to similar PBPs inside bacteria.

Cephalosporins have a broad spectrum of bacteria they can destroy, and this is directly related to the chemical changes that have been made to their basic cephalosporin structure. Broadly they are active against many gram-positive bacteria, some gram-negative bacteria, and some anaerobic bacteria. They are active against fungi and viruses. The cephalosporins have thus far been divided into three generations of agents according to the differences in their antimicrobial activity. Each generation has certain chemical similarities and thus similar spectrums of bacteria that they kill. In general, the first-generation cephalosporins have the best gram-positive coverage but poor gram-negative coverage. On the other hand, the third-generation cephalosporins have the best gram-negative coverage but poor gram-positive coverage. The currently available parenteral and oral cephalosporin antibiotics are listed in the box on the next page.

The safety profiles, contraindications, and pregnancy ratings of the cephalosporins are very similar to those of the penicillins. The most frequently reported side effects include mild diarrhea, abdominal cramps or distress, rash, pruritus, redness, and edema. Because cephalosporins are chemically very similar to penicillins, a person who has had an allergic reaction to penicillin may also have an allergic reaction to a cephalosporin. This is referred to as cross-sensitivity. Various investigators have observed that the incidence of cross-sensitivity between penicillins and cephalosporins is between 1% and 18%. However, only those patients who have had a serious anaphylactic reaction to penicillin should not be given cephalosporins. As a class the cephalosporins are very safe and effective antibi-

❦ PHARMACOKINETICS

Carbenicillin indanyl sodium (Geocillin): 382-mg film-coated tablets			
HALF-LIFE	**ONSET**	**PEAK**	**DURATION**
0.8-1 hr	Variable	0.5-2 hr*	6 hr

Mezlocillin sodium (Mezlin): 1-, 2-, 3-, 4-, and 20-g vials for injection			
HALF-LIFE	**ONSET**	**PEAK**	**DURATION**
0.7-1.3 hr	Variable	IM: 49-90 min*	Variable

Piperacillin sodium (Pipracil): 2-, 3-, 4-, and 40-g vials for injection			
HALF-LIFE	**ONSET**	**PEAK**	**DURATION**
0.6-1.3 hr	Variable	IM: 0.5 hr*	Variable

Ticarcillin disodium (Ticar): 1-, 3-, 6-, and 20-gm vials for injection			
HALF-LIFE	**ONSET**	**PEAK**	**DURATION**
0.9-1.3 hr	Variable	IM: 0.5-1 hr*	Variable

*Serum.

Cephalosporins: Parenteral and Oral Preparations

FIRST GENERATION		SECOND GENERATION		THIRD GENERATION	
IV	**PO**	**IV**	**PO**	**IV**	**PO**
⚓Cefazolin	Cefadroxil	Cefamandole	Cefaclor	Cefoperazone	Cefixime
Cephalothin	Cephalexin	Cefoxitin	Cefuroxime	Cefotaxime	Cefpodoxime proxetil
Cephradine	Cephradine	Cefuroxime	Cefprozil	Ceftizoxime	
Cephapirin		Cefonicid		Ceftriaxone	
		Ceforanide		Ceftazidime	
		Cefmetazole		Moxalactam	
		Cefotetan			

otics, and they should not be unnecessarily avoided out of overly cautious concern about possible cross-sensitivity.

The penicillins and the cephalosporins are practically identical in their mechanism of action, drug effects, therapeutic effects, side effects and adverse effects, and drug interactions. For that reason this information is not repeated for the cephalosporins and the reader is referred to the pertinent discussion in the section on the penicillin agents. Cephalosporins of all generations are very safe agents that are categorized as pregnancy category B drugs. They are contraindicated in patients who have shown a hypersensitivity to them and in infants younger than 1 month old. The prototypical first-, second-, and third-generation cephalosporins are described in the drug profiles.

Dosages

For the recommended dosages of selected cephalosporin agents, see the dosages table on p. 554.

*D*RUG *P*ROFILES

First-Generation Cephalosporins

First-generation cephalosporins are usually active against gram-positive bacteria and have limited activity against gram-negative bacteria. They are available both in parenteral and oral forms. One of the most frequently used parenteral first-generation cephalosporins is cefazolin; cephalexin is a very frequently used oral first-generation cephalosporin.

⚓ CEFAZOLIN SODIUM

Cefazolin (Ancef, Kefzol) is a prototypical first-generation cephalosporin. As with all the first-generation cephalosporins, it has excellent coverage against gram-positive bacteria but limited coverage against gram-negative bacteria. It is only available in a parenteral formulation that comes as 500- and 1000-mg vials for IM or IV injection. Commonly recommended dosages are given in the dosages table on the next page.

✺ PHARMACOKINETICS

HALF-LIFE	ONSET	PEAK	DURATION
1.2-2.2 hr	Variable	1-2 hr	Variable

CEPHALEXIN

Cephalexin (Keflex, Keftab) is a prototypical oral first-generation cephalosporin. It also has excellent coverage against gram-positive bacteria but limited coverage against gram-negative bacteria. It is only available in oral formulations—250- and 500-mg capsules (Keflex pulvules); a 125– and 250–mg/5 ml oral suspension; 250-mg film-coated tablets (Keflex); and 250- and 500-mg tablets (Keftab). Commonly recommended dosages can be found in the dosages table on the next page.

✺ PHARMACOKINETICS

HALF-LIFE	ONSET	PEAK	DURATION
0.5-1.2 hr	Variable	1 hr	6-12 hr

Second-Generation Cephalosporins

The second-generation cephalosporins have similar coverage against gram-positive organisms as the first-generation cephalosporins but enhanced gram-

DOSAGES

SELECTED CEPHALOSPORIN AGENTS

AGENT	PHARMACOLOGIC CLASS	DOSAGE RANGE	PURPOSE
⚓Cefazolin sodium (Ancef, Kefzol)	1st-generation cephalosporin	*Pediatric* IM/IV: 25-50 mg/kg/day in 3-4 doses; doses up to 100 mg/kg/day be required. *Adult* IM/IV: 250 mg–1 gm q8-12h; doses up to 1.5 g q6h may be required.	Antiinfective
Cephalexin (Keflex, Keftab)	1st-generation cephalosporin	*Pediatric* PO: 25-50 mg/kg/day divided; doses up to 100 mg/kg/day may be required *Adult* PO: 1-4 g/day divided	Antiinfective
⚓Cefoxitin (Mefoxin)	2nd-generation cephalosporin	*Pediatric* IM/IV: 80-160 mg/kg/day in 4-6 equal doses *Adult* IM/IV: 1-3 g q4-8h	Antiinfective
Cefuroxime (Ceftin, Kefurox, Zinacef)	2nd-generation cephalosporin	*Pediatric >3 mo* IM/IV: 50-100 mg/kg/day in 3-4 doses *Adult* IM/IV: 0.75-1.5 g q6-8h	Antiinfective
Cefixime (Suprax)	3rd-generation cephalosporin	*Pediatric* PO: 8 mg/kg/day as a single dose or 4 mg/kg q12h *Adult* PO: 400 mg/day as a single dose or 200 mg q12h	Antiinfective
Ceftriaxone (Rocephin)	3rd-generation cephalosporin	*Pediatric* IM/IV: 50-75 mg/kg/day divided q12h *Adult* IM/IV: 1-4 g/day as a single dose or divided	Antiinfective
⚓Ceftazidime (Ceptaz, Fortaz, Tazidime, Tazicef)	3rd-generation cephalosporin	*Neonate* IV: 30 mg/kg q12h *Infants/Children* IV: 30-50 mg/kg q8h *Adult* IV: 2 g q8-12h	Antiinfective

negative coverage. They include both parenteral and oral formulations. Like the first-generation agents, the second-generation cephalosporins are also excellent prophylactic antibiotics. The qualities that make them excellent prophylactic agents are their favorable safety profile, the broad range of organisms they can kill, and their relatively low cost. Currently there are seven parenteral second-generation cephalosporins: cefamandole, cefoxitin, cefuroxime, cefonicid, ceforanide, cefmetazole, and cefotetan, and three oral agents: cefaclor, cefuroxime axetil, and cefprozil. These agents differ slightly with regard to their antibacterial coverage. Cefoxitin and cefotetan may have better coverage against various anaerobic bacteria such as *Bacteroides fragilis, Peptostreptococcus* spp., and *Clostridium* spp. than the other agents in this class. Three of the second-generation agents (cefoxitin, cefmetazole, and cefotetan) are structurally different from the other agents in the class by having a methoxy group rather than a hydrogen group on the beta-lactam ring of the cephalosporin nucleus. They are called cephamycins. Their unique structure enables them to kill certain bacteria that the other second-generation agents cannot.

⚕ CEFOXITIN

Cefoxitin (Mefoxin) is a parenteral second-generation cephalosporin that because of its unique structure is a cephamycin. By being a second-generation cephalosporin it has excellent gram-positive coverage and better gram-negative coverage than the first-generation agents. Because it is a cephamycin, it can kill anaerobic bacteria. Cefoxitin has been used extensively as a prophylactic antibiotic in patients undergoing such surgical procedures as abdominal or colorectal operations because it can kill the bacteria that usually reside in these areas—gram-positive and gram-negative bacteria and anaerobes. Like the other cephalosporins, it is very safe and is rated as a pregnancy category B agent. Its contraindications are the same as those of the other cephalosporins. Cefoxitin is only available in parenteral preparations: 1-, 2-, and 10-gm vials for injection and a 20- and 40-mg/ml frozen powder for injection. Commonly recommended dosages can be found in the dosages table on the previous page.

🐝 PHARMACOKINETICS

HALF-LIFE	ONSET	PEAK	DURATION
30-60 min	Variable	20-30 min	Variable

CEFUROXIME

Cefuroxime sodium (Kefurox, Zinacef) is the parenteral form of this second-generation cephalosporin. The oral form is a different salt of cefuroxime, cefuroxime axetil (Ceftin). Cefuroxime is a very versatile second-generation cephalosporin. It is also highly used as a prophylactic antibiotic for various surgical procedures. It has more activity against gram-negative bacteria than the first-generation cephalosporins but a narrower spectrum of activity against gram-negative bacteria than the third-generation cephalosporins. It differs from the cephamycins such as cefoxitin in that it does not kill anaerobic bacteria. Cefuroxime axetil is a prodrug. It has little antibacterial activity until it is hydrolyzed in the liver to its active form. It is available as 125-, 250-, and 500-mg film-coated tablets. Ce-

furoxime sodium is available as 750-mg, 1.5-gm, and 7.5-gm vials for injection. Commonly recommended dosages can be found in the dosages table on the previous page.

🐝 PHARMACOKINETICS

HALF-LIFE	ONSET	PEAK	DURATION
1.2 hr	Variable	2.2-3 hr	6-8 hr

Third-Generation Cephalosporins

The third-generation cephalosporins (cefoperazone, cefotaxime, ceftizoxime, ceftriaxone, ceftazidime, and cefixime) are the most potent of the three generations of cephalosporins in fighting gram-negative bacteria, but they generally have less activity than the first- and second-generation agents when it comes to destroying gram-positive bacteria. Slight changes in the chemical structure have endowed specific agents with certain advantages over the others.

Because of specific changes in their basic cephalosporin structure, cefoperazone and ceftazidime have significant activity against *Pseudomonas* spp. In fact, these two third-generation agents have the best activity of all the cephalosporins against this difficult-to-treat gram-negative bacteria. Cefoperazone differs from ceftazidime in that it is principally excreted in the bile rather than the kidneys, as ceftazidime is. Ceftriaxone is an extremely long acting third-generation agent that can be given only once a day in the treatment of most infections. It also has the unique characteristic of being able to pass easily through the blood-brain barrier. For this reason, it is one of the few cephalosporins that is indicated for the treatment of meningitis, an infection of the meninges of the brain. Cefixime is the only third-generation cephalosporin that comes as an oral preparation. All the other third-generation agents are only available in parenteral forms.

CEFIXIME

Structurally cefixime (Suprax) is similar to cefotaxime, ceftizoxime, and ceftriaxone, but it differs from these three agents in that one aspect of its structure allows for better gastrointestinal absorption. It has better activity against gram-negative bacteria than other oral cephalosporins such as cefaclor, cefuroxime axetil, or cefprozil, but its gram-negative activity is less than that of many of the other parenterally administered third-generation cephalosporins, especially against Enterobacteriaceae such as *Enterobacter* and *Pseudomonas* spp. Cefixime is a prescription-only drug that has the same pregnancy rating and contraindications as the other cephalosporins. Cefixime comes as a 100–mg/5 ml oral suspension and as 200- and 400-mg film-coated tablets. Commonly recommended dosages can be found in the dosages table on p. 554.

⬡ PHARMACOKINETICS

HALF-LIFE	ONSET	PEAK	DURATION
2.4-4 hr	Variable	3-4.4 hr	12 hr

CEFTRIAXONE

Ceftriaxone (Rocephin) is a parenterally administered third-generation cephalosporin that differs from the other agents in that it has a very long half-life that allows it to be given once a day. Structurally it resembles other third-generation agents such as cefotaxime and ceftizoxime, but it has an acidic enol group that distinguishes it from these other agents. This is believed to be responsible for the long serum half-life of the drug. Ceftriaxone's spectrum of activity is similar to that of the other third-generation agents cefotaxime, ceftazidime, and ceftizoxime. It can be given both intravenously and intramuscularly. In some cases of infections one IM injection can eradicate the infection. Ceftriaxone is 93% to 96% bound to plasma protein, an amount higher than that of many of the other cephalosporins. It can also easily pass through the meninges and diffuse into the cerebrospinal fluid, making it an excellent agent for the treatment of CNS infections. Ceftriaxone is available as an injection that can be given either IM or IV. It comes as 250-mg, 500-mg, 1-gm, 2-gm, and 10-gm vials. Commonly recommended dosages can be found in the dosages table on p. 554.

⬡ PHARMACOKINETICS

HALF-LIFE	ONSET	PEAK	DURATION
4.3-8.7 hr	Variable	IM: 2-4 hr	6-8 hr

⚓ CEFTAZIDIME

Ceftazidime (Ceptaz, Fortaz, Tazidime, Tazicef) is a parenterally administered third-generation cephalosporin with excellent coverage against difficult-to-treat gram-negative bacteria such as *Pseudomonas* spp. It differs from its closest third-generation relative cefoperazone in that it is eliminated renally as opposed to by the biliary route. It is the third-generation cephalosporin of choice for many indications because of its excellent spectrum of activity and safety profile. It can be given either IM or IV and to children as well as adults. It is available as 500-mg, 1-gm, 2-gm, 6-gm, and 10-gm vials for injection. Ceptaz was created so that the amount of gas produced when it is reconstituted is decreased. The gas produced can be so great that it

expels the needle directly out of the vial. Commonly recommended dosages are given in the dosages table on p. 554.

⬡ PHARMACOKINETICS

HALF-LIFE	ONSET	PEAK	DURATION
2 hr	Variable	IM: 1 hr	8-12 hr

TETRACYCLINES

The tetracyclines are a small chemically related group of five antibiotics, three of which are naturally occurring and two of which are semisynthetic. They are derivatives of *Streptomyces* organisms. The tetracyclines can only inhibit the growth of bacteria; they cannot kill bacteria. Therefore they are considered *bacteriostatic.* The three naturally occurring tetracyclines are demeclocycline, oxytetracycline, and tetracycline. The two semisynthetic tetracyclines are doxycycline and minocycline. The available tetracycline antibiotics and a brief description of them is given in the box below.

The tetracyclines are chemically and pharmacologically similar. The most significant chemical characteristic of these agents is their ability to bind (chelate) to divalent (Ca^{2+}, Mg^{2+}) and trivalent metallic (Al^{3+}) ions to form insoluble complexes. Therefore their coadministration with milk, antacids, or iron salts causes a considerable reduction in the oral absorption of the tetracycline. In addition, their strong affinity for calcium usually precludes their use in pediatric patients younger than 8 years of age, pregnant women, and nursing mothers (tetracyclines are present in breast milk).

The tetracyclines primarily differ in their:
- Oral absorption rates: all are adequately absorbed, but doxycycline and minocycline are absorbed the most.
- Body tissue penetration: doxycycline and minocy-

Available Tetracycline Antibiotics

TETRACYCLINE PRODUCT	DESCRIPTION
Natural tetracyclines	
Demeclocycline Oxytetracycline Tetracycline	Are all chemically derived from *Streptomyces* spp. by a fermentation process.
Semisynthetic Tetracyclines	
Doxycycline	Chemical derivative of oxytetracycline.
Minocycline	Chemical derivative of tetracycline.

cline possess the best penetration potential (brain and CSF).

■ Half-life and resulting dosage schedule: see the dosages table on p. 558 and pharmacokinetics information in the drug profiles section.

Mechanism of Action

Tetracyclines work by inhibiting protein synthesis in susceptible bacteria. For this synthesis to occur, transfer RNA must bind to the messenger RNA ribosome. The tetracyclines obstruct this synthesis by binding to that portion of the ribosome called the *30S subunit.* This in turn shuts down many of the bacteria's essential functions, ones such as growth and repair, so that eventually the bacteria stops growing and dies.

Drug Effects

Tetracyclines are used primarily for their antibiotic effects. They inhibit the growth of and kill a very wide range of *Rickettsia, Chlamydia,* and *Mycoplasma* organisms, as well as a variety of gram-negative and gram-positive bacteria. They are also useful in the treatment of spirochetal infections such as syphilis and Lyme disease. Demeclocycline possesses a unique drug effect in that it inhibits the action of antidiuretic hormone, making it useful in the treatment of the syndrome of inappropriate antidiuretic hormone (SIADH). Another drug effect of the tetracyclines is their ability to cause inflammation that results in fibrosis in the lungs. This is a useful property in patients with pleural or pericardial effusions caused by metastatic tumors, thoracentesis, or thoracastomy tubes because when instilled into the pleural space of the lungs, they cause scar tissue to form, thereby reducing the fluid accumulation.

Therapeutic Uses

The tetracyclines have a wide range of activity and as a class have essentially the same antimicrobial spectrum. They inhibit the growth of many gram-negative and gram-positive organisms and even some protozoa. They are considered the drugs of choice for the treatment of the following infections caused by susceptible organisms:

■ *Chlamydia:* lymphogranuloma venereum, psittacosis, and nonspecific endocervical, rectal, and urethral infections.
■ *Mycoplasma: Mycoplasma* pneumonia
■ *Rickettsia:* Q fever, rickettsial pox, Rocky Mountain spotted fever, scrub typhus, typhus.
■ *Other Bacteria:* acne control, brucellosis, chan-

croid, cholera, granuloma inguinale, shigellosis, and spirochetal relapsing fever. In addition, it is used for the treatment of Lyme disease and as part of the treatment regimen for *Helicobacter pylori* infections associated with peptic ulcer disease. It is also used as an alternative agent in penicillin-allergic patients for treatment of gonorrhea and syphilis.

■ *Protozoa:* balantidiasis.

Besides these antibiotic-related indications, as already noted, demeclocycline is also used to treat SIADH as well as pleural and pericardial effusions.

Side Effects and Adverse Effects

The tetracyclines cause similar side effects and adverse effects. They can cause discoloration of the permanent teeth and tooth enamel hypoplasia in both fetuses and children and possibly retard fetal skeletal development if taken during pregnancy. Other clinically significant undesirable effects include photosensitivity, with the highest incidence of this seen in patients taking demeclocycline, and alteration of the intestinal flora, resulting in:

■ The overgrowth of nonsusceptible organisms (superinfection), especially *Monilia* and pediatric staphylococcal enteritis.
■ Diarrhea.
■ Reduced bacterial vitamin K synthesis.
■ Pseudomembranous colitis.

They can also alter the vaginal flora, resulting in moniliasis; cause reversible bulging fontanelles in neonates; precipitate thrombocytopenia, possible coagulation irregularities, and hemolytic anemia; and exacerbate systemic lupus erythematosus. Other effects include gastric upset, enterocolitis, and maculopapular rash.

Interactions

There are several significant drug interactions associated with the use of tetracyclines. When taken with antacids, antidiarrheal agents, dairy products, or iron preparations, the oral absorption of the tetracycline is reduced. Nephrotoxicity may occur when they are taken with methoxyflurane. Their use with oral anticoagulants requires caution, and they can also antagonize the effects of bactericidal antibiotics.

In addition, depending on the dose, they can cause the BUN levels to be increased.

Dosages

For dosage information for selected tetracyclines, see the dosages table on the next page.

DOSAGES

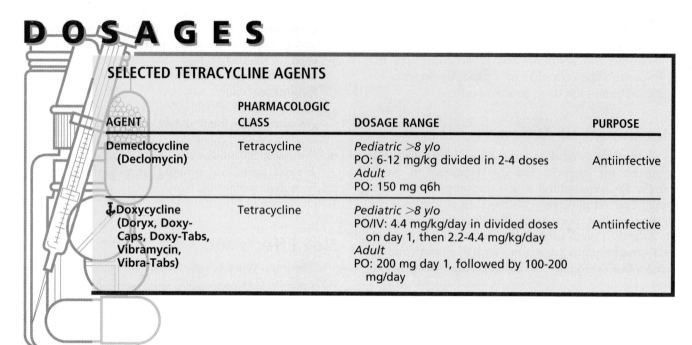

SELECTED TETRACYCLINE AGENTS

AGENT	PHARMACOLOGIC CLASS	DOSAGE RANGE	PURPOSE
Demeclocycline (Declomycin)	Tetracycline	*Pediatric >8 y/o* PO: 6-12 mg/kg divided in 2-4 doses *Adult* PO: 150 mg q6h	Antiinfective
⚓**Doxycycline** (Doryx, Doxy-Caps, Doxy-Tabs, Vibramycin, Vibra-Tabs)	Tetracycline	*Pediatric >8 y/o* PO/IV: 4.4 mg/kg/day in divided doses on day 1, then 2.2-4.4 mg/kg/day *Adult* PO: 200 mg day 1, followed by 100-200 mg/day	Antiinfective

DRUG PROFILES

The tetracyclines were one of the first class of antibiotics capable of a wide range of antibiotic coverage. They are also unique in that they are useful in the treatment of conditions other than bacterial infections. In this regard they are used for the treatment of SIADH and as sclerosing agents in the treatment of pleural effusions. They are prescription-only drugs that are potentially harmful to children younger than 8 years of age and that should not be given to pregnant women because by binding to calcium they can prevent normal bone growth and cause tooth enamel hypoplasia in the child or the fetus. They are also contraindicated in patients who have had hypersensitivity reactions to them in the past and in lactating women. Resistance to one tetracycline implies resistance to all tetracyclines. They are classified as pregnancy category D agents.

DEMECLOCYCLINE

Demeclocycline (Declomycin) is a naturally occurring tetracycline antibiotic that is derived from strains of *Streptomyces.* It is used both for its antibacterial action and for its ability to inhibit the inappropriate secretion of antidiuretic hormone (SIADH). Demeclocycline has

all the characteristics of this class of tetracyclines. It is only available orally as 150- and 300-mg film-coated tablets. Commonly recommended dosages can be found in the dosages table above. Pregnancy category D.

❇ PHARMACOKINETICS

HALF-LIFE	ONSET	PEAK	DURATION
10-17 hr	Variable	3-4 hr	6-12 hr

⚓ DOXYCYCLINE

Doxycycline (Doryx, Doxy-Caps, Doxy-Tabs, Vibramycin, Vibra-Tabs) is a semisynthetic tetracycline antibiotic that was made by altering the naturally occurring tetracycline oxytetracycline. Doxycycline comes in the following three different salt forms: calcium, hyclate, and monohydrate. It is useful in the treatment of *rickettsial infections* such as Rocky Mountain spotted fever, *chlamydial and mycoplasmal infections, gonorrhea, spirochetal infections,* and many gram-negative infections. Doxycycline may also be used as a sclerosing agent in the treatment of pleural effusions.

It comes orally as a 25– and 50–mg/5 ml oral suspension; 50- and 100-mg capsules; 100-mg delayed-release capsules; and 100-mg film-coated tablets. It is also available as a parenteral agent in the form of 100- and 200-mg injections. Commonly recommended dosages can be found in the dosages table above. Pregnancy category D.

PHARMACOKINETICS

HALF-LIFE	ONSET	PEAK	DURATION
14-24 hr	Variable	1.5-4 hr	Up to 12 hr

AMINOGLYCOSIDES

The aminoglycosides are a group of natural and semisynthetic antibiotics that destroy bacteria rather than inhibit their growth, so they are **bactericidal.** They are similar to the tetracyclines in that they are derived from *Streptomyces* organisms. The aminoglycoside antibiotics available for clinical use are listed in the box below. These agents can be given by several different routes, but are not given orally because of their poor oral absorption.

The aminoglycosides are very potent antibiotics and are capable of potentially serious toxicities. As a result they are generally reserved for the treatment of more serious or life-threatening infections. They can kill both gram-positive and gram-negative bacteria but are customarily used to kill gram-negative bacteria such as *Pseudomonas* spp., *E. coli, Proteus* spp., *Klebsiella* spp., *Serratia* spp., and others because there are other less toxic antibiotics that are effective against the gram-positive bacteria they can kill. Often they are used in combination with other antibiotics such as cephalosporins, penicillins, or vancomycin in the treatment of various infections because the combined effect of the two antibiotics is greater than that of either agent alone, a phenomenon known as a synergistic effect.

The aminoglycosides work in a way that is similar to that of the tetracyclines in that they also bind to ribosomes and thereby prevent protein synthesis in bacteria. The three aminoglycosides most commonly used for the treatment of systemic infections are gentamicin, tobramycin, and amikacin. The serious toxicities of the aminoglycosides are renal failure and hearing loss (ototoxicity). Certain optimal drug blood levels are strived for to prevent these toxicities from occurring and to optimize the antibiotic killing power. Following are the levels for a few of these agents:

	Peak	Trough
Gentamicin and tobramycin	5-12 µg/ml	<2 µg/ml
Amikacin	20-35 µg/ml	<10 µg/ml

The ototoxicity associated with aminoglycoside use involves both auditory impairment and vestibular damage and is thought to be due in part to damage to the eighth cranial nerve inflicted by the agents proper. Symptoms include dizziness, tinnitus, and hearing loss. The nephrotoxicity, or renal failure, is manifested by urinary casts, proteinuria, and increased BUN and serum creatinine levels. In light of these potentially serious toxicities, patients receiving aminoglycosides should be monitored for the signs and symptoms of renal failure (rising BUN and creatinine levels) and hearing loss (fullness in ears, ringing in ears, and dizziness). The risk of these toxicities is greatest in patients with preexisting renal impairment, patients already receiving other renally toxic drugs, and patients on high doses of or prolonged aminoglycoside therapy.

Aminoglycosides should be administered with caution in premature and full-term neonates because of the renal immaturity of these patients, which can result in prolonged actions of the aminoglycosides and a greater risk of toxicities. The aminoglycosides have been shown to cross the placenta and cause fetal harm when administered to pregnant women. There have been several reports of total, irreversible bilateral congenital deafness in the children of women taking aminoglycosides during pregnancy. Therefore aminoglycosides should be used in pregnant women only in the event of life-threatening situations or severe infections when safer drugs either cannot be used or are ineffective. The pregnancy categories of the various aminoglycosides are as follows: gentamicin, C; tobramycin, D; amikacin, D; kanamycin, D; neomycin, C; netilmicin, D; and streptomycin, B. These antibiotics

Available Aminoglycoside Antibiotics

ORIGIN	AMINOGLYCOSIDE PRODUCT	DESCRIPTION
Natural	Gentamicin Kanamycin Neomycin Paromomycin Streptomycin Tobramycin	Are all chemically derived from *Streptomyces* spp. by a fermentation process.
Semisynthetic	Amikacin Netilmicin	Chemical derivative of kanamycin. Structurally related to gentamicin.

are also distributed in breast milk, so their use should be avoided in lactating women. Aminoglycosides are contraindicated in patients with a known hypersensitivity or a history of a serious toxic reaction to them.

Mechanism of Action

As already mentioned, the aminoglycosides kill bacteria by binding to and disrupting protein synthesis in bacteria. Specifically they do this by binding to both the 30S and 50S ribosomal subunits, structures that need to be functioning for protein synthesis to occur. When this process is disrupted, the bacterial cell eventually dies.

Drug Effects

The drug effects of the aminoglycosides are primarily limited to their ability to kill bacteria. They are active against many aerobic gram-negative bacteria and some aerobic gram-positive bacteria, but they are relatively inactive against fungi, viruses, and most anaerobic bacteria. Some aminoglycosides, for example, streptomycin, are active against *Mycobacterium* spp. Other agents such as paromomycin are active against protozoal infections.

Therapeutic Uses

The toxicity associated with aminoglycosides restricts their use to the treatment of serious gram-negative infections and specific conditions involving gram-positive cocci, in which case gentamicin is usually given in combination with a penicillin. Paromomycin is used to treat amebic dysentery, a protozoal intestinal disease.

The selection of an aminoglycoside is based on the susceptibility of the causative organism. Serious *Pseudomonas* infections are treated with a suitable aminoglycoside and an extended-spectrum penicillin. Refer to the box below for the antibacterial spectrums of specific aminoglycosides.

Side Effects and Adverse Effects

The most significant adverse effects of the aminoglycosides are ototoxicity and nephrotoxicity. Other undesirable effects include headache, paresthesia, neuromuscular blockade, dizziness, vertigo, skin rash, fever, and overgrowth of nonsusceptible organisms.

Interactions

There are several significant drug interactions associated with aminoglycoside use. Their use with neurotoxic or nephrotoxic drugs such as colistimethate, ethacrynic acid, furosemide, polymyxin B, and vancomycin should be avoided. The concurrent administration of dimenhydrinate can mask aminoglycoside toxicity, and the coadministration of a neuromuscular blocking agent can increase their activity. Calcium salts can be administered to reverse the blockade. In addition, their use with oral anticoagulants can increase the anticoagulant activity because they decrease intestinal vitamin K synthesis.

Aminoglycosides: Specific Antibacterial Spectrums

AMINOGLYCOSIDE	SPECTRUM
Amikacin sulfate	*Acinetobacter* spp., *Enterobacter aerogenes, Escherichia coli, Klebsiella pneumoniae, Proteus* spp., *Providencia* spp., *Pseudomonas* spp., *Serratia* spp., *Staphylococcus* infections.
⬇Gentamicin sulfate	*E. aerogenes, E. coli, Klebsiella pneumoniae, Proteus* spp., *Pseudomonas* spp., *Salmonella* spp., *Serratia* spp. (nonpigmented), *Shigella* spp.
Kanamycin sulfate	*Acinetobacter* spp., *E. coli, Klebsiella pneumoniae, Proteus* spp., *Serratia marcescens.* It is administered orally for the treatment of cirrhotic patients in hepatic coma caused by nitrogen-producing bacteria and for intestinal antisepsis.
Neomycin sulfate	Toxicity limits use to GI tract (hepatic coma, *E. coli* diarrhea, and antisepsis) and as a topical antibacterial.
Netilmicin sulfate	*Citrobacter* spp., *Enterobacter* spp., *E. coli, Klebsiella pneumoniae, Proteus* spp., *Pseudomonas aeruginosa, Serratia* spp.
Paromomycin sulfate	Amebic dysentery.
Streptomycin sulfate	Granuloma inguinale, plague, tularemia, TB, nonhemolytic *Streptococcus* endocarditis.
Tobramycin sulfate	*Citrobacter* spp., *Enterobacter* spp., *E. coli, Kebsiella* spp., *Proteus* spp., *Providencia* spp., *Pseudomonas aeruginosa, Serratia* spp.

DOSAGES

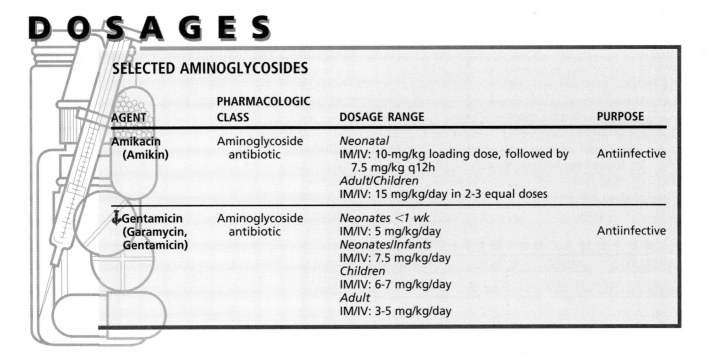

SELECTED AMINOGLYCOSIDES

AGENT	PHARMACOLOGIC CLASS	DOSAGE RANGE	PURPOSE
Amikacin (Amikin)	Aminoglycoside antibiotic	*Neonatal* IM/IV: 10-mg/kg loading dose, followed by 7.5 mg/kg q12h *Adult/Children* IM/IV: 15 mg/kg/day in 2-3 equal doses	Antiinfective
⚓Gentamicin (Garamycin, Gentamicin)	Aminoglycoside antibiotic	*Neonates <1 wk* IM/IV: 5 mg/kg/day *Neonates/Infants* IM/IV: 7.5 mg/kg/day *Children* IM/IV: 6-7 mg/kg/day *Adult* IM/IV: 3-5 mg/kg/day	Antiinfective

Dosages

For recommended dosages of selected aminoglycosides, see the dosages table above.

DRUG PROFILES

There are seven aminoglycoside antibiotics, but only three are commonly administered systemically. These are gentamicin, tobramycin, and amikacin. These agents should be used with extreme caution if at all in pregnant women and nursing mothers. Infants can tolerate aminoglycosides, but they should be given in smaller doses, the drug levels should be tightly monitored, and the infants should be closely watched for the occurrence of side effects. Aminoglycosides are frequently given in combination with other antibiotics such as penicillins, cephalosporins, and vancomycin.

AMIKACIN

Amikacin (Amikin) is a semisynthetic aminoglycoside antibiotic derived by chemically altering kanamycin, a naturally occurring aminoglycoside. As previously noted, it differs from gentamicin and tobramycin in that its therapeutic drug levels are much higher than those of the other two agents. The peak levels should be between 20 and 35 µg/ml and the trough level, less than 10 µg/ml. Aiming for blood drug levels in this range accomplishes two essential goals. First, it ensures that there will be sufficient antibiotic present to destroy the maximum amount of bacteria, and second, it prevents the unwanted nephrotoxicity and ototoxicity sometimes associated with aminoglycoside therapy.

Amikacin has the same contraindications as those already mentioned for the aminoglycosides in general and is considered a pregnancy category D agent. It is available as a 50- and 250-mg/ml injection for intravenous administration. Commonly recommended dosages can be found in the dosages table above.

☣ PHARMACOKINETICS

HALF-LIFE	ONSET	PEAK	DURATION
2-3 hr	Variable	1 hr	8-12 hr

⚓ GENTAMICIN

Gentamicin (Garamycin, Gentamicin) is a naturally occurring aminoglycoside that is obtained from cultures of *Micromonospora purpurea*. It is one of the aminoglycosides most commonly used in clinical practice today. It has the same contraindications as the other aminoglycosides and is classified as a pregnancy C agent. It can be given either intravenously or intramuscularly, with the dosage the same for both routes. It is indicated for the treatment of several susceptible gram-positive and gram-negative bacteria. As already discussed, the common therapeutic drug levels for gentamicin and tobramycin are lower than those for tobramycin. Gentamicin is available in several dosage forms. It comes as a 10- and 40 mg/ml injection for IM or IV use; a 2-mg/ml injection for intrathecal use; and a 10-, 60-, 80-, and 100-mg/ml injection for intravenous infusion. It is also available as a 3% solution or ointment for ophthalmic use, and in this form is used for the treatment of eye infections. Gentamicin also comes as a 0.1% ointment for topical application on superficial skin infections, burns, and skin ulcers. Commonly recommended dosages can be found in the dosages table on the previous page.

⬡ PHARMACOKINETICS

HALF-LIFE	ONSET	PEAK	DURATION
2 hr	Variable	0.5-2 hr	8-12 hr

QUINOLONES

The quinolone antibiotics are very potent broad-spectrum antibiotics. They kill bacteria rather than inhibit their growth and are therefore bactericidal. The first of these agents to come available were cinoxacin and nalidixic acid. These two agents have narrower spectrums of activity (kill fewer kinds of bacteria) than the newer, more potent, and less toxic quinolones, and are therefore seldom used anymore. The newer quinolone antibiotics include, in order of their release onto the market, norfloxacin, ciprofloxacin, enoxacin, ofloxacin, lomefloxacin, and perfloxacin. A fluorine atom was added onto the basic quinolone structure to create these newer agents, and this increased their antibacterial potency and made them able to kill a broader range of bacteria. Because of this chemical change, these agents are sometimes called fluoroquinolones.

The fluoroquinolones are active against a wide variety of gram-negative and selected gram-positive bacteria. Ciprofloxacin, norfloxacin, and ofloxacin are effective against an extensive spectrum of gram-negative bacteria. Enoxacin and lomefloxacin are effective against slightly fewer gram-negative bacteria, and of the gram-positive bacteria, they are only effective against *Staphylococcus* spp. The characteristics of the fluoroquinolone antibiotics and their therapeutic effects are summarized in the box below.

With the exception of norfloxacin, these antibiotics have excellent oral absorption. In fact, their oral absorption is in many cases as good as the rapidity with which the intravenous formulation is available. However, the concurrent use of antacids with the fluoroquinolones causes their oral absorption to be greatly reduced. The fluoroquinolones are primarily excreted by the kidneys, which contain a high percentage of unchanged drug. This together with the fact that they have extensive gram-negative coverage makes them suitable for treating UTIs. Their use in children is not currently recommended because they have been shown to suppress growth in laboratory animals. The risks versus the benefits must of course always be weighed when deciding whether to use a drug in this setting.

Mechanism of Action

The quinolone antibiotics destroy bacteria by altering their DNA, and they accomplish this by interfering with the DNA gyrase, the enzyme necessary for the synthesis of bacterial DNA. If bacteria cannot produce DNA, they die. The quinolones do not seem to affect the mammalian enzyme and therefore do not inhibit the production of human DNA.

Fluoroquinolone Antibiotic Characteristics

FLUOROQUINOLONE	BACTERIA KILLED	INDICATIONS
⚓Ciprofloxacin (Cipro)	Extensive gram-negative and selected gram-positive bacterial	Lower respiratory tract infections, bone and joint infections, infectious diarrhea, urinary tract infections, skin infections
Enoxacin (Penetrex)	Reduced gram-negative and gram-positive bacterial (*Staphylococcus*) coverage	Urinary tract infections, sexually transmitted diseases
Lomefloxacin (Maxaquin)		Lower respiratory tract and urinary tract infections
Norfloxacin (Noroxin)	Gram-negative and some gram-positive bacterial coverage	Urinary tract infections, sexually transmitted diseases
Ofloxacin (Floxin)	Extensive gram-negative and selected gram-positive bacterial coverage	Urinary tract and lower respiratory tract infections, sexually transmitted diseases

Drug Effects

The drug effects of the quinolone antibiotics are mostly limited to their effects on bacteria. They kill susceptible strains of mostly gram-negative organisms, and they are also capable of killing some gram-positive organisms. Some of the quinolones are also believed to diffuse into and concentrate themselves in human neutrophils, where some bacteria such as *Staphylococcus aureus, Serratia marcescens,* and *Mycobacterium fortuitum* reside. If they can do so to a sufficient extent, they can kill these bacteria.

Therapeutic Uses

The quinolone antibiotics are used in the treatment of various bacterial infections. The particular bacteria and the body site infected determine which quinolone is selected. The box on p. 562 lists the available fluoroquinolone antibiotics, the broad range of bacteria they kill, and the indications for their use according to body site.

Side Effects and Adverse Effects

The fluoroquinolones are capable of causing some both serious and bothersome adverse effects, the most common of which are listed in Table 36-4. Bacterial overgrowth is another possible complication of quinolone therapy, but this is more commonly associated with long-term use.

Interactions

There are several drugs that interact with the fluoroquinolones, with significant consequences. Their use with antacids, iron or zinc preparations, or sucralfate causes the oral absorption of the fluoroquinolone to be greatly reduced. Probenecid can reduce the renal excretion of the fluoroquinolone, and the use of fluoroquinolones with theophylline may increase the toxicity of the bronchodilator. Nitrofurantoin can antagonize the antibacterial activity of the fluoroquinolones, and oral anticoagulants should be used with caution in patients receiving fluoroquinolones because of the antibiotic-induced alteration of the intestinal flora, which affects vitamin K synthesis.

DRUG PROFILES

The quinolones are broad-spectrum synthetic antibiotics with bactericidal activity. They are very effective in both their oral and parenteral forms and are used to treat a variety of infections, including urinary tract, lower respiratory tract, bone and joint, and skin and skin structure infections, as well as sexually transmitted diseases. Because of their excellent oral bioavailability, the oral forms of many of these quinolones are just as effective as their parenteral counterparts when given to patients with a functioning gastrointestinal tract. The quinolones are prescription-only agents that are classified as pregnancy category C agents. They are contraindicated in patients with a known hypersensitivity to them.

✠ CIPROFLOXACIN

Ciprofloxacin (Cipro) was one of the first of the newer broad-coverage, potent fluoroquinolones to come available. It was first marketed in an oral form and as such has the advantage and convenience of an oral medication, plus, because of its excellent bioavailability, it can work as well as many intravenous antibiotics. It is also capable of killing a wide range of gram-negative bacteria and is even effective against traditionally difficult to kill gram-negative bacteria such as *Pseudomonas*. Some anaerobic bacteria as well as atypical organisms such as *Chlamydia, Mycoplasma,* and Mycobacterium can also be killed by ciprofloxacin. It is available in both oral and parenteral forms. Orally it comes as 250-, 500-, and 750-mg oral film-coated tablets. Parenterally it comes in doses of 200 and 400 mg contained in premixed bags for intravenous infusion or in a 10-mg/ml concentrate for intravenous injection.

Table 36-4	Fluoroquinolones: Common Adverse Effects
BODY SYSTEM	**SIDE/ADVERSE EFFECTS**
Central nervous system	Headache, dizziness, fatigue, insomnia, depression, restlessness, convulsions
Gastrointestinal	Nausea, constipation, increased SGOT and SGPT (liver function tests), flatulence, heartburn, vomiting, diarrhea, oral candidiasis, dysphagia, pseudomembranous colitis
Skin	Rash, pruritus, urticaria, photosensitivity (with lomefloxacin), flushing
Other	Fever, chills, blurred vision, tinnitus

The common adult dosage of ciprofloxacin is 250 to 750 mg q12h.

⚕ P H A R M A C O K I N E T I C S

HALF-LIFE	ONSET	PEAK	DURATION
3-4.8 hr	Variable	1-2.3 hr	Up to 12 hr

MACROLIDES

The macrolides are a large group of antibiotics that first came available in the early 1950s with the introduction of erythromycin. The macrolides are considered bacteriostatic, although, in high enough concentrations, the macrolides may be bactericidal in some susceptible bacteria. As with many of the other classes of antibiotics, the macrolides inhibit the growth of bacteria by inhibiting protein synthesis, specifically by binding to the 50S ribosomal subunit.

There are four main macrolide antibiotics: azithromycin, clarithromycin, erythromycin, and troleandomycin. Azithromycin and clarithromycin are the two newest agents in the class. Although their spectrum of antibacterial activity is similar to that of erythromycin, they have longer durations of action than erythromycin, which allows them to be given less often; they produce fewer and less severe gastrointestinal tract side effects than erythromycin, and they need to be given for shorter lengths of time than many of the erythromycin products. They also exhibit better efficacy in eradicating various bacteria and are capable of better tissue penetration.

Because erythromycin has a bitter taste and is quickly degraded by the acidity of the stomach, several salt forms and many dosage formulations were developed to circumvent these problems. These various salt forms and dosage formulations and the benefits of each are briefly summarized in the box at right.

Mechanism of Action

The mechanism of action of the macrolide antibiotics is similar to that of other antibiotics. As already mentioned, they bind to the 50S ribosomal subunit inside the cells of bacteria and by doing so prevent the production of the bacterial protein needed for the bacteria to grow, with the result that the bacteria eventually die. This action can immediately kill some susceptible strains of bacteria if the concentration of the macrolide is high enough.

Drug Effects

The drug effects of the macrolide antibiotics are limited to their actions within bacteria. The macrolides are effective in the treatment of a wide range of infections. These include various infections of the upper and lower respiratory tract, skin, and soft tissue caused by some strains of *Streptococcus* and, *Haemophilus;* spirochetal infections such as syphilis and Lyme disease; gonorrhea; *Chlamydia* and *Mycoplasma* infections; and *Listeria monocytogenes and Corynebacterium* infections. Because of its gastrointestinal tract–irritating properties, erythromycin affects the motility of the gastrointestinal tract. This property has been studied experimentally and may prove to be of benefit in increasing gastrointestinal motility in conditions such as delayed gastric emptying in diabetics.

Therapeutic Uses

The therapeutic effects of the macrolide antibiotics are mostly limited to their antibacterial actions. Infections caused by *Streptococcus pyogenes* (group A beta-hemolytic streptococci) are inhibited by the macrolides, as are mild to moderate upper and lower respiratory tract infections caused by *Haemophilus influenzae.* Spirochetal infections that are treated with the erythromycins and other macrolides are syphilis and Lyme disease. Various forms of gonorrhea and *Chlamydia* and *Mycoplasma* infections are also susceptible to the effects of the macrolides.

As already noted, a therapeutic effect of erythromycin outside its antibiotic actions is its ability to irritate the gastrointestinal tract, which stimulates the secretion of a substance in the stomach called motilin. This in turn increases the motility of the gastrointestinal tract, which may be of benefit to patients who have decreased gastrointestinal motility. It has also been

---

⚓ Erythromycin Formulations

Salt Forms	Benefit
Stearate salt Estolate Ethylsuccinate ester	Developed to overcome bitter taste of erythromycin

Dosage Formulations

Film coated Enteric coated (pellets and particles)	Developed to overcome bitter taste and to protect the erythromycin from acid degradation in the stomach.

Structural Changes

Semisynthetic ⚓macrolides: 　Azide group 　(azithromycin) 　Methylation of hydroxy group 　(clarithromycin)	Developed to improve resistance to acid degradation in the stomach and increase tissue penetration in order to improve antibiotic efficacy.

shown to be of some benefit for facilitating the passage of feeding tubes from the stomach into the small bowel.

Side Effects and Adverse Effects

Many of the older macrolide products, primarily erythromycin derivatives, have many side effects. Most affect the gastrointestinal tract, though the two newest macrolides, azithromycin and clarithromycin, seem to be associated with a lower incidence of these gastrointestinal tract complications. The most common of these adverse effects are listed in Table 36-5.

Interactions

Common drug interactions, their mechanisms, and the result of the interaction are listed in Table 36-6. Two properties of macrolides that are the source of many of these interactions are that they are highly protein bound and they are metabolized in the liver. Drugs that are bound to protein are usually bound to albumin in the blood, making them inactive. When they are displaced from these binding sites on albumin and are then free and unbound, they become active. Therefore when a patient is given two or more drugs that compete for the same binding sites on albumin in the blood, one will not successfully bind, with the result that it is free in the blood and active. That drug will then have a greater action or effect in the body. A similar situation arises when two drugs are competing for metabolism in the liver. The result is a delay in the drugs' metabolism and thus a prolonged drug effect.

Dosages

For dosage information on selected macrolide antibiotics, see the dosages table on the next page.

*D*RUG PROFILES

The macrolide antibiotics are used to treat a variety of infections ranging from Lyme disease to Legionnaire's disease. Of the four macrolide agents currently available, erythromycin has been around the longest and has been the mainstay of the treatment for various infections for more than four decades. Within the past 5 years, two new macrolides, azithromycin and clarithromycin, have come available that have been improved over the older agents in terms of having fewer side effects and a better pharmacokinetics profile.

All macrolides are prescription-only drugs and are rated as a pregnancy category C agents. They are contraindicated in patients with a known hypersensitivity to macrolides or with preexisting liver disease. As already noted, because these agents are highly protein bound and metabolized in the liver, they may interfere

Table 36-5	Macrolides: Common Adverse Effects
BODY SYSTEM	**SIDE/ADVERSE EFFECTS**
Central nervous system	Headache, dizziness, vertigo, somnolence
Cardiovascular	Palpitations, chest pain
Gastrointestinal	Nausea, hepatotoxicity, heartburn, vomiting, diarrhea, stomatitis, flatulence, cholestatic jaundice, anorexia
Skin	Rash, pruritus, urticaria, thrombophlebitis (IV site)
Other	Hearing loss, tinnitus

Table 36-6	Macrolides: Drug Interactions	
DRUG	**MECHANISM**	**RESULT**
Carbamazepine	Inhibit hepatic metabolism	Increased carbamazepine effect
Cyclosporin		Increased cyclosporin effect
Theophylline	Decreased clearance	Increased theophylline effect
Astemizole and terfenadine	Inhibit hepatic metabolism	Toxic effects (ventricular tachycardia)
Warfarin		Enhanced warfarin effects, prolonged prothrombin time

D O S A G E S

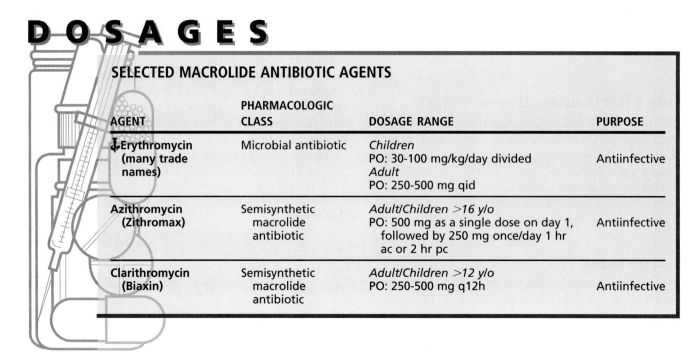

SELECTED MACROLIDE ANTIBIOTIC AGENTS

AGENT	PHARMACOLOGIC CLASS	DOSAGE RANGE	PURPOSE
⚓Erythromycin (many trade names)	Microbial antibiotic	*Children* PO: 30-100 mg/kg/day divided *Adult* PO: 250-500 mg qid	Antiinfective
Azithromycin (Zithromax)	Semisynthetic macrolide antibiotic	*Adult/Children >16 y/o* PO: 500 mg as a single dose on day 1, followed by 250 mg once/day 1 hr ac or 2 hr pc	Antiinfective
Clarithromycin (Biaxin)	Semisynthetic macrolide antibiotic	*Adult/Children >12 y/o* PO: 250-500 mg q12h	Antiinfective

with other drugs that are also highly protein bound or hepatically metabolized.

⚓ ERYTHROMYCIN

Erythromycin, which goes by many product names, is the most frequently prescribed macrolide antibiotic. It comes in several different salt and dosage forms that were developed to circumvent some of the drawbacks it has chemically. (See the box on p. 564 on erythromycin formulations that summarizes these benefits).

The absorption of oral erythromycin is enhanced if it is taken on an empty stomach, but because of the high incidence of stomach irritation associated with its use, many of the agents are taken after a meal or snack. The various salt forms and dosage formulations, their strengths, and product names are listed in the box on p. 567.

AZITHROMYCIN AND CLARITHROMYCIN

Azithromycin (Zithromax) and clarithromycin (Biaxin) are semisynthetic macrolide antibiotics that differ structurally from erythromycin and as a result have advantages over erythromycin. These include better side effect profiles and pharmacokinetic properties. They also cause less GI tract irritation. Both have very similar spectrums of activity that differ only slightly from that of erythromycin, and the two agents are used for the treatment of both upper and lower respiratory tract and skin and skin structure infections.

Azithromycin is capable of excellent tissue pene-

tration, allowing it to reach high concentrations in infected tissues. It also has a long duration of action, allowing it to be dosed once daily. Azithromycin is only available orally as 250-mg capsules and should be given at least 1 hour before or 2 hours after a meal. Food decreases both the rate and extent of gastrointestinal absorption. Azithromycin is recommended for use in adults and children 16 years of age or older. The safety and efficacy of this agent in younger patients has not been established. Commonly recommended dosages can be found in the dosages table above.

Clarithromycin can be given only twice daily and is recommended for use in adults and children 12 years of age or older. Its safety and efficacy in younger patients has not been established. It is also only available orally as 250- and 500-mg film-coated tablets. Common dosages are found in the dosages table above.

☇ PHARMACOKINETICS

Azithromycin			
HALF-LIFE	**ONSET**	**PEAK**	**DURATION**
6-8 hr	Variable	2.5 hr	Up to 24 hr
Clarithromycin			
HALF-LIFE	**ONSET**	**PEAK**	**DURATION**
3-7 hr	Variable	2 hr	Up to 12 hr

MISCELLANEOUS ANTIBIOTICS

There are many categories of antibiotics, with the aminoglycosides, cephalosporins, macrolides, penicillins, tetracyclines, quinolones, and sulfonamides represent-

⚓Erythromycin Dosage Forms and Product Names

FORM	STRENGTH	PRODUCT NAME
Erythromycin Base (PO)		
Capsules		
Delayed release (enteric-coated pellets)	250 mg	ERYC, ERYC Sprinkle
Tablets		
Delayed release (enteric-coated particles)	333 and 500 mg	PCE Dispertab
Delayed release (enteric coated)	250, 333, and 500 mg	E-mycin, Ery-Tab, and E-base
Film coated	250 and 500 mg	Erythromycin Base Filmtab
Erythromycin Estolate (PO)		
Capsules	250 mg	Ilosone Pulvules
Tablets	500 mg	Ilosone
Suspension	125 and 250 mg/5 ml	Ilosone Liquid
Erythromycin Ethylsuccinate (PO)		
Tablets		
(chewable)	200 mg	Eryped
(film-coated)	400 mg	E.E.S. 400 Filmtab
Suspension		
(drops)	100 mg/2.5 ml	Eryped Drops
(oral suspension)	200 and 400 mg/5 ml	Eryped 200 and 400
(oral liquid)	200 and 400 mg/5 ml	E.E.S. 200 and 400
Erythromycin Gluceptate (IV)		
Parenteral	1 gm	Ilotycin Gluceptate Intra Venous
Erythromycin Lactobionate (IV)		
Parenteral	500 mg and 1 gm	Erythrocin Lactobionate IV, Erythrocin Piggyback
Erythromycin Stearate (PO)		
Tablets		
(film-coated)	250 and 500 mg	Erythrocin Stearate Filmtab

ing the bulk of the antibiotics used in clinical practice. There are, however, some other important antibiotics that deserve quick mention, and these are aztreonam, clindamycin, dapsone, imipenem, polypeptide antibiotics, and vancomycin.

AZTREONAM

Aztreonam (Azactam) is a synthetic monobactam antibiotic that is primarily active against aerobic gram-negative bacteria. Aztreonam is a bactericidal antibiotic, and it destroys bacteria by inhibiting bacterial cell wall synthesis, resulting in lysis. Aztreonam is indicated for the treatment of moderately severe systemic and urinary tract infections.

Aztreonam is a prescription-only drug that can be given either intramuscularly or intravenously. It is classified as a pregnancy category B agent and is contraindicated in patients with a known hypersensitivity

to it, penicillin, or the cephalosporins. Only 6% to 16% of the agent is metabolized by the liver, with most of it excreted unchanged by the kidneys. Aztreonam is associated with no significant drug interactions worth mentioning. It is only available in a parenteral form and comes in 500-mg, 1-gm, and 2-gm vials for injection. Common dosages are found in the dosages table on p. 569.

☣ PHARMACOKINETICS

HALF-LIFE	ONSET	PEAK	DURATION
1.5-2 hr	Variable	IM: 1 hr	6-12 hr

CLINDAMYCIN

Clindamycin (Cleocin, Cleocin Pediatric, Cleocin Phosphate) is a semisynthetic derivative of lincomycin, an older antibiotic. Like many semisynthetic derivatives, it was improved over its predecessor agents through the addition of certain chemical groups to the basic structure, with the result that it is more effective and causes fewer adverse effects than its parent compound.

Clindamycin can be either bactericidal or bacteriostatic, depending on the concentration of the drug at the site of infection and on the infecting bacteria. It inhibits protein synthesis in bacteria by binding to the 50S ribosomal subunit, the same site as erythromycin. It is indicated for the treatment of chronic bone infections, genitourinary tract infections, intraabdominal infections, anaerobic pneumonia, septicemia caused by streptococci and staphylococci, and serious skin and soft tissue infections caused by susceptible bacteria. Most aerobic gram-positive bacteria, including staphylococci, streptococci, and pneumococci are susceptible to clindamycin's actions. It is also active against several anaerobic organisms.

Clindamycin is classified as a pregnancy category B agent and is contraindicated in patients with a known hypersensitivity to it, those with ulcerative colitis or enteritis, and infants younger than 1 month old. Gastrointestinal tract side effects are the most common and include nausea, vomiting, abdominal pain, diarrhea, pseudomembranous colitis, and anorexia. Clindamycin is available in both an oral and parenteral form. Orally it comes as 75-, 150-, and 300-mg capsules and as a 75–mg/5 ml oral suspension. Parenterally it comes in 300-, 600-, and 900-mg vials for injection. Common dosages are found in the dosages table on p. 569.

☙ PHARMACOKINETICS

HALF-LIFE	ONSET	PEAK	DURATION
2.4 hr	Variable	45 min	6 hr

IMIPENEM-CILASTATIN

Imipenem-cilastatin (Primaxin) is a fixed combination of imipenem, which is a semisynthetic carbapenem antibiotic similar to beta-lactam antibiotics, and cilastatin, an inhibitor of an enzyme that breaks down imipenem. Imipenem has a wide spectrum of activity against gram-positive and gram-negative aerobic and anaerobic bacteria. Cilastatin is a unique drug in that it inhibits an enzyme in the kidneys called *dihydropeptidase,* which if not inhibited quickly, would break down the imipenem. Cilastatin also blocks the renal tubular secretion of imipenem, which also prevents imipenem from being metabolized by the kidneys, the primary route of excretion of the agent.

Imipenem exerts its antibacterial effect by binding to penicillin-binding proteins inside bacteria, which in turn inhibits bacterial cell wall synthesis. Imipenem kills bacteria and is therefore bactericidal. Unlike many of the penicillins and cephalosporins, imipenem is very

resistant to the antibiotic-inhibiting actions of beta-lactamases. There are no significant drug interactions associated with imipenem use. The most serious adverse effect of imipenem therapy are seizures, which have been reported to occur in 1.5% of the patients receiving high doses of the agent (>500 mg q6h).

Imipenem is indicated for the treatment of bone, joint, skin, and soft tissue infections; bacterial endocarditis caused by *S. aureus;* intraabdominal bacterial infections; pneumonia; urinary tract and pelvic infections; and bacterial septicemia caused by susceptible bacterial organisms. Imipenem is classified as a pregnancy C agent and is contraindicated in patients with a known hypersensitivity to it or to local anesthetics of the amide type. Imipenem is only available parenterally and comes as 250- and 500-mg vials for intravenous injection and as 500- and 750-mg vials for intramuscular injection. Common dosages are given in the dosages table on p. 569.

☙ PHARMACOKINETICS

HALF-LIFE	ONSET	PEAK	DURATION
2-3 hr	Variable	2 hr	6-8 hr

⚓ VANCOMYCIN

Vancomycin (Lyphocin, Vancocin, Vancoled) is a natural bactericidal antibiotic structurally unrelated to any other commercially available antibiotics. It destroys bacteria by binding to the bacterial cell wall, producing immediate inhibition of cell wall synthesis and death. This mechanism differs from that of the penicillins and cephalosporins.

It is the antibiotic of choice for the treatment of methicillin-resistant *S. aureus* (MRSA) infection and infections caused by many other gram-positive bacteria. It is not active against gram-negative bacteria, fungi, or yeast. Oral vancomycin is indicated for the treatment of antibiotic-induced pseudomembranous colitis *(Clostridium difficile)* and for the treatment of staphylococcal enterocolitis. Because the oral formulation is poorly absorbed from the gastrointestinal tract, it is used for its local effects on the surface of the GI tract. The parenteral form is indicated for the treatment of bone and joint infections and bacterial bloodstream infections caused by *Staphylococcus* spp. Resistance to vancomycin has been noted with increasing frequency in patients with infections caused by *Enterococcus* organisms. These strains have been isolated most often from GI tract infections but have also been isolated from skin, soft tissue, and bloodstream infections.

Vancomycin is classified as a pregnancy category B agent and is contraindicated in patients with a known hypersensitivity to it. It should be used with caution in those with preexisting renal dysfunction or hearing loss, as well as in elderly patients and neo-

DOSAGES

SELECTED MISCELLANEOUS AGENTS

AGENT	PHARMACOLOGIC CLASS	DOSAGE RANGE	PURPOSE
Aztreonam (Azactam)	Monobactam antibiotic	*Adult* IM/IV: 500 mg–2 g q6-12h	Antiinfective
Clindamycin (Cleocin, Cleocin Pediatric, Cleocin Phosphate)	Lincosamide antibiotic	*Neonates* IM/IV: 15-20 mg/kg/day in 3-4 equal doses *Pediatric >1 mo* IM/IV: 20-40 mg/kg/day in 3-4 equal doses *Pediatric <10 kg* PO: 37.5 mg tid *Pediatric* PO: 8-25 mg/kg/day in 3-4 equal doses *Adult* PO: 150-450 mg q6h IV: 600-2700 mg/day in 2-4 equal doses	Antiinfective
Imipenem-cilastatin (Primaxin)	Antibiotic combination	*Adult* IV: 250 mg–1 g q6-8h	Antiinfective
⚓Vancomycin (Lyphocin, Vancocin, Vancoled)	Glycopeptide antibiotic	*Neonate* IV: 15 mg/kg, followed by 10 mg/kg q12h for first week and q8h thereafter up to 1 mo of age *Pediatric* IV: 40 mg/kg/day divided PO: 40 mg/kg/day in 3-4 divided doses for 7-10 days *Adult* PO: 0.5-2 g/day in 3-4 divided doses for 7-10 days	Antiinfective

nates. Vancomycin is similar to the aminoglycosides in that there are very specific drug levels in the blood that are safe. If the levels are too low (<5 μg/ml), there is a risk of their being subtherapeutic, with the result that their antibacterial efficacy is decreased. If the blood levels are too high (>26 μg/ml), this may cause toxicities, the two most severe of which are ototoxicity (hearing loss) and nephrotoxicity (kidney damage). Optimal blood levels of vancomycin should be a peak level of 18 to 26 μg/ml and a trough level of 5 to 10 μg/ml. If these levels are obtained, then the antibacterial effect of the vancomycin will be optimal and the side effects minimal. Vancomycin is available in both oral and parenteral forms. Orally it comes as 125- and 250-mg capsules and a 1- and 10-gm solution. Parenterally it comes in 500-mg and 1-gm vials for intravenous infusions. Common dosages are given in the dosages table above.

PHARMACOKINETICS

HALF-LIFE	ONSET	PEAK	DURATION
4-6 hr	Variable	1 hr	Up to 12 hr

NURSING PROCESS

The discussion of the nursing process will focus on each major classification of antibiotics so that there is an awareness of general and specific information about the various antibiotics.

ASSESSMENT

Before the administration of any antibiotic, it is crucial to ensuring the effectiveness and appropriateness of treatment for the nurse to collect data on the patient regarding his or her age; hypersensitivities to drugs; hepatic, renal, and cardiac function (i.e., pertinent laboratory test results); culture and sensitivity results; and CBC, Hgb, and Hct values. The status of the patient's immune system and his or her 'overall' condition is also important, because if the immune system is deficient in some way, the patient's ability to physically resist infection will be diminished. It is also important to obtain and document a list of all prescribed and over-the-counter medications the patient is taking so that drug interactions can be averted.

Penicillins

Contraindications to the use of penicillins include a known hypersensitivity to them. Cautious use is generally recommended in neonates and in pregnant or lactating women. The patient must also be assessed for a history of asthma, a sensitivity to multiple allergens, or a sensitivity to cephalosporins, because a person with any of these conditions may also be allergic to penicillin agents. In addition, a patient who is to be given a procaine penicillin should be assessed for any procaine hypersensitivity. The drugs that interact with these agents are listed in Table 36-3.

Cephalosporins

Before receiving any of the cephalosporins, the patient should be assessed thoroughly for the existence of any hypersensitivity, including a hypersensitivity to penicillins. Cautious use is recommended in patients who have a history of any type of drug allergy or who have impaired renal or liver function. In addition, cautious use, with careful and frequent monitoring of the patient's vital signs and any complaints of dyspnea, hives, and so on, is recommended for patients who are also taking furosemide, ethacrynic acid, colistin, or aminoglycosides. (See Table 36-3, which gives information on the drug interactions associated with the penicillins, but which are the same for the cephalosporins.)

Sulfonamides

Any patient who is to receive a sulfonamide agent should first be assessed for any drug allergies. Other contraindications include pregnancy, lactation, severe hepatitis, glomerular nephritis, and uremia. Cautious use is recommended in patients with impaired liver or renal function, severe allergies, or bronchial asthma, and in patients also taking anticoagulants or oral antidiabetic agents of the sulfonylurea group.

Tetracyclines

Contraindications to the use of tetracylcines include pregnancy and hypersensitivity. They should also not be given to children under 8 years of age. Cautious use is recommended in lactating women and in patients with renal or hepatic disease. Drugs and substances that interact with tetracyclines include antacids, dairy products, penicillins, and oral anticoagulants.

Aminoglycosides

Aminoglycosides should be used with caution in patients with impaired liver function. There are also many medications that interact with aminoglycosides and that should *not* be given in conjunction with this antibiotic group. These agents include oral anticoagulants, diuretics, cephalothins, skeletal muscle relaxants, and general anesthetic agents. The aminoglycosides are also ototoxic and nephrotoxic, so baseline hearing tests and renal function studies (BUN and serum and urine creatinine levels) should be performed and the results documented. Nephrotoxic effects are manifested by decreased urine creatinine clearance and increased serum creatinine levels.

Clindamycin

Hypersensitivity to either clindamycin or to its parent agent lincomycin is a contraindication to its use. It is also contraindicated in patients with ulcerative colitis or enteritis and in infants below 1 month of age. Cautious use of clindamycin is recommended in patients with renal disease, liver disease, or GI disorders; in elderly patients; and in pregnant or lactating women. Drugs that interact with it include muscle relaxants, chloramphenicol, and erythromycin.

Quinolones

The quinolone antibiotics are mostly used for the treatment of UTIs and should not be used in patients who are allergic to any of the agents. Cautious use is recommended in patients who have seizure disorders or renal disease, in the elderly, and in children. They should also be used cautiously in pregnant or lactating women.

Macrolides

The macrolides are contraindicated in patients with a known allergy to drugs. They should be used cautiously in patients with impaired liver function and in patients also receiving theophylline.

Vancomycin

Vancomycin, a tricyclic glycopeptide, is contraindicated in patients with hearing loss and also those who are allergic to the medication. Cautious use is recommended for the elderly, neonates, pregnant or lactating women, and patients with compromised renal function. Drugs that interact or are incompatible with vancomycin include the aminoglycosides, cephalosporins, polymyxin, cisplatin, and amphotericin B. The combined use of these agents with vancomycin may precipitate nephrotoxicity or ototoxicity. It is also important that vancomycin *not* be mixed with alkaline solutions or in syringes containing alkaline solutions.

NURSING DIAGNOSES

Nursing diagnoses appropriate to patients receiving any of the antibiotics include:
- Risk for infection related to the patient's compromised immune system status before treatment.
- Risk for injury stemming from side effects of medications, such as ototoxicity and nephrotoxicity, from other side effects, or from weakened state resulting from infection.
- Pain related to infection and adverse reaction to medications.
- Knowledge deficit related to lack of information and experience with the medication regimen.
- Noncompliance related to the need to take medication as prescribed (often more than 5 days and more often than once a day).

PLANNING

Goals of nursing care in patients receiving antibiotics include:
- Patient will be free of the signs and symptoms of infection once therapy is completed.
- Patient will experience minimal side effects of antibiotic therapy.
- Patient will remain compliant with therapy.
- Patient will return for follow-up visits as recommended.
- Patient will complete medical regimen of entire course of antibiotics as ordered.

Outcome Criteria

Goals related to the administration of all antibiotics are:

- Patient will experience increased sense of well-being related to resolving infection.
- Patient will state the signs and symptoms of an infection (e.g., fever, pain, malaise) and report them if they occur while on antibiotics.
- Patient will be able to identify the side effects of antibiotic therapy such as GI upset, nausea, and diarrhea (specific to each class).
- Patient will experience increased periods of comfort and improved energy levels related to a resolving infectious process and minimal side effects of therapy.
- Patient will state the reasons for compliance with therapy (i.e., to adequately irradicate bacteria).
- Patient will state the measures to take to minimize the GI distress associated with antibiotic therapy, such as taking with yogurt or other foods, *as appropriate.*
- Patient will keep follow-up appointments with the physician or other health care provider to be evaluated for therapeutic effects or complications of therapy.

IMPLEMENTATION

There are some common nursing interventions that apply to the antibiotics as a whole as well as some very different interventions that apply to specific classes or agents.

Any patient taking a penicillin should be carefully monitored for at least 30 minutes after its administration so that an allergic reaction will not go undetected. Penicillin G binds to food and is poorly absorbed in an acidic medium, so it should be given 1 hour before or 2 hours after meals. In addition, the effectiveness of oral penicillins is decreased when they are taken concurrently with caffeine, citrus fruit, cola beverages, fruit juices, or tomato juice. The IM administration of a penicillin such as penicillin G benzathine may cause irritation to localized tissue, so it should be administered into a large muscle mass. IM medications should be diluted well in the diluent recommended by the manufacturer and the sites rotated. When administering IV ampicillin, it should be diluted according to the manufacturer's guidelines and infused over the recommended time. The IV sites should be assessed frequently and changed every 48 hours, or as dictated by institutional policy. IV administration is to be *avoided*, except for agents such as ampicillin, nafcillin, and methicillin, and the nurse should always double-check to make sure that, if the medication has been ordered to be given IV, it indeed can be given by this route.

Should the patient experience an anaphylactic reaction to a penicillin, management often includes the IV or SC administration of epinephrine, maintenance of the patient's airway, and other supportive treatment

Patient Teaching TIPS

Antibiotics

✔ Patients should take any antibiotic exactly as prescribed and for the time specified.

✔ All oral antibiotics are absorbed better if taken with at least 6 to 8 ounces of water.

✔ Medic-Alert tags, bracelets, or necklaces should be worn at all times by patients with drug allergies!

✔ Oral forms of **penicillins** are better absorbed if taken with 6 to 8 ounces of water and on an empty stomach. Patients should know to report any sore throat, fever, muscle weakness, or joint pain to the physician immediately.

✔ **Cephalosporins** should be taken with meals, when taken orally, to minimize GI irritation and *not* taken concurrently with alcohol or alcohol-containing products (some cough syrups and mouth washes) because of the Antabuse-type reactions that can occur. Drugs that interact with cephalosporins include tetracyclines, erythromycin, aminoglycosides, probenecid, furosemide, and vancomycin. Yogurt or buttermilk products may be taken to help decrease the diarrhea that occurs secondary to the destruction of the normal intestinal flora. The medication should be taken exactly as prescribed and for the specified time. Should sore throat, bruising, bleeding, or joint pain develop, the patient should notify the physician of this immediately because this may indicate the occurrence of a blood dyscrasia.

✔ **Sulfonamides** should be taken with at least 2400 ml of fluid per day, unless contraindicated. Patients should avoid sunlight and using tanning beds because of the photosensitivity they cause. OTC medications should be avoided, especially vitamin C and aspirin, because these drugs interact with the sulfonamides. Patients taking oral contraceptives should use another form of contraception because sulfonamides decrease the contraceptive

effect. Patients should know to take the full course of medication and in accordance with the physician's directions. The patient should notify the physician if fever, sore throat, mouth sores, easy bruising, or skin rash occurs.

✔ **Tetracyclines** cause photosensitivity, so patients taking them should avoid sun exposure and using tanning beds. Milk products, iron preparations, antacids, and other dairy products should be avoided because of the chelation that occurs, which decreases the effectiveness of the medication. All medications should be taken with at least 6 to 8 ounces of fluids, preferably water.

✔ **Quinolones** such as norfloxacin should be taken with at least 3 liters of fluids per day, unless otherwise specified by the physician. This helps to prevent crystallization of the drug in the kidneys. Should dizziness occur, the patient may need assistance in ambulating and performing other activities of daily living. The patient should notify the physician if rash, fever, sore throat, headache, agitation, or confusion occurs.

✔ Oral forms of **lincomycin** should be taken with plenty of fluids and with food to minimize GI distress. Patients should be informed of the importance of complying with therapy and of taking the full course of therapy. Sore throat, fever, or excessive fatigue should be reported to the physician. This drug is usually ordered to be taken around the clock to maintain therapeutic blood levels.

✔ **Vancomycin** should be taken exactly as prescribed and for the number of days specified to ensure that the infecting organism is destroyed. The medication should be administered around the clock to maintain steady blood levels. The patient should report any fever, sore throat, or rash to the physician.

---

such as the administration of steroids, vasopressors, or oxygen or implementation of cardiopulmonary resuscitation.

Orally administered cephalosporins should be given with food to decrease GI upset, even though this will delay absorption. IM injections may be very irritating and so should be given deep in a large muscle mass. If accidental SC injection occurs, sterile abscesses may form. When cephradine is being given by infusion, it should not be mixed with lactated Ringer's solution. IV sites of administration should be assessed frequently for redness, swelling, and heat and changed every 48 hours, or as dictated by institutional policy. Alcohol, when used with some of the cephalosporins, may result in antabuse-like reactions, so always check

for this contraindication before giving the medication.

Sulfonamides should always be given with plenty of fluids (at least 2000 to 2400 ml per day) to prevent the crystalluria that can occur with the oral forms. Oral forms will cause less GI upset if taken with milk or food.

Tetracyclines should not be given with dairy products, antacids, sodium bicarbonate, kaolin-pectin, or iron, because these chelate or bind with the tetracycline, resulting in a decreased antibiotic effect. These foods and drugs can be given 2 hours before or 3 hours after the tetracycline. IM forms should be given deep in a large muscle mass and with no more than 2 ml of the injectant per injection site.

The quinolones should be taken exactly as prescribed and for the full course of treatment. The patient should limit his or her intake of alkaline foods and drugs such as antacids, dairy products, peanuts, vegetables, and sodium bicarbonate. Any of the quinoline agents should be administered only after culture and sensitivity testing has been done on a fresh urine sample from the patient. Fluid intake of up to 3 liters per day should be encouraged, unless contraindicated.

If an IV infusion of lincomycin is ordered, 1 gm of the medication should be diluted in 100 ml or more of D5W or NS, but not to the extent that a rate of infusion of 100 ml/hr would be exceeded. IM injections should be given deep in the muscle and the sites rotated. Oral forms should be given with at least 8 ounces (240 cc) of fluid and on an empty stomach.

Vancomycin should be reconstituted for IV administration according to the manufacturer's guidelines and should be infused over at least 60 minutes. Extravasation may cause local skin irritation and damage, so frequent monitoring of the IV tube and site is needed.

Clindamycin should be administered as ordered and if given IV should be given by infusion, not by an IV push. No more than 1200 mg should be infused in a single 1-hour infusion, and the usually recommended dilution and dosage is 300 mg per 50 ml of compatible fluids delivered over more than 10 minutes. IM injections of the agent should be given deep in a large muscle mass and the sites rotated. Oral forms should be given with at least 8 ounces (240 cc) of fluids.

Teaching guidelines applicable to patients receiving antibiotics are listed in the box on p. 572.

EVALUATION

The therapeutic effects of antibiotics in general include a decrease in the signs and symptoms of the infection; a return to normal vital signs, including temperature and negative results of culture and sensitivity tests; a decrease to a normal CBC; and improved appetite, energy level, and sense of well-being.

Common adverse reactions to monitor for in patients taking penicillins include rash, dermatitis, fever, joint pain, or itching. Patients taking cephalosporins should be watched for the occurrence of diarrhea, abdominal pain, colitis symptoms, headache, fever, chills, nausea, vomiting, rash, or dyspnea. Adverse reactions to the sulfonamides to monitor for include leukopenia, nausea, vomiting, abdominal pain, hepatitis syndrome, renal failure, nephrosis, and the Stevens-Johnson syndrome. The tetracyclines may cause diarrhea, hepatotoxicity, nausea, stomatitis, pericarditis, rash, fever, headache, and oral candidiasis or other superinfections. The quinolones may cause lethargy, dizziness, or confusion. Vancomycin may cause hearing

TAKE HOME POINTS

Antibiotic Classes

- These seven main classes of antibiotic agents: sulfonamides, penicillins, cephalosporins, macrolides, quinolones, aminoglycosides, and tetracyclines.
- Classes of antibiotics differ in the way in which they destroy bacteria.

Antibiotic Characteristics

- Antibiotics are either bacteriostatic or bactericidal.
- *Bacteriostatic* means that the antibiotic inhibits the growth of the bacteria but does not directly kill it.
- *Bactericidal* means that the antibiotic directly kills the bacteria.
- Most antibiotics work by inhibiting bacterial cell wall synthesis in some way.

Bacteria Characteristics

- Bacteria have survived for years because they can adapt to their surroundings.
- If a bacteria's surroundings include an antibiotic, over time it can mutate in such a way that it can survive an attack by an antibiotic.
- The production of beta-lactamases is one way in which bacteria can fend off the effects of antibiotics.

Cephalosporins

- There are many oral and parenteral cephalosporins.
- They can be broken down into three generations of agents.
- Each generation of agents has specific bacteria that can and cannot kill.
- As a general rule, as one goes from the first to third generations of agents, gram-negative coverage is gained and gram-positive coverage is lost.

Nursing Considerations

- The most common side effects of antibiotics are nausea, vomiting, and diarrhea.
- Antibiotics should always be taken for the length of time prescribed.
- A therapeutic response to antibiotic treatment includes disappearance of fever, lethargy, drainage, and redness.
- Each class of antibiotics has specific side effects and drugs that the agents interact with.

Critical Thinking **A C T I V I T I E S**

1. Your patient is scheduled for colorectal surgery tomorrow. He is not septic, his WBC is normal, he has no fever, and he is otherwise in good health. The GI surgeon asks you to recommend a cephalosporin for prophylaxis. What generation of cephalosporin would you recommend and why?
   a. A first-generation cephalosporin because it kills the bacteria that are most common in this surgical field.
   b. A second-generation cephalosporin because it kills the bacteria that are most common in this surgical field.
   c. A third-generation cephalosporin because it is the most potent.
   d. A second-generation cephalosporin because it is the least toxic.

2. You are caring for a 34-year-old man who has been admitted for the treatment of Rocky Mountain spotted fever (RMSF). He is placed on doxycycline, a tetracycline antibiotic, but is now complaining of GI tract upset. The physician orders Maalox to be taken after each dose of the doxycycline. You call the physician and inform him that the GI upset is caused by _____ and that the Maalox will result in _____ if continued.
   a. the RMSF / toxic shock syndrome
   b. the doxycycline / increased doxycycline efficacy
   c. the doxycycline / aluminum toxicity
   d. the doxycycline / decreased doxycycline efficacy

3. The quinolone antibiotics such as Cipro and Floxin are unique in their mechanism of action in that they _____ .
   a. bind to penicillin-binding proteins.
   b. bind to 30S and 50S ribosomal subunits.
   c. interfere with DNA gyrase.
   d. prevent the synthesis of folic acid.

4. The two newest macrolide antibiotics, azithromycin and clarithromycin, differ from the prototype macrolide, erythromycin, in that they have _____ .
   a. a longer duration of action.
   b. better efficacy.
   c. better tissue penetration.
   d. all of the above.

5. Ms. Smith is taking an aminoglycoside for the treatment of a recurrent UTI. What conditions should be assessed for or laboratory studies performed before the initiation of therapy?

6. What symptoms would alert you to the fact that a patient is suffering from a superinfection or overgrowth of normal flora stemming from the use of tetracycline?

▲▲

loss and ringing or roaring in ears, and its use should be discontinued if these symptoms appear. The physician should be notified if any unusual side effects occur or if fever, sore throat, restlessness, wheezing, or tightness in the chest arises. Treatment with clindamycin, although an agent in a different class of antibiotics, requires similar nursing interventions, and the patient education guidelines are also similar. Chloramphenicol may produce severe bone marrow depression with pancytopenia, optic neuritis, blindness, abdominal pain, nausea and vomiting, colitis, rash, headache, depression, and confusion, and patients receiving this medication should be closely monitored for the occurrence of these signs and symptoms.

BIBLIOGRAPHY

Albanese J, Nutz P: *Mosby's 1995 nursing drug cards*, St Louis, 1995, Mosby.

Johnson KB: *Harriet Lane handbook*, ed 13, St Louis, 1993, Mosby.

Keen JH: *Critical care and emergency drug reference*, St Louis, 1994, Mosby.

Knoben JE, Anderson PO: *Handbook of critical drug data*, ed 6, Hamilton, Ill, 1988, Drug Intelligence Publications.

McEvoy GK: *AHFS drug information*, Bethesda, Md, 1994, American Society of Hospital Pharmacists.

Powers MJ and Co, (eds): *All about drugs*, Am J Nurs 10:32, 1995.

Chapter 37

Antiviral Agents

Objectives

When you reach the end of this chapter, you will be able to:

1 Discuss the effects of viruses on the human body.

2 Describe the process of immunosuppression in patients afflicted with viral infections, specifically human immunodeficiency virus.

3 Discuss the indications for; contraindications and cautions to; and routes, mechanism of action, side effects, toxicity, and therapeutic effects of antiviral agents.

4 Identify the various antiviral agents and their specific indications.

5 Develop a comprehensive nursing care plan that includes patient education as it relates to patients receiving antiviral agents.

CHAPTER OUTLINE

Antiviral Therapy
Mechanism of Action
Drug Effects
Therapeutic uses
Side effects and adverse effects
Interactions
Dosages
Drug Profiles
⚓ Acyclovir
  Ganciclovir
⚓ Amantadine
  Ribavirin
  Trifluridine
⚓ Zidovudine

Nursing Process
Assessment
Nursing Diagnoses
Planning
  Outcome criteria
Implementation
Evaluation

Glossary

Antiviral agent Drug that destroys viruses. (p. 575)

Deoxyribonucleic acid (de ok′ se ri′ bo noo kle′ ik) Nucleic acid composed of a sugar, a phosphate group, and a purine or pyridine nucleoside that carries genetic information and is found principally in the chromosomes of the nucleus of a cell. (p. 576)

Ribonucleic acid Nucleic acid composed of a sugar, a phosphate group, and a purine or a pyridine nucleoside that transmits genetic information and is found in both the nucleus and the cytoplasm of cells. (p. 576)

Synthetic purine nucleoside analogue (pu rēn noo′ kle o sīd an′ ə log) Substance that is both chemically made and a purine nucleoside and that resembles another in terms of its structure or constituents but has different effects. (p. 576)

ANTIVIRAL THERAPY

The **antiviral agents** kill viruses by inhibiting their ability to replicate, but there are currently only about a dozen such agents that can destroy only a few of the known viruses. Some of these viruses are:

- Cytomegalovirus (CMV)
- Herpes simplex virus (HSV)
- Human immunodeficiency virus (HIV)
- Influenza A ("the flu")
- Respiratory syncytial virus (RSV)

One reason why only a few viruses can now be killed with the agents currently available is that often by the time the signs and symptoms of a viral illness appear, the virus has finished replicating. Because it is only during viral replication that antiviral agents can work, it is then too late for them to be effective. So, even if there were effective agents to kill these viruses, unless this silent process can be detected and therapy instituted in time, they would otherwise be of no use. Another reason why there are so few agents is that because viruses live inside the body's cells and use them to replicate, any drug that kills a virus could also kill healthy cells. So, for an antiviral agent to be effective *and* safe, it must kill only the virus and not unduly harm the body's cells, and there are few agents that have met these criteria.

As already mentioned, the antiviral agents work by inhibiting viral replication. For a virus to replicate, it must first attach to and enter the healthy cell, where it makes use of the cell's energy to generate both DNA- and RNA-synthesizing pathways as well as its own protein-synthesizing pathways to make more viruses (Fig. 37-1). Antiviral agents inhibit this process in various ways. Some antiviral drugs are able to enter the same cells that the viruses enter and then once inside interfere with viral nucleic acid synthesis, its regulation, or both. Other antiviral drugs work by keeping a virus from binding to the cells. If a virus cannot then get into the cells, it cannot replicate and it dies. Other antiviral agents stimulate the body's immune system to kill the virus.

The best antiviral response is seen in persons with a competent, well-functioning immune system. Such an immune system can work with the agent to eliminate or effectively destroy viruses. Those patients who become a host for virus are frequently immunocompromised. Cancer patients with leukemia or lymphoma, organ transplant recipients, and AIDS patients are all examples of patients who are immunocompromised. These patients are prone to frequent and often severe viral infections, which may recur when antiviral drug therapy is stopped.

Most of the antivirals agents are synthetic purine nucleoside analogues, which means that they are chemically made **(synthetic) purine nucleosides** (adenine or guanine that are chemically similar (**analogues**). There are two types of nucleic acid—**deoxyribonucleic acid** (DNA), which consists of a sugar (deoxyribose), a phosphate group, and a purine (adenine or guanine) or a pyridine (cytosine or thymine) nucleoside, and **ribonucleic acid** (RNA), which is made up of a sugar (ribose), a phosphate group, and a purine (adenine or guanine) or a pyridine (cytosine or uracil) nucleoside. The differences between DNA

Host cell

1. Attachment to host cell
2. Uncoating of virus
3. Control of DNA, RNA, and/or protein production
4. Production of viral subunits
5. Assembly of virions
6. Release of virions

▼ **FIG. 37-1** Virus replication. Some viruses integrate into host chromosome with development of latency. (Modified from Wingard et al: *Human pharmacology*, ed 1, St Louis, 1991, Mosby.)

DNA and RNA Characteristics

CHARACTERISTIC	DNA	RNA
Type of sugar	Deoxyribose	Ribose
Nucleoside pairing	Cytosine with guanine	Cytosine with guanine
	Adenine with thymine	Adenine with uracil

Purines: adenine and guanine; pyridines: cytosine, thymine, and uracil.

and RNA are listed in the box on p. 576, and the currently available antiviral agents their nucleoside type (purine verses pyridine), and their antiviral activity are summarized in Table 37-1.

Mechanism of Action

The different antiviral agents vary in the way in which they kill viruses. To replicate, the virus first attaches to and diffuses into the cell, then once in the cell it has its genetic makeup copied, after which the nucleus of the infected cell utilizes its DNA and RNA to make new viruses. An antiviral agent can work at any of these steps: attachment, the reading of the virus' genetic makeup, and the making of new virus. The overall effect of these agents, however, is the inhibition of viral replication. Many antivirals accomplish this by interfering with viral DNA polymerase; others inhibit reverse transcriptase.

Drug Effects

The antiviral agents are used to treat a variety of virus-related disorders ranging from HSV to HIV, but the agents exert varying degrees of activity against viruses. These drug effects, or antiviral activity, are

summarized for the different agents in the box on p. 578.

Therapeutic Uses

The therapeutic effects of the antiviral agents vary greatly depending on the particular agent and its spectrum of activity. The increasing public awareness of one of the most deadly viruses known to humankind, HIV, has stimulated much research into antiviral agents. This has led to the development of many new and improved agents, though many of these agents also produce significant toxicities. The therapeutic effects of the various agents are also summarized in the box on p. 578.

Side Effects and Adverse Effects

The side effects and adverse effects of the antiviral agents are as different as the agents themselves. Each has its own specific side effect profile. Because viruses reproduce in human cells and therefore have many of the same features as these cells, it makes it much harder to target a unique enzyme or feature of the virus. Selective killing is difficult, and as a result, more good human cells are killed in the process, resulting in

Table 37-1	**Antiviral Agents: Characteristics**	
ANTIVIRAL AGENT	**NUCLEOSIDE ANALOGUE OF**	**ANTIVIRAL ACTIVITY**
Purine nucleosides		
⚓Acyclovir	Guanine	HSV 1 and 2, VZV
Didanosine (ddI)	Adenosine	HIV
Ganciclovir (DHPG)	Guanine	CMV retinitis and systemic CMV infection
Ribavirin (RTCD)	Guanine	Influenza type A and B, RSV, LV, HV
Vidarabine (Ara-A)	Adenosine	HSV, herpes zoster
Pyridine nucleosides [cytosine (C), thymine (T), and uracil (C)]		
Idoxuridine (IDU)	Thymine	HSV
Trifluridine	Thymine	HSV
Zalcitabine (ddC)	Cytosine	HIV
⚓Zidovudine (AZT)	Thymine	HIV
Others		
⚓Amantadine	Synthetic adamantine derivative, related to rimantadine	Influenza A
Rimantadine		
Foscarnet	Pyrophosphate	CMV retinitis

CMV, cytomegalovirus; *HIV*, human immunodeficiency virus; *HSV*, herpes simplex virus (types 1 and 2); *HV*, hantavirus; *LV*, lassa virus; *RSV*, respiratory syncytial virus; *VZV*, varicella zoster virus.

Antiviral Therapeutic Effects

ANTIVIRAL	VIRAL ACTIVITY	THERAPEUTIC EFFECT
⚓Amantadine and rimantadine	Influenza A	Used for the treatment and prophylaxis of influenza A but ineffective against influenza B; most effective if given before exposure or within 48 hours of development of symptoms; reduces fever and palliates symptoms of influenza.
⚓Acyclovir and vidarabine	HSV 1 and 2, varicella-zoster virus	Vidarabine was used primarily in treatment of herpes simplex encephalitis, disseminated or CNS herpes infections in the newborn, herpes keratitis (topically), and herpes zoster, but has been generally replaced by acyclovir; acyclovir is used topically, orally, and intravenously for treatment of herpes simplex encephalitis and most other significant herpes infections; it is more efficacious and less toxic than vidarabine; administration as soon as possible produces the best results; these agents reduce viral shedding, decrease local symptoms, and decrease severity and duration of illness
Ganciclovir and foscarnet	CMV	Ganciclovir is the older and more studied of these two agents; it has been shown to be effective for not only CMV retinitis but also other CMV infections such as GI infection and pneumonitis; the primary dose-limiting toxicity of ganciclovir is bone marrow toxicity; foscarnet is not toxic to the bone marrow but can cause renal failure
Ribavirin	Influenza A and B, RSV, Lassa virus, Hantavirus	Used as an aerosol for treatment of severe RSV bronchopneumonia; shown to improve oxygenation, decrease viral shedding, and alleviate pneumonia symptoms; inhalation treatment has also been shown to be effective in influenza A and B infections; orally and parenterally effective for Lassa fever virus as well as Hantavirus
Didanosine, zalcitabine, zidovudine	HIV	Approved for the treatment of HIV infections in the setting of AIDS and AIDS-related complex; they produce a significant reduction in mortality and incidence of opportunistic infections, improve physical performance, and significantly improve T-cell counts.
Idoxuridine and trifluridine	HSV	Used to treat herpes simplex keratitis; are only used topically because of significant liver and bone marrow toxicity

more serious toxicities. These serious adverse effects are listed by agent in Table 37-2.

Interactions

The significant drug interactions that occur with the antiviral agents involve those agents administered systemically. Many of the antivirals are applied topically to the eye or body, and the incidence of drug interactions associated with these agents is low. The antiviral agents, the drugs they interact with, and the result of the interaction are as follows:

⚓**Acyclovir** with:
Zidovudine: increased risk of neurotoxicity
Probenecid: increased acyclovir levels by decreasing renal clearance
Antifungal agents: increased antiviral effects
Interferon: additive antiviral effects
Methotrexate: increased neurotoxicity

Table 37-2	Antivirals: Adverse Effects
ANTIVIRAL AGENT	**SIDE/ADVERSE EFFECTS**
Acyclovir	Most common are nausea, vomiting, diarrhea, headache, transient burning when topically applied
Amantadine and rimantadine	CNS: insomnia, nervousness, lightheadedness; GI: anorexia, nausea; anticholinergic effects
Didanosine	GI: pancreatitis; CNS: peripheral neuropathies, seizures
Foscarnet	CNS: headache, seizures; MET: hypocalcemia, hypophosphatemia, hyperphosphatemia, hypokalemia; GU: acute renal failure; HEM: bone marrow suppression; GI: nausea, vomiting, diarrhea
Ganciclovir	HEM: bone marrow toxicity; GI: nausea, anorexia, vomiting; CNS: headache, seizures
Idoxuridine	Nothing significant
Ribavirin	Rash, conjunctivitis, anemia
Trifluridine	Burning, swelling, stinging, photophobia, pain
Vidarabine	GI: nausea, vomiting, diarrhea, anorexia, weight loss; CNS: dizziness, weakness, tremors, ataxia, hallucinations
Zalcitabine	Peripheral neuropathy, rash, ulcers
Zidovudine	Bone marrow suppression, nausea, headache

CNS, Central nervous system; *GI,* gastrointestinal tract; *GU,* genitourinary system; *HEM,* hematologic; *MET,* metabolic.

↓**Amantadine** with:
Anticholinergic drugs: increased adverse anticholinergic effects
CNS stimulants: additive CNS stimulant effects
Didanosine with:
Antacids: increased absorption of didanosine, which is a positive effect
Dapsone: may interfere with GI absorption of dapsone
Itraconazole and ketoconazole: didanosine decreases their absorption, give 2 hours before
Quinolones: didanosine decreases absorption of some quinolone antibiotics
Tetracyclines: decreased absorption of tetracyclines; give 2 hours before tetracyclines
Zalcitabine: additive toxicity (peripheral neuropathies); avoid giving together

Zidovudine: additive and synergistic effect against HIV
Ganciclovir with:
Zidovudine: increased risk of hematologic toxicity, (i.e., bone marrow suppression)
Foscarnet: additive or synergistic effect against CMV and HSV-2
Imipenem: increased risk of seizures
Zalcitabine with:
Drugs associated with pancreatic, peripheral neuropathy, and renal toxicities: should be avoided because of additive toxicities
Zidovudine: additive or synergistic effect against HIV
↓**Zidovudine** with:
Acyclovir: increased neurotoxicity
Didanosine, zalcitabine, foscarnet, and interferon alpha: additive or synergistic effect against HIV
Ganciclovir, ribavirin: antagonize the antiviral action of zidovudine

Dosages

See the dosages table on the following page for recommended dosages for selected antiviral agents.

DRUG PROFILES

There have been many new agents recently added to the antiviral drug class. This has in part been prompted by the growing concern over the devastating effects HIV infection (AIDS) has had on our population. Many new and improved antiviral agents have been developed—some with improved actions but greater toxicities; others with similar actions but improved side effect profiles. Some of the prototypical antiviral agents are discussed here.

↓ ACYCLOVIR

Acyclovir (Zovirax) is a synthetic analogue of guanine that is mainly used to suppress the replication of HSV 1 and 2 as well as the varicella-zoster virus, commonly known as *chickenpox* and *shingles.* Acyclovir is considered the drug of choice for the treatment of both initial and recurrent episodes of both these viral infections. It is the synthetic analogue of the natural nucleoside guanine. Another antiviral agent with properties similar

DOSAGES

SELECTED ANTIVIRAL AGENTS

AGENT	PHARMACOLOGIC CLASS	DOSAGE RANGE	PURPOSE
⚓Acyclovir (Zovirax)	Purine nucleoside analogue antiviral	Topical: apply ointment q3h 6 times/day	HSV cutaneous infection
		Pediatric PO: 20 mg/kg qid for 5 days IV: 250 mg/m² for 1 hr for 7 days 500 mg/m² q8h for 10 days	Chickenpox HSV-1, HSV-2 infection HSV encephalitis and shingles
		Adult PO: 200 mg q4h 5 times/day for 10 day 800 mg q4h 5 times/day for 7-10 days	HSV-2 (genital herpes) Shingles
Ganciclovir (Cytovene)	Purine nucleoside analogue antiviral	*Adult* IV: 5 mg/kg q12h for 14-21 days; maintenance dose, 5 mg/kg over 1 hr/day or 6 mg/kg/day for 5 days every wk	CMV retinitis in immunocompromised patients
⚓Amantadine (Symmetrel)	Antiviral	*Pediatric* PO: 1-9 y/o: 2-4 mg/lb/day once daily or divided into 2 daily doses 9-12 y/o: 100 mg bid *Adult* PO: 100 mg bid or 200 mg once/day	Prophylaxis and treatment of influenza A
Ribavirin (Virazole)	Purine nucleoside analogue antiviral	*Infants/Pediatric* Aerosol: treatment with SPAG-2 for 12-18 hr/day with drug concentration of 20 mg/ml in drug reservoir of unit; average aerosal concentration for 12 hr pd, 190 µg/L of air. Treatment should last at least 3 days and not more than 7 days.	Selected infant and pediatric patients with RSV infections
Trifluridine (Viroptic)	Pyrimidine nucleoside analogue antiviral	Ophthalmic solution: 1 gtt q2h to affected eye to maximum of 9 gtts	HSV 1 and 2 keratoconjunctivitis, recurrent epithelial keratitis
⚓Zidovudine (Retrovir)	Pyrimidine nucleoside analogue antiviral	*Pediatric 3 mo-12 y/o* PO: 180 mg/m² q6h (720 mg/m²/day); do not exceed 200 mg q6h *Adult* PO: asymptomatic cases, 500 mg/day divided; symptomatic cases, 600 mg/day divided IV: 1-2 mg/kg infused over 1 hr q4h	HIV infections
		Maternal/Fetal Mother: PO: 100 mg 5 times/day after 14 weeks of pregnancy; during labor switch to 2 mg/kg IV over 1 hr, followed by continuous infusion of 1 mg/kg/hr until cord is clamped Infant: PO: 2 mg/kg q6h starting within 12 hr after delivery and continued for 6 wk	Fetal HIV prophylaxis

SPAG, small particle aerosol generator.

to those of acyclovir is vidarabine. It was one of the first effective antiviral drugs available in an injectable formulation but differs from acyclovir in that it is an analogue of adenine.

Acyclovir is available in both oral and parenteral formulations. It comes orally as 200-mg capsules, a 200-mg/5 ml suspension, and 800-mg tablets. Parenterally it comes as a 500-mg and 1-gm injection for intravenous infusion. Acyclovir is classified as a pregnancy category C drug and is contraindicated in patients hypersensitive to it. It is a prescription-only drug. Commonly recommended dosages can be found in the dosages table on the previous page.

☙ PHARMACOKINETICS

HALF-LIFE	ONSET	PEAK	DURATION
2.1-5 hr	Unknown	PO: 1.5-2 hr	4-5 hr

GANCICLOVIR

Like acyclovir, ganciclovir (Cytovene) is also a synthetic analogue of guanine but it has a much different spectrum of antiviral activity. Ganciclovir and foscarnet are the two antiviral agents that are used in the treatment of CMV infections. They also have activity against HSV 1 and 2, Epstein-Barr virus, and varicella-zoster virus, but are not used for the treatment of infection caused by these viruses because there are other less toxic antiviral agents that are just as effective in inhibiting them.

Of the two antivirals, ganciclovir is the one more frequently used in the treatment of CMV infections. The most common site of CMV infections in the immunocompromised patient is the eye, and the result is CMV retinitis, a devastating viral infection that can lead to blindness. Disseminated CMV infections such as GI tract infections and pneumonitis are other indications for ganciclovir treatment.

A dose-limiting toxicity of ganciclovir treatment is bone marrow suppression; that of foscarnet is renal toxicity. These toxicities should be kept in mind when deciding on which agent is more appropriate in a particular patient. For example, a heart transplant recipient who contracts CMV retinitis is immunocompromised because of immunosuppressant drug therapy and is most likely taking cyclosporine, which is nephrotoxic. Therefore using foscarnet in this patient is more dangerous than using ganciclovir. On the other hand, a patient who contracts a CMV infection and is immunocompromised because of a bone marrow transplant would be better treated using foscarnet.

Ganciclovir is only available in a parenteral formulation and comes as a 500-mg injection for intravenous infusion. It is classified as a pregnancy category C agent and is contraindicated in patients with a hy-

persensitivity to either it or acyclovir. Commonly recommended dosages can be found in the dosages table on the previous page.

☙ PHARMACOKINETICS

HALF-LIFE	ONSET	PEAK	DURATION
2.5-3.6 hr	Unknown	Variable	Variable

⚓ AMANTADINE

Amantadine (Symmetrel) has a narrow antiviral spectrum in that it is only active against influenza A viruses. It is used both prophylactically as well as therapeutically. It has been shown to be very effective, if not lifesaving, when used prophylactically in, for instance, elderly, chronically ill, or immunocompromised patients in whom an influenza A infection can be particularly devastating.

Rimantadine is a structural analogue of amantadine that has the same spectrum of activity, mechanism of action, and clinical indications. However, it differs from amantadine in that it has a longer half-life, may be dosed less frequently, and causes less CNS toxicity. However, it causes more GI side effects that are also more serious.

Amantadine is classified as a pregnancy category C agent and is contraindicated in patients with a known hypersensitivity to it, lactating women, children under 12 months of age, and patients with an eczematic rash. Amantadine is only available orally as a 50-mg/5 ml solution and 100-mg liquid-filled capsules. Commonly recommended dosages can be found in the dosages table on the previous page.

☙ PHARMACOKINETICS

HALF-LIFE	ONSET	PEAK	DURATION
24 hr	Unknown	Unknown	12-24 hr

RIBAVIRIN

Ribavirin (Virazole) is a unique antiviral agent in that it is only given by oral or nasal inhalation. It is a synthetic nucleoside analogue of guanosine, as are many of the other antiviral agents, but it has a spectrum of antiviral activity that is broader than that of other currently available antiviral agents. It interferes with both RNA and DNA synthesis and as a result inhibits both protein synthesis and viral replication.

Ribavirin is used for the treatment of severe lower respiratory tract infections caused by RSV. It is also useful in the treatment of both influenza A and B infections as well as Lassa fever and Hantavirus infections.

Because ribavirin may cause fetal toxicity when administered to pregnant women, it is a pregnancy category X agent. It is therefore contraindicated in pregnant women with RSV infections because the risk of teratogenic or embryocidal effects far outweighs any benefits to be gained in the treatment of these generally self-limiting infections. Ribavirin is only available in an inhalation form that is given either nasally or orally. Commonly recommended dosages can be found in the dosages table on p. 580.

✿ PHARMACOKINETICS

HALF-LIFE	ONSET	PEAK	DURATION
1.4-2.5 hr*	Unknown	End of inhalation period	Variable

*In respiratory secretions.

TRIFLURIDINE

Trifluridine (Viroptic) is an analogue of thymidine and is very similar to the antiviral agent idoxuridine (Stoxil and Herplex), differing only slightly in its chemical structure. Both are used to treat herpes simplex keratitis, but trifluridine is also indicated for the treatment of herpes simplex keratoconjunctivitis. They are applied only topically to the eye because of the significant liver and bone marrow toxicities they can cause when given orally.

Trifluridine is classified as a pregnancy category C agent and is contraindicated in patients with a known hypersensitivity to it. It is only available as a 1% ophthalmic solution. Commonly recommended dosages can be found in the dosages table on p. 580.

✿ PHARMACOKINETICS

HALF-LIFE	ONSET	PEAK	DURATION
Unknown	Unknown	Immediate	2 hr

⚓ ZIDOVUDINE

Zidovudine (AZT, ZDV, Retrovir) is a synthetic analogue of thymidine that has had an enormous impact on the treatment and quality of life of patients infected with HIV who have AIDS. HIV requires a reverse transcriptase for viral replication, and this process is inhibited by zidovudine plus two other antivirals, zalcitabine (Hivid) and didanosine (Videx). To date the only antiviral agent used to treat HIV infections that has been shown to prolong survival has been zidovudine. Zalcitabine and didanosine have been reserved for those patients who have failed zidovudine treatment or cannot tolerate the agent.

Besides its antiviral activity, zidovudine also has activity bactericidal activity against some gram-negative bacteria, particularly many Enterobacteriaceae.

These three antiviral agents are all approved for the treatment of HIV infections in patients with AIDS or ARC (AIDS-related complex). Treatment leads to a significant reduction in mortality and the incidence of opportunistic infections, improves patient's physical performance, and significantly improves T-cell counts.

Zidovudine's major dose-limiting adverse effect is bone marrow suppression, and this is often the reason why a patient with an HIV infection has to be switched to another anti-HIV agent such as zalcitabine or didanosine. Some patients may be taking a combination of two of these agents to maximize their actions but also to cut back on the dose of both agents, thus decreasing the likelihood of toxicity.

Zidovudine is classified as a pregnancy category C agent and is contraindicated in patients with a known hypersensitivity to it. It is available in both oral and parenteral formulations. Parenterally it comes as a 10-mg/ml injection for IV infusion. Orally it comes as 100-mg capsules and a 50-mg/5 ml solution. Commonly recommended dosages can be found in the dosages table on p. 580.

✿ PHARMACOKINETICS

HALF-LIFE	ONSET	PEAK	DURATION
0.78-1.93 hr	Unknown	0.4-1.5 hr	3-5 hr

Nursing Process

ASSESSMENT

Before administering an antiviral agent the nurse should perform a thorough assessment to find out what underlying diseases the patient may have and his or her past medical history. This is important to ensuring safe medication use. The nurse should also find out whether the patient has any known allergies to the medication or whether he or she has suffered any side effects of the medication in the past. It is important to assess the patient's nutritional status and baseline vital signs as well because of the profound effects viral illnesses can have on them, especially if the patient is also immunosuppressed. Contraindications to the use of most of the antiviral agents include herpes zoster infection in immunosuppressed patients, and cautious use, with careful monitoring, is recommended in patients who have renal or hepatic disease, who are de-

RESEARCH
Costs Decline for Treating
HIV-Infected Children

Acquired immunodeficiency syndrome (AIDS) had affected 4030 children under the age of 13 in the United States by 1992, many of whom relied on Medicaid to pay for their health care. Children with AIDS used services of $37,928 per year, compared with $32,508 per year for adults with AIDS, whereas HIV-infected children without diagnoses of AIDS generated only one fourth of the annual charges, $9382. These findings are in sharp contrast with the high costs of care for HIV-infected children reported in earlier studies. Children with AIDS are currently hospitalized an average of 10.6 days per admission, compared with 14 to 20 days from the mid 1980s. Over half of the children studied by Hsia, Fleishman, and Hellinger reported no inpatient admissions at all over the 18-month study period. Furthermore, the results of this study showed that children with AIDS averaged 1.4 hospitalizations, 18 outpatient care days, 15 professional home health care visits, and one dental visit per year.

From Hsia DC, Fleishman JA, Hellinger F: Pediatric human immunodeficiency virus infection, *Arch Pediatr Adolesc Med*, p. 489, AHCPR Publication #95-R007, 1995.

hydrated or in electrolyte imbalance, who are pregnant or lactating, or who have seizure disorders.

Amantadine is contraindicated in children under 1 year of age and should be used cautiously in patients suffering from congestive heart failure (because of the cardiovascular side effects it causes) or orthostatic hypotension. Laboratory results that should also be obtained before the start of therapy include WBC, RBC, BUN, CPK, LDH, and creatinine clearance. Culture and sensitivity testing should also be done. Zidovudine has been used in patients with HIV infections, but it is associated with many side effects and is capable of significant drug interactions that may increase the risk of toxicity. The agents it interacts with in this way are vincristine, adriamycin, amphotericin B, and interferon. Some of the NSAIDS, such as probenecid and indomethacin, as well as acetaminophen and aspirin may interact with it as well, also enhancing the potential for toxicity.

NURSING DIAGNOSES

Nursing diagnoses appropriate to patients receiving antiviral agents include:
- Pain related to the signs and symptoms of a viral infection.

- Risk for injury related to side effects of medication.
- Knowledge deficit regarding the viral infection, its transmission, and treatment.
- Risk for altered mobility (decreased) related to impact of viral infection.

PLANNING

Goals pertaining to patients receiving antiviral agents include:
- Patient will be free of symptoms of viral infection once therapy is completed.
- Patient remains compliant with therapy.
- Patient experiences improved energy and appetite and improved ability to engage in activities of daily living.
- Patient states the rationale for therapy for any sexual partners if diagnosed with genital herpes.
- Patient experiences minimal side effects of antiviral agent.

Outcome Criteria

Outcome criteria for patients receiving antiviral agents include:
- Patient will experience increased periods of comfort as the result of successful treatment of viral infection.
- Patient will state the effect of a viral infection on his or her state of health (e.g., compromised immune system) and need for appropriate treatment.
- Patient states the rationale for treatment of self and any sexual partners if diagnosed with genital herpes, as well as the importance of compliance with the treatment to prevent worsening of symptoms and decrease severity of episodes.
- Patient will identify possible side effects of antiviral agent such as diarrhea, headache, nausea, and insomnia.

IMPLEMENTATION

Nursing interventions pertinent to patients receiving antiviral agents include use of the appropriate technique of application or administration of ointment, aerosol powders, IV, or oral forms of medication. Handwashing before and after administration of the medication is necessary to prevent contamination of the site and spread of infection to others. In addition, strict adherence to universal precautions is important to the safety of both the patient and the nurse.

Topical antiviral agents such as acyclovir should be applied in accordance with the manufacturer's guidelines or physician's orders, and gloves must be used to prevent the spread of infection to others. Intravenously administered acyclovir should be diluted in recommended solutions such as sterile water for injection or in the solutions recommended by the manufacturer. IV administration is usually done over 1 hour, but all sources of drug information should be consulted first to make sure that this and not some other timing is called for.

Most antivirals should be administered with caution in those patients who have renal or hepatic dysfunction. Because zidovudine suppresses bone marrow functioning, it should not be used in conjunction with other agents that do the same because of the resulting additive adverse effects. Other drugs that interact with zidovudine include aspirin, acetaminophen, benzodiazepines, cimetidine, morphine, and sulfonamides.

Acyclovir and many of the other antiviral agents also interact with several drugs, and these have been enumerated earlier in the section on drug interactions. Fluid intake of at least 2400 ml per day should be encouraged in patients receiving acyclovir, unless contraindicated. This is to prevent crystalluria and is also applicable to patients receiving it intravenously. IV infusions should be administered slowly over at least 1 hour and the IV sites watched closely for the devel-

Patient Teaching TIPS

Antiviral Therapy

✔ Tell patients the importance of taking these medications exactly as prescribed and for the full course of therapy.

✔ Some antivirals may cause dizziness, so the patient should be cautioned about driving or participating in activities requiring alertness.

✔ Patients should consult the physician before taking any other prescribed or OTC medications.

✔ Patients in immunosuppressed states should avoid crowds and persons with infections.

✔ Universal precautions and safe sex should be advocated in patients who are HIV positive.

✔ Patients using acyclovir ointment for treatment of herpes simplex infection should not use any other additional creams or ointments on the site. The patient should wear a glove or finger cot when applying topical solutions to affected areas, which should be kept clean and dry.

✔ Patients with any type of viral infection should practice good hygiene.

✔ Inform patients that antiviral agents are not cures but do help to manage the related symptoms.

TAKE HOME POINTS

Viruses
■ Current viruses killed by antivirals: CMV, HSV, HIV, influenza A, RSV.
■ Difficult to kill because they live inside human cells.
■ Drugs work by inhibiting viral replication.

Antiviral Drugs
■ Are synthetic purine and pyridine nucleoside analogues.
■ They trick virus into thinking that they are either a purine (adenine or guanine) or a pyridine (cytosine or thymine) and then are taken up by the virus, which tries to use them to replicate itself and in doing so ends up dying.
■ Must be able to enter cells infected with virus, interfere with viral nucleic acid synthesis, interfere with ability of virus to bind to cells, and stimulate body's immune system.

Purine Analogue Antivirals
■ Are synthetic analogues of purine nucleosides such as adenine and guanine.
■ Most common examples are acyclovir, didanosine, and ganciclovir.

Pyridine Analogue Antivirals
■ Are synthetic analogues of pyridine nucleoside such as cytosine and thymine.
■ Most common examples are zalcitabine, zidovudine, and trifluridine.

Nursing Considerations
■ Antiviral agents should be administered only after all physician orders are read and understood and after a thorough nursing assessment that includes an examination of the patient's nutritional status and baseline vital signs.
■ Contraindications to the use of antiviral agents include herpes zoster in immunosuppressed patents.
■ Cautious use is recommended in patients with renal, hepatic, or seizure disorders; pregnant or lactating women; and patients who are dehydrated or in electrolyte imbalance.
■ There are many drugs that interact with the antiviral agents, so the nurse should always check to make sure the patient is taking none of these agents before administering the antiviral agent.

opment of redness, swelling, or heat. Acyclovir capsules may be given with food. Acyclovir sodium should not be administered SC, IM, PO, or ophthalmically. There are many IV agents and solutions that are incompatible with IV acyclovir, and the nurse should check and recheck this before proceeding with the coadministration of other agents or solutions.

Orally administered didanosine should be given every 12 hours, or as ordered, and on an empty stomach 1 hour before meals or 2 hours after meals. Antifungals are incompatible with didanosine. Buffered powder solutions for oral administration should be mixed in at least 4 ounces of water, not fruit juice or acid-containing juices, and the solution should be drunk immediately after mixing. See the box on p. 584 for more information on antivirals and associated patient education guidelines.

EVALUATION

The therapeutic effects of antiviral agents depend mainly on the type of viral infection and the immune and general status of the patient. This could range from delayed progression of AIDS and ARC to a decrease in flulike symptoms and the frequency of herpetic flare-ups and opportunistic infections. Herpetic lesions should crust over, and the frequency of recurrence should decrease. Adverse reactions to specific antiviral agents should be monitored for, and these specific reactions are listed in Table 37-2.

Critical Thinking **A C T I V I T I E S**

1. Treatment with antiviral agents is often more difficult than it seems because of which of the following?
   a. The virus develops a double-protein-layer wall, and this prevents penetration of the drug.
   b. Viral replication is not well understood.
   c. The virus develops a resistance to medications and a more porous permeable membrane.
   d. Often only after viral replication is finished do symptoms appear.

2. You are caring for a patient who has AIDS. He has been on AZT (zidovudine) for a year and a half and his CD4 count has just recently started to drop below 125. The physician adds didanosine (ddI) to the patient's antiviral drug regimen.
   Which of the following statements regarding the patient's drug therapy is most accurate?
   a. The combination of AZT and ddI is unnecessary because it consists of two drugs from the same class.
   b. The combination of AZT and ddI is potentially harmful because both drugs have similar side effect profiles, and this increases the chance of toxicity.
   c. The combination is appropriate because it consists of two antivirals with synergistic actions yet different side effect profiles.
   d. The combination is appropriate because it consists of an antifungal and an antiviral drug.
   A month into therapy with this combination-drug regimen a CBC reveals a low number of platelets, neutrophils, and other cells produced by the bone marrow. You recognize this as:
   a. a peripheral neuropathy induced by ddI.
   b. pancreatitis induced by AZT.
   c. bone marrow suppression induced by ddI.
   d. bone marrow suppression induced by AZT.
   This change in events prompts some adjustments in the patient's drug regimen. On the following day when you arrive to care for this patient, you notice that the physician on call over the weekend has stopped the AZT treatment and started ddC (zalcitabine) treatment. You call the physician to notify her that:
   a. ddI and ddC can both cause bone marrow suppression, and the combination is potentially dangerous.
   b. ddI and ddC are antagonist to each other, and each will reduce the effectiveness of the other agent.
   c. ddI and ddC can both cause peripheral neuropathies, and the combination is potentially dangerous.
   d. ddI is an antifungal and ddC is an antiviral, and the combination is okay.

▲▲

BIBLIOGRAPHY

Albanese J, Nutz P: *Mosby's 1995 nursing drug cards,* St Louis, 1995, Mosby.

Johnson KB: *Harriet Lane handbook,* ed 13, St Louis, 1993, Mosby.

Keen JH: *Critical care and emergency drug reference,* St Louis, 1994, Mosby.

Knoben JE, Anderson PO: *Handbook of critical drug data,* ed 6, Hamilton, Ill, 1988, Drug Intelligence Publications.

McEvoy GK: *AHFS drug information,* Bethesda, Md, 1994, American Society of Hospital Pharmacists.

Powers MJ and Co, (eds): All about drugs, *Am J Nurs* 10:32, 1995.

Reines ED, Gross PA: Antiviral agents, *Med Clin North Am* 72:691, 1988.

Chapter 38

Antitubercular Agents

Objectives

When you reach the end of this chapter, you will be able to:

1 Identify the various first-line and second-line agents used for the treatment of tuberculosis.
2 Discuss the mechanism of action, dosages, and side effects of the various antitubercular agents, as well as the indications for treatment, the cautions and contraindications to treatment, and the drug interactions.
3 Develop a nursing care plan as it relates to the nursing process for patients receiving antitubercular drugs.
4 Develop a teaching guide for patients receiving any of the various antitubercular agents.

CHAPTER OUTLINE

Tuberculosis
Antitubercular Agents
  Mechanism of action
  Drug effects
  Therapeutic uses
  Side effects and adverse effects
  Interactions
  Dosages
Drug Profiles
  Ethambutol
  ⚓ Isoniazid
  Pyrazinamide
  Rifampin
  Streptomycin

Nursing Process
Assessment
Nursing Diagnoses
Planning
  Outcome criteria
Implementation
Evaluation

Glossary

Aerobic (ā'ro' bik) Requiring oxygen for the maintenance of life. (p. 587)
Antitubercular agents (an' tĭ too bǝr' ku ler) Drugs used to treat infections caused by *Mycobacterium* spp. (p. 588)
  Bacillus (bǝ sil' us) Rod-shaped bacteria. (p. 587)
  Isoniazid (i' so ni' ǝ zid) Primary and most frequently prescribed tuberculostatic agent. (p. 588)
  Multi-drug–resistant TB Tuberculosis that demonstrates resistance to two or more drugs. (p. 588)
  Primary (first-line) drugs Class of drugs currently employed for the treatment of pulmonary tuberculosis. (p. 588)
  Primary TB infection A patient's first TB infection. (p. 588)
  Reinfection The most chronic form of tuberculosis. (p. 588)
  Secondary (second-line) drugs Class of drugs currently employed for the treatment of pulmonary tuberculosis. (p. 588)
  Slow acetylators Persons with a genetic defect that causes them to be deficient in the enzyme needed to break down isoniazid. (p. 592)
  Tubercle bacilli (too' bǝr ka'l) Rod-shaped tuberculosis bacteria. (p. 588)

TUBERCULOSIS

Mycobacterium tuberculosis is the bacteria that causes tuberculosis (TB). It is an **aerobic bacillus,** which means that it is a rod-shaped microorganism *(bacillus)* that requires a lot of oxygen for it to grow and flourish *(aerobic).* This bacteria's need for a highly oxygenated body site explains why *Mycobacterium* infections most commonly affect the lungs, the growing ends of bones, and the brain (cerebral cortex), with the kidney, liver, and genitourinary tract other less common sites.

These **tubercle** (tuberculous) **bacilli** are transmitted from one of three sources: human beings, cows (bovine), or birds (avian), though bovine and avian transmission are much less common than human transmission. The tubercle bacilli are conveyed in droplets expelled by infected persons or animals during coughing or sneezing and then inhaled by the new host. After these infectious droplets are inhaled, the infection spreads to the susceptible organ sites by means of the blood and lymphatic system. However, tuberculosis does not develop in all persons who inhale these infectious droplets. Instead, in these persons the bacteria become dormant or walled off by calcified or fibrous tissues. At the other end of the spectrum are the infected persons whose host defenses have been broken down as the result of immunosuppressive drug therapy, chemotherapy for cancer, or an immunosuppressive disease such as AIDS. In these persons the disease can inflict devastating and irreversible damage. The first infectious episode is considered the **primary TB infection; reinfection** represents the more chronic form of the disease.

Over the past decade there has been growing concern about the increasing number of cases of TB. This is evidenced by the 18% increase in the incidence of TB that took place between 1985 and 1991, such that it is now estimated that between 10 and 15 million persons worldwide have some form of tuberculous infection.

Several factors are responsible for fomenting this health care crisis, but one very important source of the problem is the increasing number of people who are particularly susceptible to the infection—homeless and undernourished or malnourished persons; AIDS victims; persons taking immunosuppressant drugs; drug abusers; and persons suffering from cancer. Those people at high risk of contracting the disease also tend to be members of minority groups (64% of all cases) and those who live in crowded and poorly sanitated facilities.

As great of a concern as the increasing number of TB cases has been the appearance of drug-resistant tuberculosis. For instance, the Centers for Disease Control (CDC), which track and monitor the epidemiologic course of many diseases, TB being one of major importance, observed that in 1991 in New York City 33% of the patients with TB were resistant to at least one antitubercular drug. Disease resistant to two or more drugs is called **multi-drug–resistant** TB (MDR-TB). There have already been outbreaks of such cases in nine institutional facilities, and the CDC has found these occurred to a great extent (20%-100%) in HIV-infected persons. They also found the mortality in these persons with MDR-TB to range between 72% and 89%.

ANTITUBERCULAR AGENTS

The agents used to treat infections caused by all forms of *Mycobacterium* are called **antitubercular agents,** and these agents fall into two categories: **primary (first-line)** and **secondary (second-line) agents.** The antimycobacterial activity, efficacy, and potential adverse and toxic effects of the various agents determine which class they belong to. **Isoniazid** (INH), a primary antitubercular drug, is the most frequently used antitubercular agent. It can be used either as the sole agent in the prophylaxis of TB or in combination with other antitubercular agents. The various first- and second-line antibiotics agents are listed in the box below.

An important consideration during drug selection is what the relative likelihood of drug-resistant organisms and drug toxicity is. Following are other key elements important to the planning and implementation of the affective therapy:

1. Drug-susceptibility tests should be performed on the first-isolated *Mycobacterium* sp. (to prevent the development of MDR-TB).
2. Before the results of the susceptibility tests are known, the patient should be started on a four-drug regimen, consisting of INH, rifampin, pyrazinamide, and ethambutol or streptomycin, which together are 95% effective in combating the infection.

First- and Second-Line Antitubercular Drugs

Primary
Ethambutol
Isoniazid (INH)
Pyrazinamide (PZA)
Rifampin
Streptomycin

Secondary*
Para-aminosalicylic acid (PAS)
Capreomycin
Cycloserine
Ethionamide
Kanamycin

Other
Rifabutin

*Multidrug regimens that include drugs such as streptomycin, kanamycin, and capreomycin, which have similar toxic effects, should include only one of these drugs.

3. Once drug susceptibility results are available, the regimen should be adjusted accordingly.
4. Patient compliance and the adverse effects of the prescribed regimen should be monitored closely because the incidence of both is high.

Despite all the agents available to combat TB and the efforts mounted to detect and treat victims of the disease, treatment has been made difficult by two problems already mentioned: patient noncompliance with therapy and the growing incidence of drug-resistant organisms.

Mechanism of Action

The mechanisms of action of the various antitubercular drugs vary depending on the agent. These drugs act on *M. tuberculosis* in one of three ways: they either inhibit protein or cell wall synthesis or work by some other means. The antitubercular agents are listed in the box below by their mechanism of action.

Drug Effects

The drug effects of the antitubercular agents are primarily limited to their ability to kill *M. tuberculosis,* but other strains of *Mycobacterium* may also be susceptible to the killing actions of these drugs. They are used as the initial treatment for patients with uncomplicated pulmonary TB and for most children and adults with extrapulmonary TB. The antitubercular drug effects have not been fully tested in pregnant women, but the combination of isoniazid and ethambutol has been used to treat pregnant women with clinically apparent TB without teratogenic complications.

Besides being used for the initial treatment of TB, antitubercular agents have also proved effective in the management of treatment failures and relapses. Infection with species of *Mycobacterium* other than *M. tuberculosis,* also called *MOTT,* as well as atypical mycobacterial infections have also been successfully treated with these agents. Nontuberculous mycobacteria (NTM) may also be susceptible to antitubercular drugs. However, in general, the antitubercular agents

Antitubercular Drugs: Mechanisms

DRUGS	DESCRIPTION
Inhibit Protein Synthesis Streptomycin Kanamycin Rifampin Capreomycin Rifabutin	Streptomycin and kanamycin work by interfering with normal protein synthesis and production of faulty proteins. Rifampin and capreomycin act at different points in the protein synthesis pathway from streptomycin and kanamycin. Rifampin inhibits RNA synthesis and may also inhibit DNA synthesis. Human cells are not as sensitive as the mycobacterial cells and are not affected by rifampin except at high drug concentrations. Capreomycin inhibits protein synthesis by preventing translocation on ribosomes.
Inhibit Cell Wall Synthesis Cycloserine ↓Isoniazid Ethionamide	Cycloserine acts by inhibiting two enzymes involved in the synthesis of cell walls. Isoniazid and ethionamide also act at least partly to inhibit the synthesis of cell wall components, but the mechanisms of these two agents are still not clearly understood.
Other Mechanisms ↓Isoniazid Ethionamide Ethambutol Pyrazinamide Para-aminosalicylic acid	Other proposed MOAs for isoniazid exist. Isoniazid is taken up by mycobacterial cells and undergoes hydrolysis to isonicotinic acid, which reacts with cofactor NAD to form a defective NAD that is no longer active as a coenzyme for certain life-sustaining reactions in the *M. tuberculosis* organism. Ethionamide directly inhibits mycolic acid synthesis, which eventually has the same deleterious effects on the TB organism as isoniazid. Ethambutol affects lipid synthesis, resulting in the inhibition of mycolic acid incorporation into the cell wall, thus inhibiting protein synthesis. Para-aminosalicylic acid acts as a competitive inhibitor of para-aminobenzoic acid in the synthesis of folate. The MOA of pyrazinamide in the inhibition of TB is unknown. It can be either bacteriostatic or bactericidal, depending on the susceptibility of the particular *Mycobacterium* organism.

MOA, mechanism of action; *NAD,* nicotinamide adenine dinucleotide.

are not as effective against other species of *Mycobacterium* as they are against *M. tuberculosis*. Some of these other species that may be of particular concern in immunocompromised patients such as AIDS patients are *M. avium-intracellulare*, *M. flavescens*, *M. marinum*, and *M. kansasii*. Additional *Mycobacterium* infections that may respond to antitubercular agents are those caused by *M. fortuitum*, *M. chelonei*, *M. smegmatis*, *M. xenopi*, and *M. scrofulaceum*.

Therapeutic Uses

The antitubercular drugs are primarily used for the prophylaxis or treatment of TB. The effectiveness of these agents depends on the type of infection, adequate dosing, sufficient duration of treatment, drug compliance, and the selection of an effective drug combination. The therapeutic effects of the different antitubercular drugs are listed in the box below.

Side Effects and Adverse Effects

The antitubercular agents are fairly well tolerated. The most problematic drugs and their associated adverse effects are listed in Table 38-1.

Interactions

The drugs that can interact with the antitubercular agents can cause significant effects. See Table 38-2 for

---

Antitubercular Drugs: Therapeutic Effects

DRUG	THERAPEUTIC EFFECT
Para-aminosalicylate sodium	■ Used in combination with other antitubercular agents for the treatment of pulmonary and extrapulmonary *M. tuberculosis* infection.
Capreomycin	■ Used for treatment of pulmonary TB caused by *M. tuberculosis* after primary agents fail, drug resistance appears, or drug toxicity occurs.
Cycloserine	■ Used for treatment of active pulmonary and extrapulmonary TB after failure of primary agents.
Ethambutol	■ Indicated as a primary agent for the treatment of TB.
Ethionamide	■ Used in conjunction with other antitubercular agents in the treatment of clinical TB and other mycobacterial diseases.
⚓Isoniazid	■ Used alone or in combination with other antitubercular agents in the treatment and prevention of clinical TB.
Pyrazinamide	■ Used in conjunction with other antitubercular agents in the treatment of clinical TB.
Rifabutin	■ Used to prevent or delay the development of *M. avium-intracellulare* bacteremia and disseminated infections in patients with advanced HIV infections.
Rifampin	■ Used in conjunction with other antitubercular agents in the treatment of clinical TB.
	■ Used in treatment of diseases caused by mycobacteria other than *M. tuberculosis*.
	■ Used for preventive therapy in persons exposed to isoniazid-resistant *M. tuberculosis*.
	■ Used to eliminate meningococci from the nasopharynx of asymptomatic *Neisseria meningitidis* carriers when the risk of meningococcal meningitis is high.
	■ Used for chemoprophylaxis in contacts of patients with *Haemophilus influenzae* type B (Hib) infection.
	■ Used in conjunction with at least one other antiinfective agent in the treatment of leprosy.
	■ Used in the treatment of endocarditis caused by methicillin-resistant staphylococci, chronic staphylococcal prostatitis, and multiple-antiinfective–resistant pneumococci.
Streptomycin	■ Used in combination with other antitubercular agents in treatment of clinical TB and other mycobacterial diseases.
Kanamycin	■ Used in combination with other antitubercular agents in treatment of clinical TB. It is not intended for long-term use.

a summary of these interactions. Besides these drug interactions, isoniazid can cause a false-positive Clinitest reading and an increase in the serum levels of the alanine aminotransferase (ALT) and aspartate aminotransferase (AST).

Dosages

For the recommended dosages of selected antitubercular agents, see the dosages table on the next page.

DRUG PROFILES

The antitubercular drugs can only be obtained by prescription and are indicated for the treatment of many different *Mycobacterium* infections, including *M. tuberculosis,* the organism that causes TB. They are available in many different dosage forms, including orally, intravenously, and intramuscularly administered agents. Some of the primary and secondary agents that are commonly used in the treatment of TB are discussed here.

Ethambutol

Ethambutol (Myambutol) is a primary bacteriostatic agent used in the treatment of TB that is believed to work by diffusing into the mycobacteria and suppressing RNA synthesis, thereby inhibiting protein synthesis. Ethambutol is included with isoniazid, strepto-

mycin, and rifampin in many TB combination-drug therapies. It may also be used to treat other mycobacterial diseases. It is classified as a pregnancy category D agent and is contraindicated in patients with a hypersensitivity to it, those with optic neuritis, and children less than 13 years of age. It is available only in

Table 38-1	Antitubercular Drugs: Common Adverse Effects
DRUG	**SIDE/ADVERSE EFFECTS**
Para-aminosalicylatic acid	GI tract disturbances, hepatotoxicity
Capreomycin	Ototoxicity, nephrotoxicity
Cycloserine	Psychotic behavior, seizures
Ethambutol	Retrobulbar neuritis, blindness
Ethionamide	GI tract disturbances, hepatotoxicity
⚓Isoniazid	Peripheral neuritis, hepatotoxicity
Kanamycin	Hepatotoxicity, ototoxicity, nephrotoxicity
Pyrazinamide	Hepatotoxicity, hyperuricemia
Rifabutin	GI tract disturbances, rash, neutropenia, discolored urine
Rifampin	Hepatitis
Streptomycin	Hepatotoxicity, ototoxicity, nephrotoxicity, blood dyscrasia

Table 38-2	Antituberculars: Drug Interactions	
DRUG	**MECHANISM**	**RESULTS**
Aminosalicylate		
Probenecid	Reduces excretion	Increased aminosalicylate levels
Salicylates	Additive effects	Aminosalicylate toxicity
⚓Isoniazid		
Antacids	Reduces absorption	Decreased isoniazid effects
Cycloserine, ethionamide, and rifampin	Additive effects	Increased CNS toxicity
Phenytoin	Decreases metabolism	Increased phenytoin effects
Streptomycin		
Nephrotoxic and neurotoxic drugs	Additive	Increased toxicity
Oral anticoagulants	Alter intestinal flora	Increased bleeding tendencies

DOSAGES

SELECTED ANTITUBERCULAR AGENTS

AGENT	PHARMACOLOGIC CLASS	DOSAGE RANGE	PURPOSE
Ethambutol (Myambutol)	Synthetic primary antimycobacterial	*Adult* PO: 15 mg/kg as a single dose	
⚓**Isoniazid** (INH) (Laniazid, Nydrazid)	Synthetic primary antimycobacterial	*Adult* PO: 300 mg once/day for prophylaxis and 5-10 mg/kg/day for active TB	
Pyrazinamide (none)	Synthetic primary antimycobacterial	*Adult* PO: 15-30 mg/kg/day	For active TB
Rifampin (Rifadin, Rimactane)	Semisynthetic primary antimycobacterial antibiotic	*Adult* PO: 600 mg/day	
Streptomycin (many product names)	Antimycobacterial aminoglycoside antibiotic	*Adult* IM: 1 g/day	

oral forms as a 100-mg tablet and a 400-mg film-coated tablet. The usual recommended dosages are given in the dosages table above.

⚓ PHARMACOKINETICS

HALF-LIFE	ONSET	PEAK	DURATION
3.3 hr	Variable	2-4 hr	Up to 24 hr

⚓ Isoniazid

Isoniazid (Laniazid, Nydrazid) is not only the mainstay in the treatment of TB but also is the most widely used antitubercular agent. It may be given either as a single agent for prophylaxis or in combination with other antitubercular drugs for the treatment of active TB. It is a bactericidal agent that kills the mycobacteria by disrupting cell wall synthesis as well as essential cellular functions.

Isoniazid is metabolized in the liver through a process called *acetylation,* which requires a certain enzymatic pathway to break down the drug. However, some persons have a genetic deficiency of the enzymes needed for this to occur. Such persons are called **slow acetylators.** When INH is taken by slow acetylators, the INH accumulates because there is not enough of the enzymes to break down the INH. Therefore the

dosages of INH may need to be adjusted downward in these patients.

Isoniazid is available in both oral and parenteral formulations. Orally it comes as a 50-mg/5 ml solution and as 50-, 100-, and 300-mg tablets. Parenterally it comes in a strength of 100 mg/ml for intravenous injection. There is also an oral formulation of INH called *Rifamate* that includes rifampin. It comes as a fixed-dose capsule, and the respective amounts of INH and rifampin are 150 mg and 300 mg.

Isoniazid is classified as a pregnancy category C agent. It is contraindicated in patients with a hypersensitivity to it and in those with optic neuritis. The usually recommended dosages of INH are given in the dosages table above.

⚓ PHARMACOKINETICS

HALF-LIFE	ONSET	PEAK	DURATION
1-4 hr	Variable	1-2 hr	Up to 24 hr

PYRAZINAMIDE

Pyrazinamide is an antitubercular drug that can be either bacteriostatic or bactericidal, depending on its concentration at the site of infection and the particular susceptibility of the mycobacteria. It is frequently used in combination with other antitubercular drugs for the treatment of TB. Its mechanism of action is unknown, but it is believed to work by inhibiting lipid and nucleic acid synthesis in the mycobacteria. Pyrazinamide is only available as an oral formulation—a 500-mg tablet and a 500-mg/5 ml syrup. It is classified as a pregnancy category C agent and is contraindicated in patients who have had a hypersensitivity reaction to it. The usually recommended dosages are given in the dosages table on the previous page.

♨ P H A R M A C O K I N E T I C S

HALF-LIFE	ONSET	PEAK	DURATION
9-10 hr	Variable	2 hr	Up to 24 hr

RIFAMPIN

Rifampin (Rifadin, Rimactane) is a synthetic antibiotic with activity against many forms of *Mycobacterium* as well as against meningococcus, *Haemophilus influenzae* type B, and leprosy. It is a broad-spectrum bactericidal agent that kills the offending organism by inhibiting protein synthesis. Rifampin is used either alone in the prevention of TB or in combination with other antitubercular agents in its treatment.

Rifampin is available in both oral and parenteral formulations and, as already mentioned, in combination with isoniazid (Rifamate). As an oral agent it comes as a 150- and 300-mg oral capsule. In its parenteral formulation it comes in a vial for injection that contains 50 mg of the agent. Rifampin is classified as a pregnancy category C agent and is contraindicated in patients with a known hypersensitivity to it. The usual recommended dosages are given in the dosages table on the previous page.

♨ P H A R M A C O K I N E T I C S

HALF-LIFE	ONSET	PEAK	DURATION
3 hr	Variable	2-4 hr	Up to 24 hr

STREPTOMYCIN

Streptomycin is an aminoglycoside antibiotic that goes by many trade names. Introduced in 1944, it was the very first antitubercular drug to come available that could effectively treat TB. Mostly because of its toxicities it is today most frequently used only in combination-drug regimens for the treatment of MDR-TB infections.

Streptomycin is only available in a parenteral formulation: a 1- and 5-gm injection as well as a 400-mg/ml injection. Streptomycin is classified as a pregnancy category B agent and is contraindicated in patients hy-

persensitive to it. The usually recommended dosages are given in the dosages table on the previous page.

♨ P H A R M A C O K I N E T I C S

HALF-LIFE	ONSET	PEAK	DURATION
2-3 hr	Variable	1-2 hr	Up to 24 hr

NURSING PROCESS

ASSESSMENT

Before administering any of the primary or secondary antitubercular agents, to ensure the safe and effective use of these medications, the nurse should obtain a thorough medical history on the patient and perform a complete assessment. Liver function studies should be performed in patients who used to receive INH or rifampin because of the hepatic impairment these agents can cause. This is especially important in elderly patients and patients who consume alcohol daily because of the greater likelihood of liver disorders in such patients. A thorough neurologic assessment is also called for because of the increased incidence of peripheral neuropathies of the feet and hands in patients taking INH. It is also important to check the patient's CBC, Hgb level, and Hct value before administering INH because of the hematologic disorders they can cause. Renal studies, such as the creatinine and BUN levels as well as urinalysis, should also be performed both at the start of INH or rifampin therapy and during therapy. Contraindications to the use of rifampin include hypersensitivity. Contraindications to the use of INH include hypersensitivity and optic neuritis. The drugs that interact with these agents are listed in Table 38-1. Sputum cultures are routinely done as part of the workup in patients, so the nurse should always check these results before administering the specific antitubercular drugs to confirm that the appropriate agent is being given.

Pyrazinamide, ethambutol, and streptomycin are the other primary agents used in the treatment of TB. Baseline liver function tests should be performed in patients who are to be given pyrazinamide because of the hepatotoxicity it can cause. It can also cause hyperuricemia, so gout or flare-ups of gout may occur in susceptible patients. The Hgb levels and Hct values should also be checked. Contraindications to the use of any of these three agents include hypersensitivity.

Ethambutol may cause a decrease in visual acuity resulting from optic neuritis, so a thorough eye examination may be called for before the institution of therapy. In addition, the patient's baseline liver function status, Hgb levels, and Hct values should be determined before the initiation of therapy. Contraindications to the use of ethambutol include hypersensitivity and optic neuritis. Cautious use is called for in patients with liver or renal disease, hematologic disorders, or diabetes.

Streptomycin is contraindicated in patients with renal disease or those with a hypersensitivity to the agent. The patient's BUN and creatinine levels should be measured and urinalysis performed before the start of therapy. It should be used very carefully in the elderly and in patients with hearing disorders because of the ototoxicity it can cause.

The assessment aspect of the nursing care in patients being given any of the other secondary agents (see box on therapeutic effects, p. 590) is very similar.

NURSING DIAGNOSES

Nursing diagnoses pertaining to patients receiving antitubercular agents include:
- Risk for injury as the result of drug side effects and poor living conditions.
- Noncompliance with therapy because of lack of knowledge and experience with a long-term treatment regimen.
- Knowledge deficit regarding the disease and the medication treatment.

PLANNING

Goals for patients receiving antitubercular agents are focused on patient safety and compliance with therapy, and these include:
- Patient experiences minimal side effects of the treatment for TB.
- Patient takes medication regularly and for the length of time prescribed.
- Patient remains free of injury related to drug interactions with the antitubercular drugs.
- Patient remains free of toxic effects or report them to the physician immediately.
- Patient remains compliant with the drug therapy.

Outcome Criteria

The outcome criteria for patients receiving antitubercular agents are also focused on patient safety and compliance. These include:

- Patient states the therapeutic effects (improved signs and symptoms and killing of mycobacterium) as well as possible side effects (neuropathies, GI upset) of the treatment.
- Patient states the importance of taking the medication regularly and for the length of time prescribed to prevent complications, relapses, or recurrences.
- Patient states the drugs that interact with the antitubercular agent such as salicylates, antacids, and anticoagulants.
- Patient reports toxic effects such as renal or liver dysfunction, hearing loss, and blindness to the physician, should they occur.
- Patient shows improvement of disease state with a decreased cough, fever, and normal laboratory values.

IMPLEMENTATION

Because drug therapy is the mainstay of the treatment of TB and often lasts for up to a 24 months, patient education (see the box on p. 595) is critical, with a special emphasis on compliance. Simple, clear, and concise instructions should be given to the patient. This should include the fact that multiple drugs are generally used and that 90% cure rates can be achieved with combination therapy consisting of isoniazid and rifampin—if the patient is strictly compliant with therapy. All antitubercular agents should be given exactly as ordered and at the same time every day. Consistent use and dosing is critical to maintaining steady blood levels and to minimizing the chances of resistance to the drug therapy.

Generally speaking, the oral preparations should be given with meals to diminish the GI tract upset, even though it is often recommended that they be given either 1 hour before or 2 hours after meals. An antiemetic may be necessary in some patients. Intramuscularly administered agents such as streptomycin, capreomycin sulfate and kanamycin should be given deep in a large muscle mass and the sites rotated. Pyridoxine in doses of 200 to 300 mg per day may be ordered in patients taking cycloserine or isoniazid to prevent the associated neurotoxicity.

EVALUATION

The nurse should always document patients' response, or lack of it, to therapy! The therapeutic response to antitubercular therapy is reflected by a decrease in the symptoms of TB, such as cough and fever, and by weight gain. The results of laboratory studies (culture and sensitivity tests) and the chest x-ray findings should confirm the clinical findings. Patients with drug-resistant disease do not show a clinical response to the therapy, and laboratory findings will confirm this.

Patients also need to be monitored for the occurrence of adverse reactions to the antitubercular agents. These include fatigue, nausea, vomiting, numbness and tingling of the extremities, fever, loss of appetite, depression, and jaundice. The physician should be notified if they occur and the incident documented accordingly.

Patient Teaching TIPS

Antitubercular Agents

✔ Patients should be told to take all medications directly as ordered by the physician.

✔ Patients should know that compliance with therapy means taking the medication as ordered and for the ordered length of time and that compliance is essential for achieving a cure. This includes keeping follow-up appointments with the physician.

✔ Patients should not consume alcohol while they are receiving these medications and should always check with their physician before taking any other type of medication.

✔ Diabetic patients taking isoniazid should monitor their blood glucose levels using a glucometer because of the hyperglycemia this medication can cause.

✔ Patients should take pyridoxine as prescribed by the physician to prevent some of the neurologic side effects of isoniazid such as numbness and tingling of extremities.

✔ Patients taking INH or rifampin should report the following side effects to the physician immediately: fever, nausea, vomiting, loss of appetite, yellow tint to skin or eyes, unusual bleeding, or numbness and tingling of extremities.

✔ Women taking oral contraceptives who are prescribed rifampin must be switched to another form of birth control, because oral contraceptives become ineffective when given with rifampin.

✔ Patients who are taking rifampin should be told that their urine, stool, saliva, sputum, sweat, or tears may become reddish orange, and even contact lenses may be stained.

✔ Patients should see their health care provider at least monthly during treatment.

✔ Patients must be reminded that they are contagious during the initial period of the illness and its diagnosis, so they should make every effort to wash their hands and cover their mouths when coughing or sneezing. They should also be careful about where they throw away dirty tissues.

✔ Patients being treated for TB need to always take care of themselves. This includes adequate nutrition, rest, and relaxation.

✔ Patients should keep all medications away from children.

✔ Patients should always wear a Medic-Alert tag or bracelet naming the antitubercular medications they are taking.

Critical Thinking ACTIVITIES

1. Women taking oral contraceptives in conjunction with Rifampin should
   a. have an annual pap smear.
   b. expect reddish-brown vaginal discharge.
   c. switch to an alternate form of birth control.
   d. experience increased energy level and breast discharge.
2. Patients are considered contagious
   a. during the postictal phase of tuberculosis.
   b. any time period up to 18 months post-therapy.
   c. during the initial period of the illness and its diagnosis.
   d. any phase of the illness.

▲▲

BIBLIOGRAPHY

Albanese J, Nutz P: *Mosby's 1995 nursing drug cards,* St Louis, 1995, Mosby.

Block AB et al: Nationwide survey of drug-resistant tuberculosis in the United States, *JAMA* 271(9):665, 1994.

Center for Disease Control: Outbreak of multi-drug resistant tuberculosis at a hospital—New York City, *MMWR* 42(22): 1993.

Elpern EH, Girzadas AM: Tuberculosis update: new challenges of an old disease, *Medsurg Nurs* 2(3): 1993.

Greenblatt D et al: Interaction of triazolam and ketoconazole, *Lancet* 345:191, 1995.

Johnson KB: *Harriet Lane handbook,* ed 13, St Louis, 1993, Mosby.

Keen JH: *Critical care and emergency drug reference,* St Louis, 1994, Mosby.

Knoben JE, Anderson PO: *Handbook of critical drug data,* ed 6, Hamilton, Ill, 1988, Drug Intelligence Publications.

Malseed RT: Drug-resistant tuberculosis: treatment protocols, *Medsurg Nurs* 2(3): 1993.

McEvoy GK: *AHFS drug information,* Bethesda, Md, 1994, American Society of Hospital Pharmacists.

Skidmore-Roth L: *Mosby's 1995 nursing drug reference,* St Louis, 1995, Mosby.

Chapter 39

Antifungal Agents

Objectives

When you reach the end of this chapter, you will be able to:

1 Identify the various antifungal medications.

2 Describe the mechanisms of action of the antifungal medications, the indications for and contraindications to their use, the routes of administration and side and toxic effects of these agents, and the drug interactions associated with their use.

3 Develop a comprehensive nursing care plan for patients taking antifungal medications.

4 Develop educational guidelines for patients receiving antifungal medications.

5 List appropriate outcome criteria for patients receiving antifungal medications.

CHAPTER OUTLINE

Fungal Infections
Antifungal Agents
  Mechanism of action
  Drug effects
  Therapeutic uses
  Side effects and adverse effects
  Interactions
  Dosages
Drug Profiles
  ⚓ Amphotericin B
  ⚓ Fluconazole
  Nystatin

Nursing Process
Assessment
Nursing Diagnoses
Planning
  Outcome criteria
Implementation
Evaluation

Glossary

Antimetabolite (an' tĭ mə tab' o lĭt) Drug or other substance that is an antagonist or that resembles a normal human metabolite and interferes with its function in the body, usually by competing for the metabolite's receptors or enzymes. (p. 599)

Ergosterol (er gos' tə rol') Unsaturated hydrocarbon of the vitamin D group isolated from yeast, mushrooms, ergot, and other fungi; the main sterol in fungal membranes. (p. 599)

Flucytosine (floo si' to sēn) An antimetabolite that constitutes one of the four major groups of antifungal agents. It works by being taken up into the needed cellular metabolic pathway, thereby causing a malfunction in the normal pathway, which in turn shuts down the pathway. (p. 599)

Fungi (fun' ji) A very large and diverse group of eukaryotic, thallus-forming microorganisms that require an external carbon source. Fungi consist of yeast and molds. (p. 598)

Griseofulvin (gris' e o ful' vin) One of the four major groups of antifungal agents. It acts by preventing susceptible fungi from reproducing. (p. 599)

Imidazoles (im' id az ōlz) One of the four major groups of antifungal agents. They include ketoconazole, miconazole, clotrimazole, econazole, and fluconazole and work by inhibiting a needed enzyme in susceptible fungi. (p. 599)

Molds Multicellular fungi characterized by long, branching filaments called *hyphae,* which entwine to form a mycelium. (p. 598)

Mycosis (mi ko' sis) Infection caused by fungi. (p. 598)

Oral candidiasis (kan' di di' e sis) Overgrowth of *Candida albicans* occurring in the tissues of the mouth (also called *thrush*). (p. 598)

Pathologic fungi Fungi that cause mycoses. (p. 598)

Polyenes (pol e' ēnz) One of the four major groups of antifungal agents. It includes amphotericin B and nystatin. Polyenes work by binding to sterols in fungal membranes, allowing potassium and magnesium ions to leak out of the cell and altering fungal cellular metabolism, which leads to death of the organism. (p. 599)

Sterol (ster' ol) Substance in the cell membranes of fungi to which polyenes bind. (p. 599)

Yeast Single-celled fungi that reproduce by budding. (p. 598)

Yeast infection Vaginal candidiasis. (p. 598)

FUNGAL INFECTIONS

Fungi are a very large and diverse group of microorganisms that comprise both yeast and molds. **Yeast** are single-celled fungi that reproduce by budding and are actually very useful organisms. They are used in baking and alcoholic beverages. **Molds** are multicellular and are characterized by long, branching filaments called *hyphae,* which entwine to form a "mat" called a *mycelium.* Some fungi are part of the normal flora of the skin, mouth, intestines, and vagina.

The infection caused by a fungus can also be called a **mycosis,** but there are very few fungi that cause such infections. Those that do are termed **pathologic fungi,** and the infections they cause range in severity from being mild and superficial to severe and life-threatening. These infections can be contracted by several different routes. They can be ingested orally, they can become implanted under the skin after injury, or if the fungal spores are airborne, they can be inhaled. There are four general types of mycotic infections: systemic, cutaneous, subcutaneous, and superficial. Many fungal infections are superficial and the symptoms primarily annoying; others are systemic and can be life-threatening. The most severe systemic fungal infections generally afflict persons whose host defenses are compromised. Commonly these are patients who have received organ transplants and are on immunosuppressive drug therapy, cancer patients who are immunocompromised as the result of their chemotherapy, and patients with AIDS. In addition, the use of antibiotics, antineoplastics, or immunosuppressants such as corticosteroids may result in an overgrowth of *Candida albicans,* followed by the development of a systemic infection. When this affects the mouth, it is referred to as **oral candidiasis** or thrush. It is common in newborns and immunocompromised patients. Vaginal candidiasis, commonly called a **yeast infection,** frequently afflicts pregnant women, women with diabetes mellitus, and women taking oral contraceptives. The characteristics of some of the systemic, cutaneous, and superficial mycotic infections are summarized in Table 39-1.

Table 39-1	**Mycotic Infections**				
MYCOSIS	**FUNGUS**	**ENDEMIC LOCATION**	**RESERVOIR**	**TRANSMISSION**	**PRIMARY TISSUE AFFECTED**
Systemic infection					
Blastomycosis	*Blastomyces dermatitidis*	North America	Soil, animal droppings	Inhalation	Lungs
Coccidioidomycosis	*Coccidioides immitis*	Southwestern U.S.	Soil, dust	Inhalation	Lungs
Cryptococcosis	*Cryptococcus neoformans*	Universal	Soil, pigeon droppings	Inhalation	Lungs
Histoplasmosis	*Histoplasma capsulatum*	Universal	Soil, bird and chicken droppings	Inhalation	Lungs
Cutaneous infection					
Candidiasis	*Candida albicans*	Universal	Humans	Direct contact, non-susceptible antibiotic overgrowth	Mucous membrane, skin
Dermatophytes, tinea	*Epidermophyton* spp., *Microsporum* spp., *Trichophyton* spp.	Universal	Humans	Direct and indirect contact with infected persons	Scalp, skin
Superficial infection					
Tinea versicolor	*Malassezia furfur*	Universal	Human	Unknown*	Skin

Malassezia spp. are a usual part of the normal human flora and appear to cause infection in only select individuals.

ANTIFUNGAL AGENTS

The drugs used to treat fungal infections are called *antifungal* agents. Systemic mycotic infections and some cutaneous or subcutaneous mycoses are treated with oral or parenteral agents, but these constitute a fairly small group of agents, only three or four of which are commonly used. There are few such agents because the fungi that cause these infections have proved to be very difficult to kill, and research into new and improved agents has occurred at a slow pace, with few important advances yielded so far. One difficulty that has slowed the development of new agents is that frequently the chemical concentrations required for these experimental agents to be effective cannot be tolerated by human beings. Following is a list of those agents that have met with success in the treatment of systemic and severe cutaneous or subcutaneous mycoses:

- Amphotericin B
- Fluconazole
- Flucytosine
- Griseofulvin
- Itraconazole
- Ketoconazole
- Miconazole
- Nystatin

Topical antifungal agents are primarily used for the treatment of cutaneous or subcutaneous mycoses and are discussed in detail in Chapter 41 on topical antimicrobials and disinfectants. Following is a list of those topical antifungals approved for clinical use.

- Amphotericin B
- Butoconazole
- Ciclopirox
- Clioquinol
- Clotrimazole
- Econazole
- Haloprogin
- Ketoconazole
- Miconazole
- Natamycin
- Nystatin
- Oxiconazole
- Sodium thiosulfate
- Sulconazole
- Terbinafine
- Terconazole

Topical antifungals are most commonly used in the treatment of oral and vaginal candidiasis, though occasionally a systemic antifungal is used in the management of severe cases.

The antifungal agents can be broken down into four major groups based on their chemical structures: the polyenes (amphotericin B and nystatin), flucytosine, the imidazoles (ketoconazole, miconazole, clotrimazole, econazole, and fluconazole), and griseofulvin.

Mechanism of Action

The mechanisms of action of the various antifungal agents differ depending on which of the four groups of agents they belong to. The **polyenes** act by binding to **sterols** in the cell membranes of fungi, the main sterol in fungal membranes being **ergosterol.** Human cell membranes also have sterols in their cell membranes, but in this case it is cholesterol. Polyene antifungals do not bind to human cell membranes, and therefore do not kill human cells, because polyenes have a stronger affinity for ergosterol than for cholesterol. Once the polyene binds to the ergosterol, a channel forms in the fungal cell membrane that allows potassium and magnesium ions to leak out of the cell. This loss of ions causes fungal cellular metabolism to be altered, and hence death of the cell.

Flucytosine, also known as *5-fluorocytosine,* acts in much the same way as the antiviral agents. It is an **antimetabolite,** which is a drug that is taken up into needed cellular metabolic pathways. Once it is taken up into these pathways, it causes the normal pathway to malfunction and the pathway subsequently shuts down. Flucytosine works by being taken into susceptible fungi, after which it is deaminated by cytosine deaminase to 5-fluorouracil. Because human cells do not have this enzyme, they are not harmed by this antimetabolite. Once the 5-fluorouracil is inside the fungal cell, it interferes with DNA synthesis by incorporating itself into the fungal pathway that produces DNA, with the result that the DNA needed for fungal cell metabolism is lacking and the cell dies.

Imidazoles act as either fungistatic or fungicidal agents, depending on their concentration in the fungus. They are most effective in combating rapidly growing fungi and work by inhibiting a needed enzyme in susceptible fungi. In this case the enzyme is cytochrome P-450, and it is needed to produce ergosterol. When the production of ergosterol is inhibited, another sterol, called *lanosterol,* is made instead. This results in the same problem caused by the polyene antifungals, namely a leaky cell membrane that allows needed potassium to escape. The fungi die because they cannot carry on cellular metabolism.

Griseofulvin works by preventing susceptible fungi from reproducing. It enters the fungal cell through an energy-dependent transport system and inhibits fungal mitosis, or reproduction, by binding to microtubules. This disrupts the cell's mitotic spindle structure, which arrests the metaphase of cell division. It has also been proposed that griseofulvin causes the production of defective DNA, which is then unable to replicate.

Drug Effects

The drug effects of the antifungals are limited to their ability to kill or inhibit the growth of fungi. Some of the fungi susceptible to these agents are the cutaneous, subcutaneous, and systemic mycoses listed in the box below.

Therapeutic Uses

The therapeutic effects of the various antifungals are specific to the individual agents. The side effects of the newer antifungals are fewer and less serious than those of the older agents. However, the agent of choice for the treatment of many severe systemic fungal infections remains one of the oldest antifungals, amphotericin B. **Amphotericin B** inhibits a wide range of fungi. It is given with flucytosine in the treatment of *Candida* and cryptococcal infections because of the synergy of the two agents. It is also effective for treating aspergillosis, blastomycosis, candidiasis, coccidiodomycosis, cryptococcosis, fungal endocarditis, histoplasmosis, fungal septicemia, and many other systemic fungal infections. **Nystatin**'s activity is similar to that of amphotericin B, but its usefulness is limited because of its toxic effects when given in the doses required to accomplish the same antifungal actions as those of amphotericin B. It is also not available in a parenteral form.

Fluconazole and **itraconazole** are synthetic imidazole antifungals. Fluconazole can pass into the CSF and inhibit cryptococcal fungi. This makes it effective in the treatment of cryptococcal meningitis. It is also active against oropharyngeal and esophageal *Candida* infections. Itraconazole, on the other hand, is capable of only poor CSF penetration but can be widely distributed throughout other areas of the body. It is indicated for the treatment of fungal infections in immunocompromised and nonimmunocompromised persons with disseminated candidiasis, histoplasmosis, and perhaps, invasive aspergillosis. The other systemic imidazole, **ketoconazole,** inhibits many dermatophytes and fungi that cause systemic mycoses, but it is not active against *Aspergillus* organisms or phycomycetes such as *Mucor* spp. **Miconazole,** another systemic imidazole antifungal, has a spectrum of activity similar to that of ketoconazole. Of the imidazoles, fluconazole is the most effective one for combating infections with *Candida, Cryptococcus, Blastomyces,* and *Histoplasma* organisms.

Flucytosine inhibits *Cryptococcus neoformans, Candida albicans,* and many *Cladosporium* and *Phialophora* spp. It does not inhibit *Aspergillus, Sporothrix, Blastomyces,* or *Histoplasma* spp., or *Coccidioides immitis.*

Griseofulvin inhibits dermatophytes of *Microsporum, Trichophyton,* and *Epidermophyton* spp. It has no effect on filamentous fungi such as *Aspergillus,* yeasts such as *Candida* spp., or dimorphoric species such as *Histoplasma.*

Side Effects and Adverse Effects

The major side effects and clinical problems with antifungal agents are encountered most frequently in conjunction with amphotericin treatment. Drug interactions and hepatotoxicity are the primary concerns in patients receiving other antifungal agents, but the intravenous administration of amphotericin B is associated with a multitude of adverse effects. The most common and problematic of the side effects of the various antifungal agents are listed in Table 39-2.

Interactions

There are many important drug interactions associated with the use of antifungal agents, some of which can be life-threatening. A common underlying source of the problem is the fact that many of the antifungal drugs as well as other agents are metabolized by a highly utilized enzyme system in the liver called the cytochrome P-450 system. The result of the coadministration of two agents that are both broken down by this system is that they compete for the limited amount of enzymes, and one of the drugs ends up accumulating. The drugs that interact with the various antifungal agents and the consequences of the interactions are summarized in Table 39-3.

Dosages

For the recommended dosages of selected antifungal agents, see the dosages table on p. 603.

Fungi Susceptible to Antifungal Agents

Cutaneous and Subcutaneous Mycoses
Epidermophyton *spp.*
Microsporum *spp.*
Sporothrix *spp.*
Trichophyton *spp.*

Systemic Mycoses
Aspergillus *spp.*
Candida *spp.*
Blastomyces dermatitidis
Cryptococcus neoformans
Coccidioides immitis
Histoplasma capsulatum

Table 39-2 | Antifungals: Common Adverse Effects

BODY SYSTEM	SIDE/ADVERSE EFFECTS
⇓Amphotericin B	
Kidneys	Renal toxicity, potassium loss, hypomagnesemia
CNS	Neurotoxicity; visual disturbances; hand or feet numbness, tingling, or pain; convulsions
Cardiovascular	Cardiac dysrhythmias
Pulmonary	Pulmonary infiltrates, other respiratory difficulties
Other (infusion-related)	Fever, chills, headache, malaise, nausea, occasionally hypotension
⇓Fluconazole	
Gastrointestinal	Nausea, vomiting, diarrhea, stomach pain
Other	Increased AST and ALT levels
Flucytosine	
CNS	Headache, confusion, dizziness, sedation, vertigo
Gastrointestinal	Nausea, vomiting, anorexia, diarrhea, abdominal distention, cramps, enterocolitis
Hematologic	Thrombocytopenia, agranulocytosis, anemia, leukopenia, pancytopenia
Other	Increased BUN, creatinine, ALT, and AST levels; rash; increased alkaline phosphatase activity
Griseofulvin	
Skin	Rash, urticaria, photosensitivity, angioedema
CNS	Headache, peripheral neuritis, paresthesias, confusion, dizziness, fatigue, insomnia, psychosis
EENT	Blurred vision, oral candidiasis, furry tongue, transient hearing loss
Genitourinary	Proteinuria, precipitate porphyria
Gastrointestinal	Nausea, vomiting, anorexia, diarrhea, cramps, dry mouth, flatulence, increased thirst
Hematologic	Leukopenia, granulocytopenia, neutropenia, monocytosis
Itraconazole	
Genitourinary	Gynecomastia, impotence, decreased libido
Skin	Pruritus, fever, rash
CNS	Headache, dizziness, insomnia, somnolence, depression
Gastrointestinal	Nausea, vomiting, anorexia, diarrhea, cramps, abdominal pain, flatulence, GI bleeding, hepatotoxicity
Other	Edema, fatigue, malaise, hypertension, hypokalemia, tinnitus
Ketoconazole	
Genitourinary	Gynecomastia, impotence
Skin	Pruritus, fever, chills, photophobia, rash, dermatitis, purpura, urticaria
CNS	Headache, dizziness, somnolence
Gastrointestinal	Nausea, vomiting, anorexia, diarrhea, abdominal pain, hepatotoxicity
Hematologic	Thrombocytopenia, leukopenia, hemolytic anemia
Miconazole	
Cardiovascular	Tachycardia, dysrhythmias
CNS	Drowsiness, headache, lassitude
Gastrointestinal	Nausea, vomiting, anorexia, diarrhea, cramps
Genitourinary	Vulvovaginal burning, itching, pelvic cramps
Hematologic	Decreased Hct, thrombocytopenia, hyponatremia, hyperlipidemia
Skin	Pruritus, fever, flushing, anaphylaxis, hives
Nystatin	
Skin	Rash, urticaria
Gastrointestinal	Nausea, vomiting, anorexia, diarrhea, cramps

Table 39-3	Antifungal Drugs: Drug Interactions
DRUG	**POSSIBLE EFFECTS**
Amphotericin B	
Thiazide diuretics	Severe hypokalemia or decreased adrenal cortex response to corticotropin
Nephrotoxic drug	Additive nephrotoxicity
Digitalis glycosides	Amphotericin B-induced hypokalemia may increase the potential for digitalis toxicity.
Fluconazole, Itraconazole, and Miconazole	
Cyclosporine and phenytoin	Increased plasma concentrations of both agents
Oral hypoglycemics	Reduced metabolism of hypoglycemic agents
Oral anticoagulants	Increased effects of anticoagulants seen as increases in PT
Griseofulvin	
Oral anticoagulants	Decreased effects of anticoagulants seen as decreases in PT
Contraceptives and estrogen-containing products	Decreased effectiveness of these agents
Ketoconazole and Miconazole	
Alcohol and other hepatotoxic drugs	Increased risk of hepatotoxicity
Cyclosporine	Increased cyclosporine levels and potential for nephrotoxicity
Antacids, anticholinergics, H_2-blockers, and omeprazole	Increased GI tract pH, which can reduce absorption of ketoconazole
Isoniazid or rifampin	Decreased serum levels of ketoconazole
Terfenadine and astemizole	Elevated terfenadine and astemizole levels and cardiotoxicity

DRUG PROFILES

⚓ AMPHOTERICIN B

As already mentioned, amphotericin B (Amphocin, Fungizone) remains the agent of choice for the treatment of severe systemic mycoses. It may be given with flucytosine in the treatment of many types of fungal infections because the two agents work synergistically. The main drawback of amphotericin B therapy is that the agent causes many adverse effects. Almost all patients given the agent intravenously experience fever, chills, hypotension, tachycardia, malaise, muscle and joint pain, anorexia, nausea and vomiting, and headache. For this reason, pretreatment with an antipyretic (acetaminophen), antihistamines, and antiemetics may be given to decrease the severity of this infusion-related reaction.

Amphotericin B is a prescription-only drug that is available in both a parenteral and a topical formulation. It is classified as a pregnancy category B agent and is contraindicated in patients who have shown hypersensitivity reactions to it and in those suffering from severe bone marrow suppression. It comes as a 50-mg vial for injection and as a 3% cream, lotion, or ointment for topical application. The recommended dosages are given in the dosages table on the next page.

⚗ PHARMACOKINETICS

HALF-LIFE	ONSET	PEAK	DURATION
24 hr	Variable	Variable	Variable

⚓ FLUCONAZOLE

Fluconazole (Diflucan) has proved to represent a significant improvement in the area of antifungal treatment. It has a much better side effect profile than that of amphotericin B, and it also has excellent coverage against many different fungi. In fact, it is often preferred to amphotericin B because of these qualities. Fluconazole is a prescription-only antifungal agent that is available in both an oral and a parenteral formulation. It is classified as a pregnancy category B agent and is contraindicated in patients hypersensitive to it. It comes as a 50-, 100-, and 200-mg tablet as well as a 200- and 400-mg intravenous injection. The recommended dosages are given in the dosages table on the next page.

⚗ PHARMACOKINETICS

HALF-LIFE	ONSET	PEAK	DURATION
22-30 hr	PO: <1 hr	PO: 1-2 hr	Variable

NYSTATIN

Nystatin (Nystat, Nilstat, Mycostatin, and Nystex) is a polyene antifungal agent that is often applied topically for the treatment of candidal diaper rash, as prophylaxis against candidal infections during periods of iat-

DOSAGES

SELECTED ANTIFUNGAL AGENTS

AGENT	PHARMACOLOGIC CLASS	DOSAGE RANGE	PURPOSE
⚓Amphotericin B (Amphocin, Fungizone)	Polyene antifungal antibiotic	*Pediatric/Adult* IV: initial daily dose, 0.25 mg/kg; total daily dose, 1-1.5 mg/kg. Do not exceed 1-1.5 mg/kg.	Broad spectrum of fungal infections
		Topical: apply cream, lotion, or ointment several times a day	Topical candidiasis
⚓Fluconazole (Diflucan)	Synthetic triazole antifungal	*Adult* IV or PO: 200 mg/day, followed by 100 mg/day for 2-5 wk. Doses of 400 mg/day may be required.	Oropharygeal and esophageal candidiasis
		400 mg/day, followed by 200 mg/day for 4-6 wk	Systemic candidiasis
		400 mg/day, followed by 200 mg once/day for 10-12 wk after negative CSF cultures	Cryptococcal meningitis
Nystatin (Nystant, Nilstat, Mycostatin, Nystex)	Polyene antifungal antibiotic	*Infant* 200,000 U (oral suspension) in oral cavity qid	Oral candidiasis
		Pediatric/Adult 400,000 U (oral suspension) in oral cavity qid	Oral candidiasis
		Adult PO: 0.5-1 million U (tablet) tid	Intestinal candidiasis
		Topical: apply 2-3 times/day	Topical candidiasis
		Vaginal: Insert 1 vaginal tablet once/day for 2 wk	Vaginal candidiasis

rogenic neutropenia in patients receiving immunosuppressive therapy, and for the treatment of oral and vaginal candidiasis. It is not available in a parenteral form but does come in several oral and topical formulations. It comes in a powdered suspension for oral administration in doses of 50, 150, 250, and 500 million units as well as 1, 2, 5, and 10 billion units. It is also available as a nonpowdered suspension in a dose of 100,000 unit/ml and as film-coated tablets containing 500,000 units. As a topical preparation it comes in a 100,000-unit cream, ointment, powder, spray, and vaginal tablet. Nystatin is classified as a pregnancy category B agent and is contraindicated in patients with a known hypersensitivity to it. The recommended dosages are given in the dosages table above.

⚕ PHARMACOKINETICS

HALF-LIFE	ONSET	PEAK	DURATION
Unknown	2 hr	Unknown	Unknown

NURSING PROCESS

ASSESSMENT

Before administering amphotericin B or any of the other antifungal agents, it is important for the nurse to identify any contraindications to the medication, such as hypersensitivity. Cautious use of these agents is recommended in pregnant or lactating women. Griseofulvin is contraindicated in patients with a hypersensitivity to it or with porphyria, hepatic disease, or lupus. Cautious use is recommended in patients known to be hypersensitive to penicillin and in pregnant women. The contraindications to ketoconazole use are hypersensitivity, pregnancy, lactation, and meningitis, with cautious use recommended in patients who have renal or hepatic disease. Miconazole is contraindicated in patients with a known hypersensitivity to it and should be used cautiously in pregnant women or patients with renal or hepatic disease.

The nurse should also assess the patient's vital signs and check the baseline CBC, Hgb level, Hct value, and RBC. Patients who are to receive ketoconazole should have their liver function assessed because of the hepatotoxicity it can cause. Miconazole use is associated with adverse cardiovascular effects, so patients' pulse, blood pressure, and ECG should be checked and any history of cardiac disease documented. Griseofulvin may precipitate severe blood dyscrasias, so it is important to assess patients' CBC. Patients' baseline renal and liver function and weight should also be assessed before the administration of any of the antifungals.

NURSING DIAGNOSES

Nursing diagnoses appropriate to patients receiving antifungals include:
- Pain related to symptoms of the infectious process.
- Knowledge deficit related to lack of information and experience with the antifungal and any other medication.
- Risk for injury stemming from side effects of the medications.

PLANNING

Goals for patients receiving antifungals include:
- Patient states the rationale for compliance with medication therapy.
- Patient states the common side effects of the specific antifungal medication.
- Patient experiences minimal side effects in signs and symptoms of the infection.
- Patient exhibits relief of the symptoms of the fungal infection.
- Patient states the importance of follow-up appointments.

Outcome Criteria

Outcome criteria relevant to patients receiving antifungal agents include:
- Patient will be free of the complications of suffer or minimal side effects of the antifungal agents such as nausea, vomiting, and GI upset.
- Patient remains compliant with the medication and experiences relief of infection and its signs and symptoms related to effective therapy such as normal cultures and no fever. .

- Patient experiences improved appetite and energy level after taking the antifungal agents for the prescribed time.
- Patient returns to the physician regularly as recommended by the health care provider for complete blood count with differential.

IMPLEMENTATION

The nursing interventions appropriate to patients receiving antifungal agents vary depending on the agent. Amphotericin B given intravenously must be diluted properly according to the manufacturer's guidelines. Sterile water or normal saline is recommended for its reconstitution, and normal saline or 5% dextrose in water may be used for infusion, with a test dose of 1 mg per 20 ml of 5% dextrose in water infused over 30 minutes. IV infusion pumps are recommended, the most distal veins should be used, and the IV site should be checked hourly to make sure extravasation has not occurred.

Fluconazole is administered either orally or intravenously, and when given intravenously, it should be diluted exactly according to the manufacturer's instructions. Because of the necrosis that results from extravasation of the agent at the IV site, the nurse should check the site hourly to make sure this has not happened. Griseofulvin must be given carefully and the patient frequently checked during infusions. Oral forms should be given with meals to decrease GI upset.

Patients receiving ketoconazole should not take alkaline products or antacids for at least 2 hours before or after dosing, and it should not be taken with coffee, tea, or acidic fruit juices. Just as with any other orally administered antifungal agents, taking it with food helps minimize GI upset. Miconazole often causes nausea and vomiting, so use of an antiemetic may be helpful, if ordered, to decrease these problems. Often a physician will order a test dose to be given to the patient so that any untoward reactions can be identified.

It is often necessary to check the vital signs of patients receiving any of the antifungals every 15 to 30 minutes during infusion. In addition, it is important to monitor the intake and output amounts, urinalysis findings, and specific gravity of the urine in patients receiving these medications to identify any deleterious drug effects on the kidneys. It is also important to weigh patients weekly and to document these weights because a gain of more than 2 pounds (1 kg) in a week may indicate medication-induced renal damage. Patient teaching tips are presented on p. 605.

EVALUATION

The therapeutic effects of antifungals include an easing of the symptoms of the infection, with ultimately com-

Patient Teaching TIPS

Antifungal Agents

✔ Patients receiving **amphotericin B** should be told about the need for long-term treatment (i.e., weeks, months) and the importance of taking the medication exactly as prescribed. Side effects include tinnitus, blurred vision, burning and itching at the infusion site, headache, rash, fever, chills, hypokalemia, GI upset, and various anemias. Patients should weigh themselves weekly and notify the physician if they gain more than 2 pounds (1 kg) in a week.

✔ Patients should wear gloves when applying topically administered **clotrimazole** to prevent further infection. To prevent drug interactions, they should avoid applying OTC creams, lotions, or ointments to the site unless otherwise instructed by the physician. Women taking this medication for the treatment of vaginal infections should abstain from sexual intercourse until the treatment is completed and the infection resolved. Women should also be told to continue to take the medication while actively menstruating. Skin sites where the agent is applied should be covered with an occlusive dressing. Patients should notify the physician if symptoms persist.

✔ Patients should wear gloves when applying miconazole, and should wash their hands before and after application of the medication. Often it is recommended that an occlusive dressing be placed over the skin site. Patients should be encouraged to notify the physician if symptoms persist.

✔ **Griseofulvin** is often taken for about 2 to 6 weeks until the infection clears. Patients should wash their hands before and after application and should wear gloves when applying the medication. Alcohol consumption should be avoided because of the Antabuse-type reaction that occurs in patients taking this agent. This agent also causes photosensitivity, and so patients should either avoid sunlight or use sunscreen whenever they anticipate prolonged exposure to the sun. They should be told to notify the physician should skin rash, fever, or sore throat occur.

✔ It is critical to the effectiveness of treatment with any of these agents to encourage the patient to take all medications as prescribed and for the prescribed length of time.

TAKE HOME POINTS

Fungi
- Very large and diverse group of microorganisms.
- Consist of yeast and molds.
- Yeast are single-celled fungi that may be harmful (causing infections) or helpful (baking and the brewing of beer).
- Molds are multicellular and characterized by long, branching filaments called *hyphae.*

Candidiasis
- An opportunistic fungal infection caused by *Candida albicans.*
- Occurs in patients on broad-spectrum antibiotics, antineoplastics, or immunosuppressants and in immunocompromised persons.
- When occurs in mouth = oral candidiasis or thrush; seen mostly in newborns or immunocompromised persons.
- Vaginal candidiasis = yeast infections; seen mostly in patients with diabetes mellitus, women taking oral contraceptives, and pregnant women.

Antifungals
- Can either be systemically or topically administered.
- Most common systemic antifungals are amphotericin B, fluconazole, itraconazole, and ketoconazole.
- Most common topical antifungals are clotrimazole, miconazole, and nystatin.
- Several chemical categories of both the topical and systemic agents, each with its own unique way of killing fungi.

Nursing Considerations
- Before administering any antifungals, the nurse must thoroughly assess patients to find out whether they have a known hypersensitivity to the medication, what other drugs (prescribed and OTC) are being taken, and what the status of their renal and liver function is.
- Amphotericin B must be properly diluted according to the manufacturer's guidelines and administered using an IV infusion pump
- Tissue extravasation of fluconazole at the IV site leads to tissue necrosis, so site should be checked hourly.
- Therapeutic effects include improved energy levels, normal temperature, and normal vital signs.

plete resolution seen in patients who are fully compliant with the therapy. Improved energy levels and normal temperature and other vital signs also indicate a therapeutic response. Side effects to monitor for in patients receiving these agents are listed in Table 39-2.

Critical Thinking A C T I V I T I E S

1. What laboratory data and other assessment data should be considered before administering any of the systemic antifungals? Specify the data and identify the reason for their importance.

2. The nurse should monitor which of the following laboratory parameters in patients receiving amphotericin B?
   a. Potassium   b. Chloride   c. Serum creatinine   d. Hematocrit

3. Infections caused by fungi, commonly referred to as *mycoses*, can be broken down into those caused by _____ and _____.
   a. Intracellular and extracellular fungi   b. Erythrocytic and exoerythrocytic fungi
   c. Yeast and molds   d. Flatworms and tapeworms

4. Oral candidiasis, or thrush, is caused by _____ and is commonly seen in _____ and _____.

   1. *Aspergillus*   2. *Candidia albicans*   3. *Mycobacterium tuberculosis*
   4. middle-aged patients   5. newborns   6. immunocompromised patients
   a. 3, 4, and 5   b. 2, 5, and 6   c. 1, 4, and 5   d. 3, 5, and 6

5. Of the four classes of antifungals, _____ belongs to the polyenes, which work by binding to a _____ in the cell membranes of fungi. This _____, called _____, is very similar to human _____.

   1. ergosterol   2. protein   3. amphotericin B   4. ketoconazole
   5. fluctyosine   6. cholesterol   7. RNA   8. sterol
   a. 3, 8, 8, 1, and 6   b. 4, 8, 8, 1, and 6   c. 3, 2, 2, 6, and 7   d. 5, 7, 7, 1, and 6

6. The imidazole antifungals such as _____ work by inhibiting the _____ enzyme system in the fungi, which is required for them to produce a substance needed to make their cell walls.

   1. flucytosine   2. amphotericin B   3. fluconazole
   4. acetylcholinesterase   5. cytochrome P-450   6. phosphodiesterase
   a. 1 and 5   b. 2 and 6   c. 3 and 5   d. 1 and 4

▲▲

BIBLIOGRAPHY

Albanese J, Nutz P: *Mosby's 1995 nursing drug cards,* St Louis, 1995, Mosby.

Gonzales-Delgado P et al: Hypersensitivity to ketoconazole, *Am Allergy* 73:326, 1994.

Greenblatt D et al: Interaction of triazolam and ketoconazole, *Lancet* 345:191, 1995.

Johnson KB: *Harriet Lane handbook,* ed 13, St Louis, 1993, Mosby.

Keen JH: *Critical care and emergency drug reference,* St Louis, 1994, Mosby.

Knoben JE, Anderson PO: *Handbook of critical drug data,* ed 6, Hamilton, Ill, 1988, Drug Intelligence Publications.

McEvoy GK: *AHFS drug information,* Bethesda, Md, 1994, American Society of Hospital Pharmacists.

Skidmore-Roth L: *Mosby's 1995 nursing drug reference,* St Louis, 1995, Mosby.

Chapter 40

Antimalarial, Antiprotozoal, and Antihelmintic Agents

Objectives

When you reach the end of this chapter, you will be able to:

1 Identify the various antimalarial, antiprotozoal, and antihelmintic agents.

2 Identify the signs and symptoms of malarial, protozoal, and helminthic infection.

3 Discuss the mechanism of, action of, indications for, cautions and contraindications to, and side effects and routes of administration of each antimalarial, antihelmintic, and antiprotozoal agent, as well as the relevant nursing interventions in patients receiving them.

4 Develop a comprehensive nursing care plan, including patient education, pertinent to patients receiving antimalarial, antiprotozoal, or antihelmintic agents.

CHAPTER OUTLINE

Malaria

Antimalarial Agents
  Mechanism of action
  Drug effects
  Therapeutic uses
  Side effects and adverse effects
  Interactions
  Dosages

Drug Profiles
  Chloroquine
  ⚓ Primaquine
  Mefloquine
  Pyrimethamine

Protozoal Infections

Antiprotozoal Agents
  Mechanism of action
  Drug effects
  Therapeutic uses
  Side effects and adverse effects
  Interactions
  Dosages

Drug Profiles
  Atovaquone
  Iodoquinol

  ⚓ Metronidazole
  Paromomycin
  ⚓ Pentamidine

Helminthic Infections

Antihelmintic Agents
  Mechanism of action
  Drug effects
  Therapeutic uses
  Side effects and adverse effects
  Interactions
  Dosages

Drug Profiles
  Diethylcarbamazine
  ⚓ Mebendazole
  Niclosamide
  Pyrantel
  Praziquantel

Nursing Process
Assessment
Nursing Diagnoses
Planning
  Outcome criteria
Implementation
Evaluation

Glossary

4-Aminoquinoline derivatives (ə mē′ no kwin′ o lēn) Antimalarial agents that bind to nucleoproteins and interfere with protein synthesis. (p. 608)

Antihelmintic (an′ tĭ hel min′ tik) Drug used to treat parasitic worm infections. (p. 618)

Antimalarial (an′ tĭ mə lar′ e əl) Drug that destroys or prevents the development of plasmodia in human hosts. (p. 608)

Antiprotozoal (an′ tĭ pro′ tə zo′ əl) Drug that destroys or prevents the development of single-celled microorganisms of the subkingdom protozoa in human hosts. (p. 613)

Erythrocytic phase Phase of the asexual cycle of the parasite that occurs inside the erythrocyte. (p. 608)

Exoerythrocytic phase Phase of the asexual cycle of the parasite that occurs outside the erythrocyte. (p. 608)

Helminthic infection (hel min′ thik) Parasitic worm infection. (p. 617)

Malaria (mə lar′ e ə) Most significant protozoal disease in terms of morbidity and mortality. (p. 608)

Parasite (par′ ə sīt) Organism that feeds on another living organism. (p. 612)

Parasitic protozoa (pro′ to zo′ ə) Protozoa that live on or in human beings. (p. 608)

Plasmodium (plaz mo′ de əm) Genus of protozoa that causes malaria. (p. 608)

There are more than 28,000 known types of protozoa. Those that live on or in humans are termed **parasitic protozoa**. Billions of people worldwide are infected with these organisms, and as a result, these infections are considered a serious health problem. Some of the more common protozoal infections are malaria, leishmaniasis, trypanosomiasis, amebiasis, giardiasis, and trichomoniasis. They are relatively uncommon in the United States but are becoming increasingly prevalent among immunocompromised persons, including those with AIDS. Protozoal diseases are especially prevalent among people living in tropical climates because it is easier for them to survive and be transmitted in these year-round warm and humid environments. Even though the population of the United States is relatively free of many of these protozoal infections, international travel and the immigration of persons from other countries where such infections are endemic are providing opportunities for increased exposure.

Malaria

The most significant protozoal disease in terms of morbidity and mortality is **malaria**. In Africa alone it accounts for more than 1 million infant deaths a year. It is caused by a particular genus of protozoa called **Plasmodium**, and there are four species of organisms within this genus, each with its own characteristics and its own ability to resist being killed by antimalarials. Most commonly, malaria is transmitted by the bite of an infected female mosquito. However, malaria can also be transmitted by blood transfusions, congenitally, or through the use of contaminated needles by drug abusers. Despite the combined efforts of many countries to eradicate malaria, it remains the most devastating infectious disease in the world. Many lives are lost, and the cost of treating and preventing the disease imposes a tremendous economic burden on countries, many of which are very poor.

The life cycle of the malarial parasite, the plasmodium, is quite diverse and involves many stages. It has two interdependent life cycles: the **sexual cycle**, which takes place in the mosquito, and the **asexual cycle**, which occurs in the human host. In addition, the asexual cycle of the parasite consists of a phase outside the erythrocyte called the **exoerythrocytic phase** and a phase inside the erythrocyte called the **erythrocytic phase**. The malarial parasite undergoes many changes during these two phases.

ANTIMALARIAL DRUGS

Antimalarial agents cannot affect the parasite during the sexual cycle when it resides in the mosquito, but during the asexual cycle, which takes place within the human body and is a particularly vulnerable stage, the parasite can be affected by antimalarial drugs. Chloroquine, hydroxychloroquine, quinine, and mefloquine kill the malarial parasite during the erythrocytic stage; primaquine kills the parasite during the exoerythrocytic phase. Often these drugs are given in various combinations to achieve an additive or synergistic protozoacidal effect. Other antibiotics that may be given with these agents are pyrimethamine and sulfadoxine.

Mechanism of Action

The mechanisms of action of the various antimalarial agents differ depending on the chemical family of agents they belong to. The **4-aminoquinoline derivatives** (chloroquine and hydroxychloroquine) work by binding to nucleoproteins in the organisms and interfering with protein synthesis. They also inhibit DNA and RNA polymerase, an enzyme essential to the production of DNA and RNA. Both of these actions eventuate in the destruction of the parasite by preventing the manufacture of vital parasite-sustaining substances. They are also believed to raise the pH within the parasite, which has the effect of interfering with the parasite's ability to metabolize and utilize erythrocyte hemoglobin and is one reason why they are ineffective during the exoerythrocytic phase. **Quinine** and **mefloquine** are thought to be similar to the 4-aminoquinoline derivatives in their actions, in that both are believed to raise the pH within the parasite.

The **diaminophyrimidines** (pyrimethamine and trimethoprim) work by inhibiting dihydrofolate reductase, an enzyme that is needed for the production of certain vital substances in malarial parasites. Specifically, inhibiting this enzyme blocks the synthesis of tetrahydrofolate, a precursor of purines, pyrimidines, and certain amino acids essential for the growth and survival of the parasite. These two agents are also only effective during the erythrocytic phase and are often used with a sulfonamide or sulfone (sulfadoxine or dapsone) because of the resulting synergistic effects exerted by the agents. Together they block sequential steps in the same metabolic pathway for purine, pyrimidines, and amino acid synthesis in plasmodia.

Primaquine has the ability to bind to and alter DNA and is one of the few agents that is effective in the exoerythrocytic phase.

Sulfonamides, tetracyclines, and clindamycin may all be used in combination with some of the antimalarial agents named to further augment the protozoacidal effect.

Drug Effects

The drug effects of the antimalarial agents are mostly limited to their ability to kill parasitic organisms, most of which are *Plasmodium spp.* Some of these agents do, however, have other drug effects. Chloroquine and hydroxychloroquine also have antiinflammatory effects and may be beneficial in the treatment of rheumatoid arthritis and lupus erythematosus. Quinine and quinidine, two plant alkaloids, can also decrease the excitability of both cardiac and skeletal muscles. They also have local anesthetic actions as well as analgesic, antipyretic, and oxytocic effects.

Therapeutic Uses

The antimalarial agents are used to kill *Plasmodium* organisms, the parasites that cause malaria. As already mentioned, different antimalarial agents work during different phases of the parasite's growth inside the human. Those antimalarials exerting the greatest effect on *Plasmodium* organisms during the erythrocytic phase are chloroquine, hydroxychloroquine, and pyrimethamine. Because they are ineffective during the exoerythrocytic phase, however, they cannot prevent infection. Chloroquine and related compounds remain the drugs of choice for the treatment of susceptible strains of malarial parasites. They are highly toxic to all the species of *Plasmodium* except *P. falciparum*, which has proved to be resistant to chloroquine in people with malaria caused by this species of *Plasmodium* who live in many areas of the world—Asia, Africa, and South America.

Quinine, which is available in both an oral and a parenteral form, is only indicated for the treatment of mild attacks, when the oral agent is used and for the management of acute attacks of multiple-drug–resistant *P. falciparum*, which causes a type of malaria that affects the cerebral hemispheres. A sulfonamide or tetracycline antibacterial agent is always combined with quinine to take advantage of their synergistic protozoacidal effects.

Pyrimethamine is another antimalarial antibiotic that is commonly used in combination with other antibiotics, in most cases a sulfonamide. It is also used in combination with sulfadoxine for the prophylaxis of chloroquine-resistant *P. falciparum* and *P. vivax*. Mefloquine is a newer antimalarial agent that may also be used for the prophylaxis of falciparum malaria.

The most effective antimalarial agent for eradicating the parasite during the exoerythrocytic phase is primaquine. Quinacrine, trimethoprim, clindamycin, and dapsone may also be beneficial or work synergistically with these antimalarial agents in the killing of various parasites.

Side Effects and Adverse Effects

The antimalarial agents cause diverse side effects and adverse effects, and these are listed for each drug in Table 40-1.

Interactions

Of the half dozen or so antimalarial agents, only mefloquine and primaquine are associated with any significant drug interactions. These are listed in Table 40-2.

Dosages

For the recommended dosages for selected antimalarial agents, see the dosages table on p. 611.

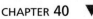

Table 40-1	Antimalarial Drugs: Common Adverse Effects
BODY SYSTEM	**SIDE/ADVERSE EFFECT**
Quinine	
Gastrointestinal	Diarrhea, nausea, vomiting, abdominal pain or discomfort
CNS	Visual disturbances, dizziness, severe headaches, tinnitus, hearing loss
Other	Rash, pruritus, hives, respiratory difficulties, wheezing
Chloroquine and Hydroxychloroquine	
Gastrointestinal	Diarrhea, anorexia, nausea, vomiting, abdominal distress
Other	Alopecia, dizziness, increased anxiety, rash, pruritus
Mefloquine	
Gastrointestinal	Stomach pain, anorexia, nausea, vomiting
CNS	Headache, dizziness, insomnia, visual disturbances, increased anxiety, convulsions, depression, psychosis
⚓**Primaquine**	
Gastrointestinal	Nausea, vomiting, abdominal distress
Other	Headaches, pruritus, dark discoloration of urine, hemolytic anemia due to G6PD deficiency
Pyrimethamine	
Gastrointestinal	Anorexia; vomiting; taste disturbances; soreness, redness, swelling, or burning of tongue; diarrhea; throat pain; swallowing difficulties; sores, ulcerations, or white spots in mouth; sore throat
Other	Fever, increased bleeding, increased weakness, rash

DRUG PROFILES

CHLOROQUINE

Chloroquine (Aralen) is a synthetic antimalarial agent that is a 4-aminoquinoline derivative. It is also effective against other parasitic infections such as amebiasis and because of its antiinflammatory actions is used in the treatment of rheumatoid arthritis and lupus erythematosus. It is a prescription-only product, and its safety in pregnant women has not been established, though it is generally thought that the drug should be used in pregnant women only when clearly needed. It is classified as a pregnancy category C agent, and hypersensitivity to it, retinal field changes, and porphyria are contraindications to its use. Hydroxychloroquine is also a 4-aminoquinoline derivative with characteristics very similar to those of chloroquine.

Chloroquine is available in both a parenteral and an oral formulation. Chloroquine hydrochloride is used in the parenteral form, coming in a strength of 40 mg/ml for injection. Chloroquine phosphate is used in the oral form, which comes as 150- and 300-mg tablets. Commonly recommended dosages are listed in the dosages table on the next page.

☣ PHARMACOKINETICS

HALF-LIFE	ONSET	PEAK	DURATION
Variable	8-10 hr	2 hr	Variable

⚓ PRIMAQUINE

Primaquine is very similar to both of the 4-aminoquinolines, chloroquine and hydroxychloroquine, but it is an 8-aminoquinolone. It has many of the same characteristics as the 4-aminoquinolines. However, as already noted, it is one of the few antimalarial agents that can destroy the malarial parasites while they are in their exoerythrocytic phase. It is indicated for the treatment of malaria caused by various species of *Plasmodium: P. falciparum, P. malariae, P. ovale,* and *P. vivax.*

Primaquine is classified as a pregnancy category C agent and is contraindicated in patients with a known hypersensitivity to it, as well as in those with anemia, lupus erythematosus, methemoglobinemia, porphyria, rheumatoid arthritis, methemoglobin reductase deficiency, and G6PD deficiency. It comes as a 15-mg tablet that is administered orally. Commonly recommended dosages are listed in the dosages table on the next page.

☣ PHARMACOKINETICS

HALF-LIFE	ONSET	PEAK	DURATION
4-7 hr	<2 hr	1-2 hr	24 hr

MEFLOQUINE

Mefloquine (Lariam) is an analogue of quinine that is indicated for the management of mild to moderate

D O S A G E S

SELECTED ANTIMALARIAL AGENTS

AGENT	PHARMACOLOGIC CLASS	DOSAGE RANGE	PURPOSE
Chloroquine PO4 (Aralen PO4)	Synthetic antimalarial, antiamebic	*Pediatric* PO: 5 mg/kg/wk	Malaria prophylaxis
		Adult PO: 500 mg/wk	Malaria prophylaxis
		Pediatric PO: Total dose of 25 mg/kg administered over 3 days	Malaria treatment
		Adult PO: Total dose of 2.5 g administered over 3 days	Malaria treatment
		Adult PO: 1 g/day for 2 days, followed by 500 mg/day for 2-3 wk	Extraintestinal amebiasis
⚓Primaquine PO4	Synthetic antimalarial	*Pediatric* PO: 0.5 mg/kg/day for 14 days	Malaria treatment
		Adult PO: 26.3 mg/day for 14 days	Malaria treatment
Mefloquine (Lariam)	Synthetic antimalarial	*Adult* PO: 1250 mg as a single dose with 8 oz of H_2O	Malaria treatment
		PO: 250 mg once weekly	Malaria prophylaxis
Pyrimethamine (Daraprim)	Folic acid antagonist, antimalarial, antitoxoplasmotic agent	*Pediatric* PO: <4 y/o, 6.25 mg once weekly 4-10 y/o, 12.5 mg once weekly	Malaria prophylaxis
		Adult/Pediatric >10 y/o PO: 25 mg once weekly	Malaria prophylaxis
		Pediatric 4-10 y/o PO: 25 mg for 2 days	Malaria treatment
		Adult PO: 25-50 mg for 2 days	Malaria treatment
		Pediatric PO: 1 mg/kg/day in 2 doses for 2-4 days, reduced to one-half for 1 mo with appropriate sulfa drug	Toxoplasmosis
		Adult PO: 50-75 mg/day with 1-4 g/day of a sulfa drug for 1-3 wk	Toxoplasmosis

Table 40-2	Antimalarial Agents: Drug Interactions	
DRUG	**MECHANISM**	**RESULT**
Mefloquine		
Beta-blockers, calcium-channel blockers, quinidine, quinine	Unknown	Increased risk of dysrhythmia, cardiac arrest, seizures
Chloroquine	Decreased seizure threshold	Increased seizure activity
Divalproex, valproic acid	Decreased serum levels of valproic acid	Loss of seizure control
↓Primaquine		
Other hemolytic agents	Unknown	Increased risk for myelotoxic effects (Monitor for muscle weakness)
Quinacrine	Potentiates the toxicity of antimalarial drugs like primaquine	Increased primaquine toxicity

acute malaria and for the prevention and treatment of chloroquine-resistant malaria and multiple-drug–resistant strains of *P. falciparum,* which as already noted is a very difficult species of *Plasmodium* to kill. Mefloquine is classified as a pregnancy C agent and is contraindicated in patients with a known hypersensitivity to it. It is available in 250-mg tablets, taken orally. Commonly recommended dosages are listed in the dosages table on the previous page.

⬡ PHARMACOKINETICS

HALF-LIFE	ONSET	PEAK	DURATION
Days to weeks	<24 hr	7-24 hr	Variable

PYRIMETHAMINE

Pyrimethamine (Daraprim) is a synthetic antimalarial agent that is structurally related to trimethoprim. These two agents are sometimes referred to as *diaminophyrimidines.* There is a fixed-combination product called *Fansidar* that contains 500 mg of sulfadoxine and 25 mg of pyrimethamine. Pyrimethamine is classified as a pregnancy category C agent and is contraindicated in patients with a known hypersensitivity to it and in those with chloroquine-resistant malaria or with megaloblastic anemia caused by folate deficiency. It is only available in an oral formulation as a 25-mg tablet. Commonly recommended dosages are listed in the dosages table on the previous page.

⬡ PHARMACOKINETICS

HALF-LIFE	ONSET	PEAK	DURATION
80-95 hr	<6 hr	1.5-8 hr	Up to 2 wk

Protozoal Infections

There are several other common protozoal infections besides malaria. Some of the most common ones are amebiasis, giardiasis, pneumocystosis, toxoplasmosis, and trichomoniasis, and like malaria, these are also more prevalent in tropical regions. The protozoal parasites that cause the most serious infections are *Cryptosporidium sp., Isospora belli, Pneumocystis carinii,* and *Toxoplasma gondii.*

The protozoa that cause these infections are **parasites,** or organisms that feed on another living organism. They can be transmitted in a number of ways: from person to person, through the ingestion of contaminated water or food, through direct contact with the parasite, or by the bite of an insect (mosquito or tick). Parasitic infections can be classified according to where they occur in the body. They can be **systemic** and occur almost anywhere in the body; they can affect the **gastrointestinal** tract, as in the case of amebiasis; or they can affect **dermatologic** sites, as in the case of lice.

The more common protozoal infections are listed in Table 40-3 along with a brief description of the infection and the antiprotozoal agents commonly used in their treatment. Patients whose immune system is compromised, such as those with leukemia, those with transplanted organs who are on immunosuppressive drugs, and those with AIDS, are at particular risk for acquiring a protozoal infection. Often such infections are fatal in these patients.

Table 40-3	Protozoal Infections: Types	
PROTOZOAL INFECTION	**DESCRIPTION**	**ANTIPROTOZOAL AGENT**
Amebiasis	An infection that mainly resides in the large intestine but can also migrate to other parts of the body, such as the liver; it is produced by the protozoal parasite, *Entamoeba histolytica.* Usually transmitted in contaminated food or water.	Metronidazole, paromomycin, iodoquinol
Giardiasis	Caused by *Giardia lamblia.* It is the most common intestinal protozoal infection, usually residing in the intestinal mucosa (most commonly the duodenum). May cause diarrhea, bloating, and foul-smelling stools. Transmitted by contaminated food or water or by contact with stool from infected persons.	Metronidazole, quinacrine, tinidazole
Pneumocytosis	Pneumonias caused by *Pneumocystis carinii* that occur exclusively in immunocompromised persons; always fatal if left untreated.	Trimethoprim-sulfamethoxazole, dapsone, atovaquone, pentamidine
Toxoplasmosis	Caused by *Toxoplasma gondii;* can produce systemic infection in both immunocompetent and immunocompromised hosts. Domesticated animals, usually cats, serve as intermediate host for parasites, passing infective oocysts in their feces.	Sulfonamides with pyrimethamine, clindamycin, metronidazole
Trichomoniasis	A sexually transmitted disease caused by *Trichomonas vaginalis.*	Metronidazole

Antiprotozoal Agents: Mechanism of Action

ANTIPROTOZOAL AGENT	**MECHANISM OF ACTION**
Atovaquone	Protozoal energy is generated in mitochondria; atovaquone selectively inhibits mitochondrial electron transport, resulting in no energy and cell death; it also inhibits pyrimidine synthesis, causing the protozoa to be unable to make life-sustaining substances.
⚓Metronidazole	Bactericidal, amebicidal, and trichomonacidal; it can also kill anaerobic bacteria, which it accomplishes by disrupting DNA synthesis as well as inhibiting other nucleic acid synthesis, two substances needed for the survival of many organisms.
⚓Pentamidine	Inhibits production of much-needed substances such as DNA and RNA; it can bind to and aggregate ribosomes; it is directly lethal to *P. carinii*, by inhibiting glucose metabolism, protein and RNA synthesis, and intracellular amino acid transport.
Iodoquinol	Called a *luminal* or *contact amebicide* because it acts primarily in the intestinal lumen of the infected host and directly kills the protozoa.
Paromomycin	Also a luminal or contact amebicide; it is a direct-acting agent and kills by inhibiting protein synthesis in susceptible bacteria by binding to the 30S ribosomal subunit.

ANTIPROTOZOAL AGENTS

The most commonly used **antiprotozoal** agents are:

- Iodoquinal, metronidazole, and paromomycin—used for the treatment of intestinal amebiasis
- Chloroquine and metronidazole—used for the treatment of extraintestinal amebiasis
- Atovaquone, pentamidine, pyrimethamine, and quinacrine—used for the treatment of other infections

Mechanism of Action

The mechanisms of action of the antiprotozoal agents are as different as the agents themselves. The most commonly used of these agents together with a brief description of their mechanisms of action are given in the box above. Pyrimethamine and quinacrine have been discussed earlier in this chapter and are therefore not included.

Antiprotozoal Agents: Drug Effects

ANTIPROTOZOAL AGENT	DRUG EFFECTS
Atovaquone	Used for the treatment of acute, mild to moderately severe P. carinii pneumonia in patients who cannot tolerate cotrimoxazole.
↓Metronidazole	An antibacterial (including anaerobes), antiprotozoal, and antihelmintic agent.
↓Pentamidine	Used for the treatment of pneumonia caused by P. carinii.
Iodoquinol	Indicated for the treatment of intestinal amebiasis in asymptomatic carriers of E. histolytica; it has also been used for the treatment of G. lamblia and T. vaginalis infections.
Paromomycin	Indicated for the treatment of acute and chronic intestinal amebiasis and as adjunct therapy in management of hepatic coma.

Table 40-4 Antiprotozoal Agents: Adverse Effects

BODY SYSTEM	SIDE/ADVERSE EFFECTS
Atovaquone	
Cardiovascular	Hypotension
Hematologic	Anemia, leukemia
Integumentary	Pruritus, urticaria, rash, oral candidiasis
Gastrointestinal	Anorexia, increased AST/ALT, acute pancreatitis, nausea, vomiting, diarrhea, constipation, abdominal pain
CNS	Dizziness, headache, anxiety
Metabolic	Hyperkalemia, hyperglycemia, hyponatremia
↓Metronidazole	
CNS	Headache, dizziness, confusion, fatigue, convulsions
EENT	Blurred vision, sore throat, dry mouth, metallic taste
Gastrointestinal	Abdominal cramps, pseudomembranous colitis, nausea, vomiting, diarrhea
Genitourinary	Darkened urine, dysuria
Hematologic	Leukopenia, bone marrow depression
Integumentary	Rash, pruritus, urticaria, flushing
↓Pentamidine	
Cardiovascular	Hypotension, dysrhythmias
Hematologic	Anemia, leukopenia, thrombocytopenia
Integumentary	Pain at injection site, pruritus, urticaria, rash
Genitourinary	Acute renal failure
Gastrointestinal	Increased AST/ALT levels, acute pancreatitis, metallic taste, nausea, vomiting, diarrhea
CNS	Disorientation, hallucinations, dizziness, confusion
Respiratory	Cough, shortness of breath, bronchospasm
Metabolic	Hyperkalemia, hypocalcemia, hypoglycemia
Other	Fatigue, chills, night sweats
Iodoquinol	
Hematologic	Agranulocytosis
Integumentary	Rash; pruritus; discolored skin, hair, nails
CNS	Headache, agitation, peripheral neuropathy
EENT	Blurred vision, sore throat
Gastrointestinal	Anorexia, gastritis, abdominal cramps, nausea, vomiting, diarrhea
Other	Fever, chills, vertigo
Paromomycin	
Gastrointestinal	Stomach cramps, nausea, vomiting, diarrhea
CNS	Hearing loss, dizziness, tinnitus

Drug Effects

The drug effects of these antiprotozoal agents are primarily limited to their ability to kill various forms of protozoal parasites, but these differ from agent to agent. The drug effects of the antiprotozoal agents that have not yet been mentioned are summarized in the box on the preceding page.

Therapeutic Uses

The antiprotozoal agents are used to treat various protozoal infections, ranging from intestinal amebiasis to pneumocystosis. Atovaquone and pentamidine are used for the treatment of *P. carinii* infection. Iodoquinol and paromomycin are effectively able to kill intestinal forms of *E. histolytica* and are used for the treatment of intestinal infections with this parasite. Metronidazole is effective against many forms of bacteria, including anaerobic bacteria, as well as against protozoa and helminths, infection with the latter being discussed later in the chapter.

Side Effects and Adverse Effects

The side effects and adverse effects of the antiprotozoal agents vary greatly depending on the agent, and the ones specific to the common antiprotozoal agents are listed in Table 40-4.

Interactions

The common drug and laboratory test interactions associated with the use of antiprotozoal agents are listed in Table 40-5. Some of these interactions can result in severe toxicities, and it is therefore important to know of them and to understand the mechanism involved.

Dosages

For dosage information on selected antiprotozoal agents, see the dosages table on the next page. Pregnancy category C.

DRUG PROFILES

The antiprotozoal agents are used for a number of indications, and these include *P. carinii* and *T. vaginitis* infections, amebic dysentery, toxoplasmosis, giardiasis, and anaerobic bacterial infections. All are prescription-only drugs because of the potential adverse effects

Table 40-5	Antiprotozoal Agents: Drug and Laboratory Test Interactions	

ANTIPROTOZOAL AGENT	MECHANISM	RESULT
Atovaquone	Complete for binding on protein, resulting in free, active Atovaquone	Highly protein-bound drugs; may increase drug concentrations and drug effects
↓Metronidazole	Increased plasma acetaldehyde concentration following ingestion of alcohol by decreasing the absorption of vitamin K from the intestines by eliminating the bacteria needed to absorb vitamin K	Alcohol: causes a "disulfiram reaction." Warfarin: may increase action of warfarin
↓Pentamidine	Additive nephrotoxic effects	Use with an aminoglycoside, amphotericin B, colistin, cisplatin, methoxyflurane, polymyxin B, or vancomycin may result in nephrotoxicity
Iodoquinol	May interfere with certain thyroid function test results	Increases protein-bound serum iodine concentrations, reflecting a decrease in iodine 131 uptake
Paromomycin	Additive nephrotoxic effects	Use with an aminoglycoside, amphotericin B, colistin, cisplatin, methoxyflurane, polymyxin B, or vancomycin may result in nephrotoxicity

DOSAGES

SELECTED ANTIPROTOZOAL AGENTS

AGENT	PHARMACOLOGIC CLASS	DOSAGE RANGE	PURPOSE
Atovaquone (Mepron)	Synthetic anti-PCP agent	*Adult* PO: 750 mg with food tid for 21 days	PCP
Iodoquinol (Yodoxin, Di-Quinol)	Amebicide	*Pediatric* PO: 40 mg/kg/day in 3 divided doses pc for 20 days; do not exceed 1.95 gm/day. *Adult* PO: 650 mg tid pc for 20 days	Amebiasis
⚓**Metronidazole (Metric 21, Protostat, Flagyl)**	Amebicide, antibacterial, trichomonacide	*Pediatric* PO: 30-50 mg/kg/day in 3 divided doses for 10 days *Adult* PO: 750 mg tid for 5-10 days. PO: 375 mg bid for 7 days or 2 g for 1 day. PO: 7.5 mg/kg q6h for 7-10 days. Do not exceed 4 g/day. IV: 15 mg/kg infused over 1 hr, followed by 7.5 mg/kg infused over 1 hr q6h. IV: 15 mg/kg infused over 30-60 min and completed 1 hr preop. and followed by 7.5 mg/kg infused over 30-60 min at 6 and 12 hr after initial dose.	Amebiasis Amebiasis, amoebic liver abscess Trichomoniasis Bacterial infection Bacterial infection Surgical bacterial prophylaxis
Paromomycin (Humatin)	Antiamebic and antibacterial aminoglycoside antibiotic	*Pediatric/Adult* PO: 25-35 mg/kg/day in 3 divided doses with meals for 5-10 days *Adult* PO: 4 g/day in 2-4 divided doses for 5-6 days	Amebiasis Hepatic coma
⚓**Pentamidine isethionate (Nebupent, Pentam)**	Synthetic anti-PCP agent	*Pediatric/Adult* IM/IV: 4 mg/kg once/day infused over 1 hr for 14 days. *Adult* Inhal: 300 mg once every 4 wk	PCP PCP prophylaxis

PCP, P. carinii pneumonia.

that can arise if they are used inappropriately. These drugs are available in a wide variety of dosage forms, including oral, parenteral, and aerosol preparations. All antiprotozoal agents except for metronidazole are classified as pregnancy category C agents, with metronidazole classified as a category B agent.

ATOVAQUONE

Atovaquone (Mepron) is a synthetic antiprotozoal agent indicated for the treatment of mild to moderate *P. carinii* pneumonia in patients cannot tolerate cotrimoxazole (trimethoprine-sulfamethoxazole). Atovaquone appears to kill protozoa by inhibiting the production of vital substances such as nucleic acids and ATP.

Atovaquone is contraindicated in patients with a hypersensitivity to it and in those who have had a life-threatening allergic reaction to any component of the formulation. It is only available orally as a 250-mg film-coated tablet. Commonly recommended dosages are given in the dosages table above. Pregnancy category C.

✦ PHARMACOKINETICS

HALF-LIFE	ONSET	PEAK	DURATION
2-3 days	8-24 hr	24-96 hr	Unknown

IODOQUINOL

Iodoquinol (Yodoxin, Di-Quinol) is considered a luminal or contact amebicide (killer of intestinal protozoa infections) because it acts primarily in the intestinal lumen. It is indicated for the treatment of intestinal amebiasis.

It is contraindicated in patients with a known hypersensitivity to it or to iodine as well as in those with renal disease, hepatic disease, severe thyroid disease, or a preexisting optic neuropathy. Iodoquinol is available only in an oral preparation—210- and 650-mg tablets. Commonly recommended dosages are given in the dosages table on the preceding page. Pregnancy safety information has not been established.

PHARMACOKINETICS

HALF-LIFE	ONSET	PEAK	DURATION
Unknown	Unknown	Unknown	Unknown

METRONIDAZOLE

Metronidazole (Metric 21, Protostat, Flagyl) is an antiinfective agent that not only has antibacterial activity against microorganisms, which include anaerobic bacteria, but also has antiprotozoal and antihelmintic activity. The therapeutic uses of metronidazole are many and varied and range from the treatment of trichomoniasis, amebiasis, and giardiasis to that of anaerobic infections and antibiotic-associated pseudomembranous colitis. It can directly kill intestinal protozoa and kills all other organisms by preventing DNA synthesis.

The contraindications to metronidazole use include hypersensitivity, renal disease, hepatic disease, blood dyscrasias, various CNS disorders, and pregnancy (during first trimester). Thus, it is classified as a pregnancy category B agent. It is available as an oral preparation in the form of 250- and 500-mg tablets and film-coated tablets and parenterally in the form of a 5-mg/ml injection for IV infusion and a 500-mg vial for injection. Commonly recommended dosages are given in the dosages table on the previous page.

PHARMACOKINETICS

HALF-LIFE	ONSET	PEAK	DURATION
8-12 hr	<1.5 hr	PO: 1-2 hr	Variable

PAROMOMYCIN

Paromomycin (Humatin) is an aminoglycoside antibiotic that is used for the treatment of amebiasis and intestinal protozoal infections. It directly kills intestinal protozoa when it comes in contact with them. Its bactericidal activity appears to be related to its ability to inhibit protein synthesis in susceptible organisms by binding to the 30S ribosomal subunit.

The contraindications to its use include hypersensitivity to it, renal disease, and gastrointestinal obstruction. It is only available in an oral formulation—a 250-mg capsule. Commonly recommended dosages are given in the dosages table on the previous page. Pregnancy category C.

PHARMACOKINETICS

HALF-LIFE	ONSET	PEAK	DURATION
Unknown	Unknown	Unknown	Unknown

PENTAMIDINE

Pentamidine (Nebupent, Pentam) is an antiprotozoal agent that is used mainly for the management of *P. carinii* pneumonia. It is also effective in combating many other protozoal infections, and it kills these protozoa by inhibiting protein and nucleic acid synthesis. It is used for both the treatment and prophylaxis of *P. carinii* pneumonia in patients at high risk for initial or recurrent infection.

Hypersensitivity to the agent, especially when administered by inhalation, is the sole contraindication to its use. It is classified as a pregnancy category C agent. However, it should be used with caution in patients with blood dyscrasias, hepatic or renal disease, diabetes mellitus, cardiac disease, hypocalcemia, or hypertension. Pentamidine comes as a 300-mg oral inhalation solution and also as a 300-mg injection for IV administration. Commonly recommended dosages are given in the dosage table on the previous page. Pregnancy category C..

PHARMACOKINETICS

HALF-LIFE	ONSET	PEAK	DURATION
6-9 hr	0.5-1 hr	<1 hr	Variable

Helminthic Infections

Parasitic **helminthic infections** (worm infections) are a worldwide problem. No country is spared. It has been estimated that one third of the world's population is infected with these parasites, but those people living in undeveloped countries where sanitary conditions are often poor are by far the most common victims. The incidence of worm infections in the inhabitants of developed countries where sewage treatment is adequate is much lower, and usually only a few select helminthic diseases are the source of the problem.

Helminthic Infections

INFECTION	ORGANISM AND OTHER FACTS
	Nematoda (various intestinal and tissue roundworms)
Ascariasis	Caused by *Ascaris lumbricoides* (giant roundworm); resides in small intestine; treated with pyrantel or mebendazole
Enterobiasis	Caused by *Enterobius vermicularis* (pinworm); resides in large intestine; treated with pyrantel or mebendazole
Platyhelminthes (Intestinal tapeworm or flatworms)	
Diphyllobothriasis	Caused by *Diaphyllobothrium latum* (fishworm); acquired from fish; treated with niclosamide or paromomycin
Hymenolepiasis	Caused by *Hymenolepis nana* (dwarf tapeworm); treated with niclosamide or paromomycin
Taeniasis	Caused by *Taenia saginata* (beef tapeworm); acquired from beef; treated with niclosamide or paromomycin
	Caused by *Taenia solium* (pork tapeworm); acquired from pork; treated with niclosamide, quinacrine, or paromomycin

The most prevalent helminthic infection in the populace of the United States is enterobiasis.

Helminths that are parasitic in humans are classified in the following way:

I. Platyhelminthes (flatworms)
   A. Cestodes (tapeworms)
   B. Trematodes (flukes)
II. Nematoda (roundworms)

The characteristics of a few of the most common of the many helminthic infections are summarized in the box above. There are essentially three types of helminths: **cestodes** (tapeworms), **nematodes** (roundworms), and **trematodes** (flukes). These usually reside in the intestines of their host but can also reside in other tissues.

ANTIHELMINTIC AGENTS

Unlike the protozoa, the helminths are large and have complex cellular structures, and it is by disrupting these structures that the **antihelmintic** agents destroy these organisms. The currently available antihelmintic drugs are very specific in the worms they can kill. For this reason the causative worm should be accurately identified before the start of treatment, and this can usually be done by analyzing samples of feces, urine, blood, sputum, or tissue from the infected host for the presence of the particular parasite ova or larvae.

There are over a half dozen antihelmintics that are commonly used in the treatment of these infections, and these include:

- Diethylcarbamazine (Hetrazan)
- Mebendazole (Vermox)
- Niclosamide (Niclocide)

- Oxamniquine (Vansil)
- Piperazine
- Praziquantel (Biltricide)
- Pyrantel (Antiminth)
- Thiabendazole (Mintezol)

As just mentioned, the antihelmintics are very specific in their actions. Only **mebendazole** can be used to treat both tapeworms and roundworms. **Oxamniquine** and **praziquantel** are the only agents that can kill flukes (trematodes). The most commonly used antihelmintics and the specific class of worms they are effective in killing are summarized in Table 40-6.

Mechanism of Action

The mechanisms of action of the various antihelmintics vary greatly from agent to agent, though there are some similarities among the agents used to kill similar types of worms. The various antihelmintic agents and their respective mechanisms of action are listed in the box on p. 619.

Drug Effects

The drug effects of the antihelmintic agents are limited to their ability to kill various forms of worms and flukes. They have no other drug effects.

Therapeutic Uses

The antihelmintic agents are used to treat infections with roundworms, tapeworms, or flukes. The antihelmintic agents and the particular helminthic infections they are used in the treatment of are listed in the box on p. 619.

Table 40-6	Antihelminitics: Class of Worms Killed			
		CLASS OF WORMS		
ANTIHELMINTIC DRUG	**CESTODES**	**NEMATODES**		**TREMATODES**
Diethylcarbamazine and thiabendazole	No	Yes (tissue and some intestinal)		No
Piperazine and pyrantel	No	Yes (giant worm and pin worm)		No
⚓Mebendazole	Yes	Yes		No
Niclosamide	Yes	No		No
Oxamniquine and praziquantel	No	No		Yes

Antihelmintics: Mechanisms of Action

ANTIHELMINTIC DRUG	MECHANISM OF ACTION
Diethylcarbamazine	Inhibits the rate of embryogenesis of nematodes.
Thiabendazole	Inhibits the helminth-specific enzyme, fumarate reductase.
Piperazine and pyrantel	Blocks acetylcholine at the neuromuscular junction, resulting in paralysis of the worm; the paralyzed worms are then expelled from the GI tract by normal peristalsis.
⚓Mebendazole	Selectively and irreversibly inhibits the uptake of glucose and other nutrients; results in the depletion of endogenous glycogen stores, eventual autolysis of the parasitic worm, and death.
Niclosamide	Inhibits mitochondrial oxidative phosphorylation; also decreases generation of ATP by inhibiting the uptake of glucose; cestodes are then dislodged from the GI wall; the worm is digested in the intestine and subsequently expelled from the GI tract by normal peristalsis.
Oxamniquine and praziquantel	Increase permeability of the cell membrane of susceptible worms to calcium, resulting in the influx of calcium ions; this causes the worms to be dislodged from their usual site of residence in the mesenteric veins to the liver; here they are killed by host tissue reactions; dislodgement of worms is the result of contraction and paralysis of their musculature and subsequent immobilization of their suckers, which causes the worms to detach from the blood vessel wall and be passively dislodged by normal blood flow.

Antihelmintics: Therapeutic Uses

ANTIHELMINTIC DRUG	THERAPEUTIC USES (INDICATIONS)
Diethylcarbamazine	Bancroft's filariasis, loiasis, onchocerciasis, tropical eosinophilia
⚓Mebendazole	Trichuriasis (whipworm), enterobiasis, ascariasis, *Ancylostoma* infection (common hookworm), *Necator* infection (American hookworm)
Niclosamide	*Taenia saginata* infection, diphyllobothriasis, *hymenolepiasis*
Oxamniquine	Schistosomiasis (blood fluke)
Piperazine	Enterobiasis, ascariasis
Praziquantel	Schistosomiasis, opisthorchiasis (liver fluke), clonorchiasis (Chinese or Oriental liver fluke)
Pyrantel	Ascariasis, enterobiasis, other helminthic infections
Thiabendazole	Cutaneous larva migrans (creeping eruption), strongyloidiasis, trichinosis

Side Effects and Adverse Effects

The adverse effects of mebendazole therapy are limited to drug-induced tissue necrosis, diarrhea, and abdominal pain. Those of niclosamide include nausea, vomiting, diarrhea, rectal bleeding, drowsiness, headache, weakness, skin rash, and anal pruritus. Piperazine's adverse effects comprise headache, EEG changes, vertigo, paresthesia, seizures, hives, erythema multiforme, bronchospasm, blurred vision, and cataracts. Pyrantel's adverse effects include headache, dizziness, insomnia, and skin rashes, but more common effects include anorexia, cramps, diarrhea, nausea, and vomiting.

Interactions

The concurrent use of pyrantel with piperazine is not recommended, and it should be used cautiously in patients with hepatic impairment.

Dosages

For dosage information for selected antihelmintic agents, see the dosages table on the next page.

DRUG PROFILES

The antihelmintics only come as oral preparations and are available only by prescription. The primary antihelmintic agents used to treat infections with intestinal nematodes (roundworms) are pyrantel and mebendazole; diethylcarbamazine is the primary agent used to treat nematode infection in tissue. Thiabendazole and piperazine are used as alternative agents because the indications for their use are limited. Mebendazole may be used to treat infection with either cestodes or nematodes, and as already mentioned, it is the only agent that can kill organisms in more than one class of helminths. The only other antihelmintic that may be used to treat cestode infection is niclosamide. Paromomycin and quinacrine are alternative agents, the former used in the treatment of either beef or pork tapeworm infection and the latter in the treatment of only infection with pork tapeworm.

DIETHYLCARBAMAZINE

Diethylcarbamazine (Hetrazan, Pec-Dec) is an antihelmintic agent indicated primarily for the treatment

of tissue infection with nematodes. It is contraindicated in patients with a known hypersensitivity to it, and its pregnancy safety has not been established. It is generally not recommended for use in pregnant women. It is available in orally administered 50- and 60-mg tablets. Commonly recommended dosages are listed in the dosages table on the next page.

PHARMACOKINETICS

HALF-LIFE	ONSET	PEAK	DURATION
8 hr	<1 hr	PO: 1-2 hr	Variable

⚕ MEBENDAZOLE

Mebendazole (Vermox) is a synthetic antihelmintic agent that may be used in the treatment of many types of nematode and a few types of cestode infection. It is classified as a pregnancy category C agent, but it should be used in pregnant women only when the potential benefits justify the possible risks to the fetus. It is contraindicated in patients hypersensitive to it and is only available in an oral formulation—a 100-mg chewable tablet. Commonly recommended dosages are listed in the dosages table on the next page.

PHARMACOKINETICS

HALF-LIFE	ONSET	PEAK	DURATION
6-12 hr	<2 hr	2-4 hr	Variable

NICLOSAMIDE

Niclosamide (Niclocide) is a synthetic antihelmintic agent that is structurally different from any of the other antihelmintics. It is primarily indicated for the treatment of infection with cestodes (beef, fish, and dwarf tapeworms). It is classified as a pregnancy category B agent and is contraindicated in patients with a known hypersensitivity to it. It is only available in an oral formulation—a 500-mg chewable tablet. Commonly recommended dosages are listed in the dosages table on the next page.

PHARMACOKINETICS

HALF-LIFE	ONSET	PEAK	DURATION
Unknown	Unknown	Unknown	Unknown

PYRANTEL

Pyrantel (Antiminth, Reese's Pinworm Medicine) is a pyrimidine-derived antihelmintic agent that is indicated for the treatment of infection with intestinal nematodes, such as ascariasis, enterobiasis, and other helminthic infections. It is classified as a pregnancy cat-

DOSAGES

SELECTED ANTIHELMINTIC AGENTS

AGENT	PHARMACOLOGIC CLASS	DOSAGE RANGE	PURPOSE
Diethylcarbamazine (Hetrazan)	General antihelmintic	*Pediatric* PO: 6-10 mg/kg tid for 7-10 days *Adult* PO: 13 mg/kg/day for 7 days 2 mg/kg tid pc for 3-4 wk	Roundworms Roundworms Bancroft's filariasis
⚓Mebendazole (Vermox)	Nematode antihelmintic	*Pediatric/Adult* PO: 100 mg once daily 100 mg in AM and PM for 3 days	Enterobiasis Hookworms, roundworms, whipworms
Niclosamide (Niclocide)	Cestode antihelmintic	*Pediatric* PO: 11-34 kg: 1 g as a single dose 1 g on day 1, then 0.5 g for next 6 days >34 kg: 1.5 g as a single dose 1.5 g on day 1, then 1 g for next 6 days *Adult* PO: 2 g as a single dose 2 g/day for 7 days	Beef, fish tapeworm Dwarf tapeworm Beef, fish tapeworm Dwarf tapeworm Beef, fish tapeworms Dwarf tapeworm
Pyrantel (Antiminth, Reese's Pinworm Medicine)	Nematode antihelmintic	*Pediatric/Adult* PO: 11 mg/kg as a single dose to maximum of 1 g	Enterobiasis, roundworms
Praziquantel (Biltricide)	Trematode antihelmintic	*Pediatric ≥4 y/o/Adult* PO: 60 mg/kg in 3 equally divided doses for 1 day 75 mg/kg in 3 equally divided doses for 1 day	Schistosomiasis Clonorchiasis, opisthorchiasis

egory C agent and is contraindicated in patients who are hypersensitive to it. It only comes in an oral formulation—a 250–mg/5 ml suspension. Commonly recommended dosages are listed in the dosages table above.

✖ PHARMACOKINETICS

HALF-LIFE	ONSET	PEAK	DURATION
Unknown	<1 hr	1-3 hr	Unknown

PRAZIQUANTEL

Praziquantel (Biltricide) is one of the primary antihelmintic agents used for the treatment of fluke (trematode) infections, specifically by schistosomiasis, opisthorchiasis, and clonorchiasis. It is classified as a pregnancy category B agent. It is contraindicated in patients who are hypersensitive to it and in lactating women. It only comes in an oral formulation as a 600-mg film-coated tablet. Commonly recommended dosages are listed in the dosages table above.

PHARMACOKINETICS

HALF-LIFE	ONSET	PEAK	DURATION
4-5 hr	<1 hr	1-2 hr	Variable

NURSING PROCESS

ASSESSMENT

Before administering an antimalarial agent to a patient, the nurse should take a thorough nursing and medication history and document the findings. Contraindications to assess for include pregnancy, porphyria, and G6PD deficiency as well as a history of drug allergy to these medications. Baseline vital signs should be checked and the malarial symptoms—fever, chills, profound sweating, headache, nausea, joint aching, and fatigue to exhaustion—assessed. Signs of malaria include periodic diaphoresis and a remittent fever as high as 104° to 105° F (40° to 40.5° C). Baseline visual status and electrocardiogram are also important to assess and the findings documented, as ordered.

It is important to assess patients who are to receive antiprotozoal agents for a history of hypersensitivity to the medications and for the presence of underlying renal, cardiac, thyroid, or liver disease. These and pregnancy are contraindications to the use of these agents. Patients' baseline visual acuity should also be determined and documented.

Before administering any antihelmintic agent, the nurse should assess patients for a history of hypersensitivity and pregnancy, because these are contraindications to the use of these agents. Patients' energy levels, activities of daily living, weight, appetite, and other symptoms should be assessed and documented as well.

NURSING DIAGNOSES

Nursing diagnoses applicable to patients receiving any of the antimalarials, antiprotozoals, or antihelmintics include:
■ Risk for self-injury related to medication side effects.
■ Risk for altered nutrition (less than body requirements) related to the disease process and side effects of medication.

■ Knowledge deficit concerning the infection and its treatment.
■ Risk for altered body image related to the disease process.
■ Risk for noncompliance with therapy related to the side effects of medication.

PLANNING

Goals for patients being treated with any of the antiparasitic medications include:
■ Patient will be free of self-injury related to the side effects of medication.
■ Patient will maintain normal body weight during drug therapy.
■ Patient will remain compliant with therapy for prescribed length of time.
■ Patient will experience minimal body image changes related to disease.
■ Patient will state side effects of medication as well as symptoms or adverse reactions to report to the physician.

Outcome Criteria

Outcome criteria for patients receiving any of the antiparasitic medications include:
■ Patient will state measures to take to minimize self-injury related to the side effects of medication such as dosing, time of day, and drug interactions.
■ Patient will list foods from the four food groups to be included in his or her diet to improve overall health.
■ Patient will state the symptoms of the infection such as fever, lethargy, loss of appetite.
■ Patients will understand the rationale for treatment for prescribed length of time.
■ Patient will state the symptoms to report to the physician such as worsening of infection, anorexia, fever.
■ Patient will verbalize feelings about altered body image openly with health care professional.
■ Patient will state importance of complying with therapy and returning for follow-up visits to the physician to monitor progress and for adverse reactions.

IMPLEMENTATION

Chloroquine and hydroxychloroquine are administered orally and should be given exactly as prescribed. At the start of the treatment for malaria the patient is given a loading dose, followed by half the dose on the next 2 days. In the prophylaxis of malaria, treatment with these agents is usually started 2 weeks before the person is exposed to the malarious areas and for 8 weeks after the person has left the area; the medication is taken once weekly on the same day of the week during this time span. Chloroquine can be given IM in the treatment of severe infection, or when the drug's absorption is questionable or nausea and vomiting are severe.

Some of these medications, such as thiabendazole, may give the urine an asparagus-like odor or the skin an unusual odor, so patients should be warned of these. Any syrup forms of these agents should be stored in tight and closed containers to prevent chemical changes from occurring in the medication. Quinine sulfate, an antiprotozoal, must be administered intact because it is very irritating to the GI mucosa.

See the box at right for patient teaching tips in patients receiving any of these antiprotozoal agents.

EVALUATION

The nurse should monitor the patient for the therapeutic effects of the antimalarials, antiprotozoals, and antihelmintic agents, such as the resolution of all symptoms. If prolonged therapy is necessary with antimalarials, CBC and urinalysis should be performed regularly and the patient observed for the signs and symptoms of hemolysis. An ECG may be desirable before and during treatment if the patient has or has had a cardiac disease. An eye examination should be done if the patient experiences visual disturbances. Side effects to watch for consist of visual changes, possible irreversible retinal damage, cardiac dysrhythmias, and thrombocytopenia. These antimalarial medications may precipitate hemolysis in patients with G6PD deficiency (mostly black patients and those of Mediterranean ancestry), so such patients should be closely monitored for its occurrence. With antiprotozoal agents, the patient should be monitored for visual disturbances, GI distress, blurred vision, and altered hearing.

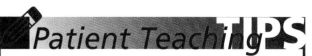

Patient Teaching **TIPS**

Antimalarials, Antiprotozoals, and Antihelmintics

Antimalarials

✔ Patients should take all the medication as prescribed and not stop the medication when they feel as though the symptoms have abated.

✔ The physician or other health care provider should be notified immediately if the patient experiences ringing (tinnitus) in the ears, a hearing decrease, or visual difficulties.

✔ GI upset can be decreased if oral forms are taken with food. The physician should be notified if nausea, vomiting, profuse diarrhea, or abdominal pain occur.

✔ This, and all medications, should be kept out of the reach of children.

✔ Quinidine products may cause dizziness, visual blurring, or yellow discoloration of the skin.

✔ Patients taking medication should exercise caution while driving because of the dizziness the agent can cause.

✔ Alert patients to the possible recurrence of the symptoms of malaria so that they will know to then seek immediate treatment.

Antiprotozoals

✔ Patients should be instructed to take the entire course of the medication and to report any side effects to the physician, such as the symptoms of cinchonism—visual disturbances, dizziness, headache, tinnitus, GI distress, blurred vision, and altered auditory acuity.

Antihelmintics

✔ These agents should be taken exactly as prescribed and the importance of compliance emphasized. Patients should also be encouraged to notify the physician immediately if they experience fatigue, fever, pallor, anorexia, darkened urine, and abdominal, leg, or back pain, which could indicate a sudden decrease in RBCs, the Hgb level, or WBCs.

TAKE HOME POINTS

Malaria

- Caused by a particular genus of protozoa = Plasmodium.
- Transmitted by the bite of an infected female mosquito.
- Must attack the parasite when it is inside the RBC (erythrocytic phase).
- Primaquine attacks the parasite when it is outside the RBC (exoerythrocytic phase).

Protozoal Infections

- Other common protozoal infections are amebiasis, giardiasis, pneumocytosis, toxoplasmosis, and trichomoniasis.
- The most toxic protozoal infections are those caused by *Cryptosporidium* spp., *Isospora belli, Pneumocystis carinii,* and *Toxoplasma gondii.*
- Protozoa are parasites that are transmitted by:
  1. Person-to-person contact
  2. Ingestion of contaminated water or food
  3. Direct contact with the parasite
  4. The bite of an insect (mosquito or tick)

Antiprotozoals

- Atovaquone and pentamidine are used to treat *P. carinii* infections.
- Metronidazole is an antibacterial, antiprotozoal, and antihelmintic.
- Iodoquinol and paromomycin directly kill protozoa such as *Entamoeba histolytica.*

Antihelmintics

- Drugs used to treat parasitic worm infections caused by:
  1. Cestodes (tapeworms)
  2. Nematodes (roundworms)
  3. Trematodes (flukes)
- Important to identify the causative worm—done by finding the parasite ova or larvae in feces, urine, blood, sputum, or tissue.
- Drugs may kill parasite directly or cause it to be expelled from the body.

Nursing Considerations

- Contraindications to the use of antimalarial agents include pregnancy, psoriasis, porphyria, G6PD deficiency, and a history of drug allergy.
- Baseline vital signs should be checked and documented.
- Contraindications to the use of the antiprotozoals include hypersensitivity; underlying renal, cardiac, thyroid, or liver disease; and pregnancy.
- Contraindications to the use of antihelmintics include a history of hypertension; hypersensitivity; visual difficulty; intestinal obstruction; inflammatory bowel disease; malaria; severe hepatic, renal, or cardiac disease; and pregnancy.

Critical Thinking **A C T I V I T I E S**

1. *Entamoeba histolytica* infection has been diagnosed in one of your migrant worker patients, a 25-year-old man. This parasitic protozoal infection of the large intestines is termed:
   a. toxoplasmosis.
   b. amebiasis.
   c. balantidiasis.
   d. giardiasis.

2. The antimalarial drugs are used to treat persons with infections caused by which genus and species of protozoa?
   a. *Candida albicans*
   b. *Mycobacterium tuberculosis*
   c. *Plasmodium* spp.
   d. *Pneumocystis carinii*

3. The antimalarial drug primaquine binds to and alters DNA during the _____ phase of the *Plasmodium* life cycle.
   1. exoerythrocytic   2. erythrocytic   3. first   4. second
   a. 1, 2, and 3   b. 2, 4, and 6   c. 1, 4, and 6   d. 4, 5, and 6

4. A 25-year-old man has *Pneumocytis carinii* pneumonia, for which he is taking a drug that is directly lethal to this protozoan. This drug inhibits DNA and RNA synthesis as well as glucose metabolism, protein synthesis, and intracellular amino acid transport. Which antiprotozoal is it?
   a. Iodoquinol
   b. Metronidazole
   c. Atovaquone
   d. Pentamidine

5. Antihelmintics are drugs that are used to treat infections caused by:
   1. mosquitoes.   2. tapeworms.   3. ticks.
   4. roundworms.   5. earthworms.   6. flukes.
   a. 1, 2, and 5   b. 2, 4, and 6   c. 1, 4, and 6   d. 4, 5, and 6

▲▲▲

BIBLIOGRAPHY

Albanese J, Nutz P: *Mosby's 1995 nursing drug cards,* St Louis, 1995, Mosby.

Johnson KB: *Harriet Lane handbook,* ed 13, St Louis, 1993, Mosby.

Keen JH: *Critical care and emergency drug reference,* St Louis, 1994, Mosby.

Knoben JE, Anderson PO: *Handbook of critical drug data,* ed 6, Hamilton, Ill, 1988, Drug Intelligence Publications.

Kuzma EC: Drug response: all bodies are not created equal, *Am J Nurs* 92 (12): 48, 1992.

McEvoy GK: *AHFS drug information,* Bethesda, Md, 1994, American Society of Hospital Pharmacists.

Skidmore-Roth L: *Mosby's 1995 nursing drug reference,* St Louis, 1995, Mosby.

United States Pharmacopeial Convention: Drug information for the health care professional, ed 14, Rockville, Md, 1995, United States Pharmacopeial Convention.

Chapter 41

Antiseptic and Disinfectant Agents

Objectives

When you reach the end of this chapter, you will be able to:

1 Identify the differences between disinfectants and antiseptics.
2 Identify the most commonly used and prescribed disinfectants and antiseptics.
3 Develop a comprehensive nursing care plan pertaining to the administration of disinfectants and antiseptics that includes patient education guidelines.

CHAPTER OUTLINE

Community-Acquired and Nosocomial Infections
Topical Antimicrobials
Mechanism of action
Drug effects
Therapeutic uses
Side effects and adverse effects
Interactions
Dosages
Drug Profiles
Acid Agents
Alcohol Agents
Aldehyde Agents
Biguanide Agents
Dyes
Chlorine Compounds
Mercurial Agents
Iodine Compounds
Oxidizing Agents
Phenolic Compounds
Surface-active Agents
Nursing Process
Assessment
Nursing Diagnoses
Planning
Outcome criteria
Implementation
Evaluation

Glossary

Acid (as' id) A compound that yields hydrogen ions when dissociated in solution. (p. 630)

Aldehyde (al' də hīd) Any of a large category of organic compounds derived from a corresponding alcohol by the removal of two hydrogen atoms, as in the conversion of ethyl alcohol to acetaldehyde. (p. 631)

Antiseptic (an' tĭ sep' tik) A substance that inhibits the growth and reproduction of microorganisms without necessarily killing them. (p. 627)

Benzyl (ben' zəl) Used as a topical antiseptic, keratolytic, antiseborrheic, and mild irritant to treat acne. (p. 633)

Community-acquired infection An infection acquired from the environment, including infections acquired indirectly through the use of medications. (p. 627)

Disinfectant (dis' in fek' tənt) A chemical applied to nonliving objects to destroy microorganisms. (p. 627)

Hexachlorophene (hek' sə klor' o fēn) A topical antiinfective and detergent. (p. 633)

Hydrogen peroxide (hi' dro jən pər ok sīd) A topical antiinfective. (p. 633)

Nosocomial infection (nos' o ko' me əl) An infection acquired at least 72 hours after hospitalization, often caused by *Candida albicans*, *Escherichia coli*, hepatitis viruses, herpes zoster virus, *Pseudomonas* organisms, or *Staphylococcus* spp.; also called *hospital-acquired infections.* (p. 627)

Resorcinol (rə sor' sĭ nol) An antiseptic used as a keratolytic agent in the treatment of dermatoses. It is also used in dyes and pharmaceuticals and as a chemical intermediate. (p. 633)

Topical antimicrobials (tap' ĭ kəl an' tĭ mi kro' be əl) A substance applied to any surface that either kills microorganisms or inhibits their growth or replication. (p. 627)

COMMUNITY-ACQUIRED AND NOSOCOMIAL INFECTIONS

Infectious organisms—bacteria, fungi, and viruses—can be acquired from a number of different sources: hospitals, the workplace, nursing homes, and home, to name just a few. These can, however, be categorized into two main sites of origin: the community and the hospital. **Community-acquired infections** are defined as those infections that are contracted either in the home or in the community. Hospital-acquired infections, more commonly known as **nosocomial infections,** are defined as those that are contracted in a hospital or institutional setting such as a nursing home and that were not present or incubating in the patient upon admission to the hospital. In other words, they are acquired during the hospital stay and from the hospital.

Of the two types of infections, nosocomial infections are much more difficult to treat, and there are several reasons for this. However, the primary reason is that, because, at least for the bacteria involved, these microorganisms have been exposed to many strong antibiotics in the past and those that are left alive in the hospital or institutional setting are then the most drug resistant and the most virulent. The particular organisms that cause these infections have changed over time, however, and these various pathogens and the reasons for their prevalence are summarized by the different time periods in Table 41-1.

Nosocomial infections develop in 5% to 10% of hospitalized patients, and the cost of treating them because of the extra hospitalization required amounts to nearly five billion dollars annually. Most of these infections (70% or more) consist of urinary tract infections and postoperative wound infections. Often they are acquired from various devices, such as mechanical ventilators, intravenous infusion lines, catheters, and dialysis equipment, to name just a few. Areas of the hospital where the risk of acquiring a nosocomial infection is particularly high are the critical care, dialysis, oncology, transplant, and burn units, and this is because the host defenses of the patients in these areas are typically compromised, making them more vulnerable to infection. It is therefore obvious from the foregoing discussion that it is important for the nurse to be aware of these infections and the methods used to reduce their incidence.

TOPICAL ANTIMICROBIALS

Topical antimicrobials are agents that can be used to reduce the risk of nosocomial infections. They are substances that are applied to any surface for the purpose of either inhibiting or killing as many microorganisms as possible in a given pathogen population. There are two categories of these agents—antiseptics and disinfectants. **Disinfectants** are able to kill organisms and are used only on nonliving objects to destroy organisms that may be present on them. They are sometimes called "cidal" agents. **Antiseptics** can primarily only inhibit the growth of microorganisms but not necessarily kill them and are applied exclusively to living tissue. They are also called "static" agents. Often the terms *disinfectant* and *antiseptic* are used interchangeably and their actions and uses confused. However, as just noted, not only are these agents not the same from the standpoint of their uses and actions but they can be very harmful if used for the same purposes. The differences between disinfectants and antiseptics in a clinical sense are summarized in Table 41-2. In chemical terms, some agents differ from disinfectants in their chemical makeup; others may simply be a diluted version of a disinfectant. Table 41-3 contains a listing of these agents classified according to their chemical structure.

Mechanism of Action

The mechanisms of action of the various antiseptics and disinfectants vary greatly. Some are strong ox-

Table 41-1	Changing Prevalence of Nosocomial Pathogens	
Period	**Cause for Change**	**Pathogen**
Before 1940	No antibiotics	Group A streptococci
Mid-1950s	Antibiotic era	Coagulase-positive *Staphylococcus aureus*
Today	New antibiotics	Gram-negative bacilli (*Pseudomonas* spp.), fungi or yeast (*Candida albicans*), herpes virus

Table 41-2	Antiseptics Versus Disinfectants	
	Antiseptics	**Disinfectants**
Where used	Living tissue	Nonliving tissue
Toxic	No	Yes
Potency	Less	More
Activity against organisms	Primarily inhibits growth (bacteriostatic)	Kills (bactericidal)

Table 41-3	Disinfectants and Antiseptics: Chemical Categories	
AGENTS	**ANTISEPTIC**	**DISINFECTANT**
Acids		
Acetic	X	X
Benzoic	X	
Boric	X	
Lactic	X	
Alcohols		
Ethanol	X	X
Isopropanol	X	X
Aldehydes		
Formaldehyde		X
Glutaraldehyde		X
Dyes		
Gentian violet	X	
Carbol-fuchsin	X	
Halogens		
Chlorine Compounds		
Sodium hypochlorite	X	X
Halazone		X
Iodine Compounds		
Iodine (tincture and solution)	X	X
Iodophors (povidone)	X	
Mercurials		
Merbromin	X	
Thimersol	X	
Yellow mercuric oxide	X	
Silver		
Silver nitrate	X	
Oxidizing agents		
Benzoyl peroxide	X	
Hydrogen peroxide	X	X
Potassium permanganate	X	
Phenolic compounds		
Cresol		X
Hexachlorophene	X	
Hexylresorcinol	X	
Resorcinol	X	
Surface-active agents		
Benzalkonium chloride	X	
Cetylpyridinium chloride	X	
Biguanides		
Chlorhexidine gluconate	X	
Nitrofurazone	X	

idizing or alkylating agents; others work by damaging microbial cell walls. The various mechanisms are discussed by drug class in the drug profiles, but for the purpose of clarity the mechanisms by which the various agents either kill or inhibit the growth of microorganisms are summarized in Table 41-4.

Drug Effects

The antimicrobial agents either inhibit the growth of microorganisms or destroy them, but the extent to which they do this depends on the number and type of microorganisms present, the concentration of the agent, the patient's temperature, and the time of exposure to the agent.

Therapeutic Uses

Living tissue such as skin and mucous membranes cannot be sterilized. However, the risk of infection can be minimized by reducing the numbers of microorganisms on such tissues. Antiseptics are applied to such living tissues to inhibit the growth of the microorganisms that typically reside there and that can do harm if they get into the body through an incision in the skin or by means of an injection. As a result these agents are contained, for example, in the presurgical scrubs (soaps) used by members of surgical teams to wash their hands in preparation for surgery. They are also applied to the patient's skin before the incision is made. The degerming action is only temporary, however, and limited to the surface. As mentioned in Chapter 36, systemic agents are sometimes administered to surgical patients as prophylaxis against infection caused by microorganisms living in the internal body environment. Besides these soaps and topical solutions, antiseptics are also contained in salves, ointments, mouthwashes, and douches.

Inanimate objects such as tabletops and surgical equipment may be treated with disinfectants as well as autoclaving, radiation, heat, and so on. Disinfectants are also used on instruments and other inanimate objects (fomites) that may harbor pathogens and are therefore a vehicle by which infectious organisms can be introduced into a new host. These instruments acquire these microbes by being placed or inserted into anatomic sites in patients where many organisms naturally dwell (e.g., thermometers, which are placed orally, rectally, or under the axilla, and proctoscopes, which are inserted into the lower GI tract to visualize the interior of the structure). Before their use in other patients, the bacteria, fungi, viruses, and spores must be removed from their surfaces to prevent their transmission to others.

The therapeutic effects of the antiseptics and disinfectants vary from class to class. Some agents are

Table 41-4	Antiseptics and Disinfectants: Mechanism of Action	
AGENT	**MECHANISM OF ACTION**	**COMMENTS**
Alcohols	Denature or essentially destroy the microorganism's protein; some may directly lyse the microorganism.	60% to 70% concentration, most effective; >95% or <60% concentration, ↓ bactericidal activity.
Halogens	Precipitate protein and oxidize essential enzymes by binding to and changing the structure of proteins.	Iodine compounds = bactericidal; mercurials = bacteriostatic; chlorine compounds = bactericidal.
Aldehydes	Act via alkylation, inhibiting the formation of the essential amino acid methionine.	Bacteriostatic or bactericidal depending on concentration.
Phenolic compounds	Interrupt bacterial electron transport (cellular respiration of microorganisms) and inhibit other membrane-bound enzymes; high concentrations rupture bacterial membranes.	Bacteriostatic or bactericidal depending on concentration.
Biguanides	Disrupt bacterial cytoplasmic membranes and inhibit membrane-bound ATPase (inhibit cell wall synthesis).	Chlorhexidine.
Surface-active agents	Denature or essentially destroy the microorganism's protein, cell membrane, and cytoplasm components.	↓ Concentrations = bacteriostatic; ↑ concentrations = bactericidal and fungicidal.
Oxidizing agents	Attack membrane lipids, DNA, and other essential components of the cell.	3% to 6% concentration = bactericidal and virucidal; 10% to 25% concentration = sporicidal.

Table 41-5	Antiseptics and Disinfectants: Therapeutic Effects				
	THERAPEUTIC EFFECTS				
AGENT	**BACTERIA**	**TUBERCLE**	**FUNGI**	**VIRUSES**	**SPORES**
Alcohols	X	X	X	X	
Iodine compounds	X	X	X	X	x
Mercurial compounds	x				
Chlorine compounds	X	X	x	X	
Aldehydes	X	X	X	X	X
Phenolic compounds	X	X	X	X	
Chlorhexidine	X		X		
Surface-active agents	X		X	x	
Oxidizing agents	X			X	x
Silver compounds	X				
Dyes	X				

X, "static" or "cidal" activity; x, some activity if high concentrations of agent and lengthy exposure.

very potent and are effective against many types of microorganisms. Others are less potent and have limited activity against only a few microorganisms. The range of microorganisms these agents are effective against is indicated for the various chemical classes of antimicrobial agents in Table 41-5.

Side Effects and Adverse Effects

Antiseptics and disinfectants are very safe agents, relatively speaking, and when used in the appropriate manner, they are very effective. Some of them are however, capable of causing some side effects and adverse effects, mostly comprising topical skin irritations. The others have no known adverse effects but at the very most may cause some skin irritation if used in exceedingly high concentrations. The agents and their side effects and adverse effects are summarized in Table 41-6.

Interactions

There are very few drugs that interact with the antiseptics, though other topical agents that also irritate the skin may produce an additive effect when given in combination with one of them. In addition, a topical agent that augments the systemic absorption of an antiseptic may increase the likelihood of systemic toxicity from these agents. However, because most of these agents are used for short periods, there is very little

Table 41-6	Antiseptic and Disinfectant Agents: Adverse Effects
BODY SYSTEM	**SIDE/ADVERSE EFFECTS**
Alcohols	
Integumentary	Excessive dryness of the skin.
Iodine compounds	
Integumentary	*Iodine* at concentrations >3% may produce skin blistering; burns may appear with *tincture of iodine* when the treated area is covered with an occlusive dressing; it may stain skin and cause irritation and pain at wound sites.
Aldehydes	
Integumentary	Burns to skin or mucous membranes.
Hexylresoreinol	
Hepatic	Toxicity resulting from systemic absorption from the skin.
Cardiovascular	Myocardial toxicity resulting from systemic absorption from the skin.
Integumentary	May produce burns on skin or mucous membranes.
Hexachlorophene	
CNS	Use as a preoperative scrub or as washes for neonates and burn patients has been stopped because absorption from the skin into systemic circulation has resulted in serious CNS toxicity.
Chlorhexidine gluconate	
Integumentary	Rarely causes dermatitis, photosensitivity, and irritation of mucosal tissue.
Surface-active agents	
Integumentary	Chemical burns if left in contact with skin for too long, as in wet packs or occlusive dressings.

opportunity for them to interact with other agents. Because disinfectants are not used for direct topical application to patients, there is of course no opportunity for drug interactions to occur.

Dosages

For information on the recommended dosages and concentrations for selected antimicrobial agents, see the dosages table on the following page.

DRUG PROFILES

Following are descriptions of the various chemical categories of antimicrobials.

ACID AGENTS

Acetic acid (vinegar), along with benzoic, boric, and lactic acid, are all members of the **acid** family of antiseptic and disinfectant agents. It is very commonly used because of its practicality, availability, and low cost. All these acid agents either kill microorganisms or inhibit their growth by creating an acidic environment for organisms that require a neutral or alkaline medium in order to live and grow.

Acetic acid in a 5% solution kills many organisms. In this concentration it is used as a vaginal douche for antisepsis and as a mild antiseptic-deodorant for the collection containers of indwelling urinary drainage catheters, for bladder irrigation, and for diaper soaks. The 1% solution may be used as a topical antiseptic for certain surgical wounds and burns. See the dosages table on the following page for dosage and concentration information.

ALCOHOL AGENTS

Isopropanol (isopropyl alcohol) and ethanol are both members of the alcohol category of antiseptics. The alcohol solutions are most effective at a concentration of 60% to 70%; at a concentration of more than 95% or less than 60% their "cidal" activity dramatically decreases. These agents kill microorganisms by either denaturing their proteins or directly lysing them. Both isopropyl and ethyl alcohol are able to kill bacteria, tubercle bacilli, fungi, and viruses. See the dosages table on the following page for the concentration information on isopropanol.

ALDEHYDE AGENTS

Formaldehyde and glutaraldehyde are members of the **aldehyde** category of agents. These disinfectants act by means of alkylation, inhibiting the formation of the es-

sential amino acid methionine. This either kills organisms or inhibits their growth, depending on the concentration of the solution.

The aldehydes, such as formaldehyde and glutar-

DOSAGES

SELECTED ANTISEPTIC AND DISINFECTANT AGENTS

AGENT	PHARMACOLOGIC CLASS	CONCENTRATION/DOSAGE RANGE	PURPOSE
Acetic acid (otic: Domeboro, Vosol Otic; irrigation solution)	Antibacterial, antifungal acid antimicrobial	Otic solution 2%; 4-6 gtt 3-4/day · Irrigation solution: 0.25%; 500-1500 ml/24 hr	Antibacterial, antifungal Bladder irrigation
Isopropanol (isopropyl alcohol)	General alcohol antiseptic/ disinfectant/ astringent	Solution: 70%	Skin astringent, cleansing agent, utensil disinfectant
Formaldehye	Broad-spectrum aldehyde antimicrobial	Solution: 37% Solution/spray: 1%	General disinfectant Skin-drying agent
Chlorhexidine gluconate (Hibiclens)	Broad-spectrum biguanide antimicrobial	Liquid: 4%	Cleanser, surgical scrub
Gentian violet (crystal violet)	Antibacterial/ antifungal dye	Solution: 1%, 2%; apply 1-2 times/day	Topical antiinfective
Sodium hypochlorite (Dakin's solution)	Broad-spectrum antimicrobial	Solution: 0.25%, 0.5%	Topical antiseptic
Thimerosal (Mersol)	Organomercurial antiseptic	Solution/spray/tincture: 1:1000; apply 1-3 times/ day	Topical antiseptic
Iodine	Broad-spectrum iodine antimicrobial	Solution/tincture: 2%, 5%, 7%; apply 1-2 times/day	Topical antiseptic
Povidone-iodine (Betadine)	Broad-spectrum iodine antimicrobial	Aerosol: 5%, solution: 10% Mouthwash: 0.5% Surgical scrub: 7.5%	Topical antiseptic Topical antiseptic
Hydrogen peroxide	Oxidizing agent	Solution 3%	Wound cleansing, antiseptic
Cresol	Phenolic disinfectant	Solution: 2%, 5%, 50%	Concurrent/terminal disinfectant
Carbolic acid (phenol; Chloroseptic)	Phenolic antiseptic	Spray: 0.5% Gargle: 1.4%	Oral antiseptic Local anesthetic
Benzalkonium chloride (Zephiran)	Broad-spectrum cationic detergent, surface-active antimicrobial	Solution concentrate: 17%; for preparing dilutions from 1:750 to 1:40,000 Tincture/spray: 1:750	Skin cleanser, antiseptic irrigation solution, instrument storage

aldehyde, are active against all types of microorganisms, including bacteria, tubercle bacilli, fungi, viruses, and spores. Because these agents are somewhat caustic, they can cause burns to the skin or mucous membranes if used as antiseptics. For this reason they are used mostly as disinfectants. Formaldehyde comes as formalin in a 37% concentration, and glutaraldehyde (Cidex) comes in a 2% solution. Both agents are commonly used as disinfectants for instruments. Cidex is used in particular to disinfect and sterilize surgical equipment. See the dosages table on the previous page for the concentration information for formaldehyde.

BIGUANIDE AGENTS

Chlorhexidine gluconate (Hibiclens) is a biguanide agent with antiseptic activity. Biguanides act by disrupting bacterial cytoplasmic membranes and inhibiting membrane-bound ATPase, which results in the inhibition of cell wall synthesis. Chlorhexidine is active against both gram-positive and gram-negative bacteria. It is used as a bactericidal skin cleansing solution and is useful as a surgical scrub, a hand-washing agent for health care personnel, and as a skin wound cleanser. It may also be used to treat aphthous ulcers of the mouth and for the prevention of dental caries. When used as directed, it causes few side effects. See the dosages table on the previous page for concentration information.

DYES

Gentian violet, crystal violet, methyl violet, brilliant green, and fuchsin are all rosaniline dyes. These are basic dyes that are currently used only occasionally as antiseptic or antiprotozoal agents. Gentian violet is typically used only topically as a 1% to 2% preparation, and it has both antibacterial and antifungal activity. See the dosages table on the previous page for dosage information.

CHLORINE COMPOUNDS

Chlorine compounds actively kill bacteria, tubercle bacilli, and viruses but are only partially active against fungi. They have no activity against spores. Sodium hypochlorite (Dakin's solution) is one of the chlorine compounds that is commonly used as a bleaching agent. Its antibacterial action is due to the hypochlorous acid, that forms when chlorine reacts with water. Hypochlorous acid is rapidly antibacterial.

Sodium hypochlorite in a 5% solution is commonly used to disinfect utensils, walls, furniture, floors, and swimming pools; in a 0.5% solution it is used on skin surfaces for the treatment of fungous infections such as athletes's foot. The strength of most household

bleach solutions is 5.25%. Intravenous drug users who frequently share needles and are at increased risk for acquiring HIV are being given small bottles of bleach to use as a disinfectant for their injection equipment and thus prevent the spread of the virus. See the dosages table on the previous page for dosage information.

Halazone is a chloramine compound. Chloramines are chlorine-related compounds but are more stable, less irritating, and slower and more prolonged in their action than their chlorine cousins. Halazone is the only chloramine product used in the United States. It is available in tablet form for sanitizing drinking water. Adding 1 or 2 tablets to a liter of water can kill all the pathogens usually found in water within 30 to 60 minutes.

MERCURIAL AGENTS

Topical mercurial antiseptics are relatively weak in their actions. They are primarily bacteriostatic agents whose effectiveness is enhanced by the vehicle in which they are contained. Inorganic mercury compounds such as ammoniated mercury ointment owe their effectiveness primarily to these vehicles, which sustain the bacteriostatic action of the agent. Organic mercurial agents such as thimerosal (Merthiolate) are more bacteriostatic, less irritating, and less toxic than the inorganic mercurials. Other examples of mercury compounds that are used as topical antiinfectives are merbromin, yellow mercuric oxide, and triclosan (Septisol).

The mercurial antiseptics probably act by inhibiting bacterial sulfhydryl enzymes, but they may also inhibit tissue enzymes as well, which reduces their usefulness. Ammoniated mercury is used for the treatment of psoriasis, impetigo, dermatomycoses, pediculosis pubis, seborrheic dermatitis, and superficial pyodermas. Skin irritations, as well as hypersensitivity to the agents, have been reported as side effects of these compounds. See the dosages table on the previous page for the dosage information for thimerosal.

IODINE COMPOUNDS

Iodine (tincture and solution) is a nonmetallic element that readily forms salts when combined with many other elements. Although it is a nonmetallic element, it has a bluish black, metallic luster and a characteristic odor. It is only slightly soluble in water but is completely soluble in alcohol and in aqueous solutions of sodium iodide and potassium iodide. Iodine tincture and solution are both active against and kill all forms of microorganisms—bacteria, tubercle bacilli, fungi, viruses, and spores. Their activity against spores depends on the concentration and the timing of admin-

Table 41-7	Iodine Formulations	
IODINE FORMULATION	**COMPOSITION**	**USES**
Aqueous solution	(5% Iodine and 10% potassium iodine)	These forms of iodine are used preoperatively to disinfect the skin. They are applied topically for their antimicrobial effects against bacteria, fungi, viruses, protozoa, and yeasts.
Iodine topical solution	2% Iodine	
Iodine tincture	2% Iodine in alcohol solution	
Strong iodine solution	5% Iodine in water	
	7% Iodine in alcohol	
Strong iodine tincture		
Povidone-iodine (Betadine, Operand, Pharmadine)	Iodine with polyvinylpyrrolidone	Used as a 10% applicator solution or as a 2% scrub, spray, foam, vaginal gel, ointment, mouthwash, perineal wash, or whirlpool concentrate.
Tincture of iodine	2% Iodine and 2.4% sodium iodide in 46% ethyl alcohol	For cutaneous infections caused by bacteria and fungi. Even a 1% tincture will kill almost an entire bacterial population in 1.5 min. Three drops in 1 quart (≈1 liter) of drinking water will reduce ameba and bacteria counts in 15 min without impairing palatability.
Iodophors (Betadine, Prepodyne)	Iodine compounds with a carrier that acts as a sustained-release pool of iodine.	Widely used as antiseptics.

istration. There are actually many forms of iodine, and some of these are listed in Table 41-7. See the dosages table on p. 631 for the recommended dosages and concentrations of a few of them.

OXIDIZING AGENTS

Hydrogen peroxide is one of three members of the oxidizing family of antiseptic agents, the other agents being benzoyl peroxide and potassium permanganate. The oxidizing agents work by attacking membrane lipids, DNA, and other essential components of the microorganism's cell. In concentrations of 3% to 6% they are bactericidal and virucidal; at 10% to 25% they are sporicidal.

Hydrogen peroxide is used as a 3% solution to irrigate suppurating wounds and some extensive traumatic wounds. It is used for wound cleansing, before Hickman catheter dressing changes, for the surgical repair of cleft lip, as an irrigation solution for use after some radical head and neck surgeries, for some oral lesions, and for oral cleansing (Peroxyl mouth rinse). **Benzyl** peroxides are used as a topical antiseptic, keratolytic, antiseborrheic, and mild irritant to treat acne.

PHENOLIC COMPOUNDS

Cresol, carbolic acid (phenol), and Lysol are all phenolic compounds that are used only as disinfectants. Because these agents cause burning and possibly blistering, they should not be allowed to come in contact with the skin in concentrations stronger than 2% and never in contact with areas where the skin is broken.

The phenolic compounds work by interrupting bacterial electron transport (cellular respiration of microorganisms) and inhibit other membrane-bound enzymes. At high concentrations they rupture bacterial membranes. Depending on the concentration of the phenolic compound they can be either "static" or "cidal" in their actions. The phenolic compounds are active against bacteria, tubercle, fungi, and viruses, but not spores. See the dosages table on p. 631 for concentration information on cresôl and carbolic acid.

Hexachlorophene and **resorcinol** are two other phenolic compounds. Hexachlorophene is available by prescription only and is used as a surgical scrub as well as a bacteriostatic skin cleanser. Resorcinol is bactericidal and fungicidal and is about a third as effective as carbolic acid. It is used to treat acne, ringworm, eczema, psoriasis, seborrheic dermatitis, and similar skin lesions.

SURFACE-ACTIVE AGENTS

Benzalkonium chloride (Zephiran) and cetylpyridinium chloride are surface-active agents. They work by denaturing the microorganism or essentially destroying its protein, cell membrane, and cytoplasm components. At low concentrations they are bacteriostatic and at high concentrations they are bactericidal and fungicidal. These agents are used to treat bacteria, fungi, and some viral topical infections.

Certain substances, when used in combination with surface-acting agents, will absorb the active ingredient and thereby weaken the surface-acting agent. Substances such as organic matter, soaps, anionic detergents, and tap water that contains metallic ions are a few examples. See the dosages table on p. 631 for concentration information on benzalkonium chloride.

*N*URSING *P*ROCESS

ASSESSMENT

When any type of topical medication such as an antiseptic is to be administered, the concentration of the medication, length of exposure to the skin, condition of the skin, size of area affected, and hydration status of the skin must be taken into consideration because they have a significant impact on the action of the medication. Before applying any topical medication, it is important for the nurse to find out whether the patient has any drug allergies or has shown any previous sensitivity to antiseptics or other topical agents. If an iodine-based agent such as povidone-iodine is being applied, the nurse should question the patient about allergies to iodine or seafood, because these are contraindications to its use. Patients being treated with peroxide agents should be asked about previous allergies and local reactions to the medication.

The risk of reactions to the antibacterial topical agents is greater because of the sensitivity of patients to antibiotics in different dosage forms. Should a patient have an allergy to a particular type of antibacterial agent, that specific agent should not be used topically, regardless of the dosage form. If a culture and sensitivity test has been ordered, the results should be known before the first application of the antibacterial agent.

NURSING DIAGNOSES

Nursing diagnoses appropriate to the use of antiseptics include:

■ Risk for infection related to compromised skin integrity.
■ Risk for infection related to skin trauma or injury resulting from adverse reactions to the topical agent.
■ Knowledge deficit concerning topical agents and their proper use.

PLANNING

Goals related to the administration of antiseptics include:

■ Patient will remain free of adverse reactions to the agent when used for the treatment of skin injury or infection.
■ Patient will show evidence of resolution of infection.
■ Patient will be compliant with the medication regimen.
■ Patient will experience minimal to no adverse reactions to medication.
■ Patient will return for follow-up visits with physician.

Outcome Criteria

Outcome criteria in patients treated with antiseptics include:

■ Patient will experience minimal discomfort (such as stinging, itching, burning) resulting from the use of the agent in the treatment of a skin injury or infection.
■ Patient will experience maximal therapeutic effects of medication once therapy complete with resolution of symptoms, such as intact skin, no redness, or no drainage.
■ Patient will demonstrate proper technique for applying topical antiseptic with applicator, tongue blade, gloved hand, and proper handwashing technique.
■ Patient will state those situations—adverse reactions to medication or worsening of symptoms of infection—when the physician should be notified of immediately.

IMPLEMENTATION

Before applying any topical agent, the nurse should check the physician's order to make sure he or she knows exactly what is required, gather the needed supplies, and wash his or her hands. Universal precautions should be followed when giving nursing care

Patient Teaching TIPS

Antiseptics Administration

✔ Patients should be instructed to wash their hands before and after applying any topical medication. This is important in preventing the spread of infection and the gross contamination of a wound.

✔ Patients should learn how to properly apply the medication, dressings, and bandage and how to change any dressings so that they can do these things at home after discharge. The instructions the nurse has given and the patients' caretaker's ability to carry them out should also be documented. The patient should also be given written instructions, pamphlets, and other aids that help to clarify the procedure and reinforce the importance of doing them correctly.

✔ Make sure patients have all the supplies needed at home to apply the medication, such as tape, gauze dressings and pads, tongue blades, cotton-tipped applicators, and gloves.

✔ Patients should be told to follow the physician's orders regarding the application and use of the topical medication. They should know to apply lotions gently but firmly by tapping the skin surface area. Lotions need to be shaken well before use. A tongue blade or cotton-tipped applicator may be used to apply creams or ointments. Patients should be encouraged to wash their hands before and after applying the medication and to note any unusual color of the skin, odor, or drainage.

TAKE HOME POINTS

Topical Antimicrobials
- Used to reduce risk of nosocomial infections.
- Applied to topical surfaces to inhibit or kill as many microorganisms as possible.
- Consist of antiseptics and disinfectants.

Disinfectants
- Antimicrobials that are used only on non-living objects
- Kill any organisms on these objects.
- They are not the same as antiseptics.

Antiseptics
- Antimicrobials that are used only on living tissues.
- Primarily only inhibit growth and reproduction of microorganisms.

Categories of Antiseptics and Disinfectants
- Categorized by their chemical makeup.
- Alcohols, halogens, aldehydes, phenolic compounds, biguanides, surface-active agents, acid agents, dyes, oxidizing agents, and nitrofurazone.

Nursing Considerations
- The nurse should always observe universal precautions whenever applying topical agents.
- Always apply agent to clean, dry skin unless otherwise ordered or specified.
- Instruct patients concerning the proper application technique before their discharge home.

that entails direct contact with a patient or possible exposure situations. If the skin is intact and it is not otherwise indicated, the nurse should wear nonsterile gloves, but if the skin is not intact or the nurse judges it appropriate, sterile gloves and technique should be used. Often there are specific directions regarding the application of the agent; for example, the order may specify that the agent be applied with a tongue depressor or that an occlusive dressing be placed. The nurse should follow these directions as well. As with any procedure the nurse should *always* ensure the patient's privacy and comfort. The skin site should be thoroughly cleansed and any other specific directions, such as removing water or alcohol-based topicals with soap and water or normal saline, should be followed. In general, before applying additional doses of a topical medication, the site should be cleansed not only of any debris but of any residual medication.

When using lotions, the nurse should store it un-

der the conditions recommended by the manufacturer and shake it well before using. Creams and ointments are often applied with a sterile cotton-tipped applicator or tongue blade. Any dressings should be applied as ordered and special attention paid to the directions for the application of occlusive, wet, or wet-to-dry dressings. Patient education about the medication and dressings is important to the safe and effective use of these agents (see the box above left). The nurse should make sure to document the site of application and any drainage from the site, whether there is any swelling, the temperature and color of the site, and any painful or other sensations that may occur.

After the medication has been administered, the nurse should wash his or her hands, dispose of contaminated dressings, record the nature of the procedure and findings, and maintain asepsis (surgical asepsis if the wound is open in any way or if the skin is not intact). The nurse should always make sure that the patient is in no danger of causing harm to the site.

EVALUATION

When using antiseptics, the patient's therapeutic response may be manifested by improved healing of affected area, decreased symptoms of inflammation or infection, or even prevention of infection for which the agent was ordered, such as preoperatively. In addition, when using these agents on inanimate objects, be sure to constantly monitor for patient safety from exposure to the agent. It is also important to evaluate patients for any side effects or adverse reactions (see Table 41-6).

Critical Thinking **A C T I V I T I E S**

1. Which of the following statements about the dermal layer of the skin is correct? It:
   a. forms a protective covering for the body.
   b. is the site of the formation of keratin.
   c. provides the skin with support because of the blood vessels it contains.
   d. is the site of the germination of blood cells.
2. What is the main purpose of using antiseptics and disinfectants?
3. Can disinfectants and antiseptics be used interchangeably? Why or why not?

BIBLIOGRAPHY

Albanese J, Nutz P: *Mosby's 1995 nursing drug cards,* St Louis, 1995, Mosby.

Johnson KB: *Harriet Lane handbook,* ed 13, St Louis, 1993, Mosby.

Keen JH: *Critical care and emergency drug reference,* St Louis, 1994, Mosby.

Knoben JE, Anderson PO: *Handbook of critical drug data,* ed 6, Hamilton, Ill, 1988, Drug Intelligence Publications.

McEvoy GK: *AHFS drug information,* Bethesda, Md, 1994, American Society of Hospital Pharmacists.

Skidmore-Roth L: *Mosby's 1995 nursing drug reference,* St Louis, 1995, Mosby.

Thibodeau GA, Patton KT: *Anatomy and physiology,* ed 2, St Louis, 1993, Mosby.

Chapter 42

The NSAIDs (Nonsteroidal Antiinflammatory Drugs)

Objectives

When you reach the end of this chapter, you will be able to:

1 Discuss the inflammatory response and the part it plays in the generation of pain.

2 Describe how NSAIDs basically work to decrease pain.

3 List the various NSAIDs.

4 Discuss the mechanism of action, indications, side effects, dosage ranges, cautions, contraindications, and drug interactions associated with the use of NSAIDs.

5 Develop a comprehensive nursing care plan that includes the nursing process and education for the patient receiving an NSAID.

6 Discuss nonpharmacologic approaches to the management of pain.

CHAPTER OUTLINE

The Arachidonic Acid Pathway
The NSAIDs
 Mechanism of action
 Drug effects
 Therapeutic uses
 Side effects and adverse effects
  Toxicity and management of overdose
 Interactions
 Dosages
Drug Profiles
Carboxylic Acids
 ⚓ Aspirin
Acetic Acids
 ⚓ Indomethacin
Propionic Acids
 ⚓ Ibuprofen
  Ketorolac
Enolic Acids, Fenamic Acids, and the Nonacidic
 Compounds
Miscellaneous Agents
 Antigout agents
  ⚓ Allopurinol
  Colchicine
  Probenecid
  Sulfinpyrazone
 Gold compounds
  Auranofin
  Aurothioglucose and Gold Sodium Thiomalate

Analgesic and antipyretic agents
 ⚓ Acetaminophen
Nursing Process
Assessment
Nursing Diagnoses
Planning
 Outcome criteria
Implementation
Evaluation

Glossary

Acute salicylate overdose (sal′ ĭ sil′ āt) Produces signs and symptoms similar to those of chronic intoxication but the effects are often more pronounced and occur more quickly. (p. 642)

Chronic salicylate intoxication A toxic condition caused by the ingestion of salicylate, most often in aspirin or oil of wintergreen. (p. 642)

Done nomogram (nom′ o gram) A graph on which a number of variables are plotted so that the value of a dependent variable can be read on the appropriate line when the values of the other variables are given. (p. 642)

Misoprostol (mi so pros′ tol) Used in the prevention of gastric ulcers in patients receiving NSAIDs. (p. 641)

Nonsteroidal antiinflammatory drugs A large and chemically diverse group of drugs that possess analgesic, antiinflammatory, and antipyretic activity. (p. 638)

Salicylism (sal′ ĭ sil′ iz əm) A syndrome of salicylate toxicity. (p. 642)

The **nonsteroidal antiinflammatory drugs** (NSAIDs) are among the most frequently prescribed drugs: every year approximately 70 million prescriptions are written for these agents. This represents over 5% of all prescriptions. There are now more than 23 different NSAIDs commonly used, plus many more that have limited use. The NSAIDs comprise a large and chemically diverse group of drugs that possess analgesic, antiinflammatory, and antipyretic activity. They are also used for the relief of mild to moderate headaches, myalgia, neuralgia, and arthralgia; for the alleviation of postoperative pain; for the inhibition of platelet aggregation; for the relief of the pain associated with arthritic disorders such as rheumatoid arthritis, juvenile arthritis, ankylosing spondylitis, and osteoarthritis; and for the treatment of gout and hyperuricemia. The list of uses for these versatile drugs is as lengthy as the list of agents.

The use of plants containing salicylates as medicinal agents goes back more than a thousand years. North American Indians used willow bark juice as an antipyretic, and South African Hottentots used a similar mixture as an antirheumatic. Willow and poplar were used as sources of medicinal compounds by both Greek and Roman physicians. Such notable physicians as Hippocrates, Pliny the Elder, and Celsus all chronicled the beneficial effects of these salicylate-containing agents in the treatment of such diverse ailments as gout, fever, sciatica, and earache.

The most common and very first drug in this class was salicylic acid, and it was Hermann Kolbe who devised an economical procedure for the manufacture of a synthetic form of salicylic acid, which made its mass production, and hence availability, possible. Subsequently, in 1899, the most famous descendent of salicylic acid, acetylsalicylic acid (ASA; aspirin), was marketed, and it rapidly became the most widely used drug in the world. The success of aspirin established the importance of drugs with antipyretic, analgesic, antiinflammatory, and antirheumatic properties—the properties that all the NSAIDs share. However, along with aspirin's widespread use came evidence of its potential for causing major toxicologic effects. Gastrointestinal intolerance, bleeding, and renal impairment became major factors limiting its long-term administration. As a result, efforts were mounted to develop agents that did not have the side effects of aspirin, and this led to the discovery of other NSAIDs, which in general are associated with a lower incidence of and less serious toxicities and are also better tolerated than aspirin in patients with chronic diseases.

Before getting into the in-depth discussion of these agents, however, it is first important to explain the arachidonic acid pathway and how it functions because the analgesic and antiinflammatory activity of the

NSAIDs is thought to result primarily from the inhibition of this pathway.

THE ARACHIDONIC ACID PATHWAY

When arachidonic acid is released from phospholipids in cell membranes in response to a triggering event (e.g., an injury), it is metabolized by either the prostaglandin pathway or the leukotriene pathway, both of which are "branches" of the arachidonic acid pathway, as shown in Fig. 42-1. Both of these pathways result in inflammation and pain.

In the prostaglandin pathway the arachidonic acid is converted by cyclooxygenase into various prostaglandins such as prostacyclin (prostaglandin I_2) as well as into thromboxane A_2 (TXA_2). The prostaglandins indirectly mediate and perpetuate inflammation by inducing vasodilation as well as enhance vasopermea-

---

NSAIDs and Their Structural Groups

Acetic Acids

Diclofenac sodium	(Voltaren)
Diclofenac potassium	(Cataflam)
Etodolac	(Lodine)
⬇Indomethacin	(Indocin)
Sulindac	(Clinoril)
Tolmetin	(Tolectin)

Carboxylic Acids
Acetylated

⬇Aspirin	(many)
Choline magnesium trisalicylate	(Trilisate)
Diflunisal	(Dolobid)

Nonacetylated

Salicylamide	(many)
Salsalate	(Disalcid)
Sodium salicylate	(many)

Propionic Acids

Fenoprofen	(Nalfon)
Flurbiprofen	(Ansaid)
⬇Ibuprofen	(Motrin, others)
Ketoprofen	(Orudis)
Ketorolac	(Toradol)
Naproxen	(Naprosyn)
Oxaprozin	(DayPro)

Enolic Acids

Phenybutazone	(Butazolidin)
Piroxicam	(Feldene)

Fenamic Acids

Meclofenamic Acid	(Meclomen)
Mefenamic Acid	(Ponstel)

Nonacidic Compounds

Nabumetone	(Relafen)

▼ FIG. 42-1 Arachidonic acid pathway.

bility. These effects in turn potentiate the action of proinflammatory substances, such as histamine and bradykinin, in the production of edema and pain. The leukotriene pathway utilizes lipoxygenases to metabolize the arachidonic acid and convert it into various leukotrienes. Although the actions of these compounds have not been characterized as well as those of the prostaglandins, they also appear to be mediators of inflammation. Some leukotrienes promote vasoconstriction, bronchospasms, and vascular permeability.

Pain, headache, fever, and inflammation are all the final consequences (symptoms) of the activation of the arachidonic acid pathway.

It has been shown that prostaglandins produce headache and pain because, when these substances are injected into test subjects, these are the symptoms that appear. They accomplish this by producing a hyperalgesia state in which the person's nerve endings are sensitized to painful stimuli. Consequently what may not have been a painful stimulus becomes one.

Fever results when prostaglandin E_2 is synthesized in the preoptic hypothalamic region, that area of the brain that regulates temperature.

The inflammatory response is mediated by a host of endogenous compounds, including proteins of the complement system, histamine, serotonin, brady-

kinin, leukotrienes, and prostaglandins, the latter two being major contributors to the symptoms of inflammation.

THE NSAIDs

As a single class of agents the NSAIDs constitute an exceptional variety of drugs, and they are used for an equally wide range of indications. Although as many as seventy agents are on the market and new agents are constantly becoming available, they can all be placed into one of six structurally and historically related groups, and these various agents are listed in the box on p. 638 according to the structural group to which they belong. The carboxylic acid agents are more commonly called *salicylates* and, as already noted, were the first nonsteroidal antiinflammatory agents to be isolated and used therapeutically. They may or may not be included in the NSAID category, however, depending on the particular reference. In this chapter they *are* included because their chemical and physiologic effects are so similar to those of the agents strictly considered NSAIDs.

Currently, at least one NSAID has been approved for each of the therapeutic indications listed in the box on p. 640, and an NSAID is considered the drug of

---

NSAIDs: Indications

FDA-Approved Indications
Acute gout
Acute gouty arthritis
Acute painful shoulder
Ankylosing spondylitis
Bursitis
Fever
Mild to moderate pain
Osteoarthritis
Primary dysmenorrhea
Rheumatoid arthritis
Juvenile rheumatoid arthritis
Tendinitis

Non–FDA-Approved Indications
Pericarditis
Periodontal disease
Glomerulonephritis
Nephrotic syndrome
Sunscreening
Symptomatic treatment of sunburn
Prophylaxis of migraine headache
Premature labor
Various ophthalmic uses

---

choice for the treatment of most of these conditions. This list of indications will continue to grow as more is learned about the mechanisms by which pain and inflammation are modified. Almost all NSAIDs are used for the treatment of rheumatoid arthritis and degenerative joint disease.

Mechanism of Action

NSAIDs relieve *pain and headache* by blocking the undesirable effects of prostaglandins. Specifically, aspirin and the other agents inhibit the enzyme cyclooxygenase and thereby prevent the formation of prostaglandins (see Fig. 42-1). This differs from the opioids, which relieve pain by interfering with its recognition in the brain.

NSAIDs reduce *fever* by inhibiting prostaglandin E_2, specifically by inhibiting its biosynthesis within the preoptic hypothalamic region, which regulates body temperature.

NSAIDs relieve *inflammation* by inhibiting the leukotriene pathway, the prostaglandin pathway, or both. The lipoxygenase (leukotriene) pathway is inhibited by some antiarthritic agents but not by salicylates. Several antiinflammatory drugs block the prostaglandin pathway as well as the leukotriene pathway, while others only weakly inhibit cyclooxygenase but primarily inhibit the lipoxygenases.

Drug Effects

The drug effects of the NSAIDs are wide and varied. There are numerous actions of the drugs within this class. The main drug effects of the NSAIDs are those of analgesic, antiinflammatory, and antipyretic effects. Some of the agents in this class of drugs may have all these effects as well as a few others, such as inhibiting platelet aggregation. Although agents may only affect inflammation and pain, the NSAIDs are used principally in the symptomatic treatment of mild to moderate pain, fever, inflammatory diseases, and rheumatic fever.

Therapeutic Uses

The therapeutic effects of the nonsteroidal antiinflammatory drugs chiefly stem from their ability to inhibit the arachidonic acid pathway, thus preventing the release of some of the harmful products of this pathway (i.e., prostaglandins and leukotrienes). Some of the more noted therapeutic uses of this broad class of agents are listed in the box at left, but they are primarily used for their analgesic, antigout, antiinflammatory, and antipyretic effects; for the relief of vascular headaches; and for platelet inhibition.

The NSAIDs are most commonly used for the treatment of rheumatoid arthritis and osteoarthritis, as well as other inflammatory conditions. In this regard, these agents have proved to be highly effective while at the same time do not adversely affect preexisting conditions. They have also proved to be extremely beneficial as adjunctive pain relief medications in patients with chronic syndromes. For the relief of pain they are sometimes combined with an opioid narcotic. This can provide pain relief mediated by a mechanism of action different from that of the narcotics. They also do not cause many of the undesirable effects of the narcotics, mainly respiratory depression. However, unlike the narcotics their effectiveness is limited by a ceiling effect, in that any further increase in the dose beyond a certain level increases the risk of adverse effects without a corresponding increase in the therapeutic effect.

The salicylates have further beneficial properties that most of the NSAIDs do not in that they have potent effects on both the aggregation properties of platelets and the thermoregulatory center in the brain. For this reason they are more commonly used for the treatment of various types of fevers as well as arterial and, possibly, venous thrombosis. Other NSAIDs, such as phenybutazone, are commonly used in the treatment of gout, which is caused by the overproduction of uric acid or decreased uric acid secretion, or by both processes. This can often result in hyperuricemia (too much uric acid in the blood), a condition that causes

NSAIDs Suggested for Patients with Particular Medical Conditions	
MEDICAL CONDITION	**RECOMMENDED NSAID**
Risk for nephrotoxicity	Sulindac, nonacetylated salicylate, nabumetone, etodolac, diclofenac, oxaprozin
Hypertension	Sulindac, nonacetylated salicylate, ibuprofen, etodolac
Hepatotoxicity	Tolmetin, naproxen, ibuprofen, piroxicam, the fenamates
Diabetic neuropathy	Sulindac
Dysmenorrhea	Fenamates, naproxen, naproxen sodium
Headaches	Naproxen, naproxen sodium, ketorolac
Warfarin therapy	Sulindac, tolmetin, naproxen, ibuprofen, oxaprozin
History of aspirin or NSAID allergy	Avoid if possible; if not, consider nonacetylated salicylate
Risk for gastrointestinal toxicity	Nonacetylated salicylate, enteric-coated aspirin, diclofenac, nabumetone, etodolac, ibuprofen, oxaprozin
Gout	Indomethacin, naproxen, naproxen sodium, sulindac
Ankylosing spondylitis	Indomethacin, diclofenac
Osteoarthritis	Acetaminophen, diclofenac, oxaprozin, indomethacin

joint pain as a result of the deposition of needlelike crystals of urate precipitate in tissues and the joints.

The appropriate selection of an NSAID calls for a consideration of the patient's history, including any prior medical conditions; the intended use of the agent; the patient's previous experience with NSAIDs; the patient's preference; and the cost. The NSAIDs of choice recommended for use in patients with certain underlying medical conditions are listed in the box above.

Side Effects and Adverse Effects

One of the more common complaints and potentially serious adverse effects of the NSAIDs is gastrointestinal distress. This can range from mild symptoms such as heartburn to the most severe gastrointestinal complication—GI bleeding. In fact, the adverse effects of salicylates mainly involve the GI tract and, besides bleeding, include symptomatic GI disturbances and mucosal lesions (e.g., erosive gastritis, gastric ulcer). These problems apparently are more frequently associated with aspirin use than with the use of other NSAIDs. The potential adverse effects of NSAIDs listed in Table 42-1 do not apply to all agents, but they do apply to many of them.

Many of the side effects and adverse effects of the NSAIDs are secondary to their inactivation of protective prostaglandins that help to maintain the normal integrity of the stomach lining. When the formation of these beneficial prostaglandins is inhibited, as occurs with NSAIDs, this protective barrier is eliminated. This sets up a perfect environment for ulceration and GI bleeding. To further complicate matters, because NSAIDs prolong bleeding times by inhibiting TXA_2 production, this can exacerbate GI bleeding. However,

Table 42-1	NSAIDs: Side Effects and Adverse Effects
BODY SYSTEM	**SIDE/ADVERSE EFFECT**
Gastrointestinal	Most frequent: dyspepsia, heartburn, epigastric distress, nausea Less frequent: vomiting, anorexia, abdominal pain, GI bleeding, mucosal lesions (erosions or ulcerations)
Renal	Reduction in creatinine clearance, acute tubular necrosis with renal failure
Hepatic	Acute reversible hepatotoxicity
Cardiovascular	Moderate to severe noncardiogenic pulmonary edema
Hematologic	Altered hemostasis through effects on platelet function
Other	Skin eruption, sensitivity reactions, tinnitus, hearing loss

an agent called **misoprostol** (Cytotec) has proved successful in preventing the gastric ulcers and hence GI bleeding that can occur in patients receiving NSAIDs. It is a synthetic prostaglandin E_1 analogue that potently inhibits gastric acid secretion, which it does by directly inhibiting the function of parietal cells. It also has a cytoprotective component, though the mechanism responsible for this action is unclear. It may prevent disruption of the gastric mucosal barrier, stimulate mucous secretion, stimulate alkaline (bicarbonate) secretion, or enhance mucosal blood flow.

The kidneys are also dependent to some extent on prostaglandins, especially in the patient who is already renally compromised, because these organs rely on the prostaglandins produced by them for stimulating vasoconstriction and increased renal blood flow. If NSAIDs inhibit this compensatory mechanism, this may be enough to precipitate acute or chronic renal failure, depending on the patient's prior renal function.

Toxicity and Management of Overdose

There are both chronic and acute manifestations of salicylate toxicity. Chronic salicylate intoxication is known as **salicylism** and results from either high doses or prolonged therapy with high doses. The most common signs and symptoms of **chronic salicylate intoxication** are listed in Table 42-2.

The most frequent manifestations of chronic intoxication in adults are tinnitus and hearing loss. Those in children are hyperventilation and CNS effects such as giddiness, drowsiness, and behavioral changes. These effects usually arise when serum salicylate concentrations exceed 300 µg/ml. Metabolic complications such as metabolic acidosis and respiratory alkalosis are usually present in the setting of chronic intoxication. Metabolic acidosis can also occur in the setting of acute intoxication, but is usually less severe than that in patients with chronic intoxication. Hypoglycemia is also likely to occur and can be life-threatening.

The treatment of chronic intoxication is based on the presenting symptoms. Serum salicylate concentrations may be determined but are not as useful in estimating the severity, as severe intoxication can occur with a concentration as low as 150 µg per ml. The suggested treatment for chronic salicylate intoxication is summarized in the box, below right.

The signs and symptoms of **acute salicylate overdose** are similar to those of chronic intoxication, but the effects are often more pronounced and occur more quickly. It results from the ingestion of a single toxic dose, and its severity can be estimated based on the estimated amount (in milligrams per kilogram of body weight) ingested, as follows:

Little or no toxicity: <150 mg/kg
Mild to moderate toxicity: 150-300 mg/kg
Severe toxicity: 300-500 mg/kg
Life-threatening: >500 mg/kg

A serum salicylate concentration measured 6 hours or more after the ingestion may be used in conjunction with the **Done nomogram** to estimate the severity of intoxication and help guide treatment. (This is a graph on which a number of variables are plotted so that the value of a dependent variable can be read on the appropriate line when the other variables are given.) This nomogram is only intended for gauging the severity of acute intoxications, however, and not that of chronic salicylate intoxication.

The pathophysiologic mechanism of salicylate overdose is complex because of the variety of toxic effects produced by salicylates, although the principal ones are extensions of the agents' pharmacologic actions. These are:

- Local GI tract irritation
- Direct CNS stimulation of respiration
- Altered glucose metabolism (stimulation of gluconeogenesis and lipid metabolism)
- Increased tissue glycolysis
- Interference with hemostatic mechanisms

The treatment of acute toxicity stemming from a salicylate overdose involves intensive symptomatic and supportive therapy. The treatment goals should consist of removing salicylate from the GI tract and

Table 42-2	Chronic Salicylate Intoxication: Signs and Symptoms
BODY SYSTEM	**SIGNS AND SYMPTOMS**
CNS	Tinnitus, hearing loss, dimness of vision, headache, dizziness, mental confusion, lassitude, drowsiness
Metabolic	Sweating, thirst, hyperventilation
Gastrointestinal	Nausea, vomiting, diarrhea
Cardiovascular	Increased heart rate

Chronic Salicylate Intoxication: Treatment

SEVERITY	TREATMENT
Mild	1. Dosage reduction or discontinuation or salicylates. 2. Symptomatic and supportive therapy.
Severe	1. Discontinuation of salicylates. 2. Intensive symptomatic and supportive therapy. 3. Dialysis if: high salicylate levels, unresponsive acidosis (pH <7.1), impaired renal function or renal failure, pulmonary edema, persistent CNS symptoms (e.g., seizures, coma), progressive deterioration despite appropriate therapy.

preventing its further absorption; correcting fluid, electrolyte, and acid-base disturbances; and implementing measures to enhance salicylate elimination. The measures to be taken to achieve these treatment goals are listed in the box below.

An acute overdose of NSAIDs causes effects similar to those of salicylate overdose, but they are generally not as extensive. The symptoms comprise central nervous system toxicities such as drowsiness, lethargy, mental confusion, paresthesias, numbness, aggressive behavior, disorientation, and seizures and gastrointestinal toxicities such as nausea, vomiting, and GI bleeding. Intense headache, dizziness, cerebral edema, cardiac arrest, and death have also been known to occur in extreme cases. Treatment should consist of the immediate removal of the ingested agent by inducing emesis with either syrup of ipecac or gastric lavage. This should be followed by the administration of activated charcoal, with supportive and symptomatic treatment initiated thereafter. Hemodialysis appears to be of no value in enhancing the elimination of NSAIDS.

Interactions

The drug interactions associated with the use of salicylates and other NSAIDs can result in significant complications and morbidity. Some of the more common of these are listed in Table 42-3.

These agents can also interfere with laboratory test results. Specifically, the salicylates can cause the serum levels of ALT, AST, and alkaline phosphatase to be increased. The hematocrit values, the hemoglobin levels, and the red blood cell counts can all be decreased in patients suffering from GI bleeding stemming from the use of salicylates or other NSAIDs. NSAID use can also cause the serum levels of potassium to be elevated and the serum levels of sodium to be lowered.

Dosages

For the recommended dosages of various NSAIDs, see the dosages table on the next page.

DRUG PROFILES

CARBOXYLIC ACIDS

The salicylates are classified as carboxylic acids and can be either acetylated (aspirin, magnesium choline salicylate, and diflunisal) or nonacetylated (salicylamide, salsalate, and sodium salicylate). Although aspirin is the most commonly used of all these agents, the others have many of the same beneficial effects as aspirin. Most salicylates are available OTC,

---

Chronic Salicylate Intoxication: Treatment Goals

TREATMENT GOAL	MEASURE
Reduce salicylate absorption	Syrup of ipecac (if patient is alert and awake). Gastric lavage.* Activated charcoal.
Treat fluid and electrolyte imbalance	Appropriate fluid replacement and electrolyte therapy should be implemented promptly, based on fluid, acid-base, and electrolyte status. Therefore arterial pH and blood gases and the serum levels of Na, K, Cl, HCO₃, serum creatine, BUN, and blood glucose should be determined.
Enhance salicylate elimination	Alkaline diuresis: IV administration of sodium bicarbonate to alkalinize the urine to a pH of 7.5 or more with sufficient urine flow. Hemodialysis: the same considerations as those that apply to chronic intoxication.
Provide symptomatic and supportive measures	Hypotension and/or hemorrhagic complications: fluids and transfusions, along with possible vitamin K injections. Respiratory depression: may require assisted pulmonary ventilation and oxygen. Seizures: IV administration of a benzodiazepine or short-acting barbiturate.

*Effective up to 3-4 hours after acute ingestion and maybe up to 10 hours after ingestion in the event of massive overdose.

Table 42-3	Salicylates and Other NSAIDs: Drug Interactions	
DRUG	**MECHANISM**	**RESULT**
Alcohol	Additive effect	Increased GI bleeding
Anticoagulants	Platelet inhibition, hypo-prothrombinemia	Increased bleeding tendencies
Aspirin and other salicylates with NSAIDs	Reduce NSAID absorption Additive GI toxicities	Increased GI toxicity with no therapeutic advantage
Corticosteroids and other ulcerogenic agents	Additive toxicities	Increased ulcerogenic effects
Uricosurics	Antagonism	Decreased uric acid excretion
Protein-bound drugs	Competite for binding	More pronounced drug actions
Hypotensive agents and diuretics	Inhibit prostaglandin synthesis	Reduced hypotensive and diuretic effects
Cyclosporin	Inhibit renal prostaglandin synthesis	May increase the nephrotoxic effects of cylcosporine

D O S A G E S

SALICYLATES AND OTHER NSAIDS

AGENT	PHARMACOLOGIC CLASS	DOSAGE RANGE	PURPOSE
Salicylic Acid Derivatives			
⚓Aspirin (acetylsalicylic acid [ASA]; many product names)	Salicylate	*Pediatric* PO/rectal: 10-16 mg/kg 4-6 times/day	Antipyretic, analgesic
		60-90 mg/kg/day divided *Adult*	Antirheumatic
		PO/rectal: 325-650 mg 4-6 times/day	Antipyretic, analgesic
		3.2-6 g/day divided	Antirheumatic
		325-650 mg 2-4 times/day	Antithrombotic
Indole			
⚓Indomethacin (Indocin)	NSAID	*Infant* <48 hr old: (doses at 12-24 hr intervals) IV: 0.2 mg/kg, followed by 0.1 mg/kg for 2 doses 2-7 days old: IV: 0.2 mg/kg for all 3 doses >7 days old: IV: 0.2 mg/kg, followed by 0.25 mg/kg for 2 doses	Patent ductus arteriosus
		Pediatric/Adult PO: 150-200 mg/day	Antirheumatic
		50 mg tid and tapered to cessation as soon as possible	Gout
Propionic Acids			
⚓Ibuprofen (Motrin, many others)	NSAID	*Pediatric 6 mo-12 yr old* PO: 5 mg/kg if <102.5° F (39.1° C) 10 mg/kg if >102.5° F (39.1° C)	Antipyretic

continued

SALICYLATES AND OTHER NSAIDS—cont'd

AGENT	PHARMACOLOGIC CLASS	DOSAGE RANGE	PURPOSE
Ibuprofen—cont'd		*Adult* PO: 200-400 mg q4-6h	Antipyretic, analgesic, dysmenorrhea
		400-800 mg 3-4 times/day; do not exceed 3.2 g/day.	Antirheumatic
Ketorolac (Toradol)	NSAID	*Adult* PO: 10 mg q4-6h prn; do not exceed 40 mg/day IM: 30-60 mg, followed by 15-30 mg q6h	Analgesic
Analgesic/Antipyretic ⚓Acetaminophen (Tylenol)	Paraaminophenol	*Adult/Pediatric >10 yr* PO: 235-650 mg q4h prn, not to exceed 4 g/day; REC: 325-650 mg q4h prn, not to exceed 4 g/day *Pediatric 0-3 mo:* 40 mg/dose *Pediatric 4-11 mo:* 80 mg/dose	Analgesic

the exceptions being choline magnesium trisalicylate (Trilisate), diflunisal (Dolobid), and salsalate (Disalcid). The salicylates are usually available in oral preparations. They are generally rated as pregnancy category C agents, except for aspirin, which is rated as a pregnancy category D agent because it has been shown to be both teratogenic and embryocidal in animals.

⚓ ASPIRIN

Aspirin (acetylsalicylic acid [ASA] and many product names) is known chemically as *acetylsalicylic acid*. It is the prototype salicylate and NSAID and is the most widely used drug in the world. First introduced in the late 1800s, it remains a mainstay of many drug treatment regimens. Aspirin is capable of many beneficial therapeutic effects; these include analgesic, antiinflammatory, and antipyretic effects. It has also been shown to have an antithrombotic effect, which is the result of its ability to inhibit platelet aggregation by blocking cyclooxygenase. This action has made it, along with the thrombolytics, a primary drug in the treatment of acute myocardial infarctions as well as many other thromboembolic disorders. Aspirin may be used to treat the pain associated with headache, neuralgia, myalgia, and arthralgia, as well as other pain syndromes resulting from inflammation. These include arthritis, pleurisy, and pericarditis. Patients with systemic lupus erythematosus may also benefit from aspirin therapy.

Aspirin is available in many dosage forms. It comes in chewing gum, tablets, chewable tablets, delayed-release enteric-coated tablets, extended-release tablets, film-coated tablets, tablets for solution, capsules, and rectal suppositories. It is also contained in many different combination products, some of the more popular combinations being aspirin, acetaminophen, and caffeine combinations, such as Goody's Headache Powder and Excedrin, and aspirin combined with various antacids (Ascriptin and Bufferin). Aspirin also comes in special dosage forms such as enteric-coated aspirin (Ecotrin). These many dosage formulations and strengths have been developed over the years in response to a need to decrease the GI toxicities associated with aspirin use, to incorporate the beneficial therapeutic effects of aspirin with those of other agents, and to provide the exact dose needed for certain indications.

Aspirin is contraindicated in patients with a known hypersensitivity to salicylates; those with GI bleeding, bleeding disorders, vitamin K deficiency, or a peptic ulcer; children younger than 12 years of age; and children with flulike symptoms. As already mentioned, it is classified as a pregnancy D agent and its use should be avoided in nursing mothers. Commonly recommended dosages are listed in the dosages table on p. 644.

PHARMACOKINETICS

HALF-LIFE	ONSET	PEAK	DURATION
5-9 hr	15-30 min	1-2 hr	4-6 hr

ACETIC ACIDS

INDOMETHACIN

Indomethacin (Indocin) is one of the six commonly used acetic acid NSAIDs, the others being diclofenac sodium, diclofenac potassium, etodolac, sulindac, and tolmetin. All are structurally related. Like the other NSAIDs, indomethacin has analgesic, antiinflammatory, and antipyretic properties. Its therapeutic actions are of particular use in the treatment of rheumatoid arthritis, ankylosing rheumatoid spondylitis, acute gouty arthritis, and the closure of patent ductus arteriosus in premature infants.

Because of its potent actions, indomethacin is available only by prescription. It can be administered by three different routes—orally, rectally, and intravenously. The oral dosage forms are a 25- and 50-mg capsule, a 75-mg extended-release capsule, and a 25–mg/5 ml suspension. The rectal suppositories contain 50 mg of the agent, and parenterally indomethacin comes as a 1-mg injection. Indomethacin is considered as a pregnancy category B agent for women in the first or second trimester of pregnancy, but its use during the last trimester is not recommended because it may inhibit prostaglandin synthesis in the fetus. For the same reason it is also not recommended for use in nursing women because it may inhibit prostaglandin synthesis in the infant. Hypersensitivity to it, asthma, severe renal and hepatic disease, and ulcer disease are all contraindications to its use. Commonly recommended dosages are listed in the dosages table on p. 644.

PHARMACOKINETICS

HALF-LIFE	ONSET	PEAK	DURATION
1.5-2 hr	<30 min	0.5-3 hr	4-6 hr

PROPIONIC ACIDS

IBUPROFEN

Ibuprofen (Motrin and many others) is the prototype NSAID in the propionic acid category, which also includes fenoprofen, flurbiprofen, ketoprofen, ketorolac, naproxen, and oxaprozin. However, ibuprofen is the most frequently used of the propionic acid agents because of the numerous indications for its use and because of its safe side effects and adverse effect profile.

Ibuprofen is also available OTC, either alone or in combination with other agents, of which there are many such products. To reduce toxicity and prevent some of the dose-related side effects of ibuprofen, the maximum strength of the OTC ibuprofen preparations is 200 mg.

Because of the therapeutic actions of ibuprofen, it is an excellent drug for the treatment of rheumatoid arthritis, osteoarthritis, primary dysmenorrhea, gout, dental pain, and musculoskeletal disorders. Ibuprofen is available only in oral formulations: a 100–mg/5 ml suspension; 200-, 300-, 400-, 600-, and 800-mg film-coated and regular tablets; and a combination product containing 200 mg of ibuprofen and 30 mg of pseudoephedrine. Some of the OTC products are Advil, Midol IB, Motrin IB, and Nuprin.

Ibuprofen is considered a pregnancy category B agent for women in their first or second trimester of pregnancy. It is not recommended for women in the last trimester because it can inhibit prostaglandin synthesis in the fetus. It is also not recommended for nursing women because it can inhibit prostaglandin synthesis in the infant. Hypersensitivity, asthma, and severe renal and hepatic disease are contraindications to its use. Commonly recommended dosages are listed in the dosages table on p. 644.

PHARMACOKINETICS

HALF-LIFE	ONSET	PEAK	DURATION
2-2.5 hr	<30 min	0.6-2 hr	4-6 hr

KETOROLAC

Ketorolac (Toradol) is another of the propionic acid NSAIDs but is unique from the other NSAIDs in that it has very little antiinflammatory action but a very potent analgesic action. As proof of this the analgesic potency of ketorolac is similar to that of the narcotic analgesics such as morphine and meperidine. It is indicated for the treatment of mild to moderate pain but not for that of osteoarthritis or rheumatoid arthritis because of its limited antiinflammatory effects. A particular advantage of ketorolac is that it may be given parenterally by either the intravenous or intramuscular route as well as orally and ophthalmically. It is the only NSAID that can be given by all these routes. Ketorolac is available as a 10-mg film-coated tablet; a 15-, 30-, and 60-mg parenteral form; and a 0.5% ophthalmic solution.

Ketorolac is available only by prescription. There are many other nonapproved uses for ketorolac, the reason for this lack of approval being that they have not been systematically evaluated by the FDA. The contraindications to ketorolac use are similar to those of the other NSAIDs, and it is classified as a pregnancy category C agent. Commonly recommended dosages are listed in the dosages table on p. 645.

⚗ PHARMACOKINETICS

HALF-LIFE	ONSET	PEAK	DURATION
5-7 hr	0.5-1 hr	1.5-3 hr	6 hr

ENOLIC ACIDS, FENAMIC ACIDS, AND THE NONACIDIC COMPOUNDS

The last three chemical categories of NSAIDs consist of the smallest number of agents, and the indications for their use are limited. Both **phenylbutazone** (Butazolidin) and **piroxicam** (Feldene) belong to the enolic acid family of NSAIDs. These are very potent agents that have been observed to produce severe GI toxicities. They are commonly used in the treatment of mild to moderate osteoarthritis, rheumatoid arthritis, and gouty arthritis. They are both available only in oral dosage formulations. Phenylbutazone is classified as pregnancy category D agent and piroxicam as a pregnancy category C agent. They both have contraindications similar to those of the other NSAIDs.

Meclofenamic acid (Meclomen) and **mefenamic acid** (Ponstel) are fenamic acid NSAIDs that are older agents and not used as commonly as the other NSAIDs. They are indicated for the treatment of mild to moderate pain, osteoarthritis, and rheumatoid arthritis. Mefenamic acid is pregnancy category C; meclofenamic acid use is *not* recommended during pregnancy.

Nabumetone (Relafen) is a relatively new NSAID that is better tolerated than some of the other agents by persons intolerant to the other NSAIDs because of the GI tract side effects. It is classified as a nonacidic compound and at present is the only such agent. Currently it is indicated only for the treatment of osteoarthritis and rheumatoid arthritis. It has contraindications similar to those of the other NSAIDs. It is a pregnancy category C agent, and the pregnancy and lactation precautions to nabumeton use are the same as those for ibuprofen use. Commonly recommended dosages for these agents can be found in the dosages table on p. 648.

MISCELLANEOUS AGENTS

The agents discussed in this section are ones that are not structurally related to NSAIDs but are used to treat some of the same conditions, such as the various forms of arthritis and gout. These agents can be classified broadly as the antigout agents, the gold compounds, and acetaminophen. They have unique characteristics that make them different from the NSAIDs and for this reason are discussed separately.

Antigout Agents

Gout is a condition that results from inappropriate uric acid metabolism. Persons with gout either overproduce or underexcrete uric acid, an end-product of purine metabolism. Purines are part of the normal dietary intake and are used to make the essential nucleoside analogues DNA and RNA. During their metabolism they are converted from hypoxanthine to xanthine and eventually to uric acid. (The normal pathway for the purine metabolism is depicted in Fig. 42-2.) When there is too much uric acid, deposits of uric acid crystals collect in tissues and joints, and this causes the pain of gout because these crystals are like small needles that jab and stick into sensitive tissues and joints.

The antigout agents consist of such drugs as allopurinol (Zyloprin), colchicine, probenecid (Benemid), and sulfinpyrazone (Anturane), and they are targeted at the underlying defect in uric acid metabolism, causing either the underexcretion or overproduction of uric acid.

☘ ALLOPURINOL

The beneficial effect of allopurinol (Zyloprin) in the relief of gout is the inhibition of the enzyme, xanthine oxidase, which thereby prevents uric acid production. Allopurinol is indicated for those persons whose gout is caused by the excess production of uric acid. Oxypurinol, a metabolite of allopurinol, also prevents uric acid production.

Allopurinol is contraindicated in patients with a hypersensitivity to it. Significant adverse effects to the agent include agranulocytosis, aplastic anemia, and serious and potentially fatal skin conditions such as exfoliative dermatitis, Stevens-Johnson syndrome, and toxic epidermal necrolysis. Azathioprine and mercaptopurine both interact with allopurinol, and because of the important interactions that can result, their doses may have to be adjusted.

Allopurinol is available only in oral preparations: a 100- and 300-mg tablet. The recommended adult dosage is 200 to 600 mg per day, to a maximum of 800 mg per day. Allopurinol is a pregnancy category C drug.

COLCHICINE

Colchicine is an antigout medication that has weak antiinflammatory activity, no effect on the urinary excretion of uric acid, and no analgesic activity. It appears to be effective in the treatment of gout by reducing the inflammatory response to the deposits of urate crystals

D O S A G E S

ENOLIC ACIDS, FENAMIC ACIDS, AND THE NONACIDIC COMPOUNDS

AGENT	PHARMACOLOGIC CLASS	DOSAGE RANGE	PURPOSE
Phenylbutazone	Pyrazolone NSAID	*Adult* PO: 300-600 mg/day in 3-4 divided doses 400 mg, followed by 100 mg q4h for up to 4-7 days	Rheumatoid arthritis Gout
Piroxicam (Feldene)	NSAID	*Adult* PO: 20 mg/day in a single daily dose; adjust according to response.	Rheumatoid arthritis, osteoarthritis
Meclofenamic acid (Meclomen)	Fenamate NSAID	*Adult* PO: 200-400 mg/day in 3-4 doses 40-100 mg q4-6h 100 mg tid	Rheumatoid arthritis, osteoarthritis Pain Primary dysmenorrhea
Mefenamic acid (Ponstel)	Fenamate NSAID	*Pediatric >14 y/o/Adult* PO: 500 mg, followed by 250 mg q6h with food	Acute pain, dysmenorrhea
Nabumetone (Relafen)	Nonacidic NSAID	*Adult* PO: 1000-2000 mg/day	Rheumatoid arthritis, osteoarthritis

in joint tissue. There are many possible explanations for its ability to do this, but the one favored by most is that it inhibits polymorphonuclear leukocyte metabolism, mobility, and chemotaxis.

Colchicine is a powerful inhibitor of cell mitosis and is extremely toxic, and for this reason it is available by prescription only. It is the drug of choice for the treatment of acute attacks of gout. Hypersensitivity is the only contraindication to its use. The drug is available in 0.5-, 0.6-, or 0.65-mg tablets to be taken orally. The usual adult dosage is an initial dose of 0.6 to 1.2 mg, then 0.6 mg every 1 to 2 hours until the pain disappears or until nausea, vomiting, or diarrhea develops. Colchicine is rated as a pregnancy category D agent.

PROBENECID

The beneficial effect of probenecid (Benemid) in the treatment of gout is the increased excretion of uric acid in the urine. Drugs that promote this excretion are known as uricosurics. In patients whose gout is due to the underexcretion of uric acid, urate crystals form because uric acid is not being excreted in the urine in sufficient quantities. Instead, most of the uric acid is being resorbed from the renal tubules back into the bloodstream and then conveyed throughout the body. Probenecid works by preferentially binding to the special transporter that takes uric acid from the urine and places it back into the blood. The probenecid rather than the uric acid is then resorbed back into the bloodstream while the uric acid remains in the urine and is excreted.

Besides its use for the treatment of the hyperuricemia associated with gout and gouty arthritis, it also has the ability to delay the renal excretion of penicillin, thus increasing the serum levels of penicillin and prolonging its effect. Probenecid is available as a 500-mg oral tablet. The usual adult dosage is 250 mg twice a day with food, milk, or antacids for 1 week. After that the dose should be adjusted to maintain normal uric acid levels. It is a pregnancy category B agent.

SULFINPYRAZONE

Sulfinpyrazone (Anturane) works similarly to probenecid. It is also a uricosuric agent. It is chemically related to the NSAID, phenylbutazone, and, like it, can also cause ulcers. It is therefore contraindicated

▼ FIG. 42-2 Uric acid production. *XO,* xanthine oxidase.

in patients with peptic ulcer disease. Sulfinpyrazone is available in 100-mg tablets and 200-mg capsules. The usual adult dosage is 100 to 200 mg twice a day for 1 week. The subsequent adjusted maintenance dosage is 200 to 400 mg daily. It is a pregnancy category C agent.

Gold Compounds

Gold compounds suppress arthritic inflammation and are therefore used in the treatment of rheumatoid arthritis. They exhibit antiinflammatory, antiarthritic, and immunomodulating effects and work by inhibiting the movement of various cells into an inflamed, damaged area, such as a joint. These cells (neutrophils, monocytes, and macrophages) are responsible for causing many of the deleterious effects of chronic rheumatoid arthritis. By preventing the accumulation of these cells in the area of the diseased joint, the gold compounds prevent progression of the disease. These agents are also believed to be effective in the treatment of such diseases as rheumatoid arthritis by modulating or controlling the involvement of the immune system. The three most commonly used gold compounds are auranofin, aurothioglucose, and gold sodium thiomalate. Gold compounds are available by prescription only and are rated as pregnancy category C agents.

AURANOFIN

Auranofin (Ridaura) is an orally active gold compound. Twenty-nine percent of it is gold, and like all gold compounds, it has antiinflammatory, antiarthritic, and immunomodulating effects. It is poorly absorbed orally, with only about 25% being absorbed from the GI tract into the blood. Auranofin is contraindicated in patients with a history of gold-induced necrotizing enterocolitis, pulmonary fibrosis, exfoliative dermatitis, bone marrow aplasia, or other types of

blood dyscrasia. It is available in 3-mg capsules for oral use. The normal recommended adult dosage is 6 mg once per day or 3 mg twice per day. The dosage can be increased to 9 mg after 6 months if the response is inadequate. Auranofin is a pregnancy category C agent.

AUROTHIOGLUCOSE AND GOLD SODIUM THIOMALATE

Aurothioglucose (Solganol) and gold sodium thiomalate (Myochrysine) are parenterally administered gold compounds. These products are made by complexing gold with thioglucose and thiomalate via a sulfur atom. Like other gold compounds they have antiinflammatory, antiarthritic, and immunomodulating effects. Aurothioglucose is available as a 50-mg/ml injection; gold sodium thiomalate is available as an injection in strengths of 25 and 50 mg/ml. The normal adult dosage of aurothioglucose is 10 mg per week, increasing to 50 mg per week. The usual maintenance dosage is 25 mg per week. The recommended adult dosage of gold sodium thiomalate is somewhat similar to that of aurothioglucose. It is recommended that it be started at a dose of 10 mg, followed by a second weekly dose of 25 mg. The third and subsequent doses are 50 mg weekly for 14 to 20 weeks. After 0.8 to 1 g has been administered and there is improvement in the patient's condition and no noted toxicity, the maintenance dose should be 50 mg given at 2-week intervals for four doses, followed by 50 mg given monthly. It is a pregnancy category C agent.

Analgesic and Antipyretic Agents

ACETAMINOPHEN

Acetaminophen (Tylenol and many others) is a synthetic, nonopioid drug that has both analgesic and antipyretic effects and is indicated for the treatment of mild to moderate pain and fever. Its mechanism of action is similar to that of salicylates. It may cause pain impulses to be blocked peripherally in response to the inhibition of prostaglandin synthesis it produces. Acetaminophen is believed to lower the body temperature in patients with fever but rarely does so in patients with normal body temperatures. It accomplishes this by acting on the hypothalamus, the structure in the brain that regulates body temperature. Heat is dissipated as the result of the vasodilation and increased peripheral blood flow that occur.

Acetaminophen is a very safe and effective agent. It is therefore available OTC and in many combination prescription drugs. It is classified as a pregnancy category B agent and is contraindicated in patients with a hypersensitivity to it or an intolerance to tartrazine (yellow dye no. 4), alcohol, sugar, or saccharin. Its use should be avoided in patients who are anemic or who have renal or hepatic disease.

The ingestion of large amounts, as in an acute overdose, can cause hepatic necrosis. This is the most serious acute toxic effect. Acute ingestion of acetaminophen doses of 150 mg/kg or more may result in hepatic toxicity. The long-term ingestion of large doses is more likely to result in nephropathy. Because the reported or estimated quantity of drug ingested is often inaccurate and not a reliable guide to the therapeutic management of the overdose, a serum acetaminophen concentration should be determined for this purpose no sooner than 4 hours after the ingestion. If a serum acetaminophen level cannot be obtained or a time since ingestion cannot be determined, it should be assumed that the overdose is potentially toxic and treatment with acetylcysteine (the recommend antidote for acetaminophen toxicity) should be started. Acetylcysteine works by preventing the hepatotoxic metabolites of acetaminophen from forming. The treatment regimen consists of an initial loading dose of 140 mg/kg orally, followed by 70 mg/kg every 4 hours for 17 additional doses. If the patient vomits within 1 hour of receiving a dose of acetylcysteine, then that dose should be given again immediately. *All 17 doses must be given to prevent hepatotoxicity from occurring, regardless of what the subsequent acetaminophen serum levels are.*

Acetaminophen is available in many oral and rectal dosage formulations. It comes in the form of capsules, a solution, granules, a suspension, tablets, chewable tablets, film-coated tablets, tablets for solution, and rectal suppositories. It is available in numerous strengths, depending on whether it is intended for use in children or adults. The adult dose is 325 to 650 mg every 4 hours as needed, not to exceed 4 g per day or 2.6 g per day if used for an extended time. The recommended pediatric oral or rectal dose is as follows (to be given every 4 to 6 hours):

0-3 mo	40 mg
4-11 mo	80 mg
1-2 yr	120 mg
2-3 yr	160 mg
4-5 yr	245 mg
6-8 yr	320 mg
9-10 yr	400 mg
11-12 yr	480 mg

NURSING PROCESS

ASSESSMENT

Before administering any of the NSAIDs, the nurse must assess the patient for the following contraindications to their use: allergies to any of the classes of NSAIDs, GI lesions or peptic ulcer disease, and bleeding disorders. Cautious use, with careful monitoring of the patient for the occurrence of side effects or toxicity, is recommended in pregnant women; patients with renal, cardiac, or hepatic disease; patients with glaucoma (i.e., enolic agents such as phenylbutazone); the elderly; and patients with psychiatric illnesses (i.e., indomethacin, sulindac, tolmetin).

A thorough medication history is needed to determine whether the patient is taking any drugs that can interact with the NSAIDs. Indole agents (e.g., indomethacin, sulindac) are ulcerogenic and should not be given with corticosteroids and aspirin agents. They should be given cautiously with anticoagulants. Enolic agents (phenylbutazone) enhance the effects of oral anticoagulants, insulin, and oral antidiabetic agents and also inhibit the action of steroids and sex hormones. Phenylpropionic agents (ibuprofen, naproxen) should be used cautiously with anticoagulants, and their concurrent use with aspirin may decrease the antiinflammatory effects of the NSAID.

Laboratory tests assessing cardiac, renal, and liver function as well as an RBC, Hgb level, Hct, and platelet count should also be determined and the results documented before the use of NSAIDs. In addition, laboratory studies that assess the status of other diseases (inflammatory-type diseases) may be ordered, such as an evaluation of rheumatoid factors.

NURSING DIAGNOSES

Nursing diagnosis relevant to the use of NSAIDs should always take into consideration the specific indication for the agents and the patient's medical di-

Patient Teaching TIPS

Use of NSAIDS

✔ Patients should understand that NSAIDS are used for the treatment of pain, an injury, or a disease process and that they work by decreasing the inflammation that leads to pain.

✔ Patients should know the various and most common side effects of the NSAIDS, which are listed below:

> Indomethacin: headache, nausea, vomiting, GI upset, ulcers, hemorrhage, hemolytic anemias, epistaxis, blurred vision, rash, leukopenia
>
> Sulindac and tolmetin: GI upset, GI discomfort, ulcers, rash, tinnitus, diarrhea, nausea
>
> Piroxicam: GI upset, elevated BUN level, dizziness, vertigo, edema, tinnitus
>
> Ibuprofen: heartburn, GI upset, ulcers, nausea
>
> Naproxen: vomiting, blurred vision, decreased Hgb level and Hct value.

✔ These medications should be taken on an empty stomach 1 hour before or 2 hours after meals. However, they generally cause GI distress and are often better tolerated if taken with food, milk, or an antacid.

✔ Patients should monitor their stools for bleeding because of the risk of GI ulcerations.

✔ Drug interactions are many, so patients should be given information about the following interactions:

> Indomethacin and tolmetin: corticosteroids, phenylbutazone, salicylates, anticoagulants
>
> Sulindac: aspirin
>
> Phenylbutazone: oral anticoagulants, oral antidiabetic agents, insulin, penicillin, sulfonamides, barbiturates, sex hormones, steroids
>
> Ibuprofen, naproxen, and fenoprofen: anticoagulants, aspirin, steroids, phenylbutazone
>
> Meclofenamate sodium: same as above

TAKE HOME POINTS

Nonsteroidal Antiinflammatory Drugs (NSAIDs)

- One of the most frequently prescribed categories of drugs.
- First drug in this category to be synthesized was salicylic acid.
- Now more than 70 different NSAIDs, but only 20 are commonly used.

Mechanism of Action

- Work in the arachidonic acid pathway.
- Inhibit cyclooxygenase and/or lipooxygenase, thereby preventing prostaglandin and/or leukotriene synthesis.

Therapeutic Effects

- Analgesic, antiinflammatory, and antipyretic.
- Also used in the treatment of gout, osteoarthritis, juvenile arthritis, rheumatoid arthritis, and dysmenorrhea.

Side Effects

- Three main ones:
  1. GI intolerance
  2. Bleeding
  3. Renal impairment
- Misoprostol (Cytotec) may be given to prevent GI intolerance.
- Misoprostol is a prostaglandin analogue.

Nursing Considerations

- Many contraindications to the use of NSAIDs such as GI tract lesions, peptic ulcers, allergies to them, and bleeding disorders.
- Most NSAIDS are better tolerated orally if taken with food to minimize GI upset.
- Patients should be closely monitored for the occurrence of bleeding such as blood in the stools or emesis.
- Therapeutic effects in patients with arthritis usually occur within 3 to 4 weeks.

agnosis. The following nursing diagnoses may be appropriate:

- Pain related to disease process or injury.
- Altered mobility related to disease process or injury.
- Risk for injury to self related to altered movement, disease process, injury, or side effects of medication.
- Risk for noncompliance related to side effects of medication and delayed onset of therapeutic effects.
- Knowledge deficit related to first-time drug therapy for pain or disease process.

PLANNING

Goals pertinent to patients receiving NSAIDs include:

- Patient will be able to describe the use of the medication as it relates to the relief of inflammation and pain.
- Patient will experience pain relief or relief of symptoms within expected period of time.
- Patient will use nonpharmacologic measures to decrease pain in addition to other therapies.

■ Patient will report adverse effects to the physician as indicated.

■ Patient will remain compliant with medication therapy.

Outcome Criteria

Outcome criteria for patients receiving NSAIDs include:

■ Patient will state that pain is characteristic of inflammation, injury, or related disease and will decrease with therapy.

■ Patient will identify factors that aggravate or alleviate pain such as movement, activity, noises, and so on.

■ Patient will state nonpharmacologic measures to use to promote comfort such as hot or cold packs, physical therapy, or relaxation therapy.

■ Patient will state side effects of NSAIDs such as GI upset, heartburn, nausea and vomiting, or anorexia.

■ Patient will discuss symptoms to report to the physician immediately, such as epigastric distress, nausea and vomiting, abdominal pain, dyspnea, and bleeding or easy bruising.

■ Patient states the importance of correct dosing and of consistency in the self-administration of medication.

■ Patient returns for follow-up visits with the physician.

IMPLEMENTATION

The patient should be educated about the various side effects of the NSAIDs (see Table 42-1 for those of the most commonly used agents). Should side effects become severe or intolerable or bleeding or GI pain occur, the physician must be contacted immediately. Most of these medications should be taken on an empty stomach (1 hour before or 2 hours after a meal); however, because they generally cause GI distress. They are often better tolerated if taken with food, milk, or an antacid. Patients should be watched closely for the occurrence of any unusual bleeding, such as in the stool, because of the risk of GI ulcerations. In addition, it is important to explain to the patient the difference between their onset of action for the relief of acute pain as opposed to their more delayed effect when used for the relief of arthritis pain; in the latter instance the therapeutic effects may not be realized for 3 to 4 weeks.

EVALUATION

The therapeutic response to NSAIDs may vary and comprise a decrease in acute pain; a decrease in swelling, pain, stiffness, and tenderness of a joint or muscle area; or a return to normal of such laboratory values as the CBC, RBC, Hgb level, Hct, sedimentation rates, and other arthritis-related laboratory test results. Monitoring for the occurrence of side effects is also essential to their safe and effective use (see Table 42-1).

Critical Thinking **A C T I V I T I E S**

1. What are the three most common toxicities of aspirin that prompted the development of the other NSAIDs?

   1. Stevens-John-son syndrome
   2. Gastrointestinal intolerance
   3. Agranulocytosis
   4. Bleeding
   5. Renal impairment
   6. Alopecia

   a. 1, 3, and 6   b. 2, 4, and 5   c. 1, 3, and 4   d. 2, 3, and 6

2. The NSAIDs work by inhibiting the enzymes _____ and _____ preventing the _____ and _____ pathways from causing inflammation.

   1. angiotensin-converting enzyme
   2. lipooxygenase
   3. prostaglandin
   4. phosphodiesterase
   5. angiotensin
   6. cyclooxygenase
   7. leukotriene
   8. folic acid

   a. 1, 4, 5, and 8   b. 4, 6, 5, and 3   c. 6, 2, 3, and 7   d. 2, 4, 5, and 8

3. What are the three primary therapeutic effects of NSAIDs?

   1. Antihypertensive
   2. Analgesic
   3. Antianginal
   4. Antiinflammatory
   5. Antitussive
   6. Antipyretic

   a. 1, 3, and 5   b. 1, 2, and 3   c. 4, 5, and 6   d. 2, 4, and 6

4. What drug may be given to prevent the gastrointestinal side effects of NSAIDs?
   a. Metoprolol (Lopressor)
   b. misoprostol (Cytotec)
   c. Metoclopramide (Reglan)
   d. Propulside (Cisapride)

5. Which one of the following is an adverse reaction common to the use of any of the NSAIDs?
   a. Visual disturbances
   b. Insomnia
   c. Chronic constipation
   d. Dysphagia

▲▲

BIBLIOGRAPHY

Albanese T, Nutz P: *Mosby's 1995 nursing drug cards,* St Louis, 1995, Mosby.

Horowitz M: IV ketorolac: getting to the route of a problem, *Nursing* 23(3):62, 1993.

Johnson KB: *Harriet Lane handbook,* ed 13, St Louis, 1993, Mosby.

Keen JH: *Critical care and emergency drug reference,* St Louis, 1994, Mosby.

Knoben JE, Anderson PO: *Handbook of critical drug data,* ed 6, Hamilton, Ill, 1988, Drug Intelligence Publications.

Lilley L, Guanci B: Med Errors: adverse effects of NSAIDs, *Am J Nurs* 17, 1995.

McEvoy GK: *AHFS drug information,* Bethesda, Md, 1994, American Society of Hospital Pharmacists.

Miller C: What's new with NSAIDs? *Geriatr Nurs* 13(4):227, 1992.

Skidmore-Roth L: *Mosby's 1995 nursing drug reference,* St Louis, 1995, Mosby.

PART 9

THE IMMUNE SYSTEM AND BIOLOGIC AND CHEMOTHERAPEUTIC MODIFIERS: STUDY SKILLS BRIEF

Time Management

The first step in preparing for a chapter or part exam is to plan for the time needed. Let us begin by assuming that the next test you have will be a test covering the chapters in Part 9. First examine the material to determine just how much there is to cover. Look at the chapter outline, the objectives, the glossary, and the number of pages of text in each chapter. This will help you determine just how big a task you face. As you are doing this also consider how much study time you have been devoting to these chapters in the days before the exam. If you have been doing regular study with frequent review sessions, then the demand on your time in the day or two just before the exam will be less than if you have to do a major "cram" session to try to catch up on study that has been put off. The basic question to answer here is a simple one. "How much time do I need to schedule for exam preparation?" The answer varies with each student. Some will need six, eight, or more hours of preparation time in the two to three days before the exam. Others will find that three, four, or five hours will be adequate. You must assess your own learning and prior success to determine what time is necessary for you, but you must set time aside and use it effectively.

There is one thing that should play a major role in helping you to determine the time you will need to set aside. Evaluate your performance on prior exams. How have you been doing? How much time have you been spending to achieve that level? If you are not achieving according to your capabilities, then you should certainly consider spending more time preparing for the next exam. If you are achieving at a satisfactory level, then plan on devoting about the same amount of time to test preparation.

The next step in preparing for an exam is to organize the time. Write down what you are going to study and when and how much time you will spend. Consider the following example based on the materials in Chapters 45 and 46:

1. Review Chapter 45 objectives. Monday, 4:00 to 4:30 PM.
   Note objectives that are unclear for further review.
2. Question and Answer review, Chapter 45 outline. Monday, 4:30 to 5:15 PM.
   Note outline topics that need rereading for better understanding.
3. Self-test, Chapter 45 glossary. Monday, 6:30 to 7:00 PM.
   Note terms that need further review for mastery.
4. Review Chapter 46 objectives. Monday, 7:00 to 7:30 PM.
5. Question and Answer review, Chapter 46 outline, Monday, 7:30 to 8:00 PM.
6. Self-test, Chapter 46 glossary. Monday, 8:00 to 8:30 PM.

The advantage to this test preparation model is that you now know where you must focus in the days before the exam.

Evaluate Prior Performance

As you begin preparing to review for any exam take some time to look back at previous exams. Evaluate your performance, and use that evaluation to improve on subsequent tests. As you look at prior tests consider the following factors:

1. What type of errors did I make?

As students we often find that there are certain question types or forms that are missed consistently. Assess your errors and try to pinpoint any recurring patterns in your mistakes. Did you miss questions that contained an exemption in the multiple choice stem? Question stems that state "all of the following except" and "Which of the following would not be . . ." are exemption questions. Questions like this are often missed because they contain too many apparently correct responses. Remember that an exemption stem means you are looking for the one response choice that is "wrong." The stem asks you to identify the inappropriate response, and it is the best choice.

2. Did I have trouble with questions that required mastery of terminology?

As part of the evaluation of prior tests also look at questions that demanded mastery of the terms from the chapters. If you missed more than one or two questions of that type, then you know you need to spend more time in review of terminology.

3. Did I miss concept questions?

If the question asked you to apply a principle, evaluate a drug response, or in some other way apply knowledge from the course, you are dealing with concepts rather than facts. If you missed a number of concept questions, then you should spend more of your review time studying applications and principles than memorizing facts and terms.

4. Did I make errors because I did not know the material?

This question focuses on the quality of your learning. If you miss one or two questions on an exam because you did not learn (or did not remember) the material, it is not a major problem. There will almost always be one or two questions that we do not remember. If you are analyzing past performance and find that there are several questions on which you guessed because you did not recall any information that seemed relevant to the question, it may be necessary to put more time into review. It may be doing more oral rehearsal so that the material is stored in long-term memory. Whatever the cause it is essential that you acknowledge to yourself that you have missed questions because you did not know the material.

Once you have acknowledged the problem, take steps to correct it.

Anticipate the Test

Do not wait until exam time to find out what you should know. As you do your review try to think like the instructor. Generate questions that you think might be a part of the test. This does not mean you need to try to write multiple choice stems and choices, but you should be trying to focus your review in a way that will facilitate learning and long-term memory.

Here are some examples of questioning that you might use based on material found in Chapter 46.

1. What are biologic response modifiers (BRMs)?
2. What is the role of BRMs in the care of patients with cancer?
3. What is the role of the immune system in treating cancer?

The sample questions were drawn from just the first few pages of the chapter. These questions focus on literal comprehension and are relatively easy to generate. Being able to answer them is important, but if all of your questions are literal in nature, it may be difficult to answer questions that require application of principles and concepts. For that reason it is essential that some questions require analysis, synthesis, and/or evaluation of the material. Question 3 is an example of this type of question. Answers to these questions require the learner to put together the literal information and relate the terms to the concepts being explained.

Plan for Distributed Study

One of the major problems that many students encounter when trying to review for a test is waiting too long to begin the review. This forces students into a review pattern of long hours of intensive study all packed into the last day or two before the exam. This is known as cramming, and although cramming does work to some degree, it is not the most effective way to learn. A better model is to distribute the review over a period of several days with short, 30-minute to 1-hour study sessions several times each day. Distributing practice in this way allows time for you to think about what you have been learning, and it fosters long-term memory.

One important consideration for review is spending more of the review time doing oral rehearsal (ask and answer sessions) than simply rereading material. Oral rehearsal encourages active learning, which enhances your ability to concentrate, improves comprehension and memory, and thus improves test performance.

Chapter 43

Immunosuppressant Agents

Objectives

When you reach the end of this chapter, you will be able to:

1 Discuss the role of immunosuppressive therapy in the treatment of autoimmune diseases.

2 Discuss the mechanism of action, contraindications, cautions, side effects, and toxicity associated with the most commonly used immunosuppressives.

3 Develop a comprehensive nursing care plan as it relates to the patient receiving immunosuppressants.

4 Discuss the education guidelines for patients receiving an immunosuppressant agent.

CHAPTER OUTLINE

Mechanism of Action
Drug Effects
Therapeutic Uses
Side Effects and Adverse Effects
Interactions
Dosages
Drug Profiles
   Azathioprine
  ⚓ Cyclosporine
   Muromonab-CD3

Nursing Process
Assessment
Nursing Diagnoses
Planning
  Outcome criteria
Implementation
Evaluation

Glossary

Autoimmune diseases (aw′ to ĭ mūn′) A large group of diseases characterized by the subversion or alteration of the function of the immune system, where the immune response is directed against normal body tissue(s) of the body resulting in pathologic conditions. (p. 656)

Immunosuppressant (im′ u no sə pres′ ənt) Agent that decreases or prevents an immune response. (p. 656)

Immunosuppressive therapy Drug treatment used to suppress the immune system. (p. 656)

Murine antibodies (mu′ rin) Monoclonal immuno-globulins. *Monoclonal* refers to a protein from a single clone of cells, all the molecules of which are the same. *Murine* refers to the family Muridae, to which mice belong. An antibody is a protective protein that counters the actions of antigens, substances that cause sensitivity or an allergic response. Thus murine antibodies are protective proteins obtained from mice. Muromonab-CD3 is a murine antibody used to reverse graft rejection. (p. 659)

The human body is under constant attack by invading microorganisms, but it possesses several mechanisms with which to fight off these foreign invaders; one is the immune system. This system defends the body against invading pathogens, foreign antigens, and its own cells that become cancerous or neoplastic. Besides these beneficial functions, however, this highly sophisticated system can also sometimes attack itself and cause what is known as **autoimmune diseases**. It also participates in hypersensitivity, or anaphylactic, reactions, which can be life-threatening. The rejection of kidney, liver, and heart (whole organ) transplants is directed by the immune system as well. From this it is easy to see that the immune system is capable of having many beneficial and detrimental effects.

Agents that decrease or prevent an immune response, and hence suppress the immune system, are known as **immunosuppressants**. Treatment with such drugs is referred to as **immunosuppressive therapy**, and it is used to selectively eradicate certain cell lines that play a major role in the rejection of a transplanted organ. These cell lines must be targeted and selectively altered or suppressed, or organ rejection will occur. The primary immunosuppressant drugs are the corti-

<table>
<tr><td colspan="2">Selected Immunosuppressants: Mechanism of Action</td></tr>
<tr><td>AGENT</td><td>MECHANISM OF ACTION</td></tr>
<tr><td>Azathioprine</td><td>Suppresses delayed hypersensitivity and antibody responses. Antagonizes purine metabolism (decreased DNA, RNA, and protein synthesis. Blocks cellular metabolism. Inhibits mitosis.</td></tr>
<tr><td>⇩Cyclosporine</td><td>Inhibits interleukin-2 release from T-lymphocytes (CD4).</td></tr>
<tr><td>Muromonab-CD3</td><td>Prevents T-cells from recognizing foreign antigens.</td></tr>
<tr><td>Prograf</td><td>Inhibits interleukin-2 release from T-lymphocytes.</td></tr>
</table>

costeroids (see Chapter 33), cyclophosphamide (see Chapter 45), azathioprine, methotrexate, cyclosporine, muromonab-CD3, and prograf (also known as FK-506). This chapter focuses on azathioprine, cyclosporine, muromonab-CD3, and prograf.

MECHANISM OF ACTION

All the immunosuppressants have similar mechanisms of action because they all selectively suppress certain lymphocyte cell lines, thereby preventing their involvement in the immune response. This results in a pharmacologically immunocompromised state similar to that in a cancer patient whose bone marrow and immune cells have been destroyed as the result of chemotherapy or that in a patient with AIDS. Each agent differs in the exact way in which it suppresses certain cell lines involved in an immune response. The mechanisms of action for the immunosuppressants discussed in this chapter are summarized in the box above.

The primary mechanism of action of azathioprine in the prevention of organ rejection is its ability to incorporate itself into the normal production pathway for purine nucleotides, which are substances such as DNA and RNA. These substances are vital to the production (synthesis) of such cells as lymphocytes (T cells). Thus, when azathioprine incorporates itself into the normal pathway for the production of DNA and RNA, it creates a faulty end-product that results in a cell that cannot function in the normal immune response.

Cyclosporine and prograf work by inhibiting the release of a substance called *interleukin-2* (IL-2) from specific T-lymphocytes called *CD4 cells* or *T-helper cells.* When IL-2 is released from T-helper cells, it stimulates cytotoxic T-cells, which in turn attack cells that are believed to be foreign cells, such as those of a transplanted organ. They destroy these cells by boring holes through them, resulting in cell lysis and death. These cytotoxic T-cells are believed to be the primary cells responsible for graft rejection. By preventing the release of IL-2 from T-helper cells, cyclosporine and pro-

graf keep these T-cells from being activated and as a result the transplanted organ from being attacked by the immune system.

Muromonab-CD3, also known as OKT3, works by binding to the CD3 receptor on mature circulating T-cells, which is located next to the T-cell antigen recognition site. This receptor is involved in the recognition of foreign invaders such as a transplanted organ. By binding to the CD3 receptor, OKT3 therefore prevents the T-cells from being stimulated by foreign antigens and thus inhibits both the generation and function of cytotoxic T-cells—the cells responsible for causing graft rejection. After the initial dose of OKT3, T-cells virtually disappear from the circulation within minutes to hours.

DRUG EFFECTS

Because of their ability to modify the immune system, the immunosuppressants are used in the treatment of organ rejection, rheumatoid arthritis, and other conditions that may have an immunologic cause.

THERAPEUTIC USES

The therapeutic uses of the immunosuppressants are multiple and vary from agent to agent. They are primarily indicated for the prevention of organ rejection. Only muromonab-CD3 works once rejection of a transplanted organ is under way. Azathioprine is used as an adjunct medication to prevent the rejection of kidney transplants and to ameliorate severe rheumatoid arthritis. Cyclosporine is the primary immunosuppressant agent used in the prevention of kidney, liver, heart, and bone marrow transplant rejection. It may also have beneficial effects in the treatment of other conditions with an immunologic cause such as certain types of arthritis, psoriasis, and irritable bowel disease.

Prograf has many of the same therapeutic effects as cyclosporine, but it is currently indicated only for the prevention of liver transplant rejection, though it has shown promise in preventing the rejection of other transplanted organs as well.

Muromonab-CD3 is indicated for the treatment of acute organ transplant rejection and is usually given in combination with azathioprine, cyclosporine, or corticosteroids, or with various combinations of these agents, for an additive therapeutic effect.

SIDE EFFECTS AND ADVERSE EFFECTS

Many of the side effects of the immunosuppressants can be devastating to the transplant patient. Although not strictly a side effect, a heightened susceptibility to opportunistic infections is a major risk factor in immunosuppressed patients. Other side effects and adverse effects are limited to the particular agents, and the common ones are listed in Table 43-1.

INTERACTIONS

The drug interactions associated with immunosuppressant use mostly involve cyclosporine. Cyclosporine is capable of many drug interactions, several of which can be very harmful. Drugs that may increase its action are amphotericin B, cimetidine, and ketoconazole. Drugs that may decrease its effects are phenytoin and rifampin. Although these are the most significant interactions, there are many more of lesser significance. It is also not recommended that azathioprine be given with allopurinol because allopurinol inhibits azathioprine's metabolism, and thereby increases its effects.

DOSAGES

For the recommended dosages of selected immunosuppressant agents, see the dosages table on the next page.

DRUG PROFILES

As previously stated, the primary use for the immunosuppressant agents discussed in this chapter is the prevention of organ rejection. Other immunologic disorders may also be treated by these agents. The agents of most importance are azathioprine, cyclosporine, muromonab-CD3, and prograf. These substances are all dispensed by prescription only.

AZATHIOPRINE

Azathioprine (Imuran) is a chemical analogue of the physiologic purines such as adenine and guanine. It is available in both an oral and parenteral formulation—a 50-mg tablet and a 100-mg injection, respectively. It is classified as a pregnancy category D agent and is contraindicated in patients who have shown a hypersensitivity to it. Commonly recommended dosages are listed in the dosages table.

PHARMACOKINETICS

HALF-LIFE	ONSET	PEAK	DURATION
1 hr	2-4 days	1-2 hr	Unknown

⚓ CYCLOSPORIN A

Cyclosporin A (Sandimmune) is an immunosuppressant agent that is indicated for the prevention of organ rejection. It is a very potent immunosuppressant and the principal agent in many immunosuppressive drug regimens. Like azathioprine, it may also be used for the treatment of other immunologic disorders, such as various forms of arthritis, psoriasis, and irritable bowel disease.

Cyclosporin A is classified as a pregnancy category C agent and is contraindicated in patients with a

Table 43-1	Immunosuppressants: Common Adverse Effects

BODY SYSTEM	SIDE/ADVERSE EFFECTS
Azathioprine	
Hematopoietic	Leukopenia, thrombocytopenia.
Hepatic	Hepatotoxicity is a common side effect.
⚓ Cyclosporine	
Renal	Nephrotoxicity is common and dose limiting.
Hepatic	Hepatotoxicity with cholestasis and hyperbilirubinemia.
CNS	Neurotoxicity including tremors in about 20% of patients.
Cardiovascular	Moderate hypertension in as many as 50% of patients.
Other	Hypersensitivity reactions to the vehicle.
Muromonab-CD3	
CNS	Pyrexia, chills, tremors.
Respiratory	Dyspnea, wheezing, pulmonary edema.
Cardiovascular	Chest pain
Gastrointestinal	Vomiting, nausea, diarrhea.
Other	Flulike symptoms, fluid retention.

known hypersensitivity to it. It is available in both oral and parenteral forms. Orally it comes as a 25- and 100-mg liquid-filled capsule as well as a 100-mg/ml solution. Parenterally it comes as a 50-mg/ml injection. Commonly recommended dosages are listed in the dosages table.

☣ PHARMACOKINETICS

HALF-LIFE	ONSET	PEAK	DURATION
1-2 hr, then 10-27 hr	Unknown	3-5 hr	Unknown

MUROMONAB-CD3

Muromonab-CD3 (Orthoclone OKT3) is the only agent indicated for the reversal, and not just the prevention, of graft rejection. It is unique in that it is a monoclonal antibody, and it is very similar to the antibodies naturally produced by the body, that is, immunoglobulin IG, IM, ID, IA, and IE. It specifically targets the binding sites on the T-cells that recognize foreign invaders such as a transplanted organ. It differs from human antibodies in that it comes from mice. These types of antibodies are commonly referred to as **murine antibodies**, hence the name *muromonab,* with 'muro-' standing for *murine;* '-mon-' for *monoclonal,* which means they come from the same clone; and '-ab' for *antibody.*

OKT3 is classified as a pregnancy category C agent and is contraindicated in patients with a hypersensitivity to murine products as well as those who are experiencing fluid overload. It is available only in a parenteral formulation—a 5-mg/5 ml injection. Commonly recommended dosages are listed in the dosages table.

☣ PHARMACOKINETICS

HALF-LIFE	ONSET	PEAK	DURATION
Unknown	Very rapid	~3 days	Unknown

DOSAGES

SELECTED IMMUNOSUPPRESSANT AGENTS

AGENT	PHARMACOLOGIC CLASS	DOSAGE RANGE	PURPOSE
Azathioprine (Imuran)	Purine antagonist immunosuppressive	*Pediatric/Adult* IV/PO: 3.5 mg/kg/day starting on day of transplant and/or 1-3 days before procedure; usual PO maintenance dose, 1-2 mg/kg/day.	Renal transplants
		Adult PO: Start with 1 mg/kg/day as a single dose or divided; may be increased by 0.5 mg/kg/day after 6-8 wk to a maximum of 2.5 mg/kg/day.	Arthritis
⚓**Cyclosporin A (Sandimmune)**	Polypeptide antibiotic immunosuppressive	*Pediatric/Adult* PO: 15 mg/kg as a single dose 4-12 hr before surgery. Continue initial daily dose (postop) for 1-2 wk, then reduce by 5%/wk to a maintenance dose of 5%-10%/wk. IV: Dose is 1/3 PO dose: 5-6 mg/kg as a single dose 4-16 hr before surgery and continued daily postop until patient can be switched to PO dose.	Liver, heart, kidney transplants
Muromonab-CD3 (Orthoclone OKT3)	Immunoglobin (IgG$_{2a}$) immunosuppressive	*Adult* IV: 5 mg/day in a single bolus injection for 10-14 days	Renal transplants, steroid-resistant cardiac and hepatic transplant rejection

NURSING PROCESS

ASSESSMENT

Before administering any of the immunosuppressants, (azathioprine, cyclosporine, or muromonab-CD3), the nurse should perform a thorough patient assessment and document the findings, including the following data: renal function (BUN and creatinine levels; information about urinary function and normal patterns of elimination); liver function (alkaline phosphatase, AST, ALT, and bilirubin levels; determining whether jaundice, edema, or ascites is present); cardiovascular function (baseline ECG, blood pressure, and pulse; documentation of any cardiovascular disease or history of dysrhythmias, chest pain, or hypertension); CNS baseline assessment (motor function and seizure disorders); and respiratory assessment (any complaints of dyspnea or wheezing; as documentation of pulmonary disorders or pulmonary edema) (see Table 43-1 for information on other systems affected by the specific agents).

Contraindications to and cautions regarding the use of these agents include the following: Azathioprine is contraindicated in patients who are hypersensitive to it and in pregnant women; cautious use is recommended in those patients with severe renal or hepatic disease. Cyclosporine is contraindicated in patients with a hypersensitivity to it; cautious use is recommended in patients with severe renal or hepatic disease and in pregnant women. Muromonab-CD3 is contraindicated in patients with a hypersensitivity to substances with a murine origin or in patients suffering from fluid overload, cautious use is advised in pregnant women and in children under 2 years of age or who are febrile.

Laboratory studies (e.g., Hgb level, Hct, WBC, and platelet count) should be performed and the results documented before, during (monthly), and after therapy. If the leukocyte count should drop below 3000/mm^3, the drug should be discontinued.

NURSING DIAGNOSES

Nursing diagnoses pertinent to patients receiving immunosuppressants include:
- Risk for injury related to disease.
- Risk for injury related to side effects of the immunosuppressant.
- Risk for infection related to disease.

Patient Teaching TIPS

Immunosuppressants

✔ Patients taking any of the immunosuppressants should be encouraged to avoid crowds to minimize the risk of infection. Patients should also be encouraged to report any fever, sore throat, chills, joint pain, or fatigue to the physician because this may indicate severe infection.

✔ It is recommended that women receiving immunosuppressants use some form of contraception during treatment and for up to 12 weeks after the end of therapy.

✔ It may take 3 to 4 months for a therapeutic response to azathioprine to be experienced in patients with rheumatoid arthritis.

✔ Azathioprine interacts with allopurinol, such that the effects of the immunosuppressant are reduced.

✔ Patients who are to undergo transplant surgery and who are receiving cyclosporine should know that several days before surgery they may be told to take it with corticosteroids and they may be also given an oral antifungal as prophylaxis for *Candida* infections.

✔ Patients taking the oral form of cyclosporine should be told to take it with meals or mixed with chocolate milk to prevent GI upset.

✔ Patients taking azathioprine or muromonab-CD3 should be informed that, several days before transplant surgery, they should take all their medication by the oral route, if possible, to avoid its having to be given by IM injections, as this carries the risk of causing infection. They should be told to take the immunosuppressant with food to help decrease the associated GI upset.

✔ Side effects of azathioprine include hepatotoxicity, leukopenia, and thrombocytopenia.

✔ Side effects of cyclosporine include nephrotoxicity, neurotoxicity, and moderate hypertension.

✔ Side effects of muromonab-CD3 include chills, fever, tremors, dyspnea, wheezing, pulmonary edema, chest pain, vomiting, nausea, and diarrhea.

- Risk for infection related to immunosuppressant therapy.
- Pain, myalgias, and arthralgias related to medication-induced side effects.
- Knowledge deficit related to initiation of new treatment regimen.
- Noncompliance with therapy related to side effects of medication.

TAKE HOME POINTS

Immunosuppressants
- Agents that decrease or prevent the body's immune response.
- Examples are corticosteroids, cyclophosphamide, azathioprine, methotrexate, cyclosporine, muromonab-CD3, and prograf.
- Suppress the action of various cells of the immune system.

Azathioprine
- Suppresses delayed hypersensitivity and antibody responses.
- Antagonizes purine metabolism (DNA, RNA, and protein synthesis).
- Blocks cellular metabolism.
- Inhibits mitosis.

Cyclosporine and Prograf
- Inhibit interleukin-2 release from T-lymphocytes (CD4).
- Used in organ transplant recipients to prevent organ rejection.
- If recipient's immune system cannot recognize the organ as being foreign, it will not mount an immune response against it.

Muromonab-CD3
- Prevents T-cells from recognizing foreign antigens.
- Used in transplant recipients suffering from acute rejection of the donated organ.
- Used to prevent acute rejection.
- Potent immunosuppressant.

Nursing Considerations
- Laboratory studies (e.g., Hgb level, Hct, WBC, and platelet count) should be performed and the results documented before, during (monthly), and after therapy; should the leukocyte count drop below 3000/mm^3, the drug should be discontinued.
- Any of these agents being taken orally should always be taken with food to minimize GI upset.
- Because of the immunosuppressed state of the patients receiving immunosuppressants, oral forms of the drugs should be used whenever possible to decrease the risk of infection associated with IM injections.
- Oral antifungals are usually also given with these medications to treat the oral candidiasis common in these patients.
- Patients should be encouraged to report any fever, sore throat, chills, joint pain, or fatigue, which may indicate severe infection.

PLANNING

Goals in patients receiving immunosuppressants include:
- Patient experiences minimal complications during immunosuppressant therapy.
- Patient experiences maximal comfort during drug therapy.
- Patient remains compliant with drug therapy and comes in for follow-up visits with the physician.
- Patient states symptoms of adverse reactions to therapy or of exacerbation of illness to report to physician.

Outcome Criteria

Outcome criteria for patients receiving immunosuppressants include:
- Patient experiences minimal problems of immunosuppressant such as myalgias, fever, nephrotoxicity, and hypertension.
- Patient experiences a decrease in disease-related symptoms.
- Patient is compliant to follow-up visits with physician to monitor therapeutic (decreased symptomology) and adverse reactions to medication (myalgias, arthralgias).
- Patient notifies physician immediately if fever, rash, sore throat, or fatigue develops.
- Patient states measures to implement to enhance comfort while on immunosuppressant therapy such as use of nonaspirin analgesics, rest, and biofeedback.

IMPLEMENTATION

When these agents are being taken orally, it is always important to take them with food to minimize GI upset. It is also important, considering the immunosuppressed state of patients receiving immunosuppressants, that oral forms of the drugs be used whenever possible to decrease the risk of infection associated with IM injections. An oral antifungal medication is usually given with these agents to treat the oral candidiasis common in these patients.

When given intravenously, cyclosporine should be diluted as recommended in the manufacturer guidelines and given according to the standards of care and institutional policy regarding its administration. Cyclosporine is normally diluted with normal saline or 5% dextrose in water in a concentration of 50 mg of the drug to 20 to 100 ml of diluting solution, which should be infused over 2 to 6 hours using an infusion pump. Intravenously administered muromonab IV is usually given over 1 minute, and only after the medication is withdrawn through a 0.2 to 0.22 low protein–binding micron filter. A new needle must be used after the medication is withdrawn. It is usually recommended that methylprednisone sodium succinate be administered before and hydrocortisone sodium succinate a half hour after the muromonab injection to minimize reactions to medication. See the patient teaching tips on p. 660.

EVALUATION

Therapeutic response to the immunosuppressants includes no rejection of a transplanted organ or graft and no obvious immunosuppression in patients with autoimmune disorders. The nurse should also check the patient for drug-specific side effects and toxicity (see Table 43-1).

Critical Thinking **ACTIVITIES**

K.J. is a 58-year-old heart transplant recipient who is currently taking cyclosporine to prevent his immune system from rejecting his transplanted heart. A cytomegalovirus (CMV) infection has developed, for which he is receiving ganciclovir.

1. How does cyclosporine prevent this patient's immune system from attacking his transplanted heart?

2. What type of infection is this CMV infection in this heart transplant recipient on immunosuppressants?
   a. Surgical wound infection
   b. Opportunistic infection
   c. Nosocomial infection
   d. Community-acquired infection

3. It is recommended that patients taking immunosuppressants should:
   a. use some form of contraception during treatment and for up to 12 weeks after the end of therapy.
   b. be given some other treatment, because it may take 6 to 9 months for a therapeutic response to occur.
   c. maintain long-term corticosteroid use just as a precaution to prevent drug side effects.
   d. use oral forms of the agents to prevent the occurrence of oral candidiasis.

BIBLIOGRAPHY

Albanese J, Nutz P: *Mosby's 1995 nursing drug cards,* St Louis, 1995, Mosby.

Johnson KB: *Harriet Lane handbook,* ed 13, St Louis, 1993, Mosby.

Keen JH: *Critical care and emergency drug reference,* St Louis, 1994, Mosby.

Knoben JE, Anderson PO: *Handbook of critical drug data,* ed 6, Hamilton, Ill, 1988, Drug Intelligence Publications.

McEvoy GK: *AHFS drug information,* Bethesda, Md, 1994, American Society of Hospital Pharmacists.

Skidmore-Roth L: *Mosby's 1995 nursing drug reference,* St Louis, 1995, Mosby.

Chapter 44

Immunizing Agents

Objectives

When you reach the end of this chapter, you will be able to:

1 Discuss the importance of immunity as it relates to the various immunizing agents.

2 Identify the diseases that the toxoids and vaccines now available immunize persons against.

3 Discuss the mechanism of action of each toxoid and vaccine, the indications for their use, the cautions to be taken in persons given them, contraindications to their use, their side effects, the routes of administration of the agents, and the related nursing interventions called for in persons receiving them.

4 Develop a comprehensive nursing care plan, including patient education, pertaining to the administration of immunizing agents.

CHAPTER OUTLINE

Immunity and Immunization

Active Immunization
  Toxoids
  Vaccines
Passive Immunization

Immunizing Agents

Mechanism of action
Drug effects
Therapeutic uses
Side effects and adverse effects
Interactions
Dosages

Drug Profiles

Active Immunizing Agents
  Bacillus Calmette-Guérin Vaccine
  Diphtheria and Tetanus Toxoids Adsorbed
    and Tetanus and Diphtheria Toxoids
    Adsorbed
  Haemophilus Influenzae Type B Conjugate
    Vaccine
  Hepatitis B Virus Vaccine Inactivated
  Measles, Mumps, and Rubella Virus Vaccine
    Live
  Poliovirus Vaccine Live Oral

Passive Immunizing Agents
  Hepatitis B Immune Globulin
  Immune Globulin
  Rh$_0$ (D) Immune Globulin
  Tetanus Immune Globulin

Nursing Process

Assessment
Nursing Diagnoses
Planning
  Outcome criteria
Implementation
Evaluation

Glossary

Active immunization (im′ u nĭ za′ shən) A process that causes a complete and long-lasting immunity to infection to develop through exposure of the body to a relatively harmless form of the antigen. This imprints a memory on the body's immune system and stimulates the body's defenses to fend off any subsequent exposure to the pathogen. (p. 664)

Antibody (an′ tĭ bod′ e) Molecules used by the cell-mediated immune system to attack and kill all substances foreign to the body. (p. 666)

Antibody titer (ti′ tər) Amount of an antibody needed to react with a specific antigen. (p. 666)

Antigen (an′ tĭ jən) A substance, usually a protein, that causes the formation of an antibody and reacts specifically with that antibody. (p. 664)

Biological A substance of biologic origin used to prevent, treat, or cure infectious diseases. (p. 664)

Booster shot An antigen, such as a vaccine or toxoid, that is usually administered in an amount smaller than that in the original immunization. It is given to maintain the immune response at an appropriate level. (p. 664)

Cell-mediated immune system Part of the immune system stimulated by active immunizing agents. (p. 666)

Herd immunity Resistance to a disease in an entire community or population because a large proportion of its members are immune to it. (p. 667)

Immunizing biological Toxoid or vaccine targeted against an infectious microorganism. (p. 664)

Immunoglobulin (im' u no glob'u lin) A glycoprotein used by the cell-mediated immune system to attack and kill all substances foreign to the body. (p. 666)

Passive immunization A process that fights infection but by bypassing the immune system. It involves giving a person serum or concentrated immune globulins obtained directly from humans or animals that directly give that person the means to fight off the invading microorganism. The person's immune system does not have to manufacture them. (p. 664)

Passive immunizing agents Agents containing antibodies that can kill or inactivate pathogens. These are directly injected into a person and provide them with the means to fend off infection, bypassing their own immune system. (p. 667)

Toxoid (tok' soid) Antigenic (foreign) preparation or gram-positive exotoxin that is detoxified with chemicals or heat. (p. 666)

Vaccine (vak' sen') A suspension of live, attenuated, or killed microorganisms that can promote an artificially cultivated active immunity against a particular microorganism. (p. 664)

Immunity and Immunization

Centuries ago it was noticed that persons who suffered a certain disease acquired an immune tolerance to it, so that, when exposed to it again, they did not suffer a second bout. This basic observation prompted scientists to investigate ways of artificially producing this tolerance. Along with this came an understanding of the way in which the normal immune system functions, a knowledge important to an understanding of how immunizing agents work. Briefly, when the body first comes in contact with an invading organism **(antigen),** some specific information is imprinted into a memory bank so that the body can effectively repel any later invasion by that same organism. It is because of this process that persons rarely suffer twice from certain diseases such as mumps, chickenpox, and measles. Instead they have a complete and long-lasting immunity to those infections.

There are two ways of cultivating this immunity— actively and passively. In **active immunization** the body is exposed to a relatively harmless form of the antigen (foreign invader), which imprints this information on the body's memory bank and stimulates the body's defenses to resist any subsequent exposure, but without actually causing the infection. In **passive immunization,** serum or concentrated immune globulins

obtained from humans or animals are injected into a person, directly giving that person the substance needed to fight off the invading microorganism. This type of immunization bypasses the immune system. The major differences between active and passive immunity are summarized in Table 44-1 and discussed in greater depth in the following sections.

ACTIVE IMMUNIZATION

Toxoids and vaccines are known as **immunizing biologicals.** In general **biologicals** are substances such as antitoxins, serum, toxoids, vaccines, or similar preparations that are used to prevent, treat, or cure infectious diseases. Immunizing biologicals are toxoids or vaccines that target a particular infectious microorganism.

Toxoids

Toxoids are antigenic (foreign) preparations or gram-positive exotoxins that are detoxified (attenuated) with chemicals or heat, rendering them nontoxic and unable to revert back to a toxic form, but nonetheless highly antigenic. In other words, toxoids are diluted, changed, or altered substances (exotoxins) that are normally secreted from bacteria. When injected into a person, this causes the person's immune system to mount an immune response by producing a specific antibody (an antitoxic antibody) against this antigen, which can then neutralize tissue-destroying bacterial exotoxins that may subsequently be introduced into the body. First developed in 1923 at the Pasteur Institute by Ramon and his associates, the toxoids now available are effective against the toxin-producing diseases diphtheria and tetanus.

Vaccines

Vaccines are suspensions of live, attenuated (weakened), or killed (inactivated) microorganisms that can artificially promote the acquisition of active immunity against the particular organism. These slight alterations in the bacteria and viruses prevent the person injected with the substance from contracting the disease, but are able to promote active immunization against the pathogen. Persons vaccinated with live bacteria or virus enjoy lifelong immunity against that particular disease. Only partial immunity is conferred on those vaccinated with killed bacteria or virus, and for this reason they must be given periodic **booster shots** to maintain the protection of the immune system against infection with this bacteria or virus. One exception to this is the smallpox vaccine because it utilizes live cowpox virus instead of the more virulent smallpox virus.

Table 44-1	Active Versus Passive Immunity	
DIFFERENCES	ACTIVE	PASSIVE
Type of immunization	Toxoid or vaccine.	Immune globulin or antitoxin.
Mechanism of action	Causes an Ag-Ab response; similar to exposure to natural disease process.	Results from direct administration of exogenous Ab; the Ab concentration will decrease over time, so if reexposure is expected, it is wise to continue passive immunizations.
Indication	Minimizes or entirely avoids active infection. Provides long-lasting or permanent immunity.	For persons who are immunodeficient, have a contraindication to active immunization, have been exposed to disease, or anticipate exposure to the disease; it provides temporary protection; it does not stimulate an Ab response in the host.

Ab, antibody; *Ag,* antigen.

In fact, some of the first work in the development of vaccines was done in the area of smallpox immunization, starting with Lady Mary Montagu, who in 1718 introduced the Eastern practice of inoculating against the smallpox virus by applying it to the nasal membranes. In 1774 Benjamin Jesty was the first to use cowpox virus inoculations to prevent smallpox. Edward Jenner, an English physician who noticed that milkmaids who had suffered cowpox infections were rarely victims of smallpox, was the first to study the relationship of cowpox to smallpox immunity. This observation led to the development of the smallpox vaccine, which utilizes the cowpox virus. In 1796 he successfully immunized a young boy against smallpox by vaccinating him with cowpox virus obtained from a cowpox vesicle on an infected cow.

With the help of the modern version of this vaccine, smallpox has now been eradicated since 1980. The advent of vaccines in general has dramatically changed the way in which we deal with public health problems. Today there are more than twenty infectious diseases for which there are vaccines, and the past decade alone has witnessed the appearance of nine new or improved vaccines.

These newer vaccines contain some extract or synthetic extract of the pathogen rather than the actual microbe and are produced by genetic engineering methods. The vaccines yielded are actually viral or bacterial antigenic preparations, and these are the substances that cause the immune system to produce antibodies against them and hence induce immunity. Examples of viral vaccines (antigenic preparations) include hepatitis B and influenza, the latter also possibly containing the whole virus or the split virus particle. Bacterial vaccines against meningitis (meningococcus), *haemophilus influenzae,* and pneumococcus contain selected bacterial capsular polysaccharides

(bacterial particles) that are taken from the respective microbes.

The process of attenuating or killing infectious microbes that are otherwise extremely virulent renders them safe for use in immunizing vaccines by removing that portion of them that causes infection. The advantage to such vaccines is that they have much greater antigenicity and produce more effective and longer-lasting immunity than inactivated vaccines. The attenuating or killing agent is usually a chemical such as formaldehyde or a physical mechanism such as heat. Attenuation may also be accomplished by the repeated passage of the microbe through some medium such as a fertile hen egg or a special tissue culture. The currently available immunizing vaccines are listed later in the box on the next page. Besides the individual active immunizing agents, there are several combinations of various vaccines and toxoids, and these are used especially in infants. Examples are the diphtheria and tetanus toxoid with pertussis vaccine (DTP) and the measles, mumps, and rubella vaccine (MMR).

The search for new and better agents is a never-ending one. One that is the current focus of worldwide research is the development of a safe and effective vaccine against the human immunodeficiency virus, which causes AIDS, an endeavor that is proving very difficult and time-consuming. An effective immunizing biological effective against malaria is also being sought. Indeed, an immunizing biological effective against every infectious disease is the ultimate goal.

PASSIVE IMMUNIZATION

As already mentioned, passive immunization bypasses the host's immune system and consists in inoculating the person with serum or immune globulins obtained

Available Immunizing Agents

Serums

Antivenin (Crotalidae) polyvalent
Antivenin (*Latrodectus mactans*)
Antivenin (*Micrurus fulvius*)
Digoxin Immune Fab
Diphtheria antitoxin
Hepatitis B immune globulin
Immune globulin
Rabies immune globulin
Rh$_0$(D) immune globulin
Tetanus immune globulin
Varicella-zoster immune globulin
Widow spider species antivenin

Toxoids

Diphtheria and tetanus toxoids
Tetanus and diphtheria toxoids
Tetanus toxoid

Vaccines

BCG vaccine
Cholera vaccine
Haemophilus influenzae type b conjugate vaccine
Hepatitis B virus vaccine inactivated
Influenza virus vaccine
Japanese encephalitis virus vaccine
Measles virus vaccine live
Mumps virus vaccine live
Plague vaccine
Pneumococcal vaccine, polyvalent
Poliovirus vaccine live oral
Rabies vaccine
Rubella virus vaccine live
Smallpox vaccine
Typhoid vaccine
Yellow fever vaccine

cause their immune systems are too suppressed to do so. Persons who already have the disease the passive immunizing agent targets are also candidates for these agents, especially those with diseases that are rapidly fatal, such as rabies and hepatitis. Because these diseases are so rapidly fatal, the body does not have time to mount an adequate defense against them, with death occurring before it can do so. The passive immunization of these people confers a temporary protection that is usually sufficient to keep the invading organism from killing them, even though it does not stimulate an antibody response.

The passive immunizing agents consist of three groups of agents—the antitoxins, the immune globulins, and snake and spider antivenins. The antitoxins are purified antiserums that are usually obtained from horses inoculated with the toxin. The immune globulins represent concentrated preparations containing predominantly immunoglobulin G and are harvested from a large pool of blood donors. Antivenins are serums obtained from animals (usually horses) that have been injected with the particular venom. The serum contains immunoglobulins that can neutralize the toxic effects of the venoms.

Immunizing Agents

Mechanism of Action

Active immunizing agents consist of vaccines and toxoids that can be administered either orally or intravenously and that work by stimulating that part of the immune system known as the **cell-mediated immune system**. The system makes use of substances called **immunoglobulins**, of which there are five, designated IgM, IgG, IgA, IgE, and IgD, to attack and kill the foreign substances that invade the body. These foreign substances are called antigens, and the immunoglobulins are called **antibodies.**

Vaccines contain substances that trigger the formation of these antibodies against specific pathogens. Sometimes these substances are the actual live, attenuated (weakened) pathogen or they are a killed pathogen and the amount of antibodies they cause to be produced can be measured in the blood. The **antibody titer** is the amount needed to effectively protect the body against the particular pathogen. Sometimes the levels of these antibodies decline over time. When this happens, a second dose of the vaccine is given to restore the antibody titers to a level that can protect the person against the infection. This second dose is referred to as a booster shot.

Toxoids are altered forms of bacterial toxins that

from humans or animals. These substances give the person the means to fight off the invading organism. Passive immunization can occur naturally between a mother and the fetus or the nursing infant when the mother passes maternal antibodies directly either through the placenta to the fetus or through breast milk to the nursing infant. This is called *naturally acquired passive immunity,* but because it can occur only between a mother and the unborn fetus or between the mother and her nursing infant, other ways have had to be found of accomplishing it by artificial means. Such passive immunization is called *artificially acquired passive immunity*. It differs from active immunization in that it is a comparatively transitory (short-lived) immune state.

As noted in Table 44-1, there are specific populations that can benefit from passive immunization but not from active immunization. Such persons are those rendered immunodeficient for whatever reason (e.g. drugs, disease) and who therefore cannot develop immunity in response to a toxoid or vaccine injection be-stimulate the production of antibodies in the same way as vaccines.

Because both toxoids and vaccines rely on the immunized host to mount an immune response, the host's immune system must be intact. Therefore patients who are immunocompromised, such as those undergoing immunosuppressive chemotherapy, those receiving immunosuppressive therapy to prevent the rejection of transplanted organs, and those with immunosuppressive diseases such as AIDS, and who as a result usually cannot mount an immune response, should not receive vaccines or toxoids.

As already explained, **passive immunizing agents** are the actual antibodies (immunoglobulins) that can kill or inactivate the pathogen. The process is called "passive" because the person's immune system does not participate in it. However, because of this, immunity acquired in this way generally endures for much less time than that produced by active immunization, lasting only until the injected immunoglobulins are removed from the person's immune system by the reticuloendothelial system.

Drug Effects

Vaccines and toxoids are the active immunizing agents that have been developed for the prevention of many illnesses caused by bacteria and their toxins as well as those caused by various viruses. Antivenins, antitoxins, and immune globulins comprise the passive immunizing agents. Such agents can inactivate spider and snake venom, bacterial toxins (exotoxins), and potentially lethal viruses. A list of the currently available immunizing agents is given in the box on p. 666.

Therapeutic Uses

Active immunization is used to prevent infection caused by bacterial toxins or viruses, and as previously noted, it confers long-lasting or permanent immunity. If a person immunized against a particular pathogen is then exposed to that foreign invader, this causes a prompt and significant increase in the person's immunoglobulin (antibody) level. However, there is an interesting phenomenon that occurs in terms of the number of people immunized, in that the successful immunization of 95% or more of a population confers protection on the entire population majority of the population cannot contract the disease. This is called **herd immunity**.

As already noted, passive immunizing agents consist of antivenins, antitoxins, and immune globulins. Antivenins, also known as *serums,* are used to prevent or minimize the effects of poisoning by the venoms of crotalids (rattlesnakes, copperheads, and cotton-

mouths), black widow spiders, or coral snakes, some of which can be lethal. Most healthy adults do not die from the bites of spiders and snakes if prompt and appropriate treatment (i.e., the administration of the appropriate antivenin) is instituted. However, very young children and elderly people with health problems are particularly susceptible to the effects of the venoms of some of these animals. In either situation an antivenin is needed in order to give the person who has been bitten the substance needed to overcome the effects of the venom.

As is well known, certain viruses are very potent and even potentially lethal, hepatitis B and rabies being examples of such viruses. They can do major harm very quickly before the infected person can mount an effective immune response against them. The passive immunization of the person with the appropriate immune globulin gives them the antibody needed to fend off the harmful effects of the virus. There are also immune globulins available for protection against some bacterial infections, two examples being pertussis and tetanus.

The antitoxins are used for protection against certain very harmful bacteria such as those that cause botulism and diphtheria.

Side Effects and Adverse Effects

The undesirable effects of the various immunizing agents can range from mild and transient to more serious and even life-threatening ones. The minor and more severe ones are listed in Table 44-2. The minor reactions can be treated with acetaminophen and rest. More severe reactions such as fever higher than 103° F (39.4° C) should be treated with acetaminophen and sponge baths. Serum sickness sometimes occurs after repeated injections of equine-made immunizing agents. The signs and symptoms consist of edema of the face, tongue, and throat; rash; urticaria; arthritis; adenopathy; fever; flushing; itching; cough; dyspnea; cyanosis; vomiting; and cardiovascular collapse. This is best treated with analgesics, antihistamines, ephedrine, or corticosteroids.

The various types of severe reactions that can occur in response to immunizing agents and the time frames involved are summarized in Table 44-3.

Interactions

Immunosuppressive agents such as corticosteroids and cancer chemotherapy agents block generation of active immunity. Isoniazid may diminish the response to Bacillus Calmette-Guérin (BCG) vaccine. Hepatitis B immune globulin has a drug interaction with live vaccines; defer for 3 months after dose of immune globulin.

Dosages

For the recommended dosages of selected immunizing agents, see the dosages table on p. 669.

DRUG PROFILES

Some of the more commonly used vaccines, toxoids, and immunoglobulins are described in the following sections. All the available immunizing agents are listed in the box on p. 666.

ACTIVE IMMUNIZING AGENTS
BACILLUS CALMETTE-GUÉRIN VACCINE

Bacillus Calmette-Guérin (BCG Vaccine or TICE BCG) vaccine is used to promote active immunity to tuberculosis (TB). It is a live, attenuated vaccine derived from a slightly weakened Calmette-Guérin strain of *Mycobacterium bovis.* There are several bacterial strains of this bacteria; the particular strain used in the United States is the Tice substrain. Because this strain is similar to *Mycobacterium tuberculosis,* vaccination with BCG causes a natural infection that promotes cell-mediated immunity against TB through the production of antibodies targeted against this foreign invader.

The BCG vaccine may also be used as a nonspecific immunotherapeutic agent for the treatment of superficial bladder tumors. When used for this purpose it is directly injected into the bladder, a process called *local treatment.* It may also be used for the treatment and possible prevention of recurrent tumors in patients with bladder cancer.

BCG vaccine is available for percutaneous injection using a multiple-puncture device. It is not known whether the vaccine is harmful to the fetus of pregnant women or if it can affect reproduction. It should therefore be used in pregnant women only when absolutely necessary. BCG vaccine is contraindicated in patients with a hypersensitivity to it, those showing a significant positive reaction to tuberculin, those who have recently received smallpox immunizations, burn patients, and those with hypogammaglobulinemia, a congenital immunodeficiency, sarcoidosis, leukemia, lymphoma, a generalized malignant condition, HIV infection, or any other disorder involving an altered natural immune response, such as is the case in patients who are on immunosuppressive therapy. The recommended dosages for the vaccine are given in the dosages table on the next page.

DIPHTHERIA AND TETANUS TOXOIDS ADSORBED AND TETANUS AND DIPHTHERIA TOXOIDS ADSORBED

Diphtheria and tetanus toxoids adsorbed (DT) for pediatric use and tetanus and diphtheria toxoids adsorbed (Td) for adult use are toxoids obtained from the bacteria *Corynebacterium diphtheriae.* To make the agents, diphtheria and tetanus toxins are taken from these bacteria, attenuated into toxoids, and adsorbed onto aluminum hydroxide, aluminum phosphate, or potassium alum. They are given by injection to infants and children (DT) (6 weeks to 6 years old) and older children and adults (Td) (7 years of age and older) with functioning immune systems. They promote immunity to diphtheria and tetanus by inducing the production of specific antitoxins.

Table 44-2	Immunizing Agents: Minor and Severe Adverse Effects
BODY SYSTEM	**SIDE/ADVERSE EFFECT**
Minor effects	
CNS	Fever, adenopathy
Integumentary	Minor rash, soreness at injection site, urticaria, arthritis
Severe effects	
CNS	Fever >103° F (39.4° C), encephalitis, convulsions, peripheral neuropathy, anaphylactic reactions, shock, unconsciousness
Integumentary	Urticaria, rash
Respiratory	Dyspnea
Other	Cyanosis

Table 44-3	Time Frame of Serious Reactions
REACTION	**TIME FRAME**
Anaphylaxis	Within 24 hr of immunization
Encephalopathy	Within 7 days of DTP or 15 days of MMR
Shock-collapse or hyporesponsive period	Within 7 days of DTP
Death	No time limit

DTP, diphtheria and tetanus toxoid with pertussis vaccine; *MMR,* measles, mumps, and rubella vaccine.

DOSAGES

SELECTED IMMUNIZING AGENTS

AGENT	PHARMACOLOGIC CLASS	DOSAGE RANGE	PURPOSE
Active Immunizing Agents			
Bacillus Calmette-Guérin vaccine (BCG vaccine or TICE BCG)	Live attenuated cow TB vaccine	*Pediatric <1 mo* Half adult dose administered percutaneously multiple puncture disk. WHO recommends admin. by intradermal injection. *Pediatric >1 mo/Adult* 0.2-0.3 ml on skin by percutaneous administration	TB prophylaxis
Diphtheria and tetanus toxoids adsorbed (DT = pediatric)	Mixed toxoid	*Infants* IM: 0.5 ml, followed by 0.5 ml in 6-8 wk and 0.5-ml booster after 1 yr	Diphtheria and tetanus prophylaxis
Tetanus and diphtheria toxoids adsorbed (TD = adult)	Mixed toxoid	*Adult* IM: 0.5 ml, followed by 0.5 ml in 4-8 wk and 0.5 ml in 6-12 mo	Diphtheria and tetanus prophylaxis
Haemophilus influenzae type b conjugate vaccine (Hib)	Bacterial capsular antigenic extract vaccine	*Infants 2-6 mo* IM: three 0.5-ml injections about 2 mo apart	*H. influenzae* type b prophylaxis
Hepatitis B virus vaccine inactivated (Recombivax HB, Engerix-B)	Viral surface antigen	*Pediatric to 10 y/o* IM: 2.5 or 5 μg doses at birth, then at 1-2 mo and at 6-18 mo of age	Hepatitis B virus prophylaxis
Measles, mumps, and rubella virus vaccine live (MMR II)	Live, attenuated mixed viral vaccine	*Pediatric >12 mo/Adults* SC: 0.5 ml and a booster at 4-6 yr	Measles, mumps, rubella prophylaxis
Poliovirus vaccine live oral (Orimune)	Live, attenuated viral vaccine	*Infants* PO 0.5 ml at 6-12 wk of age 0.5 ml 6-8 wk later 0.5 ml at about 12 mo of age	Polio prophylaxis
Passive Immunizing Agents			
Hepatitis B immune globulin (H-BIG, Hep-B-Gammagee, HyperHep)	IgG immune globulin	*Infants* IM: 0.5 ml within 12 hr after birth *Adult* IM: 0.06 mg/kg after exposure and repeated in 30 days	Passive hepatitis B prophylaxis
Immune globulin IV (Gammagard, Gammar IV, Iveegam, Polygam, Sandoglobulin, Venoglobulin)	Mixed immune globulins	IV: Refer to current manufacturer's dosage recommendations for products not listed. Gammagard: 100-400 mg/kg once monthly. Sandoglobulin: 200-300 mg/kg once monthly.	Immune deficiency syndrome
		Gammagard: 1 g/kg. Up to 3 doses on alternate days Sandoglobulin: 400 mg/kg on 2-5 consecutive days	Idiopathic thrombocytopenic purpura
		Gammagard: 400 mg/kg every 3-4 wk	Infections secondary to B cell lymphocytic leukemia

continued

SELECTED IMMUNIZING AGENTS—cont'd

AGENT	PHARMACOLOGIC CLASS	DOSAGE RANGE	PURPOSE
Rh$_0$ (D) immune globulin (Hyp●Rho-D Mini-Dose, MICRhoGAM, Gamulin)	Immunosuppressant globulin	*Adult female* IM: inject total contents of a single vial within 72 hr after delivery Micro-dose-IM: inject full contents of a single vial after abortion/pregnancy termination up to 12 wk of gestation	Postpartum antibody suppression
Tetanus immune globulin-TIB	Immune globulin (Hyper-Tet)	IM: 250 U as a single dose	Postexposure passive tetanus prophylaxis
		IM: 3000-6000 U	Tetanus treatment

It has been recommended that children younger than 7 years also receive immunization against pertussis. Therefore diphtheria and tetanus toxoids with whole-cell pertussis vaccine adsorbed (DTP) and diphtheria and tetanus toxoids with acellular pertussis vaccine adsorbed (DTaP) are the preferred preparations for primary and booster immunization against these diseases in children 6 weeks to 6 years of age, unless the pertussis component is contraindicated.

Tetanus, diphtheria and pertussis are prevalent in the populations of many developing countries throughout the world, and as a result, the risk of contracting one of these diseases may be high there. Full immunization against these diseases with DTP or DtaP is recommended for both travelers to these areas as well as the inhabitants. Td is used in persons 7 years of age or older requiring a primary or booster immunization against tetanus for routine wound management. Emergency booster doses of Td (for adult use) are unnecessary when the wound is clean and minor (not tetanus prone) and the patient has received a primary or booster immunization against tetanus within the past 10 years.

These toxoids (DT, Td, DTP, and DTaP) are available only as parenteral preparations to be given as deep intramuscular injections. They are contraindicated in persons who have had a prior systemic hypersensitivity reaction or a neurologic reaction to one of the ingredients. Some manufacturers state that use is contraindicated in the setting of concurrent acute or active infections but not in the setting of minor illness. Although there have been very few, if any, studies documenting the safety of their use in pregnant women, it is generally considered safe to give diphtheria, tetanus, and pertussis toxoids after the first trimester, but optimally during the second or third trimesters. The

Hib Combination Products

HIB COMBINATION INGREDIENTS	TRADE NAME
Hib polysaccharide conjugate (diphtheria toxoid conjugate) vaccine	ProHIBit
Hib polysaccharide conjugate (meningococcal protein conjugate) vaccine	Pedvax HIB
Hib polysaccharide conjugate (tetanus toxoid conjugate) vaccine	OmniHIB
Hib oligosaccharide conjugate (diphtheria CRM197 protein conjugate) vaccine	HibTITER

Hib, haemophilus influenzae *type b.*

recommended dosages for these toxoids are given in the dosages table on p. 669.

HAEMOPHILUS INFLUENZAE TYPE B CONJUGATE VACCINE

H. influenzae type b (Hib) vaccine is a noninfectious, bacteria-derived vaccine. It is made by extracting *H. influenzae* particles that are antigenic (cause an antigen-antibody reaction) and are then attached to a protein carrier. They are given by injection to adults and children considered at high risk of acquiring the *H. influenzae* infection. Such patients commonly have one of the following conditions: no spleen, sickle cell anemia, an immunodeficiency syndrome, or Hodgkin's disease.

The Hib vaccine may be combined with toxoids to make various combination products. Some examples of these combination products are listed in the box above. All these products are parenteral products that are administered intramuscularly. These vaccines are contraindicated in persons who have had a previous hypersensitivity reaction to any one of the ingredients. It is not known whether the vaccines can cause fetal harm when administered to pregnant women or whether they can affect fertility. As a result, the administration of any of the vaccines during pregnancy is not recommended. The recommended dosages for the vaccine are given in the dosages table on p. 669.

HEPATITIS B VIRUS VACCINE INACTIVATED

Hepatitis B virus vaccine inactivated (Recombivax HB and Engerix-B) is a noninfectious viral vaccine made from yeast fed the genetic code of the hepatitis B surface antigen (HBsAg). The yeast then produces this antigenic substance in mass quantities. After this it is attached to a substance called *alum* and made into the injection that is used to vaccinate persons against hepatitis B. This is an example of recombinant DNA technology at work. This antigenic HBsAg is used to promote active immunity to hepatitis B infection in persons considered at high risk for potential exposure to the hepatitis B virus or HbsAg-positive materials (e.g., blood, plasma, serum).

The vaccine is contraindicated in persons who are hypersensitive to yeast. Pregnancy is not considered a contraindication to use. The potential for exposure to hepatitis B infection in a pregnant woman and the potential for the development of chronic infection in the neonate are both good reasons to give the vaccine. The vaccine is administered by intramuscular injection. There are three main formulations designed for three different populations: a *pediatric formulation* for neonates, infants, children, and adolescents; an *adult formulation* for persons older than 20 years of age; and a *dialysis formulation* for predialysis and dialysis patients or for other immunocompromised persons. The recommended dosages for this vaccine are given in the dosages table on p. 669.

MEASLES, MUMPS, AND RUBELLA VIRUS VACCINE LIVE

The measles, mumps, and rubella vaccine (MMR II) is a live, attenuated virus preparation consisting of live measles, mumps, and rubella viruses that are weakened (attenuated). They promote active immunity to measles, mumps, and rubella by inducing the production of virus-specific IgG and IgM antibodies. The antibody response to initial vaccination resembles that caused by primary natural infection.

The measles vaccine or any of the combination products that include the virus are contraindicated in persons with a history of anaphylactic, anaphylactoid, or some other immediate reaction to egg ingestion. It is also contraindicated in persons who have had an

Measles Vaccine Combination Products	
MEASLES VACCINE COMBINATION PRODUCTS	**TRADE NAME**
Measles virus vaccine live (more attenuated Enders' line)	Attenuvax
Measles and rubella virus vaccine live	MRVAX II
Measles, mumps, and rubella virus vaccine live	MMR II

anaphylactic reaction to topically or systemically administered neomycin. These vaccines should not be administered to pregnant women, and pregnancy should be avoided for 3 months after measles virus vaccination and 30 days after vaccination with a rubella-containing (MR or MMR) measles virus vaccine. This precaution is based on the theoretic risk of the live virus vaccine causing a fetal infection.

These vaccines are available only in the parenteral form and should be given only by subcutaneous injection. There are several combination products containing the live measles virus vaccine, and these are listed in the box above. The recommended dosages for this vaccine are given in the dosages table on p. 669.

POLIOVIRUS VACCINE LIVE ORAL

The poliovirus vaccine live oral (OPV; Orimune) is derived from live, attenuated types 1, 2, and 3 poliovirus obtained from monkey kidney tissue cultures. OPV promotes immunity to polio by causing the production of antibodies against the injected live, attenuated virus in the lymphatic tissues surrounding the intestinal tract. This occurs because the vaccine is taken orally. The intestinal tract is the normal portal of entry of poliovirus, and this intestinal immunity may reduce the number of temporary carriers and hence dissemination of the virus.

The poliovirus vaccine is available in a parenteral form as well. Unlike the OPV, which is a live, attenuated virus vaccine, this vaccine contains an inactivated form of the virus. The poliovirus vaccine inactivated (IPV) is administered subcutaneously. The various advantages and disadvantages of OPV and IPV and the different indications for their use are listed in Table 44-4. It is classified as pregnancy category B. The recommended dosages for this vaccine are given in the dosages table on p. 669.

PASSIVE IMMUNIZING AGENTS

The currently available antivenins, antitoxins, and immune globulins that comprise the passive immunizing

Table 44-4 Advantages, Disadvantages, and Indications for IPV and OPV

TYPE OF VACCINE	ADVANTAGES AND DISADVANTAGES	INDICATIONS
IPV	*Advantage:* enhanced inactivated poliovirus vaccine, which will result in more permanent immunity. *Disadvantages:* safe but gastrointestinal immunity is not induced, and immunity is not permanent; must be given every 5 yr; side effects include tenderness and fever.	IPV for healthy adults who have never received polio vaccine and who are in close contact with an infant who is to receive TOPV.
OPV	*Advantages:* easy to administer, relatively inexpensive, and effectively induces immunity against all types of polio (GI included). *Disadvantages:* live virus is shed in stool for 6-8 wk after immunization; there is potential for transmission to nonimmunized persons; exposed nonimmunized adults or immunosuppressed persons may contract inactive disease.	TOPV in those >18 yr old (but NOT in those who are functionally or pharmacologically immunosuppressed). TOPV for the nonimmunized adults traveling to an endemic area.

TOPV, trivalent oral polio vaccine.

agents are listed in the box on p. 666. Those that are more frequently used are described in the following profiles.

HEPATITIS B IMMUNE GLOBULIN

Hepatitis B immune globulin (H-BIG₂ Hep-B-Gammagee, and HyperHep) is used to provide passive immunity to hepatitis B infection in the prophylaxis and postexposure treatment of persons exposed to hepatitis B virus or HbsAg-positive materials (e.g., blood, plasma, serum). It is prepared from the plasma of human donors with high titers of antibody to HbsAg. All donors are tested for the antibody to HIV to prevent transmission of the virus.

H-BIG is contraindicated in persons who have exhibited hypersensitivity to it. Because of the possible devastating consequences of exposure to hepatitis B infection, pregnancy is not considered a contraindication to the use of H-BIG when there is a clear need for it. H-BIG is available only in a parenteral form that is administered intramuscularly. The recommended dosages for hepatitis B immune globulin are given in the dosages table on p. 669.

IMMUNE GLOBULIN

Immune globulin (Gammagard, Gammar, Iveegam, Polygam, Sandoglobulin, Venoglobulin) can be administered intramuscularly or intravenously. They are used to provide passive immunity by increasing antibody titer and antigen-antibody reaction potential. The agents are available only parenterally and called *immune globulin IM* (IGIM) and *immune globulin IV* (IGIV), which designates the route of administration. They are given to help prevent certain infectious diseases in sus-

---

Uses of Immune Globulins

FDA-Approved

IV:
Primary immunodeficiency diseases
Idiopathic thrombocytopenic purpura (ITP)
Chronic lymphocytic leukemia (CLL)
IM:
Hepatitis A
Immune deficiencies
Measles
Varicella

Non–FDA-Approved
Kawasaki syndrome
Neonatal sepsis
Respiratory syncytial virus (RSV)
Other viral infections
AIDS
Autoimmune disorders
Asthma
Epilepsy
Cystic fibrosis

---

ceptible persons or to ameliorate the diseases in those already infected with them. Immune globulins are pooled from the blood of at least 1000 human donors. This plasma is prepared by cold alcohol fractionation and usually washed with a detergent to destroy any harmful viruses such as hepatitis or HIV. There are many FDA-approved and non–FDA-approved uses for immune globulins. These are listed in the box above. Immune globulins are contraindicated in patients hypersensitive to them and are classified as pregnancy category C agents. The recommended dosages for the immune globulins are given in the dosages table on p. 669.

Rh₀(D) IMMUNE GLOBULIN

$Rh_0(D)$ immune globulin (Rhesonativ, HypRho-D Mini-Dose, MICRhoGAM, Gamulin Rh) is used to suppress the active antibody response and the formation of anti-$Rh_0(D)$ in the $Rh_0(D)$-negative person exposed to Rh-positive blood. Because an $Rh_0(D)$-negative person reacts to Rh-positive blood as if it were a foreign, "non-self," product, an immune response develops against it and an antigen-antibody reaction occurs. This can be fatal, and the administration of this immune globulin helps prevent the reaction, and hence this dire outcome.

$Rh_0(D)$ immune globulin is prepared from the plasma or serum of adults with a high titer of anti-$Rh_0(D)$ antibody to the red blood cell antigen $Rh_0(D)$. This product is available only in a parenteral formulation and is given by intramuscular injection. This immune globulin is contraindicated in persons who have been previously immunized with this drug and in $Rh_0(D)$-positive/D^u–positive patients. The recommended dosages for $Rh_0(D)$ immune globulin are given in the dosages table on p. 669.

TETANUS IMMUNE GLOBULIN

Tetanus immune globulin (TIG; Hyper-Tet) is a passive immunizing agent effective against tetanus. It contains tetanus antitoxin antibodies that neutralize the exotoxin produced by *Clostridium tetani*, the organism that causes tetanus. TIG is prepared from the plasma of adults hyperimmunized with the tetanus toxoid and is given as prophylaxis to persons with tetanus-prone wounds. It may also be used to treat tetanus. Hypersensitivity, active infection, a poliomyelitis outbreak, and immunosuppression are contraindications to its use, and it is classified as a pregnancy category C agent. TIG is available only as a parenteral drug that is given by intramuscular injection. The recommended dosages for TIG are given in the dosages table on p. 670.

NURSING PROCESS

ASSESSMENT

Before administering a toxoid or vaccine, the nurse should gather complete information about the patient's health history, including information on allergies, the patient's present health status, previous reactions and responses to these agents, any allergy test

Patient Teaching TIPS

Toxoids and Vaccines

✔ It is not uncommon for patients to experience a localized reaction to the injection of toxoid, vaccine, or passive immunizing agent. They should be told that they can relieve the discomfort by placing warm compresses on the injection site, resting, and taking acetaminophen. Instructions for the care of infants or children suffering such reactions should be provided by the child's health care provider.

✔ Patients or the parents or caregiver of the child should notify the physician should high or prolonged fever, rash, itching, or shortness of breath occur.

✔ Patients or parents should always keep a double record (two copies kept in separate places) of all the medications being taken.

results, the use of any immunosuppressants, the presence of autoimmune or immunosuppressing disease, infection, and the pregnancy status. In children who are to receive a vaccine or toxoid, the immunization schedule and the dose ordered by the physician must be followed.

Because passive immunizing agents may precipitate serum sickness, patients with chronic illness or who are elderly or debilitated need to be assessed carefully before treatment (i.e., vital signs, intake and output, ECG, and baseline assessment). Contraindications to the use of passive immunizing agents include hypersensitivity to them and patients with active infections or who are immunosuppressed.

Contraindications to the administration of immunizing agents include active infections, febrile illnesses, a history of reactions or serious side effects to the agent, and pregnancy. Patients who are already immunosuppressed, such as those with AIDS, elderly patients, patients with chronic diseases or cancer, and neonates are at increased risk for experiencing serious side effects to toxoids or vaccines, so cautious use of these agents is called for in such patients.

NURSING DIAGNOSES

Nursing diagnoses related to the administration of immunizing agents include:

■ Risk for injury related to possible side effects of or allergic reactions to the immunizing agent.

■ Altered comfort related to local pain or systemic effects caused by injection of toxoid, vaccine, or passive immunizing agent.

- Noncompliance with therapy related to fears of reactions.
- Knowledge deficit concerning the use of toxoids, vaccines, or passive immunizing agents.

PLANNING

Goals for patients receiving immunizing agents include:

- Patient states side effects of medication.
- Patient manages minimal discomfort stemming from the administration of a toxoid, vaccine, or passive immunizing agent.
- Patient remains compliant with therapy.
- Patient returns for follow-up injections and booster injections and for follow-up visits with the physician.

Outcome Criteria

Outcome criteria related to the use of immunologic agents include:

- Patient experiences minimal side effects of or allergic reactions to the immunizing agent such as fever, chills, myalgias, and bronchospasms (allergic).
- Patient uses measures such as nonaspirin analgesics or diphenhydramine (as recommended by physician) to relieve localized discomfort or to alleviate any reactions.
- Patient remains compliant with therapy for prevention of illness or disease through following up with physician.
- Patient will state the problems to report immediately to the physician such as fever higher than 101° F, infection, wheezing, or increasing weakness.

TAKE HOME POINTS

Antibodies and Antigens

- Foreign substance to the body is termed an *antigen;* the body creates a substance called an *antibody* to specifically bind to it.
- The body has cells called *plasma cells* that remember what that particular antigen looks like.
- These plasma cells manufacture the antibodies and will mass produce clones of the antibodies upon reexposure to a particular antigen.

Immunization

- Two types: active and passive.
- Different types of agents used in each.
- Are indicated for use in different patient populations.

Active Immunization

- Utilizes a toxoid or a vaccine.
- Involves exposing the body to a relatively harmless form of the antigen (foreign invader) to imprint memory and stimulate the body's defenses against any subsequent exposure.
- The person receiving must have an active, functioning immune system.
- Provides long-lasting or permanent immunity.

Passive Immunization

- Utilizes immune globulins, antitoxins, or antivenins.
- Takes serum or concentrated immune globulins obtained from humans or animals.
- Injected into the person, directly giving him or her the ability to fight off the invading microorganism.
- For patients who are immunocompromised, been exposed to disease, or anticipate exposure to the disease.
- Provides temporary protection.
- Does not stimulate an antibody response in the host.

Nursing Considerations

- Patients who should *not* receive immunizing agents include those with active infections, febrile illnesses, or a history of a previous reaction or serious side effects to the agent. They are also usually contraindicated in pregnant women.
- Patients who are immunosuppressed are at greater risk for suffering serious side effects from immunizing agents.
- Parents should keep updated records of their children's and their own immunizations with any toxoids or vaccines.

IMPLEMENTATION

When administering immunologic agents, it is always important to recheck the specific protocols concerning their administration and the schedules of administration. In addition, it is always important to check and follow the manufacturer's recommendations concerning how the drug should be stored and administered, the routes and site of administration, the dosage, precautions pertaining to its use, and contraindications to its use. Parents of young children must be encouraged and told how to maintain an accurate journal of the child's immunization status. Patient teaching tips are presented on p. 673.

EVALUATION

Therapeutic responses in patients receiving immunizing agents are the prevention or amelioration of the disease. Adverse reactions to monitor for in patients receiving immunizing biologicals include localized swelling, redness, discomfort, and heat. Acetaminophen is recommended for the relief of these side effects in patients of all age groups. Warm compresses on the injection site may also help to ease some of the discomfort. The physician should be notified immediately if fever, rash, itching or shortness of breath occur, because these are the symptoms of an allergic reaction.

Critical Thinking A C T I V I T I E S

1. You are caring for a 56-year-old man who has recently been admitted because he is in a state of acute rejection of his transplanted heart, which he received over a year ago. This patient has been on cyclosporine, azathioprine, and prednisone at home and has now had muromonab (OKT-3) added to help stop the acute rejection. There has been an outbreak of the influenza virus at your hospital. One of your co-workers suggests vaccinating your patient with the flu vaccine that employee health has been administering to the employees. How should you respond to this co-worker.

2. Which of the following is a severe rare reaction to the influenza vaccine?
   a. Guillain-Barré syndrome
   b. Renal failure
   c. Hepatotoxicity
   d. Cardiomegaly

BIBLIOGRAPHY

Albanese J, Nutz P: *Mosby's 1995 nursing drug cards,* St Louis, 1995, Mosby.

Igoe JB, Goodwin LD: Meeting the challenge of immunizing the nation's children, *Pediatr Nurs* 17(6):583, 1991.

Johnson KB: *Harriet Lane handbook,* ed 13, St Louis, 1993, Mosby.

Keen JH: *Critical care and emergency drug reference,* St Louis, 1994, Mosby.

Knoben JE, Anderson PO: *Handbook of critical drug data,* ed 6, Hamilton, Ill, 1988, Drug Intelligence Publications.

McEvoy GK: *AHFS drug information,* Bethesda, Md, 1994, American Society of Hospital Pharmacists.

Skidmore-Roth L: *Mosby's 1995 nursing drug reference,* St Louis, 1995, Mosby.

Zanga JR: Should there be universal childhood vaccination against Hepatitis B? II. A rebuttal, *Pediatr Nurs* 19(5):447, 1993.

Chapter 45

Antineoplastic Agents

Objectives

When you reach the end of this chapter, you will be able to:

1 Discuss the purpose of antineoplastic agents in the treatment of cancer.
2 Classify antineoplastic agents by their mechanism of action.
3 List the common side effects of and adverse reactions to antineoplastic agents.
4 Discuss the mechanism of action of antineoplastic agents, cautions and contraindications to their use, the routes by which they are administered, and the drug interactions associated with their use.
5 Develop a comprehensive nursing care plan for the patient receiving antineoplastic agents.
6 Identify patient education issues and home referral or community services for patients receiving antineoplastic agents.

CHAPTER OUTLINE

Etiology of Cancer

Age- and Sex-related Differences
Genetic and Ethnic Factors
Oncogenic Viruses
Occupational and Environmental Carcinogens
Drugs
Radiation
Immunologic Factors

Cell Growth Cycle

Alkylating Agents
  Mechanism of action
  Drug effects
  Therapeutic uses
  Side effects and adverse effects
    Toxicity and management of overdose
  Interactions
  Dosages
Drug Profiles
    Mechlorethamine
  ⚓ Cyclophosphamide
  ⚓ Cisplatin
    Carmustine

Antimetabolites

Mechanism of Action
  Folic acid antagonism
  Purine antagonism
  Pyrimidine antagonism
Drug Effects

Therapeutic Uses
Side Effects and Adverse Effects
  Toxicity and management of overdose
Interactions
Dosages
Drug Profiles
Folate Antagonists
  ⚓ Methotrexate
Purine Antagonists
    Mercaptopurine
Pyrimidine Antagonists
    Cytarabine

Cytotoxic Antibiotics

  Mechanism of Action
  Drug Effects
  Therapeutic Uses
  Side Effects and Adverse Effects
    Toxicity and management of overdose
  Interactions
  Dosages
Drug Profiles
Anthracycline Cytotoxic Antibiotics
  ⚓ Doxorubicin
Other Cytotoxic Antibiotics
    Bleomycin

Mitotic Inhibitors

  Mechanism of Action
  Drug Effects

continued

Therapeutic uses
Side effects and adverse effects
    Toxicity and management of overdose
Interactions
Dosages
Drug Profiles
    Etoposide
    ⚓ Paclitaxel
    Vincristine

Miscellaneous Antineoplastics
Mechanism of action
Drug effects
Therapeutic uses
Side effects and adverse effects
Interactions
Dosages
Drug Profiles
    Altretamine
    Asparaginase
    Hydroxyurea
Nursing Process
Assessment
Nursing Diagnoses
Planning
    Outcome criteria
Implementation
Evaluation

■

Glossary

Alkylation (al′ kə la′ shən) Chemical reaction in which an alkyl group is transferred from an alkylating agent. When such organic reactions occur with a biologically significant cellular constituent such as DNA, they result in interference with mitosis and cell division. (p. 684)

Benign (be nīn′) Noncancerous and therefore not an immediate threat to life, even though treatment eventually may be required for health or cosmetic reasons. (p. 678)

Bifunctional Refers to alkylating agents that have two reactive alkyl groups that are able to alkylate two DNA molecules. (p. 684)

Carcinoma (kahr′ sĭ no′ mə) Malignant epithelial neoplasm that tends to invade surrounding tissue and to metastasize to distant regions of the body. (p. 678)

Cell cycle nonspecific Antineoplastic drugs that are cytotoxic in any phase of the cycle. (p. 681)

Cell cycle specific Antineoplastic drugs that are cytotoxic during a specific life cycle phase. (p. 681)

Dose-limited side effects Side effects that prevent the antineoplastic agent from being given in higher doses, often limiting the effectiveness of the drug. (p. 682)

Emetic potential (ə me′ tik) Potential of a substance to kill the cells of the stomach, resulting in nausea and vomiting. (p. 682)

Extravasation (ek stra ve′ ə sa′ shən) Passage or escape into the tissues, usually of blood, serum, or lymph but, in the context of antineoplastic treatment, of the agent. (p. 686)

Growth fraction Percentage of cells in mitosis at any given time. (p. 681)

Leucovorin rescue (loo′ ko vo′ rin) The use of leucovorin to reverse methotrexate-induced toxicity. (p. 690)

Leukemia (loo ke′ me ə) A malignant neoplasm of blood-forming tissues characterized by the diffuse replacement of bone marrow with proliferating leukocyte precursors, abnormal numbers and forms of immature white cells in the circulation, and the infiltration of lymph nodes, the spleen, and liver. (p. 678)

Lymphoma (lim fo′ mə) A neoplasm of lymphoid tissue that is usually malignant but in rare cases may be benign. (p. 678)

Malignant (mə lig′ nənt) Tending to worsen and cause death; anaplastic, invasive, and metastatic. (p. 678)

Metastasis (mə tas′ tə sis) The process by which a cancer spreads from the original site of growth to a new and remote part of the body. (p. 678)

Mitosis (mi to′ sis) Process of cell reproduction occurring in somatic cells and resulting in the formation of two genetically identical daughter cells containing the diploid number of chromosomes characteristic of the species. (p. 681)

Mitotic index (mi to′ tik) Number of cells per unit (usually 1000) undergoing mitosis during a given time. (p. 681)

Nadir (nā′ dər) Lowest point, such as the blood count after it has been depressed by chemotherapy. Regarding antineoplastic agents, this term refers to the time frame in which they kill bone marrow cells. (p. 683)

Paraneoplastic syndrome (PNS) (par′ ə ne′ o plas′ tik) Signs and symptoms of cancer located at a distance from the tumor or its metastatic sites. (p. 679)

Polyfunctional Refers to the action of alkylating agents which can perform several alkylation reactions. (p. 684)

Sarcoma (sahr′ ko′ mə) A malignant neoplasm of the soft tissues arising in fibrous, fatty, muscular, synovial, vascular, or neural tissue, usually first presenting as a painless swelling. (p. 678)

Tumor (too′ mor) A new growth of tissue characterized by a progressive, uncontrolled proliferation of cells. (p. 678)

Cancer is a broad term embracing a group of diseases that are characterized by uncontrolled cellular growth and possible invasion into surrounding tissue as well as by metastasis to new sites distant from the original body site. This cellular growth differs from normal cell growth in that cancerous cells do not possess a growth control mechanism, and the resulting cell usually has no physiologic function. Cancerous cells will continue to grow and invade adjacent structures or they may break away from the original tumor mass and travel by means of the blood or lymphatic system to establish a new clone (metastatic lesion) elsewhere in the body.

Metastasis refers to the spreading of a cancer (uncontrolled cell growth) from the original site of growth to a new and remote part of the body (secondary growth). The terms *malignancy, neoplasm,* and *tumor* are often used as synonyms for cancer. However, they all have their own meaning. A neoplasm is a mass of new cells that exhibit uncontrolled cellular reproduction. It is another term for **tumor.** There are two types of neoplasms, or tumors—benign and malignant. A **benign** tumor is one that is of a uniform size and shape and that displays no invasive or metastatic properties. The terms *nonmalignant* and *benign* suggest that tumors may be harmless, which in most cases they are, but a benign tumor can be lethal if it grows in vital tissue and interrupts normal function. **Malignant** neoplasms typically consist of cancerous cells that invade surrounding tissues and metastasize to other tissues and organs, where they form metastatic tumor deposits. Some of the various respective characteristics of benign and malignant neoplasms, or tumors, are listed in Table 45-1.

There are over a hundred types of malignant neoplasms that affect humans. They are usually classified by their primary anatomic (organ) location and the type of cell from which the neoplasm develops. Common body sites for malignant neoplasm growth are:

- Bladder and kidney
- Colon
- Prostate gland
- Uterus
- Blood-producing tissue
- Lymphatic system
- Rectum
- Breast
- Lung
- Skin

Tumors are classified according to their tissue of origin, and the various categories are sarcomas, carcinomas, lymphomas, leukemias, and tumors of nervous tissue origin. A list of common malignant tumors and their tissue of origin can be found in the box below. It is important to know the tissue of origin because this determines the type of chemotherapy used, the likely response to therapy, and the prognosis.

Carcinomas arise from epithelial tissue, which is located throughout the body. It covers or lines all body surfaces, both inside and outside the body. Examples are the skin, the mucosal lining of the entire gastrointestinal tract, and the bronchial tree (lungs). The purpose of these epithelial tissues is to protect the body's vital organs.

Sarcomas are malignant tumors that arise from connective tissues. This tissue is the most abundant and widely distributed of all tissues and can be found in bone, cartilage, muscle, blood, lymphatic, and vascular tissue. Its purpose is to support and protect other tissues.

Lymphomas arise from the lymphatic tissue, and **leukemias** arise from the various types of leukocytes. These two types of tumors differ from carcinomas and

---

Table 45-1 Tumor Characteristics: Benign and Malignant

CHARACTERISTIC	BENIGN	MALIGNANT
Potential to metastasize	No	Yes
Encapsulated	Yes	No
Similar to tissue of origin	Yes	No
Rate of growth	Slow	Unpredictable and unrestrained
Recurrence after surgical removal	Rare	Common

Tumor Classification Based on Specific Tissue of Origin

TISSUE OF ORIGIN	MALIGNANT TISSUE
Epithelial = Carcinomas	
Glands or ducts	Adenocarcinomas
Respiratory tract	Small- and large-cell carcinomas
Kidney	Renal cell carcinoma
Skin	Squamous cell, epidermoid, and basal cell carcinoma
Connective = Sarcomas	
Fibrous	Fibrosarcoma
Cartilage	Chondrosarcoma
Bone	Osteogenic sarcoma (Ewing's tumor)
Blood vessels	Kaposi's sarcoma
Peripheral nerve	Neuroblastoma
Lymphatic = Lymphomas	
Lymph tissue	Lymphomas (Hodgkin's disease and multiple myeloma)
Synovia	Synoviosarcoma
Mesothelium	Mesothelioma
Nerve	
Glial	Glioma
Adrenal medulla	Pheochromocytoma
Blood	
White blood cells	Leukemia

sarcomas in that the cancerous cells do not form solid tumors but are interspersed throughout the lymphatic or circulatory system and interfere with the normal functioning of these systems. The last (fifth) type of tumor is that which originates from neural tissue.

Cancers may produce signs and symptoms caused by changes in tissues remote from the tumor or its site of metastasis. This symptom complex is referred to as the **paraneoplastic syndrome** (PNS), and some of the various disorders produced are listed in the box below. The syndrome is believed to result from the effects of biologically or immunologically active substances secreted by the tumors. Some patients may also exhibit generalized symptoms, such as anorexia, weight loss, fatigue, and fever.

Etiology of Cancer

The etiology of cancer remains a mystery for the most part, and cancer researchers have made slow progress toward identifying possible causes. In recent years certain etiologic factors have come to light, however, and some of these and the cancers they cause are listed in the box at right. In addition, radiation, oncogenic viruses, and immunologic, ethnic, genetic, and age- and sex-related factors have also been identified.

AGE- AND SEX-RELATED DIFFERENCES

The probability of a neoplastic disease developing in a person generally increases with advancing age, but lymphocytic leukemia and Wilms' tumor are exceptions to this. The incidence of these decreases with age. On the other hand, lymphocytic and myelocytic leu-

kemia and colon and lung cancer usually develop during middle and old age. These cancers are rare in young children.

With the exception of cancers affecting the reproductive system, few cancers exhibit a sex-related difference in their incidence. Lung and urinary cancers are more common in men than in women, but this may have more to do with exogenous factors such as smoking patterns and exposure to environmental toxins than to sex-related causes. The incidence of colon, rectal, pancreatic, and skin cancers as well as leukemia is almost equal between the sexes.

GENETIC AND ETHNIC FACTORS

There are few cancers that appear to be inherited on a genetic basis, breast, colon, and stomach cancers being the exception. These cancers often show a familial pattern of inheritance. Burkitt's lymphoma is an example of a cancer that shows a racial pattern of inheritance. The disease in more common in young African chil-

---

Cancer: Proposed Etiologic Factors

RISK FACTOR	ASSOCIATED CANCER
Environment	
Radiation (ionizing)	Leukemia, breast, thyroid
Radiation (ultraviolet)	Skin, melanoma
Viruses	Leukemia, lymphoma, nasopharyngeal
Life-Style	
Alcohol	Esophagus, liver, stomach, larynx
Tobacco	Lung, mouth, esophagus, larynx
Reproductive History	
Late first pregnancy	Breast
No children	Ovary
Sexual promiscuity	Cervix, uterus
Occupational	
Asbestos	Lung, mesothelioma
Aniline dye	Bladder
Benzene	Leukemia
Vinyl chloride	Liver
Food	
Aflatoxin	Liver
Dietary factors	Colon, breast, endometrium, gallbladder
Medical Drugs	
Diethylstilbestrol (DES)	Vaginal in offspring
Estrogens	Endometrial
Alkylating agents	Leukemia, bladder

Paraneoplastic Syndrome Associated with Some Cancers

PARANEOPLASTIC SYNDROME	ASSOCIATED CANCER
Hypercalcemia, sensory neuropathies, SIADH	Lung
Disseminated intravascular coagulation	Leukemia
Cushing's syndrome	Lung, thyroid, testes, adrenal
Addison's syndrome	Adrenal, lymphomas

SIADH, syndrome of inappropriate antidiuretic hormone secretion.

Carcinogens

CHEMICAL	DESCRIPTION
Aflatoxins	A group of toxic/carcinogenic products produced by the mold *Aspergillus,* which contaminates peanuts and grains; aflatoxins are associated with the development of liver cancers.
Asbestos	Associated with the development of lung cancer and mesothelioma; asbestos is found in pipe and fire insulation, especially in older buildings.
Benzene	Associated with the development of acute myelogenous leukemia
Chimney soot	One of the first carcinogens to be identified (in English chimney sweepers); it is associated with the development of scrotal cancer.
Naphthalene dyes (aniline dyes)	Associated with the development of bladder cancer.
Polyvinyl chloride (PVCs)	Associated with the development of liver sarcomas.
Printer's ink	Associated with the development of liver and bladder cancer.
Smoked fish and meats	Diets rich in smoked foodstuffs is associated with the development of stomach cancer.
Tobacco	Smoking (cigarettes, pipe) and chewing tobacco are associated with the development of respiratory tract cancers.

Drug Carcinogens

DRUG	ASSOCIATED CARCINOGENIC ACTIVITY
Acetophenetidin (obsolete analgesic also known as phenacetin)	Renal cancer
Anabolic steroids	Liver cancer
Antineoplastics	Leukemia and cancer of the bladder, GI tract, skin
Coal tar preparations	Skin cancer
Diethylstilbestrol (DES)	Vaginal adenocarcinoma in female offspring of mothers who took DES during pregnancy
Estrogens	Vaginal and cervical cancer and post-menopausal endometrial cancer
Reserpine	Possible link to breast cancer

dren and children of African descent than in non-African children. Another example of an ethnic predisposition is the high incidence of nasopharyngeal cancer in persons of Chinese extraction.

ONCOGENIC VIRUSES

Extensive research has indicated that there are cancer-causing (oncogenic) viruses than can affect most mammalian species. The various cat leukemias, the Rous* sarcoma virus in chickens, and the Shope* papilloma in rabbits are a few examples.

The most common example of viral oncogenic activity in humans is the herpes viruses. The one that

causes infectious mononucleosis (the Epstein-Barr virus) is associated with the development of Burkitt's lymphoma and nasopharyngeal cancer. In addition, there is evidence indicating an association between the development of cervical cancer and infection with the herpes simplex type 2 virus (herpes genitalis).

OCCUPATIONAL AND ENVIRONMENTAL CARCINOGENS

A carcinogen is a physical or chemical agent that can induce the development of a cancer or accelerate its growth. The box above left contains a selected listing of such agents.

DRUGS

Many drugs that were once considered safe have proved to be carcinogenic. For this reason, FDA regulations now mandate that carcinogenic studies be done before any new drug is approved for use. However, no amount of clinical testing can fully reveal all the possible carcinogenic and mutagenic effects. One reason for this is that testing for drug carcinogenic activity is difficult and current test methods are not very satisfactory. Besides this there can be species-related differences in a particular drug; carcinogenic activity, such that these effects are not observed in the laboratory animals the agent has been tested on, and only become obvious when used in human subjects. Refer to the box above for a partial listing of carcinogenic drugs.

---

*Doctors P. Rous and R. Shope were early investigators of oncogenic viruses.

RADIATION

Radiation is a well-known and potent carcinogenic agent. In fact, several scientists who studied radiation or who worked on the development of the first atomic bomb* were victims of cancer. There are two basic types of radiation: (1) ionizing, or high-energy, radiation and, (2) nonionizing, or low-energy, radiation. Both types can be carcinogenic. Ionizing radiation is very potent and can penetrate deeply into the body. It is called *ionizing* because it causes the formation of ions within living cells. This type of radiation (e.g., x-ray studies, radium implants) is used to treat (irradiate) cancerous tumors. Nonionizing radiation is much less potent and cannot penetrate deeply into the body. Sunlight and ultraviolet light are examples of this type of radiation. Sunlight is a major cause of skin cancer, and ultraviolet light, which was used for the treatment of skin conditions of the head and neck, is known to cause thyroid cancer.

IMMUNOLOGIC FACTORS

Observations in patients undergoing cancer chemotherapy; organ transplant patients receiving immunosuppressive therapy to prevent organ rejection, especially those with renal transplants; patients suffering from immunologic impairment or disease; and patients with AIDS strongly indicate that the immune system plays an important role in cancer surveillance and the elimination of neoplastic cells. This is shown by the fact that there is a much higher incidence of cancer in immunocompromised persons. It has been suggested that neoplastic cells develop in everyone but that the immune system in healthy persons recognizes them as abnormal and eliminates them by means of cell-mediated immunity.

This relationship between cancer and a suppressed immune system has also been noted in cancer patients being treated with immunotherapy consisting of interferon derivatives, the bacillus Calmette-Guérin (BCG) vaccine, and lymphokines.

Cell Growth Cycle

Normal cells in the body divide (proliferate) in a controlled and organized fashion, and this growth is regulated by means of various mechanisms. In contrast, cancer cells lack regulatory mechanisms and they pro-

liferate uncontrollably, though some modulation of cancer cell proliferation may occur if blood flow to the cancer is disrupted. Their growth is usually also constant. Thus an important characteristic of malignant tumors is the time it takes for the tumor to double in size. This doubling time varies greatly for various types of cancers and is directly related to and important in determining the anticipated survival time in a patient. Cancer treatment that cannot destroy every neoplastic cell does not retard the regrowth of the tumor, and the time it takes for regrowth to occur depends on the doubling time of the particular cancer. For instance, Burkitt's lymphoma has an extremely short doubling time, whereas multiple myeloma has one of the longest.

The cell growth characteristics for normal and neoplastic cells are similar. Both types of cells go through five distinct growth phase cycles: G_0, the resting phase; G_1, the first growth phase or the postmitotic phase; S, the DNA synthesis phase; G_2, the second growth phase or the premitotic phase; and M, the **mitosis** phase (cell reproduction). Two identical daughter cells are the final product of this process in one cell. A complete cycle from one mitosis to the next is called the *generation time*, and it is different for all tumors, ranging from hours to days. The cell growth cycle and the events that occur in the various phases are summarized in the box on the next page.

The activity of a mass of tumor cells can also be characterized, and it has an important bearing on the killing power of chemotherapy. The percentage of cells undergoing mitosis at any given time is called the **growth fraction** of the tumor mass. The number of cells that are in the M phase of the cell cycle is called the **mitotic index**. Chemotherapy is most effective when the greatest number of cells are dividing, that is, when both the growth fraction and mitotic index are high.

Drugs used for chemotherapy are called *antineoplastic agents,* and they can be subdivided into two main groups of agents based on where in the cell cycle they work. Antineoplastic drugs that are cytotoxic in any phase of the cycle are called **cell cycle–nonspecific** (CCNS) agents. Those agents that are cytotoxic during a specific life cycle phase are called **cell cycle–specific** (CCS) agents. CCNS agents are effective against large, slowly growing tumors. CCS agents are effective against rapidly growing tumors. Some examples of CCNS and CCS antineoplastic agents are listed in the box on the next page, and Fig. 45-1 shows where in the general phase of the cell cycle the primary chemotherapeutic agents kill the cancerous cells.

The ultimate goal of any anticancer regimen is to kill every neoplastic cell and produce a cure, but this goal is not achieved in most cases, for a variety of reasons, one of which is that antineoplastic agents are usu-

---

*Enrico Fermi, a nuclear physicist who worked on the development of the atomic bomb, died of leukemia.

Cell Cycle Phases

PHASE	DESCRIPTION
G_0 The resting phase	Most normal human cells exist predominantly in this phase. Cancer cells in this phase are not susceptible to the toxic effects of chemotherapy.
G_1 The postmitotic phase	Enzymes necessary for DNA synthesis are produced.
S The DNA synthesis phase	DNA synthesis takes place, from DNA separation to DNA replication.
G_2 The premitotic phase	RNA and specialized proteins are made.
M The mitosis phase	Divided into four phases: prophase, metaphase, anaphase, and telophase.

CCNS and CCS Antineoplastics

ANTINEOPLASTIC	CELL CYCLE TYPE
Alkylating agent	Cell cycle nonspecific
Antimetabolites	Cell cycle specific in the S phase
Mitotic inhibitors	Cell cycle specific in the M phase

ally cytotoxic and not tumoricidal. That is, they can only kill cells while they are dividing, not all the cancer cells regardless of where they are in the cell growth cycle when exposed to the antineoplastic agent. Other factors that affect the chances of cure and the length of survival include the cancer stage at the time of diagnosis, the type of neoplasm and its doubling time, the efficacy of the cancer treatment, the development of drug resistance, and the general health of the patient. When total cure is not possible, the primary goal of therapy is then to control the growth of the neoplasm while maintaining the best life-style for the patient.

No antineoplastic agent is effective against all types of neoplasms, and they also have a low therapeutic index. However, one important discovery yielded by clinical experience is that a combination of agents is usually more effective than single-agent therapy. The reason for this is that, because drug-resistant cells often develop in tumors as the result of the tumor's genetic instability, exposure to multiple drugs with multiple mechanisms and sites of action will destroy more such subpopulations of malignant cells. The delayed onset of resistance to a particular antineoplastic agent is thus a benefit of combination drug therapy. To be most effective, however, the drugs used in such a combination regimen should be those that:

- Are effective as sole agents in the treatment of the particular type of cancer.
- Have different mechanisms of action, so that the cytotoxic effect is maximized.
- Possess different cytotoxic properties, so that each drug in the combination can be administered in a full therapeutic dose.

One major drawback to the use of these agents is that nearly all of them cause side effects and adverse effects. Many of these effects are severe or toxic and stem from the fact that these agents are harmful to all rapidly growing cells—both the harmful cancer cells and beneficial human cells. Three types of such rapidly growing beneficial human cells are hair follicles, gastrointestinal cells, and bone marrow cells. Because the antineoplastic agents cannot differentiate between the cancer cells and these healthy cells, the latter are also killed, with hair loss, nausea and vomiting, and myelosuppression the undesirable consequences, respectively. These effects are called **dose-limiting side effects** because they prevent the antineoplastic agent from being administered in the high doses ideally needed to kill the entire population of cancer cells.

Some antineoplastic agents are more disruptive or harmful to the beneficial cells of the stomach, a property known as the **emetic potential** because it represents the extent to which an agent produces nausea and vomiting. Unfortunately, to prevent these side effects requires that the agent be given in doses that may be relatively ineffective when it comes to destroying the cancer cells. The emetic potentials of the various antineoplastic drugs are summarized in the box on the next page.

The myelosuppression, or bone marrow suppression (BMS), is another unwanted effect of certain antineoplastics and results from the fact that certain cells in the bone marrow, such as granulocytes, lympho-

▼ FIG. 45-1 Cell cycle specificity of antineoplastics. General phase of the cell cycle with corresponding action of specific antineoplastic agents to produce cancerous cell kill.

Antineoplastics: Relative Emetic Potential

High (>90%)
↓Cisplatin
Dacarbazine
Mechlorethamine
Streptozocin
Cytarabine*

Moderately High (60%-90%)
Carmustine
Lomustine
↓Cyclophosphamide
Actinomycin-D
Mithramycin
Procarbazine
Methotrexate†

Moderate (30%-60%)
5-Fluorouracil
↓Doxorubicin
Daunorubicin
L-Asparaginase
Mitomycin-C

Moderately Low (10%-30%)
Bleomycin
Hydroxyurea
Melphalan
Etoposide
Teniposide
Cytarabine‡
6-Mercaptopurine
↓Methotrexate§
Thiotepa
Vinblastine

Low (<10%)
Busulfan
Chlorambucil
6-Thioguanine
Vincristine
Estrogens
Progestin
Corticosteroids
Androgens

*>500 mg/m².
†Doses >200 mg/m².
‡Standard doses.
§Low doses.

cytes, and platelets, are also destroyed. The specific hematologic disorder resulting from the myelosuppression depends on the particular cell line affected. For instance, if the cells in the bone marrow that make platelets are killed, the patient's platelet count will decrease and he or she will be more susceptible to bleeding. The time frame in which each antineoplastic agent kills these bone marrow cells differs. This property is called the **nadir.**

ALKYLATING AGENTS

Mustard gas and the derivatives of the nitrogen mustards were the first alkylating agents, with nitrogen mustard (mechlorethamine) the prototypical agent. It was in the 1940s that its antineoplastic activity was discovered, and since that time, many analogues of the agent have been synthesized and introduced into use for the treatment of cancer.

The alkylating agents commonly used in clinical practice in the United States today consist of three categories of agents: the classic alkylators; the alkylator-like agents, which have a different chemical structure but work by alkylation; and the nitrosoureas, which also have a different chemical structure but work by alkylation. The agents in each category are listed below: These antineoplastics are generally considered CCNS agents, and they are used to treat a wide spectrum of malignancies, but especially solid tumors and hematologic malignancies.

Commonly Used Alkylating Agents

Classic alkylators

- Busulfan
- Chlorambucil
- Cyclophosphamide
- Ifosfamide
- Mechlorethamine
- Melphalan
- Thiotepa (triethylene thiophosphoramide)

Alkylator-like agents

- Carboplatin
- Cisplatin
- Dacarbazine
- Procarbazine

Nitrosoureas

- Carmustine
- Lomustine
- Streptozocin

Mechanism of Action

The alkylating agents are CCNS antineoplastics that are effective at any stage in the growth cycle of cancer cells and are most effective against rapidly growing cancer cells and normal body cells. These agents work by preventing the cancer cells from reproducing, and they have a unique way of accomplishing this. Specifically, they work by interfering with the chemical structure of the DNA essential to the reproduction of any cell, and they do this by causing alkyl groups rather than hydrogen atoms to be attached to the nucleic acid. This process is called **alkylation.** Very special bonds are needed for a normal DNA to assume its double-helix form, so that during the normal process of reproduction the double helix can uncoil and RNA transcription can occur, resulting in the creation of a new cell with the same DNA sequence and thus the same characteristics. When these alkyl groups are attached to the DNA, abnormal chemical bonds form between the adjacent DNA molecules, resulting in the formation of defective nucleic acids that cannot then perform the normal cellular reproductive functions mentioned earlier.

The alkylating agents can also be characterized by the number of alkyl groups they possess and thus the number of alkylation reactions they can perform. **Bifunctional** alkylating agents have two reactive alkyl groups that are able to alkylate two DNA molecules. There are also **polyfunctional** alkylating agents that can perform several alkylation reactions. The sites on DNA most vulnerable to this reaction are position N7 on guanine, positions 1, 3, and 7 on adenine, and position N3 on cytosine. The alkylating agents that bind to guanine appear to be the most lethal agents. Figure 45-2 shows the location along the DNA double helix where the alkylating agents work.

Drug Effects

The alkylating agents in most common use today are those that are effective against a wide spectrum of malignancies, including both solid tumors and hematologic malignancies. Alkylating agents are frequently included in combination regimens because of their CCNS killing ability.

Therapeutic Uses

As just noted, because of their CCNS killing ability, alkylating agents are frequently included in

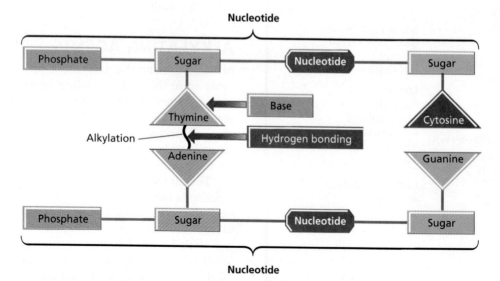

▼ **FIG. 45-2** Organization of DNA and site of action of alkylating agents.

combination regimens and can therefore be used to treat a variety of cancers. The various types of cancer and the different alkylating agents commonly used in their treatment are listed in the box at left.

Side Effects and Adverse Effects

The alkylating agents are capable of causing all the dose-limiting side effects described earlier. The relative emetic potential of the various agents is given in the box on p. 683, and the degree of BMS produced by some of these agents, along with the cell line affected and the radius, are summarized in Table 45-2, which includes data only on those agents that cause moderate to severe suppression. There are also major undesirable effects unique to these agents, and these are listed in Table 45-3. These side effects are important because of their severity, but they can be prevented through the use of prophylactic measures. For instance, nephrotoxicity can be prevented by adequately hydrating the patient with intravenously administered fluids, and careful observation and periodic monitoring can prevent pulmonary fibrosis or cardiomyopathy (heart failure) from occurring.

Specific Alkylating Agents: Therapeutic Uses

AGENT	TYPE OF CANCER
Classic Alkylators	
Busulfan	Chronic myelocytic leukemia
Chlorambucil	Chronic lymphocytic leukemia, lymphomas, multiple myeloma
⬇Cyclophosphamide	Lymphomas, many solid tumors including those of breast, ovaries, and lung
Ifosfamide	Germ cell testicular cancer
Mechlorethamine	Hodgkin's disease
Melphalan	Lymphomas, breast and ovarian carcinomas, multiple myeloma
Thiotepa	Superficial bladder cancer, combination therapy for breast cancer
Alkylator-Like Agents	
Carboplatin	Testicular, ovarian, head and neck, and lung cancers
⬇Cisplatin	Testicular, ovarian, head and neck, and lung cancers
Dacarbazine	Melanomas, Hodgkin's disease, some sarcomas
Procarbazine	Hodgkin's disease, other lymphomas, occasionally brain tumors
Nitrosoureas	
Carmustine	Malignant lymphomas, melanomas, gastrointestinal tumors
Lomustine	
Streptozocin	

Table 45-3   Alkylating Agents: Severe Adverse Effects

ALKYLATING AGENT	SEVERE SIDE/ADVERSE EFFECTS
⬇Cisplatin	Nephrotoxicity, peripheral neuropathy, ototoxicity
Carboplatin	Less nephrotoxicity and neurotoxicity but more BMS
Busulfan	Pulmonary fibrosis
⬇Cyclophosphamide	Hemorrhagic cystitis

Table 45-2   Alkylating Agents: Bone Marrow Suppression

DRUG	DEGREE OF BMS	CELL LINE	NADIR (DAYS)
Busulfan	Moderate-severe	G	21
Carboplatin	Moderate	P and G	17
Carmustine	Severe	G and P	21
Chlorambucil	Moderate-severe	G and L	21
⬇Cyclophosphamide	Moderate	G	14
Ifosfamide	Moderate	G	10
Mechlorethamine	Moderate	G and P	14
Melphalan	Moderate	G and P	21
Procarbazine	Moderate	G and P	14
Thiotepa	Moderate-severe	G and P	21

G, granulocytes; *L*, lymphocytes; *P*, platelets.

Alkylating Agent Extravasation: Specific Antidotes

ALKYLATING AGENT	ANTIDOTE PREPARATION	METHOD
Mechlorethamine	Mix 4 ml of 10% sodium thiosulfate with 6 ml of sterile water for injection.	1. Inject 5-6 ml IV through the existing line along with multiple SC injections into the extravasated site. 2. Repeat SC injections over the next few hours. 3. Apply *cold* compresses. 4. No total dose established.
Carmustine	Mix equal parts of 1 mEq/ml sodium bicarbonate (premixed) with sterile normal saline (1 hr 1 solution); resulting solution is 0.5 mEq/ml.	1. Inject 2-6 ml IV through the existing line along with multiple SC injections into the extravasated site. 2. Apply *cold* compresses. 3. Total dose not to exceed 10 ml of 0.5-mEq/ml solution.

Toxicity and Management of Overdose

One of the most devastating consequences of chemotherapy is the loss of a limb or the need for skin grafting because an antineoplastic drug has extravasated into the surrounding tissue during intravenous administration. Most antineoplastic agents are administered intravenously, and so this is a constant danger in any cancer patient undergoing chemotherapy. Such **extravasation** can result in permanent damage to nerves, tendons, and muscles, with skin grafting and even amputation needed to manage the damage. Good, attentive nursing care can do much to prevent a large proportion of these incidents, and if extravasation does occur, timely intervention can prevent the most serious consequences just mentioned. There are certain basic steps involved in treating the extravasation of any drug, but specific antidotes and additional measures are required when treating the extravasation of antineoplastics.

If extravasation is suspected, administration of the agent must be stopped immediately, but the IV tube should be left in place and any residual drug or blood aspirated from it if possible. The requisite antidote must then be prepared and instilled through the existing IV tube, after which the needle should be removed. If the residual agent cannot be aspirated from the IV tube, the antidote should not be instilled through it. A sterile occlusive dressing that covers the entire area should be placed, and warm or cold compresses applied, depending on the extravasated agent. The affected limb should then be elevated and allowed to rest. The antidotes recommended to reverse the effects of carmustine and mechlorethamine, the methods of administration, and other measures to be instituted are summarized in the box above.

Interactions

The significant drug interactions associated with the alkylating antineoplastics are listed in Table 45-4. There are only a few agents capable of causing significant drug interactions. The most important rule of thumb for preventing such drug interactions is to not administer them with any agent capable of causing similar toxicities. For example, a major adverse effect of cisplatin is nephrotoxicity. Therefore it should not be administered with an agent such as an aminoglycoside (gentamicin, tobramycin, or amikacin) because of the resulting additive nephrotoxic effect, and hence increased likelihood of the development of renal failure.

Dosages

For the recommended dosages of selected alkylating agents, see the dosages table on the next page.

DRUG PROFILES

MECHLORETHAMINE

Mechlorethamine (Mustine, Mustargen; nitrogen mustard) is a nitrogen analogue of sulfur mustard. It was the very first alkylating antineoplastic drug discovered. Its beneficial effects in the treatment of various cancers were discovered after World War I when the

Table 45-4	Alkylating Antineoplastics: Significant Drug Interactions	
DRUG	**MECHANISM**	**EFFECT**
Mechlorethamine and ⇩cyclophosphamide		
BMS drugs or radiation	Additive toxicities	Increased BMS
Probenecid and sulfinpyrazone	Competes for elimination	Hyperuricemia and gout
⇩Cisplatin		
BMS drugs or radiation	Additive toxicities	Increased BMS
Probenecid and sulfinpyrazone	Competes for elimination	Hyperuricemia and gout
Nephrotoxic or ototoxic drugs	Additive toxicities	Increased risk of nephrotoxicity and ototoxicity

DOSAGES

SELECTED ALKYLATING AGENTS

AGENT	PHARMACOLOGIC CLASS	DOSAGE RANGE	PURPOSE
Mechlorethamine (nitrogen mustard; Mustargen)	Alkylating agent	*Adult* IV/intercavitary: 0.4 mg/kg as a single dose or divided for each course	Hodgkin's disease; chronic lymphocytic or myelocytic leukemia; polycythemia vera; bronchogenic carcinoma; pleural, peritoneal, and metastatic cancer; mycosis fungoides
⇩Cyclophosphamide (Cytoxan, Neosar)	Alkylating agent	*Pediatric* PO/IV: loading dose, 2-8 mg/kg/day divided for ≥ 6 days PO: maintenance, 2.5 mg/kg twice/wk *Adult* PO/IV: loading dose, 1-5 mg/kg/day or 40-50 mg/kg divided for 2-5 days PO: maintenance, 1-5 mg/kg/day IV: maintenance, 10-15 mg/kg every 7-10 days or 3.5 mg/kg twice/wk	Breast cancer; follicular lymphoma; leukemias, including acute lymphoblastic, monocyctic, or myelogenous and chronic granulocytic or lymphocytic; malignant lymphomas; lymphocytic lymphosarcoma; multiple myeloma; mycosis fungoides; neuroblastoma; recticulum cell sarcoma; ovarian cancer; retinoblastoma
⇩Cisplatin (DDP; Platinol)	Alkylating agent	*Pediatric/Adult* IV: 20 mg/m²/day for 5 days every 3 wk for 3 courses 100 mg/m² once every 4 wk 50-70 mg/m² every 3-4 wk	Testicular Ovarian Bladder cancer
Carmustine (BCNU; BiCNU)	Alkylating agent	*Adult* IV: 150-200 mg/m² every 6 wk as a single dose or divided	Brain tumor, Hodgkin's disease, multiple myeloma, non-Hodgkin's lymphoma

agent, going by the name *mustard gas,* was used for chemical warfare. Some of the cancers it is used in the treatment of are Hodgkin's disease, lymphomas, and chronic leukemia. It is the prototypical alkylating agent.

Mechlorethamine is a bifunctional alkylating agent capable of forming cross-linkage between two DNA nucleotides, thereby interfering with RNA transcription and preventing cell division and protein synthesis. Mechlorethamine is available in a parenteral form only to be administered intravenously or by an intracavitary route such as intrapleurally or intraperitoneally.

Mechlorethamine is considered a pregnancy category D agent, and hypersensitivity, lactation, myelosuppression, and an acute herpes zoster attack are contraindications to its use. It is available as a 10-mg parenteral injection. Commonly recommended dosages are listed in the dosages table on the previous page.

✿ PHARMACOKINETICS

HALF-LIFE	ONSET	PEAK	DURATION
Several min	Several hr	2-3 days	10 wk

⚓ CYCLOPHOSPHAMIDE

Cyclophosphamide (Cytoxan, Neosar, Procytox) is a nitrogen mustard derivative that was discovered during the process of research to improve mechlorethamine. It is a polyfunctional alkylating agent and is used in the treatment of cancers of the bone and lymph as well as solid tumors. Various leukemias, Hodgkin's and non-Hodgkin's lymphoma, multiple myeloma, and some sarcomas may also respond to cyclophosphamide therapy.

It is classified as a pregnancy category D agent and is contraindicated in lactating women. It is available in both oral and parenteral formulations—as 25- and 50-mg oral tablets and 100-, 200-, 500-, 1000-, and 2000-mg vials for parenteral injection. Commonly recommended dosages are listed in the dosages table on the previous page.

✿ PHARMACOKINETICS

HALF-LIFE	ONSET	PEAK	DURATION
3-12 hr	Unknown	2-3 hr	Unknown

⚓ CISPLATIN

Cisplatin (DDP; Platinol) is an alkylator-like antineoplastic agent that contains platinum. Chemically cisplatin consists of a platinum atom surrounded by two chloride atoms and two ammonia molecules. It is classified as an alkylator-like antineoplastic agent because

it destroys cancer cells in the same way as the traditional alkylating agents—by forming cross-links with DNA and thereby preventing its replication. It is considered a bifunctional alkylating agent.

Cisplatin is classified as a pregnancy category D agent and is contraindicated within 1 month of radiation therapy or of chemotherapy with another agent. It is also contraindicated in patients with thrombocytopenia and after a recent smallpox vaccination. It is used for the treatment of many solid tumors such as bladder, testicular, and ovarian tumors. It is available only in a parenteral formulation—10- and 50-mg injections for intravenous infusion. Commonly recommended dosages are listed in the dosages table on the previous page.

✿ PHARMACOKINETICS

HALF-LIFE	ONSET	PEAK	DURATION
0.3-0.5 hr	Unknown	IV injection immediate	Unknown

CARMUSTINE

Carmustine (BCNU, BiCNU) is one of the three currently available nitrosoureas (carmustine, lomustine, and streptozocin). Because they act by alkylation, they are classified as alkylating agents. Carmustine is able to cross the blood-brain barrier and is thus useful in the treatment of primary brain tumors. It may also be used to treat Hodgkin's disease, non-Hodgkin's lymphomas, multiple myeloma.

Carmustine is classified as a pregnancy category D agent and is contraindicated in patients with a hypersensitivity to it as well as in those suffering from leukopenia or thrombocytopenia. It is available only in a parenteral preparation—a 100-mg vial for intravenous infusion. Commonly recommended dosages are listed in the dosages table on the previous page.

✿ PHARMACOKINETICS

HALF-LIFE	ONSET	PEAK	DURATION
15 min	Unknown	Several wk	Unknown

Antimetabolites

Antineoplastic antimetabolites are CCS agents that are structurally similar to normal cellular metabolites and work by mimicking the actions of important natural precursors that are required for the synthesis of DNA and RNA. They are most effective against solid tumors such as colon, rectum, breast, stomach, lung, ovarian, liver, bladder, and pancreas cancer.

Mechanism of Action

The antimetabolites interfere with the biosynthesis of precursors essential to cellular growth by mimicking folic acid, pyrimidines, and purines, thereby interfering with the normal synthesis of nucleic acids in one of two ways: (1) by falsely substituting for purines, pyrimidines, or folic acid or (2) by inhibiting critical enzymes involved in nucleic acid or folic acid synthesis. Thus, they affect DNA, RNA, and protein synthesis, and, ultimately, cellular replication. The antimetabolites work in the S phase of the cell cycle, during which DNA synthesis occurs. The available antimetabolites and the metabolites they mimic are listed below, and following this is a discussion of the specific actions of the agents in the different categories.

Purine antagonist
- Fludarabine (F-AMP)
- Mercaptopurine (6-MP)
- Thioguanine (6-TO)

Pyrimidine antagonist
- Cytarabine (ARA-C)
- Floxuridine (FUDR)
- Fluorouracil (5-FU)

Folic acid antagonist
- Methotrexate (MTM)

Folic Acid Antagonism

The antimetabolite antineoplastic agent methotrexate is an analogue of folic acid and inhibits dihydrofolate reductase, an enzyme responsible for converting folic acid to a reduced folate. This inhibition prevents the formation of the reduced folate that is needed for the synthesis of DNA and hence for cell reproduction. The end result is that DNA is not produced and the cell dies.

Purine Antagonism

The purine bases present in DNA and RNA are adenine and guanine, and they are required for the synthesis of the purine nucleotides which are incorporated into the nucleic acid molecules. Mercaptopurine and fludarabine are synthetic analogues of adenine, and thioguanine is a synthetic analogue of guanine. These agents work by getting themselves incorporated into the metabolic pathway in lieu of these two nucleosides. Once there, they interrupt the synthesis of the DNA and RNA.

Pyrimidine Antagonism

Of the pyrimidine bases, two, cytosine and thymine, make up DNA and two, cytosine and uracil, make up RNA. These bases are essential for DNA and RNA synthesis. Floxuridine and fluorouracil are syn-

thetic chemical analogues of uracil, and cytarabine is a synthetic analogue of cytosine. These agents act in a way that is very similar to that of the purine antagonist, getting themselves incorporated into the metabolic pathway for the synthesis of DNA and RNA and thereby interrupting synthesis of the nucleic acids. This stops the formation of the DNA and RNA needed for the cancer cells to live.

Drug Effects

The antimetabolite antineoplastic agents are used for the treatment of a variety of solid tumors as well as some hematologic cancers. They may also be used in combination chemotherapy regimens to enhance the overall cytotoxic effect. Because these agents are available in both oral and topical preparations, they are utilized for low-dose maintenance and palliative cancer therapy.

Therapeutic Uses

Antimetabolites are used for the treatment of a more defined and limited group of cancers. The commonly used agents and their therapeutic uses are listed in the box below.

Specific Antimetabolites: Therapeutic Uses

AGENT	TYPE OF CANCER
Folic Acid Antagonists	
⚓Methotrexate	Solid tumors (breast, head and neck, and lung cancers), acute lymphocytic leukemia, non-Hodgkin's lymphomas
Pyrimidine Antagonists	
Cytarabine	Leukemias (acute and chronic myelocytic, and acute lymphocytic), non-Hodgkin's lymphomas
Floxuridine	Solid tumors (breast, head, neck, liver, brain, gallbladder, and bile duct), GI adenocarcinoma that has metastasized to the liver
Fluorouracil	Solid tumors (breast, colon, rectum, stomach, lung, ovarian, liver, bladder, and pancreas)
Purine Antagonists	
Mercaptopurine	Leukemias (acute lymphoblastic and myelogenous and chronic myelocytic)
Fludarabine	Chronic lymphocytic leukemia
Thioguanine	Leukemias, lymphomas, multiple myelomas, solid tumors

Table 45-5	Antimetabolites: Bone Marrow Suppression		
DRUG	DEGREE OF BMS	CELL LINE	NADIR (DAYS)
Cytarabine	Severe	G and P	10
Mercaptopurine	Moderate	G and L	10-14
Fludarabine	Moderate-severe	G and L	13

G, granulocytes; *L*, lymphocytes; *P*, platelets.

Table 45-6	Antimetabolites: Severe Adverse Effects
ANTIMETABOLITE AGENT	SEVERE SIDE/ADVERSE EFFECTS
Cytarabine	Liver, kidney, lung, stomach, and heart toxicities
Floxuridine Fludarabine Fluorouracil	Kidney and stomach toxicities
Mercaptopurine	Liver and kidney toxicities
⚓Methotrexate	Liver, kidney, and stomach toxicities
Thioguanine	Liver and kidney toxicities

Side Effects and Adverse Effects

Like all the antineoplastic agents, the antimetabolites cause hair loss, nausea and vomiting, and myelosuppression. The emetic potentials for some of these agents have already been given in the box on p. 683. Those antimetalotites that cause moderate to severe BMS and the cell lines most affected are given in Table 45-5. Major side effects and adverse effects specific to antimetabolite agents are listed in Table 45-6 by the individual agents.

Toxicity and Management of Overdose

High-dose methotrexate therapy can be very toxic to beneficial human cells, but such toxicity can be reversed by what is called **leucovorin rescue.** Chemically, leucovorin is a reduced form of folic acid and is involved in the synthesis of purine and pyrimidines into nucleic acids. Because of its ready conversion to other tetrahydrofolic acid derivatives, it is a potent antidote to the toxic effects of folic acid antagonists such as methotrexate. It is believed that, in some cancers, leucovorin works by entering and "rescuing" normal cells, as opposed to cancer cells, from the toxic effects

of folic acid antagonists. It is able to do this because of a difference in the membrane transport mechanisms between human and cancer cells.

Interactions

Most of the drug interactions associated with the antimetabolite antineoplastic agents can be summarized in one general statement: The coadministration of any other drug that causes a toxicity similar to that of the antimetabolite will result in additive toxicities. Therefore the respective risks and benefits should be carefully weighed before the initiation of therapy with either the antimetabolite or the other agent. Because the concurrent administration of nonsteroidal antiinflammatory agents with methotrexate may result in severe methotrexate toxicity, this combination should be avoided. In addition, cytarabine may decrease the effects of oral digoxin and the coadministration of mercaptopurine and allopurinol may lead to an additive bone marrow toxicity because both agents are metabolized by xanthine oxidase.

Dosages

For information on the dosages of selected antimetabolite chemotherapeutic agents, see the dosages table on the next page.

FOLATE ANTAGONISTS

Methotrexate (Folex PFS, Rheumatrex) is the prototype antimetabolite antineoplastic of the folate antagonist

DOSAGES

SELECTED ANTIMETABOLITES

AGENT	PHARMACOLOGIC CLASS	DOSAGE RANGE	PURPOSE
↓Methotrexate (MTx; Folex, Folex PFS, Rheumatrex)	Folic acid antagonist antimetabolite	*Adult/Pediatric* PO/IM: 15-30 mg/day for 5 days repeated 3-5 times PO/IM: 3.3 mg/m² with prednisone PO: 10-25 mg/hr for 4-8 days for several courses Intrathecal: 12 mg/m² every 2-5 days PO: 2.5-10 mg for weeks or months	Trophoblastic tumor Lymphoblastic leukemia Lymphoma Meningeal leukemia Mycosis fungoides
Mercaptopurine (6-MP; Purinethol)	Purine antagonist antimetabolite	*Adult/Pediatric* PO: 2.5-5 mg/kg/day with a maintenance dose of 1.5-2.5 mg/kg/day	Acute lymphatic and myelogenous leukemia, CNS leukemia
Cytarabine (Ara-C; Cytosar-U, Tarabine PFS)	Pyrimidine antagonist antimetabolite	*Adult/Pediatric* IV: usual combination dose is 100 mg/m²/day as a continuous infusion for days 1-7 or 100 mg/m² q12h for days 1-7 Intrathecal: 5-75 mg/m² administered once a day for 4 days then once every 4 days	Nonlymphocytic leukemia

group and is currently the only antineoplastic folate antagonist used clinically. It has proved useful for the treatment of solid tumors such as breast, head and neck, and lung cancers as well as for the management of acute lymphocytic leukemia and non-Hodgkin's lymphomas. Methotrexate also has immunosuppressive activity because it can inhibit lymphocyte multiplication, and for this reason it may be useful for the treatment of rheumatoid arthritis. Its combined immunosuppressant and antiinflammatory properties may make it useful for the treatment of many other immune-mediated diseases or inflammatory conditions as well.

Methotrexate is classified as a pregnancy category D agent and is contraindicated in patients who have shown a hypersensitivity to it; those with leukopenia, thrombocytopnia, or anemia; and psoriatic patients with severe renal or hepatic disease. It is available in both oral and parenteral formulations. For oral administration it is available as a 2.5-mg tablet. It also comes in a strength of 25 mg/ml for parenteral injection as well as a preservative-free parenteral injection in doses of 20, 50, and 1000 mg or 25 mg/ml. Commonly recommended dosages are given in the dosages table above.

PHARMACOKINETICS

HALF-LIFE	ONSET	PEAK	DURATION
8-10 hr	Unknown	1-4 hr PO serum	Unknown

PURINE ANTAGONISTS

The currently available purine antagonists are fludarabine, mercaptopurine, and thioguanine. Of the three, mercaptopurine and thioguanine are administered orally. Fludarabine is the only purine antagonist that is available in a parenteral formulation.

MERCAPTOPURINE

Mercaptopurine (6-MP; Purinethol) is used primarily for the treatment of leukemias (acute lymphoblastic and myelogenous and chronic myelocytic). It is classified as a pregnancy category D agent. It is contraindicated in patients who have shown resistance to the drug as well as in those with leukopenia, thrombocytopenia, or anemia. It is available only in an oral formulation as a 50-mg tablet. Commonly recommended dosages are given in the dosages table above.

♆ P H A R M A C O K I N E T I C S

HALF-LIFE	ONSET	PEAK	DURATION
21-47 min	Unknown	2 hr serum	Unknown

PYRIMIDINE ANTAGONISTS

The currently available antimetabolite antineoplastics that are members of the pyrimidine antagonist family are cytarabine, floxuridine, and fluorouracil. They are available only in parenteral formulations. Floxuridine and fluorouracil are classified as pregnancy category D agents and cytarabine as a category C agent.

CYTARABINE

Cytarabine (Ara-C; Cytosar-U) is primarily used in the treatment of leukemias (acute myelocytic and lymphocytic and chronic myelocytic) and non-Hodgkin's lymphomas. As already noted, it is available only as a parenteral agent—as 20-, 100-, 500-, 1000-, and 2000-mg/ml vials to be given either by intrathecal or subcutaneous injection. Commonly recommended dosages are given in the dosages table on p. 691. Pregnancy category D.

♆ P H A R M A C O K I N E T I C S

HALF-LIFE	ONSET	PEAK	DURATION
10 min, then 1-3 hr	Unknown	20-60 min serum	Unknown

Cytotoxic Antibiotics

The cytotoxic antibiotics consist of a group of natural antibiotics produced by the mold *Streptomyces* as well as of two synthetic cytotoxic antibiotics not produced by this mold. They are used only for the treatment of cancer because they are too toxic for the treatment of infections. The cytotoxic antibiotics differ in the toxicities they cause, but they all produce BMS, with the exception of bleomycin, which causes pulmonary toxicity (pulmonary fibrosis and pneumonitis). Other severe toxicities associated with the use of cytotoxic antineoplastics are congestive heart failure (daunorubicin) and rare acute left ventricular failure (doxorubicin). The available cytotoxic antibiotics are listed below by the specific subclass they belong to.

Anthracyclines
- Daunorubicin
- Doxorubicin
- Idarubicin

Other cytotoxic antibiotics
- Bleomycin
- Dactinomycin
- Mitomycin
- Mitoxantrone
- Pentostatin
- Plicamycin

Mechanism of Action

The cytotoxic antibiotic antineoplastic agents are CCNS agents, although some, such as daunorubicin, are more active in the S phase. In most cases, however, the agents are active during all phases of the cell cycle. By virtue of their source of origin (i.e., the *Streptomyces* mold), they all also have antibacterial activity and can kill certain bacteria; some may even kill viruses. Most act either by the process of alkylation, which has already been explained for the alkylating agents, or by a process called *intercalation*, which involves the insertion of the drug molecule between the two strands of DNA, a process that is very similar to the way in which the antimetabolites work in that ultimately DNA synthesis is blocked. Specifically, it involves the binding of the agent to the nucleotide pairs of the DNA helix, causing the shape of the DNA helix to change and in turn making it unstable so that it begins to unwind. The end result is the blockade of DNA, RNA, and protein synthesis. Some cytotoxic antibiotic agents can do all three, but others affect DNA synthesis only. Agents such as the anthracyclines work by intercalation.

Drug Effects

The cytotoxic antibiotic antineoplastic agents are used to treat a variety of solid tumors as well as some hematologic malignancies. They may also be used in combination chemotherapy regimens to enhance the overall cytotoxic effect.

Therapeutic Uses

The cytotoxic antibiotic antineoplastics are used to treat a wide variety of cancers, and these and the agents used to treat them are given in the box on the next page.

Side Effects and Adverse Effects

As with all the antineoplastic agents, the cytotoxic agents have the undesirable effect of causing hair loss, nausea and vomiting, and myelosuppression. The emetic potentials of the various agents in this category are given in the box on p. 683, and those cytotoxic agents that cause moderate to severe BMS and

Specific Cytotoxic Antibiotics: Therapeutic Uses

AGENT	TYPE OF CANCER
Anthracyclines	
Daunorubicin	Myelogenous monocytic and acute nonlymphocytic leukemia, Ewing's sarcoma, Wilms' tumor, neuroblastoma, rhabdomyosarcoma
⬇Doxorubicin	Solid tumors (of every major organ), Wilms' tumor, neuroblastomas, lymphomas, sarcomas, Hodgkin's disease, lymphoblastic leukemia
Idarubicin	Acute myelocytic leukemia (in combinations of antineoplastics)
Other Cytotoxic Antibiotics	
Bleomycin	Solid tumors (head, neck, penis, cervix, and vulva of squamous cell origin), Hodgkin's disease, sarcomas (lymphosarcoma, reticulum cell, and testicular)
Dactinomycin	Sarcomas, melanomas, trophoblastic tumors in women, testicular cancer, Wilms' tumor, rhabdomyosarcoma
Mitomycin	Solid tumors (pancreas, stomach, head and neck, breast)
Mitoxantrone	Leukemias (acute nonlymphocytic and relapsed leukemia), breast cancer
Pentostatin	Alpha-interferon–refractory hairy cell leukemia
Plicamycin	Testicular cancer, hypercalcemia, hypercalciuria; symptomatic treatment of advanced neoplasms

Cytotoxic Antibiotics: Bone Marrow Suppression

DRUG	DEGREE OF BMS	CELL LINE	NADIR (DAYS)
Dactinomycin	Severe	G and P	10
Daunorubicin	Severe	G and P	10
⬇Doxorubicin	Moderate	G	14
Idarubicin	Severe	G and P	10
Mitomycin	Moderate	G and P	28
Mitoxantrone	Moderate-severe	G and P	12
Pentostatin	Moderate-severe	G and L	15

G, granulocytes; *L*, lymphocytes; *P*, platelets.

Table 45-7 Cytotoxic Antibiotics: Severe Adverse Effects

CYTOTOXIC ANTIBIOTIC AGENT	SEVERE SIDE/ADVERSE EFFECTS
Bleomycin	Pulmonary fibrosis, pneumonitis
Dactinomycin	Liver toxicities, extravasation
Daunorubicin	Liver toxicities, extravasation
⬇Doxorubicin	Liver and cardiovascular toxicities
Idarubicin	Liver and cardiovascular toxicities
Mitomycin	Liver, kidney, and lung toxicities
Mitoxantrone	Cardiovascular toxicities
Pentostatin	Genitourinary toxicities
Plicamycin	Genitourinary toxicities, extravasation

the cell lines most affected are listed in the box above right. Major side effects specific to these agents are given in Table 45-7.

Toxicity and Management of Overdose

Because all cytotoxic antibiotic antineoplastics are administered intravenously, extravasation of the agent with its devastating consequences is a constant danger. The basic steps involved in the treatment of extravasation have already been discussed in the section on alkylating agents. Specific antidotes and additional steps required for the treatment of extravasation of specific cytotoxic agents are given in the box on the following page.

Interactions

The cytotoxic antibiotics that are used as chemotherapeutic agents interact with many drugs. They all tend to produce increased toxicities when used in combination with other chemotherapeutic agents or with irradiation. Some agents, most notably bleomycin and doxorubicin, have been known to cause the serum digoxin levels to increase.

Dosages

For recommended dosages of selected cytotoxic agents see the dosages table on p. 695.

Cytotoxic Antibiotic Agent Extravasation: Specific Antidotes

CYTOTOXIC ANTIBIOTIC AGENT	ANTIDOTE PREPARATION	METHOD
Mitomycin	Mix 4 ml of 10% sodium thiosulfate with 6 ml of sterile water for injection.	1. Inject 5-6 ml IV through the existing line and multiple SC injections into the site of extravasation. 2. Repeat SC dosing over the next few hours. 3. Apply *cold* compresses. 4. No total dose established.
⚓Doxorubicin	—	1. Cooling of site to patient tolerance for 24 hr. 2. Elevate and rest extremity for 24-48 hr, then have patient resume normal activity as tolerated. 3. If pain, erythema, or swelling persists beyond 48 hr, discuss with the physician the need for surgical intervention.

DRUG PROFILES

ANTHRACYCLINE CYTOTOXIC ANTIBIOTICS

Three of the older cytotoxic antibiotics are the anthracycline antibiotics, doxorubicin, daunorubicin, and idarubicin. They all have similar pharmacologic actions in that they all work through the process of intercalation. In addition, they are effective in all phases of the cell growth cycle. These agents are used for the treatment of a wide range of cancers but come only in parenteral formulations. All are classified as pregnancy category D agents.

⚓ DOXORUBICIN

Doxorubicin (Adriamycin RDF, Adriamycin PFS, Rubex) is a very potent and effective chemotherapeutic agent, and for this reason, it is used in many combination chemotherapy regimens. It is contraindicated in patients with a known hypersensitivity to it, lactating women, and patients with systemic infections (pregnancy [first trimester] category D). It comes only in 10-, 20-, 50-, 100-, and 150-mg vials as well as in a 2-mg/ml strength for injection. Commonly used dosages are given in the dosages table on the next page.

PHARMACOKINETICS

HALF-LIFE	ONSET	PEAK	DURATION
Up to 36 hr	Unknown	Very rapid	Unknown

OTHER CYTOTOXIC ANTIBIOTICS

The other cytotoxic antibiotics have characteristics similar to those of the anthracyclines. They are also CCNS agents that are effective against a wide range of cancers. All are available only in parenteral formulations. There are currently six agents in this class: bleomycin, dactinomycin, mitomycin, mitoxantrone, pentostatin, and plicamycin.

BLEOMYCIN

Bleomycin (Blenoxane) is active against both gram-positive and gram-negative bacteria as well as fungi, but because of its cytotoxicity its use as an antibiotic is prohibited. It kills cancer cells in all phases of the cell cycle in much the same way as the alkylating agents do—by inhibiting the incorporation of a nucleotide base, thymidine, into DNA. The end result is that cancer cells cannot produce the needed DNA and protein, and they die.

Bleomycin is used to treat a variety of cancers. However, it is very toxic, one of its most harmful toxicities being its effect on the lungs. Pulmonary fibrosis and pneumonitis are the consequences. It is classified as a pregnancy category D agent and is contraindicated in patients with a hypersensitivity to it. The doses are measured in units as opposed to milligrams. It is available as a 15-unit vial, which is administered subcuta-

DOSAGES

SELECTED CYTOTOXIC ANTIBIOTICS

AGENT	PHARMACOLOGIC CLASS	DOSAGE RANGE	PURPOSE
⚓Doxorubicin (ADR, Adriamycin RDF, Adriamycin PSF, Rubex)	Antineoplastic cytotoxic antibiotic	*Adult* IV: 60-75 mg/m^2 every 21 days or 30 m^2 for 3 days, then either repeat every 4 wk or give 20 mg/m^2/wk	Breast, bladder, ovarian, thyroid cancer; bronchogenic cancer; Hodgkin's and non-Hodgkin's lymphomas; acute lymphoblastic/myeloblastic leukemia; neuroblastoma; soft-tissue/bone sarcoma; Wilms' tumor
Bleomycin (BLM; Blenoxane)	Antineoplastic cytotoxic antibiotic	*Adult* IM/IV/SC: 0.25-0.5 U/kg 1-2 times/wk	Hodgkin's disease, lymphosarcoma, recticulum cell sarcoma, squamous cell cancer, testicular cancer

neously, intravenously, or intramuscularly. Commonly used dosages are given in the dosages table above.

PHARMACOKINETICS

HALF-LIFE	ONSET	PEAK	DURATION
2 hr	Unknown	30-60 min	Unknown

*IM: time to reach peak serum levels.

Mitotic Inhibitors

The mitotic inhibitors consist of natural products obtained from the periwinkle plant (*Catharenthus roseus*, formerly called *Vinca rosea*) and of semisynthetic agents obtained from the mandrake plant (May apple). The periwinkle plant yields two antineoplastic alkaloids. These are vinblastine (VLB) and vincristine (VCR), and they are known as *vinca alkaloids*. Etoposide (VP-16) and teniposide (ETP) are semisynthetic derivatives of podophyllotoxin, which is obtained from the resinous extract of the mandrake plant. A new agent has been discovered recently that also comes from a plant source and affects mitosis. This is paclitaxel

(Taxol), and it comes from the bark of the slow-growing Western (Pacific) yew. These agents and their plant sources are listed below:

Vinca alkaloids (periwinkle)
- Vinblastine
- Vincristine

Podophyllotoxin derivatives (may apply)
- Etoposide
- Teniposide

Pacific yew tree
- Paclitaxel

Mechanism of Action

The plant alkaloids vary in their site of action in the cell cycle. They all affect the cell cycle shortly before or actually during mitosis. This entire family of antineoplastics in as yet some unknown way prevents mitosis from occurring and thus stops the cell cycle by disrupting the mitotic spindles crucial to the success of metaphase. It is for this reason that they are called *mitotic inhibitors*.

The vinca alkaloids (vincristine and vinblastine) kill cancer cells by binding to tubulin during the metaphase of mitosis (the M phase). This prevents the assembly of the microtubules, which results in the dissolution of the mitotic spindle. Without these mitotic spindles, dividing cells cannot then multiply and divide appropriately. This causes cell division and DNA,

RNA, and protein synthesis to be inhibited. Without these substances, all cells, including cancer cells, die.

The podophyllotoxin derivatives (etoposide and teniposide) exert their cytotoxic effects by damaging DNA and thereby inhibiting or altering DNA synthesis. They have also been shown to directly induce single- and double-stranded DNA breaks. These agents are considered CCS agents because they appear to kill during the late S phase and the G_2 phase of the cell cycle.

The Pacific yew tree derivative (paclitaxel) works in the late G_2 phase and M phase of the cell cycle. It is therefore a CCS agent and works by causing the formation of a nonfunctional microtubule. These microtubules are needed for mitotic spindles to function properly. Therefore paclitaxel halts mitosis in metaphase.

Drug Effects

The mitotic inhibitors are CCS agents that are used to treat a variety of solid tumors as well as some hematologic malignancies. Depending on the particular agent they can work in any phase of the cell cycle (late S phase, throughout G_2 phase, and M phase), but they work primarily in metaphase during mitosis. Mitotic inhibitors may also be used in combination chemotherapy regimens to enhance the overall cytotoxic effect.

Therapeutic Uses

The commonly used mitotic inhibitor antineoplastic agents and their therapeutic uses are listed in the box below left.

Side Effects and Adverse Effects

As is the case for all the antineoplastic agents, the mitotic inhibitor antineoplastic agents cause hair loss, nausea and vomiting, and myelosuppression. The emetic potentials of some of the agents are given in the box on p. 683, and those agents that cause moderate to severe BMS and the cell lines most affected are listed in the box below. Major side effects specific to these agents are summarized in Table 45-8.

Toxicity and Management of Overdose

All of the mitotic inhibitor antineoplastics are administered intravenously, making extravasation of the agents and its serious consequences a constant threat. The basic steps to be taken in the treatment of the extravasation of any drug have already been discussed in the section on alkylating agents. Specific antidotes and additional measures to be taken for the treatment of the extravasation of the mitotic inhibitors are given in the box on the next page.

Specific Mitotic Inhibitors: Therapeutic Uses

Vinca Alkaloids

AGENT	TYPE OF CANCER
Vinblastine	Lymphomas, including Hodgkin's and non-Hodgkin's lymphomas; neuroblastoma; Kaposi's sarcoma; mycosis fungoides; histiocytosis; solid tumors (breast and testicular cancers)
Vincristine	Lymphomas, Hodgkin's disease, neuroblastoma, leukemias; rhabdomyosarcoma, osteogenic, and other sarcomas; solid tumors (breast and lung cancers); Wilms' tumor

Podophyllotoxin Derivatives

Etoposide	Leukemias, lymphomas, neuroblastoma, melanoma, solid tumors (lung, testicular, and ovarian cancer)
Teniposide	Childhood acute lymphoblastic leukemia

Pacific Yew Tree Derivative

⇩Paclitaxel	Metastatic ovarian cancer not responsive to other chemotherapy; ever-expanding therapeutic uses

---

Mitotic Inhibitors: Bone Marrow Suppression

DRUG	DEGREE OF BMS	CELL LINE	NADIR (DAYS)
⇩Paclitaxel	Severe	G, P, and L	10-14
Teniposide	Moderate	G and P	14
Vinblastine	Moderate-severe	G and P	10

G, granulocytes; *L*, lymphocytes; *P*, platelets.

Table 45-8 Mitotic Inhibitors: Severe Adverse Effects

ANTIBIOTIC AGENT	SEVERE SIDE/ADVERSE EFFECTS
Etoposide	Liver and kidney toxicities
Teniposide	Liver toxicities
Vinblastine	Liver, kidney, and lung toxicities, convulsions
Vincristine	Liver toxicities, convulsions

Interactions

There are many notable drug interactions associated with the mitotic inhibitors, the most common of which are listed in Table 45-9.

Dosages

For the recommended dosages of selected mitotic inhibitors, see the dosages table on the following page.

DRUG PROFILES

The mitotic inhibitors consist of three groups of agents that are derived from plant sources: vinca alkaloids (perwinkle), podophyllotoxin derivatives (May apple), and the Pacific yew tree. They are all available in a parenteral form and are all classified as pregnancy category D agents. Etoposide is the only agent available in an oral formulation as well.

ETOPOSIDE

Etoposide (VP-16, VePesid) is a semisynthetic podophyllotoxin derivative with a structure, mechanism of action, and side effect profile similar to those of teniposide. As previously noted, it is believed to kill cancer cells in the late S phase and the G_2 phase of the cell cycle. It is indicated for the treatment of small-cell lung cancer and testicular cancer.

Hypersensitivity, bone marrow depression, severe hepatic or renal disease, and bacterial infection are the contraindications to its use. It is available in an oral formulation as a 50-mg liquid-filled capsule and as a

20-mg/ml injection for intravenous infusion. Commonly recommended dosages are listed in the dosages table on the next page. Pregnancy category D.

Table 45-9	Mitotic Inhibitors: Drug Interactions	
DRUG	**MECHANISM**	**RESULT**
Etoposide Warfarin	Competes for protein binding	Increased prothrombin time
Paclitaxel	Additive toxicities	Increased myelosuppression
↓**Cisplatin** Ketoconazole	Decreases metabolism of paclitaxel	Accumulation of paclitaxel
Teniposide ↓Methotrexate	Increases methotrexate clearance	Decreased methotrexate duration
Sodium salicylate, sulfamethoxazole, and tolbutamide	Additive	Increased toxicity
Vinblastine ↓Methotrexate	Increases action of methotrexate	Greater methotrexate potency
Bleomycin	Additive	Synergistic antineoplastic action
Phenytoin	Decreases absorption and/or increases metabolism	Decreased phenytoin levels

Mitotic Inhibitor Extravasation: Specific Antidotes		
MITOTIC INHIBITOR AGENT	**ANTIDOTE PREPARATION**	**METHOD**
Etoposide Teniposide Vinblastine Vincristine	Hyaluronidase (Wydase) 150 U/ml: add 1 ml NaCl (150 U/ml)	1. Inject 1-6 ml into the extravasated site along with multiple SC injections. 2. Repeat SC dosing over the next few hours. 3. Apply *warm* compresses.* 4. No total dose established.

*Important: corticosteroids and topical cooling appear to worsen toxicity.

DOSAGES

SELECTED MITOTIC INHIBITORS

AGENT	PHARMACOLOGIC CLASS	DOSAGE RANGE	PURPOSE
Etoposide (VP-16; VePesid)	Mitotic inhibitor	*Adult* IV: 50-100 mg/m²/day on days 1-5 to 100 mg/m²/day on days 1, 3, and 5	Testicular cancer
		IV: 35 mg/m²/day for 4 days to 50 mg/m²/day for 5 days PO: twice the IV dose rounded to the nearest 50 mg	Small-cell lung cancer
⚓Paclitaxel (Taxol)	Mitotic inhibitor	*Adult* IV: 135 mg/m² infused over 24 hr and repeated every 3 wk as tolerated	Metastatic ovarian cancer
Vincristine (LCR, VCR; Oncovin, Vincasar PFS)	Mitotic inhibitor	*Pediatric* IV: 2 mg/m² at weekly intervals *Adult* IV: 1.4 mg/m² at weekly intervals	Acute leukemia, Hodgkin's disease, lymphosarcoma, recticulum cell sarcoma, rhabdomyosarcoma, neuroblastoma, Wilms' tumor

❖ PHARMACOKINETICS

HALF-LIFE	ONSET	PEAK	DURATION
0.2-19 hr	Unknown	1-1.5 hr*	Unknown

*PO: time to reach peak serum levels.

⚓ PACLITAXEL

Paclitaxel (Taxol) is a natural mitotic inhibitor that is obtained from the bark of the Pacific yew tree. It is currently approved for the treatment of metastatic ovarian cancer that is not responsive to other chemotherapy (usually platinum-containing regimens). However, because of its excellent clinical effectiveness, it is also being used for the treatment of many other types of cancers. Paclitaxel is extremely water insoluble (hydrophobic), and for this reason, it is put into a solution containing oil rather than water. The particular oil is a type of castor oil called Cremophor EL, the same oil in which cyclosporin is mixed and which many patients cannot tolerate, showing hypersensitivity reactions similar to anaphylactic reactions. For this reason, before patients receive paclitaxel they are premedicated with a steroid, antihistamine, and an H_2 antagonist (cimetidine, ranitidine, famotidine, or nizatidine).

Paclitaxel is contraindicated in patients with a hypersensitivity to either it or the castor oil base. It is available only in a parenteral formulation—a 6-mg/ml concentrate for intravenous infusion. Common dosage recommendations are listed in the dosages table above. Pregnancy category D.

❖ PHARMACOKINETICS

HALF-LIFE	ONSET	PEAK	DURATION
13.1-52.7 hr	Unknown	Variable	7-8 mo

VINCRISTINE

Vincristine (VCR; Oncovin, Vincasar PFS) is an alkaloid isolated from the periwinkle plant that is indicated for the treatment of lymphomas, Hodgkin's disease, neuroblastoma, leukemias, rhabdomyosarcoma, osteogenic and other sarcomas, solid tumors (breast and lung), and Wilms' tumor. It is contraindicated in patients with a hypersensitivity to it and in infants. It is available only in a parenteral formulation as a 1-mg/ml injection. Common dosage recommendation are listed in the dosages table above. Pregnancy category D.

❖ PHARMACOKINETICS

HALF-LIFE	ONSET	PEAK	DURATION
10-155 hr	Unknown	Rapid	Unknown

Table 45-10	Miscellaneous Antineoplastics: Mechanisms of Action	
AGENT	CELL CYCLE	MECHANISM OF ACTION
Altretamine	CCNS	Inactivates DNA.
Asparaginase	CCS (G$_1$ phase)	Catalyzes the conversion of the amino acid asparagine to aspartic acid and ammonia; some leukemic cells are unable to produce the asparagine that is required for the synthesis of DNA and essential proteins and survival of the cells.
Cladribine	CCNS	Inhibits DNA synthesis and repair in a way similar to that of antimetabolites but has cytotoxic effects on resting as well as proliferating lymphocytes.
Hydroxyurea	CCS (S phase)	Interferes with DNA synthesis by inhibiting the incorporation of thymidine into DNA.
Mitotane	CCNS	Covalently bonds to mitochondrial proteins, causing a direct cytotoxic effect and resulting in the inhibition of adrenocortical function; it is an adrenocortical cytotoxic agent.

Miscellaneous Antineoplastics

The miscellaneous antineoplastic agents are those that, because of their unique structure and mechanisms of action, cannot be classified into the previously described categories. These agents consist of:

- Altretamine
- Asparaginase
- Cladribine
- Hydroxyurea
- Mitotane

Mechanism of Action

The antineoplastic drugs that fall in the miscellaneous category are a very diverse group of agents that kill cancer cells by a variety of mechanisms. The proposed mechanisms of action of these various agents are given in Table 45-10.

Drug Effects

The miscellaneous antineoplastics cited consist of both CCS and CCNS agents, and depending on the particular agent, they can work in any phase of the cell cycle. They are used to treat a variety of solid tumors as well as some hematologic malignancies and may also be used in combination chemotherapy regimens to enhance the overall cytotoxic effect.

Therapeutic Uses

The miscellaneous antineoplastics are used for the treatment of a wide variety of cancers. The agents and their therapeutic uses are listed in the box above right.

Specific Miscellaneous Antineoplastics: Therapeutic Uses

AGENT	TYPE OF CANCER
Altretamine	Palliative treatment of recurrent, persistent ovarian cancer
Asparaginase	Acute lymphocytic leukemia
Cladribine	Active hairy cell leukemia, chronic lymphocytic leukemia, non-Hodgkin's lymphomas, acute myeloid leukemia, autoimmune hemolytic anemia
Hydroxyurea	Chronic myelocytic leukemia, recurrent or metastatic ovarian cancer, squamous cell carcinoma of the head and neck
Mitotane	Adrenocortical carcinoma

Miscellaneous Antineoplastics: Bone Marrow Suppression

DRUG	DEGREE OF BMS	CELL LINE	NADIR (DAYS)
Hydroxyurea	Severe	G	7

G, granulocytes.

Side Effects and Adverse Effects

Like all the antineoplastic agents, the miscellaneous agents also cause hair loss, nausea and vomiting, and myelosuppression. The emetic potentials of some of these agents are given in the box on p. 683. The only agent that causes BMS in the moderate to severe range is hydroxyurea, and the characteristics of the BMS it causes are summarized in the box above. Major side effects specific to these agents are given in Table 45-11.

Interactions

There are many notable drug interactions associated with the miscellaneous antineoplastics, the most common of which are listed in Table 45-12.

Dosages

For information on recommended dosages of the agents in the miscellaneous category, see the dosages table on the following page.

DRUG PROFILES

The various agents in the miscellaneous category of antineoplastics are used to treat a wide range of neoplasms, ranging from recurrent, persistent ovarian cancer and hairy cell leukemia to adrenocortical carcinoma. Altretamine and hydroxyurea are administered orally, and asparaginase, cladribine, and mitotane are available only in parenteral preparations.

ALTRETAMINE

Altretamine (Hexalen) is a CCNS agent that is used for the palliative treatment of recurrent, persistent ovarian cancer after the completion of first-line treatment with cisplatin or alkylating agent–based combination therapy. Its mechanism of action appears to be the production of metabolites that bind to precursors of DNA, thus preventing its formation and leading to cell death.

It is contraindicated in patients with a hypersensitivity to it and in those suffering from either severe BMS or severe neurologic toxicity. Altretamine is available only in an oral formulation—50-mg capsules. Common dosage recommendations are listed in the dosages table on the following page. Pregnancy category D.

♦ PHARMACOKINETICS

HALF-LIFE	ONSET	PEAK	DURATION
4.7-10.2 hr	Unknown	0.5-3 hr*	2-36 mo

*In plasma.

ASPARAGINASE

Asparaginase (Elspar) is used for the treatment of acute lymphocytic leukemia. Its mechanism of action is slightly different from that of traditional antineoplastics in that it is an enzyme which catalyzes the conversion of the amino acid asparagine to aspartic acid and ammonia. Leukemic cells are then unable to synthesize the asparagine required for them to synthesize

Table 45-11	Miscellaneous Agents: Severe Adverse Effects

ANTIBIOTIC AGENT	SEVERE SIDE/ADVERSE EFFECTS
Altretamine	Liver and CNS toxicities
Asparaginase	Liver, kidney, lung, and CNS toxicities
Cladribine	Hematologic toxicities
Hydroxyurea	CNS toxicities
Mitotane	Genitourinary and lung toxicities

Table 45-12	Miscellaneous Antineoplastic: Drug Interactions	

DRUG	MECHANISM	RESULT
Altretamine		
Cimetidine	Additive	Possible increased altretamine toxicity
Asparaginase		
Mercaptopurine, ↓methotrexate, and prednisone	Additive	Additive hepatotoxicity
Prednisone	Additive effect on pancreas	Hyperglycemia
Mitotane		
Barbiturates, warfarin, and phenytoin	Induces hepatic microsomal enzymes	Increased metabolism of these drugs
CNS depressants	Additive	Combined CNS depression

DNA and other essential proteins necessary for cell survival.

Asparaginase is contraindicated in patients who are hypersensitive to it, as well as in infants, lactating women, and patients with pancreatitis. It is available only in a parenteral form as a 10,000-IU dosage for injection. Common dosage recommendations are listed in the dosages table below. Pregnancy category C.

PHARMACOKINETICS

HALF-LIFE	ONSET	PEAK	DURATION
8-30 hr	Unknown	Several days plasma	23-33 days

HYDROXYUREA

Hydroxyurea (Hydrea) most closely resembles the antimetabolite antineoplastics in its actions. It interferes with the synthesis of DNA by inhibiting the incorporation of thymidine into DNA. It works in the S phase of the cell cycle, making it a CCS agent.

Hypersensitivity, leukopenia, thrombocytopenia, and anemia are the contraindications to its use. It is a potent inhibitor of bone marrow cell production, and thus causes severe BMS. Its maximum destruction of granulocyte cell lines (nadir) occurs about 1 week after the start of therapy. Hydroxyurea is available only in an oral formulation—500-mg capsules. Common dosage recommendations are listed in the dosages table below.

PHARMACOKINETICS

HALF-LIFE	ONSET	PEAK	DURATION
~7.5 hr	Unknown	2 hr serum	Unknown

NURSING PROCESS

Discussion of the nursing process applicable to patients receiving antineoplastic agents will be broken down according to the different classes of agents.

ASSESSMENT

Antimetabolite agents such as fluorouracil are contraindicated in patients who have recently had or been exposed to chickenpox or herpes zoster because they may exacerbate the subsequent or residual symptoms of these diseases. Fluorouracil and other agents that cause bone marrow suppression should be used cautiously in patients with renal, cardiac, or hepatic dysfunction; bone marrow dysfunction; or infiltration of the malignancy to the bone marrow. Baseline vital signs, complete blood counts, and the patient's overall health status, renal and liver function, intake and output, and weight should all be assessed and the findings recorded.

Before administering methotrexate, another antimetabolite, the nurse should check the patient to make sure he or she does not have ascites, pleural effusion, or renal dysfunction, as these are contraindications to its use. Cautious use is recommended in patients suffering from BMS, infection, stomatitis, peptic ulcer disease, or ulcerative colitis. If the patient has had or has

DOSAGES

SELECTED MISCELLANEOUS ANTINEOPLASTIC AGENTS

AGENT	PHARMACOLOGIC CLASS	DOSAGE RANGE	PURPOSE
Altretamine (Hexalen)	Cytotoxic antineoplastic	*Adult* PO: 260 mg/m²/day in 4 divided doses pc and hs for 14 or 21 days in a 28-day treatment cycle	Ovarian cancer
Asparaginase (Elspar)	Antineoplastic enzyme	*Adult/Pediatric* IV: 200 IU/kg/day for 28 days	Acute lymphocytic leukemia
Hydroxyurea (Hydrea)	Urea-derived antineoplastic	*Adult* PO: 20-30 mg/kg/day as a single dose or 80 mg/kg as a single dose every 3rd day 20-30 mg/kg/day as a single dose	Solid tumors Chronic myelocytic leukemia

been exposed to chickenpox, exposure to methotrexate may cause the subsequent or residual disease process to become more generalized. It can also further increase the hyperuricemia that occurs in patients with gout or renal stones. Cautious use is recommended as well in patients who are receiving other cytotoxic agents or irradiation plus in elderly, debilitated, or very young patients. It is important to get a list of the current medications the patient is taking so that drug interactions can be avoided (see earlier discussion of the drugs that interact with the antimetabolites).

Cautious use of mechlorethamine is recommended in patients who are pregnant or breastfeeding. Cautious use is also recommended in patients suffering from BMS, infection, herpetic infections, or chickenpox; in those with a history of gout or renal stones; and in those who have had previous chemotherapy or radiotherapy because of the compounding of adverse reactions that can occur. It is important to obtain and document the baseline BUN level, urinalysis findings, renal function study results, the CBC, and the results of audiometric testing so that other problems or complications of therapy can be watched for and prevented.

Cyclophosphamide is contraindicated in lactating women and nitrosoureas are contraindicated in patients with leukopenia and thrombocytopenia. Cautious use of cyclophosphamide and the nitrosoureas is recommended in pregnant or lactating women and in patients with renal or hepatic dysfunction, BMS, infection, or tumors infiltrating the bone marrow.

The cautions applicable to cyclophosphamide treatment also pertain to cisplatin therapy. If the patient has recently had chickenpox, shingles, or infection with a live virus, caution is indicated. In addition to the routine baseline assessment, the patient's audiometric and neurologic status should also be tested and the findings documented. The contraindications and cautions that apply to doxorubicin use are the same as those that apply to cyclophosphamide therapy.

Mitotic inhibitors such as vinblastine and vincristine are contraindicated in persons who have had chickenpox or shingles.

NURSING DIAGNOSES

General nursing diagnoses pertinent to patients receiving antineoplastic agents, regardless of the class, include:

- Risk for impaired skin integrity and oral mucous membranes as the result of stomatitis from drug therapy.
- Pain related to neoplastic process and GI side effects such as anorexia, nausea, and vomiting.
- Impaired skin integrity related to effects of antineoplastic therapy.

- Risk for self-injury related to effects of BMS.
- Body-image disturbance related to alopecia or other effects of the antineoplastic agent and the neoplasm.
- Diarrhea related to effects of the antineoplastic agents.
- Risk for infection related to BMS and resultant neutropenia.
- Following are the diagnoses specific to the use of various agents:

Methotrexate
- Impaired skin integrity related to dermatologic side effects of the drug, with resultant vasculitis or photosensitivity

Mechlorethamine
- Sensory-perceptual loss (hearing loss) resulting from the effects of the antineoplastic.
- Impaired skin integrity resulting from extravasation.

Cyclophosphamide and **nitrosoureas**
- Body image disturbance related to disturbed gonadal functioning and growth, alopecia, and darkened skin.
- Risk for altered cardiac tissue perfusion related to toxicity of medication
- Altered urinary elimination (hemorrhagic cystitis, nephrotoxicity) related to cyclophosphamide use.

Cisplatin
- Activity intolerance related to anemia-induced fatigue.
- Sensory-perceptual disturbances (hearing loss, optic neuritis) related to ototoxicity.
- Risk for injury resulting from loss of reflexes and numbness of hands and feet and ataxia stemming from neurotoxicity.

Doxorubicin
- Risk for altered cardiac tissue perfusion related to cardiotoxicity.

Vinblastine and **vincristine**
- Risk for altered urinary patterns related to hyperuremia, uric acid nephropathy, and neurotoxicity with joint and back pain.

PLANNING

Goals related to the administration of antineoplastic agents, regardless of the class, include:

- Patient regains normal or prechemotherapy level of oral mucosa integrity with minimal discomfort and problems stemming from stomatitis.
- Patient experiences increased comfort levels during antineoplastic therapy.
- Patient experiences minimal breaks in skin integrity during antineoplastic therapy.
- Patient experiences minimal to no self-injury during antineoplastic therapy.

- Patient maintains a positive self-concept during antineoplastic therapy.
- Patient regains normal or prechemotherapy bowel elimination patterns.
- Patient has minimal problems with infection during chemotherapy.

Following are the goals specific to the use of various antineoplastic agents:

Methotrexate
- Patient's skin remains intact while receiving antineoplastic agents.

Mechlorethamine
- Patient experiences minimal sensory-perceptual loss (hearing loss) resulting from the effects of the antineoplastic therapy.
- Patient states measures to minimize side effects and adverse effects to chemotherapy.

Cyclophosphamide and nitrosourea
- Patient verbalizes feelings frequently.
- Patient regains prechemotherapy activity and energy levels.
- Patient experiences minimal alterations in urinary elimination patterns.

Cisplatin
- Patient maintains energy levels or near normal energy levels.
- Patient experiences minimal problems associated with possible neurotoxicity.

Doxorubicin
- Patient remains free of or has minimal cardiac difficulties.

Vinblastine and vincristine
- Patient maintains normal fluid volume status during chemotherapy.

Outcome Criteria

Outcome criteria pertinent to patients receiving antineoplastic agents, regardless of the class, include:
- Patient uses measures to minimize alterations in mucous membranes caused by stomatitis such as frequent mouthcare with toothettes and/or use of alcohol-based mouthwash.
- Patient uses nonpharmacologic and pharmacologic methods such as relaxation therapy, music therapy, and biofeedback to control pain related to neoplastic processes and to manage the GI side effects such as anorexia, nausea, and vomiting.
- Patient uses measures to enhance skin integrity while undergoing antineoplastic therapy such as keeping skin clean, dry, and lubricated.
- Patient states methods to use to minimize risk for self-injury related to effects of BMS such as avoiding crowds (i.e., patients with leukopenia), straight razors, venipuncture, and injections, if possible (i.e., patients with decreased platelets).

RESEARCH

Where Do Women Receive Their Health Care and How Effective Is the Screening in These Settings?

According to a recent study supported by the Agency for Health Care Policy and Research (HS06910), African-American women are twice as likely as white women to have breast cancer diagnosed at a later stage, after it has already spread to the lymph nodes. Differences in clinical breast examination or breast self-examination do not explain this racial difference in diagnoses of breast cancer, and dissimilar histories of mammography screening among women accounted for only about 10% of the variation. In a retrospective study at Yale University Medical School, African-American women in the study were nearly twice as likely to have breast cancer diagnosed before the age of 50 and three times as likely to be obese when diagnosed (N = 322). The same study showed that black women were significantly more likely than white women to have never had a mammogram or to have had one in the three-year period before symptom development or diagnoses. The researchers in this study cite many variables that contribute to effective mammographic screening and the inconsistent quality of such screening documented at the national level. They expressed the need for an evaluation of the settings in which women receive health care to further determine if African-American and white women benefit equally from this screening technology.

From Jones S, Curnen M et al: Can mammography screening explain the race difference in stage diagnoses of breast cancer? *Cancer* (75):2103, 1995.

- Patient verbalizes openly his or her concerns and fears regarding any self-concept disturbances related to alopecia and other effects of the antineoplastic therapy and the neoplasm.
- Patient uses nonpharmacologic methods (diet, fluids, exercise) and pharmacologic methods (e.g., bulk-forming laxatives) to regain normal or prechemotherapy bowel elimination patterns.
- Patient minimizes risk for infection by adhering to methods of preventing infection such as consuming a high-protein diet and avoiding crowds while blood counts are decreased.

Following are outcome criteria specific to the use of various antineoplastic agents:

Methotrexate
- Patient uses sunscreen and other skin protection to avoid skin injury while experiencing the derma-

(Text continued on p. 706.)

Nursing Implications: Antineoplastics

ANTINEOPLASTIC AGENT	CLASSIFICATION	NURSING IMPLICATIONS
Fluorouracil	Antimetabolite	Administer IV undiluted through a stopcock or Y-tube; give over 1-3 min or dilute in NS or D5W and give over 2-8 hr in an IV infusion. Antiemetic therapy 30 min to 1 hr before therapy (as ordered) to prevent nausea. Antibiotics may be needed to prevent infection. Antispasmodic may be needed to manage diarrhea. Use strict asepsis with patients. Increase fluids up to 3 liters per day, unless contraindicated, to prevent dehydration. IV site changed q48h. Mouth care with water and club soda or with soft-bristle toothbrush or cotton-tipped applicator. Encourage diet high in iron and vitamins, low in fiber, and including few dairy products, especially if patient also undergoing irradiation.
⚓Methotrexate	Folic acid antagonist	Administer after diluting in sterile water for injection at a concentration of 5 mg/2 ml and give through a Y-tube or three-way stopcock at a rate of ≤10 mg/1 min. Antacids given before oral agent may help minimize GI upset. Antiemetic given 30 to 60 min before therapy. Allopurinol may be ordered to help control serum uric acid levels. Encourage intake of up to 3 liters of fluids per day, unless contraindicated. Leucovorin rescue is ordered within 12 hr to prevent tissue damage and severe side effects of MTX.
Mechlorethamine	Alkylating agent	Use guidelines for administering cytotoxic agent and give IV after diluting with 10 mg/10 ml of sterile water or NaCl; leave needle in the vial and withdraw dose; give through stopcock or Y-tube. Slow IV infusion is often done using 21-, 23-, or 25-gauge needle; constant monitoring of IV site is necessary to prevent extravasation and the resulting necrosis. With extravasation, it is important to discontinue solution, leave needle in place, infuse with isotonic sodium thiosulfate, and apply ice pack for 6-12 hr or follow hospital policy guidelines. Encourage fluid intake of up to 3 liters per day to prevent formation of urate deposits in the urine; also encourage adequate diet, special skin and mouth care, and diet low in purines, organ meats, and dried beans.
⚓Cyclophospha-mide	Alkylating agent	Same instructions as for mechlorethamine. Administer IV or PO with forced fluid intake because adequate hydration is needed to prevent hemorrhagic cystitis. Allopurinol may also be needed to maintain normal uric acid levels and prevent alkalinization of the urine. Administer IV after diluting to a concentration of 100 mg/5 ml of sterile water; shake and let stand until clear then may dilute more in up to 250 ml of D5W or NS; give via Y-tube or three-way stopcock at ≤100 mg/min

continued

Nursing Implications: Antineoplastics—cont'd

ANTINEOPLASTIC AGENT	CLASSIFICATION	NURSING IMPLICATIONS
Carmustine and lomustine	Nitrosoureas	Always check IV site for extravasation and use 21-, 23-, or 25-gauge needle. Give as early in the AM as possible so can be eliminated before bedtime. Diet low in purine, high in iron and vitamins. Give IV after proper dilutional guidelines have been followed, usually diluting 100 mg of drug into 3 ml of ethyl alcohol (usually provided that way); then further dilute in 27 ml of sterile water for injection followed by further dilution in 100-500 ml of 0.9% NaCl or D5W; give over 1 hr or more; discontinue infusion if discomfort occurs. Antiemetic use 30-60 min before infusion. Increase fluids up to 3 liters per day, unless contraindicated, to prevent urate deposits from forming in urine. Follow above guidelines for mouth care. Apply warm compresses to IV site to relieve inflammation, and reduce flow rate if burning sensation occurs; monitor site continuously.

Patient Teaching TIPS

Antineoplastic Agents

✔ Patients should report black tarry stools, chills, fever, sore throat, or shortness of breath to the physician immediately.

✔ Patients receiving **5-fluorouracil** should be told about the importance of observing protective isolation and of eating foods high in iron and vitamins. They should avoid consuming foods high in fiber as well as foods containing citric acid, foods that are hot or cold, and foods that have a rough texture. Patients should be told to report the symptoms of stomatitis, which consist of any bleeding, white spots or patches, and ulcerations of the mouth. Patients should be told to examine their mouths daily and to report any problems immediately to the nurse or physician. They should also know to report headache, fatigue, faintness, shortness of breath (anemia), bleeding and easy bruising (drop in platelet count), and sore throat and fever (infection) at the first sign of these symptoms. Women will need an alternative form of nondrug contraception during therapy. Patients should also be told to avoid taking aspirin or aspirin-containing products as well as products containing ibuprofen.

✔ Patients receiving **antineoplastics** will need to purchase or rent a wig or hairpiece because of the hair loss that occurs during treatment. The hair loss is temporary however. The American Cancer Society often has some wigs available and usually at no cost, so patients should be told to contact the local chapter for information on this. Patients should avoid using alcohol and aspirin, razors, and commercial mouthwash during treatment with MTX and most antineoplastic agents.

✔ Sterility and amenorrhea may occur in patients on **mechlorethamine** or **cyclophosphamide** therapy, but these are reversible once therapy is discontinued. Patients taking these agents should know to report the usual symptoms of infection, anemia, and bleeding, as already mentioned. Hair loss is possible, so patients may wish to wear a wig or hairpiece.

✔ Patients receiving **carmustine** or **lomustine** should follow the guidelines already given concerning protective isolation and mouth care, and they should know to report bleeding and the signs or symptoms of anemia or infection. They should also be told to avoid using aspirin, ibuprofen, alcohol, commercial mouthwashes, and razors.

✔ Patients receiving **etoposide** or **teniposide**, as well as their family members, should be warned about the possible complications of therapy, such as infection, anemia, and bleeding disorders, and told to report any complaints, side effects, or changes in breathing to the physician. Hair loss is expected, so patients should consider getting hairpieces or wigs before the start of therapy. Patients should be told to change positions slowly because of the hypotension that can occur.

tologic side effects of the drug, with resultant vasculitis or photosensitivity.

Mechlorethamine

- Patient reports any changes in hearing ability stemming from the effects of the antineoplastic therapy to the physician immediately.
- Patient immediately reports any unusual changes in the skin surrounding the IV insertion site in order to prevent impaired skin integrity related to extravasation.

Cyclophosphamide and nitrosourea

- Patient verbalizes feelings openly about any disturbance of self-concept related to disturbed gonadal functioning and growth, alopecia, and darkened skin.
- Patient adheres to activity restrictions because of the altered cardiac output related to the toxicity of the medication but maintain some approximation of normal activity or of the prechemotherapy level of activity.
- Patient states measures to take to prevent or minimize hemorrhagic cystitis or nephrotoxicity related to cyclophosphamide use, such as forcing liquids (2000 cc/day) before, during, and after chemotherapy.

Cisplatin

- Patient conserves energy throughout the day when experiencing anemia-induced fatigue but maintains activities of daily living during chemotherapy.
- Patient states ways to prevent or minimize the loss of reflexes, the numbness of the hands and feet, and the ataxia related to neurotoxicity.

Doxorubicin

- Patient reports any cardiac difficulty such as shortness of breath, dysrhythmias, or chest pain resulting from possible cardiotoxicity

Vinblastine and vincristine

- Patient forces fluids (at least 2000 ml/day) within the restrictions specified by the physician to prevent or minimize hyperemia, uric acid nephropathy, or neurotoxicity with joint and back pain.

IMPLEMENTATION

The nursing actions appropriate to treatment with each antineoplastic agent are presented in the box on p. 704 and the corresponding patient teaching tips are given on p. 705. The respective drug interactions and side effects associated with the various agents are described in the section devoted to the discussion of the individual classes of agents. Home health guidelines appear in the box above right.

HOME HEALTH POINTS
Antineoplastic Agents

- The home health care of cancer patients requires the skills of an astute, well-prepared, and experienced nurse who can react quickly to critical situations yet remain empathic during the terminal stages of the disease.
- The home health care nurse should be certified to administer chemotherapy and to follow the specific policies established by the agency as well as the accepted standards of care for home health nursing.
- Documentation is a critical part of the nursing care of home health patients, and this should be done in accordance with the agency's policy. It is very important that the nurse document the location of the IV injection site, the details concerning the infusion of the chemotherapeutic agent, and the response of the patient, along with any problems with extravasation and the actions initiated to counter the effects. Should extravasation occur, accepted nursing actions should be initiated and documented and the physician contacted. Photographs of the site should be taken, if possible, so that the degree of damage can be adequately recorded. All patient and family responses to all aspects of care should also be documented.
- Antineoplastic therapy can be successfully carried out at home if the patient and family members are adequately and sufficiently taught regarding the medications used, their action, side effects, toxic effects, and procedures for administration.

EVALUATION

Therapeutic responses to antineoplastic therapy include a decrease in the tumor size and in the spread of malignancy as well as improved energy levels, activities of daily living, and quality of life after chemotherapy. It is also important to monitor patients for bleeding tendencies and the signs and symptoms of infection or anemia during and after therapy. The oral mucosa should be examined daily to look for dryness, sores, ulcerations, white patches, and bleeding of the gums. Oral discomfort and difficulty swallowing are other problems to watch for. Any abnormal changes should be reported to the physician. Yellowing of the skin, abdominal pain, fever, sore throat, decreased urine production, dehydration, rapid respirations, poor skin turgor, loss of weight and appetite, skin lesions, rashes, and restlessness should also be reported immediately to the physician.

TAKE HOME POINTS

Cancer

- A group of diseases that are characterized by uncontrolled cellular growth.
- Can invade into surrounding tissue and metastasize to new sites distant from the original body site.
- Metastasis is the spreading of a cancer from the original site of growth.
- A neoplasm or tumor is a mass of new cells that exhibit uncontrolled cellular reproduction.
- Paraneoplastic syndromes consist of signs and symptoms that arise at a distance from the tumor or its sites of metastasis.

Benign Tumors

- Tumors that are characterized by uniform size and shape.
- Show no invasiveness or metastatic properties.

Malignant Tumors

- *Malignancy* specifically refers to a neoplasm that is malignant as opposed to benign.
- Typically composed of cancerous cells.
- They invade surrounding tissues, metastasize, and migrate to other tissues and organs, where they form metastatic tumor depostits.

Tumor Classification by Tissue of Origin

- Epithelial = carcinoma
  Connective = sarcoma
  Lymphatic = lymphoma
  Blood = leukemia.

Antineoplastics

- Cell cycle–specific (CCS) and cell cycle–nonspecific (CCNS) agents.
- CCS agents kill cancer cells during specific phases of the cell growth cycle.
- CCNS agents kill cancer cells during any phase of their cell growth cycle.

Nursing Considerations

- Chemotherapy may be used in many situations and requires very astute and prudent nursing care as well as critical decisions concerning its administration.
- Assessment of baseline vital signs, complete blood counts, and assessment of overall health status, renal and liver function, intake and output, and weights should be performed and the findings recorded before the start of any chemotherapy.
- The hair that regrows after alopecia may be a different color and consistency than it was originally, and the patient should be warned about this and other possible side effects before the start of therapy.
- Oral hygiene should be performed at least once every 8 hours, sometimes more frequently, to prevent stomatitis.
- A holistic approach to the care of the cancer patient must focus on the patient's strengths and minimize the weaknesses at this time in his or her life.
- Patients receiving cisplatin are at risk for suffering seizures, reduced urinary output, nephrotoxicity, and neurotoxicity and require frequent monitoring and astute nursing care to prevent or treat these problems in a timely fashion.
- Antimetabolite agents such as fluorouracil are contraindicated in patients with a recent history of or recent exposure to chickenpox or herpes zoster because of the risk of exacerbation of the subsequent or residual symptoms of the disease.

NURSING ▪ CARE ▪ PLAN

Breast Cancer

Mrs. E.S., a 65-year-old woman with a recent diagnosis of estrogen receptor positive breast tumor, has begun life-long chemotherapy with tamoxifen citrate therapy as an adjunct to surgical therapy with a modified radical mastectomy of the left breast. Vital parameters are as follows: Hgb and Hct within normal limits, WBC 4500, platelets 100,000, vital signs within normal limits. Other data pertinent to Mrs. E.S. include complaints of metallic taste, some nausea, and decreased energy levels with a problem some days of taking in only very minimal amounts of food. No antiemetics, antacids, vitamins, iron supplements, or nutritional supplements are being taken.

Assessment with nursing diagnoses	Planning with goals and outcome criteria	Implementation and patient education	Evaluation
Subjective "I just hate these hot flashes." "Everything tastes so metallic." "Do I really have to take this all the time?" "I just don't feel like eating most of the time . . . nothing tastes good anymore . . ." **Objective** Breast cancer diagnosed 2 mo ago 65 yr in otherwise good health Estrogen receptor positive breast tumor WBC 4500 Platelets 100,000 No weight loss Takes tamoxifen citrate 10 mg bid Decreased energy level but able to carry out ADLs	**Goals** Patient will maintain diet of six frequent feedings with Ensure snacks within 2 wk **Outcome criteria** Patient will show improved appetite as evidenced by: Energy level Intake of foods within the basic food groups No weight loss Decreased complaints of diminished appetite	Encourage use of antiemetic 30-60 min before dosing of tamoxifen, as ordered, to prevent nausea and vomiting if a problem Weekly weights at home Antacid before medication, with physician's order, and give PM dose of medication after evening meal unless contraindicated Encourage patient to try cola, Jell-O, dry toast, or crackers if unable to tolerate other regular food products until nausea subsides Encourage fluid intake of at least 2-3 L/day to prevent dehydration unless contraindicated Encourage and give sample menus of a diet high in iron and vitamins such as green leafy vegetables, organ meats, nutritional supplements such as Ensure, and iron or vitamin supplements as ordered Encourage increased activity, as tolerated, to help increase appetite Encourage patient to keep daily journal of meals and nutritional intake Patient to call the physician should dietary intake decrease and nausea and vomiting occur	Patient will show improved nutritional status as evidenced by: Energy level No weight loss Normal lab values such as Hgb, Hct, BUN, protein levels Nausea and vomiting Dietary intake with nutritional supplements Improved appetite <complaints of poor taste

Critical Thinking **A C T I V I T I E S**

1. It is crucial for the patient receiving cyclophosphamide to:
   a. attain adequate hydration before the start of therapy.
   b. have his or her ECG and arterial line pressures monitored during therapy.
   c. be adequately anesthetized before infusion of the drug.
   d. receive instructions about the life-threatening complications stemming from the neurotoxicity it can cause.

2. A patient would be in danger of contracting an infection if his or her absolute granulocyte count declined to less than:
   a. 100,000 cells/mm^3
   b. 10,000 cells/mm^3
   c. 1,000 cells/mm^3
   d. 100 cells/mm^3

3. Side effects of mechlorethamine include which of the following?
   a. Sensory-perceptual loss (hearing loss)
   b. Chronic inflammatory bowel disorders
   c. Disturbed gonadal function and growth
   d. Darkened skin

4. Two broad categories of drugs used to treat cancer are cell cycle–specific agents and cell cycle–non-specific agents. Explain the difference between the two categories of drugs based on their mechanisms of action.

5. G.B. is a 45-year-old woman who has just been diagnosed with breast cancer. She has agreed to undergo chemotherapy and will begin a course of combination chemotherapy consisting of a CMF regimen, as follows:

   Cyclophosphamide, 100 mg/m^2: po days 1-14
   Methotrexate, 40 mg/m^2: IVB days 1 and 8
   Fluorouracil, 600 mg/m^2: IVB days 1 and 8
   Repeat cycle every 28 days.

   She weighs 135 pounds and is 5 feet, 4 inches tall. From the body surface area (BSA) nomogram in the appendix, calculate what doses of cyclophosphamide, methotrexate, and fluorouracil she should receive.

▲▲

BIBLIOGRAPHY

Albanese J, Nutz P: *Mosby's 1995 nursing drug cards,* St Louis, 1995, Mosby.

Cancer update: *Nursing* 23(4):59, 1993.

Johnson KB: *Harriet Lane handbook,* ed 13, St Louis, 1993, Mosby.

Keen JH: *Critical care and emergency drug reference,* St Louis, 1994, Mosby.

Knoben JE, Anderson PO: *Handbook of critical drug data,* ed 6, Hamilton, Ill, 1988, Drug Intelligence Publications.

McEvoy GK: *AHFS drug information,* Bethesda, Md, 1994, American Society of Hospital Pharmacists.

McKenry L, Salerno E: *Mosby's pharmacology in nursing,* ed 19, St Louis, 1995, Mosby.

Meyer C: New drugs on the oncology front, *Am J Nurs* 93(3):63, 1993.

Rutherford, C: Position paper: administration of antineoplastic agents, *J Intrav Nurs* 15(1):8, 1992.

Skidmore-Roth L: *Mosby's 1995 nursing drug reference,* St Louis, 1995, Mosby.

Studva KV: Programmed instruction: cancer chemotherapy, *Canc Nurs* 16(2):145, 1993.

Chapter 46

Biologic Response Modifiers

Objectives

When you reach the end of this chapter, you will be able to:

1 Discuss the use of biologic response modifiers in the treatment of neoplasms.

2 Classify the biologic response modifiers by specific classification grouping.

3 List the side effects, adverse reactions, and toxic effects associated with the biologic response modifiers.

4 Discuss the mechanism of action, cautions, contraindications, routes of administration, and drug interactions associated with biologic response modifiers.

5 Develop a comprehensive nursing care plan using the nursing process and including patient education for patients receiving biologic response modifiers.

CHAPTER OUTLINE

Immune System
 Humoral immune system
 Cellular immune system
Interferons
 Mechanism of action
 Drug effects
 Therapeutic uses
 Side effects and adverse effects
 Interactions
 Dosages

Drug Profiles
Interferon-α Products
  Interferon alfa-2a, Interferon alfa-2b,
   Interferon alfa-n3
Interferon-β Products
  ⚓ Interferon beta-1b
Interferon-γ Products
  Interferon gamma-1b
Interleukins
 Mechanism of action
 Drug effects
 Therapeutic uses
 Side effects and adverse effects
 Interactions
 Dosages

Drug Profiles
  ⚓ Aldesleukin
Colony-stimulating Factors

Mechanism of action
Drug effects
Therapeutic uses
Side effects and adverse effects
Interactions
Dosages

Drug Profiles
 ⚓ Epoetin alfa
 ⚓ Filgrastim
  Sargramstim

Nursing Process
Assessment
Nursing Diagnoses
Planning
 Outcome criteria
Implementation
Evaluation

Glossary

Antibody (an' tĭ-bod' e) An immunoglobulin that binds to antigens to form an antibody-antigen complex. (p. 712)

Antigen (an' tĭ-jen) Substance that is foreign to the human body. (p. 712)

B-cells Cells of the humoral immune system that attack foreign invaders; synonymous with lymphocytes. (p. 712)

Biologic response modifiers (BRMs) Agents whose primary site of action is the immune system. (p. 711)

Cellular immunity One of the two major components of the immune system; acts in accordance with humoral immunity to recognize and destroy foreign particles and cells. (p. 711)

Colony-stimulating factors (CSFs) Cytokines that regulate the growth, differentiation, and function of bone marrow stem cells. (p. 712)

Cytokines (si″ to-kīn) Immune system protein that directs the actions and communications between the cellular and humoral divisions of the immune system and augments or enhances the immune response. (p. 715)

Cytotoxic T-cells (si″ to-tok′ sik) Cells that directly kill their target cells without the help of other immune system cells. (p. 712)

Humoral immunity (hu′ mər-əl) One of the two major components of the immune system; acts in accordance with cellular immunity to recognize and destroy foreign particles and cells. (p. 711)

Interferon (in″ tən-fēr′ on) Biologic response modifier that enhances the activity of macrophages and natural killer cells. (p. 712)

Lymphokine-activated killer (LAK) cell Cell resulting from the multiplication of T-cells that recognizes cancer cells and ignores normal cells. (p. 717)

Memory cells Cells involved in the humoral immune system that remember the exact characteristics of a particular foreign invader or antigen. (p. 712)

Monoclonal (mon″ o-klōn′ əl) A group of identical cells or organisms derived from a single cell. (p. 712)

Plasma cells Lymphoid or lymphocyte-like cells found in the bone marrow, connective tissue, and sometimes blood; they produce antibodies. (p. 712)

Stem cells Precursors of mature blood cells; they bind to specific receptors and direct the growth and differentiation of distinct cell lines. (p. 720)

T-helper cells Cells that direct the actions of most of the other cells of the immune system. (p. 712)

T-lymphocytes Workhorses of the cellular immune system that are differentiated by their function in the immune system. (p. 712)

T-suppressor cells Cells that regulate and limit the immune response; opposite of T-helper cells. (p. 712)

Tumor antigens Chemical compounds expressed on the surfaces of tumor cells; they tell the immune system that these cells do not belong in the body, labeling the tumor cells as foreign. (p. 711)

In the past, care of patients with cancer required an understanding of three treatment modalities: surgery, radiation, and chemotherapy. Although these are highly sophisticated methods of cancer treatment, many cancer patients still are not cured. Surgery and radiation therapy are, at best, local or regional treatments, and, as discussed in the preceding chapter, adjuvant therapy is needed to destroy undetected distant micrometastases. The advantage of cytotoxic chemotherapy with antineoplastics is that these agents attack tumor cells throughout the body. However, this advantage is at the same time the greatest limitation, because all normal cells are exposed to the cytotoxic drug effects as well. Toxicity to normal cells may cause the

administration of many other drugs to correct antineoplastic-induced side effects, or chemotherapy doses may have to be reduced to decrease side effects. This will simultaneously reduce their effectiveness.

Over the last two decades medical technology has developed a group of agents whose primary site of action is the immune system. These agents are collectively known as **biologic response modifiers** (BRMs). BRMs make up the fourth type of cancer therapy. The current modalities available to treat cancer are surgery, radiation, chemotherapy, and biologic response modifiers.

Biologic response modifiers can be broadly defined as agents that modify the body's own immune system (biologic response) so that it can destroy bacteria, viruses, and cancerous cells. The immune system is thought of primarily as our defense system against disease-carrying bacteria and viruses, but it is also an effective antitumor defense system. An intact immune system can identify cells as malignant and destroy them. In contrast to chemotherapy, the immune system can distinguish between tumor cells and normal body tissues. Normal cells are recognized as "self" and are not destroyed.

There are three major mechanisms by which BRMs work. The first mechanism augments, restores, or modifies the host defenses against the tumor. The second mechanism uses agents that are directly toxic to tumors (kill tumors). The third mechanism modifies the tumor's biology. To better understand this important class of anticancer drugs, a quick review of the immune system is beneficial.

IMMUNE SYSTEM

The immune system is an intricate biologic defense network of cells that are capable of distinguishing an unlimited variety of substances as being either foreign ("nonself") or being our own ("self"). When one of these foreign substances such as a bacteria or virus enters the body, the cells of the immune system recognize it as being nonself and eliminate or neutralize the invader. Tumors are not truly foreign substances because they arise from cells of normal tissues that have undergone uncontrolled growth. However, tumor cells do express chemical compounds on their surfaces that signal the immune system that these cells do not belong in the body. These chemical markers, called **tumor antigens** (Ag), label the tumor cells as abnormal cells.

The two major components of the body's immune system are **humoral immunity** and **cellular immunity**. These two systems act together to recognize and destroy humoral foreign particles and cells. Communication between these two divisions is vital to the success of the immune system. Attack of tumor cells by

antibodies produced by the humoral immune system prepares those tumor cells for destruction by the white blood cells of the cellular immune system. This is just one example of the effective way these two divisions of the immune system function and communicate.

Humoral Immune System

The specific "soldiers," or cells, of the humoral immune system that attack foreign invaders are the lymphocytes, also known as **B-cells**, so named because they originate from the bone marrow, or bursa. B-cells (B-lymphocytes) are cells that are specific for production of antibodies. They remain dormant until that particular foreign substance antigen is detected.

B-lymphocytes are transformed in several steps into plasma cells. **Plasma cells** can be considered factories for the production of antibodies. Antibodies (Ab) are also known as immunoglobulins (Ig). They belong to and are made by the body. These cells bind to **antigens** to form an antibody-antigen complex. The antibodies that a particular plasma cell makes are all identical, therefore they are called **monoclonal**. They are made specifically to kill or neutralize the particular foreign antigen that the B-cell initially recognizes as being nonself. There are five major types of immunoglobulins: IgA, IgD, IgE, IgG, and IgM. These different types have different structures and functions and are found in different areas of the body. As the B-lymphocytes are transformed to plasma cells, some become memory cells. **Memory cells** "remember" the exact characteristics of the particular foreign invader or antigen. The cells of the humoral immune system are shown in Fig. 46-1.

▼ **FIG. 46-1** Cells of the humoral immune system. *Ab*, antibody; *Ag*, antigen; *Ig*, immunoglobulin.

Cellular Immune System

The workhorses of the cellular immune system are the **T-lymphocytes**, also called T-cells. They are referred to as T-cells because one of their sites of origin is the thymus gland. There are three distinct populations of T-cells: **cytotoxic T-cells**, **T-helper cells**, and **T-suppressor cells**. They can be differentiated by the function they perform when working for the immune system. The cytotoxic T-cells directly kill their targets without the help of other immune system cells. They do this by causing cell lysis. The T-helper cells are considered the master controllers of the immune system. These cells direct the actions of most of the other cells of the immune system, such as lymphokines (interferons, interleukins, tumor necrosis factor, and monoclonal antibodies). The T-suppressor cells have the opposite effect on the immune system. The T-suppressor cells regulate the immune response. Their role is to limit the immune response. They have the most important negative influence on antitumor actions of the immune system. Overactive T-suppressor cells may be responsible for and permit tumor growth. A healthy immune system has about twice as many T-helper cells as T-suppressor cells at any one time.

The cells of the cellular immune system are believed to be the major cells that are involved in destruction of cancer cells. The cancer-killing cells that make up the cellular immune system are the macrophages, several types of T-cells, natural killer cells, and polymorphonuclear leukocytes. Figure 46-2 shows the components of the cellular immune system.

Therapy with biologic response modifiers combines the knowledge of several disciplines, including biology, genetics, immunology, pharmacology, medicine, and nursing. The therapeutic effects of BRMs are as follows:

- Regulation or augmentation of the immune response
- Cytotoxic or cytostatic activity directed toward cancer cells
- Inhibition of metastases, prevention of cell division, or inhibition of cell maturation

The box on the following page lists the currently available BRMs that are used in the treatment of cancer or as adjunctive agents for patients receiving chemotherapy. They are classified according to biologic effects. There are many other types of BRMs, but those listed are the ones that are most commonly used in clinical practice.

INTERFERONS

Before the commercial use of the **colony-stimulating factors** (CSFs), the interferons were the best studied and most widely used of the BRMs. **Interferons** (IFNs) are biologic response modifiers that enhance the activ-

▼ **FIG. 46-2** Cells of the cellular immune system.

Biologic Response Modifiers

INTERFERONS (IFNs)

| Interferon-alpha | Interferon-beta | Interferon-gamma |

COLONY-STIMULATING FACTORS (CSFs)

| Granulocyte CSF (G-CSF) | Granulocyte-macrophage CSF (GM-CSF) | Erythrocyte CSF (EPO) |

INTERLEUKINS (ILs)   **VACCINES**

| Interleukin-2 (IL-2) | Bacillus Calmette-Guérin vaccine (BCG) |

ity of macrophages and natural killer cells. These are the cells of the immune system that kill cancer cells. They are proteins that have three basic properties: antiviral, immune-modulating, and antitumor. Chemically they are glycoproteins (glyco = sugar and protein = amino acids). There are three different groups of interferons, each with different antigenic and biologic activity. They can be separated into alpha (α), beta (β), and gamma (γ) interferons. Their greatest activity is in the treatment of hematologic malignancies or cancers. They can be manufactured from genetically modified *Escherichia coli* bacteria *(E. coli)* by recombinant DNA (rDNA) technology. In addition, interferons are also obtained from pooled human leukocytes that have been stimulated (challenged) with various natural and synthetic inducers (antigens). The box at the top of the next page lists the available interferon preparations.

Mechanism of Action

The interferons possess both antiviral and antineoplastic effects. Their effects on cancer cells are believed to be a combination of direct inhibitory effects on DNA and protein synthesis and multiple effects on the host's immune system. The IFNs increase the cytotoxic activity of natural killer cells (NK cells) and the phagocytic ability of macrophages. It is important to note that these characteristics of IFNs are ineffective at high doses. Unlike that of conventional cytotoxic antineoplastics, the optimal biologic dose of INFs is not necessarily the maximum dose tolerated by the patient. The IFNs are also believed to increase the expression of cancer cell antigens on the cell surface, which enables the immune system to recognize them more easily.

Drug Effects

The interferons are recombinantly made natural substances that are identical to the interferons that are present within our own bodies. Therefore they have the same properties of the interferons in our own immune system. They protect our cells from virus attack by enabling our own cells to produce proteins (enzymes) that stop virus replication and prevent viruses from penetrating healthy cells. They prevent cancer

---

Interferon Preparations

INTERFERON-α	**INTERFERON-β**	**INTERFERON-γ**
IFN alfa-2a (recombinant)*	⚓IFN beta-1b (recombinant)*	IFN gamma-1b (recombinant)*
IFN alfa-2b (recombinant)*		
IFN alfa-n3†		

*Recombinant refers to the origin, (i.e., made by rDNA technology).
†The agent has been made with pooled human leukocytes.

Interferon: Therapeutic Uses

ANTIVIRAL USES	**ANTINEOPLASTIC USES**	**IMMUNOMODULATORY USES**
Rhinovirus	Hairy cell leukemia	Multiple sclerosis
Papillovirus	Kaposi's sarcoma	Other autoimmune disorders
Retrovirus	Multiple myeloma	
Hepatitis	T-cell lymphoma	
Condyloma	Chronic myeloid leukemia	
	Renal cell carcinoma	
	Melanoma	
	Bladder cancer	

---

cells from dividing and replicating and increase the activity of other cells in the immune system such as macrophages, monocytes, and natural killer cells. Interferons have three different effects on the immune system. They can restore its function if it is impaired. They can augment (amplify) the immune system's ability to function as the body's defense. Finally, they can inhibit the immune system from working. This is especially useful if the immune system has become dysfunctional, such as in an autoimmune disorder like systemic lupus erythematosis (SLE). Inhibiting the dysfunctional immune system prevents further damage to the body.

Therapeutic Uses

The beneficial actions of the interferons (antiviral, antineoplastic, and immunomodulatory) make them excellent agents for the treatment of viral infections, various cancers, and some autoimmune disorders. The box above lists the currently accepted indications for the use of interferons.

Side Effects and Adverse Effects

The most common side effects and adverse effects can be broadly classified as flulike effects: fever, chills,

Table 46-1	Interferons: Adverse Effects
BODY SYSTEM	**SIDE/ADVERSE EFFECT**
Gastrointestinal	Nausea, diarrhea, vomiting, anorexia, taste alterations, dry mouth
CNS	Mild confusion, somnolence, irritability, poor concentration, seizures, hallucinations, paranoid psychoses
Cardiovascular	Tachycardia, cyanosis, tachypnea, ECG changes, rare MI, orthostatic hypotension
Renal/hepatic	Increased BUN, creatinine, proteinuria, liver function tests (transaminases)
Hematopoietic	Neutropenia, thrombocytopenia

headache, malaise, myalgia, and fatigue. The major dose-limiting side effect of the interferons is fatigue. In high doses patients become so exhausted that they are essentially confined to bed. Other side effects and adverse effects that can be seen with interferons include anorexia, dizziness, nausea, vomiting, and diarrhea.

Table 46-1 lists the common side effects and adverse effects seen with the IFNs.

Interactions

Drug interactions are seen with both IFN-α products (2a and 2b) when used with drugs such as aminophylline that are metabolized via the cytochrome P-450 enzyme system. The combination results in decreased metabolism and increased accumulation of these drugs, which leads to toxicity. There is also some evidence that concomitant use of IFNs and antiviral agents such as zidovudine enhances the activity of both. Interferon-gamma can produce additive toxic effects to the bone marrow when used with other myelosuppressive agents.

Dosages

For recommended dosages, see the dosages table on the next page.

DRUG PROFILES

The three major classes of IFNs, IFN-α, IFN-β, and IFN-γ, vary in their antigenic makeup, biologic actions, and pharmacologic properties. The best known IFN is alpha. It can be made recombinantly with *E. coli* or collected from pooled human leukocytes.

INTERFERON-α PRODUCTS

The interferon products are biologic response modifiers that can be broadly classified as cytokines. **Cytokines** are immune system proteins that serve two essential functions. Cytokines direct the actions and communication between the cellular and humoral divisions of the immune system and augment or enhance the immune response. Other cytokines are tumor necrosis factor, interleukins, colony-stimulating factors, and transfer factor. In 1957 they were found to have antiviral activity; their beneficial effects in treating cancer were discovered much later.

The IFNs are all classified as pregnancy category C agents and are contraindicated in hypersensitivity. With the exception of the colony-stimulating factors, they are the most well studied and most widely used of the biologic response modifiers. There are three alpha-IFNs, one beta-IFN, and one gamma-IFN.

INTERFERON ALFA-2a, INTERFERON ALFA-2b, INTERFERON ALFA-n3

The most widely used of the three interferon products are the alpha interferons. They are also referred to as leukocyte interferons because they are produced from human leukocytes. The two interferon products, 2a (Roferon-A) and 2b (Intron A), are pure clones of single alpha subtypes manufactured by recombinant DNA technology. This means that they are consistent from lot to lot. These two products differ in the sequence of two amino acids. The other alpha interferon, n3 (Alferon N), is a polyclonal mixture of all alpha subtypes. It is the product of pooled human leukocytes.

Interferons are classified as pregnancy category C agents and are contraindicated in hypersensitivity. They are most commonly given by either intramuscular (IM) or subcutaneous (SC) routes of administration. However, interferons have been given by intravenous and intraperitoneal routes as well. Alpha interferons are available only parenterally as 3-, 6-, 10-, and 36-million U/ml solutions (Roferon-A); 3-, 5-, 10-, 18-, 25-, and 50-million U/ml solutions (Intron A); and a 5-million U/ml solution (Alferon-N). Commonly recommended dosages are listed in the following dosages table.

P H A R M A C O K I N E T I C S

HALF-LIFE	ONSET	PEAK	DURATION
2a: 3.7-8.5 hr	3-4 hr	IM: 3.8-7.3 hr	24 hr
2b: 2-3 hr	3-4 hr	IM: 2-3 hr	Variable

INTERFERON-β PRODUCTS

⚕ INTERFERON BETA-1b

Interferon beta (Betaseron) is one of the three available IFNs. It is manufactured from cultures of *E. coli* by means of recombinant DNA technology and is identical to the body's IFN-beta. The *E. coli* has been modified to include a plasmid that incorporates the gene for human interferon-beta. The *E. coli* then mass produces the exact genetic sequence for IFN-beta. As with the other IFNs it has antiviral, antineoplastic, and immunomodulating activities. IFN-beta is indicated to reduce the frequency of neurologic exacerbations of relapsing-remitting multiple sclerosis and is classified as a pregnancy category B agent. It is available only parenterally as a 9.6-million-unit vial for subcutaneous injection. Commonly recommended dosages are listed in the following dosages table.

P H A R M A C O K I N E T I C S

HALF-LIFE	ONSET	PEAK	DURATION
Up to 4.3 hr	3-4 hr	1-8 hr	Variable

DOSAGES

SELECTED INTERFERONS

AGENT	PHARMACOLOGIC CLASS	DOSAGE RANGE	PURPOSE
Interferon-α Products			
Interferon alfa-2a	Immunomodulator, antineoplastic	IM/SC: 3 million IU/day for 16-24 wk; maintenance dose 3 million IU 3 times/wk	Hairy cell leukemia
		IM/SC: 36 million IU/day for 10-12 wk; maintenance dose 36 million IU 3 times/wk	Kaposi's sarcoma (AIDS-related)
Interferon alfa-2b (Intron A)	Immunomodulator, antineoplastic antiviral	*≥18 yr* IM/SC: 3 million IU 3 times/wk for up to 6 mo	Chronic hepatis non-A, non-B, non-C
		IM/SC: 30-35 million IU/wk as 5 million IU/day or 10 million IU 3 times/wk for 16 wk	Chronic hepatitis B
		IM/SC: 2 million IU/m² 3 times/wk	Hairy cell leukemia
		IM/SC: 30 million IU/m² 3 times/ wk	Kaposi's sarcoma (AIDS-related)
		IM/SC: 1 million IU into each wart (lesion) 3 times/wk PM	Condylomata acuminata (genital/perianal warts)
Interferon alfa-n3 (Alferon N)	Immunomodulator, antiviral	*≥18 yr* IM/SC: 250,000 IU/wart twice/wk for up to 8 wk; do *not* exceed 2.5 million IU/treatment session	Condylomata acuminata
Interferon-β Products			
Interferon beta-1b (Betaseron)	Immunomodulator	SC: 0.25 mg (8 million IU) qod	Multiple sclerosis
Interferon-γ Products			
Interferon-gamma-1b	Immunomodulator	SC: Body surface >0.5 m²: 50 μg/ m² 3 times/wk Body surface ≤0.5 m²: 1.5 μg/kg 3 times/wk	Reducing frequency/ severity of infec- tions associated with chronic granulomatous disease

INTERFERON-γ PRODUCTS
INTERFERON GAMMA-1b

Interferon gamma-1b (Actimmune) is the last of the three currently available interferon products. It was approved by the Food and Drug Administration in 1991 for the treatment of serious infections associated with chronic granulomatous disease. Its use in the treatment of cancer has not been approved. It is similar in its characteristics to the other members of the interferon family of BRMs. It is also produced by rDNA technology. Interferon-gamma is also available parenterally only as a 3-million-unit single-dose vial for subcutaneous injection. Commonly recommended dosages are listed in the dosages table above.

❖ PHARMACOKINETICS

HALF-LIFE	ONSET	PEAK	DURATION
IM: 2.9 hr	4 hr	4 hr	24 hr

INTERLEUKINS

Interleukins are classified in the immune system as lymphokines. Lymphokines are soluble proteins that are released from activated lymphocytes (particularly from T-cells and natural killer cells). There are many interleukins (IL-2, IL-3, IL-4, IL-5, and IL-6), and more are being identified as we learn more about the immune system.

The primary interleukin currently used in clinical practice is interleukin-2 (IL-2). Interleukin-2 is produced by activated T-cells in response to macrophage-"processed" antigens and secreted interleukin-1 (IL-1). Interleukin-2 was formerly called T-cell growth factor because, among other actions, it aids in the growth and differentiation of T-lymphocytes. Interleukin-2 is not directly toxic but acts primarily as an immunomodulator and immunorestorer.

Mechanism of Action

Interleukins cause multiple effects and actions within the immune system, one of which is beneficial antitumor action. Interleukin-2 binds to receptor sites on certain white blood cells (WBCs) called T-cells, causing the T-cells to multiply. One type of cell that results from this multiplication is the **lymphokine-activated killer (LAK) cell**. The LAK cells recognize cancer cells and ignore normal cells (avoiding the toxic effects of antineoplastics). When the LAK cells come into contact with cancer cells, the cancer cells are destroyed.

Drug Effects

The drug effects of interleukin-2 are multiple. The lymphokine IL-2 both directs and enhances the function of the immune system and its cells. It is therefore said to be an immunomodulator and an immunorestorer. The drug effects of interleukin-2 are listed in the box below.

Therapeutic Uses

The best documented clinical activity is that seen in the treatment of melanomas and renal cell carcinomas. Other cancers that have shown varying degrees of response to therapy with interleukin-2 are listed in the box below.

Side Effects and Adverse Effects

Unfortunately, therapy with IL-2 is frequently complicated by severe toxicity. A syndrome known as capillary leak syndrome is responsible for the severe toxicities of IL-2. As the name implies, capillary leak syndrome refers to the condition induced by interleukin therapy in which the capillaries lose their ability to retain vital colloids such as albumin, protein, and other essential components of blood vessels. Because the capillaries are "leaky" these substances migrate into the surrounding tissues. This results in massive fluid retention (20 to 30 pounds), which can lead to the following life-threatening problems: respiratory distress, congestive heart failure, arrhythmias, and myocardial infarction. The positive side to this is that these are all reversible after discontinuation of the interleukin therapy. Close patient monitoring and vigorous supportive care are essential in the patient receiving interleukin-2 therapy. Other side effects and adverse effects that may be associated with IL-2 therapy are fever, chills, rash, fatigue, hepatotoxicity, myalgias, headaches, and eosinophilia.

Interactions

Although several interleukins have been isolated, aldesleukin is the only one that is currently available. The drug interactions with aldesleukin are listed in Table 46-2.

Dosages

For recommended dosages see the dosages table on the next page.

Interleukin-2: Drug Effects

MODULATING EFFECTS	ENHANCING EFFECTS
Proliferation of T-cells	Killer T-cell activity
Synthesis and secretion of cytokines	Amplifies effects of these cytokines
Increases production of B-cells (Abs)	Enhances the cytotoxic actions of NK cells and LAK cells
Proliferation and activation of NK cells	
Proliferation and activation of LAK cells	

Interleukin-2: Therapeutic Uses

NUMEROUS STUDIES	LIMITED STUDIES
Metastatic renal cell carcinoma	Glial tumors
Malignant melanoma	Non-Hodgkin's lymphomas
Colorectal adenocarcinoma	Hodgkin's disease
	Lung carcinoma
	Head and neck cancer
	Ovarian cancer
	Breast carcinoma

Table 46-2 Drug Interactions: Interleukin

DRUG	MECHANISM	RESULT
Antihypertensives	Additive	Hypotension
Corticosteroids	Antagonism	Reduced antitumor effectiveness
Aminoglycosides, indomethacin, cytotoxic chemotherapy, methotrexate, asparaginase, and doxorubicin	Additive	Toxicity

DOSAGES

SELECTED INTERLEUKINS AND COLONY-STIMULATING FACTORS

AGENT	PHARMACOLOGIC CLASS	DOSAGE RANGE	PURPOSE
Interleukins			
⇩Aldesleukin (Proleukin)	Lymphokine antineoplastic	*Adult* IV: 600,000 IU/kg dose by a 15 m infusion q8h for 14 doses; repeated following a 9-day period	Selected metastatic renal cell carcinoma
Colony-stimulating Factors			
⇩Epoetin alfa (Erythropoietin recombinant, Epogen, Procrit)	Erythropoietic agent	*Adult* IV/SC: 50-100 U/kg 3 times/wk, and adjust dose when the hematocrit is close to 36% IV/SC: 100 U/kg 3 times/wk for 8-12 wk SC: 150 U/kg 3 times/wk for 8 wk	Anemia associated with chronic renal failure Zrdovudine-associated anemia Chemotherapy-associated anemia
⇩Filgrastim (Neupogen)	Granulocyte colony-stimulating factor (G-CSF)	IV/SC: Usual dose of 5 µg/kg as a single daily injection with a range of 0.6-120 µg/kg/day IV/SC: 10 µg/kg/day SC: 5 µg/kg/day SC: 6 µg/kg twice/day	Chemotherapy-induced neutropenia Bone marrow transplantation Cyclic/idiopathic neutropenia Congenital neutropenia
Sargramstim (Leukine)	Granulocyte-macrophage colony–stimulating factor (CM-CSF)	IV: 250 µg/m²/day in 2-hr infusion for 14 days; may be repeated in 7 days; a third course of 500 µg/m²/day for 14 days may be required IV: 250 µg/m²/day in a 2-hr infusion starting 2-4 hr after transplant infusion for 21 days	Bone marrow transplantation delay/failure Myeloid recovery

*D*RUG PROFILES

Interleukin-2, also known as aldesleukin, is a human interleukin-2 derivative that is made by recombinant DNA technology. It is a cytokine that is produced by lymphocytes and therefore belongs to the lymphokine family of biologic response modifiers. Aldesleukin is currently FDA-approved only for the treatment of metastatic renal cell carcinoma, despite its activity in other cancers. It is recommended by the manufacturer to be administered only in a hospital setting under the supervision of a qualified physician who is experienced in the use of antineoplastic agents and only when the benefits are thought to outweigh the possible risks.

⚓ ALDESLEUKIN

Aldesleukin (IL-2) (Proleukin) is a BRM that kills cancer cells by causing the production of LAK cells, which recognize and destroy cancer cells. Although many interleukins have been identified, interleukin-2 is the only currently available interleukin. Interleukin-2 is classified as a pregnancy category C agent and is contraindicated in patients with hypersensitivity, abnormal thallium stress test or pulmonary function tests, and organ allografts. It is available only in parenteral form as a 22-million-unit vial for intravenous infusion. Although it is recommended to be given over 15 minutes by intravenous infusion, it has been given by IV bolus, continuous infusion, and subcutaneous, perilesional, intraperitoneal, intrahepatic, and intrathecal routes. Commonly recommended dosages are listed in the dosages table on the previous page.

☙ P H A R M A C O K I N E T I C S

HALF-LIFE	ONSET	PEAK	DURATION
85 min	≥4 wk*	Unknown	≥12 mo

*To reach therapeutic onset.

COLONY-STIMULATING FACTORS

The colony-stimulating factors (CSFs) are cytokines that regulate the growth, differentiation, and function of bone marrow stem cells. Stem cells are the precursors of mature blood cells such as platelets, granulocytes, and macrophages. They include the kidney-derived protein erythropoietin (EPO), granulocyte CSF (G-CSF), granulocyte-macrophage CSF (GM-CSF),

---

Colony-Stimulating Factors: Target Cell Lines	
CSF	**CELL LINE STIMULATED**
EPO (erythropoietin)	Erythrocytes (RBCs)
IL-3 (interleukin-3)	Pluripotent stem cells*
G-CSF (granulocyte CSF)	Granulocytes
GM-CSF (granulocyte-macrophage CSF)	Granulocytes and macrophages
M-CSF (macrophage CSF)	Macrophages

*The first cell involved in the production of cells that arise from the bone marrow.

---

macrophage CSF (M-CSF), and interleukin-3 (IL-3). Each binds to specific receptors and directs the growth and differentiation of distinct cell lines. The survival of the mature cells and regulation of their biologic activity is also a consequence of CSF binding. The box above lists the colony-stimulating factors and the cell lines that they stimulate.

The CSFs are not directly toxic to cancer cells, but they do have beneficial effects in the treatment of cancer. The colony-stimulating factors decrease the duration of chemotherapy-induced neutropenia, enable higher doses of chemotherapy to be given, decrease bone marrow recovery time after bone marrow transplants or radiation, and stimulate other cells in the immune system to destroy or inhibit the growth of cancer and viral- or fungal-infected cells.

Mechanism of Action

The same mechanism of action applies to all five of the CSFs (EPO, IL-3, G-CSF, GM-CSF, and M-CSF). These agents are produced by recombinant DNA technology and thus are identical to endogenously produced colony-stimulating factors. These substances work by binding to receptors on the surface of cells in the bone marrow. These particular cells are called progenitor cells and are responsible for the production of particular cell lines (red blood cells, white blood cells, platelets, etc.). When a CSF binds to the surface, the progenitor cell is stimulated to make new cells, to mature, and to become functionally active. The principal effects on the progenitor cells are proliferation, differentiation, and activation. They may also enhance certain functions of mature cell lines.

Drug Effects

The colony-stimulating factors have many potential effects. CSFs can decrease the duration of neutro-

Table 46-3	Colony-Stimulating Factors: Common Adverse Effects
BODY SYSTEM	**SIDE/ADVERSE EFFECT**
Cardiovascular	Hypertension (EPO) and edema
Gastrointestinal	Anorexia, nausea, vomiting, diarrhea
Integumentary	Alopecia and rash
Respiratory	Cough, dyspnea, sore throat
Other	Fever, blood dyscrasias, headache, bone pain

Table 46-4	Drug Interactions: Biologic Response Modifiers		
DRUG	**MECHANISM**	**RESULT**
Antineoplastics Myelosuppressive	Antagonism	Prevent BRMs from working

penia, or low neutrophil counts. This is typically seen after chemotherapy because the cytotoxic effects of the antineoplastic agents are not directed solely at the cancer cells but also kill the bone marrow cells. The CSFs also limit the severity of this toxic chemotherapy-induced effect. They prevent the decrease of neutrophil counts.

Another beneficial drug effect of the CSFs is the stimulation of certain immune cells (macrophages and granulocytes) to destroy or inhibit the growth of tumor cells and viral- or fungal-infected cells. They enhance the immune system's ability to kill off cancer cells, viruses, and fungi.

Therapeutic Uses

There are many beneficial therapeutic uses of CSFs. Because they decrease the duration of low neutrophil counts (WBCs) they reduce the incidence and the duration of infections. These infections normally appear in patients who have experienced destruction of bone marrow cells as a result of cytotoxic chemotherapy. The CSFs stimulate these cells to grow and mature and thus directly oppose the detrimental bone marrow actions of chemotherapy.

Because of the CSFs effect on the cells of the bone marrow, higher doses of chemotherapy can be given, resulting in the destruction of a greater number of cancer cells.

The effect of CSFs on the bone marrow cells also results in a decrease of the recovery time of bone marrow cells after bone marrow transplants and radiation therapy. Both bone marrow transplantation and radiation therapy are toxic to the bone marrow. When a CSF is administered, bone marrow cells return to normal counts in a drastically shortened time.

The colony-stimulating factors also enhance the cells of the immune system, such as the macrophages and the granulocytes. The result of this is enhanced

ability to kill cancer cells and inhibition of both viral- and fungal-infected cells.

Side Effects and Adverse Effects

Side effects and adverse effects associated with the use of CSFs are mild. The most common are fever, muscle aches, bone pain, and flushing. The common side effects and adverse effects associated with the CSFs are listed in Table 46-3.

Interactions

Of the currently available biologic response modifiers, G-CSF (filgrastim) and GM-CSF (sargramostim) are the only two agents that have any significant drug interactions. These are listed in Table 46-4.

Dosages

For recommended dosages see the dosages table on p. 718.

DRUG PROFILES

Colony-stimulating factors are cytokines that regulate the growth, differentiation, and function of bone marrow stem cells. **Stem cells** are the precursors of mature blood cells such as platelets, granulocytes, and macrophages. They include the kidney-derived protein erythropoietin (EPO), granulocyte CSF (G-CSF), granulocyte-macrophage CSF (GM-CSF), macrophage CSF (M-CSF), and interleukin-3 (IL-3). Each binds to specific receptors and directs the growth and differentiation of distinct cell lines. The survival of the mature cells and regulation of their biologic activity is also a consequence of CSF binding. Only three of the above-mentioned five CSFs are currently available—EPO, G-CSF, and GM-CSF.

EPOETIN ALFA

Epoetin alfa (erythropoietin recombinant, Epogen, and Procrit) is a biosynthetic form of the natural hormone erythropoietin, which is normally secreted from the kidneys in response to a decrease in red blood cells (RBCs) and many other stimuli. Epoetin is a CSF that is primarily responsible for erythropoiesis (formation of RBCs). It is made by means of recombinant DNA technology, resulting in the production of mass quantities of identical erythropoietin alfa.

Epoetin is used to correct deficiencies of endogenous erythropoietin production. These conditions are common in patients with anemia resulting from end-stage renal disease, HIV infection, and cancer. Its use is associated with two potential serious adverse effects that should be closely monitored. Its use will cause the progenitor cells in the bone marrow to manufacture more red blood cells and mature these immature RBCs more quickly. If therapy is not stopped when the hemoglobin and hematocrit (H/H) reach a certain level or if the H/H rises too quickly, hypertension and seizures can result.

Erythropoietin should be used during pregnancy only when the potential benefits justify the possible risks to the fetus. As such it is classified as a pregnancy category C agent. It is contraindicated in hypersensitivity. Erythropoietin is available only in a parenteral form as 2000-, 3000-, 4000-, and 10,000-U vials for intravenous or subcutaneous injection. Commonly recommended dosages are found in the table on p. 718.

PHARMACOKINETICS

HALF-LIFE	ONSET	PEAK	DURATION
4-13 hr	7-10 days	5-24 hr (serum)	Variable

FILGRASTIM

Filgrastim (granulocyte colony-stimulating factor, G-CSF, and Neupogen) is a human granulocyte colony-stimulating factor (G-CSF). G-CSF stimulates the cells in the bone marrow that are the precursors to the granulocytes. Granulocytes are basophils, eosinophils, and neutrophils. These are more commonly referred to as white blood cells and are the body's primary defense against bacterial and fungal infections. Filgrastim (G-CSF) has the same pharmacologic effects as endogenous human G-CSF. It affects the proliferation, differentiation, and activation of the cells that make neutrophils.

Filgrastim is indicated to decrease infections (febrile neutropenia) in patients receiving myelosuppressive antineoplastics for nonmyeloid malignancies. Fil-

grastim is classified as a pregnancy category C agent and is contraindicated in hypersensitivity and excessive myeloid blast cells (10% in the blood or bone marrow). Filgrastim is available only in a parenteral form as 300- and 480-µg vials for intravenous or subcutaneous injection. Commonly recommended dosages are found in the table on p. 718.

PHARMACOKINETICS

HALF-LIFE	ONSET	PEAK	DURATION
3-5 hr*	1 hr	2-6 hr	12-24 hr

*Highly variable.

SARGRAMSTIM

Sargramstim (granulocyte-macrophage colony-stimulating factor, CM-CSF, and Leukine) is a human granulocyte-macrophage colony-stimulating factor. GM-CSF stimulates the cells in the bone marrow that are the precursors to the granulocytes and macrophages. Sargramstim has the same pharmacologic effects as endogenous human GM-CSF. It affects the proliferation, differentiation, and activation of the cells that make granulocytes and macrophages.

Sargramstim is indicated for use in bone marrow transplantation patients for myeloid recovery (bone

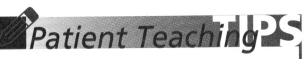

Patient Teaching TIPS

Biologic Response Modifiers

✔ Patients should avoid hazardous tasks because of CNS changes. Fatigue is a common side effect. Patients should report signs of infection such as sore throat, fever, diarrhea, and vomiting. Pregnancy is discouraged while the patient is taking biologic response modifiers.

✔ Interleukins can be self-administered, so patients should learn self-injection technique and proper disposal of equipment such as needles and syringes. A corresponding instruction sheet should be provided for the patient.

✔ Bone pain and flulike symptoms often occur with some of the CSFs and may require the use of nonopiod analgesics. Patients should report any side effects (hair loss, fever, joint pain, chills, diarrhea, edema, anemia, anorexia, fatigue, hypotension, thrombocytopenia) to their physician immediately so that dosage can be changed, corrected, or reconsidered.

marrow recovery) following autologous bone marrow transplantation in Hodgkin's and non-Hodgkin's lymphoma and acute lymphoblastic leukemia. Sargramstim is classified as a pregnancy category C agent and is contraindicated in hypersensitivity and excessive myeloid blast cells (10% in the blood or bone marrow). Sargramstim is available only in a parenteral form as 250- and 500-µg vials for intravenous or subcutaneous injection. Commonly recommended dosages are found in the table on p. 718.

☣ PHARMACOKINETICS

HALF-LIFE	ONSET	PEAK	DURATION
2 hr	4 hr*	SC: 2 hr	10 days*

*Therapeutic effect.

NURSING PROCESS

ASSESSMENT

Before administering any of the interferon agents, it is important for the nurse to rule out any of the contraindications for its use, such as hypersensitivity to the drug, egg proteins, IgG, or neomycin. Cautious use, with close monitoring, is recommended in pregnancy, lactation, children, and in patients with cardiac disease, angina, CHF, COPD, diabetes mellitus, bleeding

TAKE HOME POINTS

Cancer Treatments
- Traditional involved surgery, radiation, and chemotherapy.
- These are at best local or regional therapy.
- Often adjuvant therapy is needed to destroy undetected distant micrometastases.
- Fourth type of cancer therapy is collectively known as biologic response modifiers (BRMs).

Biologic Response Modifiers (BRMs)
- Modify a person's own immune system (biologic response) to foreign invaders.
- Body's own immune system is exploited to destroy cancerous cells.
- Can either augment, restore, or modify the host defenses against the tumor.
- May be directly toxic to tumors.
- May modify the tumor's biology.

Immune System
- Humoral and cellular immune system act together to recognize and destroy foreign particles and cells.
- Humoral immune system is composed of lymphocytes known as B-cells until they are transformed into plasma cells when they come in contact with an antigen (foreign substance).
- Plasma cells then manufacture antibodies to that antigen.
- There are five antibodies known as immunoglobulins (IgA, IgD, IgE, IgG, and IgM).
- Cellular immune system is composed of T-lymphocytes and T-cells.
- Cytotoxic, helper, and suppressor T-cells.

Interferons
- Biologic response modifiers that enhance the activity of macrophages and natural killer cells.
- Have three basic properties: antiviral, immune-modulating, and antitumor actions.
- Different from interleukins, which are lymphokines.
- Lymphokines are substances that are released from activated lymphocytes (T-cells and natural killer cells).

Colony-Stimulating Factors
- Substances that regulate the growth, differentiation, and function of bone marrow stem cells, which are the precursors of mature blood cells (platelets, granulocytes, and macrophages).

Nursing Considerations
- Nursing management associated with the administration of BRMs focuses on careful asepsis, proper nutrition, oral hygiene, and the prevention of infection.
- Nursing care of patients receiving BRMs often focuses on comfort because of the flulike symptoms associated with these agents.
- Biologic response modifiers have the ability to alter the immunologic relationship between a tumor and the patient with cancer to provide a potentially therapeutic response.
- Interferons, monoclonal antibodies, lymphokines, and cytokines are examples of BRMs.
- Side effects common to BRMs include fatigue, flulike symptoms, leukopenia, nausea, and vomiting.

disorders (hemophilia, thrombophlebitis), bone marrow depression, and convulsive disorders. In addition, baseline vital signs and an assessment of infection, CBC, level of consciousness, mental status, and any confusion should be obtained and documented.

Interleukin-1 and interleukin-2 are lymphokines that are commonly ordered biologic response modifiers. Before administering these agents, you should assess the patient for underlying diseases, such as cardiac conditions, because cautious use is recommended in these situations. Contraindications to its use include hypersensitivity to the drug and to proteins of *E. coli*. These interleukins are *not* to be given with antineoplastics. Serum laboratory values such as CBC, platelet levels, BUN, creatinine, urinalysis, aspartate transaminase (AST), and alkaline phosphatase should be checked before treatment and twice weekly during therapy. Neutrophil counts must also be obtained and documented.

NURSING DIAGNOSES

Nursing diagnoses are as follows:
- Pain related to the side effects of immunomodulators
- Altered nutrition, less than body requirements, related to GI side effects of BRMs
- Impaired tissue integrity, rash, related to side effects of BRMs
- Risk for self-injury related to weakness and fatigue from the BRMs
- Risk for altered respiratory gaseous exchange related to side effects of BRMs

PLANNING

Goals related to administration of the BRMs include the following:
- Patient will regain prechemotherapy (and as near normal as possible) nutritional status.
- Patient will experience minimal weight loss during therapy.
- Patient will maintain or regain normal GI/GU patterns.
- Patient's mucous membranes will regain and/or maintain intactness during therapy.
- Patient will be free of self-injury related to drug therapy.

Outcome Criteria

Outcome criteria related to the administration of immunomodulators are as follows:

- Patient will describe nutritional needs and a menu to follow inclusive of four food groups and other dietary changes, as prescribed (i.e., high calorie, low residue).
- Patient will state measures to minimize GI side effects such as small, frequent meals, avoiding spicy foods, etc.
- Patient will be without injured tissue during therapy because of good mouth and oral hygiene daily and as needed.
- Patient will state ways to minimize self-injury related to weakness and fatigue from the BRMs such as assistive devices, grab bars or rails, and help at home.

IMPLEMENTATION

The interferon agents are usually give SC or IM and should be given at bedtime to minimize the CNS side effects. Acetaminophen may be needed for the commonly occurring side effects of headache, fever, and joint aches. Fluids should be increased while patients are taking these medications.

Granulocyte-macrophage colony-stimulating factors and other colony-stimulating factors are immunomodulators, and response to the medication in patients who receive these should be closely monitored. Sargramstim should be administered after reconstitution with 1 ml of sterile water without preservatives for injection, and the vial should not be shaken. For IV infusions, you should dilute the medication in 0.9% NaCl. If the final concentration is <10 μg/ml you should add human albumin to the NaCl to make a final concentration of 0.1% before adding the sargramstim. This agent is to be given within 6 hours after reconstitution.

Interleukins, such as filgrastim (G-CSF), should be given with single-use vials only. This agent is generally given until absolute neutrophil count (ANC) is approximately 10,000/mm^3 after the expected chemotherapy neutrophil nadir, which is usually a 2-week time period. The vial should not be shaken when withdrawing solution. Aldesleukin, another interleukin, should be administered by IV infusion every 8 hours as ordered. See the patient teaching tips on p. 721.

EVALUATION

Therapeutic responses to the biologic response modifiers include a decrease in the growth of the lesion or mass, decreased tumor size, and ease in breathing. Possible side effects are presented in Table 46-3.

Critical Thinking **A C T I V I T I E S**

1. C.F. is to receive Neupogen following a course of carmustine and radiation for a brain tumor. C.F. weighs 132 pounds. The protocol that the oncologist has given you states that the G-CSF should be dosed at 5 µg/kg. What dose should the patient receive, and what vial should be used so as to waste as little drug as possible?

2. What is so important about the timing of the dosage of colony-stimulating factor in treatment of neoplasms?

3. Many medications, especially chemotherapy, may lead to the adverse effect of bone marrow suppression of various blood cell components. What symptoms would you expect to see if your patient had diminished production of platelets? Red blood cells? White blood cells? Explain your answers.

4. One of your patients is being prescribed leuprolide. Which of the following conditions or disorders would be a contraindication to its use?
   a. Thromboembolic disorders
   b. Dysphagia
   c. Polyuria
   d. Diagnosed vaginal bleeding

5. What is the purpose of adjuvant chemotherapy?

6. List an example of an adjuvant chemotherapy agent used in women with breast cancer.

   a. Flutamide
   b. Prednisone
   c. Tamoxifen
   d. Megestrol

7. Which of the following best describes the action of interferons in the management of malignant tumors?
   a. Interferons stimulate the production and activation of T-lymphocytes and cytotoxic T-cells.
   b. Interferons increase the production of specific anticancer enzymes.
   c. Interferons have antiviral and antitumor properties and strengthen the immune system.
   d. Interferons are retrieved from healthy donors and help improve the cell-killing action of T-cells.

▲▲

BIBLIOGRAPHY

Albanese J, Nutz P: *Mosby's 1995 nursing drug cards,* St Louis, 1995, Mosby.

Hussar DA: New drugs, *Nursing 92* 23(4):59, 1992.

Johnson KB: *Harriet Lane handbook,* ed 13, St Louis, 1993, Mosby.

Keen JH: *Critical care and emergency drug reference,* St Louis, 1994, Mosby.

Knoben JE, Anderson PO: *Handbook of critical drug data,* ed 6, Hamilton, Ill, 1988, Drug Intelligence Publications.

Mayer DK: Biotherapy: recent advances and nursing implications, *Nurs Clin of North Am* 25(2):291, 1990.

McEvoy GK: *AHFS drug information,* Bethesda, Md, 1994, American Society of Hospital Pharmacists.

McKenry L, Salerno E: *Pharmacology in nursing,* ed 19, St Louis, 1995, Mosby.

Skidmore-Roth L: *Mosby's 1995 nursing drug reference,* St Louis, 1995, Mosby.

THE GASTROINTESTINAL SYSTEM AND NUTRITIONAL AGENTS: STUDY SKILLS BRIEF

ACTIVE QUESTIONING

There is one technique for study that cannot be over-emphasized. The technique is active questioning. In the PURR study model it is critical to be able to generate questions in the PLAN, REHEARSAL, and REVIEW steps. The questions you generate when applying PURR are essential in helping you maintain concentration as you study, improving your comprehension as you read assigned material, and developing long-term memory. Active questioning is a strategy that you must practice continuously. It is a strategy that develops with practice.

WHAT ARE THE RIGHT QUESTIONS?

Some questions generated during the PLAN step will be useful and will focus on exactly the right issues for maximum learning. On the other hand, sometimes the

questions generated by looking at the chapter outline or accented material in the body of the text will be inappropriate. These questions seem logical and important when you are working with the limited amount of information available using the PLAN step, but as you read the chapter you will find that they miss the mark. Do not worry about whether each question you ask is perfectly focused. As you read, rehearse, and review the material, you can and should revise questions based on your growing understanding of the material. The important point is to ask many questions to help you maintain active involvement in the learning process and anticipate questions that will appear on exams. The more questions you ask, the more effective you will become both as an active questioner and as an active learner.

KINDS OF QUESTIONS

First, you must realize that there is more than one kind of question to be asked. Over the year there have been many different questioning hierarchies proposed by educators and scholars. The different kinds of questions vary from three or four to as many as seven or eight. I am going to take a simple approach to the issue of how many kinds of questions and limit the focus to only two.

Literal Questions

Literal questions are those that are answered directly and specifically by the text. When you were reading a story in grade school and the teacher asked, "What did Sally do when she lost her movie money?" you were able to answer easily because the question asked for specific information that was stated clearly and directly in the story. If you were reading an American History text and found a topic heading, "The First President," an obvious question would be: "Who was the first president?" The answer is one that would be stated clearly and directly in the body of this topic heading. These are examples of literal questions. A literal question usually has a single correct response. The answer is stated directly in the text and every reader will find that same information.

Interpretive Questions

Interpretive questions are more challenging questions that require the reader to interpret, synthesize, evaluate, and analyze the material. Interpretive questions require knowledge of the literal information in addition to understanding the reading material well enough to be able to select several different pieces or bits of data and put them together to formulate a response that demonstrates your understanding. In the American History example about the first president an interpretive question might be, "Why was George

Washington considered to be such an exemplary model as the first president of the new nation?" This question requires that you know not only the literal facts about Washington, but also that you are able to evaluate and judge those facts to reach a conclusion that could be supported by the literal information. Even though a question is interpretive in nature it is possible that there will be only one correct response. However, it is equally possible that there is more than one correct

response to an interpretive question. The literal information can be evaluated in a number of different ways in responding to the question, and the answers derived by different readers will vary. Both kinds of questions are essential in the learning process.

QUESTIONING APPLICATION

On the third page of Chapter 50 you will see the italicized phrase, *excessive need* or *excessive loss*. Italicization is used to gain the reader's attention and to indicate that the italicized material is especially noteworthy. Accented material should always be considered as a potential source of questions. What is excessive need? What is excessive loss? Again, we can begin the questioning with simple, literal questions, but it is essential that interpretive questions also be asked. What does excessive need and loss have to do with the care of the patient? How can we determine if there is excessive need and/or loss? What should be done to remedy excessive need or loss? These questions require that you read for broader general understanding and not just focus on the "facts."

At the end of each chapter there is a section entitled "Critical Thinking Activities." Even though this information is stated in question form, you should consider generating additional questions of your own. The first question in Chapter 50 is, "Explain why patients with a cardiac history need to have a baseline ECG and serum calcium performed before initiation of calcium supplemental therapy?" In answering it, some additional questions will help you focus your learning. What is serum calcium? How does calcium affect cardiac patients? Why? Is calcium supplemental therapy inappropriate for all cardiac patients? If not, what are the circumstances that might rule out supplemental calcium? Of what signs and symptoms should the caregiver be aware if calcium supplemental therapy is being administered to a cardiac patient?

The more active you become as a questioner the easier it will become to ask the kinds of questions that are necessary for your own learning.

Chapter 47

Antacids and Antiflatulents

Objectives

When you reach the end of this chapter, you will able to:

1 Discuss the various gastrointestinal diseases, specifically peptic ulcer disease, gastritis, spastic colon, and diverticulitis.

2 Identify the various agents used to treat peptic ulcer disease and other related gastric disorders, such as antacids, antiflatulents, and H_2 histamine-blocking agents.

3 Describe the mechanism of action, indications, cautions, contraindications, side effects, and toxicity associated with the use of antacids, antiflatulents, and H_2 histamine-blocking agents.

4 Develop a nursing care plan as related to the nursing process in the administration of antacids, antiflatulents, and H_2 histamine-blocking agents.

5 Discuss the patient education guidelines associated with the use of antacids, antiflatulents, and H_2 histamine-blocking agents.

CHAPTER OUTLINE

Acid-related Pathophysiology
Antacids
  Mechanism of action
  Drug effects
  Therapeutic uses
  Side effects and adverse effects
  Interactions
  Dosages
Drug Profiles
    Aluminum-containing Antacids
    Calcium-containing Antacids
    Magnesium-containing Antacids
H_2 Antagonists
  Mechanism of action
  Drug effects
  Therapeutic uses
  Side effects and adverse effects
  Interactions
  Dosages
Drug Profiles
  ⚓ Cimetidine
Proton Pump Inhibitors
  Mechanism of action
  Drug effects
  Therapeutic uses
  Side effects and adverse effects
  Interactions
  Dosages

Drug Profiles
  ⚓ Omeprazole
Other Drugs
Sucralfate
  Mechanism of action
  Drug effects
  Therapeutic uses
  Side effects and adverse effects
  Interactions
  Dosages
Drug Profiles
  ⚓ Sucralfate
  ⚓ Misoprostol
Nursing Process
Assessment
Nursing Diagnoses
Planning
  Outcome criteria
Implementation
Evaluation

Glossary

Activated charcoal Substance that appears to be effective in reducing breath H_2 and intestinal complaints caused by ingestion of indigestible carbohydrates. (p. 733)

Antacids (ant a' sid) Large group of prescription and

over-the-counter drugs used to correct too much acid production and hyperacidity of the stomach. (p. 729)

    Antiflatulents (an' tĭ flat μ lənt) Agents used to relieve the painful symptoms associated with gas by binding to or altering intestinal gas. (p. 729)

    Chief cells Cells that secrete the enzyme pepsinogen. (p. 729)

    Gastric gland (gas' trik) Highly specialized secretory gland composed of many different types of cells: parietal, chief, mucus, endocrine, and enterochromaffin. (p. 729)

    Gastric hyperacidity (gas' trik hi' pər ə sid' ĭ te) Overproduction of stomach acid. (p. 729)

    Hydrochloric acid (hi' dro klor' ik) Acid secreted by the parietal cells in the lining of the stomach that maintains the environment of the stomach at a pH of 1 to 4. (p. 729)

    Mucoid cell (mu' koid) Cell whose function is to secrete mucus that serves as a protective mucous coat against the digestive properties of hydrochloric acid (also called surface epithelia cells). (p. 729)

    Parietal cells (pə ri' ə təl) Cell responsible for producing and secreting hydrochloric acid; the primary site of action for many of the drugs used to treat acid-related disorders. (p. 729)

    Pepsin (pep' sin) Proteolytic enzyme responsible for breaking down proteins. (p. 729)

    Simethicone (sĭ meth' ĭ kōn) Substance that alters the elasticity of mucus-coated bubbles causing them to break. (p. 733)

One of the conditions of the stomach requiring drug therapy is hyperacidity, that is, too much acid production. Left untreated this condition can lead to such serious conditions as ulcer disease and gastric reflux. **Antacids** are a large group of prescription and over-the-counter (OTC) drugs that may be used to correct this condition. Overproduction of stomach acid is also referred to as **gastric hyperacidity.**

    Another condition or disorder of the gastrointestinal tract is gas. Gas can appear in the gastrointestinal tract as a consequence of the normal digestive process and air swallowing, or it can result from disorders such as diverticulitis, dyspepsia, peptic ulcers, postoperative gaseous distention, and spastic or irritable colon. **Antiflatulents** are agents that are used to relieve the painful symptoms associated with gas. Other drugs and their role in the treatment of gastrointestinal-related disorders will also be discussed.

ACID-RELATED PATHOPHYSIOLOGY

For a more complete understanding of the large family of drugs used to treat acid-related disorders of the stomach, a brief overview of gastrointestinal system function and the role of hydrochloric acid in digestion is beneficial. The stomach secretes many substances:

- Hydrochloric acid
- Bicarbonate
- Pepsinogen
- Intrinsic factor
- Mucus
- Prostaglandins

Each one of these substances has a specific role in the digestive process.

    The stomach, although one structure, can be divided into three functional areas. Each area has specific glands with which it is associated. These glands are composed of different cells, and these cells secrete different substances. Figure 47-1 shows three functional areas of the stomach and the distribution of the three different stomach glands.

    The three primary glands in the stomach are the cardiac, pyloric, and gastric glands. These glands are named for their position in the stomach. The cardiac glands are located around the cardiac orifice; the gastric glands are in the fundus, over the greater part of the body of the stomach; and the pyloric glands are in the pyloric region and in the transitional zone between the pyloric and the fundic zone. The gastric glands are the largest in number and are of primary importance when discussing acid-related disorders and drug therapy.

    The **gastric gland** is a highly specialized secretory gland composed of many different types of cells: parietal, chief, mucus, endocrine, and enterochromaffin. Each cell secretes a specific substance. The three primary cells are the mucoid cells, the chief cells, and the parietal cells. These cells are depicted in Fig. 47-1.

    The **parietal cells** are responsible for producing and secreting hydrochloric acid. They are the primary site of action for many of the drugs used to treat acid-related disorders. The **chief cells** secrete pepsinogen. Pepsinogen is a proenzyme that becomes pepsin when activated by exposure to acid. **Pepsin** breaks down proteins and is referred to as a proteolytic enzyme. The **mucoid cells** are mucus-secreting cells that are also called surface epithelia cells. The secreted mucus serves as a protective mucous coat against the digestive properties of hydrochloric acid. Table 47-1 lists the cells of the gastric glands and their functions.

    The three cells of the gastric gland (chief, mucoid, and parietal) play an important role in the digestive process. When the balance of these three cells and their secretions is impaired, acid-related diseases occur. The most harmful of these disorders is peptic ulcer disease (PUD). The most common is hyperacidity. Many lay terms (e.g., indigestion, sour stomach, heartburn, acid stomach) have been used to describe this condition of overproduction of hydrochloric acid by the parietal cells.

    Hydrochloric acid is an acid that is secreted by the parietal cells in the lining of the stomach. It is the primary substance secreted in the stomach that maintains the environment of the stomach at a pH of 1 to 4. There are many stimulants of hydrochloric acid secretion by the parietal cells. Some of these stimulants are normal and good. Others, such as large, fatty meals, consumption of excessive amounts of alcohol, and emotional stress, may result in hyperproduction of hydrochloric acid from the parietal cells and disorders such as PUD.

Because the parietal cell is the source of hydrochloric acid production, it is the primary target for many of the most effective drugs for the treatment of acid-related disorders. A closer look at how the pari-

etal cell receives signals to produce and secrete hydrochloric acid will enhance the understanding of the mechanism of action of many of the drugs used to treat acid-related disorders.

The wall of the parietal cell has three types of receptors: acetylcholine, histamine, and gastrin. When any one of these is occupied, the parietal cell will produce and secrete hydrochloric acid. Figure 47-2 shows the parietal cell with its three receptors. Once these receptors have become occupied, a second messenger is sent. In the case of histamine receptors, occupation

Cardiac gland

Cardiac zone

Fundic or Gastric zone

Pyloric zone

Epithelial cell

Mucous cell

Parietal cell

Pyloric gland

Gastric or Fundic gland

▼ **FIG. 47-1** The three specific zones of the stomach and the different glands.

results in the production of adenylate cyclase. Adenylate cyclase converts adenosine triphosphate (ATP) to cylic adenosine monophophate (cAMP), which provides energy for the proton pump. The proton pump is a pump for hydrogen ions located in the parietal cell. The pump requires energy to work. If energy is present the hydrogen potassium ATPase system will be activated and the pump will be able to produce hydrogen ions needed for the production of hydrochloric acid.

Rantiditine, famotidine, nizatinide, and cimetidine block hydrogen ion secretion from the parietal cells by binding to these receptors. Anticholinergic (AC, see Chapter 18) drugs such as atropine block acetylcholine receptors, resulting in decreased hydrogen ion secretion from the parietal cells. Omeprazole binds to the H^+/K^+ ATPase pump and irreversibly inhibits this enzyme, resulting in a total inhibition of hydrogen ion secretion from the parietal cells.

Table 47-1	Three Cells of the Gastric Gland
CELL TYPE	**FUNCTION**
Chief	Secretes pepsinogen → pepsin Breaks down proteins in the diet
Mucoid	Secretes mucus Provides a protective mucous coat to protect stomach from digestion of itself from hydrochloric acid
Parietal	Secretes hydrochloric acid Keeps the pH of the stomach between 1 and 4 so as to properly digest food

ANTACIDS

Antacids have been used for centuries in the treatment of patients with acid-related disorders. The ancient Greeks used crushed coral (calcium carbonate) in the first century AD to treat patients with dyspepsia. They were the principal antiucler treatment until the availability of the H_2-receptor blockers in the late 1970s. For decades the classic treatment for acid-related disorders was a combination anticholinergic/antacid regimen. With the introduction of H_2 blockers as well as proton

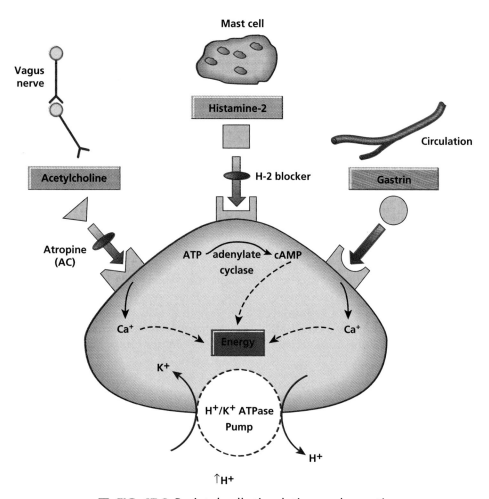

▼ **FIG. 47-2** Parietal cell stimulation and secretion.

pump inhibitors (H+/K+ ATPase inhibitors), protective agents and mucus-producing prostaglandins are rapidly replacing the anticholinergics for acid-related gastrointestinal (GI) disease. However, the antacids are still extensively used, especially on the OTC market. They are available in a variety of dosage preparations as sole antacid preparations or in multiple antacid formulations. In addition, many antacid preparations contain the antiflatulent agent simethicone, which reduces gas and bloating.

There are basically three forms of antacids: aluminum, magnesium, and calcium based. Many aluminum-based formulations combine magnesium, which contributes to the acid-neutralizing capacity and counteracts the constipating effects of aluminum. Calcium carbonate is also effective in acid neutralization but is not used frequently because it may result in kidney stones and increased gastric acid secretion. Sodium bicarbonate is a highly soluble antacid form with a quick onset but a short duration of action. It may also cause metabolic alkalosis.

Some of the available aluminum, magnesium, and calcium salts that are used in many of the antacid formulations are listed in the box above right. There are far too many individual antacid products to mention all formulations. The OTC antacid formulations are available as capsules, chewable tablets, effervescent granules and tablets, powders, suspensions, and tablets.

Mechanism of Action

As the name applies, antacids were originally believed to work by neutralization of gastric acidity. They do nothing to prevent the overproduction of acid but neutralize it once it is in the stomach. It is now believed that, especially at low doses, antacids promote gastric mucosal defensive mechanisms. They do this by stimulating mucus, prostaglandin, and bicarbonate secretion from the cells inside the gastric glands. Mucus serves as a protective barrier against the destructive properties of hydrochloric acid. Bicarbonate helps buffer the acidic properties of hydrochloric acid. Prostaglandins prevent histamine from stimulating adenylate cyclase. Without adenylate cyclase no cAMP is formed and no second messenger is available to activate the proton pump.

Drug Effects

The primary drug effect of antacids is the reduction of the symptoms associated with various acid-related disorders such as peptic ulcer disease and hyperacidity disorders. By raising the pH of the stomach from 1.3 to 1.6 (only 0.3 points), acid in the gastric juices will be 50% neutralized, and if the pH is raised

---

Aluminum, Calcium, and Magnesium Salts in Antacids

ALUMINUM SALTS	CALCIUM SALTS	MAGNESIUM SALTS
Carbonate	Carbonate	Carbonate
Hydroxide		Hydroxide
Phosphate		Oxide
		Trisilicate

---

an entire point from 1.3 to 2.3, a 90% reduction of acid will occur. This causes the pain reduction associated with acid-related disorders.

The ability of antacids to reduce the pain associated with acid-related disorders is thought to be a result of inhibition of the protein-digesting ability of pepsin, an increase in the resistance of the stomach lining to irritation, and an increase in the tone of the lower esophageal sphincter.

Therapeutic Uses

Antacids are selected for their potential acid-neutralizing capacity and their onset of action. Antacids are indicated for the relief of symptoms associated with hyperacidity related to peptic ulcer, gastritis, peptic esophagitis, gastric hyperacidity, heartburn, and hiatal hernia.

Side Effects and Adverse Effects

The side effects and adverse effects of the antacids are limited. The magnesium preparations, especially milk of magnesia (MOM), can cause diarrhea. The aluminum- and calcium-containing formulations can result in constipation. For this reason many combination antacids have been formulated with agents that have counteracting side effects in an attempt to ameliorate the effects. Excessive use of these agents can result in systemic alkalosis. This is more common with sodium bicarbonate. Another adverse effect that is more common with the calcium-containing products is rebound hyperacidity, or acid rebound, in which the patient experiences hyperacidity on discontinuation of the antacid.

Interactions

Antacids are capable of causing several drug interactions when administered with other drugs. There are four basic mechanisms by which antacids cause these interactions. Understanding these mechanisms enhances the knowledge of interactions with antacids. These mechanisms include adsorption (chelation) of

Table 47-2	Antacids: Drug-Interacting Mechanisms
MECHANISM	**DESCRIPTION**
Chelation	A chemical binding or inactivation of another drug to the antacid reducing the absorption of the other drug into the bloodstream.
Altered stomach pH	Drugs that are ionized will have reduced absorption into the bloodstream; increasing the pH of the stomach with an antacid will cause drugs that are acid salts (HCl salts) to be more ionized and less absorbed and drugs that are basic salts (sulfate salts) to be less ionized and more readily absorbed into the bloodstream.
Altered urinary pH	The same alteration in absorption in the stomach will affect excretion of basic and acidic drugs in the urine because the urinary pH will be elevated and acidic drugs will be more ionized, less absorbed, and more excreted.

other drugs to antacids, which reduces the ability of the other drug to be absorbed into the body; chemical inactivation, which produces insoluble complexes; increased stomach pH, which increases the absorption of basic drugs and decreases the absorption of acidic drugs; and increased urinary pH, which increases the excretion of acidic drugs and decreases the excretion of basic drugs. These mechanisms are further explained in Table 47-2.

Dosages

For information on dosage for selected agents, see the dosages table on the next page.

DRUG PROFILES

There are many antacids and antacid combinations. One way to categorize the large family of antacid drugs is separation by the type of metal they contain: aluminum, calcium, or magnesium. Antacids are generally considered safe for use in pregnancy if prolonged or high doses are avoided. FDA category is not established. Antacids are OTC drugs; that is, a prescription is not needed for their purchase.

ALUMINUM-CONTAINING ANTACIDS

The amount of antacid necessary to neutralize hydrochloric acid depends on the patient, the condition being treated, and the buffering capacity of the preparation used. The acid-neutralizing property of antacids varies. Examples of aluminum-containing antacids and aluminum-magnesium combination products are listed in the box on the next page.

CALCIUM-CONTAINING ANTACIDS

Calcium-containing antacids are currently being advertised as an extra source of calcium. Calcium carbonate neutralization will produce gas and possibly belching. For this reason it may be combined with an antiflatulent type of drug such as **simethicone**. Calcium-containing products have a long duration of acid action, which can cause hyperacidity rebound. One example of a calcium-containing antacid is calcium carbonate (Tums).

MAGNESIUM-CONTAINING ANTACIDS

Magnesium-containing antacids commonly cause a laxative effect, and frequent administration of these antacids alone often cannot be tolerated. The administration of magnesium-containing antacids is dangerous in patients with renal failure because the failing kidney cannot excrete the extra magnesium and accumulation may occur. Examples of magnesium-containing antacids are listed in the box on p. 735.

Other agents that may be added in antacid combination products are antiflatulents. Flatulence is the passage of gas via the rectum, a disturbing symptom for many patients but rarely an indicator of serious disease. Gas in the upper gastrointestinal tract is composed of swallowed air and is thus largely nitrogen. It is usually expelled from the body by belching. However, the composition of flatulence is determined largely by dietary intake of carbohydrates and the metabolic activity of the bacteria in the intestines. These bacteria, anaerobic bacteria, produce fermentation with the production of hydrogen (H_2), carbon dioxide (CO_2), and in some patients methane (CH_4).

Several agents have been used to bind or alter intestinal gas. **Activated charcoal** and simethicone are OTC antiflatulents and may be added to many antacid products. They are also available as sole agents. Acti-

DOSAGES

SELECTED ANTACID AGENTS

AGENT	PHARMACOLOGIC CLASS	DOSAGE RANGE	PURPOSE
ALUMINUM-CONTAINING			
Al (OH)$_3$, Mg (OH)$_2$ (Maalox)	Antacid	PO: 5-10 ml/tab 3-4 times/day and hs	Hyperacidity
Antacid Al (OH)$_3$, Mg (OH)$_2$ (Mylanta)		PO: 10-20 ml/tab 3-4 times/day and hs	Hyperacidity
CALCIUM-CONTAINING			
Calcium carbonate (Tums)	Antacid	PO: 1-2 tabs prn	Hyperacidity
MAGNESIUM-CONTAINING			
Milk of Magnesia	Antacid	PO: 5-15 ml/1-2 tabs prn; pediatric dose	Antacid
	Laxative	¼-½ adult dose PO: 20-60 ml with a full glass of water	Laxative
H$_2$ ANTAGONISTS			
⚓Cimetidine (Tagamet)	H$_2$-antihistamine	*Adult* PO: 300 or 400 mg qid with meals and hs or 800 mg hs	Ulcers
		PO: 1600 mg/day divided	GERD
		PO/IM/IV: 300 mg or higher qid with meals and hs; do not exceed 2400 mg/day	Pathologic hypersecretion
Famotidine (Pepcid)	H$_2$-antihistamine	*Adult* PO: 40 mg/day hs or 20 mg bid	Ulcers
		PO: 20-160 mg qhr	Pathologic hypersecretion
		PO: 20 mg bid	GERD
		IV: 20 mg q12h	Pathologic hypersecretion
Nizatidine (Axid)	H$_2$-antihistamine	*Adult* PO: 300 mg hs or 150 mg bid	Ulcers
		PO: 150 mg bid	GERD
Ranitidine (Zantac)	H$_2$-antihistamine	*Adult* PO: 150 mg bid or 300 mg hs	Ulcers
		PO: 150 mg bid	Pathologic hypersecretion, GERD
		PO: 150 mg qid	Erosive esophagitis
		IM/IV: 50 mg q6-8h	Any indications

Aluminum-Containing Antacids

CARBONATE SALT	HYDROXIDE SALT	PHOSPHATE SALT	COMBINATION PRODUCTS
Basaljel	AlternaGel Amphojel	Phosphajel	Gaviscon Maalox Mylanta

---

Magnesium-Containing Antacids

CARBONATE SALT	HYDROXIDE SALT	OXIDE SALT	TRISILICATE
Bisodol powder Alkets	Milk of magnesia (MOM)	Mag-Ox	Gaviscon

Currently Available H$_2$ Blockers

↓Cimetidine (Tagamet)   Famotidine (Pepcid)   Nizatidine (Axid)   Ranitidine (Zantac)

---

vated charcoal appears to be effective in reducing breath H$_2$ and intestinal complaints caused by ingestion of indigestible carbohydrates. Simethicone alters the elasticity of mucus-coated bubbles, which causes the bubbles to break. Although simethicone is frequently used, there are limited data to support its effectiveness.

H$_2$ ANTAGONISTS

Histamine type 2 receptor (H$_2$) antagonists are the prototypical acid secretory antagonists. These agents reduce but do not abolish stimulated acid secretion. They have become the most popular drugs for the treatment of many acid-related disorders, including PUD. This can be attributed to their efficacy, patient acceptance, and excellent safety profile. There are presently four FDA approved H$_2$ antagonists. They are listed in the box above.

There is little difference among the four available H$_2$ blockers from an efficacy standpoint. Their relative potencies differ, but increased potency does not necessarily confer a therapeutic advantage, provided the drugs can be administered in equipotent dose without toxicity.

Mechanism of Action

The efficacy of the H$_2$ blockers is related to their ability to competitively block the H$_2$ receptor of acid-producing parietal cells, thus rendering the cells less responsive not only to histamine but also to the stimulation of acetylcholine and gastrin. This is shown in Fig. 47-2. Up to 90% inhibition of vagal-stimulated and gastrin-stimulated acid secretion occurs by histamine blockers. However, complete inhibition has not been shown.

Drug Effects

The drug effects of the H$_2$ blockers are limited to specific blocking actions on the parietal cells of the gas-

---

H$_2$ Antagonists: Indications

SHOWN TO BE EFFECTIVE

Gastric ulcer   Duodenal ulcer
Gastroesophageal reflux   Upper GI bleeding
Hypersecretory conditions (e.g., Zollinger-Ellison
   syndrome)

MAY BE EFFECTIVE

Stress ulcers   Peptic esophagitis
Prevention and management of allergic condition
   in combination with H$_1$ blockers (e.g., urticaria
   and anaphylactic reactions)

---

tric glands in the stomach. The parietal cells are responsible for the production of hydrogen ions and ultimately hydrochloric acid. The H$_2$ blockers compete with histamine for binding sites on the surface of parietal cells. The drug effects of H$_2$ blockers are decreased hydrogen ion production from the parietal cells, which results in an increase in the pH of the stomach and relief of many of the symptoms associated with hyperacid-secreting conditions.

Therapeutic Uses

The H$_2$ blockers have many therapeutic effects related to their ability to suppress acid production in the stomach. The four currently available agents have identical mechanisms of action but vary in potency and side effect profile. Although they may differ in their formal FDA-approved indications, they all suppress acid secretion in the stomach. Some of the indications for H$_2$ blockers are listed in the box above.

Side Effects and Adverse Effects

The H$_2$ antagonists have a remarkably low incidence of side effects, less than 3%. The four available blockers are similar in many respects but have some differences in side effect profiles. Table 47-3 lists the side effects and adverse effects seen with these agents. Central nervous system side effects occur in less than 1% of patients taking H_2 antagonists. Cimetidine may induce impotence and gynecomastia. This is the result of cimetidine inhibiting estradiol metabolism and displacement of dihydrotestosterone from peripheral androgen-binding sites. All four H_2 agonists may increase the secretion of prolactin from the anterior pituitary.

Interactions

Besides the different side effect profiles of the four H_2 antagonists, differences in the drug interactions of the H_2 antagonists exist. These may be of potential clinical importance. Cimetidine binds the hepatic cytochrome P-450 microsomal oxidase system. This is a group of enzymes in the liver that metabolize many different drugs by oxidation. By inhibiting oxidation of drugs metabolized via this pathway, cimetidine may raise the blood concentrations of these drugs. Ranitidine has only 10% to 20% of the binding action of cimetidine on the P-450 system, and nizatidine and famotidine have essentially no effect. This interaction has little clinical significance for most drugs, but problems occur with medications with a narrow therapeutic-to-toxic ratio, such as theophylline, warfarin, lido-

caine, and phenytoin. All H_2 antagonists may inhibit the absorption of certain drugs, such as ketoconazole, that require an acidic gastrointestinal environment for gastric absorption.

Dosages

For dosage information see the dosages table on p. 734.

DRUG PROFILES

H_2 antagonists are the prototypical acid secretory antagonists. These agents reduce but do not abolish stimulated acid secretion. They are among the most frequently used drugs in the world. This can be attributed to their efficacy, patient acceptance, and excellent safety profile. As previously mentioned, except for relative potencies, there are only minor differences among the four currently available H_2 antagonists: cimetidine (tagamet), famotidine (pepcid), nizatidine (axid), and ranitidine (zantac). Potency and equipotent dosages of the four available H_2 antagonists are listed in Table 47-4.

All the H_2 antagonists except cimetidine (Tagamet) and famotidine (Pepcid) are currently available by prescription. This has been a topic of much discussion lately. It has been proposed that all of these products become available OTC. Each agent is available orally, and all except nizatidine are also available parenterally. The H_2 antagonists are classified as pregnancy category B agents and are contraindicated in hypersensitivity.

⚓ CIMETIDINE

In 1977 cimetidine (Tagamet) was the first agent in this class to be released on the market. It is the prototypical H_2 antagonist. Cimetidine may be given orally and intravenously either by injection or continuous intravenous infusion. Cimetidine comes as 200-, 300-, 400-,

Table 47-3	H_2 Blockers: Adverse Effects
BODY SYSTEM	**SIDE/ADVERSE EFFECT**
Central nervous system	Headache, lethargy, confusion, depression, hallucinations (<1% total)
Endocrine	Impotence, increased prolactin, gynecomastia
Gastrointestinal	Diarrhea, abdominal cramps, jaundice
Genitourinary	Increase BUN, liver function tests, creatinine
Hematopoietic	Agranulocytosis, thrombocytopenia, neutropenia, aplastic anemia
Integumentary	Urticaria, rash, alopecia, sweating, flushing, exfoliative dermatitis

Table 47-4	H_2 Antagonists: Potency and Equipotent Dosages			
	CIMETIDINE	**RANITIDINE**	**NIZATIDINE**	**FAMOTIDINE**
Relative potency	1	4-8	4-8	20-50
Equivalent dose (mg)	1600	300	300	40

and 800-mg tablets and a 300-mg/5 ml oral solution. The parenteral form of cimetidine is a 150 mg/ml injection. Common dosage recommendations are listed in the dosages table on p. 734.

⬡ PHARMACOKINETICS

HALF-LIFE	ONSET	PEAK	DURATION
2 hr	15-60 min	1-2 hr	4-5 hr

PROTON PUMP INHIBITORS

The newest drug introduced for the treatment of acid-related disorders is omeprazole. Omeprazole is the first of a new line of antisecretory drugs. The enzyme H^+/K^+ ATPase is the final common step in the acid-secretory process of the parietal cell (see Fig. 47-2). If there is energy present to run the pump, it will release hydrogen ions out of the parietal cell. Because hydrogen ions are protons (positively charged substances) the pump may also be called the proton pump. Anticholinergics and antihistamines (H_2 blockers) do not stop the action of the pump. Other substances are able to stimulate the pump even in the presence of these drugs. They are thus unable to totally inhibit acid production.

Mechanism of Action

Omeprazole irreversibly binds to H^+/K^+ ATPase. The binding of this enzyme prevents the movement of hydrogen ions out of the parietal cell into the stomach, thereby blocking all gastric acid secretion. Whereas H_2 blockers may block close to 90% of all acid secretion, proton pump inhibitors such as omeprazole effectively block all acid secretion. Because omeprazole inhibits over 90% of 24-hour acid secretion, it makes most patients achlorhydric (without acid). For acid secretion to return to normal after omeprazole has been stopped, the parietal cell must synthesize new H^+/K^+ ATPase.

Drug Effects

The proton pump inhibitor, omeprazole, is almost the ideal drug for hypersecretion of acid. Its drug effects are confined to the parietal cell and specifically to the H^+/K^+ ATPase enzyme. Although there are other proton pumps in the body, the H^+/K^+ ATPase is distinct structurally and mechanically from other H^+-transporting enzymes and appears to exist only in the parietal cell. Thus the action of omeprazole is limited to total inhibition of gastric acid secretion.

Therapeutic Uses

The ability to totally inhibit the production of acid from the parietal cells in the stomach gives omeprazole many beneficial therapeutic effects. Some concerns have been expressed regarding omeprazole's stability in the prohibition of acid secretion. Most of these concerns stem from long-term use of omeprazole in humans. Some have shown that this may produce enterochromaffin-like (ECL) cells and carcinoid tumors. Although this has not yet clearly been established, the FDA has initially approved omeprazole only for acute treatment of severe gastroesophageal reflux disease unresponsive to conventional therapy, endoscopically proven erosive esophagitis, and the chronic treatment of Zollinger-Ellison syndrome. However, omeprazole will likely be approved soon for the acute treatment of duodenal ulcer disease, at least for ulcers resistant to conventional therapy.

Side Effects and Adverse Effects

Omeprazole appears to be remarkably safe for short-term therapy. The frequency of adverse effects has been similar to that of placebo or H_2 antagonists. Omeprazole appears to inhibit a subset of the hepatic P-450 enzyme system and cause some *interactions with other drugs*. When inhibited by omeprazole this subset of the P-450 system will effectively decrease the clearance of warfarin and phenytoin but not theophylline. Some of the other less common side effects and adverse effects seen with omeprazole therapy are listed in Table 47-5.

Interactions

There are few drug interactions with the proton pump inhibitors. There is the possibility that the proton pump inhibitors may increase serum levels of di-

Table 47-5	Omeprazole: Adverse Effects
BODY SYSTEM	**SIDE/ADVERSE EFFECT**
Central nervous system	Headache, dizziness
Gastrointestinal	Diarrhea, abdominal pain, vomiting, nausea, anorexia
Genitourinary	Proteinuria, hematuria, glycosuria
Hematopoietic	Pancytopenia, thrombocytopenia, neutropenia, leukocytosis, anemia
Integumentary	Rash, dry skin, urticaria, pruritis, alopecia
Respiratory	Upper respiratory infections, cough
Other	Back pain, fever, fatigue

DOSAGES

SELECTED OMEPRAZOLE, SUCRALFATE, AND MISOPROSTOL AGENTS

AGENT	PHARMACOLOGIC CLASS	DOSAGE RANGE	PURPOSE
⚓Omeprazole (Prilosec)	Antisecretory	*Adult* PO: 20 mg/day for 4-8 wk	Esophagitis, duodenal ulcer
		PO: 60-360/day divided	Hypersecretory conditions
⚓Sucralfate (Carafate)	Antiulcer agent	*Adult* PO: 1 g qid ac	Duodenal ulcers
⚓Misoprostol (Cytotec)	Antisecretory	*Adult* PO: 200 μg qid with meals and hs for duration of NSAID therapy	Gastric ulcer prophylaxis during NSAID therapy

azepam and phenytoin. There is also the possibility that there may be an increased chance for bleeding in patients that are on both a proton pump inhibitor and warfarin.

Dosages

For recommended dosages see the dosages table above.

DRUG PROFILES

⚓ OMEPRAZOLE

Omeprazole (Prilosec) is the only currently available drug in this unique class of antisecretory drugs. It is the newest drug introduced for the treatment of acid-related disorders. Omeprazole binds to and inhibits the enzyme H^+/K^+ ATPase, which is the final common step in the acid-secretory process of the parietal cell.

The ability of omeprazole to totally prohibit the production of acid from the parietal cells in the stomach gives it many beneficial therapeutic effects. As mentioned in the section on therapeutic uses, omeprazole is currently approved only for acute treatment of severe gastroesophageal reflux disease unresponsive

to conventional therapy, endoscopically proven erosive esophagitis, and the chronic treatment of Zollinger-Ellison syndrome.

Omeprazole is available only in an oral formulation as a 20-mg sustained-release capsule. It is classified as a pregnancy category C agent and is contraindicated in hypersensitivity. Common dosage recommendations are listed in the dosages table above.

▼ PHARMACOKINETICS

HALF-LIFE	ONSET	PEAK	DURATION
Variable	2 hr	0.5-3.5 hr	24 hr

Other Drugs

Antacids, antiflatulents, H_2 antagonists, and omeprazole are some of the many commonly used drugs to treat acid-related disorders. Some of the other drugs that may be used to treat acid-related and other disorders are: sucralfate, misoprostol, bismuth, anticholinergics, and tricyclic antidepressants. Some of these agents, such as anticholinergics and tricyclics, are mentioned in other chapters. Sucralfate and misoprostol will be discussed here.

SUCRALFATE

Sucralfate (Carafate) is an agent used as an acute cytoprotective agent in the treatment of stress ulcerations and chronically in peptic ulcer disease. It works in a manner that is totally different from that of the antacids, H$_2$ antagonists, and proton pump inhibitors. A closer look at sucralfate's chemical structure provides insight into its many actions.

Mechanism of Action

Sucralfate has as its basic structure a sugar, sucrose. Sulfates and aluminum hydroxide groups are attached to that sugar in the place where there are normally hydroxyl groups. Once sucralfate comes into contact with the acid of the stomach it begins to dissociate into aluminum hydroxide and sulfate anions. Sucralfate is sometimes referred to as a cytoprotective agent. The sulfated sucrose molecules of sucralfate are attracted to and bind to the base of ulcers and erosions, forming a protective barrier over the base of this area. By binding to the exposed proteins of ulcers and erosions, sucralfate limits access of pepsin, which normally breaks down proteins, either causing ulcers or making them worse. This is believed to be the primary mechanism by which sucralfate heals ulcers and protects erosions. It has a multitude of other effects that may also explain its mechanism of action.

Drug Effects

The drug effects of sucralfate are numerous. This can be attributed to its unique structure, which contains sucrose (a sugar), sulfate anions (negatively charged particles), and aluminum hydroxide (an antacid). The many drug effects of sucralfate are listed in Table 47-6.

Therapeutic Uses

Sucralfate has many attractive characteristics that make it a beneficial agent for the treatment of such disorders as stress ulcers, erosions, and PUD.

Side Effects and Adverse Effects

Sucralfate has little absorption from the gut into the blood and is chemically inert. These characteristics make it virtually devoid of systemic toxicity. The most common side effects are constipation and nausea, which appear 2% to 3% of the time.

Interactions

Sucralfate may impair the absorption of certain drugs, particularly phenytoin and warfarin. The clinical significance of these drug interactions is rare. This can be avoided by the administration of sucralfate without any other medications. This binding property

Table 47-6	Sucralfate: Drug Effects
CHARACTERISTIC	**DRUG EFFECT**
Sulfate anions	Binds to positively charged tissue proteins that are exposed at the tissue surface of an ulcer or an erosion.
Weak base	Buffers the acidic pH of the stomach.
Epidermal growth factor	Binds and concentrates epidermal growth factor (EGF), which accelerates the healing process.
Prostaglandin synthesis	Stimulates gastric mucosal prostaglandin E$_2$ synthesis.
Stimulates mucus and bicarbonate	The aluminum salt stimulates the secretion of mucus and bicarbonate from the cells of the stomach to counteract the actions of hydrochloric acid.

of sucralfate may be used therapeutically. Sucralfate binds phosphates in the gastrointestinal tract and has been used as a phosphate binder in patients with chronic renal failure.

Dosages

For recommended dosages see the dosages table on p. 738.

*D*RUG PROFILES

⚕ SUCRALFATE

Sucralfate is available only with a prescription and comes only in an oral formulation as a 1-g oral tablet and as a 1g/10 ml oral solution. Sucralfate is classified as a pregnancy category B agent and is contraindicated in hypersensitivity. Common dosage recommendation for sucralfate is 1 g four times a day.

⬡ PHARMACOKINETICS

HALF-LIFE	ONSET	PEAK	DURATION
6-20 hr	1 hr	2-4 hr	3-6 hr

⚓ MISOPROSTOL

Misoprostol (Cytotec) is a synthetic prostaglandin analog. Prostaglandins have a wide variety of biologic activities. They are believed to inhibit gastric acid secretion and exhibit "cytoprotective" activity. They are believed to protect the gastric mucosa from injury, possibly by enhancing the local production of mucus or bicarbonate, by promoting local cell regeneration, or possibly by maintaining mucosal blood flow.

Because of their inhibitory effects on gastric acid secretion and their cytoprotective properties, synthetic analogues of prostaglandins (of the E class) have been produced. They were made with the expectation that they might be useful agents for the treatment of peptic ulcer disease. Misoprostol, an E analog, has been shown to be effective in reducing the incidence of gastric ulcers in patients taking NSAIDs. The drug has been approved by the FDA for this prophylactic use.

Although some studies show that synthetic analogues of prostaglandins promote the healing of duodenal ulcers, they must be used in doses that usually produce more disturbing side effects, such as abdominal cramps and diarrhea. Thus they are not believed to be as effective as the H₂ blockers for this indication. Pregnancy category X.

ℕURSING PROCESS

ASSESSMENT

Before administering any antacid agent, the nurse should assess the patient and gather information regarding the following: presence of congestive heart failure, hypertension, sodium restrictions, and other cardiac diseases, especially if the antacid is high in sodium content; fluid imbalances; dehydration; GI obstruction; renal disease; and pregnancy. Under these conditions, antacids, must be used cautiously. Contraindications to the use of aluminum-containing antacids include hypersensitivity to the drug.

Magnesium antacids should be used cautiously in patients who have a history of renal insufficiency and also in pregnant or lactating patients. Contraindications to the use of magnesium antacids include hypersensitivity to the medication. Calcium-containing antacids are not used as frequently because of their risk of rebound hyperacidity, milk-alkali syndrome, and changes in systemic pH, especially if the patient has abnormal renal functioning. Milk-alkali syndrome and rebound hyperacidity are also problematic with the administration of antacids containing sodium bicarbonate. Sodium bicarbonate is generally not recommended as an antacid because of the high risk of systemic electrolyte disturbances and alkalosis. Sodium content in sodium bicarbonate is high and can be problematic for patients who have hypertension, CHF, or renal insufficiency.

There are many drug interactions with antacids because of the effect on absorption of the medication that is given concurrently with the antacid. Some of the medications whose effects are increased by the use of antacids include quinidine (antiarrhythmic), pseudoephedrine (decongestant), levodopa (antiparkinson agent), valproic acid (anticonvulsant), and dicumarol (anticoagulant). Medications with decreased effects when used simultaneously with antacids include digoxin (cardiac glycoside), corticosteroids, cimetadine and rantidine (H₂ receptor-blocking agents), iron preparations, phenothiazines (antiemetics and tranquilizer), salicylates (aspirin), and isoniazid (INH, antituberculin agent). See Table 47-2 for further information on drug interactions.

Antiflatulents, such as simethicone, help in dispersing and preventing gas formation in the GI system. They have few side effects, are contraindicated with

---

Patient Teaching TIPS

Antacids, Antiflatulents, and H₂ Receptor Antagonists

✔ Patients should not take any other medications within 1 to 2 hours after taking an antacid. The antacid will affect the absorption of many medications in the stomach, so it is better to take antacids without any other medications.

✔ Patients should contact the physician immediately if they experience constipation, diarrhea, an increase in abdominal pain, or any change in symptomatology.

✔ If patients are taking enteric-coated medications, it is important for them to know that antacids may promote premature dissolving of the enteric coating. Enteric coatings are used to diminish stomach upset in irritating medications, and if the coating is destroyed early in the stomach GI upset may occur.

✔ Patients should take antiflatulents such as simethicone as recommended by manufacturer directions. Chewable forms must always be chewed thoroughly; liquid preparations should be shaken thoroughly before administration.

✔ Patients should take histamine H₂ receptor antagonists exactly as prescribed. For parenteral use, follow manufacturer guidelines.

hypersensitivity to the drug, and should be given cautiously to pregnant women and only after a physician's order.

H$_2$ receptor antagonists are contraindicated in patients with known drug allergy or who have impaired renal functioning or liver disease. Cautious use is recommended in patients who are confused, disoriented, or elderly.

NURSING DIAGNOSES

Nursing diagnoses related to the administration of antacids and antiflatulents include the following:

- Pain related to gastric hyperacidity.
- Constipation related to side effects of aluminum-containing antacids.
- Diarrhea related to side effects of magnesium-containing antacids.

TAKE HOME POINTS

Acid Physiology

- Stomach secretes many substances (hydrochloric acid, pepsinogen, mucus, bicarbonate, intrinsic factor, and prostaglandins).
- The parietal cell is responsible for the production of acid.
- In acid-related disorders there is an impairment in the balance between these substances.
- The most common impairment is hyperacidity or the overproduction of acid.
- The most harmful is peptic ulcer disease.

Drug Therapy

- Antacids have been used for centuries and were the mainstays of antiulcer therapy until the 1970s.
- In the 1970s the H$_2$ antagonists arrived on the scene.
- Later came the proton pump inhibitors.
- Other agents are sucralfate and misoprostol.

H$_2$ Antagonists

- Histamine type 2 blockers bind to and block histamine receptors located on parietal cells.
- This blockade renders these cells less responsive to stimuli and thus acid secretion.
- Up to 90% inhibition can be achieved with these agents.

Proton Pump Inhibitors

- Block the final step in the acid production pathway—H$^+$/K$^+$ ATPase
- This energy-requiring pump is needed to pump out H$^+$ ions or protons.
- Block all acid secretion.

Other Drug Therapy

- Sucralfate is a cytoprotective agent for stress ulcerations and PUD.
- Binds to exposed proteins of ulcers and thus limits pepsin's proteolytic action.
- Misoprostol is a synthetic prostaglandin analog
- Inhibits gastric acid secretion, enhances local production of mucus or bicarbonate.
- Also helps maintain mucosal blood flow.

Nursing Considerations

- Cautious use of antacids is recommended in patients with congestive heart failure, hypertension, sodium restrictions, and other cardiac diseases, especially if the antacid is high in sodium content.
- Other cautions to antacid use include fluid imbalances, dehydration, GI obstruction, renal disease, and pregnancy.
- Contraindications to the use of aluminum-containing antacids include hypersensitivity.
- There are many drug interactions with antacids because of the effect on absorption of the medication that is given concurrently with the antacid, so always check for interactions before giving the medication.
- It is best *not* to administer other medications within 1 to 2 hours after giving an antacid; but contact the physician if medication time needs to be rescheduled.
- If taking enteric-coated medications, it is important to know that antacids may result in premature dissolving of the enteric coating, and stomach upset may occur.
- Antacids containing magnesium are contraindicated in patients with renal failure; aluminum-containing antacids must be used cautiously in patients with renal failure. The recommended dosage of most antacids is usually 15 to 60 cc with water every 1 to 3 hours after meals and at bedtime.
- Antiflatulents are useful in the management of conditions associated with excessive gas production, such as postoperative flatus and bloating, diverticulitis, irritable or spastic colon, air swallowing associated with anxiety, and peptic ulcer disease.
- H$_2$ histamine antagonists are used in the management of peptic ulcer disease by elevating the gastric pH to help neutralize the effects of hyperacidic or hypersecretory states in the GI tract.

NURSING ▪ CARE ▪ PLAN

Peptic Ulcer

Dr. K.T., a 46-year-old college professor, has been diagnosed with gastritis and a small peptic ulcer after having an endoscopy today. Serum electrolytes were within normal limits; however, gastrin levels were elevated. The physician has encouraged a regular exercise program, stress management, eating a regular diet high in fiber and vegetables, and avoiding alcohol and nicotine (he is a nonsmoker and only drinks occasionally). Along with his discharge care instructions for postendoscopy, he also received a prescription for omeprazole (Prilosec).

Assessment with nursing diagnoses	Planning with goals and outcome criteria	Implementation and patient education	Evaluation

Subjective
 	
Complaint of heartburn and gastric reflux with pain waking him at night
Snacks on junkfood frequently to "soak up" acid
 	
Objective
 	
High stress job
No alcohol and does not smoke
Heartburn X 6 mo
Takes antacids daily
Recent endoscopy with diagnosis of reflux and peptic ulcer with prescription for Prilosec
 	
Nursing diagnosis
 	
Pain, epigastric related to diagnosis of reflux and peptic ulcer
	Goals
	
	Patient will experience more comfort from relief of reflux and ulcer pain within 1 wk of treatment with medications
	
	Outcome criteria
	
	Patient will state the following ways to minimize discomfort associated with reflux and PUD:
	  Take meds as prescribed
	  Proper diet
	  Decrease stress
	  Eliminate other factors that elevate gastric acid production
		Always take medication as prescribed and take before meals . . . do not open, chew, or crush capsule
		
		Report any severe diarrhea to the physician
		
		Eat diet as recommended by physician and limit gas-producing foods and those that are acidic such as orange juice, and avoid highly spicy foods
		
		Decrease food intake before bedtime to avoid reflux at night
		
		Sleep with head of bed slightly elevated
		
		Avoid alcohol, nicotine, and caffeine
		
		Exercise regularly at least 3 times/wk to help decrease stress
		
		Participate in relaxing activities and attend stress-reducing seminars at the hospital this month
		
		Eat diet high in fiber and drink at least 2-3 liters of fluid a day
		
		Avoid snacking, especially at bedtime
		
		Eat a balanced diet with all four food groups represented
		
		Follow-up with physician as ordered
		
		Contact physician should gastric pain increase
			Patient shows a therapeutic response such as:
			  Absence of epigastric pain
			  Less belching
			  Absence of abdominal fullness and swelling
			  Normal stool patterns
			  Less GI upset
			  Changes in life style that are positive in decreasing stress
			  Changes in diet
			  Better sleeping patterns
			  Taking medication as prescribed

- Knowledge deficit as related to lack of information about antacids, H_2 receptor antagonists, or antiflatulents, their use and potential side effects.

PLANNING

Goals are as follows:
- Patient has minimal to no pain during antacid or antiflatulent therapy.
- Patient experiences minimal side effects while using antacids or antiflatulents.
- Patient remains compliant to therapy.

Outcome Criteria

Outcome criteria related to the administration of antacids include the following:
- Patient experiences increased comfort as related to the use of antacids especially at night.
- Patient states expected side effects as related to the use of antacids, such as constipation or diarrhea and when to seek further assistance regarding their management.
- Patient states the importance of compliance and following administration guidelines associated with the use of antacids or antiflatulents to help decrease manifestations of disease or disorder.

IMPLEMENTATION

When giving antacids or antiflatulents always be sure that chewable tablets are well-chewed and liquid forms are thoroughly shaken before administration. Administer all antacid agents with at least 8 ounces of water to enhance absorption of the antacid in the stomach. Should constipation or diarrhea occur with single agents suggest a combination aluminum and magnesium product. It is also recommended that when you administer an antacid as ordered, do *not* administer it within 1 to 2 hours of other medications because of the effect of antacids on the absorption of medications in the stomach. For patient teaching tips see p. 740.

EVALUATION

Therapeutic response to the administration of antacids or histamine H_2 receptor antagonists includes relief of symptoms associated with hyperacidity related to the diagnosis of peptic ulcer, gastritis, esophagitis, gastric hyperacidity, or hiatal hernia. Side effects to check for in patients on antacids or antiflatulants include nausea, vomiting, abdominal pain, and diarrhea. Constipation, milk-alkali syndrome, and acid rebound are complications associated with sodium bicarbonate and calcium antacids. Therapeutic response to antiflatulents includes a decrease in the occurrence of flatus.

Critical Thinking A C T I V I T I E S

1. One of your patients, a 30-year-old business executive, is taking simethicone for excessive flatus associated with diverticulitis. Which of the following actions best describes the mechanism of action in reducing flatus by simethicone?
   a. It disperses and prevents gas formation in the stomach.
   b. It neutralizes gastric pH, thereby preventing gas.
   c. It decreases gastric acid secretion and minimizes flatus.
   d. It buffers the effects of pepsin on the gastric wall.

2. Digoxin preparations and adsorbers should not be given simultaneously. As a nurse you are aware that if these agents are given simultaneously one of the following will occur. Which will occur?
   a. Increased absorption of the adsorbent
   b. Decreased absorption of the adsorbent
   c. Increased absorption of the digoxin
   d. Decreased absorption of the digoxin

3. One of your patients is receiving digitalis orally and is also to receive an antacid at the same time. Your most appropriate action, based on the pharmacokinetics of antacids, would be to:
   a. administer both medications as ordered and document in the nurses notes
   b. contact the physician regarding the drug interaction and request a change in the time dosing of the drugs
   c. delay the digitalis for 1 to 2 hours until the antacid is absorbed
   d. give the antacid at least 2 to 4 hours before administering the digitalis

4. One of your patients, a 30-year-old business executive, is taking simethicone for excessive flatus associated with diverticulitis. Which of the following actions best describes the mechanism of action in reducing flatus by simethicone?
   a. It disperses and prevents gas formation in the stomach.
   b. It neutralizes gastric pH, thereby preventing gas.
   c. It decreases gastric acid secretion and minimizes flatus.
   d. It buffers the effects of pepsin on the gastric wall.

BIBLIOGRAPHY

Albanese J, Nutz P: *Mosby's 1995 nursing drug cards,* St Louis, 1995, Mosby.

Fledman M et al: Treating ulcers and reflux. what's new? *JA Patient Care,* ed 4, St Louis, 1992, Mosby.

Holmgren C: Perfecting the art of abdominal assessment, *RN* 55(3):28, 1992.

Johnson KB: *Harriet Lane handbook,* ed 13, St Louis, 1993, Mosby.

Keen JH: *Critical care and emergency drug reference,* St Louis, 1994, Mosby.

Knoben JE, Anderson PO: *Handbook of critical drug data,* ed 6, Hamilton, Ill, 1988, Drug Intelligence Publications.

McEvoy GK: *AHFS drug information,* Bethesda, Md, 1994, American Society of Hospital Pharmacists.

McQuaid KF, Isenberg JI: Medical therapy of peptic ulcer disease, *Surg Clin North Am* 72(2):285, 1992.

Richter JE: Gastroesophageal reflux: diagnosis and management, *Hosp Pract* 27(1):39, 1992.

Rubin W: Medical treatment of peptic ulcer disease, *Med Clin North Am* 75(4):981, 1991.

Skidmore-Roth L: *Mosby's 1995 nursing drug reference,* St Louis, 1995, Mosby.

Chapter 48

Antidiarrheals and Laxatives

Objectives

When you reach the end of this chapter, you will be able to:

1 Identify the various agents used as antidiarrheals, laxatives, and cathartics.

2 Define the terms antidiarrheal, cathartic, and laxative.

3 Discuss the mechanisms of action, indications, cautions, contraindications, side effects, and dosages associated with the use of antidiarrheals, laxatives, and cathartics.

4 Develop a nursing care plan as it relates to the nursing process in the administration of antidiarrheals, cathartics, and laxatives.

5 Discuss patient education guidelines associated with the use of antidiarrheals, laxatives, and cathartics.

CHAPTER OUTLINE

Antidiarrheals
  Mechanism of action
  Drug effects
  Therapeutic uses
  Side effects and adverse effects
  Interactions
  Dosages
Drug Profiles
Adsorbents
    Bismuth Subsalicylate
    Attapulgite
Anticholingerics
    Belladonna-alkaloid Combinations
Opiates
    Diphenoxylate and Atropine
  ⚓ Loperamide
Intestinal Flora Modifiers
    Lactobacillus Acidophilus
Laxatives
  Mechanism of action
  Drug effects
  Therapeutic uses
  Side effects and adverse effects
  Interactions
  Dosages
Drug Profiles
Bulk-Forming Laxatives
  ⚓ Methylcellulose

    Psyllium
Emollient Laxatives
    Mineral Oil
  ⚓ Docusate Salts
Hyperosmotic Laxatives
    Polyethylene Glycol
    Lactulose
    Glycerin
Saline Laxatives
    Magnesium Salts
Stimulant Laxatives
    Phenolphthalein

Nursing Process
Assessment
Nursing Diagnoses
Planning
  Outcome criteria
Implementation
Evaluation

Glossary

Acute diarrhea (ə kūt' di' ə re'ə) Diarrhea that is sudden in onset in a previously healthy individual, lasting anywhere from 3 days to 2 weeks. (p. 746)

Adsorbent (ad sor' bənt) Antidiarrheal agent that acts by coating the walls of the gastrointestinal tract, absorbing the bacteria or toxins causing the diarrhea, and eliminating them with the stools. (p. 747)

Anticholinergic (an' tĭ ko' lin ər' jik) Antidiarrheal agent that acts by decreasing the muscular tone of the intestine and thus decreasing peristalis. (p. 747)

Bulk-forming laxatives Agents that absorb water into the intestine, which increases bulk, distending the bowel to initiate reflex bowel activity and promoting a bowel movement. Bulk-forming laxatives act in a manner similar to that of fiber naturally contained in the diet. (p. 753)

Chronic diarrhea Diarrhea that lasts for over 3 to 4 weeks, associated with recurring passage of diarrheal stools, fever, loss of appetite, nausea, vomiting, weight reduction, and chronic weakness. (p. 746)

Constipation (kon' stĭ pā' shən) A condition of abnormally infrequent and difficult passage of feces through the lower gastrointestinal tract. (p. 752)

Diarrhea (di' ə re' ə) Abnormal frequent passage of loose stools. (p. 746)

Emollient laxatives (e mol' e ənt) Agents often referred to as *stool softeners* and *lubricant laxatives.* The fecal softeners work by lowering the surface tension of fluids resulting in more water and fat being absorbed into the stool and the intestines. The lubricant type of emollient laxatives works by lubricating the fecal material and the intestinal walls. This prevents water from leaking out of the intestines and softens and expands the stool. (p. 753)

Intestinal flora modifiers (flor' ə) Product obtained from bacterial cultures, most commonly *Lactobacillus* organisms. (p. 747)

Laxative (lak' sə tiv) Agent that promotes bowel evacuation by increasing the bulk of the feces, softening the stool, or lubricating the intestinal wall. (p. 753)

Opiate (o' pe ət) Antidiarrheal agent that acts by decreasing motility of the bowel, causing constipation and sedation, and often reducing pain associated with diarrhea. (p. 747)

Saline laxative (sa' lin) Agent that works primarily in the small intestines by preventing water from being absorbed. (p. 753)

Stimulant laxative Agent that stimulates movement of the intestines by stimulating the nerves that innervate the intestines, resulting in increased peristalsis activity in the intestinal tract. (p. 753)

Diarrhea and the diseases commonly associated with it are among the leading causes of death and morbidity in third world nations, accounting for 5 to 8 million deaths per year in infants and small children. Diarrheal disorders also have a financial impact on our society. Outpatient costs and loss of time from work because of acute infectious diarrhea have been estimated to cost $23 billion per year or $106 per person in the United States. To the gastroenterologist, diarrhea is one of the "big three" symptoms of gastrointestinal disease: abdominal pain, nausea and/or vomiting, and diarrhea.

Diarrhea is defined as the abnormal frequent passage of loose stools or, more specifically, the abnormal passage of stools with increased frequency, fluidity, and weight, or with increased stool water excretion. **Acute diarrhea** refers to diarrhea that is sudden in onset in a previously healthy individual. It lasts anywhere from 3 days to 2 weeks and is self-limiting, resolving without sequelae. **Chronic diarrhea** lasts for over 3 to 4 weeks and is associated with recurring passage of diarrheal stools, fever, loss of appetite, nausea, vomiting, weight reduction, and chronic weakness.

Specific treatment requires knowledge of the cause of or the condition creating the diarrhea. Possible causes of diarrhea are listed in the box below. Nonspecific treatment is directed at the cessation of the increased stool frequency associated with diarrhea, alleviation of abdominal cramps, and prevention of dehydration from fluid and electrolyte loss and weight loss and nutritional deficits from malabsorption.

ANTIDIARRHEALS

The agents used to treat diarrhea are called *antidiarrheals;* they are divided into different groups based on specific mechanisms of action: adsorbents, antimotility drugs (anticholinergics and opiates), bacterial replacement drugs (intestinal flora modifiers), antisecretory drugs, and enzymes. The specific classes and the agents in each are listed in Table 48-1.

Mechanism of Action

Antidiarrheal agents have varying mechanisms of action. It is important to know the specific mechanism of an agent to ensure that the appropriate one is being used (treating the underlying cause).

Causes of Diarrhea

Causes of Acute Diarrhea
Bacterial
Drug-induced
Viral
Nutritional
Protozoal
Other

Causes of Chronic Diarrhea
Tumors
Diabetes mellitus
Hyperthyroidism
Addison's disease
Irritable bowel syndrome
Other

Adsorbents act by coating the walls of the gastrointestinal tract; they remain in the intestine, bind to the causative bacteria or toxin, and eliminate it from the body through the stool.

Anticholinergics work by decreasing peristalsis (rhythmic contractions of the gastrointestinal (GI) tract) and the muscular tone of the intestine, thus slowing the movement of substances through the GI tract. They are often used in combination with adsorbents and opiates. Anticholinergics are discussed in detail in Chapter 18.

Intestinal flora modifiers are products obtained from bacterial cultures, most commonly *Lactobacillus* organisms. They make up the majority of the body's normal bacterial flora and are the organisms that are most commonly destroyed by antibiotics. Exogenously supplying these bacteria helps to restore the balance of normal flora and suppress the growth of diarrhea-causing bacteria.

The primary action of the **opiates** is to decrease bowel motility. Secondary mechanisms of action that make opiates beneficial in the treatment of diarrhea include reducing the pain associated with diarrhea and relieving rectal spasms. Because they decrease the transit time of food, they permit longer contact of the intestinal contents with the absorptive surface of the bowel, increasing the reabsorption of water and electrolytes from the stool and reducing stool frequency and net volume.

Drug Effects

Although all classes of antidiarrheal agents counteract diarrhea, other drug effects vary depending upon the drug class and its specific mechanism of action. Within the class of adsorbents, bismuth subsalicylate is a form of aspirin, or acetylsalicylic acid, and therefore it has many of the same drug effects as aspirin (see Chapter 42). Activated charcoal is not only helpful in coating the walls of the gastrointestinal tract and adsorbing bacteria, but it is also useful in cases of overdose because of its drug-binding properties. Colestipol and cholestyramine are anion exchange resins that are prescription antidiarrheals. Besides binding to diarrhea-causing toxins, they have the additional benefit of decreasing cholesterol.

The anticholinergics have many drug effects beyond those of diarrhea relief (see Chapter 18). Some of the antidiarrheals in the opiate family of drugs are used solely for their therapeutic effects in treating diarrhea, whereas others have analgesic properties and may be used to treat various types of pain. The drug effects of intestinal flora modifiers are limited to their antidiarrheal influence.

Therapeutic Uses

All four antidiarrheal drug families effectively combat diarrhea, though the therapeutic effects vary slightly from family to family. Because diarrhea has various causes, it is useful to know that antidiarrheals have different mechanisms of action that allow the caregiver to pick an agent that is specific to the underlying cause of the diarrhea. The box on the next page lists the four families of antidiarrheal drugs and their specific therapeutic effects.

Side Effects and Adverse Effects

The side effects and adverse effects of the antidiarrheals are also specific to each drug family. Most of these potential effects are minor and not life threatening. The major side effects of specific agents in each drug class are listed in Table 48-2.

Interactions

Many drugs are absorbed from the intestines into the bloodstream, where they are delivered to their respective sites of action. Many of the antidiarrheals have the potential to alter this normal process, either by increasing or decreasing the absorption of these other drugs. Table 48-3 lists some of the more common and more serious drug interactions of the antidiarrheals.

Dosages

For the recommended dosages of antidiarrheal agents see the dosages table on p. 750.

Table 48-1	Antidiarrheals: Drug Categories and Selected Agents
CATEGORY	**ANTIDIARRHEAL AGENT**
Adsorbents	Activated charcoal, aluminum hydroxide, attapulgite, bismuth subsalicylate, cholestyramine, kaolin-pectin, polycarbophil
Anticholinergics	Atropine, hyoscyamine, hyoscine
Opiates	Opium tincture, paregoric, codeine, diphenoxylate, ↓loperamide
Intestinal flora modifiers	*Lactobacillus acidophilus*

Antidiarrheals: Therapeutic Effects

AGENT	THERAPEUTIC EFFECT
Adsorbents	
Activated charcoal, aluminum hydroxide attapulgite, bismuth subsalicylate, cholestyramine, kaolin-pectin, and polycarbophil	Of the adsorbents, kaolin-pectin, bismuth salts, attapulgite, and aluminum hydroxide are the most commonly used. These agents act by coating the walls of the GI tract, absorbing the bacteria or toxins causing the diarrhea, and eliminating them with the stools, thus removing the substances that are actually causing the diarrhea.
Anticholinergics	
Atropine, hyoscyamine, and hyoscine	The anticholinergics decrease intestinal muscle tone and peristalsis thereby slowing the movement of fecal matter through the GI tract. They are often combined with other antidiarrheals to increase their effectiveness.
Intestinal Flora Modifiers	
Lactobacillus acidophilus	Intestinal flora modifiers suppress the growth of diarrhea-causing bacteria and help reestablish the normal intestinal flora that has been depleted by the diarrhea.
Opiates	
Opium tincture, paregoric, codeine, diphenoxylate, and loperamide	The opiates are used in the treatment of diarrhea because of their constipating effects and their therapeutic pain-relieving effects. They cause constipation by lowering the motility of the bowel and relieving rectal spasms. By slowing the time it takes to pass food through the intestines, water and electrolytes have a greater chance of being absorbed, which reduces stool frequency and volume.

Table 48-2 Antidiarrheals: Adverse Effects

AGENT	BODY SYSTEM	SIDE/ADVERSE EFFECT
Adsorbents		
Bismuth subsalicylate	Hematopoietic	Increased bleeding time
	Gastrointestinal	Constipation, dark stools
	Central nervous system	Confusion, twitching
	Eye, ear, nose, throat	Hearing loss, tinnitus, metallic taste, blue gums
Anticholinergics		
Atropine, hyoscyamine, hyoscine	Genitourinary	Urinary retention and hesitancy, impotence
	Central nervous system	Headache, dizziness, confusion, anxiety, drowsiness
	Cardiovascular	Hypotension, hypertension, bradycardia, tachycardia
	Integumentary	Dry skin, rash, flushing
	Eye, ear, nose, throat	Blurred vision, photophobia, increased pressure in the eye
Opiates		
Codeine	Central nervous system	Drowsiness, sedation, dizziness, lethargy
	Gastrointestinal	Nausea, vomiting, anorexia, constipation
	Respiratory	Respiratory depression
	Cardiovascular	Bradycardia, palpitations, hypotension
	Genitourinary	Urinary retention
	Integumentary	Flushing, rash, urticaria

Table 48-3	Antidiarrheal Agents: Drug Interactions	
ANTIDIARRHEAL	**INTERACTING DRUG**	**RESULT**
Adsorbents	Digoxin, clindamycin, quinidine	Decreased absorption
	Oral anticoagulants	Increased bleeding time, bruising
	Methotrexate	Increased toxicity
	Probenecid	Decreased probenecid effects
	Hypoglycemic agents	Decreased hypoglycemic effects
Anticholinergics	Antacids	Decreased anticholinergic effects
	Amantadine, tricyclic antidepressants, MAOIs, antihistamines	Increased anticholinergic effects
Opiates	CNS depressants, alcohol, narcotics, sedative hypnotics, antipsychotics, skeletal muscle relaxants	Increased CNS depressant effects

DRUG PROFILES

Drug therapy for diarrhea is dependent upon the cause of the diarrhea and the antidiarrheal that will best combat it. All antidiarrheals are orally administered agents available as suspensions, tablets, or capsules. Some of the antidiarrheals are over-the-counter (OTC) medications whereas others require a prescription.

ADSORBENTS

As mentioned earlier, the adsorbents bind to the diarrhea-causing bacteria and pass them out with the stool. Of the adsorbent antidiarrheals, bismuth subsalicylate, attapulgite, aluminum hydroxide, and kaolin-pectin are the most commonly used. These agents are all OTC medications and are classified in different pregnancy categories. They are contraindicated in children under 3 years of age.

BISMUTH SUBSALICYLATE

Bismuth subsalicylate (Pepto-Bismol) is a salicylate by chemical structure; therefore it should be used with caution in children and teenagers who have or are recovering from chicken pox or flu because of the attendant risk of Reye's syndrome. It can also cause all the side effects and adverse effects that are associated with an aspirin-based product. Two alarming but harmless side effects are temporary darkening of the tongue and/or stool. It is a pregnancy category C agent. Bis-

muth subsalicylate is available OTC as a 262-mg chewable tablet or a 262-mg/15 ml suspension. Commonly recommended dosages are listed in the dosages table on the next page.

PHARMACOKINETICS

HALF-LIFE	ONSET	PEAK	DURATION
24-33 hr*	0.5-2 hr	2-5 hr	Variable

*For bismuth.

ATTAPULGITE

Attapulgite (Kaopectate) has replaced the use of kaolin-pectin in this preparation. Kaolin is a naturally hydrated aluminum compound that is now rarely used as an antidiarrheal agent. However, pectin, which is extracted from apples or citrus fruit, is used in many combination products. The original Kaopectate contained 980 mg/5 ml of kaolin and 21.7 mg/5 ml of pectin.

Attapulgite is also an OTC antidiarrheal and is a pregnancy category C agent. It is available as 300-mg chewable tablets, 600-mg maximum-strength tablets, and a 600-mg/15 ml solution. Commonly recommended dosages are listed in the dosages table on the next page.

PHARMACOKINETICS

HALF-LIFE	ONSET	PEAK	DURATION
Unknown	12 hr	14-20 hr	Unknown

ANTICHOLINGERICS

The anticholinergics, atropine, hyoscyamine, and hyoscine, are used either alone or in combination with

DOSAGES

SELECTED ANTIDIARRHEAL AGENTS

AGENT	PHARMACOLOGIC CLASS	DOSAGE RANGE	PURPOSE
Bismuth subsalicylate (Pepto-Bismol)	Antimicrobial, antisecretory, antidiarrheal	*Pediatric* (repeated q30-60min not to exceed 8 doses/ day) PO: 3-6 y/o: 5 ml or ⅓ tablet 6-9 y/o: 10 ml or ⅔ tablet 9-12 y/o: 15 ml or 1 tablet *Adult* PO: 30 ml or 2 tablets	Diarrhea
Attapulgite (Kaopectate)	Adsorbent antidiarrheal	*Chewable tablets* *Pediatric* PO: 3-6 y/o: 1 tablet after each BM 6-12 y/o: 2 tablets after each BM *Adult* PO: 4 tablets after each BM *Concentrated liquid* *Pediatric* PO: 3-6 y/o: 7.5 ml after each BM 6-12 y/o: 15 ml after each BM *Adult* PO: 30 ml after each BM *Maximum strength tablet* *Pediatric* PO: 6-12 y/o: 1 tablet after each BM *Adult* PO: 2 tablets after each BM	Diarrhea
Belladonna alkaloids (Donnatal, Donnatal Extentabs, Kinesed)	Fixed-combination anticholinergic	*Adult* PO: 5-10 ml or 1-2 capsules or tablets 3-4 times/day or 1 tablet q12h (Donnatal Extentabs)	Decreased intestinal motility
⚓Loperamide hydrochloride (Imodium, Imodium A-D, Pepto-Diarrhea Control)	Opiate anti-diarrheal	*Pediatric* PO: 2-5 y/o: 1 mg tid PO: 6-8 y/o: 2 mg bid PO: 8-12 y/o: 2 mg tid *Adult* PO: 4 mg followed by 2 mg after each BM	Decreased intestinal motility
Lactobacillus acidophilus (Bacid, Lactinex)	Intestinal flora modifier	*Bacid:* PO: 2 capsules 2-4 times/day *Lactinex:* PO: 1 granule packet with liquids or food 3-4 times/day 4 tablets 3-4 times/day with liquid	Diarrhea

BM, bowel movement.

other antidiarrheals because they slow GI tract motility. These agents are commonly referred to as the belladonna alkaloids and are discussed in Chapter 18. Their safety margin is not as broad as that of many of the other antidiarrheals because they can cause serious adverse effects if used inappropriately. For this reason they are available only by prescription.

BELLADONNA-ALKALOID COMBINATIONS

The belladonna alkaloids (Donnatal, Donnatal Extentabs, Kinesed) are used to treat many GI disorders, including diarrhea. Of the belladonna-alkaloid combination products, Donnatal is the most commonly used.

The belladonna-alkaloid preparations are classified as pregnancy category C agents and are contraindicated in patients who have shown a hypersensitivity to anticholinergics, and in patients with narrow-angle glaucoma, GI obstruction, myasthenia gravis, paralytic ileus, and toxic megacolon. Donnatal tablets contain a combination of four different alkaloids: atropine (0.0194 mg), hyoscyamine (0.1037), phenobarbital (16.2 mg), and scopolamine (0.0065 mg). There are many dosage forms of this combination: oral capsules, elixir, tablets, and extended-release tablets. Donnatal No. 2 tablets contain two times as much phenobarbital (32.4 mg), and the Donnatal Extentabs contain 48.6 mg of phenobarbital and increased amounts of all the other above-mentioned alkaloids. Commonly recommended dosages are listed in the preceding dosages table.

PHARMACOKINETICS

HALF-LIFE	ONSET	PEAK	DURATION
Unknown	1-2 hr*	2-3 hr*	6-8 hr*

*Anticholinergic effects.

OPIATES

There are five opiate-related antidiarrheal agents: codeine, diphenoxylate with atropine, loperamide, paregoric, and tincture of opium. The only opiate-related antidiarrheal that is available as an OTC medication is loperamide; all others are prescription-only drugs because of the risks of respiratory depression and dependency associated with opiate use.

DIPHENOXYLATE AND ATROPINE

Diphenoxylate (Logen, Lomenate, Lofen, Lomotil) is a synthetic opiate agonist that is structurally related to meperidine (Demerol). It acts on smooth muscle of the intestinal tract, inhibiting GI motility and excessive GI propulsion. It has little or no analgesic activity. Diphenoxylate has been combined with subtherapeutic quantities of atropine to prevent deliberate overdosage. The amount of atropine present in the combination is too small to interfere with the constipating effect of diphenoxylate. However, when taken in large doses, the combination results in extreme cholinergic symptoms (e.g., dry mouth, abdominal pain, tachycardia, and blurred vision).

The combination of diphenoxylate and atropine is classified as a pregnancy category C agent. It is contraindicated in patients who have shown a hypersensitivity reaction to it and in patients suffering from di-

arrhea associated with pseudomembranous colitis or toxigenic/enterotoxin bacteria. This combination antidiarrheal is available only as oral agents in a solution or tablets. The solution form of Lomotil contains 2.5 mg/5 ml diphenoxylate and 0.025 mg/5 ml atropine; the tablets contain 2.5 mg of diphenoxylate and 0.025 mg of atropine.

PHARMACOKINETICS

HALF-LIFE	ONSET	PEAK	DURATION
2.5-4 hr*	2 hr*	2-3 hr*	4-6 hr*

*Diphenoxylate component.

⚓ LOPERAMIDE

Loperamide (Imodium, Imodium A-D) is a synthetic antidiarrheal that is similar to diphenoxylate. It inhibits both peristalsis in the intestinal wall and intestinal secretion, thereby decreasing the number of stools and the water content. Although the drug exhibits many characteristics of the opiate class, physical dependence on loperamide has not been reported. Because of its safety profile it is the only opiate antidiarrheal agent that is available as an OTC medication.

Loperamide is classified as a pregnancy category B agent and is contraindicated in patients who have shown a hypersensitivity reaction to it. It is also contraindicated in patients with severe ulcerative colitis, pseudomembranous colitis, and acute diarrhea associated with *E. coli*. Loperamide is available only in oral form as 2-mg capsules or tablets and 1-mg/5 ml solution. Commonly recommended dosages are listed in the preceding dosages table.

PHARMACOKINETICS

HALF-LIFE	ONSET	PEAK	DURATION
7-15 hr	1-3 hr	4 hr	40-50 hr

INTESTINAL FLORA MODIFIERS

Intestinal flora modifiers suppress the growth of diarrhea-causing bacteria and reestablish the normal florae that reside in the intestine. They are bacterial cultures that have been obtained from *Lactobacillus* organisms. Currently available agents are discussed below.

LACTOBACILLUS ACIDOPHILUS

Lactobacillus acidophilus (Bacid, Enterodophilus, Intestinex, Lactinex) is an acid-producing bacteria prepared in a concentrated, dried culture for oral administration. It is a normal inhabitant of the GI tract, where it creates an unfavorable environment for the overgrowth of harmful fungii and bacteria through the fermentation of carbohydrates, which produces lactic acid. *Lactobacillus acidophilus* has been used for more than 75 years in the treatment of uncomplicated diarrhea, particularly that caused by antibiotic treatment that destroys normal intestinal florae. It is available as an OTC medication in the following oral forms: a capsule (Bacid and Intestinex), an enteric-coated capsule (Enterodophilus), a 1-g powder (Lactinex granules), and tablets (Lactinex). Commonly recommended dosages are listed in the table on p. 750.

☙ PHARMACOKINETICS

HALF-LIFE	ONSET	PEAK	DURATION
Unknown	Unknown	Unknown	Unknown

LAXATIVES

Laxatives are used for the treatment of **constipation,** which is defined as a condition of abnormally infrequent and difficult passage of feces through the lower GI tract. Individuals may complain of constipation if they think they defecate too infrequently or with too much effort, if their stools are too hard or too small, if defecation is painful, or if they have a sense of incomplete evacuation. Constipation is a symptom not a disease; it is a disorder of movement through the colon and/or rectum that can be caused by a variety of diseases or drugs. Some of the more common causes of constipation are noted in the box below.

The GI tract is responsible for the digestive process that involves (1) ingestion of dietary intake, (2) digestion of dietary intake into basic nutrients, (3) absorption of basic nutrients, and (4) storage and removal of fecal material via defecation.

Ingestion→Digestion→Absorption→Storage and removal

The usual time span between ingestion and defecation is 24 to 36 hours.

The last segment of the GI tract, the large intestine, or colon, is responsible for (1) forming the stool by removing excess water from the fecal material, (2) temporarily storing the stool until defecation, and (3) extracting essential vitamins from the intestinal bacteria (especially vitamin K).

The colon is 120 to 150 cm in length and is separated from the small intestine by the ileocecal valve. The colon extends into its last segment, the rectum, which terminates at the anus. The rectum is the temporary storage site for the stool, which is composed of water and unabsorbed and indigestible material. Evacuation of the rectal contents is accomplished by bowel movements.

A bowel movement (defecation) is a reflex act that involves both smooth and skeletal muscles. The entry of feces into the rectum stimulates mass peristaltic movement that results in a bowel movement. However, voluntary initiation or inhibition of defecation is also possible via skeletal muscle pathways.

Treatment of constipation must involve an understanding of the whole patient, with special attention given to the underlying cause(s) for the constipation. Treatment should be individualized, taking into consideration the patient's age, concerns, and expectations; duration and severity of constipation; and po-

---

Causes of Constipation

CAUSES	EXAMPLES
Metabolic and endocrine disorders	Diabetes mellitus, hypothyroidism, pregnancy, hypercalcemia, hypokalemia
Neurogenic disorders	Autonomic neuropathy, intestinal pseudo-obstruction, multiple sclerosis, spinal cord lesions, Parkinson's disease, cerebrovascular accidents
Adverse drug effects	Analgesics, anticholinergics, iron supplements, aluminum antacids, calcium antacids, opiates, calcium channel blockers, Vinca alkaloids
Life-style	*Poor bowel movement habits:* Voluntary refusal to defecate resulting in constipation *Diet:* Poor fluid intake and/or low-residue (roughage) diets or excessive consumption of dairy products *Physical inactivity:* Lack of proper exercise, especially in elderly individuals *Psychologic:* Anxiety, stress, hypochondria

tential contributing factors. Treatment can be either surgical or nonsurgical; nonsurgical treatment can be separated into three broad categories of approach: dietary (e.g., fiber supplementation), behavioral (e.g., increased physical activity) and pharmacologic. Our focus is pharmacologic treatment.

Laxatives promote bowel movements by (1) affecting fecal consistency, (2) increasing fecal movement through the colon, and (3) removing stool from the rectum. Laxatives are useful in relieving constipation, in preparing for some medical procedures, and in removing unwanted substances from the body. Some of the more common indications for laxative use are listed below:

- Removal of intestinal parasites
- Inactive colon
- Reduction of ammonia absorption in hepatic encephalopathic conditions
- Treatment of drug-induced constipation
- Pregnancy and/or postobstetric period
- Poor physical activity
- Removal of toxic substances from the body
- Poor dietary habits
- Megacolon
- Preparation for colonic diagnostic procedures or surgery
- Facilitation of bowel movements with reduced pain in anorectal disorders

Of the OTC medications, laxatives are some of the most misused. Chronic and often inappropriate use of laxatives may result in laxative dependence, produce damage to the bowel, or lead to previously nonexistent problems. With the exception of the bulk-forming type, laxatives should not be used for long periods of time. All laxatives share the same general contraindications and precautions, including cautious use in the presence of acute surgical abdomen; appendicitis symptoms such as abdominal pain, nausea, and vomiting; fecal impaction (mineral oil enemas excepted); intestinal obstructions; and undiagnosed abdominal pain. They are also contraindicated in patients who have shown a hypersensitivity reaction to them.

Laxatives are divided into five major groups based on mechanism of action: bulk-forming, emollient, hyperosmotic, saline, and stimulant laxatives. Table 48-4 lists the currently available laxative agents by their respective drug family.

Mechanism of Action

All laxatives promote bowel movements but each class of laxative has a different mechanism of action. They may act by (1) affecting fecal consistency, (2) increasing fecal movement through the colon, and/or (3) removing stool from the rectum. **Bulk-forming laxatives** act in a manner similar to that of the fiber natu-

rally contained in the diet. They absorb water into the intestine, which increases bulk and distends the bowel to initiate reflex bowel activity, thus promoting a bowel movement.

Emollient laxatives are also referred to as *stool softeners* (docusate salts) and *lubricant laxatives* (mineral oil). The fecal softeners work by lowering the surface tension of GI fluids, resulting in more water and fat being absorbed into the stool and the intestines. The lubricant type of emollient laxatives work by lubricating the fecal material and the intestinal wall, preventing water from leaking out of the intestines, which softens and expands the stool.

Hyperosmotic laxatives work by increasing fecal water content, which results in distention, increased peristalsis, and evacuation. Their site of action is limited to the large intestine.

Saline laxatives increase osmotic pressure in the small intestine by inhibiting absorption and increasing water and electrolyte secretions, resulting in a watery stool; the increased distention promotes peristalsis and evacuation. Rectal enemas of sodium phosphate, a saline laxative, produce defecation 2 to 5 minutes after administration.

As the name implies, **stimulant laxatives** stimulate the nerves that innervate the intestines, resulting in increased peristalsis. They also increase fluid in the colon, which increases bulk and softens the stool. See Fig. 48-1 for a brief explanation of how and where in the intestine the various laxatives work.

Drug Effects

The drug effects of laxatives are numerous, although their action is primarily limited to the site of the intestines, and thus they have few, if any, systemic effects. Table 48-5 lists the specific drug effects of the different laxatives.

Table 48-4	Laxatives: Drug Categories and Selected Agents
CATEGORY	**LAXATIVE AGENT**
Bulk-forming	Psyllium, polycarbophil, methylcellulose
Emollient	Docusate salts, mineral oil
Hyperosmotic	Polyethylene glycol, lactulose, sorbitol, glycerine
Saline	Magnesium sulfate, magnesium phosphate, magnesium citrate
Stimulant	Castor oil, phenolphthalein, anthraquinones

Stool softener
Mechanism: Wetting agent used to soften fecal mass
Example: Docsuate
Onset of action: 1 to 3 days
Precaution Liquid dosage form may cause throat irritation; dilute in fruit juice or milk prior to administration.

Site 2 Bulk forming (high fiber)
Example: Psyllium hydrophilic
Mechanism: Absorbs water to increase bulk, distending bowel to initiate reflex bowel activity
Onset of action: 12 hours to 3 days
Precaution: Contraindicated in persons with dysphagia because esophageal obstruction may result. Avoid in dehydrated persons or individuals with limited or restricted fluid intake.

Stimulant
Example: Senna
Mechanism: Increases peristalsis via nerve stimulation in colon
Onset of action: 6 to 12 hours
Precaution: May cause discoloration of feces and urine (alkaline urine from pink, red to brown; acid urine from yellow to brown)

Site 4 Osmotic saline
Example: Magnesium citrate
Mechanism: Increases water content of feces, resulting in distention, peristalsis and evacuation. Laxation may be enhanced by release of cholecystokinin.
Onset of action: 1 to 3 hours
Precaution: Avoid use in patients who are dehydrated or whose renal function is impaired and in those with a colostomy or ileostomy. Ensure adequate fluid intake of at least 8 ounces of fluid with each dose to prevent dehydration.

Site 5 Lubricant
Example: Mineral oil
Mechanism: Coats surface of feces and colon to ease passage of stool; also softens fecal mass.
Onset of action: 6 to 8 hours
Precaution: Avoid administration within 2 hours of meals because it may reduce absorption of vitamins A, D, E, and K. Avoid use in dysphagic and bedridden persons because aspiration of mineral oil may result in lipid pneumonitis.

Site 6 Combination of stool softener and stimulant
Example: Docsuate and senna
Mechanism: Stool softener and stimulant
Onset of action: 6 to 12 hours
Precaution: As noted for individual laxatives

▼ **FIG. 48-1** Site and mechanism of action of laxatives within the intestines.

Therapeutic Uses

There are various therapeutic uses for the laxatives, ranging from common constipation to bowel preparation prior to surgery. The therapeutic effects vary by category. See Table 48-6 for specific therapeutic indications for each laxative drug class.

Side Effects and Adverse Effects

As is true for the drug and therapeutic effects of laxatives, the side effects and adverse effects of the various agents are specific to the laxative group. Most of the side effects from laxatives are confined to the site of the intestines; however, the overuse and misuse of laxatives lead to many unwanted effects that are not expected or designed to occur with appropriate use. The major side effects and adverse effects of the laxative agents are listed in Table 48-7.

Interactions

Many drugs are absorbed in some part of the intestine. Since laxatives alter intestinal function, they can interact with other drugs quite readily. Table

Table 48-5 | Laxatives: Drug Effects

DRUG EFFECT	BULK	EMOLLIENT	HYPEROSMOTIC	SALINE	STIMULANT
Increases peristalsis	Y	Y	Y	Y	Y
Causes increased secretion of water and electrolytes in small bowel	Y	Y	N	Y	Y
Inhibits absorption in small bowel	Y	Y	N	Y	Y
Increases wall permeability in small bowel	N	Y	N	N	Y
Causes wall damage in small bowel	N	Y	N	N	Y
Acts only in large bowel	N	N	Y	N	N
Increases fecal mass water	Y	Y	Y	Y	Y
Softens fecal mass	Y	Y	Y	Y	Y

Y, yes; N, no

Table 48-6 | Laxatives: Therapeutic Effects

LAXATIVE GROUP	THERAPEUTIC EFFECT
Bulk-forming	Acute constipation, irritable bowel syndrome, diverticulosis
Emollient	Acute constipation, softens fecal impacts, facilitates bowel movements in anorectal conditions
Hyperosmotic	Chronic constipation, diagnostic and surgical preparations
Saline	Constipation, removal of anthelmintics and parasites, diagnostic and surgical preparations
Stimulant	Acute constipation, diagnostic and surgical bowel preparations

Table 48-7 | Laxatives: Adverse Effects

LAXATIVE GROUP	SIDE/ADVERSE EFFECT
Bulk-forming	Impaction above strictures, fluid overload
Emollient	Skin rashes, decreased absorption of vitamins, lipid pneumonia
Hyperosmotic	Abdominal bloating, rectal irritation
Saline	Magnesium toxicity (with renal insufficiency)
Stimulant	Nutrient malabsorption, skin rashes, gastric irritation, rectal stimulation

48-8 lists the common interactions of each laxative group.

Dosages

For the recommended dosages of selected laxatives see the dosages table on p. 757.

*D*RUG PROFILES

As mentioned earlier, laxatives are used for the treatment of constipation; such treatment must involve an understanding of the whole patient. Of the five major groups of laxatives many are available as OTC medications, whereas others require a prescription for use. The following are prototypical agents from each of the laxative groups.

BULK-FORMING LAXATIVES

Bulk-forming laxatives are composed of water-retaining (hydrophilic) natural and synthetic cellulose derivatives. Psyllium is an example of a natural bulk-forming laxative, while methylcellulose is an example of a synthetic cellulose derivative. Other bulk-forming laxatives are malt-soup–extract preparations and polycarbophil preparations. The bulk-forming agents increase water absorption, resulting in greater total volume (bulk) of the intestinal contents. Unlike some of the other laxatives, bulk-forming laxatives tend to produce normal, formed stools. Their site of action is limited to the GI tract so there are few, if any, systemic effects. However, they should be taken with liberal amounts

Table 48-8	Laxatives: Drug Interactions	
LAXATIVE GROUP	**INTERACTING DRUG**	**RESULT**
Bulk-forming	Antibiotics, digoxin, nitrofurantoin, salicylates, tetracyclines, oral anticoagulants	Increased absorption
Emollient (mineral oil)	Oral anticoagulants	Increased effect of anticoagulant
	Fat-soluble vitamins (A,D,E, and K)	Decreased absorption
Hyperosmotic	Oral antibiotics	Decreased effects of lactulose
Saline	Barbiturates, general anesthetics, narcotics, antipsychotics	Increased CNS depression
	Neuromuscular blockers	Increased effects
Stimulant	Antacids, H₂ blockers*	Gastric irritation
	Antibiotics, digoxin, nitrofurantoin, salicylates, tetracyclines, oral anticoagulants†	Decreased absorption

*With bisacodyl.
†With cascara.

of water to prevent esophageal obstruction and/or fecal impaction. These laxatives are OTC medications and are classified as pregnancy category C agents. The bulk-forming laxatives are among the safest available and the only ones that are recommended for long-term use.

METHYLCELLULOSE

Methylcellulose (Citrucel) is a synthetic bulk-forming laxative that attracts water into the intestine and absorbs excess water into the stool, stimulating the intestines and increasing peristalsis. It is contraindicated in patients who have shown a hypersensitivity reaction to it and in those with GI obstruction or hepatitis. Methylcellulose is an oral agent available as 105-mg and 364-mg powders and 500-mg tablets. Commonly recommended dosages are listed in the following dosages table.

PHARMACOKINETICS

HALF-LIFE	ONSET	PEAK	DURATION
Unknown	Unknown	Unknown	Unknown

PSYLLIUM

Psyllium (Metamucil, Fiberall, Peridem) is a natural bulk-forming laxative obtained from the dried seed of the *Plantago psyllium* plant. It has many of the characteristics of methylcellulose. Psyllium is contraindicated in patients who have shown a hypersensitivity reaction to it and in those with intestinal obstruction or fecal impaction. Its use is also contraindicated in patients experiencing abdominal pain and/or nausea and vomiting. Psyllium is available as 1.7-g and 3.4-g chewable tablets and as a variety of powdered prod-

ucts with strengths ranging from 309 mg to 1000 mg. There is also a psyllium combination product combining 542 mg of psyllium and 123 mg of senna. Commonly recommended dosages are listed in the following dosages table.

PHARMACOKINETICS

HALF-LIFE	ONSET	PEAK	DURATION
Unknown	Unknown	Unknown	Unknown

EMOLLIENT LAXATIVES

Emollient laxatives either directly lubricate the stool and the intestines, as with mineral oil, or they act as fecal softeners. By lubricating the fecal material and the intestinal walls, lubricant emollient laxatives prevent water from leaking out of the intestines, which softens and expands the stool. The stool softeners (docusate salts) work by lowering the surface tension of fluids, allowing more water and fat to be absorbed into the stool and the intestines.

MINERAL OIL

Mineral oil (Agoral Plain, Fleet Mineral Oil Enema, Kondremul, Zymenol) eases passage of stool by preventing water from escaping the stool and lubricating the intestines. Mineral oil is the only lubricant laxative in the emollient category; it is a mixture of liquid hydrocarbons derived from petroleum. It is most commonly used to treat constipation associated with hard stools or fecal impaction.

Mineral oil is classified as a pregnancy category C agent and is contraindicated in patients who have shown a hypersensitivity reaction to it. Its use is also contraindicated in patients with intestinal obstruction,

D O S A G E S

SELECTED LAXATIVE AGENTS

AGENT	PHARMACOLOGIC CLASS	DOSAGE RANGE	PURPOSE
⚓Methylcellulose (Citrucel)	Bulk-forming laxative	*Adult/Pediatric >12 y/o* PO: 1 Tbs in 8 oz of water 1-3 times/day *Pediatric 6 to ≤12 y/o* PO: ½ adult dose in 4 oz of water	Constipation
Psyllium (Metamucil, Fiberall)	Bulk-forming laxative	*Adult/Pediatric ≥12 y/o* PO: 1-2 tsp in 8 oz of water 1-4 times/day *Pediatric 6 to ≤12 y/o* PO: ½ the adult dose in 4 oz of water at bedtime	Constipation
Mineral oil (Agoral Plain, Mineral Oil Enema, Kondremul, Zymenol)	Emollient laxative	*Adult/Pediatric ≤12 y/o* PO: 15-45 ml as a single daily dose *Pediatric 6-11 y/o* PO: 5-15 ml/day *Adult/Pediatric ≥12 y/o* PO: 60-150 ml as a single daily dose *Pediatric 2-11 y/o* PO: 30-60 ml/day	Constipation / Enema
Glycerin (Fleet Babylax, Glycerin, Sani-Supp)	Hyperosmotic laxative	*Rectal:* Insert one adult, child, or infant suppository into the rectum	Constipation
Magnesium salts	Saline laxative	*Citrate—Adult/Pediatric ≥12 y/o* PO: 11-25 g/day 6-11 y/o: 5.5-12.5 g/day 2-5 y/o: 2.7-6.25 g/day *Sulfate—Adult/Pediatric* PO: ≥12 y/o: 10-30 g/day 6-11 y/o: 5-10 g/day 2-5 y/o: 2.5-5 g/day	Constipation
Phenolphthalein (White: Alophen, Medilax; Yellow: Evac-U-Lax, Ex-Lax)	Stimulant/ irritant laxative	*Adult/Pediatric* PO: ≥12 y/o: 30-270 mg/day PO: 6-11 y/o: 30-60 mg/day PO: 2-5 y/o: 15-30 mg/day	Constipation
⚓Docusate (Calcium, potassium, and sodium salts)	Fecal softener	*Adult/Pediatric >12 y/o* PO: 50-360 mg/day *Pediatric 2-12 y/o* PO: 50-150 mg/day *Pediatric <2 y/o* PO: 25 mg/day	Stool softener
Polyethylene glycol (CoLyte, GoLytely, OCL)	Bowel evacuant	*Adult* PO: 4 L daily administered in 240-ml doses q10min	Bowel cleansing before examination
Lactulose (Chronulac, Constilac, Duphalac)	Disaccharid laxative	*Adult* PO: 15-30 ml/day	Constipation

abdominal pain, and nausea and vomiting. Mineral oil agents are available as enemas or as 1.4-, 2.75-, and 4.75-mg/5 ml oral suspensions. There are also many combination products that contain mineral oil such as Haley's M-O, which is a mixture of 1 mg/5 ml of mineral oil and 4 mg/5 ml of milk of magnesia. Commonly recommended dosages are listed in the preceding dosages table.

✯ PHARMACOKINETICS

HALF-LIFE	ONSET	PEAK	DURATION
Unknown	6-8 hr	Unknown	Unknown

⚓ DOCUSATE SALTS

Docusate salts (calcium, potassium, and sodium) are fecal softening emollient laxatives that facilitate the passage of water and lipids (fats) into the fecal mass, softening the stool. The currently available agents in each salt form are listed below:

Calcium salt (docusate calcium)
■ Pro-Cal-Sof capsules
■ Surfak capsules
Potassium salt (docusate potassium)
■ Diocto-K capsules
■ Kasof capsules
Sodium salt (docusate sodium)
■ Colace capsules, liquid, syrup
■ Dialose capsules, tablets
■ D.S.S. capsules
■ Modane Soft capsules
■ Regutol tablets

These agents are used to treat constipation, soften fecal impacts, and to facilitate easy bowel movements in patients with hemorrhoids and other painful anorectal conditions. In addition to the above-mentioned docusate-salt formulations, there are also combination products available. Docusate is classified as a pregnancy category C agent and is contraindicated in patients who have shown a hypersensitivity reaction to it and in those with intestinal obstruction, fecal impaction, and nausea and vomiting. Commonly recommended dosages are listed in the preceding dosages table.

✯ PHARMACOKINETICS

HALF-LIFE	ONSET	PEAK	DURATION
Unknown	1-3 days	Unknown	1-3 days

HYPEROSMOTIC LAXATIVES

The hyperosmotic laxatives, polyethylene glycol (PEG), lactulose sorbitol, and glycerine, relieve constipation by increasing the water content of feces, resulting in distention, peristalsis, and evacuation. They are most commonly used to treat constipation and to evacuate the bowels before diagnostic and surgical procedures.

POLYETHYLENE GLYCOL

Polyethylene glycol (CoLyte, GoLytely, OCL) is most commonly used before diagnostic or surgical bowel procedures because it is a very potent laxative that induces total cleansing of the bowel. Polyethylene glycol is contraindicated in patients with gastrointestinal obstruction, gastric retention, bowel perforation, toxic colitis, toxic megalocolon, or ileus. It is classified as a pregnancy category C agent. The particular PEG that is used in the products mentioned is PEG-3350; its composition is as follows (in grams per liter):

PEG 3350 60
Sodium chloride 1.46
Potassium chloride 0.745
Sodium bicarbonate 1.68
Sodium sulfate 5.68

An oral solution of PEG-3350 and electrolytes is available for gastrointestinal lavage. Diarrhea usually occurs within 30 to 60 minutes following ingestion; complete evacuation and cleansing of the bowel is accomplished within 4 hours. Commonly recommended dosages are listed in the preceding dosages table.

✯ PHARMACOKINETICS

HALF-LIFE	ONSET	PEAK	DURATION
Unknown	1 hr	2-4 hr	4 hr

LACTULOSE

Lactulose (Chronulac, Duphalac, Enulose) is a disaccharide sugar containing one molecule of galactose and one molecule of fructose (two types of sugar molecules). It is a synthetic derivative of the natural sugar lactose, which is not digested in the stomach or absorbed in the small bowel. Instead it is passed unchanged into the large intestine where it is metabolized. This process produces lactic acid, formic acid, and acetic acid, creating a hyperosmotic environment that draws water into the colon and produces a laxative effect. This drug-induced acidic environment also reduces blood ammonia levels by forcing ammonia from the blood into the colon. This has proved helpful in treating patients with systemic encephalopathy.

Lactulose is classified as a pregnancy category C agent and is contraindicated in patients who have shown a hypersensitivity reaction to it and in patients on a low galactose diet. It is available as either a 3.33-g/5 ml oral or rectal solution. Commonly recommended dosages are listed in the preceding dosages table.

✸ PHARMACOKINETICS

HALF-LIFE	ONSET	PEAK	DURATION
Unknown	24 hr	24-48 hr	Variable

GLYCERIN

Glycerin (Fleet Babylax, Glycerin, Sani-Supp) promotes bowel movements by increasing osmotic pressure in the intestine, which draws fluid into the colon. Because it is a very mild laxative, it is often used in children. Sorbitol, another hyperosmotic laxative, has similar properties. Glycerin is classified as a pregnancy category C agent and is contraindicated in patients who have shown a hypersensitivity reaction to it. It is available as a 4 ml per applicator rectal solution and as a suppository. Commonly recommended dosages are listed in the dosages table on p. 757.

✸ PHARMACOKINETICS

HALF-LIFE	ONSET	PEAK	DURATION
30-45 min	16-36 min	1 hr	2-4 hr

SALINE LAXATIVES

The saline laxatives consist of various magnesium and sodium salts. They increase osmotic pressure and draw water into the colon, producing a watery stool usually within 3 to 6 hours of ingestion. The currently available magnesium and sodium salt agents are listed below:

MAGNESIUM LAXATIVES
Sulfate
- Epsom salt

Hydroxide
- Milk of magnesia
- Phillips' Milk of Magnesia
- Haley's M-O

Citrate
- Evac-Q-Mag

SODIUM LAXATIVES
Phosphate
- Fleet Phospho-Soda
- Fleet Enema

MAGNESIUM SALTS

Magnesium saline laxatives magnesium citrate, milk of magnesia, and Epsom salts are commonly used, unpleasant tasting OTC laxative preparations. They should be used with caution or not at all in patients with renal insufficiency because they can be absorbed into the systemic circulation, causing hypermagnesemia. They are most commonly used for rapid evacuation of the bowel in preparation for endoscopic examination and to help remove unabsorbed poisons from the GI tract.

They are classified as pregnancy category B agents and are contraindicated in patients who have shown a hypersensitivity reaction to them. Their use is also contraindicated in patients with renal diseases, abdominal pain, nausea and vomiting, obstruction, acute surgical abdomen, and rectal bleeding. Magnesium hydroxide is available as a 77.5-mg/g suspension, a concentrated milk of magnesia preparation, and 300- and 500-mg tablets. It is also used in a variety of combination products such as Haley's M-O. Other magnesium products are listed in the discussion of saline laxatives. Commonly recommended dosages are listed in the dosages table on p. 757.

✸ PHARMACOKINETICS

HALF-LIFE	ONSET	PEAK	DURATION
Unknown	0.5-3 hr	3 hr	Variable

STIMULANT LAXATIVES

Stimulant laxatives, consisting of natural plant products and synthetic chemical agents, induce intestinal peristalsis. Plant-derived stimulant laxatives include bisacodyl, disacodyl tannex, and phenolphthalein (white and yellow). The anthraquinones make up another subgroup of the stimulant laxatives, including agents such as cascara sagrada, senna, aloe (casanthrol), and danthron. Their site of action includes the entire GI tract. The action of the stimulant laxatives is proportional to the dose. They are the most likely of all the laxative classes to cause dependence.

PHENOLPHTHALEIN

Phenolphthalein (White: Alophen, Medilax, Modane, Feen-A-Mint; Yellow: Feen-A-Mint, Evac-U-Lax, Ex-Lax, Lax-Pills) and bisacodyl both stimulate the intestinal nervous system to increase peristalsis. Over extended periods of time this can damage the intestines. Both of these natural stimulants are in many OTC laxative products either as a single active ingredient or as part of a combination product. They come in a variety of strengths and formulations, including liquid-filled and regular capsules; enteric-coated, chewable, and regular tablets; and chewing gum. As rectally administered agents they are available as suppositories, suspensions, and as kits to be used before a diagnostic or surgical bowel procedure. Phenolphthalein is contraindicated in patients who have shown a hypersensitivity reaction to it and in patients with GI obstruction, abdominal pain, nausea and vomiting, and fecal impaction. In addition to the contraindications of phenolphthalein, bisacodyl is contraindicated in patients with rectal fissures, appendicitis, acute surgical abdomen, ulcerated hemorrhoids, acute hepatitis, and intestinal or biliary tract obstruction. Commonly recommended dosages are listed in the dosages table on p. 757.

PHARMACOKINETICS

HALF-LIFE	ONSET	PEAK	DURATION
Unknown	6-8 hr	8 hr	Variable

NURSING PROCESS

ASSESSMENT

Before administering antidiarrheal preparations, the nurse should obtain and document a thorough history of bowel patterns, general state of health, and recent history of illness or dietary changes. The adsorbent, bismuth subsalicylate, should not be given to children under 16 years of age because of the risk of Reye's syndrome or to patients who are allergic to either of the chemical ingredients (bismuth or salicylates). Caution and careful monitoring are required with the use of adsorbents in patients who are elderly or who have a history of decreased bleeding time, clotting disorders, recent bowel surgery, or confusion.

Anticholinergics should not be administered to a patient who has a history of allergy to such medications or to patients with glaucoma, benign prostatic hypertrophy, urinary retention, recent bladder surgery, or cardiac history. Other contraindications to use include myasthenia gravis, paralytic ileus, and toxic megacolon. Cautious use is recommended in patients with a history of confusion, dizziness, hypotension, hypertension, bradycardia, tachycardia, or blurred vision.

PEDIATRIC IMPLICATIONS
Antidiarrheal Preparations

- Always check with the physician or pediatrician before administering antidiarrheal preparations to a child at home and report the symptoms in case further assessment or medical management is needed.

- Dehydration and electrolyte loss occur very rapidly in the pediatric patient.

- Always contact the physician for proper dosage of antidiarrheals for any child under 6 years of age or if you have any doubt regarding the amount to administer. Dosages are usually calculated by body weight, and the guidelines or directions provided for most OTC medications are for averaged-sized children over 12 years of age. *Never hesitate* to contact the physician with any concern or question regarding a pediatric patient.

- Abdominal distention, firm abdomen, painful abdomen, and worsening or no improvement in the diarrhea 24 to 48 hours after medication administration should be reported to the physician immediately. Measuring amounts of diarrhea by the number of diapers or number of stools per day provides important information.

- BLOODY diarrhea or a sluggish, lethargic or confused patient should always be reported immediately to a physician.

Patient Teaching TIPS

Laxatives, Cathartics, and Antidiarrheals

✔ Patients should swallow all laxative tablets whole with at least 120 cc (6 oz) of water. Make sure patients do not crush or chew tablets, especially if they are enteric coated.

✔ If taking a bulk-forming laxative such as psyllium or methylcellulose (Metamucil), patients should be sure to take it as directed by the manufacturer with at least 120 cc (6 oz) of water.

✔ Long-term use of laxatives or cathartics often results in decreased bowel tone and may lead to dependency.

✔ Patients should be honest with their physician, nurse, or any other health care provider regarding their dietary habits, fiber and fluid intake, and elimination patterns. A normal bowel pattern does not necessarily mean a bowel movement everyday.

✔ Patients should not take a laxative or cathartic if they are experiencing nausea, vomiting, and/or abdominal pain.

✔ Patients should contact their physician if they experience severe abdominal pain, muscle weakness, cramps, and/or dizziness, which may indicate possible fluid or electrolyte loss.

✔ Patients should take antidiarrheals exactly as prescribed. Stool frequency, consistency, and amount should be recorded for comparison and evaluation.

Codeine preparations should not be given to patients with an allergy to the drug or to those who are in respiratory distress or who have possible head injury. Cautious use is recommended in patients who are hypotensive or in those who are experiencing bradycardia, palpitations, or urinary retention. See Table 48-3 for drug interactions with other antidiarrheal agents.

Bulk-forming laxatives, such as psyllium preparations, are often used to treat chronic constipation and have few side effects. A thorough history of presenting symptoms and elimination patterns must be completed and documented before administering the medication to ensure patient safety. In addition, the patient's intake and output ratio and electrolytes should be assessed and documented before initiating therapy to establish baseline values for later comparison.

NURSING DIAGNOSES

Nursing diagnoses associated with the use of antidiarrheals, laxatives, and cathartics include, but are not limited to:

- Altered bowel patterns related to GI disorder.
- Risk for fluid and electrolyte disturbance due to excessive loss of water and electrolytes through stool.
- Risk for self-injury as related to weakness and dizziness from possible excessive loss of fluid and electrolytes through stool.

TAKE HOME POINTS

Diarrhea
- Leading cause of morbidity and mortality in third world countries.
- Five to 8 million deaths per year in infants and children.
- Loss of time and productivity at work has an enormous financial impact with an estimated cost of $23 billion per year or $108 per person per year in the United States.
- Acute and chronic types.

Drug Therapy
- Adsorbents, anticholinergics, opiates, and intestinal flora modifiers.
- Most acute diarrhea is self-limiting, subsiding in 3 days to 2 weeks.
- Fluid and electrolyte replacement is vital.
- Encourage patients to check and recheck dosage instructions before taking medication and note any drug-food interactions.

Anticholinergics
- Decrease muscle tone of GI tract and decrease peristalsis.
- Can cause urinary retention, headache, confusion, dry skin, rash, and blurred vision.
- Belladonna alkaloids (Donnatal) are common anticholinergic antidiarrheals.

Adsorbents
- Coat walls of GI tract, absorbing bacteria or toxins causing diarrhea, and eliminating them with stool.
- May increase bleeding, cause constipation, dark stools, and black tongue.
- Bismuth subsalicylate and attapulgite (Kaopectate) are common adsorbents.

Intestinal Flora Modifiers
- Bacterial cultures of *Lactobacillus*.
- Supply normal intestinal florae destroyed by infection or antibiotics.
- Suppress the growth of diarrhea-causing bacteria.

Opiates
- Decrease bowel motility and thus permit longer contact of intestinal contents with absorptive surface of the bowel.
- Reduce pain associated with rectal spasms.

Laxatives
- Laxatives and cathartics may cause side effects that precipitate problems in volume.
- Patients must be made aware of abuse potential and the problems associated with the misuse of laxatives.
- Encourage patient to keep a log of daily elimination patterns and any problems related to laxative use.

Nursing Considerations
- Keep these medications, as well as all other medications, out of the reach of children.
- Report abdominal distention, firm abdomen, pain and worsening (or no improvement) of diarrhea, and GI-related signs and symptoms to the physician immediately.
- Long-term use may lead to laxative dependence.

- Knowledge deficit related to possible chronic laxative abuse, side effects of laxatives and cathartics, and nonpharmacologic measures to relieve constipation.

PLANNING

Goals related to the administration of antidiarrheals, laxatives, and cathartics include:

- Patient remains free of fluid and electrolyte disturbances related to changes in bowel patterns.
- Patients is free from self-injury related to possible weakness and dizziness or from side effects of either groups of medications.
- Patient remains compliant to medication and nonpharmacologic measures.

Outcome Criteria

Outcome criteria for the patient receiving antidiarrheals, laxatives, and cathartics include, but are not limited to:

- Patient reports the signs and symptoms of fluid and electrolyte loss such as weakness, lethargy, decreased urinary output, and dizziness.
- Patient states measures to avoid side effects and injuries related to change in bowel patterns, changes in fluid and electrolyte status, or treatment such as changing positions slowly.
- Patient states methods of administration that enhance effective and safe use of antidiarrheals, laxatives, or cathartics such as taking as prescribed.
- Patient states nonpharmacologic measures to relieve constipation, flatus, and diarrhea such as forcing fluids, increasing fiber or bulk, or withdrawing irritating food sources from diet.

IMPLEMENTATION

Antidiarrheals should be taken exactly as prescribed, with strict adherence to the recommended dosage. Make sure that patients are aware of their fluid intake and any dietary changes. Patients should also be aware of the precipitating factors of the diarrhea and, if symptoms persist, they should know to contact a physician immediately. Documentation of bowel pattern changes, weight, fluid volume status, intake and output, and mucosa membrane status should be done before, during, and after the initiation of treatment.

Bulk-forming laxatives, such as psyllium and methylcellulose, must be administered as specified by package inserts, which is usually in the morning and evening. They should be given alone (i.e., not with food) and mixed with at least 120 cc of fluid and drunk immediately to prevent possible obstruction. Instructions for administering mineral oil agents are similar to those for other laxatives with the additional concern of preventing aspiration in the elderly patient. Bisacodyl and cascara sagrada should be given with water only because of interactions with milk, antacids, and cimetidine. Patient education is important to compliance and safe, effective use of laxatives or cathartics. See p. 760 for the patient teaching tips.

EVALUATION

Therapeutic response to the antidiarrheals, laxatives, and cathartics includes an improvement in the GI-related signs and symptoms reported by the patient as well as improvement in bowel sounds and no abnormal findings from an assessment of the abdomen and bowel patterns. Side effects to monitor in patients vary according to drug classification group. See the patient teaching tips on p. 760.

Critical Thinking A C T I V I T I E S

1. Side effects associated with loperamide (Imodium) include which of the following:
    a. CNS overstimulation
    b. Excessive salivation
    c. Epigastric pain
    d. Dysphagia

2. What is the bacterial organism that is replaced by intestinal flora modifiers?
    a. *Pseudomonas* b. *Streptococcus* c. *Haemophilus* d. *Lactobacillus*

3. What nonpharmacologic measures are recommended for the patient recovering from diarrhea secondary to a GI viral infection?
a. Intake of citrus juices
b. Increased exercise
c. Diluted gelatin
d. High-bulk diet

4. The long-term use of what main type of laxative group may result in harmful effects such as atrophied intestines?
    a. Bulk-forming b. Emollient c. Stimulant d. Hyperosmotic

▲▲

BIBLIOGRAPHY

Albanese J, Nutz P: *Mosby's 1995 nursing drug cards,* St Louis, 1995, Mosby.

Cooke DM: Inflammatory bowel disease: primary health care management of ulcerative colitis and Crohn's disease, *Nurse Pract* 16(8):27, 1991.

Goldfinger SE: Constipation: the hard facts, *Harv Health Lett* 16(4):1, 1991.

Johnson KB: *Harriet Lane handbook,* ed 13, St Louis, 1993, Mosby.

Keen JH: *Critical care and emergency drug reference,* St Louis, 1994, Mosby.

Knoben JE, Anderson PO: *Handbook of critical drug data,* ed 6, Hamilton, Ill, 1988, Drug Intelligence Publications.

McEvoy GK: *AHFS drug information,* Bethesda, Md, 1994, American Society of Hospital Pharmacists.

Skidmore-Roth L: *Mosby's 1995 nursing drug reference,* St Louis, 1995, Mosby.

Chapter 49

Antiemetic (Antinausea) Agents

Objectives

When you reach the end of this chapter, you will be able to:

1 Discuss the pathophysiology of nausea and vomiting.

2 Identify the neurotransmitters involved in the causation of nausea and vomiting.

3 Identify the common antiemetic drug categories and antiemetic agents in each.

4 Identify the indications for the various types of antiemetic agents and the respective mechanisms of action of the different groups of agents.

5 Discuss the contraindications to the use of the various antiemetic agents, the cautions to be observed in patients receiving them, and the drug interactions that involve these agents.

6 Develop a comprehensive nursing care plan, using the nursing process, related to the administration of antiemetic agents.

7 Cite the education guidelines for patients receiving antiemetics.

CHAPTER OUTLINE

Nausea and Vomiting
Antiemetic Agents
  Mechanism of action
  Drug effects
  Therapeutic uses
  Side effects and adverse effects
  Interactions
  Dosages
Drug Profiles
Anticholinergics
  ⬇ Scopolamine
Antihistamines
  Meclizine
Neuroleptic Agents
  ⬇ Prochlorperazine
Prokinetic Agents
  ⬇ Metoclopramide
Serotonin Blockers
Tetracannabinoids
  Dronabinol

Nursing Process
Assessment
Nursing Diagnoses
Planning
  Outcome criteria
Implementation
Evaluation

Glossary

Anticholinergic (an′ tĭ ko′ lin ər′ jik) Drug given to treat motion sickness. (p. 766)

Antiemetic (an′ te ə met′ ik) Drug given to relieve nausea and vomiting. (p. 765)

Antihistamine (an′ tĭ his′ tə mēn) Agent that works by inhibiting vestibular stimulation. (p. 766)

Chemoreceptor trigger zone (CTZ) The area in the brain that is involved with the sensation of nausea and vomiting. (p. 765)

Emesis (em′ ə sis) The forcible emptying or expulsion of gastric and, occasionally, intestinal contents through the mouth, also called *vomiting*. (p. 765)

Nausea Sensation often leading to the urge to vomit. (p. 765)

Neuroleptic agent (nur′ o lep′ tik) Drug that prevents nausea and vomiting by blocking dopamine receptors on the chemoreceptor trigger zone. (p. 766)

Prokinetic agent (pro kĭ net′ ik) Drug that prevents nausea and vomiting by blocking dopamine in the chemoreceptor trigger zone, making the zone less sensitive to impulses sent to it from the gastrointestinal tract. (p. 767)

Serotonin blocker (ser′ o to′ nin) Agent that prevents vomiting and nausea by blocking serotonin receptors located in the gastrointestinal tract, the chemoreceptor trigger zone, and the vomiting center. (p. 767)

Tetrahydrocannabinoid (tet′ rə hi′ dro kə nab′ i noid) The major psychoactive substance in marijuana. Nonintoxicating doses have been used experimentally to treat glaucoma and to relieve nausea and increase the appetite in patients receiving cancer chemotherapy. (p. 767)

Vomiting The forcible emptying or expulsion of gastric and, occasionally, intestinal contents through the mouth; also called *emesis.* (p. 765)

Vomiting center (VC) The area in the brain that is involved in stimulating the physioloigc events that lead to nausea and vomiting. (p. 765)

NAUSEA AND VOMITING

Nausea and vomiting are two gastrointestinal disorders that can be not only extremely unpleasant but also lead to other, more serious complications if not treated promptly. **Nausea** is an unpleasant feeling that often precedes vomiting. If it does not subside spontaneously or is not relieved by medication, it can lead to vomiting. **Vomiting,** which is also called **emesis,** is the forcible emptying or expulsion of gastric and, occasionally, intestinal contents through the mouth. There is a variety of stimuli that can induce nausea and vomiting, and these are foul odors or tastes, irritation of the stomach or intestines, and certain drugs (ipecac or antineoplastic agents).

Much research into the nature of nausea and vomiting has been done over the past decade, with the result that the physiology of these phenomena is now better understood. This improved understanding has included the concept of a **vomiting center (VC)** in the brain that is responsible for initiating the necessary physiologic events that lead to nausea and eventually vomiting. There are in turn several pathways that transmit stimuli to the VC and the **chemoreceptor trigger zone (CTZ),** another area in the brain involved in the causation of nausea and vomiting. These pathways communicate with the CTZ and VC by means of neurotransmitters, and thereby alert these areas of the brain to the existence of nauseating substances (nauseous stimuli) that need to be expelled from the body.

Once the VC and CTZ are stimulated, they initiate the events that stimulate the vomiting reflex. The neurotransmitters involved in this process and their respective receptors are listed in Table 49-1. The various pathways and the areas of the body that send the signals to the VC via these pathways are illustrated in Fig. 49-1.

ANTIEMETIC AGENTS

The drugs that are used to relieve nausea and vomiting are called **antiemetic agents,** and the discovery of new agents coupled with a better understanding of the way in which the older drugs work has had a dramatic impact on the way in which nausea and vomiting are now treated. All of these agents work at some site in the vomiting pathway, and there are six categories of such agents. By combining agents from these various categories, the antiemetic effectiveness of the resulting

Table 49-1	Neurotransmitters Involved in Nausea and Vomiting
NEUROTRANSMITTER	**SITE IN THE VOMITING PATHWAY**
Dopamine (D₂)	GI tract and CTZ
Histamine (H₁)	Vestibular, vomiting center, and labyrinth pathways
Prostaglandins (PG)	GI tract
Serotonin (5 HT₃)	GI tract, CTZ, and vomiting center
Acetylcholine (ACh)	Vestibular, vomiting center, and labyrinth pathways

GI, gastrointestinal; *CTZ,* chemoreceptor trigger zone.

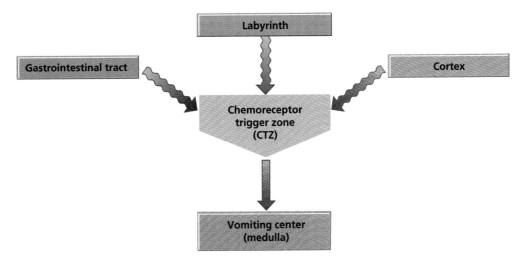

▼ **FIG. 49-1** The various pathways and areas in the body sending signals to the vomiting center.

agent is increased because it can then block more than just one of the pathways in the overall vomiting pathway. Some of the more commonly used antiemetics in the different categories are listed in Table 49-2, and the sites where they work in the vomiting pathway are shown in Fig. 49-2.

Mechanism of Action

The numerous drugs used to prevent or treat nausea and vomiting have many different mechanisms of action. Most work by blocking one of the pathways in the vomiting pathway, as shown in Fig. 49-2, and in doing so block the stimulus that induces vomiting. The mechanisms of action of the drugs in the six antiemetic drug categories are summarized in Table 49-3.

The **anticholinergics** act by binding to and blocking acetylcholine (ACh) receptors on the vestibular nuclei, which are located in the labyrinth. By preventing ACh from binding to these receptors, nauseous stimuli originating from this area cannot be transmitted to the CTZ. Anticholinergics also block receptors located in the reticular formation and by doing so prevent ACh from binding to these receptors so that nauseous stimuli originating from this area cannot be transmitted to the VC.

Antihistamines (H₁ receptor blockers) act by inhibiting vestibular stimulation in a manner that is very similar to the way in which anticholinergics work. They inhibit ACh by binding to histamine₁ receptors,

which thereby prevent cholinergic stimulation in both the vestibular and reticular systems. Nausea and vomiting occur when these areas of the brain are stimulated.

Neuroleptic agents prevent nausea and vomiting by blocking dopamine receptors on the CTZ. Many of the neuroleptics also have anticholinergic actions similar to those of the anticholinergics.

Table 49-2	Antiemetics: Common Drug Categories
ANTIEMETIC CATEGORY	**ANTIEMETIC AGENTS**
Anticholinergic (acetylcholine)	⚓Scopolamine
Antihistamine (H₁ receptor blockers)	Promethazine, meclizine, dimenhydrinate, diphenhydramine
Neuroleptic agents	Chlorpromazine, perphenazine, ⚓prochlorperazine, promethazine, thiethylperazine, triflupromazine, trimeprazine
Prokinetic agents	⚓Metoclopramide, cisapride
Serotonin blockers	Granisetron, ondansetron
Tetracannabinoids	Dronabinol

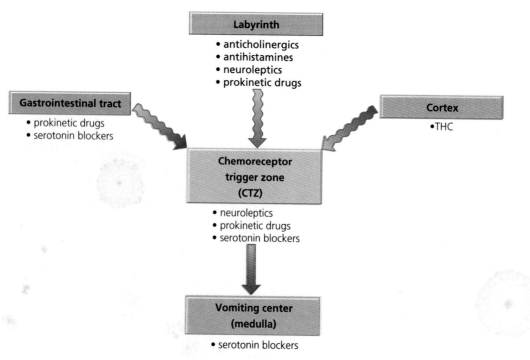

▼ FIG. 49-2 Sites of action of selected antiemetics.

Prokinetic agents, in particular metoclopramide, act by blocking dopamine in the CTZ, which causes it to be desensitized to the impulses it receives from the gastrointestinal (GI) tract. In particular, the VC and the lateral reticular formation are prevented from receiving nauseous stimuli originating from the GI tract. Cisapride is also classified as a prokinetic drug because it hastens the GI transit time, which is the rate at which food moves through the tract. Cisapride accomplishes this by stimulating cholinergic pathways (i.e., by stimulating ACh receptors), which has the effect of increasing muscle tone and contractility. The resulting enhanced gastric emptying is believed to minimize the gastric stasis that usually precedes vomiting. It is in this way that cisapride has some antiemetic properties.

Serotonin blockers work by blocking serotonin receptors located in the GI tract, the CTZ, and VC. There are many subtypes of serotonin receptors, and these various receptors are located throughout the body—in the central nervous system, smooth muscles, platelets, and GI tract. The subtype of receptor involved in the mediation of nausea and vomiting is the 5-HT$_3$ receptor, and these receptors are the site of action for the serotonin blockers such as ondansetron and granisetron.

Tetrahydrocannabinoid (THC) is the major psychoactive substance in marijuana, and in the form of the drug dronabinol (Marinol), it is occasionally used as an antiemetic because of its inhibitory effects on the reticular formation, thalamus, and cerebral cortex. These effects cause an alteration in mood and the body's perception of its surroundings, which may be beneficial in relieving nausea and vomiting. Although this particular category of antiemetics is used very rarely, there are occasionally unusual cases of nausea and vomiting that respond well to the THCs.

Drug Effects

The drug effects of the antiemetic agents are related to their mechanisms of action. As already explained, these agents act by blocking receptors that, when occupied by neurotransmitters, stimulate various vomiting pathways. These receptors are also located in areas throughout the central nervous system as well as in other areas of the body. For this reason, the antiemetics may have drug effects other than antiemetic ones. For instance, by blocking ACh and histamine receptors throughout the CNS and the GI tract, the anticholinergic drugs and antihistamines may also cause drowsiness; the drying of secretions; and the prevention of smooth muscle spasms. In addition, the neuroleptic agents calm the CNS, an effect beneficial in treating the symptoms of various psychotic disorders (anxiety, tension, and agitation).

Therapeutic Uses

The therapeutic uses of the antiemetic agents vary depending on the category of agents. There are, however, many indications for drugs in each category. These agents have a variety of therapeutic uses because of the wide distribution of dopamine, ACh, and serotonin receptors throughout the body. Most of the antiemetics act on these receptors to produce a specific physiologic response. The specific therapeutic effects of each class of antiemetic agents are listed in Table 49-4.

Side Effects and Adverse Effects

Most of the side effects and adverse effects of the antiemetics stem from their nonselective blockade of receptors. For example, the antihistamines not only bind to histamine$_1$ receptors and prevent ACh from binding to receptors in the vestibular nuclei, but they also bind to histamine receptors located elsewhere in the body, thus, for instance, causing secretion to become dry. Some of the more common side effects associated with the various categories of antiemetics are listed in Table 49-5.

Table 49-3	Antiemetics: Mechanism of Action
ANTIEMETIC CATEGORY	**MECHANISM OF ACTION**
Anticholinergic agents	Block **acetylcholine** receptors in the vestibular nuclei and reticular formation.
Antihistamine agents	Block histamine$_1$ receptors, thereby preventing **acetylcholine** from binding to receptors in the vestibular nuclei.
Neuroleptic agents	Block **dopamine** in the CTZ and may also block acetylcholine.
Prokinetic agents	Block **dopamine** in the CTZ or stimulate **acetylcholine** receptors.
Serotonin blockers	Block **serotonin** receptors in the GI tract, CTZ, and VC.
Tetrahydro-cannabinoid	Has inhibitory effects on the reticular formation, thalamus, and cerebral cortex.

CTZ, chemoreceptor trigger zone; *GI,* gastrointestinal; *VC,* vomiting center.

Table 49-4	Antiemetics: Therapeutic Effects
ANTIEMETIC CATEGORY	**THERAPEUTIC EFFECTS**
Anticholinergic	Motion sickness, secretion reduction before surgery, nausea and vomiting
Antihistamine	Motion sickness, nonproductive cough, sedation, rhinitis, allergy symptoms, nausea and vomiting
Neuroleptic agents	Psychotic disorders (mania, schizophrenia, anxiety), intractable hiccups, nausea and vomiting
Prokinetic agents	Delayed gastric emptying, gastroesophageal reflux, nausea and vomiting
Serotonin blockers	Nausea and vomiting associated with cancer chemotherapy, postoperative nausea and vomiting
Tetrahydro-cannabinoid	Nausea and vomiting associated with cancer chemotherapy

Table 49-5	Antiemetics: Adverse Effects
BODY SYSTEM	**SIDE/ADVERSE EFFECTS**
Anticholinergic	
Integumentary	Rash, erythema
Genitourinary	Difficult urination
CNS	Dizziness, drowsiness, disorientation
EENT	Blurred vision, dilated pupils, dry mouth
Antihistamine	
CNS	Dizziness, drowsiness, confusion
Genitourinary	Urinary retention
EENT	Blurred vision, dilated pupils, dry mouth
Neuroleptic agents	
Cardiovascular	Orthostatic hypotension, ECG changes, tachycardia
EENT	Blurred vision, dry eyes
GI	Dry mouth, nausea, vomiting, anorexia, constipation
Genitourinary	Urinary retention
CNS	Extrapyramidal symptoms, pseudoparkinsonism, akathisia, dystonia, tardive dyskinesia, headache
Prokinetic agents	
CNS	Sedation, fatigue, restlessness, headache, dystonia
GI	Dry mouth, nausea and vomiting
Cardiovascular	Hypotension, supraventricular tachycardia
Serotonin blockers	
CNS	Headache
GI	Diarrhea, increased AST and ALT levels
Other	Rash, bronchospasm
Tetrahydrocannabinoid	
CNS	Drowsiness, dizziness, anxiety, confusion
GI	Dry mouth
EENT	Visual disturbances

Interactions

The drug interactions associated with the antiemetic agents are also specific to the individual categories of agents. The most common and important drug interactions are listed in Table 49-6. Serotonin blockers and THCs have no significant drug interactions, and are therefore not mentioned in the table.

Dosages

For the recommended dosages of selected antiemetic agents, see the dosages table on p. 770.

DRUG PROFILES

The various antiemetics have many different therapeutic uses, but the ultimate goals of such therapy are to minimize or prevent fluid and electrolyte disturbances, to minimize deterioration in the nutritional status, and

to blunt the memory of the nausea and vomiting experience. Most of the antiemetics act by blocking receptors within the central nervous system, but some work directly in the GI tract. As already noted, there are six main classes of antiemetic agents. However, there are other agents that may also be used to treat nausea and vomiting. These are the corticosteroids (dexamethasone) and anxiolytics (lorazepam). When used in combination therapies, these latter agents plus the THCs are very beneficial in preventing the nausea and vomiting caused by cancer chemotherapy.

Table 49-6	Antiemetics: Common Drug Interactions	
DRUG	**MECHANISM**	**EFFECT**
Anticholinergic agents		
Antihistamines and antidepressants	Additive effect	Increased anticholinergic effects (drying effects)
Antihistamine		
Barbiturates, narcotics, hypnotics, tricyclic antidepressants, alcohol	Additive effect	Increased CNS depression
Neuroleptic agents		
Levodopa	Block	May cancel beneficial effects of levodopa in treatment of Parkinson's disease
Quinidine	Additive effect	Increased adverse cardiac effects
Prokinetic agents		
Alcohol	Additive effect	CNS depression
Anticholinergics and analgesics	Block	Antagonism of motility effects of metoclopramide

ANTICHOLINERGICS

⚓ SCOPOLAMINE

Scopolamine (Transderm-Scop) is the primary anticholinergic drug used as an antiemetic. It has potent effects on the vestibular nuclei, which are located in the inner ear and represent the area of the brain that controls balance. It works by blocking the binding of ACh to the cholinergic receptors in this region, thereby correcting an imbalance between the two neurotransmitters ACh and norepinephrine. These effects make scopolamine one of the most commonly used drugs for the treatment and prevention of the nausea and vomiting associated with motion sickness.

Scopolamine is classified as a pregnancy category C agent. It is contraindicated in patients with a known hypersensitivity to it and in patients with glaucoma. Scopolamine is available in many dosage formulations. The most commonly used formulation is the 72-hour transdermal patch, which releases a total of 0.5 mg of the agent. It is also available as 0.3-, 0.4-, and 1-mg/ml parenteral injections as well as a hydrobromide salt that is used for ophthalmic purposes.

⬡ PHARMACOKINETICS

HALF-LIFE	ONSET	PEAK	DURATION
Unknown	1-2 hr	6-8 hr	8 hr

Antihistamines

The antihistamine antiemetics are some of the most commonly used and most safe antiemetics, some of the popular ones being promethazine, meclizine, dimenhydrinate, and diphenhydramine. Many of them are available over-the-counter (OTC).

MECLIZINE

Meclizine (Antivert, Bonamine, Dizmiss, Ru-Vert-M) is available in several oral formulations—as 12.5-, 25-, and 50-mg tablets; as 25-mg chewable tablets; as 25-mg film-coated tablets; and as 15-, 25-, and 50-mg capsules. It is most commonly used to treat the dizziness, vertigo, and nausea and vomiting associated with motion sickness. It is classified as a pregnancy category B agent, and hypersensitivity, shock, and lactation are contraindications to its use. Commonly recommended dosages are listed in the dosages table.

⬡ PHARMACOKINETICS

HALF-LIFE	ONSET	PEAK	DURATION
6 hr	1 hr	Variable	24 hr

NEUROLEPTIC AGENTS

Prochlorperazine, chlorpromazine, perphenazine, promethazine, thiethylperazine, triflupromazine, and trimeprazine are antiemetics in the neurolytic class. Many of these agents are used to treat psychotic disorders such as mania and schizophrenia, and the associated anxiety, as well as intractable hiccups and nausea and vomiting.

⚓ PROCHLORPERAZINE

Prochlorperazine (Compazine) is classified as a pregnancy category C agent and is contraindicated in patients with a hypersensitivity to phenothiazines, those in a coma, and those suffering from seizures, encephalopathy, or bone marrow depression. It comes in

DOSAGES

SELECTED ANTIEMETIC AGENTS

AGENT	PHARMACOLOGIC CLASS	DOSAGE RANGE	PURPOSE
Anticholinergics ⚓**Scopolamine (Transderm-Scop)**	Anticholinergic solanaceous alkaloid	Apply one patch to hairless area behind ear every 3 days	Motion sickness prophylaxis
Antihistamines **Meclizine (Antivert, Bonine, Dizmiss, Ru-Vert-M)**	Anticholinergic antihistamine	*Adult* PO: 25-50 mg 1 hr before travel and repeated once daily during travel 25-100 mg/day	Motion sickness prophylaxis Vertigo
Neuroleptic agents ⚓**Prochlorperazine (Compazine)**	Phenothiazine	*Pediatric* PO/rectal: 20-29 lb (9-13 kg): 2.5 mg 1-2 times/day; 30-39 lb (13.5-17.5 kg): 2.5 mg 2-3 times/day; 40-85 lb (18-38 kg), 2.5 mg tid or 5 mg bid IM: 0.6 mg/day *Adult* PO: 5-10 mg 3-4 times/day IM: 5-10 mg q3-4h Rectal: 25 mg bid	Antiemetic
Prokinetic agents ⚓**Metoclopramide (Maxolon, Octamide, Reglan)**	Dopamine antagonist antiemetic	*Adult* IV: 1-2 mg/kg IM: 10-20 mg	Chemotherapy antiemetic Barium removal, intubation-associated emesis, postoperative nausea
Serotonin blockers **Ondansetron (Zofran)**	Antiserotonergic antiemetic	*Pediatric 4-12 y/o* PO: 4 mg tid, with first dose administered 30 min before chemotherapy, repeated 4 and 8 hr after first dose *Children 4-18 y/o* IV: 3 doses of 0.15 mg/kg, with first dose infused over 15 min and given 30 min before chemotherapy, repeated 4 and 8 hr after first dose *Adult* PO: 8 mg tid, with first dose administered 30 min before chemotherapy, repeated 4 and 8 hr after first dose, followed by 8 mg q8h for 1-2 days after completion of chemotherapy IV: 3 doses of 0.15 mg/kg, with first dose infused over 15 min and administered 30 min before chemotherapy, repeated 4 and 8 hr after first dose, *or* 32 mg infused over 15 min and administered 30 min before chemotherapy IV: 4 mg over 2-5 min	Chemotherapy antiemetic Postoperative nausea

continued

		SELECTED ANTIEMETIC AGENTS–cont'd		
AGENT	**PHARMACOLOGIC CLASS**	**DOSAGE RANGE**		**PURPOSE**
Tetracannabinoids **Dronabinol** **(Marinol)**	Marijuana- derived antiemetic	*Adult* PO: 5 mg 3-4 times/day		Chemotherapy antiemetic

many different dosage formulations: 2.5-, 5-, and 25-mg suppositories; a 5–mg/5 ml oral solution; a 5-mg/ml parenteral injection; 10-, 15-, and 30-mg extended-release capsules; and 5-, 10-, and 25-mg film-coated tablets. Commonly used dosages are listed in the dosages table.

❖ PHARMACOKINETICS

HALF-LIFE	ONSET	PEAK	DURATION
6-8 hr	2 hr	2-4 hr	4-6 hr

PROKINETIC AGENTS

The prokinetic agents promote the movement of substances through the GI tract and increase GI motility. Those prokinetic agents used to prevent nausea and vomiting are metoclopramide and cisapride.

⚓ METOCLOPRAMIDE

Metoclopramide (Maxolon, Octamide, Reglan) is the oldest and most commonly used prokinetic agent. It is available only by prescription because it can cause some severe side effects if not used correctly. Metoclopramide is also used for the treatment of delayed gastric emptying and gastroesophageal reflux. It is classified as a pregnancy category B agent and is contraindicated in patients with a seizure disorder, pheochromocytoma, breast cancer, or GI obstruction, and also in patients with a hypersensitivity to it, procaine, or procainamide.

Metoclopramide is available in both oral and parenteral formulations—as 5– and 10–mg/5 ml oral solutions, as 5- and 10-mg tablets, and as a 5-mg/ml parenteral injection. Commonly used dosages are listed in the dosages table.

❖ PHARMACOKINETICS

HALF-LIFE	ONSET	PEAK	DURATION
PO: 2.5-5 hr	PO: 15-60 min	PO: 2-3 hr	PO: 3-4 hr

SEROTONIN BLOCKERS

The serotonin blockers are also called *5-HT$_3$ receptor blockers* because they block the 5-HT$_3$ receptors in the GI tract, CTZ, and VC. Because of their specific actions, they cause few adverse effects. They are indicated for the prevention of nausea and vomiting associated with cancer chemotherapy and also for the prevention of postoperative nausea and vomiting. Currently there are only two agents available in this drug category, granisetron (Kytril) and ondansetron (Zofran). They are both available by prescription only in oral and parenteral forms and are classified as pregnancy category B agents. The only contraindication to their use is hypersensitivity. Ondansetron comes as a 2-mg/ml parenteral injection and 4- and 8-mg tablets. Commonly used dosages are listed in the dosages table.

❖ PHARMACOKINETICS

HALF-LIFE	ONSET	PEAK	DURATION
3-5.5 hr*	15-30 min*	1-1.5 hr*	6-12 hr*

*Zofran IV.

TETRACANNABINOIDS
DRONABINOL

Dronabinol (Marinol) is the only currently available THC and it is a synthetic derivative of the major active substance in marijuana. Dronabinol was approved by the FDA in 1985 for the treatment of the nausea and vomiting related to cancer chemotherapy. It is generally used as a second-line agent after treatment with other antiemetics has failed. Dronabinol is classified as a pregnancy category B agent and is contraindicated in the treatment of nausea and vomiting stemming from any cause other than cancer chemotherapy. It is available as 2.5-, 5-, and 10-mg capsules. Commonly used dosages are listed in the dosages table.

❖ PHARMACOKINETICS

HALF-LIFE	ONSET	PEAK	DURATION
4 days	30-60 min	1-3 hr	4-6 hr

NURSING PROCESS

ASSESSMENT

Before administering any antiemetic agent, the nurse should perform a thorough nursing assessment of the patient and obtain a complete history concerning the nausea and vomiting, then document the findings. Precipitating factors, weight loss, baseline vital signs, and laboratory findings such as the electrolyte levels and the fluid volume status should also be assessed and the findings documented regardless of the antiemetic agent being used.

The anticholinergic agent, scopolamine is contraindicated in patients with a hypersensitivity to it and in those with glaucoma. Cautious use with careful and close monitoring is recommended in patients suffering from blurred vision, dizziness, or benign prostatic hyperplasia (BPH). The effects of antihistamines and antidepressants are enhanced when these agents are used with the anticholinergic antiemetics, so the nurse should find out whether the patient is taking these other agents.

Antihistamines such as meclizine are often the most commonly used and safest antiemetics. Meclizine is contraindicated in patients with a hypersensitivity to it, those in shock, and lactating women. Cautious use is recommended in patients suffering from BPH, dizziness, confusion, or blurred vision. Barbiturates, narcotics, hypnotics, tricyclic antidepressants, and alcohol cause increased CNS depression when used with antihistamines, so the patient should be asked about the use of these agents and about alcohol consumption.

Neuroleptic agents such as prochlorperazine are contraindicated in patients with a hypersensitivity to them and in those suffering from coma, seizures, encephalopathy, or bone marrow depression. Cautious use is encouraged in patients with hypotension, cardiac dysrhythmias, BPH, or a CNS disorder. The effect of levodopa is decreased or absent in patients with Parkinson's disease taking neuroleptic agents. An increase in adverse cardiac effects occurs when quinidine and neuroleptic agents are taken simultaneously.

Prokinetic agents such as metoclopramide are often reserved for the treatment of the nausea and vomiting associated with chemotherapy and radiation therapy. Contraindications to its use include hypersensitivity to it or to procaine or procainamide, seizure disorders, pheochromocytoma, breast cancer and GI obstruction. Cautious use is recommended in pregnant or lactating women and in patients with congestive heart failure or GI hemorrhage. The action of metoclopramide is decreased when it is used with anticholinergics or opiates. Increased sedation occurs when prokinetic agents are used with alcohol and other CNS depressants.

Ondansetron, a serotonin blocker, increases tolerance to chemotherapy because of its very effective antiemetic properties. It is contraindicated in patients with a hypersensitivity to it, and cautious use is recommended in pregnant or lactating women, children, and the elderly. Before its use, the patient should be asked about the nature of the nausea and vomiting caused by chemotherapy and the findings documented.

The THC agent dronabinol (Marinol) is used only in patients who are undergoing chemotherapy and experiencing the attendant nausea and vomiting. Documentation of the nature of the nausea and vomiting is essential. A thorough nursing history and assessment must also be done before the start of therapy.

NURSING DIAGNOSES

Nursing diagnoses appropriate to patients receiving antiemetics include:
- Risk for injury resulting from side effects of the medication.
- Risk for injury, self, related to pathologic insult of fluid volume deficit related to nausea and vomiting.
- Activity intolerance due to weakness stemming from fluid and electrolyte disturbances.

PLANNING

Goals for patients receiving antiemetics include:
- Patient remains free of injury from nausea, vomiting, or medication therapy.
- Patient manages the side effects or identifies when to seek medical care for them.
- Patient regains normal fluid volume status and electrolyte levels.
- Patient will regain normal levels of activity.

Outcome Criteria

Outcome criteria for patients receiving antiemetics include:
- Patient states measures to implement to prevent injury such as assistance while ill, rising slowly, and changing positions slowly.
- Patient states side effects of the medication to report to the physician such as severe sedation, confusion, or lethargy.
- Patient states measures to implement in order to prevent further fluid volume deficits such as use of oral fluids, clear liquids, or chilled gelatin.

- Patient will increase activity day by day by 10 to 15 minutes.
- Time frame for goals and outcome criteria must be individualized with all patients.

IMPLEMENTATION

It is important to administer IV undiluted forms of diphenhydramine at a rate of 25-mg/1min. IM forms should be administered in large muscles, such as the gluteus maximus, and the sites rotated. Antiemetics such as prochlorperazine maleate, thiethylperazine maleate, and metoclopramide that are used to prevent nausea and vomiting in patients undergoing chemotherapy should be administered before the chemotherapy.

When metochlopramide is given orally, it should be given 30 minutes before meals and at bedtime. If given IV, it should be given slowly over 1 to 2 minutes. Parenteral infusions should not be given over less than 15 minutes. In addition, solutions for parenteral dos-

Patient Teaching TIPS

Antiemetic Administration

✔ Patients taking any of the antiemetics should be warned about the drowsiness they can cause, and as a result, told to avoid performing any hazardous tasks or driving. Patients should also be cautioned about taking antiemetics with alcohol and other CNS depressants because of the possible toxicity and CNS depression that can occur.

✔ Ondansetron hydrochloride may cause headache that can be relieved with a simple analgesic.

✔ Patients taking dronabinal should be reminded to change positions slowly to prevent the syncope or dizziness resulting from the hypotensive effects of the agent. They should also avoid taking any other CNS depressants with this antiemetic and be cautious when engaging in activities that require mental alertness.

TAKE HOME POINTS

Antiemetics
- Vomiting, or emesis, is the forcible emptying or expulsion of gastric and occasionally intestinal contents through the mouth
- Antiemetics are the drugs that relieve or prevent nausea and vomiting.
- The various categories of agents are the anticholinergics, antihistamines, neuroleptic agents, prokinetic agents, serotonin blockers, and tetracannabinoids.
- Used to prevent motion sickness, to reduce secretions before surgery, to treat delayed gastric emptying, and to prevent postoperative nausea and vomiting, as well as in the management of many other conditions

Anticholinergics and Antihistamines
- Anticholinergics work by blocking ACh receptors in the vestibular nuclei and reticular formation.
- This blockade prevents areas in the brain from being stimulated by nauseous stimuli.
- Antihistamines work by blocking histamine$_1$ receptors, which has the same effect as the anticholinergics.

Neuroleptics and Prokinetics
- Neuroleptics block dopamine in the CTZ and may also block ACh.
- Prokinetic agents also block dopamine receptors.

Serotonin blockers
- Highly effective antiemetics, most commonly used for the prevention of chemotherapy-induced nausea and vomiting.
- Work by blocking serotonin (5-HT$_3$) receptors in the GI tract, CTZ, and the VC.

Nursing Considerations
- Nausea and vomiting may be treated very effectively with antiemetics and prudent nursing care.
- Antiemetics in general should be given before any chemotherapy agent is administered, often 1 to 3 hours beforehand.
- Most antiemetics cause drowsiness.
- Ondansetron hydrochloride (Zofran) and granisetron (Kytril) are newer antiemetics that are making chemotherapy much more bearable for patients.
- Dronabinol therapy is used to prevent chemotherapy-induced nausea and vomiting and is associated with postural hypotension.
- Caution patients taking antiemetics that drowsiness and hypotension may occur, so they should avoid driving and using heavy machinery during use.

age should be kept for only 48 hours and protected from light. This agent should not be given in combination with any other medications, such as phenothiazines, which together would cause extrapyramidal reactions.

Diphenidol hydrochloride, an antiemetic used mainly for the treatment of Meniere's disease, should be administered with food, water, or milk to decrease GI upset and should not be used in conjunction with alcohol or other CNS depressants.

Thiethylperazine maleate is used for preventing the nausea and vomiting associated with surgery, radiation therapy, and chemotherapy. It should not be given IV because of the severe hypotension it can cause when given by this route. Trimethobenzamide may also produce hypotension, so it should be administered carefully, especially when given with other CNS depressants. IM injections should be given deep in the upper outer quadrant of the gluteal muscle to prevent site irritation.

The scopolamine transdermal patch should be applied behind an ear at least 4 hours before the antiemetic effect is desired. The area behind the ear should be cleansed and dried before its application. Ondansetron should be diluted in 50 ml of either 5% dextrose in water or 0.9% NaCl solution, or in the amounts specified by hospital policy or in the manufacturer's guidelines. If three doses are to be given, the individual doses should be infused over 15 minutes.

Dronobinol should be administered 1 to 3 hours before chemotherapy, even if the agent is given at home before the appointment at the oncologist's office. Granisetron, a newer antiemetic, provides 24-hour protection against chemotherapy-induced nausea and vomiting. In adult patients the agent is administered IV over 5 minutes, starting a half hour before the chemotherapy session. See also the patient teaching tips on p. 773.

EVALUATION

The therapeutic effects of antiemetics range from a decrease in to no complaints of nausea and vomiting. The patient should also be monitored for adverse effects such as GI upset, drowsiness, lethargy, weakness, extrapyramidal reactions, and orthostatic hypotension.

Critical Thinking A C T I V I T I E S

1. Chemotherapy-induced nausea and vomiting may be decreased or possibly prevented by which of the following measures?
   a. Consuming liquids at mealtimes only.
   b. Administering an antiemetic as prescribed 1 to 3 hours before the chemotherapy session.
   c. Consuming hot and cold liquids every 3 hours before and after meals.
   d. Increasing mobility before eating.

2. Explain how ondansetron hydrochloride (Zofran) decreases the nausea and vomiting associated with chemotherapy.

3. List the three areas in the body that send signals to the CTZ and cause nausea and vomiting.

4. What is the mechanism of action of Zofran and Kytril?
   a. Block Dopamine receptors.
   b. Inhibit acetylcholine.
   c. Block serotonin.
   d. Inhibit effects on reticular formation, thalamus, and cerebral cortex.

BIBLIOGRAPHY

Albanese J, Nutz P: *Mosby's 1995 nursing drug cards,* St Louis, 1995, Mosby.

Distasio S: Zofran makes chemo bearable, *RN* 56(5):56, 1991.

Johnson KB: *Harriet Lane handbook,* ed 13, St Louis, 1993, Mosby.

Keen JH: *Critical care and emergency drug reference,* St Louis, 1994, Mosby.

Knoben JE, Anderson PO: *Handbook of critical drug data,* ed 6, Hamilton, Ill, 1988, Drug Intelligence Publications.

Leibman MC: Practice corner, *Oncol Nurs Forum* 19(6):939, 1992.

McEvoy GK: *AHFS drug information,* Bethesda, Md, 1994, American Society of Hospital Pharmacists.

News: Granisetron enters antiemetic market, *Am J Hosp Pharm* 51(6):1382, 1994.

Skidmore-Roth L: *Mosby's 1995 nursing drug reference,* St Louis, 1995, Mosby.

Chapter 50

Vitamins and Minerals

Objectives

When you reach the end of this chapter, you will be able to:

1 Discuss the importance of the various vitamins and minerals.

2 Describe the nutritional states and diseases caused by vitamin and mineral hypostates and hyperstate.

3 Discuss the treatment of the various vitamin or mineral hypostates and hyperstates.

4 Discuss the indications, cautions, contraindications, dosages, recommended daily allowances (RDAs), mechanism of action, and associated measures to decrease side effects of each vitamin or mineral supplement.

5 Develop a comprehensive nursing care plan as it relates to the nursing process in the administration of vitamins and minerals.

CHAPTER OUTLINE

Vitamins
Fat-Soluble Vitamins

Vitamin A
  Mechanism of action
  Drug effects
  Therapeutic uses
  Side effects and adverse effects
    Toxicity and management of overdose
  Interactions
  Dosages
Drug Profile
  Vitamin A
Vitamin D
  Mechanism of action
  Drug effects
  Therapeutic uses
  Side effects and adverse effects
    Toxicity and management of overdose
  Interactions
  Dosages
Drug Profiles
  Calcifediol
  Calcitriol
  Ergocalciferol and Dihydrotachysterol
Vitamin E
  Mechanism of action
  Drug effects

  Therapeutic uses
  Side effects and adverse effects
  Dosages
Drug Profile
  Vitamin E
Vitamin K
  Mechanism of action
  Drug effects
  Therapeutic uses
  Side effects and adverse effects
    Toxicity and management of overdose
  Dosages
Drug Profile
  Vitamin K_1

Water-Soluble Vitamins

Vitamin B_1
  Mechanism of action
  Drug effects
  Therapeutic uses
  Side effects and adverse effects
  Interactions
  Dosages
Drug Profile
  Thiamine
Vitamin B_2
  Mechanism of action
  Drug effects
  Therapeutic uses
  Side effects and adverse effects

continued

Dosages
Drug Profile
  Riboflavin
Vitamin B₃
  Mechanism of action
  Drug effects
  Therapeutic uses
  Side effects and adverse effects
  Dosages
Drug Profile
  Niacin
Vitamin B₆
  Mechanism of action
  Drug effects
  Therapeutic uses
  Side effects and adverse effects
  Interactions
  Dosages
Drug Profile
  Pyridoxine
Vitamin B₁₂
  Mechanism of action
  Drug effects
  Therapeutic uses
  Side effects and adverse effects
  Interactions
  Dosages
Drug Profile
  Cyanocobalamin
Vitamin C
  Mechanism of action
  Drug effects
  Therapeutic uses
  Side effects and adverse effects
  Interactions
  Dosages
Drug Profile
  Ascorbic acid

Minerals

Calcium
  Mechanism of action
  Drug effects
  Therapeutic uses
  Side effects and adverse effects
    Toxicity and management of overdose
  Interactions
  Dosages
Drug Profile
  Calcium
Magnesium
  Mechanism of action
  Therapeutic uses
  Side effects and adverse effects
    Toxicity and management of overdose

Interactions
Dosages
Drug Profile
  Magnesium
Phosphorus
  Mechanism of action
  Therapeutic uses
  Side effects and adverse effects
    Toxicity and management of overdose
  Interactions
  Dosages
Drug Profile
  Phosphorus

Nursing Process
Assessment
Nursing Diagnoses
Planning
  Outcome criteria
Implementation
Evaluation

Glossary

Beriberi (ber′ e ber′ e) A disease of the peripheral nerves caused by an inability to assimilate thiamine. Symptoms are fatigue, diarrhea, appetite and weight loss, and disturbed nerve function causing paralysis and wasting of limbs, edema, and heart failure. (p. 787)

Coenzyme (ko en′ zīm) A nonprotein substance that combines with a protein molecule to form the active enzyme. (p. 777)

Enzymes (en′ zīm) Specialized proteins that catalyze chemical reactions in organic matter. (p. 777)

Fat-soluble vitamins (sol′ u bəl) Vitamins that can be dissolved (i.e., are soluble) in fat. These vitamins can be stored in large amounts in the liver and fatty tissues, thus daily ingestion of these vitamins is not necessary to maintain good health. (p. 777)

Minerals (min′ ər əlz) Inorganic substances that are ingested and attach to enzymes or other organic molecules. Minerals play a vital role in regulating many body functions. (p. 777)

Pellagra (pə lag′ rə) A disease resulting from a niacin or tryptophan deficiency or a metabolic defect that interferes with the conversion of tryptophan to niacin. It is characterized by scaly dermatitis, glossitis, inflammation of the mucous membranes, diarrhea, and mental disturbances. (p. 789)

Rhodopsin (ro dop′ sin) The purple pigmented compound in the rods of the retina, formed by a protein, opsin, and a derivative of vitamin A, retinol. (p. 779)

Rickets (rik′ əts) A condition caused by a vitamin D deficiency. Symptoms include soft, pliable bones, causing such deformities as bowlegs and knock knees; nodular enlargement on the ends and sides of the bones; muscle pain; enlarged skull; chest deformities; spinal curvature; enlargement of the liver and spleen; profuse sweating;

and general tenderness of the body when touched. (p. 782)

Scurvy (skur' ve) A condition resulting from an ascorbic acid deficiency. It is characterized by weakness, anemia, edema, spongy gums, mucocutaneous hemorrhages, and hardening of leg muscles. (p. 793)

Tocopherols (to kof' ər olz) Biologically active chemicals that make up vitamin E compounds. (p. 784)

Vitamins (vi' tə minz) An organic compound essential in small quantities for normal physiologic and metabolic functioning of the body. (p. 777)

Water-soluble vitamins (sol' u bəl) Vitamins that can be dissolved (i.e., are soluble) in water. Because water-soluble vitamins are not stored in the body for long periods, daily ingestion of these vitamins is necessary for good health. (p. 777)

Vitamins and minerals are essential in our lives whether we are conscientious in our food choices or consume whatever we desire. The importance that we as a nation place on vitamins and minerals is evidenced by the nutritional information available on any packaged food product. Under most circumstances daily requirements of vitamins and minerals are met by ingestion of fluids and regular, balanced meals. Ingesting food not only helps us to maintain adequate stores of essential vitamins and minerals, it also serves to preserve the intestinal mass and structure, to secrete hormones and enzymes, and to prevent harmful overgrowth of bacteria.

Various life events can occur that create *excessive need* or *excessive loss* of nutrients, vitamins, minerals, electrolytes, and fluids, requiring replacement or supplementation. Excessive vitamin and mineral needs can occur with almost any illness and are typically seen in burn victims and AIDS patients. Excessive loss of vitamins and minerals may be the result of poor dietary intake, because of an inability to swallow following cancer chemotherapy or radiation, or mental disorders such as anorexia nervosa. Poor dietary absorption attributable to many types of gastrointestinal (GI) disorders or alcoholism can also contribute to inadequate intake that may require vitamin and mineral supplementation.

In order for the body to heal and repair itself it needs the essential building blocks provided by carbohydrates, fats, and proteins, and vitamins and minerals are needed to efficiently utilize them. **Vitamins** are *organic* molecules needed in small quantities for normal metabolism and other biochemical functions such as growth or repair of tissue. They attach to enzymes or coenzymes and help them activate metabolic or building processes in the body. Minerals are as important as vitamins. **Minerals** are *inorganic* elements or salts found naturally in the earth. Like vitamins, mineral ions bind with enzymes or other organic molecules and help to regulate many body functions. The

collagen, hormone, and enzyme synthesis that is needed to heal wounds requires vitamins and minerals.

Although vitamins and minerals are essential to life, there are instances when we are unable to acquire these essentials compounds through diet or when a normal diet cannot meet the increased demand for them. In such cases vitamin and mineral supplementation is necessary. This chapter discusses both vitamins and minerals and their therapeutic effects.

VITAMINS

As mentioned earlier, vitamins are organic molecules needed in small amounts to carry on normal metabolism in the body. **Enzymes** are proteins secreted by cells; they act as catalysts to induce chemical changes in other substances, but they themselves remain chemically unchanged by the process. A **coenzyme** is a substance that enhances or is necessary for the action of enzymes. Vitamins function primarily as coenzymes in various metabolic pathways throughout the body. Many enzymes are totally useless without the appropriate vitamins to bind with to cause them to function properly. For example, coenzyme A (CoA) is an important carrier molecule associated with the citric acid cycle. However, it requires pantothenic acid (vitamin B_5) to complete its function in the citric acid cycle.

All known vitamins or their precursors (provitamins) are synthesized by plants. We require vitamins in specific amounts on a daily basis and obtain them from plant foods and, to a lesser extent, from animal food sources. Nondietary supplemental amounts of vitamin B complex and vitamin K are obtained from intestinal microbial synthesis. In addition, vitamin D can be synthesized by the skin with the proper precursors when exposed to sunlight. An insufficient diet will cause various nutrition-related vitamin deficiencies. As a result of extensive study, the National Academy of Science has compiled a Chart of vitamins and minerals. Table 50-1 lists the recommended daily dietary allowances (RDAs) suggested for the maintenance of good nutrition.

Vitamins are classified as either fat or water soluble. **Water-soluble vitamins** can be dissolved in water; **Fat-soluble vitamins** are dissolvable in fat. Because water-soluble vitamins (B-complex group and vitamin C) cannot be stored in the body in large amounts over long periods of time, daily intake is required to prevent the development of deficiencies. Conversely, fat-soluble vitamins (A, D, E, and K) do not need to be taken daily because they are stored in the liver and fatty tissues in large amounts. Deficiency in these vitamins occurs only after prolonged deprivation from an ade-

Table 50-1 | Recommended Daily Dietary Allowances (designed for the maintenance of good nutrition of practically all healthy people in the United States)*

	Age (Years)	Weight KG	Weight LB	Height CM	Height IN	Protein (G)	Vitamin A (µG RE)[†]	Vitamin D (µG)[‡]	Vitamin E (MG α TE)[§]
Infants	0-0.5	6	13	60	24	13	375	7.5	3
	0.5-1.0	9	20	71	28	14	375	10	4
Children	1-3	13	29	90	35	16	400	10	6
	4-6	20	44	112	44	24	500	10	7
	7-10	28	62	132	52	28	700	10	7
Males	11-14	45	99	157	62	45	1000	10	10
	15-18	66	145	176	69	59	1000	10	10
	19-24	72	160	177	70	58	1000	10	10
	25-50	79	174	176	70	63	1000	5	10
	51+	77	170	173	68	63	1000	5	10
Females	11-14	46	101	157	62	46	800	10	8
	15-18	55	120	163	64	44	800	10	8
	19-24	58	128	164	65	46	800	10	8
	25-50	63	138	163	64	50	800	5	8
	51+	65	143	160	63	50	800	5	8
Pregnant						60	800	10	10
Lactating	0-6 mo					65	1300	10	12

Water-Soluble Vitamins							Minerals					
Vitamin C (MG)	Thiamin (MG)	Ribo-flavin (MG)	Niacin (MG NE)[‖]	Vitamin B4 (MG)	Folic Acid (µG)	Vitamin B12 (µG)	Calcium (MG)	Phos-phorus (MG)	Mag-nesium (MG)	Iron (MG)	Zinc (MG)	Iodine (µG)
30	0.3	0.4	5	0.3	25	0.3	400	300	40	6	5	40
35	0.4	0.5	6	0.6	35	0.5	600	500	60	10	5	50
40	0.7	0.8	9	1.0	50	0.7	800	800	80	10	10	70
45	0.9	1.1	12	1.1	75	1.0	800	800	120	10	10	90
45	1.0	1.2	13	1.4	100	1.4	800	800	170	10	10	120
50	1.3	1.5	17	1.7	150	2	1200	1200	270	12	15	150
60	1.5	1.8	20	2	200	2	1200	1200	400	12	15	150
60	1.5	1.7	19	2	200	2	1200	1200	350	10	15	150
60	1.5	1.7	19	2	200	2	800	800	350	10	15	150
60	1.2	1.4	15	2	200	2	800	800	350	10	15	150
50	1.1	1.3	15	1.4	150	2	1200	1200	280	15	12	150
60	1.1	1.3	15	1.5	180	2	1200	1200	300	15	12	150
60	1.1	1.3	15	1.6	180	2	1200	1200	280	15	12	150
60	1.1	1.3	15	1.6	180	2	800	800	280	15	12	150
60	1.0	1.2	13	1.6	180	2	800	800	280	10	12	150
70	1.5	1.6	17	2.2	400	2.2	1200	1200	320	30	15	175
95	1.6	1.8	20	2.1	280	2.6	1200	1200	355	15	19	200

From McKenry L, Salerno E: *Mosby's pharmacology in nursing*, ed 19, St Louis, 1995, Mosby.

*The allowances are intended to provide for individual variations among most normal persons as they live in the United States under usual environmental stresses. Diets should be based on a variety of common foods in order to provide other nutrients for which human requirements have been less well defined.

[†]Retinol equivalents 1 Retinol equivalent = 1 µg retinol or 6 µg β carotene.

[‡]As cholecalciferol, 10 µg cholecalciferol = 400 IU vitamin D.

[§]α-Tocopherol equivalents. 1 mg d-α-tocopherol = 1 α TE.

[‖]NE (niacin equivalent) is equal to 1 mg of niacin or 60 mg of dietary tryptophan.

Table 50-2	Fat- and Water-Soluble Vitamins			
FAT-SOLUBLE			**WATER-SOLUBLE**	
DESIGNATION	NAME		B-COMPLEX VITAMINS	NAME
Vitamin A	Retinol		Vitamin B_1	Thiamine
Vitamin D	D_3, Cholecalciferol		Vitamin B_2	Riboflavin
	D_2, Ergocalciferol		Vitamin B_3	Niacin
Vitamin E	Tocopherols		Vitamin B_5	Pantothenic acid
Vitamin K	K_1, Phytonadione		Vitamin B_6	Pyridoxine
	K_2, Menaquinone		Vitamin B_{12}	Cyanocobalamin
			Biotin	
			Folic acid	
			Vitamin C	Ascorbic acid

quate supply or from disorders that prevent their absorption. Table 50-2 lists the fat-soluble and water-soluble vitamins.

Fat-Soluble Vitamins

The fat-soluble vitamins are A, D, E, and K. As a group they share various characteristics. They

- are present in both plant and animal foods,
- are stored primarily in the liver,
- exhibit slow metabolism or breakdown,
- are excreted via the feces, and
- they can become toxic if excessive amounts are consumed.

VITAMIN A

Vitamin A (retinol) is derived from animal fats such as those found in dairy products (butter and milk), eggs, meat, liver, and fish liver oils. The vitamin A stored in animal tissues was derived from carotenes, which are found in plants (green and yellow vegetables and yellow fruits). Carotenes or carotenoids are precursors to vitamin A and are thus called provitamin A carotenoids. They must be converted to vitamin A by enzymes in the intestinal mucosa. When beta-carotene, a major precursor of vitamin A, is consumed it is broken down to form two molecules of vitamin A. The sources of vitamin A as discussed are outlined below:

Vitamin A → animal source → dairy products, meat, liver

Provitamin A → plant source → green and yellow (carotene) vegetables, yellow fruit

Mechanism of Action

Vitamin A is an exogenous substance because it must be obtained from either plants or animals. Vitamin A is required for the growth and development of bones and teeth and is also necessary for maintaining other processes, including reproduction, integrity of mucosal and epithelial surfaces, and cholesterol and steroid synthesis. It is essential for night vision and for normal vision because it is part of one of the major retinal pigments called rhodopsin. Vitamin A (retinol) is converted to the aldehyde, *cis* retinal, which combines with opsin to form **rhodopsin,** the visual pigment that is required for normal "rod vision" in the retina.

Drug Effects

The drug effects of vitamin A are diverse. It may be used as a supplement to satisfy normal body requirements or an increased demand as in infants and pregnant and nursing women. Vitamin A may also be used to treat and correct the result of a long-term deficiency that leads to such conditions as hyperkeratosis of the skin, night blindness, retarded infant growth, and xerophthalmia. Because vitamin A is essential for healthy skin, it may be used to treat various forms of acne.

Therapeutic Uses

Therapeutic uses for vitamin A are listed in the box on the next page. As it indicates, vitamin A is primarily utilized as a dietary supplement and for treatment of deficiency states, and skin conditions. A normal diet should provide adequate amounts of vitamin A, but in cases of excessive need or inadequate dietary intake, vitamin A supplementation is indicated to avoid problems associated with deficiency. Symptoms of vitamin

Vitamin A: Indications

Dietary Supplement
Infants
Pregnant women
Nursing women

Deficiency States
Hyperkeratosis of the skin
Night blindness
Retarded infant growth
Xerophthalmia

Skin Conditions
Acne (vitamin A derivatives)
Keratosis follicularis
Psoriasis

A deficiency include night blindness, xerophthalmia, keratomalacia, hyperkeratosis, retarded growth, weakness, and increased susceptibility of mucous membranes to infection.

Side Effects and Adverse Effects

There are very few acute side effects and adverse effects associated with normal vitamin A ingestion. Only after long-term, excessive ingestion of vitamin A do symptoms appear. Side effects and adverse effects are usually noticed in bones, mucous membranes, the liver, and skin. Table 50-3 lists some of the symptoms of long-term, excessive ingestion of vitamin A.

Toxicity and Management of Overdose

The major toxic effects from vitamin A result from ingestion of excessive amounts, which occurs most commonly in children. A few hours after administration of an excess dose of vitamin A (>25,000 U/kg) irritability, drowsiness, vertigo, delirium, coma, vomiting, and/or diarrhea may occur. In infants excessive amounts of vitamin A can cause an increase in cranial pressure, resulting in symptoms such as bulging fontanelles, headache, papilledema, exophthalmos, and visual disturbances. Over several weeks a generalized peeling of the skin and erythremia may occur. These symptoms seem to disappear a few days after discontinuation of the drug, which is the only treatment necessary in situations of overdose.

Interactions

Vitamin A is absorbed to a lesser extent with the simultaneous use of lubricant laxatives and cholestyramine. In addition, the use of isotretinoin with vitamin A can result in additive effects and possibly toxicity.

Table 50-3	**Vitamin A: Adverse Effects**
BODY SYSTEM	**SIDE/ADVERSE EFFECT**
Gastrointestinal	Nausea, vomiting, anorexia, abdominal pain, jaundice
Central nervous system	Headache, increased intracranial pressure, lethargy, malaise
Integumentary	Drying of skin, pruritis, increased pigmentation, night sweats
Musculoskeletal	Arthralgia, retarded growth
Metabolic	Hypomenorrhea, hypercalcemia

Dosages

For the RDAs of vitamin A see Table 50-1. For the recommended dosages of vitamin A see the dosages table.

*D*RUG PROFILE

There are three forms of vitamin A: retinol, retinyl palmitate, and retinyl acetate. Medications containing vitamin A may require a prescription, but many OTC products such as multivitamins are also available. All vitamin A products are classified as pregnancy category A agents and are contraindicated in patients who have a hypersensitivity to vitamin A and in those with oral malabsorption syndromes.

VITAMIN A

Vitamin A (Aquasol A) is available orally as 10,000-, 25,000-, and 50,000-U capsules; 10,000-U tablets; and a 50,000-U/ml solution. It is also available parenterally as an injection. Doses for vitamin A can be expressed in USP units or μg retinol equivalents (RE). A microgram retinol equivalent can be calculated if the number of USP units of vitamin A is known: 1 USP = 0.3 μg RE. Current RDAs are listed in Table 50-1.

PHARMACOKINETICS

HALF-LIFE	ONSET	PEAK	DURATION
13 days†	42 days*	Unknown	Unknown

*Follicular hyperkeratosis resolution with 300 μg/day of retinal.
†First order, 3 compartment model, the delta half-life.

DOSAGES

SELECTED VITAMINS

VITAMIN	PHARMACOLOGIC CLASS	DOSAGE RANGE	PURPOSE
A	Fat-soluble	*Adult* PO: 10,000-50,000 U/day *Pediatric* PO: 5000 U/kg/day	Deficiency
B₂ (Riboflavin)	Water-soluble B-complex group	*Adult* PO: 5-30 mg/day *Pediatric* PO: 3-10 mg/day	Deficiency
B₃ (Niacin)	Water-soluble B-complex group	*Adult* PO: 300-500 mg/day *Pediatric* PO: ≤300 mg/day	Deficiency
B₆ (Pyridoxine)	Water-soluble B-complex group	*Adult* PO: 2.5-10 mg/day PO: 30-600 mg/day *Infants* PO: 2-100 mg/day	Deficiency Pyridoxine deficiency
B₁₂ (Cyanocobalamin)	Water-soluble B-complex group	*Adult* IM/SC: 100 µg/day *Pediatric* IM/SC: 30-50 µg/day	Deficiency
C (Ascorbic acid)	Water-soluble	*Adult* IM/PO: 100-250 mg/day *Pediatric* IM/PO: 100-300 mg/day	Deficiency
Calcifediol	Fat-soluble	*Adult/Pediatric >10 y/o* PO: 50-100 µg/day *Pediatric 2-10 y/o* PO: 50 µg/day *Pediatric ≤2 y/o* PO: 20 µg/day	Deficiency
Calcitriol	Fat-soluble D analogue	*Adult* PO: 0.25 µg/day *Adult/Pediatric ≥6 y/o* PO: 0.5-2 µg/day *Pediatric 1-5 y/o* PO: 0.25-0.75 µg/day	Dialysis deficiency Hypoparathyroidism
Dihydrotachysterol	Fat-soluble D analogue	*Adult* PO: 0.75-2.5 mg/day *Pediatric* PO: 1-5 mg/day *Adult/Pediatric* PO: 0.5-2 mg/day	Hypoparathyroidism Familial hypophosphatemia
D₂ (Ergocalciferol)	Fat-soluble	*Adult/Pediatric* PO: 25-125 µg/day *Adult* PO: 250 µg/day-1.5 mg/day *Pediatric* PO: 75-125 µg/day *Pediatric* PO: ≥1-2 mg/day	Nutritional rickets Osteomalacia Vitamin D–dependent rickets Vitamin D–resistant rickets

continued

SELECTED VITAMINS—cont'd

VITAMIN	PHARMACOLOGIC CLASS	DOSAGE RANGE	PURPOSE
D$_2$—cont'd		*Adult* PO: 6.25 μg-5 mg *Pediatric* PO: 1.25-5 mg	Hypoparathyroidism
E	Fat-soluble	*Adult* PO: 60-76 U/day *Premature Neonatal* PO: 15-30 U/day	Deficiency Retinopathy prophylaxis

VITAMIN D

Vitamin D, also called the "sunshine" vitamin, is responsible for the proper utilization of calcium and phosphorus in the body. The term "vitamin D" designates a group of analogue steroid structural chemicals with vitamin D activity. The two most important members of the vitamin D family are vitamin D$_2$ (ergocalciferol) and vitamin D$_3$ (cholecalciferol). They have different sites of origin but similar functions in the body. Ergocalciferol (vitamin D$_2$) is plant vitamin D and is therefore obtained through dietary sources. The natural form of vitamin D produced in the skin by ultraviolet irradiation (sun), 7-dehydrocholesterol, is referred to as cholecalciferol (vitamin D$_3$). This endogenous synthesis of vitamin D$_3$ usually produces sufficient amounts to meet daily requirements. Chemically the two vitamin D compounds are different, but physiologically they produce the same effect. See below:

Vitamin D$_2$ → ergocalciferol → plant vitamin D
Vitamin D$_3$ → cholecalciferol → human vitamin D

Vitamin D then is obtained through endogenous synthesis and through vitamin D$_2$-containing foods such as fish oils, salmon, sardines, and herring; fortified milk, bread, and cereals; and animal livers, tuna fish, eggs, and butter.

Mechanism of Action

The basic function of vitamin D is to regulate the absorption and subsequent utilization of calcium and phosphorus. It is also necessary for the normal calcification of bone. Vitamin D in coordination with parathyroid hormone and calcitonin regulates serum calcium levels by increasing absorption from the small intestine and extracting calcium from the bone when needed.

As ergocalciferol and cholecalciferol, vitamin D is inactive and requires transformation into active metabolites for biologic activity. Both vitamin D$_2$ and vitamin D$_3$ are biotransformed primarily in the liver by the actions of the parathyroid hormone. The resulting calcifediol is then transported to the kidney where it is converted to calcitriol, which is believed to be the most active vitamin D analogue. It is calcitriol that promotes the intestinal absorption of calcium and phosphorus and the deposition of calcium and phosphorus in the teeth and bone.

Drug Effects

The drug effects of vitamin D are very similar to those of vitamin A and essentially all vitamin and mineral compounds. It is used as a supplement to satisfy normal daily requirements or an increased demand as in infants and pregnant and nursing women. Vitamin D may also be used to treat and correct the result of a long-term deficiency that leads to such conditions as infantile **rickets,** tetany, and osteomalacia. Because of vitamin D's role in the regulation of calcium and phosphorus, it may be used to correct deficiencies of these two elements.

Therapeutic Uses

Vitamin D can be used either to supplement the present daily intake of vitamin D or to treat a deficiency of vitamin D. In the case of supplementation it is given as a prophylactic measure to prevent deficiency-related problems. Vitamin D is also used therapeutically to treat conditions resulting from long-term insufficiency. The box on the next page lists the therapeutic indications for vitamin D.

Side Effects and Adverse Effects

As with vitamin A, there are very few acute side effects and adverse effects associated with normal vitamin D ingestion. Only after long-term, excessive ingestion of vitamin D do symptoms appear. Such effects

Vitamin D: Therapeutic Effects

- ■ Rickets
- ■ Osteodystrophy
- ■ Osteoporosis
- ■ Osteomalacia
- ■ Hypocalcemia
- ■ Pseudohypoparathyroidism
- ■ Hypophosphatemia
- ■ Hypoparathyroidism
- ■ Dietary supplement

Table 50-4 Vitamin D: Adverse Effects	
BODY SYSTEM	**SIDE/ADVERSE EFFECT**
Gastrointestinal	Nausea, vomiting, anorexia, cramps, metallic taste, dry mouth
Central nervous system	Fatigue, weakness, drowsiness, convulsion, headache
Genitourinary	Polyuria, hematuria, albuminuria, renal failure
Cardiovascular	Hypertension, dysrhythmias
Musculoskeletal	Decreased bone growth, early joint pain, early muscle pain

are usually noticed in the GI tract or central nervous system and are listed in Table 50-4.

Toxicity and Management of Overdose

The major toxic effects from ingesting excessive amounts of vitamin D occur most commonly in children. Discontinuation of vitamin D and reduced calcium intake will reverse the toxic state. The amount of vitamin D considered to be too much varies considerably among individuals, but is generally thought to be 1.25 to 2.5 mg of ergocalciferol daily in adults and 25 μg daily in infants and children.

The toxic effects of vitamin D are those associated with hypertension, such as weakness, fatigue, headache, anorexia, dry mouth, metallic taste, nausea, vomiting, abdominal cramps, ataxia, and bone pain. If not recognized and treated, these symptoms can progress to impairment of renal function, osteoporosis, pancreatitis, and seizures.

Interactions

Reduced absorption of vitamin D will occur with the simultaneous use of lubricant laxatives and chole-

styramine. Patients taking digitalis preparations can develop cardiac arrhythmias as a result of vitamin D intake.

Dosages

For the RDAs of vitamin D see Table 50-1. For the recommended dosages of vitamin D see the dosages table on p. 781.

DRUG PROFILES

There are three forms of vitamin D: calcifediol, calcitriol, and dihydrotachysterol. Vitamin D is available in OTC medications, such as a multivitamin product, or by prescription. All vitamin D products are classified as pregnancy category A agents and are contraindicated in patients who have shown a hypersensitivity reaction to them and in patients with hypercalcemia, renal dysfunction, and hyperphosphatemia.

CALCIFEDIOL

Calcifediol (Calderol) is the 25-hydroxylated form of cholecalciferol (vitamin D_3). It is a vitamin D analogue primarily used for the management of hypocalcemia in patients with chronic renal failure who are undergoing hemodialysis. It is available only as 20- and 50-μg capsules. Commonly recommended dosages are listed in the dosages table on p. 781.

PHARMACOKINETICS

HALF-LIFE	ONSET	PEAK	DURATION
16 days	Variable	Unknown	Unknown

CALCITRIOL

Calcitriol (Rocaltrol, Calcijex) is the 1,25-dihydroxylated form of cholecalciferol (vitamin D_3). It is a vitamin D analogue used for the management of hypocalcemia in patients with chronic renal failure who are undergoing hemodialysis. It is also used in the treatment of hypoparathyroidism and pseudohypoparathyroidism, vitamin D–dependent rickets, hypophosphatemia, and hypocalcemia in premature infants. It is available orally as 0.25- and 0.5-μg capsules and parenterally as 1- and 2-μg/ml injections. Commonly recommended dosages are listed in the dosages table on p. 781.

♆ PHARMACOKINETICS

HALF-LIFE	ONSET	PEAK	DURATION
3-6 hr	<3 hr	3-6 hr	3-5 days

ERGOCALCIFEROL AND DIHYDROTACHYSTEROL

Dihydrotachysterol (Hytakerol, DHT Intensol, DHT Tablets) is a vitamin D analogue that is administered orally once daily for the treatment of any of the above-mentioned conditions. Ergocalciferol (Deltalin, Drisdol, and Calciferol) is vitamin D_2. Its use is indicated for patients with GI, liver, or biliary disease associated with malabsorption of vitamin D analogues.

Dihydrotachysterol is only available orally as 0.125-mg capsules, 0.125-, 0.2-, and 0.4 mg-tablets, and 0.2- and 0.25-mg/ml solutions. Ergocalciferol is available orally and parenterally. Oral agents include 1.25-mg (50,000 U) capsules, 1.25-mg (50,000 U) tablets, and a 200-μg (8000 U)/ml solution. A 12.5-mg/ml parenteral injection is available for intramuscular use. Commonly recommended dosages for both dihydrotachysterol and ergocalciferol are listed in the dosages table on p. 781. The pharmacokinetics of ergocalciferol are listed below.

♆ PHARMACOKINETICS

HALF-LIFE	ONSET	PEAK	DURATION
19 days†	30 days*	Unknown	Mo-yr

*Therapeutic effects.
†Biologic of half-life.

VITAMIN E

Four biologically active chemicals called **tocopherols**, alpha, beta, gamma, and delta, make up the vitamin E compounds. Alpha-tocopherol is the most biologically active natural form of vitamin E. Dietary plant sources of vitamin E are fruits, grains, cereals, vegetables, oils, and wheat germ. Animal sources include eggs, chicken, and meats. The exact biologic function of vitamin E is unknown, but it is believed to act as an antioxidant.

Mechanism of Action

Although vitamin E is a powerful biologic antioxidant and an essential component of the diet, its exact nutritional function has not been fully demonstrated. The only significant deficiency syndrome for vitamin E has been recognized in premature infants. In this situation vitamin E deficiency may result in irritability, edema, thrombosis, and hemolytic anemia.

Table 50-5	Vitamin E: Adverse Effects	
BODY SYSTEM	**SIDE/ADVERSE EFFECT**
Gastrointestinal	Nausea, cramps, diarrhea
Central nervous system	Fatigue, headache
Genitourinary	Gonadal dysfunction
Musculoskeletal	Weakness
Metabolic	Altered metabolism and immunity of thyroid, pituitary, and adrenal hormones

Drug Effects

The drug effects of vitamin E are not as well defined as those of the other fat-soluble vitamins. It is believed to protect polyunsaturated fatty acids, a component of cellular membranes. It has also been shown to hinder the deterioration of substances such as vitamin A and ascorbic acid (vitamin C), two substances that are highly oxygen sensitive and readily oxidized, thus acting as an antioxidant.

Therapeutic Uses

Vitamin E is most commonly used as a dietary supplement to augment present daily intake or to treat a deficiency. Those at greatest risk of complications from vitamin E deficiency are premature infants. As previously mentioned, vitamin E has recently received much attention as an antioxidant. Preventing the oxidation of various substances prevents the formation of toxic chemicals within the body, some of which are believed to cause cancer. There is a popular but unproved theory that vitamin E has beneficial effects for patients with cancer, heart disease, premenstrual syndrome (PMS), and sexual dysfunction.

Side Effects and Adverse Effects

As with vitamin D, there are very few acute side effects and adverse effects associated with normal vitamin E ingestion because it is relatively nontoxic. Side effects and adverse effects are usually noticed in the gastrointestinal tract or central nervous system and are listed in Table 50-5.

Dosages

For the RDAs of vitamin E see Table 50-1. For the recommended dosages of vitamin E see the dosages table on p. 782.

DRUG PROFILE

The four forms of vitamin E, alpha, beta, gamma, and delta tocopherol, are available as OTC medications, such as a multivitamin product, or by prescription. All vitamin E products are classified as pregnancy category A agents and are contraindicated in patients who have shown a hypersensitivity reaction to them.

VITAMIN E

Vitamin E (E-Vitamin Succinate, Vita-Plus E, Aquasol E, Phenyl-E) activity is generally expressed in USP or international units. One unit of vitamin E equals the biologic activity of 1 mg of dl-alpha-tocopheryl acetate, 1.12 mg of dl-alpha-tocopheryl acid succinate, 910 µg of dl-alpha-tocopherol, 735 µg of d-alpha-tocopheryl acetate, 830 µg of d-alpha-tocopheryl acid succinate, and 670 µg of d-alpha-tocopherol. Vitamin E is available only in an oral formulation as regular and water-miscible capsules, an oil solution, and regular and chewable tablets. Current RDAs for vitamin E are listed in Table 50-1. Commonly recommended dosages for vitamin E are listed in the dosages table on p. 782.

⬡ PHARMACOKINETICS

HALF-LIFE	ONSET	PEAK	DURATION
Variable	Unknown	Unknown	Variable

VITAMIN K

Vitamin K is the last of the four fat-soluble vitamins (A, D, E, and K). There are three types of vitamin K—phytonadione (vitamin K_1), menaquinone (vitamin K_2), and menadione (vitamin K_3). The primary dietary sources of vitamin K_1 are green leafy vegetables (e.g., cabbage, spinach), meats, and milk. The body does not store large amounts of vitamin K; however, vitamin K_2 is synthesized by the intestinal flora, thus providing an endogenous supply. (See the diagram below.)

Vitamin K_1 → phytonadione → green leafy vegetables (exogenous)
Vitamin K_2 → menaquinone → intestinal flora (endogenous)

Vitamin K is essential for the synthesis of blood coagulation factors, which takes place in the liver. Vitamin K–dependent blood coagulation factors are factors II, VII, IX, and X. Other names for these clotting factors are listed below:

Vitamin K
factor II → prothrombin
factor VII → proconvertin
factor IX → Christmas factor
factor X → Stuart-Power factor

Mechanism of Action

As mentioned earlier, vitamin K activity is essential for effective blood clotting because it facilitates the hepatic biosynthesis of factor II (prothrombin), factor VII (convertin), factor IX (Christmas factor), and factor X (Stuart-Power factor). Vitamin K deficiency results in coagulation disorders caused by hypoprothrombinemia.

Drug Effects

The drug effects of vitamin K are limited to its action on the vitamin K–dependent clotting factors produced in the liver (II, VII, IX, and X). Coagulation defects affecting these clotting factors can be corrected with administration of vitamin K. Vitamin K deficiencies are rare because intestinal flora are able to synthesize sufficient amounts. If a deficiency develops, it can be corrected with vitamin K supplementation.

Therapeutic Uses

Vitamin K is indicated for dietary supplementation and for treating deficiency states. Although rare, deficiency states can develop with inadequate dietary intake or broad-spectrum inhibition of the intestinal flora, resulting from administration of broad-spectrum antibiotics. Deficiency states can also be seen in newborns because of malabsorption attributable to inadequate amounts of bile or selected drugs, and as a result of the administration of specific anticoagulants that inhibit hepatic vitamin K activity. Coumarin- and indanedione-derivative anticoagulants thin the blood by inhibiting vitamin K–dependent clotting factors in the liver. Administration of vitamin K will override the mechanism by which the anticoagulants inhibit production of vitamin K–dependent clotting factors.

Side Effects and Adverse Effects

Vitamin K is relatively nontoxic and thus causes very few side effects and adverse effects. Severe reactions limited to hypersensitivity or anaphylaxis have occurred rarely during or immediately following IV administration. Side effects and adverse effects are usually related to injection site reactions and hypersensitivity. See Table 50-6 for a list of such major effects by body system.

Toxicity and Management of Overdose

Toxicity is primarily limited to use in the newborn. Hemolysis of red blood cells can occur, especially in infants with low levels of glucose-6-phosphate dehydrogenase. In this case replacement with blood products is indicated.

Dosages

The RDA for vitamin K is 5 to 30 μg for infants and children, 45 to 65 μg for women, and 45 to 80 μg for men. The dose of phytonadione (Aqua-MEPHYTON, Konakion, Mephyton) is 0.5 to 1 mg as a single IM dose for infants within 1 hour after delivery and 2.5 to 10 mg administered orally or parenterally as an IM or SC injection for adults.

Ⓓ RUG PROFILE

The most frequently used form of vitamin K is phytonadione (vitamin K_1). Both phytonadione and menadione (vitamin K_3) are available by prescription only in oral and parenteral forms. Menadione is classified as a pregnancy category X agent while phytonadione is a category C agent. They are both contraindicated in patients who have shown a hypersensitivity reaction to them. Their use is also contraindicated during the last few weeks of pregnancy and in patients with severe hepatic disease.

Table 50-6	Vitamin K: Adverse Effects
BODY SYSTEM	**SIDE/ADVERSE EFFECT**
Gastrointestinal	Nausea, decreased liver function tests
Central nervous system	Headache, brain damage (large doses)
Hematopoietic	Hemolytic anemia, hemoglobinuria, hyperbilirubinemia
Integumentary	Rash, urticaria

VITAMIN K_1

Vitamin K_1 (Phytonadione, Mephyton, Aqua-MEPHTYON, Konakion) is available orally as a 5-mg tablet and parenterally as 2- and 10-mg intravenous or intramuscular injections.

⬡ P H A R M A C O K I N E T I C S

HALF-LIFE	ONSET	PEAK	DURATION
Unknown	Variable	1-2 hr	Unknown

Water-Soluble Vitamins

The water-soluble vitamins include the vitamin-B-complex group and vitamin C (ascorbic acid). They are present in a variety of plant and animal food sources. The vitamin B complex is a group of 10 vitamins that are often found together in food, although they are chemically dissimilar and have different metabolic functions. Because the B vitamins were discovered in sequential order, they were grouped together as B complex vitamins. The most commonly used B complex and C vitamins are listed in the box below.

The water-soluble vitamins are a chemically diverse group sharing only the characteristic of being dissolvable in water. Like the fat-soluble vitamins, they act primarily as coenzymes or oxidation-reduction agents in important metabolic pathways. Unlike the fat-soluble vitamins, water-soluble vitamins are not stored in the body in appreciable amounts. Therefore dietary intake must be adequate and regular or deficiency states will develop. Because these vitamins are water-soluble, excess amounts are excreted in the urine. The body excretes what it does not need, which makes toxic reactions to water-soluble vitamins very rare.

Water-Soluble Vitamins: Alternate Names

Vitamin B complex	Vitamin B_1 →thiamine Vitamin B_2 →riboflavin Vitamin B_3 →niacin Vitamin B_5 →pantothenic acid Vitamin B_6 →pyridoxine Vitamin B_9 →folic acid Vitamin B_{12}→cyanocobalamine
Vitamin C	→ascorbic acid

VITAMIN B₁

Vitamin B₁ (thiamine) is present in a wide variety of foods, especially whole grains, liver, and beans. When it is combined with adenosine triphosphate (ATP) the result is thiamine pyrophosphate coenzyme, which is required for carbohydrate metabolism. A deficiency of vitamin B₁ results in the classic disease **beriberi** or Wernicke's encephalopathy (cerebral beriberi). Common findings in beriberi include brain lesions, polyneuropathy of peripheral nerves, serous effusions, and cardiac anatomic changes. Vitamin deficiency can result from poor diet, extended fever, hyperthyroidism, liver disease, alcoholism, malabsorption, and pregnancy and breast feeding.

Mechanism of Action

As mentioned, thiamine is an essential precursor for the formation of thiamine pyrophosphate. In addition to carbohydrate metabolism, there are several other metabolic pathways that require thiamine to function, including the Krebs cycle.

Drug Effects

The drug effects of vitamin B₁ (thiamine) are multiple. The integrity of the peripheral nervous system, cardiovascular system, and the gastrointestinal tract are all heavily dependent upon thiamine.

Therapeutic Uses

The beneficial drug effects and the essential role of thiamine in so many metabolic pathways make it useful in treating a variety of disorders, including thiamine deficiency and metabolic disorders. It is also used as a dietary supplement and an oral insect repellent. Some of the deficiency states treated by thiamine are beriberi, Wernicke's encephalopathy syndrome, and peripheral neuritis associated with pellagra or neuritis of pregnancy.

Thiamine is used as a dietary supplement in cases of malabsorption such as those induced by alcoholism, cirrhosis, or GI disease. Thiamine may be useful in preventing deficiency in patients with these diseases. Some metabolic disorders that benefit from thiamine treatment are subacute necrotizing encephalomyelopathy, maple syrup urine disease, and lactic acidosis associated with pyruvate carboxylase deficiency and hyper-β-alaninemia.

Other areas in which thiamine may have therapeutic value are the management of poor appetite, ulcerative colitis, chronic diarrhea, and the cerebellar syndrome.

Side Effects and Adverse Effects

Adverse effects are rare but include hypersensitivity reactions, nausea, restlessness, and pulmonary edema. Administration by intramuscular injection can produce local tenderness, and intravenous injections can produce anaphylaxis.

Interactions

Thiamine is incompatible with alkaline- and sulfite-containing solutions.

Dosages

The RDAs for thiamine are 0.3 to 1 mg for infants and children, 1.1 mg for women, and 1.2 to 1.5 mg for men. In addition, ingestion of raw fish, a high carbohydrate diet, and heavy exercise are situations in which a higher intake of thiamine is required. The usual dose for treating beriberi is 10 to 20 mg IM three times daily in addition to a multivitamin preparation. See also Table 50-1.

*D*RUG *P*ROFILE

THIAMINE

Thiamine (Betalin S, Biamine) is classified as a pregnancy category A agent (i.e., it is relatively safe to administer during pregnancy) and is contraindicated only in individuals with a prior history of a hypersensitivity reaction. Thiamine is available orally as 5-, 10-, 25-, 50-, 100-, 250-, and 500-mg tablets and parenterally as 100- and 200-mg/ml injections.

✦ P H A R M A C O K I N E T I C S

HALF-LIFE	ONSET	PEAK	DURATION
Unknown	Unknown	Unknown	24 hr

VITAMIN B₂

Vitamin B₂ (riboflavin) is found in leafy green vegetables, eggs, nuts, meats, and yeast. Riboflavin serves several important functions. In the body riboflavin is converted into two coenzymes, flavin mononucleotide (FMN) and flavin adenine dinucleotide (FAD), that are essential for tissue respiration. Another B vitamin, vitamin B_6 (pyridoxine), requires riboflavin for activation. It is also needed to convert tryptophan into niacin and to maintain erythrocyte integrity. A deficiency of riboflavin results in cutaneous, oral, and corneal changes that include cheilosis, seborrheic dermatitis, and keratitis. Alcoholism is a major cause of riboflavin deficiency.

Mechanism of Action

As previously mentioned, vitamin B_2 is an important precursor for the synthesis of FMN and FAD that are required in tissue respiration pathways. Riboflavin also plays an important part in transfer reactions, especially in carbohydrate catabolism.

Drug Effects

The drug effects of riboflavin are mainly limited to replacement therapy for deficiency states. Deficiency is rare and does not usually occur in healthy persons. However, deficiency may occur as a result of malnutrition or intestinal malabsorption or because of alcoholism or other diseases or infections.

Therapeutic Uses

Riboflavin is primarily used as a dietary supplement and to treat deficiency states. Although few disorders result because of a deficiency of riboflavin, supplementation is sufficient treatment for those disorders. Patients that may suffer from riboflavin deficiency are those with long-standing infections, liver disease, alcoholism, and malignancy and those taking probenecid. Riboflavin supplementation may be beneficial in treating microcytic anemia, acne, migraine headache, congenital methemoglobinemia, muscle cramps, and burning feet syndrome.

Side Effects and Adverse Effects

Riboflavin is a very safe and effective vitamin; to date, no side effects or toxic effects have been reported. It should be noted that in large doses riboflavin will discolor urine a yellow-green.

Dosages

For the RDAs of riboflavin see Table 50-1. For commonly recommended dosages of riboflavin see the dosages table on p. 781.

$\mathcal{D}$RUG PROFILE

RIBOFLAVIN

Riboflavin (vitamin B_2) is needed for normal respiratory reactions. It is a safe, nontoxic water-soluble vitamin with almost no adverse effects; it is classified as a pregnancy category A agent. It is available only orally as 10-, 25-, 50-, and 100-mg tablets. Commonly recommended dosages of riboflavin are listed in the dosages table on p. 781.

PHARMACOKINETICS

HALF-LIFE	ONSET	PEAK	DURATION
66-84 min	Unknown	Unknown	24 hr

VITAMIN B_3

Vitamin B_3 (niacin) can be synthesized from tryptophan, an essential amino acid obtained from protein digestion. Niacin is present in meats, beans, yeast, liver, and wheat germ. Once in the body niacin is converted to niacinamide, which is then converted into two coenzymes, nicotinamide adenine dinucleotide (NAD) and nicotinamide adenine dinucleotide phosphate (NADP). These coenzymes are needed for glycogenolysis, tissue respiration, and lipid, protein, and purine metabolism (see Fig. 50-1).

A dietary deficiency of niacin will produce the classic symptoms of pellagra as outlined below:

Mental: Various psychotic symptoms
Neurologic: Neurasthenic syndrome
Cutaneous: Crusting, erythema, and desquamation
Mucous membrane: Oral, vaginal, and urethral lesions
Gastrointestinal: Diarrhea or bloody diarrhea

Niacin is also an antihyperlipidemic agent. Niacin lowers serum cholesterol and triglyceride levels by reducing very-low-density lipoprotein (VLDL) synthesis. The principal carrier of cholesterol in the blood is low-density lipoprotein (LDL). Since VLDL is the precursor to LDL, reducing VLDL will result in reduction of LDL and, consequently, harmful plaque-forming, artery-narrowing cholesterol.

▼ **FIG. 50-1** Niacin, once in the body, is converted to NAD and NADP, which are coenzymes needed for many metabolic processes.

niacin
tryptophan → niacinamide → NAD
NADP

- glycogenolysis
- tissue respiration
- lipid metabolism

▼ **FIG. 50-2** Niacin and tryptophan combine to make niacinamide, a needed component for NAD and NADP, which are needed for many body processes.

Mechanism of Action

The actions of vitamin B_3 are not due to niacin in the ingested form but rather to the metabolic product of niacin, niacinamide (except in the function of reducing serum cholesterol). The body may also utilize dietary tryptophan to produce niacinamide by oxidizing niacin and then converting it to niacinamide. As already mentioned, niacinamide is required for lipid metabolism, tissue respiration, and glycogenolysis (see Fig. 50-2).

Drug Effects

The drug effects of niacin result from the production of NAD and NADP, which are necessary for glycogenolysis—the breakdown of stored glycogen to usable glucose. As explained already, it is also necessary for tissue respiration and lipid, protein, and purine metabolism, and it also acts as a cholesterol- and triglyceride-lowering agent by reducing VLDL synthesis.

Therapeutic Uses

Niacin is indicated for the prevention and treatment of **pellagra**, a condition caused by a deficiency of vitamin B_3 that is most commonly the result of malabsorption. As stated earlier, niacin is also an antihyperlipidemic agent that reduces VLDL synthesis, resulting in lower serum cholesterol and triglyceride levels.

Table 50-7	Niacin: Adverse Effects
BODY SYSTEM	**SIDE/ADVERSE EFFECT**
Gastrointestinal	Nausea, vomiting, anorexia, diarrhea, peptic ulcer, jaundice
Central nervous system	Headache, paresthesias, dizziness, anxiety
Integumentary	Flushing, dry skin, rash, pruritis
Cardiovascular	Postural hypotension, vasovagal attacks, dysrhythmias, vasodilation
Genitourinary	Hyperuricemia, glycosuria, hypoalbuminemia

Side Effects and Adverse Effects

Side effects and adverse effects of niacin are rare. They are most commonly associated with large initial doses when niacin is used as an antihyperlipidemic agent. Table 50-7 lists side effects and adverse effects by body system.

Dosages

For the RDAs of niacin see Table 50-1. Commonly recommended dosages of niacin are listed in the dosages table on p. 781.

DRUG PROFILE

Niacin (vitamin B_3) is used to treat pellagra, hyperlipidemias, and peripheral vascular disease. It is classified as a pregnancy category A agent and is contraindicated in patients with peptic ulcer, hepatic disease, hemorrhage, and severe hypotension. Its use is also contraindicated in patients who are lactating and in those who have shown a hypersensitivity reaction to it.

NIACIN

Niacin (Nicobid, Niac, Nia-Bid, Niacels, Niaplus, Nico-400, Nicotinex, Niacor, Slo-Niacin) is available orally as 125-, 250-, 300-, 400-, and 500-mg extended-release capsules; 150-, 250-, 500-, and 750-mg extended-release tablets; 25-, 50-, 100-, 250-, 500-mg regular-strength tablets; and as a 50–mg/5 ml elixir. For the RDAs of niacin see Table 50-1. Commonly recommended dosages of niacin are listed in the dosages table on p. 781.

✸ PHARMACOKINETICS

HALF-LIFE	ONSET	PEAK	DURATION
45 min	Variable	Serum: 45 min	Variable

VITAMIN B₆

Vitamin B$_6$ (Pyridoxine) is composed of three compounds: pyridoxine, pyridoxal, and pyridoxamine. Plant sources that contain pyridoxine include whole grains, wheat germ, nuts, and yeast. Fish and organ meats contain both pyridoxal and pyridoxamine.

Pyridoxine is taken up by red blood cells (RBCs) where it is converted into the coenzyme pyridoxal phosphate, which is necessary for many metabolic functions such as protein, carbohydrate, and lipid utilization in the body. It also plays an important part in the conversion of tryptophan to niacin or serotonin.

Deficiency of vitamin B$_6$ can lead to sideroblastic anemia, neurologic disturbances, seborrheic dermatitis, cheilosis, and xanthurenic aciduria. It may also result in epileptiform convulsions, especially in neonates and infants; hypochromic microcytic anemia; and glossitis and stomatitis. Inadequate intake or poor absorption of pyridoxine causes the development of these conditions. Vitamin B$_6$ deficiency may occur as a result of uremia, alcoholism, cirrhosis, hyperthyroidism, malabsorption syndromes, and congestive heart failure. It may also be induced by various drugs, such as isoniazid (INH), cycloserine, ethionamide, hydralazine, penicillamine, or pyrazinamide.

Mechanism of Action

Pyridoxine, pyridoxal, and pyridoxamine are all converted to the active forms of vitamin B$_6$, *pyridoxal phosphate* and *pyridoxamine phosphate* that act as coenzymes in a wide variety of reactions, including the

Table 50-8	Pyridoxine: Adverse Effects
BODY SYSTEM	**SIDE/ADVERSE EFFECT**
Central nervous system	Paresthesias, flushing, warmth, headache, lethargy
Integumentary	Pain at injection site

transamination of amino acids and the conversion of tryptophan to niacin. They are also essential in the synthesis of gamma-aminobutyric acid (GABA), an inhibitory neurotransmitter in the central nervous system. They are important in the synthesis of heme and the maintenance of the hematopoietic system. Pyridoxine deficiency principally affects the peripheral nerves, skin, mucous membranes, and the hematopoietic system.

Drug Effects

The drug effects of pyridoxine are the result of the two coenzymes pyridoxal phosphate and pyridoxamine phosphate. As already mentioned, pyridoxine is necessary for the integrity of the peripheral nerves, skin, mucous membranes, and the hematopoietic system.

Therapeutic Uses

Pyridoxine is used to prevent and treat vitamin B$_6$ deficiency. Although deficiency of vitamin B$_6$ is rare, it can occur in conditions of inadequate intake or poor absorption of pyridoxine. The situations in which this may occur were explained in a previous section. Seizures that are unresponsive to usual therapy, morning sickness during pregnancy, and various metabolic disorders may respond to pyridoxine therapy.

Side Effects and Adverse Effects

Side effects and adverse effects with pyridoxine are rare and usually do not occur with normal doses; high doses and chronic usage may produce side effects and adverse effects as listed in Table 50-8. Toxic effects are a result of very large doses sustained for several months. Neurotoxicity is the most likely result, but this will subside upon discontinuation of the pyridoxine.

Interactions

Pyridoxine exhibits several significant interactions with selected drugs. Pyridoxine will reduce the activity of levodopa, so vitamin formulations containing B$_6$ should be avoided. Drugs that have an antivitamin effect on pyridoxin include cycloserine, ethionamide, INH, pyrazinamide, and oral contraceptives.

Dosages

For the RDAs of vitamin B_6 see Table 50-1. For the commonly recommended dosages of vitamin B_6 see the dosages table on p. 781.

DRUG PROFILE

Pyridoxine is a water-soluble B complex vitamin composed of three components: pyridoxine, pyridoxal, and pyridoxamine. It has several vital roles in the body but is primarily responsible for the integrity of peripheral nerves, skin, mucous membranes, and the hematopoietic system.

PYRIDOXINE

Pyridoxine (Rodex T.D., Beesix, HexaBetalin) is classified as a pregnancy category A agent and is contraindicated in patients who have shown a hypersensitivity reaction to it. It is available in an oral form 100- and 150-mg as extended-release capsules; a 500-mg extended-release tablet; 10-, 25-, 50-, 100-, 200-, 250-, and 500-mg regular-strength tablets; and a 500-mg regular-strength capsule. For the RDAs of vitamin B_6 see Table 50-1. Commonly recommended dosages of vitamin B_6 are listed in the dosages table on p. 781.

☙ P H A R M A C O K I N E T I C S

HALF-LIFE	ONSET	PEAK	DURATION
15-20 days	Unknown	Unknown	Unknown

VITAMIN B_{12}

Vitamin B_{12} (Cyanocobalamin) is a cobalt-containing, water-soluble B complex vitamin. It is synthesized by microorganisms and is present in the body as two different coenzymes, adenosylcobalamin and methylcobalamin. Cyanocobalamin is a required coenzyme for many metabolic pathways, including fat and carbohydrate metabolism and protein synthesis. It is also required for growth, cell replication, hematopoiesis, and nucleoprotein and myelin synthesis (See Fig. 50-3).

Cyanocobalamin is present in foods of animal origin, particularly liver, kidney, fish and shellfish, meat, and dairy foods. Plants contain only minimal amounts. Vitamin B_{12} deficiency will result in GI lesions, neurologic symptoms that can result in degenerative CNS lesions, and megaloblastic anemia. The major cause of cyanocobalamin deficiency is malabsorption. Other possible but less likely causes are poor diet, chronic alcoholism, and chronic hemorrhage.

Mechanism of Action

It is essential that humans have an exogenous source of cyanocobalamin because it is required for nucleoprotein and myelin synthesis, cell reproduction, normal growth, and the maintenance of normal erythropoiesis. The cells that have the greatest requirement for vitamin B_{12} are those that divide rapidly such as epithelial cells, bone marrow, and myeloid cells.

Reduced sulfhydryl (SH) groups are required to metabolize fats and carbohydrates and to synthesize protein. Cyanocobalamin is involved in maintaining sulfhydryl (SH) groups in the reduced form that is required by many SH-activated enzyme systems. Cyanocobalamin deficiency can lead to neurologic damage that begins with an inability to produce myelin and is followed by gradual degeneration of the axon and nerve head.

Cyanocobalamin has biologic activity that is identical to that of the antipernicious factor present in liver extract called the extrinsic factor and Castle's factor. The oral absorption of cyanocobalamin (extrinsic factor) requires the presence of the intrinsic factor (gastric intrinsic factor), which is a glycoprotein secreted by gastric parietal cells. A complex is formed between the two factors and is then absorbed by the intestines. This is depicted in Fig. 50-4.

▼ FIG. 50-3 Cyanocobalamin is a required coenzyme for many metabolic pathways.

Drug Effects

The drug effects of cyanocobalamin are very much like those of the other water-soluble vitamins. It is used to treat or prevent vitamin B_{12} deficiency caused by malabsorption or strict vegetarianism. If not treated this condition can lead to megaloblastic anemia and irreversible neurologic damage. Cyanocobalamin is also useful in the treatment of pernicious anemia caused by a endogenous lack of intrinsic factor.

Therapeutic Uses

Cyanocobalamin is used to treat deficiency states that develop because of an insufficient intake of the vitamin. As mentioned this is most often the result of malabsorption or poor dietary intake. Poor dietary intake is most common in vegetarians because the primary source of cyanocobalamin is foods of animal origin. Cyanocobalamin is used to treat vitamin B_{12} deficiency states, especially pernicious anemia. It is also included in a multivitamin formulation that is used as a dietary supplement.

The use of vitamin B_{12} to treat pernicious anemia and other megaloblastic anemias results in a rapid conversion of a megaloblastic bone marrow to a normoblastic bone marrow. The preferred route of administration of vitamin B_{12} in treating megaloblastic anemias is by deep IM injection.

Side Effects and Adverse Effects

Vitamin B_{12} is nontoxic and large doses must be ingested to produce adverse effects, which include itching, transitory diarrhea, and fever. Other side ef-

fects and adverse effects are listed by body system in the Table 50-9.

Interactions

Use with anticonvulsants, aminoglycoside antibiotics, and long-acting potassium preparations will decrease the oral absorption of vitamin B_{12}. In addition it has been suggested that chloramphenicol will antagonize the hematologic response of vitamin B_{12}.

Dosages

For RDAs of vitamin B_{12} see Table 50-1. Commonly recommended dosages of vitamin B_{12} are listed in the dosages table on p. 781.

Table 50-9	Cyanocobalamin: Adverse Effects
BODY SYSTEM	**SIDE/ADVERSE EFFECT**
Central nervous system	Flushing, optic nerve atrophy
Integumentary	Itching, rash, pain at injection site
Cardiovascular	Congestive heart failure, peripheral vascular thrombosis, pulmonary edema
Gastrointestinal	Diarrhea
Metabolic	Hypokalemia

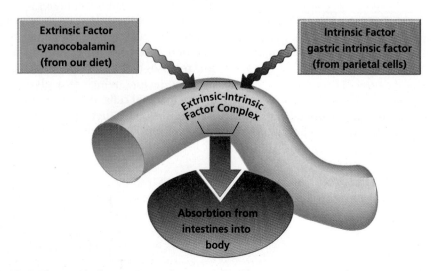

▼ **FIG. 50-4** The oral absorption of cyanocobalamin requires the presence of the intrinsic factor secreted by gastric parietal cells.

DRUG PROFILE

Cyanocobalamin is a water-soluble B complex vitamin required for maintaining body fat and carbohydrate metabolism and protein synthesis. It is also needed for growth, cell replication, blood cell production, and the integrity of normal nerve function.

CYANOCOBALAMIN

Cyanocobalamin (Redisol, Rubramin PC, Betalin-12, Sytobex, Cyanoject) is available both as OTC preparations and by prescription. Most of the OTC cyanocobalamin-containing products are multivitamin preparations, while many of the sole cyanocobalamin-containing products contain large doses for parenteral injection and are available by prescription only. Cyanocobalamin is classified as a pregnancy category A agent and is contraindicated in patients who have shown a hypersensitivity reaction to it and in those with optic nerve atrophy.

Cyanocobalamin is available orally as 25-, 50-, 100-, 250-, 500-, and 1000-μg tablets and parenterally as 30-, 100-, and 1000-μg/ml injections. Commonly recommended dosages for vitamin B_{12} are listed in the dosages table on p. 781.

☙ PHARMACOKINETICS

HALF-LIFE	ONSET	PEAK	DURATION
6 days	Unknown	Plasma: 8-12 hr	Unknown

VITAMIN C

Vitamin C (ascorbic acid) is a water-soluble vitamin present in citrus fruits and juices, tomatoes, cabbage, cherries, and liver. It can be synthesized for use as a drug and is used in many therapeutic situations. Prolonged ascorbic acid deficiency results in the nutritional disease **scurvy,** which is characterized by gingivitis and bleeding gums, loss of teeth, anemia, subcutaneous hemorrhage, bone lesions, and delayed healing of soft tissues and bones. It was recognized for several centuries, especially among sailors; in 1795 the British navy ordered the eating of limes to prevent the disease.

Mechanism of Action

Vitamin C is reversibly oxidized to dehydroascorbic acid in the body, and it acts in oxidation-reduction reactions. It is required for several important metabolic activities, including collagen synthesis and the maintenance of connective tissue; tissue repair; maintenance of bone, teeth, and capillaries; and folic acid metabolism (specifically, the conversion of folic acid into its active metabolite). Accordingly, it is essential for erythropoiesis. Vitamin C enhances the absorption of iron and is required for the synthesis of lipids, proteins, and steroids. It has also been shown to aid in cellular respiration and resistance to infections.

Drug Effects

The drug effects of vitamin C are the prevention of scurvy and dietary supplementation. Because vitamin C is an acid, it can also be used as a urinary acidifier. In larger doses vitamin C is also believed to lessen the severity of and prevent the common cold.

Therapeutic Uses

Vitamin C is used to treat diseases associated with vitamin C deficiency and as a dietary supplement. It is most beneficial in patients who require larger daily requirements because of pregnancy, lactation, hyperthyroidism, fever, stress, infection, trauma, burns, smoking, and cold exposure and the consumption of certain drugs (e.g., estrogens, oral contraceptives, barbiturates, tetracyclines, and salicylates). The benefits of other uses of vitamin C are less well documented. For example it is a common practice to take vitamin C to prevent or treat the common cold. However, most large controlled studies have shown that ascorbic acid has little or no value as a prophylactic for colds.

Side Effects and Adverse Effects

Vitamin C is usually nontoxic unless excessive dosages are consumed. Megadoses can produce nausea, vomiting, headache, and abdominal cramps and will acidify the urine, resulting in the formation of cystine, oxalate, and urate renal stones. Furthermore, individuals who discontinue taking excessive daily doses of ascorbic acid can suffer from scurvy-like symptoms.

Interactions

Ascorbic acid has the potential to interact with many classes of drugs. However, clinical experience concerning many interactions is inconclusive. For example, it has been reported that ascorbic acid can decrease the effectiveness of oral anticoagulants. This does not always happen, but practitioners should be aware of this possibility. Coadministration of acid-labile drugs such as penicillin G or erythromycin should be avoided. As already mentioned, megadoses of vitamin C can acidify the urine, which can enhance the excretion of basic drugs and delay the excretion of acidic drugs.

Dosages

The RDAs of vitamin C are listed in Table 50-1. For the commonly recommended dosages of vitamin C see the dosages table on p. 781.

DRUG PROFILE

Ascorbic acid is a water-soluble vitamin required in the prevention and treatment of scurvy. As previously explained, it is required for erythropoiesis and the synthesis of lipids, protein, and steroids.

ASCORBIC ACID

Ascorbic acid (Ascorbicap, Cebid Timecelles, Cetane, Cspan, Ce-Vi-Sol, Cecon) is available in OTC preparations such as multivitamin products and by prescription. It is classified as a pregnancy category A agent and has no contraindications.

Ascorbic acid is available orally as a 60-mg lozenge; 60-, 100-, and 500-mg/ml solutions; a 500-mg extended-release capsule; 50-, 100-, 250-, 500-, and 1000-mg tablets; 100-, 250-, 500-, and 1000-mg chewable tablets; and 500-, 1000-, and 1500-mg extended-release tablets. It is also available parenterally as a 100-, 250-, and 500-mg/ml injections. See Table 50-1 for the RDAs for vitamin C. Commonly recommended dosages are listed in the dosages table on p. 781.

PHARMACOKINETICS

HALF-LIFE	ONSET	PEAK	DURATION
Unknown	Unknown	Unknown	Unknown

Minerals

Minerals are essential nutrients that are classified as inorganic compounds. They act as building blocks for many body structures and thus are necessary for a variety of physiologic functions. They are also needed for intracellular and extracellular body fluid electrolytes.

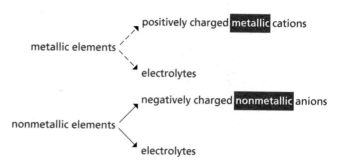

▼ **FIG. 50-5** When mineral compounds are dissolved in water, they separate into positively charged metabolic cations or negatively charged nonmetallic anions and electrolytes.

Iron is essential for the production of hemoglobin, which is necessary for oxygen transport throughout the body. Minerals are required for muscle contraction, nerve transmission, and the makeup of essential enzymes.

Mineral compounds are composed of various metallic and nonmetallic elements that are chemically combined with ionic bonds. When these compounds are dissolved in water they separate (dissociate) into positively charged metallic cations and electrolytes or negatively charged nonmetallic anions and electrolytes (see Fig. 50-5).

Ingestion of mineral nutrients provide essential elements necessary for vital bodily functions. Elements that are required in larger amounts are called *macrominerals*; those required in smaller amounts are called *microminerals* or *trace elements*. Table 50-10 lists the classification of nutrient elements as either macro- or microminerals and as metal or nonmetal.

CALCIUM

Calcium is the most abundant mineral element in the human body, accounting for approximately 2% of the total body weight. The highest concentration of calcium is in bones and teeth. Calcium is widely distributed in many foods, especially milk and dairy products. Calcium requirements are high for growing children and for women who are pregnant or breastfeeding. The efficient absorption of calcium requires adequate amounts of vitamin D.

Calcium deficiency results in hypocalcemia and affects many bodily functions. Causes of calcium deficiency include inadequate calcium intake and/or insufficient vitamin D to facilitate absorption, hypoparathyroidism, and malabsorption syndrome, especially in older persons. Calcium deficiency–related disorders include infantile rickets, adult osteomalacia, muscle cramps, osteoporosis (especially in postmenopausal females), hypothyroidism, and renal dysfunc-

Table 50-10 | Mineral Elements

ELEMENT	SYMBOL	TYPE	IONIC/ELECTROLYTE FORM
Macrominerals			
Calcium*	Ca	Metal	Ca^{+2} calcium cation
Chlorine	Cl	Nonmetal	Cl^{-1} chloride anion
Magnesium*	Mg	Metal	Mg^{+2} magnesium cation
Phosphorus*	P	Nonmetal	PO_4^{-3} phosphate anion
Potassium	K	Metal	K^{+1} potassium cation
Sodium	Na	Metal	Na^{+1} sodium cation
Sulfur	S	Nonmetal	SO_4^{-2} sulfate anion
Microminerals			
Chromium	Cr	Metal	CR^{+3} chromium cation
Cobalt	Co	Metal	Co^{+2} cobalt cation
Copper	Cu	Metal	Cu^{+2} copper cation
Fluorine	F	Nonmetal	F^{-1} fluoride anion
Iodine*	I	Nonmetal	I^{-1} iodide anion
Iron*	Fe	Metal	Fe^{++} ferrous cation
Manganese	Mn	Metal	Mn^{+2} manganese cation
Molybdenum	Mo	Metal	Mo^{+6} molybdenum cation
Selenium*	Se	Metal	Se^{+4} selenium cation
Zinc*	Zn	Metal	Zn^{+2} zinc cation

*Mineral elements that have a current RDA.

Table 50-11 | Calcium Deficiency: Causes and Disorders

CAUSE	DISORDER
Inadequate intake	Infantile rickets
Insufficient vitamin D	Adult osteomalacia
Hypoparathyroidism	Muscle cramps
Malabsorption syndrome	Osteoporosis

tion. Table 50-11 lists the possible causes of calcium deficiency and the resulting disorders.

Calcium is essential for the normal maintenance and function of the nervous, muscular, and skeletal systems as well as cell membrane and capillary permeability. It is an important catalyst in many enzymatic reactions and is essential in many physiologic processes, including transmission of nerve impulses; contraction of cardiac, smooth, and skeletal muscles; renal function; respiration; and blood coagulation. Calcium also plays a regulatory role in the release and storage of neurotransmitters and hormones, in white blood cell and harmone activity, in the uptake and binding of amino acids, and in intestinal absorption of cyanocobalamin (vitamin B_{12}) and gastrin secretion. The roles of calcium in normal physiologic processes are summarized in Table 50-12.

Mechanism of Action

Calcium participates in a variety of essential physiologic functions and is a building block for body structures. Specifically calcium is involved with the proper development and maintenance of teeth and skeletal bones. It is an important catalyst in many of the coagulation pathways in the blood. Calcium acts as a cofactor in clotting reactions involving the intrinsic and extrinsic pathways of thromboplastin. It is also a cofactor in the conversion of prothrombin to thrombin by thromboplastin and the conversion of fibrinogen to fibrin.

Drug Effects

Calcium salts are used as a source of calcium cations for the treatment or prevention of calcium depletion in patients for whom dietary measures are inad-

Table 50-12	Physiologic Processes Requiring Calcium
ROLE	**PHYSIOLOGIC INFLUENCE**
Normal maintenance and function	Nervous system Muscular system Skeletal system Cell membranes Capillary permeability
Physiologic processes	Transmission of nerve impulses Contraction of cardiac, smooth, and skeletal muscles Renal function Respiration Blood coagulation
Regulatory	Release and storage of neurotransmitters and hormones Uptake and binding of amino acids Cyanocobalamin (vitamin B_{12}) absorption Gastrin secretion

Table 50-13	Calcium Salts: Calcium Content
CALCIUM SALT	**CA CONTENT (PER GRAM)**
Phosphate tribasic	400 mg (20 mEq)
Carbonate	400 mg (20 mEq)
Phosphate dibasic anhydrous	290 mg (14.5 mEq)
Chloride	270 mg (13.5 mEq)
Acetate	253 mg (12.7 mEq)
Phosphate dibasic dihydrate	230 mg (11.5 mEq)
Citrate	211 mg (10.6 mEq)
Glycerophosphate	191 mg (9.6 mEq)
Lactate	130 mg (6.5 mEq)
Gluconate	90 mg (4.5 mEq)
Gluceptate	82 mg (4.1 mEq)
Glubionate	64 mg (3.2 mEq)

equate. There are many conditions that may be associated with calcium deficiency as listed below:
- Hypoparathyroidism
- Vitamin D deficiency
- Pregnancy and lactation
- Renal failure
- Achlorhydria
- Steatorrhea
- Menopause
- Alkalosis
- Chronic diarrhea
- Sprue
- Pancreatitis
- Hyperphosphatemia

Table 50-14	Calcium Salts: Adverse Effects
BODY SYSTEM	**SIDE/ADVERSE EFFECT**
Gastrointestinal	Constipation, obstruction, nausea, vomiting, flatulence
Cardiovascular	Hemorrhage, rebound hypertension
Metabolic	Hypercalcemia, metabolic alkalosis
Genitourinary	Renal dysfunction, renal stones, renal failure

Therapeutic Uses

Calcium is used to treat various manifestations of deficiency states, including adult osteomalacia, hypothyroidism, infantile rickets or tetany, muscle cramps, osteoporosis, and renal insufficiency. In addition, calcium is used as a dietary supplement for women during pregnancy and lactation.

There are over 12 different selected calcium salts available for treatment or nutritional supplementation. Each calcium salt contains a different amount of elemental calcium per gram of calcium salt. Table 50-13 lists the available salts and their associated calcium contents.

Side Effects and Adverse Effects

Although adverse effects and toxicity are rare, hypercalcemia can occur; symptoms include anorexia, nausea, vomiting, and constipation. In addition when calcium salts are administered by intramuscular or subcutaneous injection, mild to severe local reactions, including burning, necrosis and sloughing of tissue, cellulitis, and soft tissue calcification, may occur. Venous irritation may occur with intravenous administration. Other side effects and adverse effects associated with both oral and parenteral use of calcium salts are listed in Table 50-14.

Toxicity and Management of Overdose

Chronic and excessive calcium intake can result in severe hypercalcemia, which can cause cardiac irregularities, delirium, and coma. Management of acute hypercalcemia may require hemodialysis, whereas milder cases will respond to discontinuation of calcium intake.

Interactions

Calcium salts will complex with tetracyclines to produce an insoluble complex. Use in patients taking digitalis preparations can produce serious cardiac arrhythmias.

Dosages

For the RDAs of calcium see Table 50-1.

*D*RUG PROFILE

CALCIUM

Calcium salts are minerals that are primarily used in the treatment or prevention of calcium depletion in patients in whom dietary measures are inadequate. There are many calcium salts available, all with a different content of elemental calcium per gram of salt. Calcium is available in both oral and parenteral forms.

The calcium salts are classified as pregnancy category C agents and are contraindicated in patients who have shown a hypersensitivity reaction to them and in patients with hypercalcemia, hyperparathyroidism, and bone tumors. There are numerous dosages and names of calcium preparations. Consult manufacturer instructions for recommended dosages. The calcium salts are available in liquid-filled capsules, powders, oral suspensions, tablets, chewable tablets, film-coated tablets, oral solutions, and parenteral injections. For the RDAs of calcium see Table 50-1.

♟ P H A R M A C O K I N E T I C S

HALF-LIFE	ONSET	PEAK	DURATION
Unknown	Unknown	Unknown	Unknown

MAGNESIUM

Magnesium is one of the principal cations present in the intracellular fluid. It is an essential part of many enzyme systems associated with energy metabolism. Magnesium deficiency (hypomagnesia) is usually caused by (1) malabsorption, especially in the presence of high calcium intake, (2) alcoholism, (3) long-term IV feeding, (4) diuretics, and (5) metabolic disorders, including hyperthyroidism and diabetic ketoacidosis. Symptoms associated with hypomagnesia include cardiovascular disturbances, neuromuscular impairment, and mental disturbances.

Dietary intake from vegetables and other foods will usually prevent magnesium deficiency. However, magnesium is required in greater amounts in individuals with diets high in protein-rich foods, calcium, and phosphorous.

Mechanism of Action

The precise mechanism for magnesium has not been fully determined. Magnesium is a known cofactor for many enzyme systems. It is required for muscle contraction and nerve physiology. Magnesium produces an anticonvulsant effect by inhibiting neuromuscular transmission for selected convulsive states.

Therapeutic Uses

Magnesium is used to treat magnesium deficiency and as a nutritional supplement in total parenteral nutrition (TPN) and multivitamin preparations. It is used as an anticonvulsant in magnesium deficiency, preeclampsia, and eclampsia.

Side Effects and Adverse Effects

Adverse effects of magnesium are due to hypermagnesia, which results in (1) tendon reflex loss, (2) difficult bowel movements, (3) CNS depression, (4) respiratory distress and heart block, and (5) hypothermia.

Toxicity and Management of Overdose

Toxic effects are extensions of symptoms caused by hypermagnesia, a major cause of which is the long-term use of magnesium products (especially antacids in patients with renal dysfunction). Severe hypermagnesia is treated with a calcium salt administered IV in doses up to 10 mEq.

Interactions

Use of magnesium with neuromuscular blocking agents and CNS depressants produces additive effects.

Dosages

The RDA for magnesium is 6 to 10 mg for infants and children, 10 to 15 mg for women, and 10 to 12 mg for men. The usual dose of magnesium for treating convulsant conditions is 4 to 5 g IV or IM, repeated as required. For the RDAs of magnesium see Table 50-1.

DRUG PROFILE

MAGNESIUM

Magnesium is a mineral that has a variety of dosage forms and uses. Magnesium is an essential part of many enzyme systems. When absent or diminished in the body, cardiovascular, neuromuscular, and mental disturbances can occur.

Magnesium sulfate is the most common form of magnesium used as a mineral replacement. It is classified as a pregnancy category C agent and is contraindicated in hypersensitivity and renal disease. It is available in the parenteral form as a 4%, 8%, 10%, 12.5%, and 50% injection. For the RDA of magnesium see Table 50-1.

PHOSPHORUS

Phosphorus is widely distributed in foods, and thus a dietary deficiency is rare. Deficiency states are usually nondietary and are primarily due to (1) malabsorption, (2) extensive diarrhea or vomiting, (3) hyperthyroidism, (4) hepatic disease, and (5) long-term use of aluminum or calcium antacids.

Mechanism of Action

Phosphorus in the form of the phosphate group and/or anion (PO_4^{-3}) is a required precursor for the synthesis of essential body chemicals. In addition, the mineral is an important building block for body structures. Phosphorus is required as a structural unit for the synthesis of nucleic acid and the adenosine-phosphate compounds (adenosine monophosphate [AMP], adenosine disphosphate [ADP], and adenosine triphosphate [ATP]) responsible for cellular energy transfer. It is also necessary for the development and maintenance of the skeletal system and teeth. The skeletal bones contain up to 85% of the phosphorus content of the body. In addition, magnesium is required for the proper utilization of many B-complex vitamins, and it is an essential component of physiologic buffering systems.

Therapeutic Uses

Phosphorus is used to treat deficiency states and as a dietary supplement in many multivitamin formulations.

Side Effects and Adverse Effects

Adverse effects are usually associated with phosphorus replacement products. Effects include diarrhea, nausea, vomiting, and other GI disturbances. Other side effects include confusion, weakness, and breathing difficulties.

Toxicity and Management of Overdose

Toxic reactions to phosphorus are extremely rare and are usually restricted to the ingestion of the pure element.

Interactions

Antacids can reduce the oral absorption of phosphorus.

Dosages

The RDA for phosphorus is 300 to 800 mg for infants and children and 300 to 800 mg for adults. For the RDAs of phosphorus see Table 50-1.

DRUG PROFILE

PHOSPHORUS

Phosphorus is a very essential mineral to our well-being. It is needed to make energy in the form of adenosine diphosphate and triphosphate (ADP and ATP) for all our bodily processes. Fortunately it is present in a variety of foods and drinks, and a true dietary deficiency is rare. Phosphorus is present in a large number of drug formulations and appears as a phosphate salt (PO_4).

Phosphorus is classified as a pregnancy category C agent and should be used with caution in patients with renal impairment. It is available in both oral and parenteral formulations. Oral phosphorus comes as capsules and tablets. The capsules come as sodium phosphate and contain 250 μg of phosphorus combined with 7 mEq of sodium and 7 mEq of potassium and as potassium phosphate that contains 250 μg of phosphorus combined with 14.25 mEq of potassium. The parenteral form contains 94 μg of phosphorus with 4 mEq of sodium per milliliter. Recommended dosages vary depending on the indication. The RDA is listed in Table 50-1.

NURSING PROCESS

ASSESSMENT

Before administering any vitamins, the nurse must assess patients for any nutritional disorders with an evaluation of baseline hemoglobin (Hgb), hematocrit (Hct), white blood cell (WBC) and red blood cell (RBC) counts, and protein and albumin levels. A daily journal of dietary intake and a history of dietary patterns and meals must also be documented. To test for vitamin A deficiency a baseline assessment of the patient's vision, including night vision, and an examination of the appearance of the skin and mucous membranes must be done. Serum laboratory values of vitamin A less than 20 μg/dl in adults and 10 μg/dl in children indicate a deficiency. Interactions of vitamin A with the drug isotretinon may lead to toxicity, with manifestations such as headache, nausea, vomiting, elevated liver enzymes, and dry, cracked skin.

Vitamin D is contraindicated in patients with hypercalcemia or hypervitaminosis D. Cautious use is recommended, with close and careful monitoring in patients with arteriosclerosis, hyperphosphatemia, renal or cardiac dysfunction, and hypersensitivity to vitamin D. Baseline assessment should include a status assessment of the patient's skeletal formation and a baseline serum calcium level. Serum calcium levels under 7.5 mg/dl indicate possible vitamin D deficiency. In addition, it would be advisable to monitor baseline levels of inorganic phosphorus and serum citrate. Drug interactions may occur with antacids, high doses of calcium preparations, thiazide diuretics, and products high in vitamin D.

Before administering vitamin E, patients should be assessed for hypoprothrombinemia secondary to vitamin E deficiency. Vitamin E will aggravate those conditions and result in hematologic problems such as bleeding. Baseline assessment data include a check of skin integrity and determination of the presence or absence of edema and any muscle weakness.

Vitamin B (thiamine) hypersensitivity may cause skin rash and wheezing. Since it is rare that only one vitamin B deficiency occurs, deficiencies of all forms of vitamin B must be ruled out. Baseline assessments of vital signs, mental status, and urinary thiamine levels must be done. For adults, less than 27 μg/dl indicates deficiency.

Vitamin C is contraindicated in patients with cystinuria, oxalosis, or a history of gout or urate kidney stones. In patients with sickle cell anemia, large doses of vitamin C may precipitate a sickle cell crisis. Diabetic patients may experience abnormal glucose levels when taking large doses of vitamin C.

There are few contraindications to the administration of trace elements. However, baseline assessments of nutritional status and specific nutrition-related laboratory studies (Hgb, Hct, RBC and WBC counts, trace elemental laboratory values) should be ordered by the physician and documented before initiation of therapy. Trace elements should be administered as ordered and only after the element or mineral and reviewed laboratory studies and specific manufacturer guidelines for administration have been researched. Cautious use is recommended in any patient with liver or biliary disease.

Before administering calcium and magnesium the patients' current levels should be obtained and recorded. Calcium is contraindicated in patients who are hypercalcemic and have digitalis toxicity, ventricular fibrillation, or renal calculi. Cautious use is recommended in patients who are pregnant or breastfeeding, in children, in patients with renal or respiratory disease or failure, and in patients taking digitalis. Calcium interacts with digitalis, calcium channel blockers, amphotericin, cephalothin, digoxin, digitoxin, epinephrine, tetracycline, sodium warfarin, phosphate, and sodium bicarbonate. Baseline ECGs are often necessary in patients who have cardiac disease. If decreased QT and T wave inversion are observed, calcium is often discontinued or given in reduced dosages.

Magnesium is contraindicated in patients with hypersensitivity to it, and cautious use is recommended in patients with severe renal disease, GI bleeding, diarrhea, and possible intestinal obstruction. Magnesium interacts with tetracyclines, anticholinergics, iron salts, cimetidine, corticosteroids, and chlordiazepoxide.

NURSING DIAGNOSES

Nursing diagnoses include, but are not limited to:

Vitamin A therapy
- Sensory/perceptual deficit related to night blindness.
- Impaired sensory integrity related to nutritional deficiency.

Vitamin D therapy
- Altered comfort or pain, related to bone and skeletal deformities.
- Impaired physical mobility related to poorly developed muscles.

Vitamin E
- Impaired mobility (muscle weakness) related to vitamin E deficiency.
- Altered bowel elimination, diarrhea, related to vitamin E use.

- Risk for self-injury related to side effects of vitamin E therapy.
  Vitamin B₁ (thiamine) deficiency
- Altered thought processes with confusion and psychosis.
  Other vitamin B forms
- Impaired mobility related to poor nutrition.
  Vitamin C (ascorbic acid)
- Pain in joints related to disease.
- Impaired skin and integrity related to lack of Vitamin C.
- Altered protection to skin related to deficiency of Vitamin C.

PLANNING

Goals related to the use of vitamins and minerals are as follows:
- Patient will maintain sensory and perceptual integrity during therapy.

- Patient experiences minimal complaints related to vitamin and mineral therapy.
- Patient's skin integrity remains intact.
- Patient regains and maintains activity level considered normal for him or her.

Outcome Criteria

Outcome criteria related to the above goals include the following:
- Patient openly verbalizes fears and anxieties about possible visual changes.
- Patient keeps skin clean, dry to moist (as needed), to maintain skin intactness and prevent infection.
- Patient increases ADLs as warranted and as tolerated.
- Patient returns to pre-illness levels of functioning.

Patient Teaching TIPS

Vitamins, Minerals, and Trace Elements

✔ Patients should be provided with information and counseling about the best sources of dietary vitamin A, such as egg yolks, butter, milk, liver, kidney, cream, cheese, and fortified margarine. Carotene, the precursor to vitamin A, is found in leafy green vegetables and yellow and orange fruits and vegetables.

✔ Patients taking vitamin D should be closely monitored and should maintain regular visits to the physician for review of diet and calcium therapy. Patients should be instructed about foods high in vitamin D such as egg yolks, vitamin D–fortified milk, fish liver oils, whole grain cereals, wheat germ, liver, and vegetable oils. Unless medically contraindicated, careful exposure to the sun should be encouraged.

✔ Patients should be provided with information and counseling about necessary foods to include in their diet. Examples of such information follow.

✔ Foods high in vitamin E include vegetable oils, wheat germ, whole grain cereals, egg yolks, and liver.

✔ Vitamin B is found in many different foods. Thiamine is found in enriched cereals or whole grains, pork, nuts, fish, organ and muscle meats, poultry, rice bran, and green vegetables. Riboflavin is found in milk and other dairy products, meats, eggs, fish, poultry, and enriched grains and cereals.

✔ Niacin is found in meats, eggs, whole grain and enriched cereals, breads, flour, milk, and other diary products. Pyridoxine is found in meats, poultry, fish, eggs, whole grains, sweet potatoes, lima beans, and bananas.

✔ Patients who have had a gastrectomy or ileal resection or who have pernicious anemia should be informed of the necessity for cyanocobalamin in their diet.

✔ Patients taking up to 600 mg/day of vitamin C should be informed that they may experience a slight increase in daily urination patterns and that more than 1 g per day may lead to diarrhea. They should also be informed of foods high in ascorbic acid such as citrus fruits, tomatoes, strawberries, cantaloupe, and raw peppers.

✔ Patients taking trace elements (e.g., zinc, copper, magnesium, iodine, chromium) must take medication as prescribed. They should also know to call the physician if any unusual reactions occur.

✔ Patients who are trying to increase calcium intake should be informed of foods high in calcium, such as milk and other dairy products, shellfish, and dark green leafy vegetables. Patients taking calcium supplements should be told not to eat foods high in oxalate and zinc such as nuts, legumes, chocolate, spinach, and soy products and to avoid bran because these foods decrease the absorption of oral calcium supplementation. Patients should also know that calcium products chelate or bind with tetracyclines and thus decrease or negate their effects.

IMPLEMENTATION

Before administering vitamin A, the nurse should check and document the patient's diet and signs and symptoms of hypervitaminosis and hypercarotenemia (excess vitamin A). Vitamin D should be given with concurrent evaluations of renal functioning and serum calcium levels, especially at the beginning of therapy. The nurse should monitor growth measurements before start of therapy in children, and all patients should be assessed for signs of toxicity such as constipation, anorexia, nausea, vomiting, metallic taste, and dry mouth.

The water-miscible forms of vitamin E are more rapidly absorbed, and patients should always be encouraged to obtain adequate vitamin intake through diet. Vitamin B$_1$ (thiamine) therapy is usually administered in an oral preparation, but parenteral forms are also available. Niacin should be administered with milk or food to decrease GI upset. Oral forms of niacin are preferred. If administered IV, pyridoxine should be given at a rate of 50 mg/min and may be given with most IV fluids. Cyanocobalamin should be administered orally with meals to increase its absorption. Ascorbic acid should be administered orally, if possible; if administered IV it should be given at a rate no greater than 100 mg/min. The oral effervescent forms should be dissolved in at least 6 oz of fluid such as water or juice.

When vitamin C is prescribed for acidification of the urine, it is important to frequently assess urinary pH. If vitamin C is administered IV, it should be given as a continuous infusion (not to exceed 100 mg/min) as an additive to IV solutions. Oral effervescent tablets should be dissolved thoroughly in water before administration.

Because of venous irritation, calcium should be given via an IV infusion pump when given intravenously. The nurse should also monitor closely for hypercalcemia. Calcium should be given slowly intravenously (<1 ml/min for adults) to avoid cardiac arrhythmias and cardiac arrest, and the patient should be kept recumbent for 15 minutes after the infusion. Should extravasation occur, you should discontinue the infusion immediately. The physician may order infusion with 1% procaine or other antidote to reduce vasospasm and to dilute the effects of calcium on surrounding tissue. Follow institutional guidelines regarding treatment of calcium extravasation. Oral calcium supplements should be given 1 to 2 hours after meals.

Magnesium should be administered according to manufacturer guidelines and as ordered. Because different dosages result in different effects, always recheck the order, dosage, and intended use and therapeutic effects. For patient teaching tips see p. 800.

EVALUATION

Therapeutic responses to vitamin A therapy include restoration of normal vision and intact skin. Side effects include lethargy, night blindness, skin and corneal changes, and, in infancy, failure to thrive. Therapeutic response to vitamin D include improved bone growth and formation and an intact skeleton with decreased or no pain. Side effects include constipation, anorexia, metallic taste, and dry mouth.

Therapeutic responses to vitamin E include improved muscle strength, more intact skin, and alphatocopherol levels within normal limits. Side effects include blurred vision, dizziness, drowsiness, breast enlargement, and flulike symptoms. Therapeutic response to vitamin B (thiamine) includes improved mental status with less confusion. Therapeutic responses to riboflavin, niacin, pyridoxine, and cyanocobalamin include improved skin integrity, normal vision, improved mental status, and normal RBC, Hgb, and Hct levels. Therapeutic responses to vitamin C include improved capillary intactness, improved skin and mucous membrane integrity, and improved heal-

TAKE HOME POINTS

Nursing Considerations

■ Over the counter use of vitamins and minerals may lead to serious problems and side effects; therefore a physician should be consulted before supplementation.

■ Nurses must incorporate the nutritional status of each patient into the nursing care plan to provide "comprehensive" care during medication therapy.

■ The nurse's participation in health promotion and wellness includes providing information about dietary needs and the body's need for vitamins and minerals.

■ Patient education as related to vitamin and mineral replacement must focus on dietary sources of the specific nutrient, drug and food interactions, and side effects. Patients must be instructed about when it is necessary to contact the physician.

■ Vitamins and minerals can be dangerous to the patient if given without concern and caution for the patient's overall condition and underlying disease processes.

■ Never assume that because the drug is a vitamin or a mineral it does not have adverse reactions or toxicity—most of them can become toxic.

ing, as well as improved energy and mental state. An adverse reaction associated with vitamin C is precipitate formation in the urine with possible stone formation. Side effects for the B vitamins and ascorbic acid are included in the discussion and tables pertinent to each vitamin.

Therapeutic responses to trace elements include resolution of the deficient state and associated signs and symptoms, depending on the specific element or mineral.

Critical Thinking **A C T I V I T I E S**

1. Explain why patients with a cardiac history need a baseline ECG and serum calcium assessment performed before initiation of calcium supplemental therapy.

2. Your patient is experiencing constipation and abdominal pain since beginning calcium therapy. Your assessment reveals a distended abdomen and diminished bowel sounds. What could possibly be occurring, and what should your nursing actions be at this time?

3. Ms. Wall takes 2500 mg calcium carbonate daily in the form of an OTC calcium supplement. How much elemental calcium is Ms. Wall actually taking?

BIBLIOGRAPHY

Albanese J, Nutz P: *Mosby's 1995 nursing drug cards,* St Louis, 1995, Mosby.

Johnson KB: *Harriet Lane handbook,* ed 13, St Louis, 1993, Mosby.

Keen JH: *Critical care and emergency drug reference,* St Louis, 1994, Mosby.

Knoben JE, Anderson PO: *Handbook of critical drug data,* ed 6, Hamilton, Ill, 1988, Drug Intelligence Publications.

Margen S et al: Vitamin supplementation: fact and fancy, Hosp Med 25(4):102, 1989.

McEvoy GK: *AHFS drug information,* Bethesda, Md, 1994, American Society of Hospital Pharmacists.

McKenry L, Salerno E: *Mosby's pharmacology in nursing,* ed 17, St Louis, 1995, Mosby.

Skidmore-Roth L: *Mosby's 1995 nursing drug reference,* St Louis, 1995, Mosby.

Chapter 51

Nutritional Supplements

Objectives

When you reach the end of this chapter, you will be able to:

1 Discuss the anatomy and physiology related to the use of enteral and parenteral nurtritional feedings.

2 List the various enteral supplemental feedings and parenteral feedings and the major ingredients for both.

3 Describe the process of initiating and maintaining continuous and intermittent enteral feedings, as well as the process of initiating and maintaining total parenteral nutrition (TPN).

4 Compare the use of older nasogastric tubes versus the newer, smaller, more flexible tubes.

5 Discuss the mechanisms of action, cautions, contraindications, and associated nursing implications for the various enteral feedings and parenteral nutritional feedings.

6 Develop a comprehensive nursing care plan, including patient education for patients receiving enteral and parenteral supplemental feedings.

7 Identify home health care needs for patients receiving enteral or parenteral nutritional feedings at home.

CHAPTER OUTLINE

Enteral Nutrition

Mechanism of action
Drug effects
Therapeutic uses
Side effects and adverse effects
Interactions
Dosages

Drug Profiles
Elemental Formulations
   Vivonex
Polymeric Formulations
   Ensure
Modular Formulations
   Carbohydrate Formulation
   Fat Formulation
   Protein Formulation
Altered Amino Acid Formulations
   Amin-Aid

Parenteral Nutrition

Peripheral TPN
   Mechanism of action
   Drug effects
   Therapeutic uses

Side effects and adverse effects
Dosages
Drug Profiles
Amino Acids
   Amino Acids
   Carbohydrates
   Fats
   Lipid emulsions
Trace Elements
Central TPN
   Mechanism of action
   Drug effects
   Therapeutic uses
   Side effects and adverse effects
   Dosages

Drug Profiles

Nursing Process
Assessment
Nursing Diagnoses
Planning
   Outcome criteria
Implementation
Evaluation

Glossary

Anabolism (ə nab'ə liz' əm) Constructive metabolism characterized by the conversion of simple substances into the more complex compounds of living matter. (p. 810)

Catabolism (kə tab' o liz əm) A complex metabolic process in which energy is liberated for use in work, energy storage, or heat production by the destruction of complex substances by living cells to form simple compounds. (p. 810)

Enteral nutrition (en'ter əl) The provision of food or nutrients via the gastrointestinal tract. (p. 804)

Essential amino acids Those amino acids that cannot be manufactured by the body. (p. 810)

Essential fatty acid deficiency A condition that develops if fatty acids that the body cannot produce are not present in dietary or nutritional supplements. (p. 811)

Hyperalimentation (hi'pər al'i men ta' shən) Overfeeding or the ingestion or administration of an amount of nutrients in excess of the demands of the appetite. (p. 808)

Malnutrition (mal' noo trĭsh' ən) Any disorder of nutrition. (p. 804)

Multivitamin infusion (MVI) Vitamins and minerals added, depending on the patient's needs. (p. 811)

Nonessential amino acids Those amino acids that the body can produce without extracting from dietary intake. (p. 810)

Nutrients (noo' tre ənt) A substance that provides nourishment and affects the nutritive and metabolic processes of the body. (p. 804)

Nutritional supplements Means of providing adequate nutritional support to meet the body's nutritional needs. (p. 804)

Nutritional support Support for the body's nutritional needs. (p. 804)

Parenteral nutrition (pə ren' tər əl) The administration of nutrients by a route other than through the alimentary canal, such as subcutaneously, intravenously, intramuscularly, or intradermally. (p. 804)

Semiessential amino acids Those that can be produced by the body but not in sufficient amounts in infants and children. (p. 810)

Total parenteral nutrition The same as parenteral nutrition. (p. 808)

The integrity and normal function of all cells within the body require a constant supply of nutrients. **Nutrients** are dietary products that undergo chemical changes when ingested (metabolism) that cause tissue to be enhanced and energy to be liberated. Nutrients are required for cell growth and division, enzyme activity, protein-carbohydrate-fat synthesis, muscle contraction, neurohumoral secretion, wound repair, immune competence, gut integrity, and numerous other essential cellular functions. Providing for these nutritional needs is known as **nutritional support**. Adequate nutritional support is needed to prevent the breakdown of proteins for use as energy to sustain essential organ systems. **Malnutrition** can decrease or-

gan size and impair the function of organ systems (cardiac, respiratory, gastrointestinal, hepatic, renal, and so on). **Nutritional supplements** are a means of providing adequate nutritional support to meet the body's nutritional needs.

Malnutrition is a condition in which the body's essential need for nutrients is not met by nutrient intake. The purpose of nutritional support is the successful prevention, recognition, and management of malnutrition. Nutritional supplements are dietary products used to provide nutritional support. There are many nutritional supplement products that can be administered to patients in a variety of ways. Nutritional supplements vary in the amounts and chemical complexity of carbohydrate, protein, and fat. The electrolyte, vitamin, mineral, and osmolality of the specific product can vary as well. These nutrients may be given in a digested form, a partially digested form, or an undigested form. Nutritional supplements can also be tailored for specific disease states.

A wide variety of nutritional supplements is needed because of the wide variety of conditions for which patients require nutritional support. Patient nutrient requirements vary according to age, gender, size or weight, physical activity, preexisting medical conditions, and current medical or surgical treatment. Nutritional supplements are classified according to the method of administration. They can be classified as either enteral or parenteral. **Enteral nutrition** is the provision of food or nutrients with the gastrointestinal tract as the route of administration. Nutritional supplements may also be administered parenterally. **Parenteral nutrition** differs from enteral nutrition in the route of administration. Nutritional supplements are delivered directly into the circulation by means of intravenous infusion. The selection of either enteral nutrition or parenteral nutrition and the specific nutritional composition of the product depends on the specific patient profile and the clinical situation.

Nutritional support ↗ Enteral nutrition → Gastrointestinal tract
↘ Parenteral nutrition → Circulation

Enteral Nutrition

Enteral nutrition is the provision of food or nutrients through the gastrointestinal tract. The most common and least invasive route of administration is oral consumption. A feeding tube is used in the other five routes (see Fig. 51-1). The six routes of enteral nutrition delivery are listed in the box on the next page. Patients who may benefit from feeding tube delivery of nutri-

Nasogastric

Nasoduodenal

Nasojejunal

Gastrostomy

Jejunostomy

▼ **FIG. 51-1** Tube feeding routes. (Modified from Beare, Myers: *Principles and practice of adult health nursing,* ed 2, St Louis, 1994, Mosby.)

Routes of Enteral Nutrition Delivery

ROUTE	DESCRIPTION
Oral	Nutritional supplements delivered by mouth
Nasogastric	Feeding tube placed from the nose to the stomach
Nasoduodenal	Feeding tube placed from the nose to the duodenum
Nasojejunal	Feeding tube placed from the nose to the jejunum
Gastrostomy	Feeding tube surgically inserted directly into the stomach
Jejunostomy	Feeding tube surgically inserted into the jejunum

tional supplements are those with abnormal esophageal or stomach peristalsis, altered anatomy secondary to surgery, depressed consciousness, or impaired digestive capacity. Nutrients may be administered via the enteral or parenteral routes depending on the clinical situation. Many processes occur from the beginning of the digestive system in the mouth to the end of the digestive system in the anus. These processes have evolved over time to most effectively digest dietary nutrients. The enteral route is considered to be the superior route of administration of nutritional supplements.

There are approximately 100 different enteral formulations available. The enteral supplements have been divided into basic groups according to the basic

Enteral Formulations

ELEMENTAL FORMULATIONS

Flexical
Vital
Vivonex
Vivonex HN

Contents: dipeptides, tripeptides, or crystalline amino acids, glucose oligosaccharides, and vegetable oil or medium-chain triglycerides
Comments: minimum digestion; residue is minimal
Indications: partial bowel obstruction, irritable bowel disease, radiation enteritis, bowel fistulas, and short bowel syndrome

POLYMERIC FORMULATIONS

Complete-B
Ensure
Ensure-Plus
Isocal
Magnacal
Meritene
Osmolite
Portagen
Precision LR
Sustacal

Contents: complex nutrients (proteins, carbohydrates, and fat)
Indications: preferred over elemental for patients with fully functional gastrointestinal tracts and few specialized nutrient requirements and preferred because hyperosmolarity of elemental formulas causes more GI problems

MODULAR FORMULATIONS

Carbohydrate
 Controlyte
 Polycose
Fat
 MCT Oil
 Microlipid
Protein
 Amin-Aid
 Casec
 Hepatic-Aid
 Travasorb Renal
 Traum-Aid HBC
 Stresstein

Contents: single nutrient formulas (protein, carbohydrate, or fat)
Indications: can be added to a monomeric or polymeric formulation to provide a more individual specialized nutrient formulation

ALTERED AMINO ACID FORMULATIONS

Amin-Aid
Lonalac
''Protein'' Modular
Formulations

Contents: varying amounts of specific amino acids
Indications: patients with genetically altered metabolism problems

characteristics of the individual formulations. There are four enteral formulation groups: elemental, polymeric, modular, and altered amino acid. These are described in the box above.

Mechanism of Action

The enteral formula groups provide the basic building blocks for anabolism. Different combinations and amounts of these agents are used based on the individual patient's anabolic needs. After the body receives and absorbs these nutrients, it must process them into living matter.

Drug Effects

Enteral nutrition can be used to supplement an oral diet that is currently insufficient for a patient's

nutrient needs or used solely to meet all the patient's nutrient needs.

Therapeutic Uses

Enteral nutrition supplies complete dietary needs through the gastrointestinal (GI) tract by the normal oral route or by feeding tube. It is used for patients who are unable to consume or digest normal foods, who have accelerated catabolic status, or who are undernourished because of disease. The box on the next page lists the main types of enteral nutrition supplements and their indications.

Side Effects and Adverse Effects

The most common side effect and adverse effect from the nutritional supplements is gastrointestinal intolerance. The most common result of this intolerance is diarrhea. Infant nutritional formulations are most commonly associated with allergies and digestive intolerance. The other nutritional supplements are most commonly associated with osmotic diarrhea. Rapid feeding or bolus doses can result in dumping syndrome, which produces intestinal disturbances. In addition, tube feeding can often result in aspiration.

Interactions

Various nutrients can interact with drugs to produce significant food-drug interactions. With some exceptions, food usually delays the absorption of drugs when administered simultaneously. Table 51-1 lists some of the most common drug interactions with the nutritional supplements.

Enteral Nutrition Supplements: Therapeutic Effects

INFANT NUTRITIONAL FORMULATIONS

Therapeutic effects	1. Sole nutritional intake for premature and full-term infants 2. Supplemental nutritional intake for older infants receiving solid foods 3. Supplemental nutrition for breast-fed infants

COMPLETE NUTRITIONAL FORMULATIONS

Therapeutic effects	1. Unable to consume or digest normal foods 2. Accelerated catabolic status 3. Undernourished because of disease

INCOMPLETE NUTRITIONAL FORMULATIONS

Therapeutic effects	1. Genetic metabolic enzyme deficiency 2. Hepatic or renal impairment

Dosages

Because nutrient requirements vary greatly, dosages are individualized according to patient needs.

DRUG PROFILES

Enteral nutrition can be provided by a variety of supplements. The individual patient characteristics determine the appropriate enteral supplement. There are four basic types of enteral formulations: elemental, polymeric, modular, and altered amino acid.

ELEMENTAL FORMULATIONS
VIVONEX

Vivonex is an enteral supplement of the elemental formulation class of enteral nutrition products. It is lactose free, and the proteins it provides are from amino acids rather than peptides. It is also available as Vivonex HN, which delivers more concentrated nutrients with less fat content than the regular Vivonex. Other products in this elemental formulation category are Flexical and Vital. These products are available without a prescription, have no pregnancy category, and are contraindicated only if a patient has had a hypersensitivity reaction to them in the past. They are available in liquid formulations only.

POLYMERIC FORMULATIONS
ENSURE

Ensure is a commonly used enteral supplement from the polymeric formulation category of enteral nutrition products. It is lactose free and also comes in a higher

Table 51-1	Drug Interactions: Nutritional Supplement		
DRUG	**MECHANISM**	**RESULT**
Cephalosporins Erythromycin Penicillins	Chemical inactivation with high gastric acid content or prolonged emptying time	Decreased antibiotic effects
Adrenal steroids Vitamins A and D	Increased absorption rate in presence of fats	Increased therapeutic effects
Tetracyclines	Chemical inactivation forms an insoluble complex with calcium in foods	Decreased antibiotic effects

caloric formula called Ensure-Plus. Other polymeric formulations are Complete-B, Isocal, Magnacal, Meritene, Osmolite, Portagen, Precision LR, and Sustacal. These agents contain complex nutrients such as casein and soy protein as protein, corn syrup and maltodextrins as carbohydrates, and vegetable oil or milk fat for fat. They are available without a prescription, have no pregnancy category, and are contraindicated only if a patient has had a hypersensitivity reaction to them in the past. They are available in liquid formulations only.

MODULAR FORMULATIONS
CARBOHYDRATE FORMULATION

Centrality and Polycose are the two commonly used enteral supplements from the carbohydrate modular formulation category. Centrality is a carbohydrate supplement that supplies carbohydrates only. It has low sodium and no vitamins, minerals, or lactose. It is intended to be used as an addition to monomeric or polymeric formulations to provide a more individual specialized nutrient formulation. These products are available without a prescription, have no pregnancy category, and are contraindicated only if a patient has had a hypersensitivity reaction to them in the past. They are available in liquid formulations only.

FAT FORMULATION

Microlipid and MCT Oil are the formulations available in the fat category. Microlipid is a fat supplement supplying solely fats. It is a concentrated source of calories and contains 4.5 calories per ml. These agents are used to help individualize nutrient formulations. They may be used in malabsorption and other gastrointestinal disorders or in patients with pancreatitis. These products are available without a prescription, have no pregnancy category, and are contraindicated only if a patient has had a hypersensitivity reaction to them in the past. They are available in liquid formulations only.

PROTEIN FORMULATION

Hepatic-Aid is one of many products from the protein modular formulation category. It contains high concentrations of branched-chain amino acids and low concentrations of aromatic amino acids to correct the abnormal serum amino acid profiles seen in many patients with chronic or acute liver impairment who are in intensive care. Most of the modular formulation products are used because they have a specific nutrient makeup needed to prevent the administration of a nutrient that a critically ill patient cannot metabolize or that would be harmful. Others are formulated to de-

liver special amounts of specific nutrients that may help critically ill patients heal more quickly.

ALTERED AMINO ACID
FORMULATIONS
AMIN-AID

Amin-Aid is an altered amino acid formulation nutrition supplement. Many of the nutritional supplements in this category are also listed as modular formulations because they can be used as both single-nutrient formulas and as nutrition formulations for patients with genetic errors of metabolism. The amino acid formulations are used most commonly in patients who have metabolic disorders such as phenylketonuria, homocystinuria, and maple syrup urine disease. They are also used to supply nutritional support to patients with renal impairment, eclampsia, or congestive heart failure.

Parenteral Nutrition

Parenteral nutritional supplementation is the preferred method for patients who are unable to tolerate and maintain adequate enteral or oral intake. It is the intravenous administration of nutritional supplements. Instead of administering partially digested nutrients into the gastrointestinal tract, totally digested vitamins, minerals, amino acids, dextrose, and so on are administered intravenously directly into the circulatory system. This effectively bypasses the entire gastrointestinal system, eliminating the need for absorption, metabolism, and excretion. Parenteral nutrition is also called **total parenteral nutrition** (TPN) or **hyperalimentation.**

TPN can supply all the calories, dextrose, amino acids, fats, trace elements, and other essential nutrients needed for growth, weight gain, wound healing, convalescence, immunocompetence, and other health-sustaining functions.

Parenteral nutrition can be administered either through a peripheral vein or a central vein. Each route of delivery of parenteral nutrition has specific requirements and limitations. It is generally accepted that parenteral nutrition should be considered only when oral or enteral support is impossible or when the gastrointestinal absorptive or functional capacity is not sufficient to meet the nutritional needs of the patient. Some of the conditions that must be considered in the decision to place a patient on peripheral versus central hyperalimentation are listed in Table 51-2.

Table 51-2	Peripheral and Central Nutrition: Characteristics	
	CHARACTERISTICS	
CONSIDERATIONS	PERIPHERAL	CENTRAL
Goal of nutritional therapy (total versus supplemental)	Supplemental (total if moderate to low needs)	Total
Length of therapy	Short (<2 wk)	Long (>7-10 days)
Osmolarity	Isotonic (<600 mosm/L)	Hypertonic (2000 + mosm/L)
Fluid tolerance	Must be high	Can be fluid restricted
Dextrose	<5% to 10%	10% to 50%
Amino acids	3% to 5%	3% to 7%
Fats	10% to 20%	10% to 20%
Calories/day	500 to 700	2000 to 4000 kcal/day

PERIPHERAL TPN

Peripheral TPN is one route of administration of parenteral nutrition. A peripheral vein is used to deliver nutrients to the patient's circulatory system. It is usually a temporary method of administration. The long-term administration of nutritional supplements via a peripheral vein may lead to phlebitis and ultimately the loss of a limb. Indications for peripheral TPN are as follows:

- Procedure that imposes restriction on oral feedings
- GI illnesses that prevent oral food ingestion
- Anorexia caused by radiation or cancer chemotherapy
- Following surgery
- If a patient's nutritional deficits are minimal, but oral nutrition will not be instituted for 5 or more days

It should be considered a temporary measure to provide adequate nutrient needs in patients with mild deficits or who are restricted from oral intake and have slightly elevated metabolic rates.

Mechanism of Action

Peripheral parenteral nutrition is most valuable in patients who do not have large nutritional needs, who can tolerate moderately large fluid loads, and who need nutritional supplements only temporarily. Peripheral parenteral nutrition may be used alone or in combination with oral nutritional supplements to provide the necessary fat, carbohydrate, and protein needed by the patient to maintain health.

Drug Effects

Peripheral parenteral nutrition is used to administer nutrients to patients who need more nu-

trients than present oral intake can provide or to provide entire daily nutrition. Peripheral parenteral nutrition is meant only as a temporary means (less than 2 weeks) of delivering parenteral nutrition.

Therapeutic Uses

Conditions in which patients may benefit from the delivery of peripheral parenteral nutrition are listed below:

- Procedures that restrict oral feedings
- Anorexia caused by radiation or cancer chemotherapy
- GI illnesses that prevent oral food ingestion
- Following any type of surgery
- Nutritional deficits are minimal, but oral nutrition will not be started for more than 5 days

Side Effects and Adverse Effects

The most devastating adverse effect of peripheral parenteral nutrition is phlebitis, which is a vein irritation or inflammation of a vein. If severe enough and not treated appropriately, phlebitis can lead to the loss of a limb. However, this is rare. Another potential adverse effect is fluid overload. Peripheral parenteral nutrition is limited to lower concentrated solutions, generally less than 10%, to avoid sclerosing vein. Larger amounts of nutritional supplements are needed with lower concentrated solutions to meet a patient's daily nutritional requirements. Some patients, such as those with renal failure or congestive heart failure, cannot tolerate large fluid volume. In these patients peripheral parenteral nutrition may be contraindicated or used cautiously only if absolutely necessary.

Dosages

Dosage requirements vary from patient to patient. Age, gender, weight, and numerous other factors must be considered for proper administration of TPN. Guidelines for amino acids appear in Table 51-3.

DRUG PROFILES

The individual components of peripheral and central parenteral nutrition are the same. The difference lies in the concentrations and amounts of the components delivered per volume of nutritional supplement. There are four basic components of peripheral or central parenteral nutrition: amino acid, carbohydrate, lipid, and trace elements and electrolytes. Most of the electrolyte components are discussed in Chapter 50.

AMINO ACIDS

Amino acids have many roles in the maintenance of normal nutritional status. The primary role is protein production, or **anabolism.** Adequate amino acids in nutritional supplements reduce the breakdown of proteins **(catabolism)** and also help promote normal growth and wound healing.

Amino acids are commonly classified as essential or nonessential according to whether they can or cannot be produced by the body. **Nonessential amino acids** are those that the body produces and are therefore not needed in dietary intake. The body is able to manufacture from nitrogen sources all but eight of the available amino acids. **Essential amino acids** are those amino acids that cannot be produced by the body. Therefore it is essential that they be included in daily dietary intake. Amino acids are used as building blocks for protein that is needed for normal growth and development. Two amino acids, histidine and arginine, are not manufactured by the body in large enough quantities during rapid growth periods such as infancy or childhood. Thus they are referred to as

semiessential amino acids. The box below lists the amino acids according to their categories.

AMINO ACIDS

Amino acid crystalline solutions (Aminosyn 3%, 5%, and 10% and Free-Amine III 8.5% and 10%) can be used in either peripheral or central hyperalimentation. The two currently available amino acid solutions differ only in their respective concentrations. These drugs have no restrictions regarding pregnancy and have no contraindications to use. The dosage of these solutions varies depending on the patient's weight and requirements. Recommended dosages for healthy and traumatized patients are listed in Table 51-3.

CARBOHYDRATES

In nutritional support carbohydrates are usually supplied to patients through dextrose. Under normal circumstances both carbohydrates and lipids are used as calorie sources (see Fig. 51-2). Concentrations of dextrose in parenteral nutrition are important considerations. In peripheral TPN dextrose concentrations are kept below 10% to decrease the possibility of phlebitis. In central TPN dextrose concentrations can range from

Amino Acids: Classification

ESSENTIAL	NONESSENTIAL	SEMIESSENTIAL
Isoleucine	Alanine	Arginine
Leucine	Aspartic acid	Histidine
Lysine	Cysteine	
Methionine	Glutamine acid	
Phenylalanine	Glycine	
Threonine	Proline	
Tryptophan	Serine	
Valine	Tyrosine	

Table 51-3	Amino Acids: Recommended Dosage Guidelines	

	HEALTHY		UNDERNOURISHED
ADULT		INFANT/CHILD	OR TRAUMATIZED
0.9 g/kg		1.4 to 2.2 g/kg	3 g/kg or more

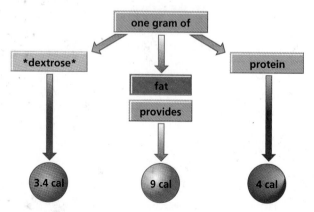

▼ **FIG. 51-2** One gram of dextrose, fat, or protein will provide varying amounts of energy as calories.

10% to 50% but are commonly 25% to 35%. Because dextrose is a sugar, supplemental insulin must be given simultaneously in nutritional supplements. A balanced nutritional supplement that contains dextrose and lipids for caloric sources decreases the need for large amounts of insulin.

FATS

The average North American diet consists of 40% fat. Of the total calories supplied, 40% to 50% of the calories are obtained through fat grams. Intravenous fat emulsions serve two functions: they supply essential fatty acids and they are a source of energy or calories. As with the amino acids, certain fatty acids are essential because the body cannot produce them. Linoleic acid cannot be synthesized by the body. It is needed to produce linolenic and arachidonic acid. If these fatty acids are not present in dietary or nutritional supplements, an essential fatty acid deficiency may develop. Clinical signs of **essential fatty acid deficiency** are hair loss, scaly dermatitis, growth retardation, reduced wound healing, decreased platelets, and fatty liver (see Fig. 51-3).

LIPID EMULSIONS

The currently available lipid emulsions, Intralipid and Liposyn, are available as either 10% or 20% emulsions. They differ in fat origin. Liposyn is made from safflower oil, and Intralipid is made from soybean oil (see Fig. 51-4).

Fat emulsions should be calibrated to deliver no more than 60% of the total daily caloric intake. Fat emulsions are beneficial when combined with dextrose

solutions. The use of fat to meet caloric needs prevents potentially harmful conditions, such as hyperglycemia, hyperinsulinemia, and hyperosmolarity, that can occur when a patient's entire caloric needs are being met solely by dextrose. A normal diet should contain 40% fat, 40% protein, and 20% carbohydrate.

TRACE ELEMENTS

Trace element solutions are available individually or in many different combinations. The following are considered trace elements:
- Zinc
- Chromium
- Copper
- Selenium
- Manganese
- Iodine
- Molybdenum

Other combination trace element formulations are listed in the box on the next page. Specific dosages and frequencies depend on the individual patient's requirements. Vitamins and minerals may also be added accordingly. A common multivitamin combination is **multivitamin infusion** (MVI).

CENTRAL TPN

In central TPN a large central vein is used to deliver nutrients directly into the patient's circulation. Usually the subclavian or internal jugular vein is used. Central TPN is generally indicated for patients who require nutritional supplements for prolonged periods of time, usually more than 7 to 10 days. It can also be used in

▼ **FIG. 51-3** Lipid emulsions supply essential fatty acids and energy.

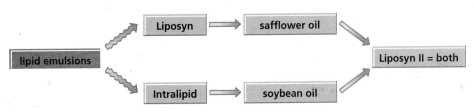

▼ **FIG. 51-4** Liposyn is made of safflower oil; Intralipid of soybean oil; and Liposyn II contains both.

Trace Element Formulations

TRACE ELEMENT COMBINATIONS	TRACE ELEMENTS WITH ELECTROLYTES (SMALL VOLUME)	TRACE ELEMENTS WITH ELECTROLYTES (LARGE VOLUME)
M.T.E. 4	Tracelyte	Hyperlyte
M.T.E. 5	Tracelyte	Lypholyte
M.T.E. 6	(with double electrolytes)	TPN electrolytes
Others		Others

the home care setting. Indications for central TPN are as follows:

■ Fluid-restricted (renal failure, CHF, etc.)
■ Large nutritional requirements (metabolic stress/hypermetabolism)
■ Nutritional support for prolonged periods (more than 7 to 10 days)

The disadvantages of central parenteral nutrition are the risks associated with insertion, use, and maintenance of the central vein. There is a greater potential for infection, more serious catheter-induced trauma and related events, metabolic alterations, and other technical or mechanical problems than with parenteral nutrition.

Mechanism of Action

Central parenteral nutrition works by delivering essential nutrients directly into the circulation via a central vein. It is most valuable in patients who have large nutritional needs, who cannot tolerate large fluid loads, and who need nutritional supplements for prolonged periods of time. Central parenteral nutrition provides the necessary fat, carbohydrate, and protein that the patient needs to maintain health.

Drug Effects

Central parenteral nutrition is used to supply nutrients to patients who cannot ingest nutrients by mouth and cannot meet required daily nutritional needs by the enteral or peripheral parenteral routes. Central parenteral nutrition can safely provide nutritional needs for extended periods of time.

Therapeutic Uses

Central parenteral nutrition delivers total dietary nutrients to patients who require nutritional supplementation. Patients who may benefit from the delivery of central parenteral nutrition include the following:

■ Fluid-restricted patients such as those with renal failure or congestive heart failure

■ Patients having large nutritional requirements (metabolic stress or hypermetabolism)
■ Patients needing nutritional support for prolonged periods (more than 7 to 10 days)

Side Effects and Adverse Effects

The most common side effects and adverse effects of central parenteral nutrition are those surrounding the use of the central vein for delivery of the parenteral nutrition. The risks associated with insertion of the infusion line, as well as the use and maintenance of the central vein for administration of parenteral nutrition, can create some complications. There is a greater potential for infection, more serious catheter-induced trauma and related events, and other technical or mechanical problems than with parenteral nutrition. There are larger and more concentrated volumes of nutritional supplements being delivered with central parenteral nutrition and therefore a greater chance for metabolic complications such as hyperglycemia.

Dosages

Administration is individualized according to patient needs.

DRUG PROFILES

The same formulations used in peripheral parenteral support are used in central parenteral support. Often the concentrations of fluids administered through the central vein are much higher than those used in peripheral nutrition supplements. Besides these minor differences the nutritional supplements used are identical.

NURSING PROCESS

ASSESSMENT

The nurse should conduct a thorough nutritional assessment with a dietary history and review. Consultation with a registered dietician is crucial to identification of the nutrients that are missing in a particular patient's diet. Laboratory studies including total protein, albumin, BUN, RBC, WBC, vitamin B_{12}, cholesterol, and Hgb will be needed. Anthropometric measurements and weights also provide much-needed data. The data collected will help the physician and other members of the health care team select the appropriate needed nutritional supplements for the patient.

Before beginning enteral nutritional supplements of elemental formulation, such as Vivonex, it must be determined if the patient has a history of allergic reaction to its contents. Polymeric formulations, such as Ensure, are contraindicated in patients with a hypersensitivity to any of its ingredients. Modular formulations such as Centrality, fat formulations such as Microlipid, and protein formulations such as Hepatic-Aid are also contraindicated in patients with known hypersensitivity. Altered amino acid formulas are contraindicated in patients who have a known hypersensitivity to the formulation. Enteral feedings are generally contraindicated in patients who are capable of oral intake or who have intestinal obstruction, severe vomiting, or esophageal fistulas.

Parenteral nutrition supplements should be given after an assessment of the patient's body weight, history of weight loss, and any signs of malnutrition. Laboratory studies such as serum albumin, electrolytes, serum transferrin, urine creatinine clearance, total lymphocyte count, Hgb, and Hct should also be obtained and documented.

NURSING DIAGNOSES

Nursing diagnoses appropriate for the patient receiving enteral or parenteral nutritional supplementation are as follows:
- Diarrhea related to the enteral feedings.
- Airway clearance, ineffective due to possible aspiration.
- Fluid volume deficit related to nutritional status.
- Risk for infection or injury related to parenteral infusions.
- Risk for noncompliance to therapy.

PLANNING

Goals related to nutritional supplements are as follows:
- Patient remains free of complications associated with enteral feedings.
- Patient regains near-normal to normal bowel patterns.
- Patient remains free of injury during nutritional support.
- Patient remains free of infection.
- Patient regains normal fluid volume status.
- Patient remains compliant and makes return visits to the physician as needed.

Outcome Criteria

Outcome criteria are as follows:
- Patient (or caregiver) states method of administration of enteral feedings through tube feedings and subsequent nursing care, such as checking enteral tube placement.
- Patient identifies measures to decrease diarrhea such as use of drug and nondrug therapies.
- Patient (or caregiver) demonstrates adequate technique for enteral tube feedings to decrease risk of aspiration with emphasis on elevated head of bed and checking tube placement.
- Patient states measures to minimize risk of infection at TPN site such as making sure site is changed as ordered and assessed for redness, swelling, or drainage.
- Patient will begin to show adequate fluid volume status with improved turgor, urinary output, return to normal lab values.
- Patient states symptoms to report to the physician such as increased lethargy, fever, shortness of breath, etc.

IMPLEMENTATION

In general, monitoring the status of the patient during and after enteral feedings is crucial to safe and prudent nursing care. Tinting tube feedings with blue food coloring helps assist the nurse in detection of aspiration in the tube-feeding substance. Gastric residual volumes should be obtained and documented before each feeding and before each medication is administered. Stop the tube feeding and aspirate stomach contents to detect any residual. If the volume is more than that from 2 hours of continuous feeding, return the aspirate, hold the feeding, and contact the physician.

For intermittent bolus feedings, if the residual amount is greater than 50% of the volume previously infused, return the aspirate, withhold the feeding, and contact the physician. Reduced feeding volume will probably be ordered by the physician. Always remember that the head of the bed should remain elevated with tube feedings to decrease the risk of aspiration. The process of tube feedings is presented in Chapter 4.

Newer tubes for nasogastric and enteral feeding are less thick and hard and are thinner (Nos. 5 through 10 French) and more pliable for better patient tolerance. However, the smaller-diameter tubes make checking for gastric aspiration more difficult. If the attempt is unsuccessful, instill air and auscultate over the gastric area. Air sound in the stomach denotes accurate placement. Place the end of the tube in water to test for air bubbles, which signify incorrect placement.

To prevent clogging of the feeding tube with formula, it is often helpful to flush the tube with 30 cc of cranberry juice (per policy) followed by 10 cc of water. The juice may help break up the formula residue and unclog the tube.

Physician-ordered enteral feeding infusion rates and concentration should be followed carefully. Usually the initial rate is 50 cc per hour at one-half strength but can be increased per patient tolerance to a rate of 25 cc per hour at three-fourth strength concentration. Although more rapid feeding increases the risk of hyperglycemia or dumping syndrome, nurses should continue to increase the patient's intake because 1000 cc to 2000 cc of the milk-based formula (1 kcal per ml) is needed to provide adequate calories and RDAs for vitamins and minerals. Tube feeding formulas should always be at room temperature. If all the necessary steps to decrease or prevent diarrhea have failed, antidiarrheal medications may be needed.

Lactose-free solutions are also available and should be used when individuals are lactose intolerant. Patients who suffer from this condition experience cramping, diarrhea, abdominal bloating, and flatulence with the ingestion of lactose. Patient teaching tips are presented in the box at right.

Infusions of TPN should be assessed every hour. The entire system as well as the condition of the patient should be included in this assessment. It is good practice to examine the patient first and then check the TPN insertion site and the tubing at the site of connection to the infusion pump. Patency should be assessed every hour as well.

Tubing should be changed every 24 hours to prevent infection. It is recommended that tubing changes occur daily with the beginning of each new infusion. A 0.22-μm filter is used to trap bacteria, including *Pseudomonas* species. The patient's temperature should be recorded every 4 hours. Any increased temperature should be reported to the physician immediately because it may be the first sign of infection. The patient should also be checked frequently for signs and symptoms of hyperglycemia, such as headache, dehydration, and weakness. IV rates should never be accelerated to increase reduced volume because this may

Patient Teaching TIPS

Nasogastric and Enteral Tube Feedings

✔ Because patients often go home with tube feedings, the patient and family should begin preparation for this procedure at least 1 week before discharge. Individualized patient teaching about the procedure and care of the tube requires at least 6 hours. More instructional time is needed if the tube is to be inserted and removed at night only.

✔ Incorrect placement is characterized by coughing, choking, difficulty in speaking, and cyanosis.

✔ The patient should have written and verbal instruction. Ross Laboratories, 625 Clinton Ave., Columbus, OH 43216, is an excellent contact for questions and explanations.

✔ Home health care may be needed if assistance is required.

✔ Physician phone numbers and those for other resources should be kept at the patient's home for immediate use when needed.

✔ The physician should be contacted if diarrhea, nausea, vomiting, fever, or any other unusual symptoms occur.

✔ Patients on home parenteral nutrition will need some support from home health care. Practice is critical to acquisition of skill by the patient and family. All procedures for storage; cleansing of site; care of site; dressing changes; irrigation of the catheter; pump function and care; and changing of the bag, filters, and tubing should also be demonstrated and practiced well before the patient is discharged.

✔ Patients on TPN should be weighed daily at the same time wearing the same clothing. Intake and output volumes should be noted and recorded.

✔ Glucose levels should be checked at home. Procedures for use of glucometers and periodically checking urine glucose should be demonstrated and practiced.

✔ Potential complications of TPN are manifested by fever, cough, chest pains, dyspnea, and chills and may indicate adverse reactions to lipid infusions. Chest pain and coughing may indicate air embolism. Restlessness, nervousness, fainting, and tachycardia are associated with hypoglycemia. Nausea, vomiting, polyuria, polydipsia, and elevated glucose levels may indicate hyperglycemia. If any of these occur, the patient should discontinue the infusion and contact the physician immediately.

precipitate hyperglycemia. Insulin replacement may be needed, so glucometer readings are important for immediate recognition and treatment of hyperglycemia.

Hypoglycemia is manifested by cold, clammy skin, dizziness, tachycardia, and tingling of the extremities. Hypoglycemia associated with TPN may be prevented by gradual reduction of the IV rate to allow the pancreas time to adapt to the changing blood glucose levels. If TPN is discontinued abruptly, rebound hypoglycemia may occur. This can be prevented with infusion of 5% to 10% glucose in situations in which TPN must be discontinued immediately.

Fluid overload may occur with TPN, manifested by weak pulse, hypertension, tachycardia, confusion, decreased urine output, and pitting edema. This can be prevented by maintaining IV rates and assessing the IV infusion every hour. If signs of overload occur, the nurse should slow the infusion rate, remain with the patient, and contact the physician immediately. A continual assessment of the patient and vital signs is also necessary at this time.

EVALUATION

Therapeutic responses to nutritional supplementation include improved well-being, energy, strength, and performance of activities of daily living, an increase in weight, and laboratory studies that reflect a more positive nutritional status. Besides evaluation of outcome criteria, evaluation of the patient and family input and participation in care are important because the patient should always be encouraged to participate in the planning and evaluation of care.

TAKE HOME POINTS

Nursing Considerations

■ A thorough nutritional assessment and possible consultation with a registered dietitian or nutritionist is essential for adequate intervention for the malnourished patient.

■ There are various enteral feedings with different nutritional content, including some that are lactose free.

■ Enteral feedings may result in complications such as hyperglycemia, dumping syndrome, and aspiration of feeding.

■ Parenteral nutrition is often administered through a central vein catheter because of the hyperosmolarity of substances used.

■ Parenteral feedings may result in air embolism, hyperglycemia, or hypoglycemia. If discontinued abruptly, infection and fluid volume overload may result.

■ Cautious and astute nursing care with enteral or parenteral nutritional supplementation may prevent or decrease the occurrence of associated complications.

Critical Thinking **A C T I V I T I E S**

1. Which nursing actions will help address the nursing diagnosis of altered bowel elimination or diarrhea as related to enteral feedings?

2. What outcome criteria will address the nursing diagnosis of fluid volume deficit related to nutritional deficit?

BIBLIOGRAPHY

Albanese J, Nutz P: *Mosby's 1995 nursing drug cards,* St Louis, 1995, Mosby.

Bockus S: When your patient needs tube feedings: making the right decisions, *Nursing 93* 23(7):34, 1993.

Johnson KB: *Harriet Lane handbook,* ed 13, St Louis, 1993, Mosby.

Keen JH: *Critical care and emergency drug reference,* St Louis, 1994, Mosby.

Knoben JE, Anderson PO: *Handbook of critical drug data,* ed 6, Hamilton, Ill, 1988, Drug Intelligence Publications.

McEvoy GK: *AHFS drug information,* Bethesda, Md, 1994, American Society of Hospital Pharmacists.

Murphy H: Tube feeding problems and solutions, *Adv Clin Care* 5(2):7, 1990.

Orr ME: Hyperglycemia during nutritional support, *Crit Care Nurs* 12(1):64, 1992.

Skidmore-Roth L: *Mosby's 1995 nursing drug reference,* St Louis, 1995, Mosby.

PART 11

MISCELLANEOUS THERAPEUTICS: HEMATOLOGIC, DERMATOLOGIC, OPHTHALMIC, AND OTIC SYSTEMS: STUDY SKILLS BRIEF

TIME MANAGEMENT

As you plan your study time for Part 11, it should be very clear that Chapter 54 will take significantly more time to complete than the other chapters. Do not let the length of the chapter overwhelm you. Apply the principles of time management to this chapter, and you will succeed. The most important aspect of time management to apply to this chapter is the use of clear goal statements and action plan steps to help you achieve the goals.

Goal Statements

Remember the criteria for goal statements. First, they must be realistic. The statements must be things you know you can accomplish. Second, they must be specific to the task. "I will study the chapter" is not a very specific goal. Specify what you expect to accomplish. "I will master the 26 terms in the chapter glossary" is a more specific goal statement. Third, there must be a time limit. How long will you spend in achieving this goal? Set a time limit for the completion of each activity for the quantity of time to be spent in each learning activity. Finally, goal state-

ments must be measurable. In the example about studying the glossary, including the number of terms contained in Chapter 54 helps to clarify the goal.

Action Planning

The second segment of time management is the use of action planning. An action plan is a series of smaller, specific activities that you will accomplish in order to meet your goal statements. Your goal is to master the 26 terms. What will you do in order to meet that goal?

Action Steps Example

1. I will spend one hour making vocabulary drill cards for the terms found in the glossary in Chapter 54 from 3:00 to 4:00 PM on Monday.
2. I will spend 15 minutes in rehearsal and review of these cards every day until the exam on this chapter is over.
3. Each time I cannot define and explain a term I will put an "x" on the card to identify it as a term needing more review.
4. I will spend one hour the night before the exam doing a comprehensive review of the terms in Chapter 54, with special emphasis on those cards that have one or more x marks.

Action steps help to assure that you are spending your study time actively focusing on what you need to learn.

PURR
Prepare Example

Chapter 54, Objective 4: "Discuss the mechanism of action, cautions, contraindications, and associated nursing implications as related to ophthalmic preparations."

Question 1. What does ophthalmic mean? (Literal question [LQ])

Question 2. What are ophthalmic preparations? (LQ)

Question 3. What is the mechanism of action of ophthalmic preparations? (LQ)

Question 4. Is there more than one mechanism of action? (LQ)

Question 5. If there is more than one mechanism of action, how are the mechanisms similar and how are they different? (Interpretive Question)

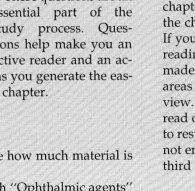

These questions are only suggestions of generated questions based on the chapter objectives. There are many more questions that can be asked about Objective 4. These questions are an essential part of the study process. Questions help make you an active reader and an active learner. The more questions you generate the easier it will be to understand the chapter.

Outline Example

1. Using the outline, decide how much material is appropriate.

The section that begins with "Ophthalmic agents" is probably too much material. Looking at the outline headings, this section could be broken down into five blocks of material. Block one would cover the material under the heading "Parasympathomimetics." Block two would be the material under the heading "Sympathomimetics." The next three blocks would be "Beta-adrenergic blockers," "Carbonic anhydrase inhibitors," and "Osmotic diuretics."

2. Apply the Prepare step to each block.

Beginning with "Parasympathomimetics," generate some questions to guide your reading. Remember that it is important to ask questions that will focus on both literal information and questions that will help you to interpret, evaluate, and analyze when you read.

3. Read the material.

As soon as you have completed the self-questioning over the first block of material, read the material in the chapter. It is important that the reading be done immediately. Read for understanding and as you read remember the questions you generated. This approach will help your concentration and comprehension.

4. Take a short break.

Once you have completed the reading of this section of the chapter, give your mind a chance to reflect and consolidate the learning. Limit the time you allow for a break and use the time for something pleasurable. Give yourself five or ten minutes to read the newspaper, get a snack, or just take a short walk.

5. Rehearse.

Before going on to the next section of the chapter it is important to spend a few minutes in rehearsal. Using the questions from Step 2, go back over the material you read and try to respond to those questions. When you find yourself unable to answer a question, put a mark in the text beside the heading that caused the difficulty and move on. The mark will serve as a reminder for future review. At this point, the objective is not complete mastery of the material. The objective is to see what you have learned so that you can move smoothly into the next section. Breaking a chapter into blocks is useful, but it is imperative that the links between sections be made as you study.

6. Review.

After completing two or three major sections of the chapter, it is time to review. Start at the beginning of the chapter. Ask your questions. Try to answer them. If you cannot formulate a clear answer, then some rereading is necessary. Also, pay attention to the marks made during the rehearsal step. Those marks indicate areas that you have already identified as needing review. When rereading, remember that the object is to read only as much of the material as needed to be able to respond to self-generated questions. There simply is not enough time to read the entire chapter a second or third time.

REPEAT THE STEPS

Prepare, read for understanding, take a short break, and then rehearse the material just read. It may seem

that this process takes an excessive amount of time and involves a lot of repetition, but in the long run this process will produce better learning. The time spent in Prepare, Understand, and Rehearsal will reduce the time needed to review. Frequent review as you move through the chapter will make the final review at exam time proceed more quickly and enable you to achieve mastery of the material.

Chapter 52

Blood-Forming Agents

Objectives

When you reach the end of this chapter, you will be able to:

1 Discuss the importance of iron, vitamin B$_{12}$, and other blood-forming agents.

2 Discuss the various conditions when the blood-forming agents may be used.

3 Discuss the mechanism of action, cautions, contraindications, uses, dosages, special administration techniques, and measures to enhance the effectiveness and decrease side effects related to the use of blood-forming agents.

4 Develop a comprehensive nursing care plan using the nursing process for the administration of blood-forming agents.

CHAPTER OUTLINE

Hematopoiesis

Types of Anemia

Iron
  Mechanism of action
  Drug effects
  Therapeutic uses
  Side effects and adverse effects
    Toxicity and management of overdose
  Interactions
  Dosages
Drug Profiles
  Ferrous Fumarate
  ⚓ Iron Dextran
Folic Acid
  Mechanism of action
  Drug effects
  Therapeutic uses
  Side effects and adverse effects
  Interactions
  Dosages
Drug Profile
  Folic Acid
Other Blood-forming Agents

Nursing Process
Assessment
Nursing Diagnoses
Planning
  Outcome criteria
Implementation
Evaluation

Glossary

Cytoplasmic maturation (si′ to plaz′ mik mach′ u ra′ shən) A type of defect that accounts for anemias secondary to maturation defects. (p. 819)

Erythrocyte (ə rith′ ro sit) Another name for red blood cell. (p. 819)

Erythropoiesis (ə rith′ ro poi e′ sis) The process of erythrocyte production involving the maturation of a nucleated precursor into a hemoglobin-filled, nucleus-free erythrocyte that is regulated by erythropoietin, a hormone produced by the kidney. (p. 819)

Fragmented (frag′ mənt ed) Composed of and resembling fragments. (p. 820)

Globin (glo′ bin) A protein chain of which there are four structural different chains: alpha-1 and alpha-2 and beta-1 and beta-2. (p. 819)

Hematopoeisis (hem′ ə to poi e′ sis) The normal formation and development of blood cells in the bone marrow. (p. 819)

Heme (hēm) The pigmented, iron-containing, non-protein portion of the hemoglobin molecule. (p. 819)

Hemoglobin (he′ mo glo′ ben) A complex protein-iron compound in the blood that carries oxygen to the cells from the lungs and carbon dioxide away from the cells to the lungs. (p. 819)

Hypochromic (hi′ po kro′ mik) Pertaining to less than normal color. The term usually describes a red blood cell and characterizes anemias associated with decreased synthesis of hemoglobin. (p. 819)

Microcytic (mī krə ′sit ik) Pertaining to smaller than normal cells. (p. 819)

Reticulocytes (rə tik′ u lo sītz′) An immature erythrocyte characterized by a meshlike pattern of threads and particles at the former site of the nucleus. (p. 819)

Spherocytes (sfēr o′ sītz) Small, globular, completely hemoglobinated erythrocytes without the usual central pallor. (p. 820)

Hematopoiesis

The formation of new blood cells is one of the primary functions of bones. Bones are also responsible for support, protection, movement, and mineral storage. They provide a framework for the body that acts as a support and also serves to protect delicate internal organs. Bones in coordination with muscles help the body move and major reservoirs of minerals, such as calcium and phosphorus, are stored in bone. However, it is the process of blood cell formation, or **hematopoiesis,** that is the focus of this chapter. Both hematopoiesis and **erythropoiesis,** the process of red blood cell (RBC) or **erythrocyte** formation, take place in myeloid tissue. This specialized tissue is located primarily in the ends or epiphyses of certain long bones, in the flat bones of the skull, in the pelvis, and in the sternum and ribs.

When red blood cells are manufactured in the bone marrow by myeloid tissue, they are released into the circulation as immature RBCs called **reticulocytes.** Once in the circulation the reticulocytes undergo a 24- to 36-hour maturation process to become mature, fully functional RBCs.

It is important to know the structural components of the red blood cell in order to understand how anemia develops and why certain drugs are used to correct it. Over one third of a red blood cell is made of **hemoglobin.** Hemoglobin is composed of two parts—heme and globin. **Heme** is a red pigment; each molecule of heme contains one atom of iron. **Globin** is a protein chain that consists of four structurally different parts or globulins: alpha-1 and alpha-2 and beta-1 and beta-2 ($\alpha_1 + \alpha_2$ and $\beta_1 + \beta_2$). Together one molecule of heme and one protein chain of globin make one hemoglobin molecule (see Fig. 52-1).

Types of Anemia

Anemias are classified into four main types based on underlying causes. Knowledge of the etiologies of anemias will help you to understand the therapies used to treat them. Anemias can be caused by maturation defects, or they can be secondary to increased destruction. There are two types of maturation defects that cause anemias—cytoplasmic maturation defects and nuclear maturation defects. Factors responsible for increased destruction can be either intrinsic or extrinsic (see Fig. 52-2).

Red blood cells in anemias associated with **cytoplasmic maturation** defects appear **hypochromic** (lighter red than normal) and **microcytic** (smaller than normal) on blood smear. All cytoplasmic maturation anemias occur as a result of abnormal hemoglobin synthesis. Since hemoglobin is synthesized from both iron and globin, a deficiency in either one can lead to a hemoglobin deficiency. (see Fig. 52-3).

Anemias associated with immature RBCs nuclear maturation defects occur secondary to defects in DNA or protein synthesis problems. DNA and protein re-

▼ **FIG. 52-1** Structure of a hemoglobin molecule.

▼ **FIG. 52-2** Underlying causes of anemia are maturation defects and factors secondary to increased destruction.

▼ **FIG. 52-3** A schematic showing the forms of abnormal hemoglobin synthesis in cytoplasmic maturation anemia.

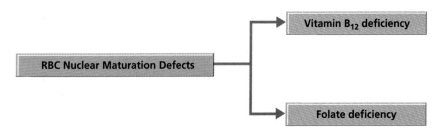

▼ **FIG. 52-4** Red blood cell *(RBC)* nuclear maturation defects occur because of vitamin B$_{12}$ or folate deficiencies.

quire vitamin B$_{12}$ and folate to be present in normal amounts for their proper production. If either of these two vitamins is absent or deficient, anemias secondary to nuclear maturation defects may develop (see Fig. 52-4). RBCs in such anemias appear to be *normochromic* (normal in color) and *macrocytic* (larger than normal) on blood smear.

Anemias secondary to increased RBC destruction can occur because of abnormalities in the RBCs themselves (intrinsic factors) as a result of factors outside (extrinsic) the RBCs. The erythrocytes in anemias attributable to intrinsic or extrinsic factors have **spherocytes** and appear to be **fragmented** when observed on blood smear. Intrinsic RBC abnormalities are usually the result of a genetic defect. Some examples are sickle cell anemia, hereditary spherocytosis, and glucose-6-phosphate dehydrogenase (G6PD) deficiency. Extrinsic mechanisms for increased RBC destruction are not attributable to abnormalities in the RBC itself. Examples of extrinsic mechanisms are drug-induced antibodies that target and destroy RBCs, septic shock that produces disseminated intravascular coagulation (DIC), and mechanical forces such as intraaortic balloon pumps and ventricular assist devices that directly damage RBCs (see Fig. 52-5).

IRON

Iron is an essential mineral for the proper functioning of all biologic systems in the body. It is an oxygen carrier in hemoglobin and myoglobin, is used for tissue respiration, and is used in many enzyme reactions in the body. Although iron is stored in many sites throughout the body (liver, spleen, and bone marrow), it is the principal nutritional deficiency in the United States, resulting in anemia. Individuals who require the greatest amount of iron are women, especially pregnant women, and children. They are also the individuals who are most likely to develop iron-deficiency anemia.

Dietary sources for iron are meats and certain vegetables and grains. This form of iron must be converted by gastric juices before it can actually be absorbed. Other foods such as orange juice, veal, fish, and ascorbic acid may help with iron absorption. Conversely, eggs, corn, beans, and many cereal products containing phytates may impair iron absorption.

Supplemental iron contained in multivitamins plus iron or iron supplements alone are indicated for the treatment of iron-deficiency anemia. Iron preparations are available as ferrous salts. See Table 52-1 for

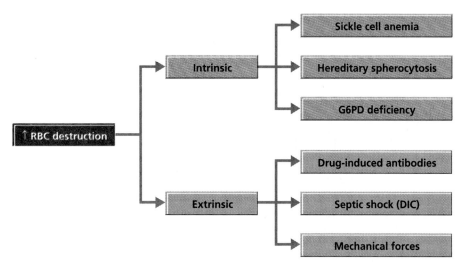

▼ FIG. 52-5 Increased RBC destruction occurs as a result of intrinsic and extrinsic factors.

Table 52-1	Ferrous Salts: Iron Content
FERROUS SALTS	**IRON CONTENT**
Ferrous fumarate	33% iron or 330 mg/g
Ferrous gluconate	12% iron or 120 mg/g
Ferrous sulfate	20% iron or 200 mg/g
Ferrous sulfate (dried)	30% iron or 300 mg/g

Table 52-2	Iron Preparations: Adverse Effects
BODY SYSTEM	**SIDE/ADVERSE EFFECT**
Gastrointestinal	Nausea, constipation, epigastric pain, black and red tarry stools, vomiting, diarrhea
Integumentary	Temporarily discolored tooth enamel and eyes, pain upon injection

a list of the currently available iron salts and their respective iron content.

Mechanism of Action

Iron is a required component of a number of enzyme systems in the body and is necessary for energy transfer in the cytochrome oxidase and xanthine oxidase enzyme systems. It is present in hemoglobin and myoglobin, which are necessary for transport and utilization of oxygen. Administration of iron corrects iron deficiency states such as anemia and soreness of the tongue, dysphagia, dystrophy of the nails and skin, and fissuring of the angles of the lips.

Drug Effects

Iron preparations are used to prevent and treat iron-deficiency syndromes. The symptoms associated with iron-deficiency anemia can be alleviated by the administration of iron. In all cases an underlying cause should be identified. Following identification of the cause, treatment should attempt to correct the cause rather than simply alleviating the symptoms.

Therapeutic Uses

As just mentioned, iron preparations are used to prevent and treat iron-deficiency syndromes because the agents replenish iron stores needed for red blood cell development and energy and oxygen transport and utilization.

Side Effects and Adverse Effects

The most frequent side effects and adverse effects associated with the iron preparations are nausea, vomiting, stomach cramps, and stomach pain. Iron is not eliminated physiologically by the body and therefore excess iron intake can lead to accumulation and iron toxicity. See Table 52-2 for a more complete listing of the undesirable effects seen with iron preparations.

Toxicity and Management of Overdose

Iron overdose is the most common cause of pediatric poisoning deaths reported to U.S. poison control centers. In 1991, there were 5144 cases of accidental ingestion of oral iron preparations reported; eleven of

Table 52-3 | Iron Preparations: Drug Interactions

DRUG	MECHANISM	EFFECT
Antacids		Decreased iron absorption
Quinolone antibiotics		Decreased quinolone absorption
Tetracyclines	Absorption	Decreased tetracycline absorption
Thyroid drugs		Decreased thyroid absorption
Ascorbic acid		Increased iron absorption

these were fatal. Toxicity from iron ingestion results from a combination of the corrosive effects on the GI mucosa and the metabolic and hemodynamic effects caused by the presence of excessive elemental iron.

Treatment is founded on good symptomatic and supportive measures, including suction and maintenance of airway, correction of acidosis, and control of shock and dehydration with IV fluids or blood, oxygen, and vasopressor. Abdominal radiographs may be helpful because iron preparations are radiopaque and may be visualized on an x-ray. Serum iron concentrations may be helpful in establishing severity of ingestion. A serum iron concentration >300 µg/dl places the patient at serious risk of toxicity. The stomach should be emptied immediately with syrup of ipecac–induced emesis or by lavage. Since many of the iron products are extended-release formulations that release contents in the intestines rather than the stomach, whole gut lavage is generally believed to be superior and more effective. This should be followed by a saline cathartic or possible surgical removal of intake iron tablets. In patients with severe symptoms of iron intoxication such as coma, shock, or seizures, chelation therapy with deferoxamine should be initiated.

Interactions

Some of the more common drug interactions with iron preparations are listed in Table 52-3.

Dosages

For the recommended dosages of iron preparations see the dosages table on the following page.

DRUG PROFILES

Iron preparations are available by prescription and as OTC medications. They are classified as pregnancy category A agents and are contraindicated in patients who have shown a hypersensitivity reaction to them. Their use is also contraindicated in patients with ulcerative colitis and regional enteritis, hemosiderosis and hemochromatosis, peptic ulcer disease, hemolytic anemia, and cirrhosis.

FERROUS FUMARATE

The ferrous fumarate iron salts (Femiron, Feostat, Hemocyte, and Span-FF) contain the largest amount of iron per gram of salt consumed. One gram of ferrous fumarate provides 33% (333 mg) of elemental iron. Ferrous fumarate is available only as an oral preparation in the following forms: a 325-mg extended-release capsule; a 45-mg/0.6 ml suspension drop and a 100-mg/5 ml suspension; a 60-, 195-, 200-, 300, 324-, and 325-mg tablet; and a 100-mg chewable tablet. Commonly recommended dosages for iron salts are listed in the dosages table.

♥ PHARMACOKINETICS

HALF-LIFE	ONSET	PEAK	DURATION
6 hr	3-10 days*	Unknown	Variable

*Increase reticulocyte values.

⚓ IRON DEXTRAN

Iron dextran (INFeD) is a colloidal solution of iron combined with low–molecular weight dextran. It is the only parenteral form of iron available. Anaphylactic reactions to iron dextran, including fatal anaphylaxis, have been reported in only 0.2% to 0.3% of patients. Because of this, a test dose of 25 mg of iron dextran should be administered by the chosen route and appropriate method of administration before injection. Although anaphylactic reactions usually occur within a few moments after the test dose, it is recommended that a period of at least 1 hour elapse before the remaining portion of the initial dose is given. Iron dextran is available as a 50 mg/ml parenteral injection for either intravenous or intramuscular use. Commonly recommended dosages for iron salts are listed in the dosages table.

DOSAGES

SELECTED IRON PREPARATIONS AND FOLIC ACID AGENTS

AGENT	PHARMACOLOGIC CLASS	DOSAGE RANGE	PURPOSE
Ferrous fumarate (Femiron, Feostat, Hemocyte, Span-FF)	Oral iron salt	Expressed in mg of elemental iron *Pediatric* PO: 4-6 mg/kg/day in 3 divided doses *Adult* PO: 50-200 mg/tid	Iron deficiency
↓Iron dextran (INFeD)	Parenteral iron salt	Expressed in mg of elemental iron. Dosages must be calculated for each patient according to manufacturer's tables. *Pediatric* IM: <5 kg: 25 mg (0.5 ml)/day <10 kg: 50 mg (1 ml)/day All other patients: 100 mg (2 mg/day)	Iron deficiency when oral iron is unsatisfactory
Folic acid	Vitamin B-complex group	*Adult/Pediatric* PO: 0.25-1 mg/day 3-15 mg/day	Folate deficiency Tropical sprue

☧ PHARMACOKINETICS

HALF-LIFE	ONSET	PEAK	DURATION
5-20 hr	Unknown	IM: 24-48 hr	≥3 wk

FOLIC ACID

Folic acid is a water-soluble B complex vitamin. It is converted to tetrahydrofolic acid in the body, which is then used for normal erythropoiesis and to produce nucleoproteins such as DNA and RNA.

Folic acid is primarily used to prevent and treat folic acid deficiency. Folic acid should not be used to treat anemias until the underlying cause and type of anemia have been determined. The potential risk involved in administering folic acid without first determining the cause is that folic acid will correct the hematologic changes of anemia but mask pernicious anemia symptoms. Pernicious anemia requires specific treatment other than folic acid. If the pernicious anemia is masked, underlying neurologic damage progresses. There are several conditions that can lead to folic acid deficiency; however, since folic acid is absorbed in the upper duodenum, malabsorption syndromes are the most common cause of deficiency.

Mechanism of Action

Dietary ingestion of folate is required for the production of nucleoproteins such as DNA and RNA. It is also essential for normal erythropoiesis. Folic acid is not active in the ingested form. It must first be converted to tetrahydrofolic acid, which is a cofactor for reactions in the biosynthesis of purines and thymidylates of nucleic acids.

Drug Effects

Folic acid is used primarily for the treatment of megaloblastic and macrocytic anemias resulting from folate deficiency. It is indicated in the treatment of nutritional macrocytic anemia; megaloblastic anemias of pregnancy, infancy and childhood; and megaloblastic anemia associated with primary liver disease, alcoholism and alcoholic cirrhosis, intestinal strictures, anastomoses, or sprue. Other types of folate deficiency that may respond to therapy with folic acid are those that result from renal dialysis or the administration of drugs such as phenytoin, primidone, barbiturates, oral contraceptives, or nitrofurantoin. Folic acid may be used in large doses in the treatment of tropical sprue. The prophylactic use of folic acid in the prevention of fetal neural tube defects is another possible use.

Therapeutic Uses

Anemias caused by folic acid deficiency can be treated by exogenous supplementation of folic acid. There is also much evidence to support the use of folic acid in the prevention of neural tube defects such as spina bifida, anencephaly, and encephalocele. It is recommended that administration should begin at least 1 month before pregnancy and through early pregnancy to reduce the risk of fetal neural tube defects. Indications for folic acid are listed below:

- Megaloblastic anemia
- Tropical sprue
- Macrocytic anemia
- Prophylaxis of neural tube defects

Side Effects and Adverse Effects

Side effects and adverse effects associated with folic acid are rare. Allergic reaction or yellow discoloration of urine may occur.

Interactions

No significant drug interactions are reported with folic acid.

Dosages

For recommended dosages of folic acid see the dosages table on p. 823.

DRUG PROFILE

Folic acid is a water-soluble B complex vitamin that is used primarily in the treatment and prevention of folic acid deficiency and anemias caused by folic acid deficiency. It is essential in the body for the production of normal red blood cells and nucleoproteins such as DNA and RNA.

FOLIC ACID

Folic acid is available as an OTC medication in multivitamin preparations and by prescription as a single agent. It is classified as a pregnancy category A agent and is contraindicated in patients who have shown a hypersensitivity reaction to it and in patients with anemias other than megaloblastic/macrocytic anemia, vitamin B_{12} deficiency anemia, and uncorrected pernicious anemia. Folic acid is available as an oral formulation in 0.4-, 0.8-, and 1-mg tablets and as 5- and 10-mg/ml parenteral injections. Commonly recommended dosages for iron salts are listed in the dosages table on the previous page.

PHARMACOKINETICS

HALF-LIFE	ONSET	PEAK	DURATION
Unknown	Unknown	60-90 min	Unknown

OTHER BLOOD-FORMING AGENTS

Other agents that may be used in the prevention and treatment of anemia are cyanocobalamin (vitamin B_{12}) and erythropoietin (Epogen or Procrit). Cyanocobalamin is discussed in detail in Chapter 50 and erythropoietin is discussed in Chapter 46.

NURSING PROCESS

ASSESSMENT

Before the nurse administers any of the iron products it is important to assess for contraindications to use such as hypersensitivity reactions, colitis, enteritis, hemochromatosis, peptic ulcer disease, hemolytic anemia, and cirrhosis. Long-term use of hemopoietic agents for treatment of anemia should be approached cautiously. Laboratory studies such as hemoglobin (Hgb), hematocrit (Hct), reticulocytes, and bilirubin levels should be obtained and documented before initiation of drug treatment. Drug interactions are presented in Table 52-3.

Folic acid has additional contraindications to use in megaloblastic/macrocytic anemias, vitamin B_{12} deficiency anemia, and uncorrected pernicious anemia. Cautious use in pregnancy is recommended. Folic acid interacts with chloramphenicol, phenobarbital, hydantoins, and methotrexate unless leucovorin rescue is possible. It is incompatible with calcium, chlorpromazine, iron sulfate, vitamin B complex with vitamin C in solution or syringe and dextrose 40% concentrations. Hgb, Hct, and reticulocyte counts as well as baseline levels of folate (6 to 15 g/ml) should be assessed before initiation of therapy.

Iron dextran is contraindicated in hypersensitivity and all anemias with the exception of iron-deficiency anemia. It is also contraindicated in patients with liver disease. Cautious use and careful monitoring is recommended in patients with acute renal disease, asthma, and rheumatoid arthritis, in pregnant or lactating women and infants under 4 months of age and in children. Iron dextran must not be mixed with other medications in syringe or solution, and it interacts with chloramphenicol and oral iron (increased toxicity).

Before the nurse administers vitamin B_{12}, it is important to obtain data about drug allergies to it. In addition, the vitamin interacts with alcohol, colchicine (an antigout drug), paraaminosalicylic acid, and some antibiotics. Treatment of vitamin B_{12} deficiencies is critical in prevention of possibly irreversible neurologic damage. Therefore, assessment of underlying symptoms before initiating drug therapy is essential for effective treatment. A thorough dietary history is important, and patients should be questioned about their intake of foods high in vitamin B_{12}, such as organ meats, clams, oysters, seafood, nonfat dry milk, and fermented cheeses. Inadequate intake of these foods may contribute to the deficiency.

NURSING DIAGNOSES

Nursing diagnoses associated with the use of blood-forming agents include, but are not limited to:

- Activity intolerance related to fatigue and lethargy associated with anemias.
- Risk for self-injury related to side effects of iron products.
- Knowledge deficit about medication therapy related to inadequate information base.
- Altered nutrition (decreased) less than body requirements.
- Noncompliance related to new drug therapy with iron products or blood-forming agents.

PLANNING

Goals for the patient receiving blood-forming agents include, but are not limited to:

- Patient maintains normal level of activity as ordered.
- Patient remains free of self-injury related to anemia or use of iron products.
- Patient discusses rationale for use, side effects, and patient education guidelines related to use of blood-forming agents.
- Patient attains normal nutritional status through use of pharmacologic and nonpharmacologic measures.

Outcome Criteria

Outcome criteria related to the administration of blood-forming agents include the following:

- Patient will be able to tolerate gradual increase in activity as ordered while taking blood-forming

agents such as ADLs to walking 10 minutes per day with increases as tolerated.

- Patient uses measures to minimize occurrence of side effects of blood-forming agents such as taking with food.
- Patient takes the medication exactly as prescribed to enhance efficacy of medication.
- Patient states symptoms to report associated with increased symptomatology related to disease process or to adverse reactions to medications such as abdominal distention, cramping, nausea, and vomiting.
- Patients keeps daily journal of dietary intake to share with health care provider every week.
- Patient uses examples of a balanced diet for daily menu planning.

Patient Teaching TIPS

Blood-Forming Agents

✔ Patients taking iron products should be informed of potential poisoning if medication is increased beyond recommended levels.

✔ Patients should be informed that iron products should not be crushed and that the tablets should be swallowed whole.

✔ All medications should be kept away and out of the reach of children.

✔ Patients should be informed that one iron product cannot be substituted for another. Each product contains different forms of the iron salt in different amounts.

✔ Patients taking iron products should avoid reclining positions for 15 to 30 minutes after taking the drug to avoid esophageal irritation or corrosion.

✔ Patients should be encouraged to continue to eat foods high in iron such as meat, dark green leafy vegetables, dried beans, dried fruits, and eggs.

✔ Patients should be informed to take oral forms of vitamin B_{12} with fruit juice and/or with meals to help disguise the taste.

✔ Patients should be informed that IM vitamin B_{12} is used to treat pernicious anemia and must be taken for life.

✔ Patients taking vitamin B_{12} should be encouraged to eat a well-balanced diet, including foods high in vitamin B_{12} such as egg yolks, fish, organ meats, oysters, dairy products, and clams. They should also avoid persons with infections because of a compromised immune system.

IMPLEMENTATION

Liquid oral forms of iron products should be taken through a plastic straw to avoid discoloration of tooth enamel and should be diluted adequately per manufacturer's guidelines. Oral forms should also be given with juice (but not antacids or milk) between meals for maximal absorption. Should GI distress occur, the iron should be taken with meals.

Iron dextran should be administered only after all oral iron preparations have been discontinued and only after a test dose of iron dextran has been ordered (usually 25 mg by preferred route with remaining dose given 1 hour later). IM iron should be administered deep in large muscle mass using a Z-track method and a 19 to 20 gauge, 2- to 3-inch needle that is long enough to administer the drug deep in the muscle mass. IV iron dextran should be given after the IV line is flushed with 10 ml of normal saline. IV iron dextran may be given undiluted or with 50 to 250 ml of normal saline. You should always check the label on the IV bottle to be sure that the vial is *without* preservatives and that IV administration is verified on the label. Epinephrine and resuscitative equipment should be available. In addition, it may be necessary for the patient to remain recumbent 30 minutes after the IV injection to prevent orthostatic hypotension. Iron dextran is *never* to be mixed with other drugs in the syringe or with 5% glucose in distilled water. Patient teaching tips are presented on p. 825.

GERIATRIC CONSIDERATIONS
Iron Agents

- Instructions on how to take oral forms of iron is crucial to safe administration. Patients should not make changes in the medication regimen such as doubling doses or discontinuing without a physician's order.

- Elderly patients should be instructed on food sources high in iron and how to include them in their menu planning. Instructions on how to steam vegetables and not to overcook foods would also be helpful to assure that foods do not lose folic acid compounds.

- Patients should be instructed to take oral iron with meals to help buffer and minimize GI distress.

- Encourage elderly patients to use community resources and provide lists to them of resources for meals, such as churches in the community that have elderly care programs or agencies such as Meals on Wheels.

EVALUATION

Therapeutic responses to iron products include increased nutritional status, increased weight, increased activity tolerance and well-being, and absence of fatigue. Side effects to look for include nausea, constipation, epigastric pain, black and tarry stools, vomiting and toxic signs and symptoms of nausea, vomiting, diarrhea (green, tarry stools), hematemesis, pallor, cyanosis, shock, and coma.

Therapeutic effects of vitamin B_{12} include decreased anorexia, dyspnea on exertion, palpitations, tachycardia, psychosis, and visual disturbances. With use of vitamin B_{12}, patients who have congestive heart failure or cardiac disorders should be closely monitored for worsening of CHF or pulmonary edema.

T A K E   H O M E   P O I N T S

Nursing Considerations

- Iron and vitamin B_{12} are very important in the treatment of many disorders and diseases, such as malignancies, to achieve RBC and Hgb formation that is as adequate as possible and to help prevent nutritional deficits that can affect all body systems, especially the immune system.

- Blood-forming agents are often used in the treatment of pernicious anemias, malabsorption syndromes, hemolytic anemias, hemorrhage, and renal and liver diseases.

- The patient must have a thorough assessment, including a head-to-toe nursing assessment, dietary history, and list of medications (including OTC agents) to rule out any major nutritional deficits. Baseline values in nutritional disorders should also be documented.

- Iron dextran, if given IM, should be administered by Z-track method.

- A doctor should be consulted before any vitamin B_{12} or iron products are administered.

- Oral iron products are not interchangeable

- Oral iron products may lead to GI and esophageal irritation.

- Lifelong vitamin B_{12} injections (IM) are needed for treatment of pernicious anemias unless contraindicated.

- Foods high in vitamin B_{12} include egg yolks, fish, organ meats, dairy products, and oysters; foods high in iron include dark leafy vegetables, dried beans, and dried fruits.

Critical Thinking **A C T I V I T I E S**

1. In your clinical area, take a 24-hour dietary intake history of any of your assigned patients. Analyze their intake, while hospitalized, for iron content. In addition, note the medications ordered to identify any supplemental vitamins or iron tablets and to identify any drug interactions. Also note any laboratory values, such as RBC, Hgb, Hct, bilirubin levels, and reticulocyte levels.

2. Discuss the importance of monitoring reticulocyte counts, Hgb, and Hct levels once oral iron therapy has been initiated.

▲▲▲

BIBLIOGRAPHY

Albanese J, Nutz P: *Mosby's 1995 nursing drug cards,* St Louis, 1995, Mosby.

Johnson KB: *Harriet Lane handbook,* ed 13, St Louis, 1993, Mosby.

Keen JH: *Critical care and emergency drug reference,* St Louis, 1994, Mosby.

Knoben JE, Anderson PO: *Handbook of critical drug data,* ed 6, Hamilton, Ill, 1988, Drug Intelligence Publications.

McEvoy GK: *AHFS drug information,* Bethesda, Md, 1994, American Society of Hospital Pharmacists.

Sharts-Hopko NC: Folic acid in the prevention of neural tube defects, *MCN* 18(4):232, 1993.

Skidmore-Roth L: *Mosby's 1995 nursing drug reference,* St Louis, 1995, Mosby.

United States Pharmacopeial Convention: *Drug information for the health care professional,* ed 14, Baltimore, 1994, The Convention.

Chapter 53

Dermatologic Agents

Objectives

When you reach the end of this chapter, you will be able to:

1 Discuss the normal actions and functions of the skin.

2 Describe the different skin disorders, infections, and conditions commonly affecting the skin.

3 Identify the various dermatologic agents that are used in treatment of skin disorders, infections, or infestations.

4 Discuss the mechanism of action, indications, contraindications, cautions, and side effects of dermatologic agents.

5 Develop a nursing care plan related to the nursing process for the patient receiving any of the dermatologic agents.

6 Identify patient teaching guidelines for the patient receiving ophthalmic agents.

CHAPTER OUTLINE

The Skin

Dermatologic Agents

Topical Antiinfectives

Drug Profiles
Antibacterial Agents
 Bacitracin
Acne Agents
 Benzoyl peroxide
 ⚓ Erythromycin
 Tretinoin
Antifungal Agents
 Clotrimazole
 ⚓ Miconazole
Antiviral Agents
Topical Anesthetic, Antipruritic, and
 Antiinflammatory Agents

Drug Profiles
Miscellaneous Dermatologic Agents
 Topical ectoparasiticidal drugs
 ⚓ Lindane
 Minoxidil
 Topical antineoplastics
 Silver Sulfadiazine

Nursing Process
Assessment
Nursing Diagnoses

Planning
 Outcome criteria
Implementation
Evaluation

Glossary

Actinic keratosis (ak tin′ ik ker′ ə to′ sis) A slowly developing, localized thickening of the outer layers of the skin resulting from long-term, prolonged exposure to the sun. Also called *solar keratosis.* (p. 837)

Dermatologic agent (dər′ mə to loj′ ik) Drug used to treat reactions or disorders of the skin. (p. 829)

Dermis (dər′ mis) The layer of the skin just below the epidermis, consisting of papillary and reticular layers and containing blood and lymphatic vessels, nerves and nerve endings, glands, and hair follicles. (p. 829)

Epidermis (ep′ ĭ dər′ mis) The superficial, avascular layers of the skin, made up of an outer, dead, cornified portion and a deeper, living, cellular portion. (p. 829)

Keratolytic (ker′ ə to lit′ ik) A drug that promotes loosening and shedding of the outer layer of the skin. (p. 832)

Pediculicides (pə dik′ u lĭ sīdz) A drug that kills lice. (p. 836)

Pediculosis (pə dik u lo′ sis) An infestation with bloodsucking lice. (p. 836)

Scabicide (ska′ bĭ sīd) Any one of a large group of drugs that destroy the itch mite, *Sarcoptes scabiei.* They are used with caution in children. (p. 836)

Scabies (skā′ bēz) A contagious disease caused by *Sarcoptes scabiei,* the itch mite, characterized by intense itching of the skin and injury to the skin (excoriation) resulting from scratching. (p. 836)

Tinea (tin′ ē ə) A group of fungal skin diseases caused by dermatophytes of several kinds and characterized by itching, scaling, and, sometimes, painful lesions. *Tinea* is a general term for infections of various causes that occur on several sites. Also called *ringworm.* (p. 833)

The Skin

The largest organ of the body is the skin. It covers the body and serves many functions, many of which we take for granted. It serves as a protective barrier for the internal organs. Without it harmful external forces such as microorganisms and chemicals would gain access to and damage or destroy many of our delicate internal organs. Part of this protection includes its ability to maintain a surface pH of 4.5 to 5.5. This weakly acidic environment discourages the growth of microorganisms that grow at a more alkaline pH of 6 to 7.5, explaining why infected skin usually has a higher pH. The skin also has the ability to sense changes in temperature (hot or cold), pressure, or pain, information that is then transmitted to nerve endings. The temperature of the environment around us changes constantly and can be extremely hot or cold. Despite this, our body maintains an almost constant temperature in any environment thanks in large part to the skin, which plays a major role in the regulation of body temperature. Heat loss and heat conservation are regulated in coordination with the blood vessels that supply blood to the skin and by means of perspiration. The skin is also able to excrete fluid and electrolytes through its sweat glands. In addition, it can store fat, synthesize vitamin D, and provide a site for drug absorption.

The skin is made up of two layers called the **dermis** and the **epidermis,** and these and many of the other structures within them are shown in Fig. 53-1. The outer skin layer, or epidermis, is itself composed of four layers. Going from the outermost to innermost layer, these are the stratum corneum, stratum lucidum, stratum granulosum, and the stratum germinativum. The respective functions of these layers are described in the box on p. 830. None of these layers has a direct

blood supply of their own. Instead all their nourishment is provided through diffusion.

The dermis lies between the epidermis and subcutaneous fat and differs from the epidermis in many ways. A major difference is that it is approximately forty times thicker than the epidermis, the reason for this being that it is composed of many types of tissues and blood vessels. Traversing the dermis is a rich supply of blood vessels, nerves, lymphatic tissue, elastic tissue, and connective tissue, all of which are meant to provide extra support and nourishment to the skin. Also contained in this layer are the exocrine glands—the eccrine, apocrine, and sebaceous glands—and the hair follicles. The functions of the various types of exocrine glands are explained in the box on p. 830.

Below the dermis is a layer of loose connective tissue called the *hypodermis.* It helps make the skin flexible. It is also here that the subcutaneous fat tissue is located, which provides thermal insulation and cushioning or padding. It is also the source of nutrition for the skin.

Dermatologic Agents

Reactions or disorders of the skin are common and numerous. The drugs used to treat these disorders can be administered directly to the site and are called **dermatologic agents.** There are many such agents, and they come in a multitude of formulations, some of the more common of which are listed below:

- Ointment
- Gel/jelly
- Oil
- Cream
- Aerosol spray
- Paste
- Aerosol foam
- Tape
- Lotion
- Powder

Each formulation has certain characteristics that make it suitable for specific indications. The formulations, their characteristics, and examples of each are summarized in Table 53-1.

There are also several categories of dermatologic agents, and these are listed below:

- Antibacterial agents
- Emollients
- Antiinflammatory agents
- Antifungal agents
- Keratolytics

▼ **FIG. 53-1** A microscopic view of the skin. The epidermis, shown in longitudinal section, is raised at one corner to reveal the ridges in the dermis. (Modified from Thibodeau: *Structure and function of the body,* ed 9, St Louis, 1992, Mosby.)

Epidermal Layers

LAYER	DESCRIPTION
Stratum corneum (horny layer)	Outer dead cells that are a converted water-repellent protein known as keratin; it is the protective layer for the entire body. After it is desquamated or shed, it is replaced by new cells from below.
Stratum lucidum (clear layer)	Layer where keratin is formed; it is translucent and contains flat cells.
Stratum granulosum (granular layer)	Cells die in this layer; granulated cells are located there, giving this layer the appearance it is named for.
Stratum germinativum	New skin cells are made in this layer; contains melanocytes, which produce melanin, the skin color pigment.

Exocrine Glands of the Skin

GLAND	FUNCTION
Sebaceous	Large lipid-containing cells that produce oil or film that covers the epidermis; it protects and lubricates skin and is water repellent and antiseptic.
Eccrine	Sweat glands that are located throughout the skin surface; help regulate body temperature and prevent skin dryness.
Apocrine	Mainly in axilla, genital organs, and breast areas; emit an odor; believed to be scent or sex glands.

Table 53-1	Dermatologic Formulations: Characteristics and Examples	
FORMULATION	**CHARACTERISTICS**	**EXAMPLES**
Aerosol foam	■ Can cover large area ■ Useful for drug delivery into a body cavity (e.g., vagina or rectum) or hairy areas	Proctofoam, Epifoam, contraceptive foams
Aerosol spray	■ Spreads thin liquid or powder film ■ Covers large areas ■ Useful when skin is tender to touch (e.g., burns)	Solarcaine, Desenex, Kenalog
Cream	■ Contains water and can be removed with water ■ Not greasy or occlusive ■ Usually white semisolid ■ Good for moist areas	Hydrocortisone cream, Benadryl cream
Gel/jelly	■ Contains water and possibly alcohol ■ Easily removed and good lubricator ■ Usually clear, semisolid substance ■ Useful when lubricant properties are desirable	K-Y jelly, Saligel, Surgilube
Lotion	■ Contains water, alcohol, and solvents ■ May be a suspension, emulsion, or solution ■ Good for large or hairy areas	Calamine lotion, Lubriderm lotion, Kwell lotion
Oil	■ Contains very little if any water ■ Occlusive, liquid ■ Not removable with water ■ Excellent emollient properties	Lubriderm bath oil
Ointment	■ Contains no water and is not removable with water ■ Is occlusive, greasy, and semisolid ■ Desirable for dry lesions because of occlusiveness	Petrolatum (Vasoline), zinc oxide ointment, A & D ointment
Paste	■ Similar properties to those of the ointments ■ Contains more powder than ointments ■ Excellent protectant properties	Zinc oxide paste
Powder	■ Slight lubricating properties ■ May be shaken on affected area ■ Promotes drying of area where applied	Tinactin powder, Desenex powder
Tape	■ Most occlusive formulation ■ Consistent topical drug delivery ■ Useful when small, straight areas require drug application	Cordran tape

- Local anesthetics
- Antiviral agents
- Debriding agents
- Antipruritic agents
- Antineoplastics
- Burn drugs
- Minoxidil

TOPICAL ANTIINFECTIVES

Topical antiinfectives consist of antibacterial, antifungal, and antiviral drugs that, as the name implies, are applied topically. The systemically administered antiinfective agents are discussed in detail in Part 8, where their specific pharmacologic characteristics are also described. Their topical uses are discussed here, as are any characteristics specific to this use. Although they have many of the same properties as the systemic forms, there are some differences in terms of the toxicities and side effects they cause. The drugs that are used to treat dermatologic parasitic infections, the pediculicides and scabicides, as well as the drugs commonly used to treat acne, are also covered in this section.

DRUG PROFILES

ANTIBACTERIAL AGENTS

Common skin disorders that are caused by various bacteria are folliculitis, impetigo, furuncles, carbuncles, and cellulitis. The bacteria responsible are most commonly *Streptococcus pyogenes* and *Staphylococcus aureus*. Dermatologic antibacterial agents are used to treat or prevent these skin infections, the most commonly used ones being bacitracin, polymyxin, and neomycin.

BACITRACIN

Bacitracin (Baciguent) is a polypeptide antibiotic that is applied topically for the treatment or prevention of local skin infections caused by susceptible aerobic and anaerobic gram-positive organisms such as staphylococci and streptococci as well as corynebacteria and clostridia. It works by inhibiting bacterial cell wall synthesis, which leads to cell death. It can be either bactericidal or bacteriostatic, depending on the causative organism.

Its antimicrobial spectrum is broadened when it is used in combination with other topical antibiotics, and there are several such combination products available. Most contain neomycin and polymyxin B. Ointment formulations of the agent are the ones most frequently used, but powders and aerosols are also available. As a single-agent product, bacitracin comes as a 500-U/gm ointment and a powder which is applied to the affected area one to three times daily.

ACNE AGENTS

Other antibacterial agents are used to treat acne, the skin infection commonly caused by *Propionibacterium acnes*. These agents include benzoyl peroxide, clindamycin, erythromycin, meclocycline, tetracycline, and the vitamin A acid called *retinoic acid*. There are also many other agents used in the treatment and prevention of acne.

BENZOYL PEROXIDE

The microorganism that most commonly causes acne, *Propionibacterium acnes*, is an anaerobic bacteria that needs an environment poor in oxygen in order to grow. Benzoyl peroxide is effective in combating such infection because it slowly and continuously liberates active oxygen, causing antibacterial, antiseptic, drying, and keratolytic actions. All these actions create an environment unfavorable for the continued growth of the *P. acnes* bacteria, and they soon die. Such drugs as benzoyl peroxide that soften scales and loosen the outer horny layer of the skin are referred to as **keratolytics**.

Benzoyl peroxide generally produces signs of improvement within 4 to 6 weeks. Side effects are infrequent and rarely a problem. Most are confined to the skin and involve peeling skin, red skin, or a sensation of warmth. Blistering or swelling of the skin is generally considered an allergic reaction to the product, and is an indication to stop treatment.

Benzoyl peroxide comes as a 5% or 10% lotion that is usually applied topically one to four times a day. It also comes as a cleansing bar that is used two or three times daily and as a cream or cleansing lotion that is applied one to two times daily. Benzoyl peroxide is rated as a pregnancy category C agent.

⚓ ERYTHROMYCIN

Erythromycin (A/T/S, EryDerm, T-stat, Erygel) is a macrolide antibiotic used for the topical treatment of acne vulgaris, a common form of acne. It usually only stops the growth of the acne-causing bacteria (bacteriostatic), but it may kill bacteria either when given in high concentrations or when the organisms are highly susceptible. It exerts its antibacterial effects by inhibiting protein synthesis in susceptible organisms.

Erythromycin topical preparations are applied to the cleansed affected areas each morning and evening. Skin reactions are the most common side effect and consist of erythema, desquamation, tenderness, dryness, pruritus, burning, oiliness, and acne. Erythromycin comes as a 1.5% or 2% solution, a 2% gel, or a 2% ointment and is classified as a pregnancy category C agent. It is contraindicated in patients with a known hypersensitivity to it.

TRETINOIN

Tretinoin (retinoic acid, vitamin A acid, Retin-A) is a derivative of vitamin A that is used to treat acne as well as to ameliorate the dermatologic changes (e.g., fine wrinkling, mottled hyperpigmentation, roughness) associated with photodamage. The drug appears to act as an an irritant on the skin, in particular the follicular epithelium. Specifically, it stimulates the turnover of epidermal cells, which results in skin peeling. While this is occurring, the free fatty acid levels are reduced and horny cells cannot then adhere to each other. Without fatty acids and horny cells, acne and its comedo, or pimple, cannot exist.

Topically administered tretinoin has been shown to enhance the repair of skin damaged by ultraviolet radiation or sunlight. It does this by increasing the formation of fibroblasts and collagen, both of which are needed to rebuild skin. The drug also may reduce collagen degradation by inhibiting the enzyme coleagenase that breaks down collagen.

As with erythromycin, tretinoin's main side effects are local inflammatory reactions, which are reversible when therapy is discontinued. Some of the most common side effects are excessively red and edematous blisters, crusted skin, and temporary alterations in skin pigmentation. Tretinoin is available in many topical formulations: a topical powder; a 0.025%, 0.05%, and 0.1% topical cream; a 0.01% and 0.025% topical gel; and a 0.05% topical solution. Because of its potential to cause severe irritation and peeling, it may initially be applied once every 2 or 3 days, preferably using the lower-concentration cream or gel.

ANTIFUNGAL AGENTS

There are a few fungi that produce keratinolytic enzymes, which allows them to live on the skin. Topical fungal infections are primarily caused by *Candida* spp. (candidiasis), dermatophytes, and *Malassezia furfur* (tinae versicolor). These fungi exist in moist, warm environments, preferably in dark areas such as the feet or groin.

Candidal infections are most commonly caused by *Candida albicans,* a yeastlike opportunistic fungus present in the normal flora of the mouth, vagina, and intestinal tract. Two significant factors that commonly predispose a person to a candidal infection are broad-spectrum antibiotic therapy, which promotes an overgrowth of nonsusceptible organism in the natural body florae, and immunodeficiency disorders such as those that occur in patients with cancer, AIDS, or organ transplants. Because these infections favor warm, moist areas of the skin and mucous membranes, they most frequently occur orally, a form commonly seen in infants and called thrush, vaginally, and cutaneously in such sites as beneath the breasts and in diaper areas. They may also cause nail infections.

Dermatophytes are a group of three closely related genera consisting of *Epidermophyton* spp., *Microsporum* spp., and *Trichophyton* spp. that utilize the keratin found on the skin for their growth. They produce superficial mycotic (fungal) infections of keratinized tissue (hair, skin, and nails). Infections due to dermatophytes are collectively called **tinea**, or ringworm, infections. The name *ringworm* comes from the fact that the infection often assumes a circular pattern at the site of infection. The tinea infections are further identified by the body location where they occur: tinea pedis (foot), tinea crusis (groin), tinea corporis (body), and

tinea capitis (scalp). Tinea infections are also known as *athlete's foot* or *jock itch.*

Fungi usually invade the stratum corneum, which is the dead layer of desquamated cells. Inflammation occurs when the fungi invade this layer; sensitivity occurs when they penetrate the epidermis and dermis.

Many of the fungi that cause topical infections are very difficult to eradicate. They are very slow growing, and antifungal therapy may be required for periods ranging from several weeks to as long as a year. There are however, many topical antifungal drugs available for the treatment of both dermatophyte infections and those caused by yeast and yeastlike fungi. Some of these agents, their dosage forms, and their uses are listed in Table 53-2.

The most commonly reported side effects of topical antifungals include local irritation, pruritus, a burning sensation, and scaling. Ciclopirox, clotrimazole, miconazole, and haloprogin are classified as pregnancy category B agents, and econazole and ketoconazole are classified as pregnancy category C agents. Hypersensitivity is the one contraindication to the use of any of these agents.

CLOTRIMAZOLE

Clotrimazole (Mycelex troche, Lotrimin, Mycelex-G) is a prescription-only medication. It comes as a lozenge for the treatment of oropharyngeal candidiasis, commonly known as *thrush.* It also comes as a cream, lotion, or solution for the treatment of dermatophytoses, superficial mycoses, and cutaneous candidiasis. Such topical preparations are also available for intravaginal administration in the treatment of both vulvovaginal candidiasis, commonly called a *yeast infection,* and vaginal trichomoniasis.

Clotrimazole is available in many topical formulations. It comes as a powder; a 10-mg oral topical lozenge; a 1% cream, lotion, and solution; a 1% vaginal cream; and a 100- and a 500-mg vaginal tablet. Different dosages and the different dosage forms are used for the treatment of the various fungal infections.

⚓ MICONAZOLE

Miconazole (Monistat, MicaTin, Monistat 7) is a topical antifungal agent that is available in several over-the-counter (OTC) and prescription products. It inhibits the growth of several fungi, including dermatophytes and yeast, as well as gram-positive bacteria and is commonly used to treat dermatophytoses, superficial mycoses, cutaneous candidiasis, and vulvovaginal candidiasis. It is in many OTC remedies for athlete's foot, jock itch, and yeast infections.

For the treatment of athlete's foot, jock itch, ringworm, and other susceptible fungal infections, micon-

Table 53-2 | Topical Antifungal Agents

DRUG	PRODUCT NAMES	DOSAGE FORMS	USE	LEGAL STATUS
Amphotericin B	Fungizone	3% cream, 3% lotion, 3% ointment	Candidiasis	Rx
Butoconazole	Femstat	2% vaginal cream	Candidiasis	Rx
Ciclopirox olamine	Loprox	1% cream, 1% lotion	Candidiasis, dermatophytoses, tinea versicolor	Rx
Clioquinol	Vioform	3% cream, ointment	Dermatophytoses	OTC
Clotrimazole	Gyne-Lotrimin	1% cream, 100- and 500-mg vaginal tablets	Candidiasis	OTC
	Lotrimin	1% cream, 1% lotion, 1% solution	Candidiasis, tinea versicolor	Rx
	Lotrimin AF	1% cream, 1% lotion, 1% solution	Dermatophytoses	OTC
	Mycelex	1% cream, 1% solution	Dermatophytoses	OTC
	Mycelex	10-mg troches	Oropharyngeal candidiasis	Rx
	Mycelex-7	1% vaginal cream, 100-mg vaginal tablets	Candidiasis	OTC
	Mycelex G	500-mg vaginal tablets	Candidiasis	Rx
Econazole nitrate	Spectazole	1% cream	Candidiasis, dermatophytoses	Rx
Haloprogin	Halotex	1% cream, 1% solution	Dermatophytoses, tinea versicolor	Rx
Ketoconazole	Nizoral	2% cream, 2% shampoo	Candidiasis, dermatophytoses, tinea versicolor	Rx
Miconazole nitrate	MicaTin	2% cream, 2% powder, 2% spray	Dermatophytoses	OTC
	Monistat Derm	2% cream,	Candidiasis, dermatophytoses, tinea versicolor	Rx
Naftifine Hcl	Naftin	1% cream, 1% gel	Dermatophytoses	Rx
Natamycin	Natacyn	5% ophthalmic suspension	Ocular fungal infections	Rx
Nystatin	Nilstat/Mycostatin	cream, ointment, powder	Candidiasis	Rx
Oxiconazole nitrate	Oxistat	1% cream, 1% lotion	Dermatophytoses	Rx
Sodium thiosulfate	None	25% solution	Tinea versicolor	OTC
Sulconazole	Exelderm	1% cream, 1% solution	Dermatophytoses	Rx
Terbinafine Hcl	Lamisil	1% cream	Dermatophytoses	Rx
Tolnaftate	ND .27	1% cream, 1% solution	Dermatophytoses	OTC
	Tinactin	1% cream, 1% solution		

Rx, prescription only; *OTC*, over the counter.

azole should be applied sparingly to the cleansed, dry, infected area twice daily, in the morning and the evening. For the treatment of yeast infections, one 200-mg suppository should be inserted in the vagina once daily at bedtime for 3 consecutive days or 100 mg (one suppository or 5 gm of the 2% cream) should be administered intravaginally once daily at bedtime for 7 days.

The most common side effects of topically administered miconazole are vulvovaginal burning and itching, pelvic cramps and rash, urticaria, stinging, burning, and contact dermatitis. It is available in a variety of topical formulations: a 2% aerosol spray and powder, a 2% powder, and a 2% cream, as well as a 2% vaginal cream and a 100- and 500-mg vaginal suppository.

ANTIVIRAL AGENTS

As noted in the chapter on antiviral agents, viral infections are very difficult to treat because they live in the body's own healthy cells and use their cell mechanisms to reproduce. The same holds true for topical viral infections. Infections caused by herpes simplex types 1 and 2 are particularly serious and are becoming more common. The only drug currently available to treat such topical viral infections is acyclovir.

Acyclovir works by inhibiting the viral enzymes necessary for DNA synthesis. It is applied topically for the treatment of initial and recurrent herpes simplex infections in immunocompromised patients, although often these topical infections can be prevented or treated more efficaciously with systemically administered antiviral agents. Topically applied acyclovir does not cure viral skin infections but does appear to decrease the healing time and associated pain.

Acyclovir is available as a 5% topical ointment that is applied every 3 hours, or six times daily, for 1 week. A finger cot or rubber glove should be worn for the application of the ointment to prevent the spread of infection. The most common side effects are stinging, itching, and rash. Acyclovir is classified as a pregnancy category C agent and is contraindicated in patients with a hypersensitivity to it.

TOPICAL ANESTHETIC, ANTIPRURITIC, AND ANTIINFLAMMATORY AGENTS

The topical anesthetic agents are drugs that are used to numb the skin. They accomplish this by inhibiting the conduction of nerve impulses from sensory nerves, thereby reducing or eliminating the pain or pruritus associated with insect bites, sunburn, and plant allergies such as poison ivy, as well as many other uncomfortable skin disorders. They are also used to numb the skin before giving a person a painful injection. Topical anesthetics are available as ointments, creams, sprays, liquids, and jellies, and have been discussed in Chapter 9.

The topical antipruritic agents contain antihistamines or corticosteroids. Many exert a combined anesthetic and antipruritic action when applied topically. The antihistamines and their therapeutic effects have been covered in Chapter 34.

The topical antiinflammatory agents are most commonly corticosteroids, and they are generally indicated for the relief of inflammatory and pruritic dermatoses. By administering them topically, many of the undesirable systemic side effects associated with the use of the systemically administered corticosteroids are averted. The beneficial drug effects of the corticosteroids are their antiinflammatory, antipruritic, and vasoconstrictor actions.

Topical Corticosteroids	
RANGE OF POTENCY	**CORTICOSTEROID**
Most potent	Betamethasone dipropionate (cream and ointment), clobetasol propionate
Very potent	Amcinonide, betamethasone dipropionate (lotion), desoximethasone (cream and ointment, 0.25%), diflorasone diacetate, fluocinolone, halcinonide, triamcinolone acetonide (cream and ointment, 0.5%)
Potent	Betamethasone, betamethasone valerate (0.1% cream, ointment, and lotion), desoximethasone (0.5% gel), fluocinolone acetonide, flurandrenolide, halcinonide, and triamcinolone acetonide
Less potent	Betamethasone valerate (reduced strength cream, 0.01%), clocortolone, desonide, fluocinolone acetonide, flurandrenolide, hydrocortisone valerate, triamcinolone acetonide (cream, ointment, and lotion, 0.1%)
Least potent	Dexamethasone, hydrocortisone, methylprednisolone

Skin penetration and thus potency is enhanced by the vehicle the steroid is in. In decreasing order of effectiveness are ointments, gels, creams, and lotions.

Topical corticosteroids have many acquired properties that have the effect of altering their relative potency, and hence the conditions they are used to treat. For instance, the corticosteroids that are fluorinated are used for the treatment of dermatologic disorders such as psoriasis. The vehicle in which the corticosteroid is contained also has the effect of altering their vasoconstrictor property and therapeutic efficacy. Ointments are generally the most penetrating, followed next by gels, creams, and lotions. Propylene glycol also enhances the penetration of the corticosteroid and its vasoconstrictor effects. Most corticosteroids come in many different topical formulations, thus offering a variety of options. The currently available topical corticosteroids along with their respective potencies are listed in the box above.

Side effects of the agents include skin reactions such as acne eruptions, allergic contact dermatitis, burning sensations, dryness, itching, hypopigmentation, purpura, hirsutism (usually facial), folliculitis, round and swollen face, and alopecia (usually of scalp). An overgrowth of a bacteria, fungus, or virus and immunosuppression are others. The usual adult dosage of these drugs is one or two applications daily, as directed. Less potent topical corticosteroids are used in children, but following the same schedule. Corticosteroids are classified as pregnancy category C agents and are contraindicated in patients with a hypersensitivity to them.

DRUG PROFILES

MISCELLANEOUS DERMATOLOGIC AGENTS

There are many other topically applied drugs. Those discussed here are the topical ectoparasiticidal drugs (scabicides and pediculicides), minoxidil, antineoplastics, and silver sulfadiazine. Many of these agents are available both OTC and by prescription.

Topical Ectoparasiticidal Drugs

Ectoparasites are insects that live on the outer surface of the body, and the drugs that are used to kill them are called ectoparasiticidal drugs.

Lice are transmitted from person to person by close contact with infested persons, clothing, combs, or towels. A parasitic infestation on the skin with lice is called **pediculosis,** and such infestations go by one of four different names, depending on the location of the infestation.

> **Pediculosis pubis** → **pubic louse** or "crabs," caused by *Phthirus pubis.*
> **Pediculosis corporis** → **body louse,** caused by *Pediculus humanus corporis.*
> **Pediculosis capitis** → **head louse,** caused by *P. humanus capitis.*

Common findings in infested persons include itching, eggs of the louse on the hair shafts (called nits), lice on the skin or clothes, and, in the case of pubic lice, sky blue macules on the inner thighs or lower abdomen. Pediculoses are treated with a class of drugs called **pediculicides,** the most commonly used one being lindane.

A second common parasitic skin infection is that caused by the itch mite, *Sarcoptes scabiei,* commonly known as scabies. **Scabies** is transmitted from person to person by close contact, such as sleeping next to an infested person. The scabies mite causes irritation and itching by boring into the horny layers of skin located in cracks and folds. Itching seems to be most common in the evening. The drugs used to treat these infestations are called **scabicides.**

Treatment of these parasitic infestations should begin with identification of the source of infestation in order to prevent reinfestation. Next, the clothing and personal articles of the infested person should be decontaminated. This is best accomplished by washing them in hot, soapy water or by dry cleaning. All close contacts of the person should be treated as well, also to prevent reinfestation. Besides lindane, malathion (Prioderm), crotamiton (Eurax), and permethrin (Nix, Elimite) are other ectoparasiticidal drugs.

⚓ LINDANE

Lindane (Kwell, Scabene) is a chlorinated hydrocarbon originally developed as an agricultural insecticide. It is both a scabicide and a pediculicide because it is effective in treating both scabies and pediculosis. It is available in three topical formulations: a 1% cream, lotion, and shampoo.

For the treatment of pubic or body lice, the cream or lotion is applied in a sufficient quantity to cover the skin and hair of the infested and surrounding areas. It is left on for 12 hours and then thoroughly washed off. A second application is seldom needed. Head lice can be treated with lindane shampoo, which should be worked into the hair and left on for 4 minutes. The hair should then be rinsed and dried, after which the nits (eggs) should be combed from the hair shafts. The treatment for scabies is similar. It involves the application of lindane over the entire body, from the neck down. It is left on for 8 to 12 hours and washed off. Side effects of lindane are an eczematous skin rash and rarely CNS toxicity, the latter is more common in young children.

MINOXIDIL

Minoxidil (Rogaine) is a vasodilating drug that is administered systemically to control hypertension. Topically it has the same vasodilating effect, but when used in this way, it is applied to the scalp to stimulate hair growth. The vasodilation it causes is one possible explanation for how it stimulates hair growth. It may also act at the level of the hair follicle, possibly stimulating hair follicle growth directly.

It can be used in both men and women suffering from baldness or hair thinning. Treatment consists of administering the agent to the affected (balding and anticipated balding) area twice daily, usually morning and evening. It generally takes 4 months before results are seen, however.

Systemic absorption of the topically applied minoxidil is possible. Therefore the side effects of topically applied minoxidil are systemic ones, such as tachycardia, fluid retention, and weight gain. Topically administered minoxidil is available as a 2% solution. Each metered dose delivers 1 ml or 20 mg of the agent.

Topical Antineoplastics

Various premalignant skin lesions and basal cell carcinomas may be treated with the topically applied antineoplastic drug fluorouracil (Efudex or Fluoroplex). It acts by destroying rapidly growing cells such as premalignant and malignant cells. It is also used topically in the treatment of solar or **actinic keratosis** and basal cell carcinomas of the skin when surgical and other techniques are impractical or unfeasible.

The adverse effects associated with the topical use of this antineoplastic are much different from those seen in association with the systemic administration of the agent. Such effects are minimal and generally limited to local inflammatory reactions such as dermatitis, stomatitis, and photosensitivity. Major adverse effects of fluorouracil topical therapy are swelling, scaling, pain, pruritus, burning, soreness, tenderness, suppuration, scarring, and hyperpigmentation.

Fluorouracil is available as a 1% and 5% topical cream and a 1%, 2%, and 5% topical solution. It can be applied with a nonmetallic applicator, clean fingertips, or gloved fingers. If the fingers are used, they should be washed thoroughly immediately after application. Either a 1% or 2% fluorouracil solution should be used for the treatment of multiple actinic keratoses of the head and neck. It should be applied twice daily to the lesions. Superficial basal cell carcinoma may be treated with 5% fluorouracil, administered twice daily for at least 3 to 6 weeks.

SILVER SULFADIAZINE

One of the concerns in burn victims is infection at the burn site, but there are two problems posed by the use of either topically or administered antiinfective agents in this setting. Because of the systemic absorption of a drug that can occur in compromised skin areas such as burns, the agent cannot be so toxic, or the quantities absorbed so toxic, that if absorbed into the circulation this leads to untoward effects. On the other hand, the blood supply to burned areas is often drastically reduced, such that systemically administered antibiotics either cannot reach the site or do so only in quantities too low to be effective. Therefore, the only way of applying these agents to ensure that they reach the burn site is to do so topically. Some of the commonly used agents that have proved both effective and safe in the prevention or treatment of infections in burns are silver sulfadiazine (Silvadene), mafenide (Sulfamylon), and nitrofurazone (Furacin).

Silver sulfadiazine is a synthetic antiinfective agent produced when silver nitrate reacts with sulfadiazine. It appears to act on the cell membrane and cell wall of susceptible bacteria and is used as an adjunct in the prevention and treatment of infection in second- and third-degree burns. The side effects of silver sulfadiazine are similar to those of other topical drugs and include pain, burning, or itching. It is available as a 1% cream and should be applied topically to cleansed, debrided, burned areas once or twice daily using a sterile-gloved hand.

NURSING PROCESS

ASSESSMENT

Before using any of the dermatologic preparations, the nurse should rule out the presence of the many conditions and problems that may be a contraindication to its use, one being a known hypersensitivity to any of the agents. It is important for the nurse to always check to make sure the patient has no drug allergies and has shown no previous sensitivity to antimicrobials or any of the other topical agents. Patients who are to be treated with benzoyl peroxide agents should be checked for allergies and previous local reactions to the medication. The antibacterial topical agents are associated with a broader risk of reactions because of the generalized sensitivity of patients to the same antibiotic in its different dosage forms. Therefore, should a patient have an allergy to a particular antibacterial agent, that agent should not be used topically either. Always be sure that, if culture and sensitivity testing has been ordered, the specimen has been collected before the first application of the antibacterial agent.

When administering any type of topical medication, such as an antimicrobial, steroid, or antiacne agent, the concentration of the medication, the length of exposure to the skin, the condition of the skin, the size of the area affected, and the hydration status of the skin should all be taken into consideration because all have a significant effect on the action of the medication.

The skin, and in particular the area affected, must be inspected thoroughly under an adequate light source and the area palpated with a gloved hand, especially in dark-skinned persons because often an erythematous area may not be visible but may be palpated as an area of warmth. All findings should be thoroughly documented and reflect a systematic and bilateral assessment of all areas.

The patient's overall health status and hygiene practices should also be assessed, and this includes whether the patient has suffered any trauma or whether his or her immune system is suppressed. Exudate or drainage material should also be obtained for culture studies before therapy is initiated, but with a physician's order. The nurse should also remember that the skin of the very young and the very old is often more permeable to some of the dermatologic preparations such as the corticosteroids.

NURSING DIAGNOSES

Nursing diagnoses pertinent to the use of dermatologic preparations include:
- Impaired skin integrity related to disease or disorder.
- Pain related to the skin condition or adverse reactions to the topical preparation.
- Self-care deficit pertaining to care of the affected area.
- Disturbed self-concept related to the patient's fear about and perception of the skin disorder.
- Knowledge deficit about the skin disorder and the recommended drug therapy.

PLANNING

Goals related to the administration of dermatologic preparations include:
- Patient's skin remains intact and healed in appearance and integrity.
- Patient remains compliant with therapy.
- Patient remains free of injury to skin while on therapy.
- Patient experiences minimal to no complications of therapy.
- Patient maintains positive self-concept.

Outcome Criteria

Outcome criteria related to the administration of dermatologic agents include:
- Patient's skin improves daily, that is, there will be less redness, drainage, discomfort, itching, rash, and the like.
- Patient has fewer complaints about localized skin discomfort (e.g., pain, itching).
- Patient demonstrates how to apply medication as

prescribed and to follow physician's orders in its application.
- Patient openly verbalizes feelings about altered self-concept and fears about social isolation or ridicule.
- Patient states the rationale for treatment, the side effects of the dermatologic preparation, and symptoms to report associated with the dermatologic therapy.
- Patient remains compliant with the medication therapy with resultant improved condition.

IMPLEMENTATION

Generally speaking, before applying any more topical medication, the nurse should cleanse thoroughly the site of any debris as well as any residual medication, making sure to follow any specific directions, such as removing water or alcohol-based topicals with soap and water.

Universal precautions should be maintained. The nurse should wear gloves, not only to prevent contamination from secretions but also to prevent absorption of the medication through his or her skin. If using lotions, they should be stored according to the manufacturer's recommendations and shaken well before using. Creams and ointments are often applied with a sterile cotton-tipped applicator or tongue blade. Any dressings should be applied as ordered and special attention paid to directions concerning occlusive, wet, or wet-to-dry dressings. Information about the site of application; about any drainage, swelling, temperature, color, and any painful or other sensations; and about the type of treatment rendered and any response should all be documented.

The manufacturer's guidelines regarding the use of any of the dermatologic preparations should always

RESEARCH ACTIVITIES
Dermatologic Preparations

Read two nursing research articles published within the past 5 years about tretinoin, and answer the following questions:

1. What is the controversy concerning the use of tretinoin in pregnant women?
2. What are the pros and cons of topical tretinoin therapy for sun-induced aged skin disorders?
3. Why are some insurers not covering tretinoin in middle-aged women?

be followed because often each medication has a different type of base solution and specific application procedures are required for different dosage forms. In addition, it is important to follow any instructions or orders regarding any adjuvant therapy. Often an occlusive or wet dressing may be needed, and medicated areas may need to be protected from exposure to air or sunlight. Strict adherence to the proper method of application and dosage of any dermatologic preparation is important to its effectiveness; however, doubling-up on dosing if a dose is missed is not recommended. See the box below for teaching tips for patients being treated with any of the various dermatologic preparations.

After completing the application procedure, the nurse should wash his or her hands, dispose of contaminated dressings, chart the procedure and findings, and maintain asepsis, surgical asepsis if the wound is open in any way or the skin is not intact. The privacy, comfort, and safety of the patient must be maintained, as it would be for any procedure. See Table 53-3 for the nursing implications pertinent to each group of dermatologic agents.

Patient Teaching TIPS

Dermatologic Preparations

✔ Instruct patients to keep their skin clean and dry and to maintain adequate general hygiene and diet during therapy for skin disorder.

✔ Patients should apply medication only as ordered and follow instructions carefully.

✔ Patients should be told to avoid exposure to sunlight, unless it is indicated.

✔ Patients should apply dressings to the area after the medication has been applied, as ordered or per the manufacturer's guidelines.

✔ Patients should be instructed to notify the physician of any unusual or adverse reactions.

✔ Patients must know that compliance with therapy is crucial to the therapeutic effectiveness of dermatologic preparations.

✔ Antifungals should be administered as ordered and consistently, because fungal infections are very difficult to treat and often require prolonged therapy.

✔ Have patients demonstrate the application technique, because this is important to ensuring effective therapy and compliance.

TAKE HOME POINTS

Pharmacologic Principles

■ Topical infections

■ Common skin disorders caused by bacteria: folliculitis, impetigo, furuncles, carbuncles, cellulitis.

■ The bacteria most frequently responsible for acne is *Propionibacterium acnes*.

■ The fungi that are responsible for causing topical fungal infections are *Candida*, dermatophytes, and *Malassezia furfur*.

■ The most common topical fungal infections are candidal infections such as yeast-infections.

■ One of the most common topical viral infections is *herpes simplex* types 1 and 2.

Topical Anesthetics

■ Used topically to numb the skin.

■ Some indications include insect bites, burns (sunburn), poison ivy, and before painful injections.

Topical Antiinflammatory Agents

■ Most commonly used are corticosteroids.

■ Indicated for relief of topical inflammatory and pruritic disorders.

■ Beneficial effects of corticosteroids include antiinflammatory, antipruritic, vasoconstrictor actions.

Topical Antineoplastics

■ Used to treat various skin lesions that are believed to be premalignant, as well as basal cell carcinomas.

■ Commonly used agent = fluorouracil.

Nursing Considerations

■ Adverse and toxic reactions to dermatologic agents *can* and *do* happen, so cautious administration, per physician's orders and manufacturer's guidelines, is critical to ensuring safe and effective treatment.

■ Adequate and correct application of these agents by the nurse is also critical to ensuring safe and effective treatment.

■ Patient education about the medication, its administration, and effectiveness is important to ensure compliance.

■ The effectiveness of the therapy is determined by whether the lesions or affected areas heal or resolve without adverse reactions.

Table 53-3 | Dermatologic Agents: Nursing Implications

CLASSIFICATION	SPECIFIC AGENT	NURSING IMPLICATIONS
Antiinfectives and antibiotics	Bacitracin, neomycin, clindamycin, erythromycin, tetracycline	■ Bacitracin is odorless and nonstaining. ■ Neomycin may cause sensitization and photosensitivity when used with topical gentamicin. ■ Apply thin film of clindamycin and assess for allergy to drug and other antibiotics. ■ Erythromycin is applied with fingertips and hands each AM and PM. ■ Tetracycline is applied until skin is wet/moist, but avoid eyes and mucous membranes because of alcohol content.
Antiinflammatories	Betamethasone benzoate, dexamethasone, fluocinolone acetonide, fluocinonide, hydrocortisone, methylprednisolone	■ All of these help to stabilize cell membranes, and the ointment bases and glycol enhance the penetration of the agent into the skin; usually are applied two times a day, and application technique depends on site; monitor serum cortisol levels every other month in patients receiving long term, until discharge; be careful with occlusive dressings because this can lead to follicle infections, heat retention, or systemic effects, but occlusive dressings are often ordered.
Antiparasitic	Lindane, malathion	■ With lindane, leave shampoo on for 4 min, then rinse and use nit comb to remove nits (eggs) from the hair shafts; cream and lotions are usually left on for 12 hr, then washed off; pubic lice treated by applying for 12 hr then washed off. ■ With malathion, there must be much care because it is flammable; need to avoid open flames and hair dryers; apply to hair and wash off after 8-12 hr.
Acne products (keratolytics)	Benzoyl peroxide, tretinoin	■ With benzoyl, see effects in 4-6 wk; applied by lotion, bar, or cream sparingly. ■ Tretinoin to be applied each night at bedtime; apply after cleansing and allow 30 min to dry; if applied to wet skin, there may be increased redness or drying; avoid ultraviolet light, weather extremes, or sunlight; avoid abrasive cleansers, other keratolytic products, etc., because of possible toxicity to the skin; wear sunscreen during therapy.
Burn products	Silver sulfadiazine	■ Apply as a 1% cream only to clean, debrided wounds and with gloved hands; apply 1/16 in thick; keep continuously covered; daily cleansing and debriding important; hemolysis may occur in patients with G6PD deficiency; if applied to extensive areas, adverse systemic reactions may occur similar to those seen for sulfonamide.
Antivirals	Acylovir	■ To be applied using a finger cot or gloved hand to prevent autocontamination; avoid contact with eyes; with genital lesions, loose covering or clothing over lesion is recommended to prevent further irritation to site; avoid sexual activity if active lesions; can be transmitted even if person asymptomatic; condom use encouraged depending on location of lesion; apply a half-inch (1.25-cm) ribbon of ointment to about a 4-inch (10 cm) area.
Antifungals	Amphotericin B, clotrimazole, haloprogin, ketoconazole, nystatin, miconazole	■ Can apply any of these very liberally to a clean, dry, affected skin area; occlusive dressings *not* recommended unless ordered; avoid contact with eyes; encourage good hygiene; keep area dry and clean; keep dry with powders to prevent maceration; keep area exposed to air to keep dry.

EVALUATION

Therapeutic responses to the various dermatologic preparations include improved condition of skin and healing of lesions or of wound; a decrease in the size of the lesions with eventual resolution of the lesions; and a decrease in swelling, redness, weeping, itching, and burning of area. The physician should be notified if a therapeutic response is not noted within an appro-priate time (for some agents, possibly 48 to 72 hours; for acne agents, often no response is seen for 1 to 2 months). Side effects to monitor for include an in-creased severity of symptoms such as redness, swell-ing, pain, and drainage; fever; or any other unusual adverse reactions. Side effects may range from slight irritation of the site where the topical agent has been applied to an allergic reaction to toxic systemic effects.

Critical Thinking **A C T I V I T I E S**

1. Develop a teaching plan for a 29-year-old mother who has a 6-year-old child newly diagnosed with head lice. Include an emphasis on how to prevent con-taminating others and preventing future episodes.

2. Do you consider tretinoin therapy beneficial for all patients? Why or why not, and support your answer.

BIBLIOGRAPHY

Albanese J, Nutz P: *Mosby's 1995 nursing drug cards,* St Louis, 1995, Mosby.

Dicken CH et al: Retinoids: what role in your practice? *Patient Care* 26(10):18, 1992.

Johnson KB: *Harriet Lane handbook,* ed 13, St Louis, 1993, Mosby.

Keen JH: *Critical care and emergency drug reference,* St Louis, 1994, Mosby.

Knoben JE, Anderson PO: *Handbook of critical drug data,* ed 6, Hamilton, Ill, 1988, Drug Intelligence Publica-tions.

McEvoy GK: *AHFS drug information,* Bethesda, Md, 1994, American Society of Hospital Pharmacists.

McKenry L, Salerno E: *Mosby's pharmacology in nursing,* ed 19, St Louis, 1995, Mosby.

Skidmore-Roth L: *Mosby's 1995 nursing drug reference,* St Louis, 1995, Mosby.

United States Pharmacopeial Convention: *USP DI: drug in-formation for the health care professional,* ed 14, Rockville, Md, 1994, The United States Pharmacopeial Convention.

Chapter 54

Ophthalmic Agents

Objectives

When you reach the end of this chapter, you will be able to:

1 Discuss the anatomy and physiology of the structures of the eye.

2 List the various opthalmic agents used within their classifications.

3 Describe the process of instilling eye drops or eye ointments.

4 Discuss the mechanism of action, cautions, and contraindications of opthalmic preparations and associated nursing implications.

5 Develop a comprehensive nursing care plan that includes education for patients receiving opthalmic agents.

CHAPTER OUTLINE

Structure of the Eye

Lacrimal Glands
Layers of the Eye

Antiglaucoma Drugs

Parasympathomimetics
  Mechanism of action
  Drug effects
  Therapeutic uses
  Side effects and adverse effects
    Toxicity and management of overdose
  Interactions
  Dosages

Drug Profiles
Direct-acting Miotics
  Acetylcholine
  ⇕ Pilocarpine
Indirect-acting Miotics
  Echothiophate and Isoflurophate
  ⇕ Physostigmine
Sympathomimetics
  Mechanism of action
  Drug effects
  Therapeutic uses
  Side effects and adverse effects
    Toxicity and management of overdose
  Interactions
  Dosages

Drug Profiles
  Apraclonidine
  Dipivefrin
Beta-Adrenergic Blockers
  Mechanism of action
  Drug effects
  Therapeutic uses
  Side effects and adverse effects
    Toxicity and management of overdose
  Interactions
  Dosages

Drug Profiles
  Betaxolol
  Timolol
Carbonic Anhydrase Inhibitors
  Drug effects
  Therapeutic uses
  Side effects and adverse effects
    Toxicity and management of overdose
  Interactions
  Dosages

Drug Profile
  Acetazolamide
Osmotic Diuretics
  Mechanism of action
  Drug effects
  Therapeutic uses
  Side effects and adverse effects
    Toxicity and management of overdose
  Interactions
  Dosages

continued

Drug Profiles

Glycerin

Mannitol

Ocular Antiinfectives

Mechanism of action

Drug effects

Therapeutic uses

Side effects and adverse effects

Interactions

Dosages

Drug Profiles

Aminoglycosides

⚓ Gentamicin

Macrolides

⚓ Erythromycin

Natamycin

Polypeptides

Bacitracin

Tetracyclines

Tetracycline

Quinolones

⚓ Ciprofloxacin

Sulfonamides

Sulfacetamide

Miscellaneous

Chloramphenicol

Silver Nitrate

Antivirals

Vidarabine

Antiinflammatory Ophthalmic Agents

Mechanism of action

Drug effects

Therapeutic uses

Side effects and adverse effects

Dosages

Drug Profiles

Flurbiprofen

⚓ Ketorolac

Dexamethasone

Topical Anesthetics

Mechanism of action

Drug effects

Therapeutic uses

Side effects and adverse effects

Interactions

Dosages

Drug Profiles

Tetracaine

Miscellaneous Drugs

Artificial Tears

⚓ Atropine sulfate

⚓ Cromolyn

Chymotrypsin

Cyclopentolate

⚓ Fluorescein

Hyperosmolar sodium chloride

Nursing Process

Assessment

Nursing Diagnoses

Planning

Outcome criteria

Implementation

Evaluation

Glossary

Accommodation (ə kom′ ə da′ shən) The state or process of adapting or adjusting one thing or set of things to another. In ophthalmology, *accommodation* refers to the adjustment of the eye to variation in distance; the elasticity of the lens allows it to change shape and focusing power. (p. 846)

Acute-angle glaucoma (glow ko′ mə) Glaucoma that occurs if the pupil in an eye with a narrow angle between the iris and cornea dilates markedly, causing the folded iris to block the exit of aqueous humor. Also called *angle-closure glaucoma*. (p. 849)

Aqueous humor (a′ kwe əs hu′mər) The clear, watery fluid circulating in the anterior and posterior chambers of the eye. (p. 846)

Bactericidal (bak ter′ i si′ dəl) Destructive to bacteria. (p. 862)

Bacteriostatic (bak tēr′ e o stat′ ik) Tending to restrain the development or the reproduction of bacteria. (p. 862)

Canal of Schlemm A tiny vein at the angle of the anterior chamber of the eye that connects with the pectinate villi, draining the aqueous humor and funneling it into the bloodstream. Also called *Schlemm's canal*. (p. 846)

Cataract (kat′ ə rakt) An abnormal progressive condition of the lens of the eye, characterized by loss of transparency. A gray-white opacity can be seen within the lens. If cataracts are untreated, sight is eventually lost. At onset vision is blurred; then, bright lights glare diffusely, and distortion and double vision may develop. (p. 846)

Cones A photoreceptive cell in the retina of the eye that enables a person to visualize colors. (p. 846)

Cornea (kor′ ne ə) The convex, transparent, anterior part of the eye. It is nonvascular and allows light to pass through it to the lens. (p. 846)

Cycloplegia (si′ klo ple′ je ə) Paralysis of the ciliary muscles, which prevents the accommodation of the lens to variations in distance. Certain ophthalmic drugs are used to induce cycloplegia to allow examination of the eye. (p. 846)

Cycloplegics (si′ klo ple′ jikz) Drugs that paralyze the ciliary muscles of the eye. (p. 846)

Dilatator muscle (dil' ə ta' tər) A muscle that contracts the iris of the eye and dilates the pupil. It is composed of radiating fibers, like spokes of a wheel, that converge from the circumference of the iris toward the center. The sympathetic nervous system controls this muscle. Also called *dilatator pupillae*. (p. 846)

Glaucoma (glaw ko' mə) An abnormal condition of elevated pressure within an eye because of obstruction of the outflow of aqueous humor. (p. 847)

Lens (lenz) The transparent, crystalline, curved structure of the eye that is located directly behind the iris and the pupil and attached to the ciliary body by ligaments. (p. 846)

Lysozyme (li so sōm) An enzyme with antiseptic actions that destroys some foreign organisms. It is normally present in tears, saliva, sweat, and breast milk. (p. 846)

Miotics (mi ot' iks) Drugs that constrict the pupil. (p. 846)

Open-angle glaucoma (glaw ko' mə) A type of glaucoma that is often bilateral, develops slowly, and is genetically determined. The obstruction that prevents outflow of aqueous humor is believed to be within the canal of Schlemm. It occurs more commonly than closed-angle glaucoma. Open-angle glaucoma is also called *chronic glaucoma*. (p. 849)

Ophthalmoscopic examinations (of thal mə skōp ik) An eye examination using an ophthalmoscope. An ophthalmoscope is a device used to examine the interior of the eye. It includes a light, a mirror with a single hole through which the examiner may look, and a dial holding several lenses of varying strengths. (p. 849)

Pupil (pu' pil) A circular opening in the iris of the eye, located slightly to the nasal side of the center of the iris. The pupil lies behind the anterior chamber of the eye and the cornea and in front of the lens. Its diameter changes with contraction and relaxation of the muscular fibers of the iris as the eye responds to changes in light, emotional states, and other kinds of stimulation. The pupil is the window of the eye through which light passes to the lens and the retina. (p. 846)

Rod One of the tiny cylindric photoreceptive elements arranged perpendicularly to the surface of the retina. Rods are especially sensitive in low-intensity light and are responsible for black and white vision. (p. 846)

Sphincter muscle (sfingk' tər) A circular band of muscle fibers that constricts a passage or closes a natural opening in the body, such as the *sphincter pupillae*. The sphincter pupillae is a muscle that expands the iris, narrowing the diameter of the pupil of the eye. The parasympathetic nervous system controls this muscle. (p. 846)

Tears A watery saline or alkaline fluid secreted by the lacrimal glands to moisten the conjunctiva. It is isotonic and contains an enzyme called *lysozyme*. Tears are also called *dacryon*. (p. 846)

Uvea (u' ve ə) The fibrous tunic beneath the sclera that includes the iris, the ciliary body, and the choroid of the eye. Also called *tunica vasculosa bulbi or uveal tract*. (p. 846)

Vitreous humor (vit' re əs) A transparent, semigelatinous substance contained in a thin membrane filling the cavity behind the crystalline lens of the eye. Also called *corpus vitreum or vitreous body*. (p. 846)

Structure of the Eye

To thoroughly understand the agents used to treat disorders of the eye, it is necessary to understand the structure and normal function of the eye. The eye is the organ responsible for the sense of sight. Figure 54-1 illustrates the structures of the eye, all of which are needed for accurate eyesight. Each eyeball is nearly spherical and approximately 1 inch in diameter. Each eye is recessed into a skull cavity in the frontal orbit of the skull. The exposed anterior (front) portion is covered by three layers: the protective external layer (cornea and sclera), the middle layer (the choroid, iris, and ciliary body), and the light-sensitive retina. All of these layers are protected by the eyelid, an external protection device.

The eye is held in place and moved by several sets of muscles that are controlled by cranial nerves. These muscles include the rectus and oblique muscles. There are four types of rectus muscles: inferior, superior, medial, and lateral. There are two types of oblique muscles: inferior and superior. These muscles are shown in Fig. 54-2. In addition to the structures associated with the sight organ, there are several accessory structures listed below:

- Eyebrow
- Eyelid
- Eyelashes
- Palpebral fissure
- Sclera
- Conjunctiva
- Iris
- Pupil
- Medial canthus
- Lacrimal carnucle
- Lateral canthus

The structure and purpose of each is listed below:

- *Eyebrow:* Rows of short hair above (superior) the upper eyelids. The eyebrow protects the eye from direct light, falling dust or other small particles, and perspiration coming from the forehead.
- *Eyelid(s):* Layer(s) of muscle and skin lined by the conjunctiva. The eyelids are moveable and can open or close. They protect the eyes when closed and allow for vision when open.
- *Eyelashes:* Two or three rows of hairs that are located on the edge (margin) of the eyelids. They help to prevent small particles from falling into the eye when it is open.
- *Palpebral fissure:* The space between the upper and lower eyelids when the eyelids are open.
- *Sclera:* A tough white coat of fibrous tissue that sur-

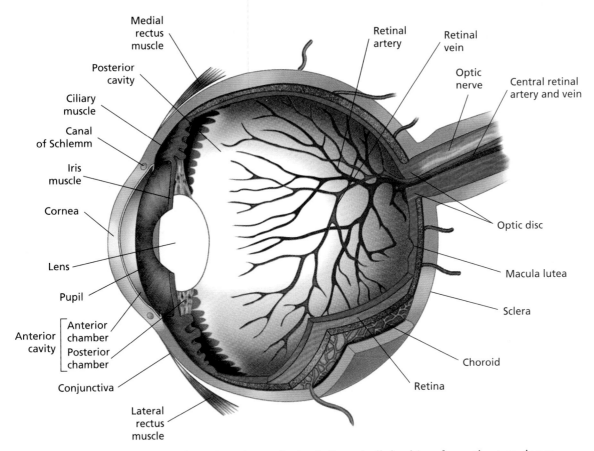

▼ **FIG. 54-1** A horizontal section through the left eyeball, looking from the top down. (Modified from Thibodeau: *Anthony's textbook of anatomy and physiology*, ed 2, St Louis, 1993, Mosby.)

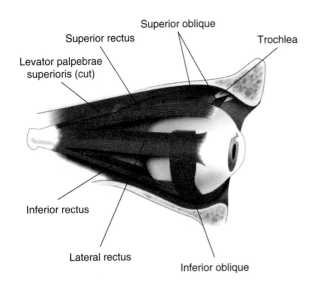

▼ **FIG. 54-2** Extrinsic muscles of the right eye. Lateral view. (Modified from Thibodeau: *Anthony's textbook of anatomy and physiology*, ed 2, St Louis, 1993, Mosby.)

rounds the entire eyeball except for the cornea. Commonly called the white of the eye.

■ *Conjunctiva:* Mucous membrane that lines the eyelids and covers the exposed surface of the eyeball.

■ *Iris:* Colored (pigmented) muscular apparatus behind the cornea.

■ *Pupil:* The variable-sized opening in the center of the iris that allows light to enter into the eyeball when the eyelids are open.

■ *Medial canthus:* The site of union near the nose for the upper and lower eyelids.

■ *Lacrimal caruncle:* A small and rounded elevation covered by modified skin at the medial palpebral commissure.

■ *Lateral canthus:* The site of union away from the nose for the upper and lower eyelids.

LACRIMAL GLANDS

The eye is kept moist and healthy by an intricate network of connected canals, ducts, and sacs. They work

▼ **FIG. 54-3** Different nervous systems control pupil size.

together to keep the eye moist. The lacrimal glands produce tears that bathe and cleanse the exposed anterior portion of the eye. **Tears** are composed of an isotonic, aqueous solution that contains an enzyme called **lysozyme,** which acts as an antibacterial to help prevent eye infections.

▼ **FIG. 54-4** Drug classes and their effects on pupil size.

LAYERS OF THE EYE

The fibrous outer layer of the eye has two parts—the sclera and the cornea. The sclera is a tough, fibrous layer that protects and maintains the shape of the eye. The **cornea** is a nonvascular transparent portion of the outer layer that allows light to enter the eye. It is pain sensitive and obtains nutrition from the **aqueous humor,** the clear watery fluid that circulates in the anterior and posterior chambers of the eye.

The vascular middle layer of the eye is composed of the anterior iris, ciliary body, and posterior choroid. These three structures are collectively called the **uvea.** The *iris* gives color to the eye and has an adjustable-sized opening in the center called the **pupil.** The main function of the iris is to regulate the amount of light that enters the eye by causing the size of the pupil to vary. Pupil size is controlled by a circular smooth muscle called the **sphincter muscle** and radial smooth muscle called the **dilatator muscle.** The circular muscles decrease pupil size, and the radial muscles increase pupil size. The parasympathetic nervous system innervates the sphincter muscles, while the sympathetic nervous system controls the dilatator muscles (see Fig. 54-3).

The anterior portion of the sclera becomes the *ciliary body,* which produces aqueous humor. The aqueous humor is removed from the anterior chamber via the **canal of Schlemm.** The *choroid* is a thin dark layer that lines most of the internal side of the sclera. The function of the choroid is to absorb light and prevent its reflection out of the eye.

The **lens** is the transparent crystalline structure of the eye, located directly behind the iris and the pupil. It is held in place by ligaments that are attached to the ciliary body. Accordingly the lens divides the interior

of the eyeball into a posterior (back) and anterior (forward) chamber. The larger posterior chamber behind the lens is filled with a jelly-like fluid called the **vitreous humor** that is constantly being formed by the ciliary body.

The transparent lens is composed of uniform layers of protein fibers that are encased by a clear connective tissue capsule. A loss of lens transparency results in a visual condition called **cataracts.** Before light images reach the retina, they are focused into a sharp image by the biconvex lens of the eye. The elasticity of the lens enables it to change its shape and focusing power. This process is called **accommodation** and is facilitated by the ciliary body. Paralysis of accommodation is called **cycloplegia.**

Mydriatics are drugs that dilate the pupil; those agents that constrict the pupil are called **miotics.** Drugs that paralyze the ciliary body are termed **cycloplegics** (see Fig. 54-4.)

The retinal layer of the eye is a thin delicate layer that contains light-sensitive receptors. It covers the choroid and is attached to the optic nerve near its center. The basic function of the retina is image formation via light-sensitive receptors called rods and cones. Both types of photoreceptors are located near the surface of the retina. **Rods** produce black and white vision, especially in low light, and **cones** are responsible for color vision (see Fig. 54-5). The function of the attached optic nerve is to connect the retina with the visual center of the brain.

This chapter focuses on the drugs used to treat disorders of the eye, which can be divided into three major groups: antiglaucoma agents, mydriatics and cycloplegics, and antiinfective/antiinflammatory agents. In

▼ FIG. 54-5 Functions of rods and cones in relation to color vision.

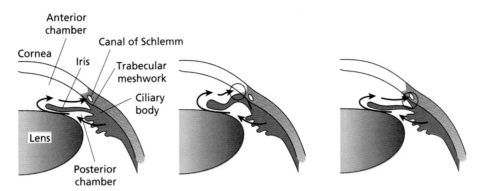

▼ FIG. 54-6 Main structures of the eye and an enlargement of the canal of Schlemm showing aqueous flow. (Modified from McKenry, Salerno: *Mosby's pharmacology in nursing*, ed 19, St Louis, 1995, Mosby.)

▼ FIG. 54-7 How increased aqueous humor can result in impaired vision.

addition to the three principal types of drugs are the diagnostic products: enzymes, irrigating solutions, eye washes, and hyperosmolar preparations.

Antiglaucoma Drugs

The aqueous humor is a nourishing liquid that is produced by the ciliary body and flows from the posterior chamber (behind the iris) to the anterior chamber (in front of the iris). It is removed via the canal of Schlemm, which is located adjacent to the union of the sclera and cornea in the anterior chamber. When the normal flow and drainage of aqueous humor is inhibited a serious ocular condition called glaucoma occurs. Figure 54-6 illustrates the main structures of the eye and an enlargement of the canal of Schlemm showing aqueous flow.

Glaucoma is an eye disorder characterized by excessive intraocular pressure (IOP) created by abnormally elevated levels of aqueous humor. This occurs when the aqueous humor is not drained through the canal of Schlemm as quickly as it is formed. The accumulated aqueous humor creates a backward pressure that pushes the vitreous humor against the retina. Continued pressure on the retina destroys its neurons, leading to impaired vision and eventual blindness (see Fig. 54-7). There are several categories of glaucoma that are classified according to underlying cause. The three main categories are primary glaucoma, secondary glaucoma, and congenital glaucoma. Table 54-1 lists the types of glaucoma and their characteristics.

Effective treatment of glaucoma involves reducing IOP either by increasing the drainage of aqueous humor or by decreasing the production of aqueous humor. Some drugs may do both. Drugs used to reduce IOP include:

1. Parasympathomimetics, also called cholinesterase inhibitors (direct or indirect acting)
2. Sympathomimetics
3. Beta blockers
4. Carbonic anhydrase inhibitors
5. Osmotic diuretics.

Refer to Table 54-2 for a drug class comparison of aqueous humor effects.

Table 54-1	Glaucoma: Types and Characteristics	
	CHRONIC OPEN-ANGLE	**ACUTE ANGLE-CLOSURE**
Primary Glaucoma		
Nature of angle	Large	Narrow
Age of onset	>30 yr African-American > white	>30 yr
Major symptoms	Blurred vision Occasional headaches	Blurred vision Severe headaches Eye pain Visual halos around lights
Treatment	Topical or systemic drugs Surgery	Topical or systemic drugs Surgery

Table 54-2	Antiglaucoma Drug Effects on Aqueous Humor	
DRUG CLASS	**INCREASED DRAINAGE**	**DECREASED PRODUCTION**
Direct parasympathomimetic	+++	+
Indirect parasympathomimetic (i.e., cholinesterase inhibitor)	+++	0
Sympathomimetic	++	+++
Beta blockers	+	+++
Carbonic anhydrase inhibitors	0	+++
Osmotic diuretics	0	+++

Direct- and Indirect-Acting Parasympathomimetic Ophthalmic Drugs

DIRECT-ACTING	INDIRECT-ACTING
Acetylcholine	Demecarium
Carbachol	Echothiophate
Pilocarpine	Isoflurophate
	Physostigmine

nervous system receptor and potentiates the normal effects of ACh. Examples of ophthalmic drugs that fall into these two drug categories are found in the box above.

Mechanism of Action

The direct-acting miotics are able to directly stimulate parasympathetic nervous system receptors because their structures closely resemble that of the PSNS neurotransmitter acetylcholine. Direct-acting miotics are administered topically to the eye. This route of administration drastically limits systemic absorption of the drug by keeping the cholinergic effects localized to the site of administration in the eye. The cholinergic response produced by these drugs causes pupillary contraction (miosis), which leads to a reduction of IOP secondary to an increased outflow of aqueous humor (see Fig. 54-8).

The indirect-acting miotics work by preventing acetylcholine breakdown. They prevent ACh from being inactivated by inhibiting cholinesterase, which results in higher levels of ACh and allows ACh to remain

PARASYMPATHOMIMETICS

Both the direct and indirect parasympathomimetic drugs cause miosis and pupillary constriction. These two types of ophthalmic agents work in different ways to *mimic* the parasympathetic nervous system (PSNS) neurotransmitter, acetylcholine (ACh), and are thus referred to as parasympatho*mimetic* drugs. The direct-acting parasympathomimetic drugs are chemically related to acetylcholine and can therefore mediate nerve impulse transmission at all cholinergic or parasympathetic nerve sites. The indirect parasympathomimetic drugs indirectly stimulate the parasympathetic nervous system by inhibiting cholinesterase, the enzyme that normally inactivates acetylcholine. This causes more ACh to be present at the parasympathetic

▼ **FIG. 54-8** The therapeutic effects of direct-acting parasympathomimetics on glaucoma.

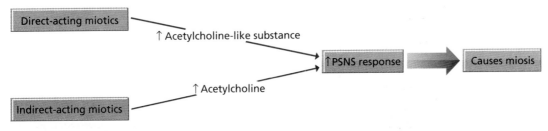

▼ **FIG. 54-9** Cholinergic response of miosis to parasympathomimetics.

at the receptor longer. The cholinergic response produced by these drugs causes miosis, which leads to reduced IOP (see Fig. 54-9).

Acetylcholine is the endogenous mediator of nerve impulses in the PSNS. It stimulates cholinergic receptors. This results in several effects: miosis, vasodilation, contraction of ciliary muscles, and reduced IOP. The action of acetylcholine is short lived. It is rapidly hydrolyzed by cholinesterases (acetylcholinesterase and pseudocholinesterase) to choline and acetic acid. Direct-acting miotics have effects similar to those of acetylcholine, but their actions are more prolonged (see Fig. 54-10).

The indirect-acting miotics bind with and inactivate cholinesterases (acetylcholinesterase and pseudocholinesterase), thus inhibiting hydrolysis of acetylcholine. As a result acetylcholine accumulates at cholinergic nerve endings. Indirect-acting agents that are organophosphates (echothiophate and isofluorophate) act by phosphorylating cholinesterase. This effect is irreversible. Pralidoxime, a cholinesterase reactivator, may reverse these effects and stimulate production of new cholinesterase enzyme by the body. This production of new enzyme may take days or even weeks.

Drug Effects

The drug effects of the miotics (direct and indirect) alter various eye muscles, IOP, aqueous humor, and vasodilation of blood vessels in and around the eye. The drug effects that alter the muscles of the eye result in contraction of the iris sphincter, which produces constriction of the pupil (miosis) and contraction of the ciliary muscle resulting in spasm of accommodation.

The drug effects that alter the pressure within the eye reduce IOP in both normal and glaucomatous eyes. They do this by facilitating aqueous humor outflow by causing contraction of the ciliary muscle, thus widening the area from which this fluid escapes. IOP is also reduced by constriction of the pupil, which causes the iris to stretch and thus relieves blockage of the area where the fluid leaves the inner eye. This effect is less pronounced in individuals with dark eyes (brown or hazel) than in those with light eyes (blue) because the pigment absorbs the drugs and dark eyes have more pigment.

The drug effects of the miotics cause vasodilation of blood vessels of the conjunctiva, iris, and ciliary body, resulting in increased permeability of the blood aqueous barrier, which may lead to vascular congestion and ocular inflammation. This congestion and inflammation is more common with long-acting anticholinesterases (indirect miotics).

Therapeutic Uses

The direct- and indirect-acting miotics are used for open-angle glaucoma, angle-closure glaucoma, ocular surgery, convergent strabismus, and ophthalmologic examinations. The miotics are used topically on the eye to reduce elevated IOP in the treatment of primary **open-angle glaucoma.** This reduction in IOP is the result of contraction of the ciliary muscle and widening of the exit route of the aqueous humor. **Acute (congestive) angle-closure glaucoma** may be relieved temporarily by pilocarpine or occasionally by carbachol to acutely decrease extremely high IOP.

Some of the miotic drugs may be used for ocular surgery. Pilocarpine, carbachol, and acetylcholine are used to reduce IOP and to protect the lens by causing miosis prior to certain types of laser surgery on the iris. Miotics may be used to counteract the mydriatic effects (dilation effects) of sympathomimetic agents such as hydroxyamphetamine and phenylephrine that are used for **ophthalmoscopic examinations.** Table 54-3 lists the miotic drugs and their indications.

▼ **FIG. 54-10** Metabolism of acetylcholine by endogenous enzymes.

Table 54-3	Miotics: Indications
MIOTIC AGENT	**INDICATIONS**
Acetylcholine	Complete and rapid miosis following cataract lens extraction, iridectomy
Carbachol	Open-angle glaucoma
Demecarium	Accommodative esotropia, obstructive aqueous humor outflow, open-angle glaucoma, following iridectomy
Echothiophate	Accommodative estropia, obstructive aqueous humor outflow, open- and closed-angle glaucoma, following iridectomy
Isoflurophate	Accommodative estropia, obstructive aqueous humor outflow, open-angle glaucoma, following iridectomy
Physostigmine	Open-angle glaucoma
Pilocarpine	Open-angle glaucoma, secondary glaucoma, following iridectomy, cycloplegic reversal

Table 54-4	Miotics: Adverse Effects
BODY SYSTEM	**SIDE/ADVERSE EFFECT**
Eye, ear, nose, throat	Visual blurring, myopia (nearsightedness), ciliary spasm, brow pain
Central nervous system	Headache
Cardiovascular	Hypotension, bradycardia, or tachycardia
Gastrointestinal	Nausea, vomiting, abdominal cramps, diarrhea
Respiratory	May precipitate asthma attacks

Side Effects and Adverse Effects

Most of the side effects and adverse effects associated with the use of cholinergic and anticholinesterase drugs (miotics) are local and limited to the eye. There are, however, some systemic effects that can occur, especially if sufficient amounts of drug pass into the bloodstream. Some common side effects and adverse effects associated with the miotics are listed in Table 54-4.

The most common *ocular side effects* that may occur with use of miotic drugs are blurred vision and accommodative spasms. Other undesirable effects include conjunctivitis, lacrimation, twitching eyelids, poor low-light vision, and pain. Prolonged use can result in iris cysts, lens opacities, and, rarely, retinal detachment.

Systemic effects that may occur with the use of miotic drugs are caused by parasympathetic nervous system stimulation. The cholinesterase inhibitors usually produce more pronounced effects than the direct-acting agents. The most common effects include bronchodilation, lacrimation, nausea, vomiting, salivation, sweating, gastrointestinal (GI) stimulation, and urinary frequency.

Toxicity and Management of Overdose

Occasionally toxic effects may develop following the use of topically applied miotic drugs. Toxicity produced by miotics is an extension of their systemic effects and is more common with prolonged use of high doses. Most severe and prolonged effects are seen with long-acting anticholinesterases. Excessive parasympathetic nervous system effects are treated with 0.4 to 2 mg of atropine administered IM or IV for adults and 0.04 to 0.08 mg/kg administered IV or IM for children. If required, repeat doses can be given every 5 minutes IV and every 15 minutes IM. In addition, pralidoxime (Protapam) may be required to reverse paralysis induced by either of the organophosphate anticholinesterases (echothiophate and isoflurophate).

Table 54-5	Miotic Drugs: Interactions	
DRUG	**MECHANISM**	**RESULT**
Topical epinephrine Topical timolol Systemic carbonic anhydrase inhibitor (CAI)	Additive effects	Additive lowering of IOP
Systemic cholinesterase inhibitors	Additive effects	Additive effects of both types of cholinesterases inhibitors (systemic and ocular)
Anesthetic agents	Potentiation	Increased anesthetic effect with the indirect-acting miotics

Interactions

The direct- and indirect-acting miotics are capable of interactions with several categories of drugs. Table 54-5 lists the possible interactions that may occur with miotic drugs.

Dosages

For recommended dosages of miotic agents see the dosages table on p. 852.

DRUG PROFILES

The direct-acting and indirect-acting miotics have a variety of uses. The principal use is that of relief of symptoms caused by glaucoma and increased IOP. The three most commonly used direct-acting miotics are acetylcholine, carbachol, and pilocarpine. These drugs have actions similar to those of acetylcholine. The four commonly used indirect-acting miotics are demecarium, echothiophate, isoflurophate, and physostigmine. These agents work by preventing cholinesterase from breaking down acetylcholine, allowing it to produce a prolonged parasympathetic nervous system response.

Since the safe use of miotics in pregnancy has not been established, many of the miotics are classified as pregnancy category C agents. Because of the potential risks of cholinesterase inhibition in general, the manufacturers of some anticholinesterase agents (e.g., demecarium and isoflurophate) state that the drugs are contraindicated in women who are or may become pregnant.

The direct-acting miotic drugs are contraindicated in patients who have shown a hypersensitivity reaction to them, in those with acute inflammatory conditions in the anterior chamber, and those with pupillary block glaucoma. The indirect-acting miotics are contraindicated in patients who have shown a hypersensitivity reaction to them and in patients with acute inflammatory conditions and glaucoma associated with iridocyclitis. In addition, echothiophate is not suitable for treatment of most cases of closed-angle glaucoma.

DIRECT-ACTING MIOTICS
ACETYLCHOLINE

Acetylcholine (Miochol) is a direct-acting parasympathomimetic agent that is used to produce miosis during ophthalmic surgery. It has very quick onset and may begin to work almost immediately. When used for ophthalmic indications, acetylcholine is administered directly into the anterior chamber of the eye before and after securing one or more sutures. It is available as a 20-mg powder for intraocular use only. Commonly recommended dosages for acetylcholine are listed in the following dosages table.

❦ PHARMACOKINETICS

HALF-LIFE	ONSET	PEAK	DURATION
Short	Instant	Instant	10 min

⚓ PILOCARPINE

Pilocarpine (Ocusert Pilo, Pilopine HS, Isopto Carpine, Pilocar, and many others) is a direct-acting parasympathomimetic agent that is used as a miotic in the treatment of glaucoma. Unlike other direct-acting miotics (acetylcholine and carbachol), which have only one formulation and limited indications, pilocarpine has a variety of uses and is available in many different formulations and strengths.

Pilocarpine is available as an ocular system formulation that offers the advantage of less frequent dosing because it may only need to be administered once per week. This may be an advantage over ophthalmic solutions with shorter durations, particularly in patients with compliance problems.

Pilocarpine is also available as a gel, solution, and some combination solutions. Pilocarpine ocular system delivers 20 μg/per hour for 7 days or 40 μg/per hour for 7 days (Ocusert Pilo-20 and Ocusert Pilo-40). It is also available as a 4% gel and 0.25%, 0.5%, 1%, 2%, 3%, 4%, 5%, 6%, 7%, 8%, and 10% ophthalmic solutions. Commonly recommended dosages for pilocarpine are listed in the dosages table below.

❖ PHARMACOKINETICS

HALF-LIFE	ONSET	PEAK	DURATION
Unknown	10-30 min	75 min	4-8 hr

INDIRECT-ACTING MIOTICS · ECHOTHIOPHATE AND ISOFLUROPHATE

Echothiophate (Phospholine Iodide) and isoflurophate (Floropryl) act indirectly and are classified as long-acting anticholinesterase miotics. Structurally both of these agents are organophosphates, which work by phosphorylating the enzyme cholinesterase. This results in an irreversible inhibition of the enzyme. Because the enzyme is permanently inactivated and the patient must synthesize new enzyme in order to reverse the drug effects, these drugs are considered long acting.

Both drugs are indicated for the symptomatic treatment of glaucoma and convergent strabismus (crossed eyes). The potential for misuse and the consequences of this misuse are very harmful. For these reasons both of these drugs are available only by prescription. They are classified as pregnancy C drugs and are contraindicated in patients who have shown a hypersensitivity reaction to them and in those with uveitis. Echothiophate is available only in 0.03%, 0.06%, 0.125%, and 0.25% ophthalmic solutions. Isoflurophate is available only as a 0.025% ophthalmic ointment. Commonly recommended dosages for echothiophate and isoflurophate are listed in the dosages table below.

❖ PHARMACOKINETICS

HALF-LIFE	ONSET	PEAK	DURATION
Long	10-30 min	30 min	1-4 wk

DOSAGES

SELECTED MIOTIC AGENTS

AGENT	PHARMACOLOGIC CLASS	DOSAGE RANGE	PURPOSE
Acetycholine (Miochol)	Direct-acting	5-70 mg	Surgical miosis
Demecarium (Humorsol) 0.125%, 0.25% solution	Indirect-acting	1-2 gtt/day	Glaucoma
Echothiophate (Phospholine Iodide) 0.03%, 0.06%, 0.125%, 0.25% solution	Indirect-acting	2 gtt/day	Glaucoma
Isoflurophate (Floropryl) (0.025% ophthalmic ointment	Indirect-acting	0.5 cm ribbon q8-72h	Glaucoma
⬇Physostigmine (Isopto Eserine) 0.25%, 0.5% solution 0.02% ophthalmic ointment	Indirect-acting	2 gtt up to 4 times/day 0.5 cm ribbon up to 3 times/day	Glaucoma
⬇Pilocarpine (Pilocar, Akarpine, IsoptoCarpine, Miocarpine) 0.25%, 0.5%, 1%, 2%, 3%, 4% solution 4% gel	Direct-acting	1-2 gtt q4-12h 1.5 cm ribbon/day hs	Glaucoma
Pilocarpine insert (Ocusert Pilo) 20 μg/h, 40 μg/h	Direct-acting	Insert 1/wk	Glaucoma

gtt, drop.

⚓ PHYSOSTIGMINE

Physostigmine (Isopto Eserine, Isopto P-ES, Eserine Sulfate) and demecarium (Humorsol) are indirect-acting miotics that are classified as anticholinesterase inhibitors. Structurally both of these agents are carbamates. They inactivate cholinesterases by carbamylation; this inactivation of cholinesterase is reversible because the enzyme is not permanently inactivated and the patient does not have to synthesize new cholinesterase to reverse the drug effects.

These two agents are classified as pregnancy category C agents and are contraindicated in patients who have shown a hypersensitivity reaction to them and in those with inflammatory disease of the iris or ciliary body. Physostigmine is available as 0.25% and 0.5% ophthalmic solutions, and demecarium is available as 0.125% and 0.25% ophthalmic solutions. Commonly recommended dosages for physostigmine and demecarium are listed in the dosages table on the previous page.

⚗ PHARMACOKINETICS

HALF-LIFE	ONSET	PEAK	DURATION
Unknown	10-30 min	Variable	12-48 hr

SYMPATHOMIMETICS

Sympathomimetic drugs apraclonidine, dipivefrin, and epinephrine are used for the treatment of glaucoma. Dipivefrin is the product of epinephrine. When instilled into the eye, it is hydrolyzed to epinephrine. Its advantage over epinephrine is that it has enhanced lipophilicity and can penetrate into the anterior chamber of the eye. On a weight basis, dipivefrin is 4 to 11 times as potent as epinephrine in reducing IOP and 5 to 12 times as potent as epinephrine in pupil dilation (mydriasis). Apraclonidine is structurally and pharmacologically related to clonidine. It is a relatively selective alpha-2 stimulant.

Because these drugs are sympathomimetic agents, they mimic the sympathetic neurotransmitters norepinephrine and epinephrine and stimulate the dilator muscle to contract. This stimulation results in increased pupil size (mydriasis) (see Fig. 54-11). Dilation is seen within minutes of instillation of the ophthalmic drops and lasts for several hours, during which time the IOP is reduced.

Mechanism of Action

These agents reduce IOP in patients with normal IOP or in patients with elevated IOP, such as those with glaucoma. Dipivefrin 0.1% reduces mean IOP approximately 15% to 25%. The exact mechanism by which the sympathomimetic drugs lower IOP is unknown. They are believed to work by stimulating both α- and β₂-receptors, causing the dilator muscle to contract resulting in mydriasis. During mydriasis there is an increase in aqueous humor outflow, resulting in a decrease in IOP. These effects appear to be dose dependent.

Apraclonidine reduces IOP 23% to 39% both peripherally and centrally. The centrally mediated effect is inhibition of adrenergic vasoconstriction in the eye. By stimulating α₂-receptors, apraclonidine prevents constriction of the blood vessels of the eye and reduces pressure, resulting in reduced aqueous humor formation.

Drug Effects

The drug effects of dipivefrin and epinephrine are the result of both α- and β₂-stimulation, which causes both ocular and systemic effects. The ocular effects of these drugs are a decrease in IOP and an increase in aqueous humor outflow (see Fig. 54-12). The decreased IOP is apparently the result of decreased aqueous humor fluid in the anterior chamber of the eye.

Dipivefrin is a more lipophilic agent and therefore has more localized effects in the eye. However, both dipivefrin and epinephrine can cause drug effects outside the eye. Because these two drugs mimic the effects of the sympathetic nervous system neurotransmitters, they can cause increased cardiovascular effects such as increased heart rate or blood pressure.

Therapeutic Uses

Both epinephrine and dipivefrin may be used to reduce elevated IOP in the treatment of chronic, open-angle glaucoma, either as initial therapy or as chronic

▼ FIG. 54-11 Increased pupil size (mydriasis).

Alpha stimulation α ──→ **Mydriasis (dilation)** ──→ ↑ **Aqueous humor outflow**

Beta stimulation β ──→ ↓ **IOP** ──→ ↓ **Aqueous humor formation**

▼ **FIG. 54-12** Ocular effects of alpha (α) and beta (β) stimulation.

therapy. Dipivefrin has been used to reduce IOP in other ocular conditions, including ocular hypertension and pseudoexfoliative, low-tension, and secondary glaucomas.

Apraclonidine is primarily used to *inhibit perioperative IOP increases.* Increases in IOP during ophthalmic surgery are usually mediated via increased catecholamine stimulation of the sympathetic nervous system. Apraclonidine stimulates the α_2-receptors, which oppose these effects, and thus corrects the surgery-induced changes in IOP. It has also been used in the treatment of open-angle glaucoma, but its effectiveness has not yet been established.

Side Effects and Adverse Effects

The side effects and adverse effects of the sympathomimetic mydriatics are primarily limited to ocular effects; however, systemic effects are possible. Ocular side effects are transient and most commonly consist of burning, eye pain, and lacrimation. Other ocular effects are conjunctival hyperemia, localized melanin deposits in the conjunctiva, and released pigment granules from the iris.

The systemic effects associated with the use of sympathomimetic mydriatics are rare. They include cardiovascular effects such as extrasystoles, tachycardia, and hypertension. Other effects that may be noticed are headache and faintness.

Toxicity and Management of Overdose

Rare toxic reactions are primarily the result of an extension of the therapeutic and adverse effects of these drugs. The most significant are cardiac arrhythmias. Discontinuation of the drugs usually alleviates the toxic symptoms.

Interactions

With sufficient topical absorption, sympathomimetic mydriatics have the potential to react with other drugs. Table 54-6 lists the most common drug interactions with these agents.

Table 54-6	Mydriatic Drugs: Drug Interactions	
DRUG	**MECHANISM**	**RESULT**
Anesthetic (halogenated general)		
Cardiac glycosides	Potentiation	Possible cardiac arrhythmias
Thyroid hormones		
Tricyclic antidepressants		

Dosages

For recommended dosages of sympathomimetic agents see the dosages table on the next page.

DRUG PROFILES

The two primary sympathomimetic agents are dipivefrin and epinephrine. Apraclonidine is also a sympathomimetic miotic drug, but it is not used as extensively as dipivefrin and epinephrine. They are believed to work by stimulating both (α- and β_2-receptors. This stimulation causes the dilator muscle to contract and results in mydriasis. During mydriasis there is an increase in aqueous humor outflow that results in a decrease in IOP.

Both epinephrine and apraclonidine are classified as pregnancy category C agents. Because of dipivefrin's lipophilicity and limited systemic absorption, it is classified as a pregnancy category B agent. These drugs are available only by prescription.

DOSAGES

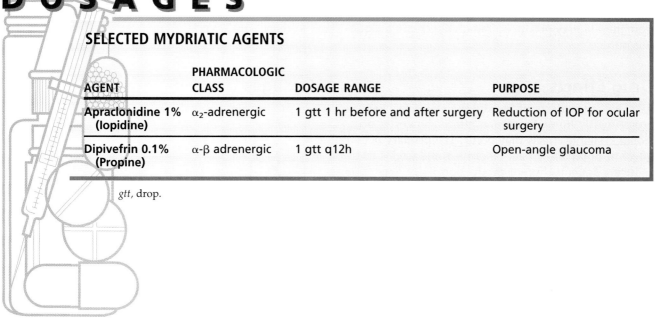

SELECTED MYDRIATIC AGENTS

AGENT	PHARMACOLOGIC CLASS	DOSAGE RANGE	PURPOSE
Apraclonidine 1% (Iopidine)	α_2-adrenergic	1 gtt 1 hr before and after surgery	Reduction of IOP for ocular surgery
Dipivefrin 0.1% (Propine)	α-β adrenergic	1 gtt q12h	Open-angle glaucoma

gtt, drop.

APRACLONIDINE

Apraclonidine (Iopidine) is structurally and pharmacologically related to the α_2 stimulant clonidine. Apraclonidine is primarily used to inhibit perioperative IOP increases. Apraclonidine stimulates α_2-receptors, which inhibits increases in IOP that occur during ophthalmic surgery. Its use in the treatment of open-angle glaucoma remains to be established.

Apraclonidine is available as a 1% ophthalmic solution. Commonly recommended dosages for apraclonidine are listed in the dosages table above.

PHARMACOKINETICS

HALF-LIFE	ONSET	PEAK	DURATION
8 hr	1 hr	3-5 hr	12 hr

DIPIVEFRIN

Dipivefrin (Propine) is a synthetic sympathomimetic miotic drug. It is a prodrug of epinephrine. The prodrug has little or no pharmacologic activity until hydrolyzed in the eye to two forms of epinephrine. These chemical alterations allow epinephrine to penetrate into the anterior chamber of the eye. The decrease in IOP is apparently the result of aqueous humor fluid outflow from the anterior chamber of the eye.

Dipivefrin is available as a 0.1% ophthalmic solution. Commonly recommended dosages for dipivefrin are listed in the dosages table above.

PHARMACOKINETICS

HALF-LIFE	ONSET	PEAK	DURATION
1-3 hr	30 min	1 hr	12 hr

BETA-ADRENERGIC BLOCKERS

The antiglaucoma beta-adrenergic blockers that reduce IOP include selective β_1 and nonselective β_1 and β_2 blockers. These drugs are believed to work by reducing intraocular pressure through reducing aqueous humor formation and increasing its outflow. The most commonly used drugs in this drug class are listed in Table 54-7.

Mechanism of Action

The ophthalmic beta blockers reduce both elevated and normal IOP. They do this without affecting pupil-

Table 54-7	Glaucoma Therapy: Beta-Adrenergic Blockers
CLASS	**BETA-BLOCKERS**
Selective β-blocker (β_1)	Betaxolol
Nonselective β-blocker (β_1 β_2)	Carteolol, levobunolol, metipranolol, timolol

lary size or accommodation. They appear to reduce IOP by reducing aqueous humor formation. In addition, timolol may produce a minimal increase in aqueous outflow.

Drug Effects

The drug effects of the ophthalmic beta blockers are primarily limited to ocular effects; however, occasional systemic effects may occur. The primary ocular effect of ophthalmic beta blockers is reduced IOP by reducing aqueous humor production. They have little or no effect on accommodation, pupil size, and night vision.

The systemic effects are primarily those associated with the adrenergic blockers as discussed in Chapter 16, specifically systemic pulmonary and cardiovascular effects. Because these drugs are administered topically, few, if any, systemic effects are expected. These agents have not been shown to affect glucose metabolism as do some of the systemic adrenergic blockers.

Therapeutic Uses

The ophthalmic beta blockers are used to reduce elevated IOP in various conditions, including chronic open-angle glaucoma and ocular hypertension. They may also be used alone or in combination with a topical miotic (e.g., echothiophate iodide or pilocarpine), topical dipivefrin, and/or systemic carbonic anhydrase inhibitors. When used in combination these agents may have an additive IOP-lowering effect. They may also be used to treat some forms of angle-closure glaucoma.

Side Effects and Adverse Effects

The side effects and adverse effects of the antiglaucoma beta blockers are primarily limited to ocular effects and limited systemic effects. The most common ocular effects are transient burning and discomfort. Other effects include blurred vision, pain photophobia, lacrimation, blepharitis, keratitis (inflammation of the cornea), and decreased corneal sensitivity. The systemic effects produced by the beta blockers include headache, dizziness, cardiac irregularities, and bronchospasm.

Toxicity and Management of Overdose

Toxic reactions to the beta blockers are rare and primarily involve the cardiovascular system. Symptoms include bradycardia, cardiac failure, hypotension, and bronchospasms. Treatment involves discontinuation of the drug and symptomatic treatment.

Interactions

With sufficient topical absorption the beta blockers can react with several categories of drugs. Table 54-8 lists some of these drug interactions.

Dosages

For recommended dosages of beta-adrenergic blockers see the dosages table on p. 857.

DRUG PROFILES

The ophthalmic beta-blocking drugs are betaxolol, carteolol, levobunolol, metepranolol, and timolol. The action of these drugs is reduction of intraocular pressure by decreased aqueous humor formation and an increase in outflow of aqueous humor.

These ophthalmic drugs are classified as pregnancy category C agents and are contraindicated in patients with bronchial asthma, cardiac failure, cardiogenic shock, obstructive breathing disorders, second- or third-degree AV block, and sinus bradycardia. They are also contraindicated in patients who have shown a hypersensitivity reaction to them. They are all available only by prescription.

BETAXOLOL

Betaxolol (Betopic, Betopic S) is a β_1 selective beta blocker. It is structurally related to the systemic adrenergic blocker metoprolol (Lopressor) that is used primarily for cardiovascular disorders. Betaxolol is one of the most potent and selective beta-blocking agents. Its ability to decrease aqueous humor formation and consequently IOP has made it an excellent agent for the

Table 54-8	Beta Blockers: Drug Interactions	
DRUG	**MECHANISM**	**RESULT**
Beta blockers (systemic) Reserpine	Additive	Increased therapeutic and side and adverse effects
Verapamil	Additive	Use with timolol can result in asystole

treatment of ocular disorders such as open-angle glaucoma and ocular hypertension. Betaxolol is available as 0.5% ophthalmic solution and a 0.25% ophthalmic suspension. Commonly recommended dosages for betaxolol are listed in the dosages table below.

❇ PHARMACOKINETICS

HALF-LIFE	ONSET	PEAK	DURATION
Unknown	0.5-1 hr	2 hr	≥12 hr

TIMOLOL

Timolol (Timoptic, Timoptic Ocudose) may differ slightly from the other ophthalmic beta blockers in that it may increase the outflow of aqueous humor as well as its formation. Timolol is indicated for the treatment of open-angle glaucoma, ocular hypertension, secondary glaucoma, and glaucoma in aphakic eyes. It is available in 0.25% and 0.5% ophthalmic solutions as both a preservative-free and a preservative-containing product. Because some patients have had allergic reactions to benzalkonium chloride, one of the preservatives that is commonly in ocular products, the preservative-free products were developed. Commonly recommended dosages for timolol are listed in the dosages table below.

❇ PHARMACOKINETICS

HALF-LIFE	ONSET	PEAK	DURATION
Unknown	15-30 min	1-5 hr	24 hr

CARBONIC ANHYDRASE INHIBITORS

The carbonic anhydrase inhibitors (CAIs) are sulfonamide derivatives that lack antimicrobial activity. The CAIs include acetazolamide, dichlorphenamide, and methazolamide. Of these, acetazolamide is the most widely used. They have many uses, but their use in ophthalmic disorders is to decrease IOP. The prototype drug of the group, acetazolamide, is also used as an adjunct anticonvulsant and as treatment for acute mountain sickness. Their ophthalmic uses include treatment for open-angle, secondary, and angle-closure glaucoma.

Drug Effects

The CAIs are administered orally as opposed to topically. The drug effects of the carbonic anhydrase inhibitors are decreased IOP through reduced aqueous humor formation; increased renal excretion of water, bicarbonate, and potassium; and urinary alkalinization through decreased excretion of ammonia.

Therapeutic Uses

The carbonic anhydrase inhibitors are used primarily in the treatment of glaucoma. Because they decrease IOP by reducing aqueous humor formation, they are excellent therapeutic agents in the treatment of such ocular disorders as open-angle glaucoma, secondary glaucoma, and closed-angle glaucoma before ocular surgery.

DOSAGES

SELECTED BETA-ADRENERGIC BLOCKERS

AGENT	PHARMACOLOGIC CLASS	DOSAGE RANGE	PURPOSE
Betaxolol (Betopic, Betopics) 0.25%, 0.5%	β1-blocker	1 gtt bid	Open-angle glaucoma, ocular hypertension
Timolol (Timoptic, Timoptic Ocudose) 0.25%, 0.5%	β1-β2-blocker	1 gtt bid	Open-angle glaucoma, ocular hypertension

gtt, drop.

Side Effects and Adverse Effects

Since the carbonic anhydrase inhibitors are administered orally, they produce systemic side effects and adverse effects. Table 54-9 lists the most common such effects associated with the carbonic anhydrase inhibitors.

Toxicity and Management of Overdose

Toxicity associated with the use of CAIs is rare. The mechanism by which these agents work predisposes the patient to possible acidotic states and electrolyte imbalances. These toxic reactions generally require only supportive care. This may include the restoration of electrolytes, especially potassium, and the administration of bicarbonate to correct the carbonic anhydrase inhibitor–induced acidotic state.

Interactions

The systemic use of CAIs can result in several significant drug interactions. Table 54-10 lists the most common and significant drug interactions that may occur with this group of ophthalmic agents.

Dosages

For recommended dosages of acetazolamide see the dosages table on p. 859.

DRUG PROFILE

The carbonic anhydrase inhibitors are the first class of ophthalmic drugs discussed thus far that can be given orally and produce therapeutic effects in the eye that are beneficial in the treatment of glaucoma. The CAIs include acetazolamide, dichlorphenamide, and methazolamide. As previously mentioned, the most commonly used CAI is acetazolamide. The carbonic anhydrase inhibitors appear to work by decreasing the production of aqueous humor, which decreases IOP.

The CAIs are classified as pregnancy category C agents and are contraindicated in patients with a history of hypersensitivity reactions to them or in patients with chronic noncongestive closed-angle glaucoma, marked kidney-liver disease, hyperchloremic acidosis, low sodium and potassium serum levels, and adrenal

Table 54-9	Carbonic Anhydrase Inhibitors: Adverse Effects
BODY SYSTEM	**SIDE/ADVERSE EFFECT**
Eyes, ears, nose, and throat	Transient myopia, tinnitus
Central nervous system	Drowsiness, confusion, parasthesias, seizures
Gastrointestinal	Anorexia, vomiting, diarrhea
Genitourinary	Polyuria, hematuria
Integumentary	Urticaria, rare photosensitivity
Metabolic	Acidotic states and electrolyte imbalance with long-term therapy

Table 54-10	Carbonic Anhydrase Inhibitors: Drug Interactions	
DRUG	**MECHANISM**	**RESULT**
Digitalis	Induced hypokalemia	Increased digitalis toxicity
Corticosteroids Diuretics	Additive potassium excretion	Severe hypokalemia
Lithium	Increased renal excretion	Decreased lithium effects
Basic drugs (e.g., amphetamines)	Decreased renal excretion	Increased drug effects

gland failure. All CAIs are available only by prescription.

The prototype CAI, acetazolamide, is also used as an adjunct anticonvulsant and for treatment of acute mountain sickness. Their ophthalmic uses include open-angle, secondary, and angle-closure glaucoma.

ACETAZOLAMIDE

Acetazolamide (Diamox, AK-Zol) is a carbonic anhydrase inhibitor that is primarily used in the treatment of glaucoma. It is available orally as 500-mg extended-release capsules and 125- and 250-mg tablets and parenterally as a 500-mg injection. Commonly recommended dosages for acetazolamide are listed in the following dosages table.

DOSAGES

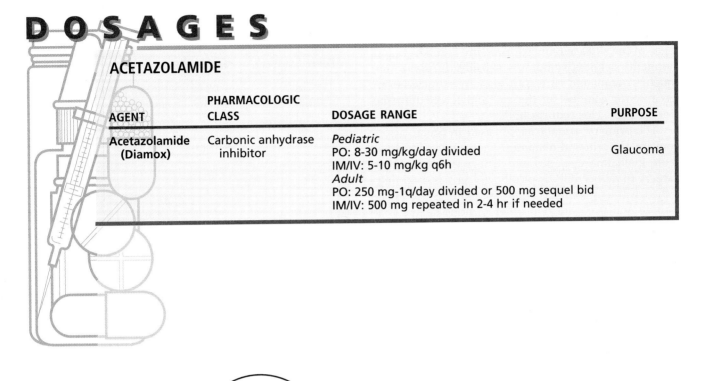

ACETAZOLAMIDE

AGENT	PHARMACOLOGIC CLASS	DOSAGE RANGE	PURPOSE
Acetazolamide (Diamox)	Carbonic anhydrase inhibitor	*Pediatric* PO: 8-30 mg/kg/day divided IM/IV: 5-10 mg/kg q6h *Adult* PO: 250 mg-1q/day divided or 500 mg sequel bid IM/IV: 500 mg repeated in 2-4 hr if needed	Glaucoma

▼ FIG. 54-13 Mechanism and ocular effects of osmotic diuretics.

PHARMACOKINETICS

HALF-LIFE	ONSET	PEAK	DURATION
2.5-6 hr	1-1.5 hr	2-4 hr	8-12 hr

OSMOTIC DIURETICS

Osmotic agents may be administered either intravenously or orally to reduce IOP. The osmotic diuretics that are most commonly used for this purpose are glycerin and mannitol. Isosorbide and urea are two other less frequently used osmotic diuretics. These drugs create ocular hypotension by producing an osmotic gradient. This causes the blood to become hypertonic in the presence of intraocular fluids. The gradient forces the water from the aqueous and vitreous humors into the bloodstream causing a reduction of volume of intraocular fluid, which results in a decrease in IOP.

Mechanism of Action

The osmotic diuretics produce an increase in the osmolarity of the blood causing it to become hypertonic. The hyperosmotic blood causes a shift of fluid from various isotonic extracirculatory fluids, especially from the cerebrospinal fluid and aqueous humor. Water via the osmotic gradient is removed, and the respective fluids in the brain and the eye are reduced in volume. This reduced volume of water decreases pressure on both the brain and the eye (see Fig. 54-13).

Drug Effects

The drug effects of the osmotic diuretics are all related to their ability to extract fluid from certain spaces and shift it into the bloodstream. This action is important in the treatment of various ocular disorders because of the resultant reduction in IOP caused by the decreased volume of aqueous humor. Osmotic diuretics promote diuresis by increasing the osmolarity of the glomerular filtrate, which results in tubular reabsorption inhibition and an increase in the renal excretion of electrolytes.

Therapeutic Uses

The therapeutic effectiveness of the osmotic diuretics is the result of the production of hypertonic blood, which causes fluid extraction from various areas. In the brain this is beneficial for the treatment of mountain sickness. When fluid from the enclosed space of the skull is reduced, pressure is relieved and mountain sickness symptoms subside. In glaucoma, aqueous humor and vitreous humor are extracted from the anterior chamber of the eye and forced into the bloodstream. This reduces IOP.

The primary osmotic agents used in ocular disorders are glycerin and mannitol. They are used to treat acute glaucoma episodes and before or after ocular surgery to reduce IOP. Typically, glycerin is used first; if the treatment is unsuccessful, mannitol is tried. Isosorbide and urea are two other osmotic agents that may also be used in similar situations. They are usually used after glycerin or mannitol has failed.

Side Effects and Adverse Effects

The most frequent reactions to osmotic diuretic agents are nausea, vomiting, and headache. The most significant adverse effects are fluid and electrolyte imbalance. Other effects include possible irritation and thrombosis at the injection site. For a list of other possible side effects and adverse effects associated with the use of osmotic diuretics see Table 54-11.

Toxicity and Management of Overdose

Toxic reactions are primarily a result of the hyperosmolarity of the blood. Hypovolemia caused by diuresis, cardiac arrhythmias, and hyperosmolar nonketotic coma are the most significant toxic reactions. Treatment involves discontinuation of the drug and general symptomatic treatment.

Interactions

No significant drug interactions have been reported, with the exception of increased lithium excretion caused by mannitol.

Dosages

For recommended dosages of osmotic agents see the dosages table on p. 861.

DRUG PROFILES

The osmotic diuretics are classified as pregnancy category C agents and are contraindicated in patients

Table 54-11	Osmotic Diuretics: Adverse Effects
BODY SYSTEM	**SIDE/ADVERSE EFFECT**
Eyes, ears, nose, throat	Loss of hearing, blurred vision, nasal congestion
Central nervous system	Dizziness, headache, convulsions, rebound increased intracranial pressure, confusion
Gastrointestinal	Nausea, vomiting, dry mouth, diarrhea
Genitourinary	Marked diuresis, urinary retention, thirst
Cardiovascular	Edema, thrombophlebitis, hypotension, hypertension, tachycardia, angina-like chest pains, fever, chills
Electrolytes	Fluid electrolyte imbalances, acidosis, electrolyte loss, dehydration

with pronounced anuria, acute pulmonary edema, cardiac decompensation, and severe dehydration. They are also contraindicated in patients who have shown a hypersensitivity reaction to them.

GLYCERIN

Glycerin (Osmoglyn, Ophthalgan) is an osmotic agent used orally to lower IOP, or topically to reduce superficial corneal edema. Glycerin can be administered orally before iridectomy to reduce IOP in individuals with acute narrow-angle glaucoma. It is used preoperatively and postoperatively in conditions such as congenital glaucoma, retinal detachment, cataract extraction, and keratoplasty (corneal transplant). It may also be used in some secondary glaucomas.

Glycerin is administered orally as a 50% hyperosmotic solution (Osmoglyn). It is also available as an ophthalmic solution (Ophthalgan). Commonly recommended dosages for glycerin are listed in the following dosages table.

PHARMACOKINETICS

HALF-LIFE	ONSET	PEAK	DURATION
30-45 min	10-30 min	0.5-2 hr	4-8 hr

MANNITOL

Mannitol (Osmitrol) is used to reduce elevated IOP when the pressure cannot be lowered by other treatment. Mannitol has been shown to be effective in treatment of acute episodes of angle-closure, absolute, or secondary glaucoma and for lowering IOP before in-

DOSAGES

SELECTED OSMOTIC DIURETICS

AGENT	PHARMACOLOGIC CLASS	DOSAGE RANGE	PURPOSE
Glycerin (Osmoglyn, Ophthalgan)	Osmotic diuretic	*Pediatric/Adult* PO: 1-2 g/kg 1-1.5 hr before surgery	Reduction of IOP
Mannitol (Osmitrol)	Osmotic diuretic	*Pediatric* IV: 1-2 g/kg by infusion over 30-60 min *Adult* IV: 1.5-2 g/kg by infusion over 30-60 min	Reduction of IOP

traocular surgery. Mannitol does not penetrate the eye and may be used when irritation is present, unlike some of the other osmotic agents such as urea. Mannitol is available as 5%, 10%, 15%, 20%, and 25% parenteral injections. Commonly recommended dosages for mannitol are listed in the dosages table above.

PHARMACOKINETICS

HALF-LIFE	ONSET	PEAK	DURATION
1.5-2 hr	0.5-1 hr	0.5-1 hr	4-6 hr

Ocular Antiinfectives

Topical antiinfectives used for treating ocular infections include a wide range of antibacterial, antiviral, and antifungal drugs. Many of these drugs are also available for systemic administration. Caution should be used in deciding to use a topical antiinfective ophthalmic drug. In general prophylactic use of antiinfective drugs is useless, wasteful, and potentially dangerous. Many of the inflammatory diseases seen in ophthalmology are caused by viruses or other agents that are not susceptible to any currently available antiinfective agents. The use of these agents in such situations is unwarranted.

Topically applied antiinfective drugs can cause sensitivity reactions. Symptoms associated with sensitivity reactions include stinging, itching, angioneu-

rotic edema, urticaria, and dermatitis. Topical application of antiinfective drugs also interferes with growth of the normal bacterial flora of the eye, which may encourage growth of other more harmful organisms.

Any of the available systemically administered antibiotics are used at indicated times to treat infections of the eye. To avoid development of resistant strains of offending organisms and possible sensitization to common systemic antiinfectives, the antibiotic of choice is often administered topically rather than systemically.

The choice of a particular ophthalmic antiinfective drug should be based on the following:
- Past clinical experience
- The sensitivity and characteristics of the organisms most likely to cause this infection
- The disease itself
- Sensitivity and response of the patient
- Laboratory results (cultures and sensitivities).

Some common eye infections that may require antibiotic therapy are listed in the box on p. 862.

Mechanism of Action

The drugs used to treat infections of the eye work in a variety of ways to destroy the invading organism. The antimicrobial effects on susceptible organisms is primarily caused by inhibition of cell wall synthesis, inhibition of protein synthesis, or alteration of cell membrane permeability. Specific mechanisms of action can be found for the individual classes of antiinfectives in Chapter 36.

Common Ocular Infections	
INFECTION	**DESCRIPTION**
Conjunctivitis	Inflammation of the conjunctiva, which is the mucous membrane lining the back of the lids and the front of the eye except the cornea. It may be bacterial or viral in nature and is often associated with common colds. When caused by *Hemophilus* organisms it is commonly called "pink eye" and is usually self-limiting.
Hordeolum (sty)	Acute localized infection of the eyelash follicles and the glands of the anterior lid; results in the formation of a small abscess or cyst.
Keratitis	Inflammation of the cornea caused by bacterial infection. Herpes simplex keratitis is caused by viral infection.
Uveitis	Infection of the uveal tract or the vascular layer of the eye, which includes the iris, ciliary body, and choroid.
Endophthalmitis	Inner eye structure inflammation caused by bacteria

Drug Effects

The drug effects of the agents used to treat ocular infections are focused on the microorganism invading the eye. Some antiinfectives destroy the causative organism (**bactericidal**), whereas others simply inhibit the organism's growth (**bacteriostatic**), allowing the body's immune system to fight the infection. Whatever the case, the final drug effect is elimination of the infecting organism.

Therapeutic Uses

The therapeutic effects of the ocular antiinfectives vary depending upon the individual antiinfective drug. The spectrum of bacteria that each drug kills is very specific to the individual agent. The therapeutic effect is elimination of ocular infections.

Side Effects and Adverse Effects

The most common side effects and adverse effects of the ocular antibiotics are local and transient inflammation, burning, stinging, and drug hypersensitivity. Other such effects, toxicities, and drug interactions are specific for the individual antiinfectives and are therefore mentioned in the drug profiles.

Interactions

The ophthalmic agents undergo very little if any systemic absorption. For this reason, there are no drug interactions to mention for this category of agents.

Dosages

For recommended dosages of ocular antiinfectives see the dosages table on p. 863.

DRUG PROFILES

A variety of infections can occur in the eye; many are self-limiting, (i.e., the body's own defense system will fight them.) They seldom result in harm. However, some infections require ocular antiinfectives to be eliminated. The most commonly used antiinfectives from the main antiinfective drug classes are discussed here.

AMINOGLYCOSIDES

The aminoglycosides are potent antiinfectives that destroy bacteria by interfering with protein synthesis in bacterial cells by binding to ribosomal subunits, which eventually leads to bacteria death. Because aminoglycosides kill bacteria, they are classified as bactericidal.

The three aminoglycosides that are used to treat ocular infections are gentamicin, neomycin, and tobramycin. They are classified as pregnancy category C agents and are contraindicated in patients who have shown a hypersensitivity reaction to them and in patients with vaccinia, varicella, mycobacterial, fungal infections of eye, epithelial herpes, and simplex keratitis.

Side effects and adverse effects include swollen eyelids, mydriasis, and local erythema. Toxic reactions are rare because of poor topical absorption. Another possible toxic reaction is the overgrowth of nonsusceptible organisms, which can lead to eye infections that are resistant to treatment.

⚓ GENTAMICIN

Gentamicin (Garamycin, Genoptic) is effective against a wide variety of gram-negative and gram-positive organisms. It is particularly useful against *Pseudomonas, Proteus,* and *Klebsiella* organisms. Gram-positive organisms that are effectively destroyed by gentamicin are

D O S A G E S

SELECTED OCULAR ANTIINFECTIVE AGENTS

AGENT	PHARMACOLOGIC CLASS	DOSAGE RANGE	PURPOSE
Bacitracin (AK-Tracin)	Antibiotic: Polypeptide	Apply ointment 1-2 times/day	Bacterial infections
Chlortetracycline	Antibiotic: Tetracycline	Apply ointment 1-2 times/day	Bacterial and chlamydial infection; apply once within 1 hr after delivery for ophthalmia neonatorum
Chloramphenicol (Chloromycetin)	Miscellaneous	Apply ointment or 1-2 gtt several times/day	Bacterial infections
↓**Ciprofloxacin** (Cipro)	Fluroquinolone	2 gtt q15min for 6 hr followed by 2 gtt q30min for the remainder of the day; then 2 gtt qh on the second day followed by 2 gtt q4h for 12 more days	Bacterial keratitis
		1-2 gtt q2h while awake for 2 days followed by 1-2 gtt q4h while awake for 5 more days	Bacterial conjunctivitis
↓**Erythromycin** (AK-Mycin)	Macrolide	Apply ointment several times/day	Bacterial and chlamydial infections; apply once within 1 hr after birth for ophthalmia neonatorum
↓**Gentamicin** (Garamycin)	Aminoglycoside	Apply ointment or 1-2 gtt several times/day	Bacterial infections
Natamycin (Natacyn)	Macrolide	1 gtt q1-2h for 3-4 days followed by 1 gtt q6-8h for 3-4 days	Fungal infections
Polymyxin B	Antibiotic: Polypeptide	1-3 gtt several times/day	Bacterial infections
Silver nitrate	Inorganic hu metal salt	2 gtt after birth	Ophthalmic neonatorum
Sulfacetamide (AK-Sulf, Bleph)	Sulfonamide	Apply ointment 1-2 gtt several times/day	Bacterial infection
Tetracycline (Achromycin)	Antibiotic: Tetracycline	Apply ointment or 1-2 gtt several times/day	Bacterial and chlamydial infections; apply ointment once within 1 hr after delivery for ophthalmia neonatorum
Vidarabine (Vira A)	Purine nucleoside	Apply ointment 5 times/day at 3-hr intervals	Viral infections

gtt, drop.

staphylococci and streptococci that have developed resistance to other antibiotics. Gentamicin is available as an ophthalmic ointment and a solution. It is also available in combination with prednisolone as a suspension and an ointment. It is available as a 0.3% ophthalmic ointment and a 0.3% ophthalmic solution. Commonly recommended dosages are listed in the preceding dosages table.

✸ PHARMACOKINETICS

HALF-LIFE	ONSET	PEAK	DURATION
Unknown	Variable	Immediate	6-12 hr

MACROLIDES

The antibacterial erythromycin is a bacteriostatic drug. In normal concentrations it will inhibit the growth of an organism but not destroy it. Erythromycin relies on the body's defense mechanisms to destroy the bacteria although in high concentrations, it will become bactericidal. It is indicated for the treatment of neonatal conjunctivitis caused by *Chlamydia trachomatous* and for the prevention of eye infections in newborns that may be caused by *Neisseria gonorrhoea* or other susceptible organisms.

The two most commonly used agents in this antibiotic category are erythromycin ophthalmic ointment and natamycin ophthalmic suspension. Eye irritation is the only rare adverse reaction reported with these two antiinfectives.

⚓ ERYTHROMYCIN

Erythromycin (AK-Mycin, Ilotycin, Ocu-Mycin) is a macrolide antibiotic indicated for the treatment of various ophthalmic infections. It is classified as a pregnancy category C agent and is contraindicated in patients who have shown a hypersensitivity reaction to it and in patients with epithelial herpes, varicella, mycobacterial or fungal infections, and simplex keratitis. It is available only as 0.5% strength ophthalmic ointment. Commonly recommended dosages are listed in the preceding dosages table.

✸ PHARMACOKINETICS

HALF-LIFE	ONSET	PEAK	DURATION
Unknown	Variable	Immediate	Variable

NATAMYCIN

Natamycin (Natacyn) is an antifungal antibiotic that is structurally a macrolide antibiotic. It is related to the other antifungal agents amphotericin B and nystatin. It destroys fungi in the eye by binding to sterols

in the fungal cell membrane, thus disrupting the protective capabilities of the cell, which results in cell death.

Natamycin is used topically in the treatment of blepharitis, conjunctivitis, and keratitis caused by susceptible fungi. The side effects and adverse effects associated with natamycin are limited to the eye and consist of temporary visual haze and overgrowth of nonsusceptible organisms. It is also classified as a pregnancy category C agent and is contraindicated in patients who have shown a hypersensitivity reaction to it. It is available as a 5% ophthalmic suspension. Commonly recommended dosages are listed in the preceding dosages table.

✸ PHARMACOKINETICS

HALF-LIFE	ONSET	PEAK	DURATION
Unknown	Variable	Immediate	Variable

POLYPEPTIDES

Bacitracin and polymyxin B are polypeptide antibiotics. These drugs are rarely used systemically because of potent nephrotoxic effects. They are bactericidal antiinfectives that inhibit protein synthesis in susceptible organisms, which leads to cell death. They are most commonly used in the treatment of surface superficial infections caused by gram-positive bacteria.

They are often used in combination with other antibiotics to broaden their spectrum of activity. Neosporin is a combination of bacitracin and gramicidin, neomycin, and polymyxin. Bacitracin is preferable to neomycin for topical use because fewer organisms are resistant to it, allergic reactions occur less frequently, and sensitization is avoided.

BACITRACIN

Bacitracin (AK-Tracin) is an ophthalmic antiinfective drug used to treat various eye infections. It is classified as a pregnancy category C agent and is contraindicated in patients who have shown a hypersensitivity reaction to it. It is available as a single ingredient product and as a combination product with polymixin or neomycin and polymyxin. These combinations were developed to make bacitracin a broad-spectrum antibiotic. Bacitracin comes as a 500-U/gram ophthalmic ointment and as two combination ophthalmic ointments. Commonly recommended dosages are listed in the preceding dosages table.

✸ PHARMACOKINETICS

HALF-LIFE	ONSET	PEAK	DURATION
Unknown	Variable	Immediate	Variable

TETRACYCLINES

Tetracycline antibiotics are used topically to treat superficial infections of the cornea and conjunctiva. They are usually bacteriostatic rather than bactericidal. They are broad-spectrum antimicrobials. The administration of tetracyclines is recommended to prevent eye infections in newborns of mothers with gonorrheal infections. Topical tetracyclines rarely cause any side effects or adverse effects. They are better tolerated than silver nitrate and have a lower incidence of conjunctivitis and eye irritation. Presently there are three tetracycline-based ophthalmic preparations—chlortetracycline, oxytetracycline, and tetracycline.

TETRACYCLINE

The prototype tetracycline antibiotic is Achromycin. It is classified as a pregnancy category D agent and is contraindicated in patients who have shown a hypersensitivity reaction to it and in patients with varicella, vaccinia, mycobacterial or fungal infections of the eye, and epithelial herpes simplex keratitis. Tetracycline is available as a 1% ointment and suspension. Commonly recommended dosages are listed in the dosages table on p. 863.

☣ PHARMACOKINETICS

HALF-LIFE	ONSET	PEAK	DURATION
Unknown	Variable	Immediate	Variable

QUINOLONES

The quinolone antibiotics are very effective broad-spectrum antibiotics. They are discussed in detail in Chapter 36. They are bactericidal, destroying a wide spectrum of organisms that are often very difficult to treat. There are currently three ophthalmic quinolones available—ciprofloxacin, norfloxacin, and ofloxacin.

They are all classified as pregnancy category C agents and are contraindicated in patients who have shown a hypersensitivity reaction to them. Significant side effects and adverse effects include corneal precipitates during treatment for bacterial keratitis. Other reactions include corneal staining and infiltrates. Toxic reactions are limited because of poor topical absorption. Those that occur are usually taste disorders and nausea. There are no significant drug interactions.

⚓ CIPROFLOXACIN

Ciprofloxacin (Cipro) is a synthetic quinolone antibiotic. It is available only by prescription. Although it is available in many systemic formulations, it is available only as a 0.3% ophthalmic solution in an ocular formulation. Cipro is indicated in the treatment of bac-

terial keratitis and conjunctivitis caused by susceptible bacteria. Commonly recommended dosages are listed in the dosages table on p. 863.

☣ PHARMACOKINETICS

HALF-LIFE	ONSET	PEAK	DURATION
1-2 hr	Variable	Immediate	Variable

SULFONAMIDES

Sulfonamides are synthetic bacteriostatic antibiotics that work by blocking the synthesis of folic acid in susceptible bacteria. Sulfacetamide sodium and sulfisoxazole are sulfonamides used to treat conjunctivitis and other ocular infections caused by susceptible bacteria.

The side effects and adverse effects are primarily limited to local reactions and include local irritation and stinging. Sulfonamide use can result in the overgrowth of nonsusceptible organisms. No significant topical toxic effects have been reported with their use. These ocular antiinfectives are classified as pregnancy category C agents and are contraindicated in infants under 2 months of age, and in patients with varicella, vaccinia, viral disease, mycobacterial and fungal infections of the eye, epithelial herpes simplex, and keratitis. They are also contraindicated in patients who have shown a hypersensitivity reaction to them. They are available in ophthalmic ointments, solutions, and suspensions.

SULFACETAMIDE

Sulfacetamide (AK-Sulf, Bleph, Sodium Sulamyd, and many others) is the most commonly used ophthalmic sulfonamide antiinfective. It is available as a solution, ointment, and suspension in ophthalmic formulations. It is also used in combination with phenylephrine or prednisolone. It comes as a 10% ophthalmic ointment and 10%, 15%, and 30% ophthalmic solutions. Commonly recommended dosages are listed in the dosages table on p. 863.

☣ PHARMACOKINETICS

HALF-LIFE	ONSET	PEAK	DURATION
Unknown	Variable	Immediate	Variable

MISCELLANEOUS

Three other ophthalmic antiinfective drugs that are commonly used are chloramphenicol, silver nitrate, and zinc sulfate. These antiinfectives have been available for many years and remain very effective for susceptible organisms.

CHLORAMPHENICOL

Chloramphenicol (Chloromycetin, AK-Chlor, Ocu-Chlor) is a bacteriostatic antiinfective that works by preventing peptide bond formation and protein synthesis in a wide variety of gram-positive and gram-negative organisms. It is extremely useful in the treatment of superficial intraocular infections. Side effects with the ophthalmic use of chloramphenicol are usually rare. As with most of the other ophthalmic antiinfectives, the most common side effects and adverse effects are burning and stinging upon instillation. Irreversible aplastic anemia has not been reported with the ophthalmic preparation of this drug. It is available as a 0.5% solution and a 1% ointment. Commonly recommended dosages are listed in the dosages table on p. 863.

▼ PHARMACOKINETICS

HALF-LIFE	ONSET	PEAK	DURATION
Unknown	Variable	Immediate	Variable

SILVER NITRATE

Silver nitrate is a topical antiinfective, astringent, and caustic agent. It also exhibits antiseptic and germicidal activity and works by inhibiting protein synthesis. It is not readily absorbed from mucous membranes and does not readily penetrate into tissues. It has had long-term use in newborns to prevent gonococcal infections of the eyes. This is required by law in many states. The U.S. Centers for Disease Control (CDC) and the American Academy of Pediatrics (AAP) currently state that topical erythromycin or a topical tetracycline may be used as an alternative to 1% silver nitrate ophthalmic solution for prophylaxis of gonococcal ophthalmia neonatorum. Silver nitrate is classified as a pregnancy category C agent and is contraindicated in patients who have shown a hypersensitivity reaction to it. It is available as a 1% ophthalmic solution. Commonly recommended dosages are listed in the dosages table on p. 863.

▼ PHARMACOKINETICS

HALF-LIFE	ONSET	PEAK	DURATION
Unknown	Variable	Immediate	Variable

ANTIVIRALS

There are three currently available antiviral ophthalmic agents—idoxuridine, trifluridine, and vidarabine. Idoxuridine and trifluridine are both pyrimidine nucleosides; vidarabine is a purine nucleoside. These agents inhibit viral replication because their metabolites block viral DNA synthesis by inhibiting viral DNA polymerase. These three antiviral ophthalmic drugs destroy herpes simplex virus types 1 and 2, varicella-zoster, cytomegalovirus, vaccinia, and hepatitis B virus. Of these agents, vidarabine has the broadest antiviral spectrum.

These antivirals are classified as pregnancy category C agents and are contraindicated in patients who have shown a hypersensitivity reaction to them. Significant side effects and adverse effects include secondary glaucoma, corneal punctate defects, uveitis, and stromal edema. The drugs exhibit no appreciable topical absorption, and no significant drug interactions have been reported.

VIDARABINE

Vidarabine (Vira-A) is an antiviral ophthalmic drug used in the treatment of herpes simplex keratitis and keratoconjunctivitis. It may also be useful in the treatment of vaccinia keratitis. Vidarabine is only available as a 3% ophthalmic ointment. Commonly recommended dosages are listed in the dosages table on p. 863.

▼ PHARMACOKINETICS

HALF-LIFE	ONSET	PEAK	DURATION
Unknown	Variable	Immediate	Variable

Antiinflammatory Ophthalmic Agents

Many of the same antiinflammatory drug classes that are used systemically may also be used ophthalmically to treat various inflammatory disorders and surgery-related pain and inflammation. Both nonsteroidal antiinflammatory drugs (NSAIDs) and corticosteroids are used ophthalmically as listed in the box below.

Ophthalmic Antiinflammatory Agents

NSAIDs	CORTICOSTEROIDS
Diclofenac	Dexamethasone
Flurbiprofen	Fluorometholone
Ketorolac	Hydrocortisone
Supiofen	Medrysone
	Prednisolone

Mechanism of Action

Both corticosteroids and NSAIDs work by inhibiting the inflammatory response. However, they differ in the mechanisms of action. The corticosteroids and NSAIDs both act on enzymes involved in arachidonic acid metabolism. The corticosteroids work in a different area of the pathway than the NSAIDs. Figure 54-14 illustrates where on this pathway the corticosteroids and NSAIDs act.

Whenever tissues are damaged their cell membranes release phospholipids as a part of the tissue-damaging process. These phospholipids are then broken down by several different enzymes and pathways that are collectively referred to as the arachidonic acid pathway. Phospholipase is one of the first enzymes involved, and it is the enzyme that is inhibited by corticosteroids.

By preventing phospholipase from breaking down phospholipids, many of the inflammatory mediators or substances that cause inflammation and pain cannot be produced. This is the action of the NSAIDs. However, they inhibit a different enzyme than the corticosteroids. NSAIDs inhibit cyclooxygenase and, to a lesser extent, lipoxygenase. In doing so, they also prevent the production of many of the substances that cause inflammation and pain.

Drug Effects

The drug effects of the corticosteroids following topical application to the conjunctiva are primarily the inhibition of the inflammatory response to mechanical, chemical, or immunologic agents. The NSAIDs exhibit antiinflammatory, analgesic, and antipyretic activity (i.e., they decrease inflammation, relieve pain, and reduce fever associated with tissue damage in the eye). This is believed to occur as a result of inhibition of the enzyme cyclooxygenase, which is the enzyme responsible for the production of prostaglandins and other inflammatory substances.

▼ **FIG. 54-14** Antiinflammatory action of corticosteroids and nonsteroidals.

Therapeutic Uses

Corticosteroids and NSAIDs are applied topically for the symptomatic relief of many ophthalmic inflammatory conditions. They may be used topically in corneal, conjunctival, and scleral injuries from chemical, radiation, or thermal burns or penetration of foreign bodies. They are used during the acute phase of the injury process to prevent fibrosis and scarring that results in visual impairment. They should not be used for minor abrasions or wounds because they may suppress the eye's ability to resist bacterial, viral, or fungal infections. This adverse effect is more notable in corticosteroids than in NSAIDs. Consequently, NSAIDs are considered less toxic and are preferred as initial topical therapy.

Corticosteroids and NSAIDs may also be used prophylactically after ocular surgery, such as cataract extraction, glaucoma surgery, and corneal transplants, to prevent inflammation and scarring. NSAIDs are used in the symptomatic treatment of seasonal allergic conjunctivitis. They may also be used prophylactically before ocular surgery to prevent or reduce intraoperative miosis that may occur secondary to surgery-induced trauma.

Side Effects and Adverse Effects

The most common adverse effect of corticosteroids is transient burning or stinging on application. Since NSAIDs have the potential to cause increased bleeding, patients should be monitored closely. The extended use of the corticosteroids may result in cataracts, increased IOP, and optic nerve damage.

Dosages

For recommended dosages of corticosteroid agents see the dosages table on p. 869.

DRUG PROFILES

The corticosteroids and NSAIDs that are used to treat ophthalmic inflammatory disorders are discussed in Chapter 33 and Chapter 42, respectively. These ophthalmic formulations share many of the same characteristics of their systemic counterparts. However, the ophthalmic derivatives do have limited systemic absorption. Thus, the majority of therapeutic and toxic effects are limited to the eye.

With the exception of diclofenac, which is classified as a pregnancy category B agent, NSAIDs are classified as pregnancy category C agents. They are contraindicated in patients who have shown a hypersensitivity reaction to them and in patients with epithelial herpes simplex keratitis. They are all available only by prescription as ophthalmic solutions.

The corticosteroid ophthalmic preparations are indicated for many of the same conditions as the NSAIDs with a few exceptions. Many of these agents are also available in systemic formulations and are discussed in Chapter 33. The corticosteroids are classified as pregnancy category C agents and are contraindicated in patients with fungal and viral ocular infections and acute epithelial herpes simplex keratitis. Systemic reactions as a result of ophthalmic absorption and drug interactions with the ophthalmic corticosteroids are rare.

FLURBIPROFEN

Flurbiprofen (Ocufen Liquifilm) is a nonsteroidal antiiflammatory drug that is available as an ophthalmic drug. It is used to treat inflammatory ophthalmic conditions such as postoperative inflammation after a cataract extraction. It is also used to inhibit intraoperative miosis that may be induced by operative trauma and tissue injury. Flurbiprofen is available as a 0.03% ophthalmic solution. Commonly recommended dosages are listed in the following dosages table.

❋ PHARMACOKINETICS

HALF-LIFE	ONSET	PEAK	DURATION
Unknown	2 hr	1-2 hr	Several hr

⚓ KETOROLAC

Ketorolac (Acular) is an NSAID that is available in many different formulations. It is the only parenteral NSAID and may be given either intravenously or intramuscularly. Ketorolac is available orally as well. Ketorolac is contraindicated in patients who have exhibited a hypersensitivity to it. The ophthalmic formulation is used to reduce certain manifestations of ocular inflammation caused by trauma, such as ocular surgery, or inflammation secondary to external agents, such as allergens and bacteria. Ketorolac is available as a 0.5% ophthalmic solution. Commonly recommended dosages are listed in the following dosages table.

❋ PHARMACOKINETICS

HALF-LIFE	ONSET	PEAK	DURATION
Unknown	Rapid	Immediate	4-6 hr

DEXAMETHASONE

Dexamethasone (AK-Dex, Decadron, and many others) is a synthetic corticosteroid that has many systemic and ophthalmic formulations. It is used to treat inflammation of the eye, eye lids, conjunctiva, and cornea, and it may also be used to treat uveitis, iridocyclitis, allergic conditions, burns, and in removal of foreign bodies. Dexamethasone is available as an ophthalmic ointment and as a 0.1% suspension. It is also contained in many combination formulations with various antibiotics. Commonly recommended dosages are listed in the dosages table below.

☙ P H A R M A C O K I N E T I C S

HALF-LIFE	ONSET	PEAK	DURATION
Unknown	Variable	Immediate	Variable

Topical Anesthetics

Topical anesthetic ophthalmic drugs are used to prevent eye pain. This is beneficial during surgery, ophthalmic examinations, removal of foreign bodies, and any extremely painful procedure or condition. The two currently available topical anesthetics used for ophthalmic purposes are proparacaine and tetracaine. The anesthetic drugs are discussed in depth in Chapter 9.

Mechanism of Action

Local anesthetics stabilize the membranes of nerves, resulting in a decrease in the movement of ions into and out of the nerve endings. Without a change in the concentrations of these ions a nerve impulse cannot be started or transmitted. Pain and many other sensory impulses are transmitted via nerves. When nerves are stabilized, as they are after application of topical anesthetics, they cannot transmit signals about painful stimuli to the brain.

Drug Effects

Usually the application of topical anesthetic drugs to the eye results in local anesthesia in less than one-half of a minute. This drug effect of numbness or the absence of the ability to feel pain is beneficial in many circumstances.

Therapeutic Uses

The ophthalmic anesthetic drugs are used to produce ocular anesthesia for short corneal and conjunctival procedures. They prevent pain during surgical procedures such as removal of sutures and foreign bodies and during certain painful ophthalmic examinations. The various procedures in which ophthalmic anesthetic drugs have been used are listed below:

- Tonometry
- Paracentesis
- Short procedures

D O S A G E S

SELECTED NONSTEROIDAL ANTIINFLAMMATORY OPHTHALMIC AGENTS

AGENT	PHARMACOLOGIC CLASS	DOSAGE RANGE	PURPOSE
Flurbiprofen (Ocufen Liquifilm)	NSAID	0.03% solution: 1 gtt q1/2h starting 2 hr before surgery	Inhibition of intraoperative miosis
⬇Ketorolac (Acular)	NSAID	0.5% solution: 1 gtt qid	Treatment of allergic conjunctivitis
Dexamethasone (AK-Dex, Decadron)	Glucosteroid	0.1% solution: Apply gtt, ointment several times/day	Treatment of corneal, conjunctiva/eyelid, sclera, and uveal tract inflammatory conditions

gtt, drop.

- Gonioscopy
- Eye examinations of painful injuries
- Irrigation of painful injuries
- Removal of foreign bodies
- Removal of sutures
- Corneal scraping for diagnostic purposes

Side Effects and Adverse Effects

Side effects and adverse effects are rare with ophthalmic anesthetic agents and are limited to local effects such as stinging, burning, redness, and lacrimation. Some of the more common side effects and adverse effects are allergic contact dermatitis, softening and erosion of corneal epithelium, pupillary dilation, cycloplegia, conjunctival congestion and hemorrhage, and stromal edema.

Interactions

Because of limited systemic absorption and short duration of action, the ophthalmic anesthetic agents have no significant drug interactions.

Dosages

Tetracaine is available as a 0.5% ophthalmic ointment and solution. The recommended dosage is application of 1.25 to 2.5 cm of the ointment or 1 to 2 gtt of solution for local anesthesia as needed. Not intended for prolonged use.

*D*RUG PROFILES

Ophthalmic anesthetic drugs are a small class of the many available ophthalmic agents. There are currently only two drugs available to treat ophthalmic conditions that require an anesthetic—proparacaine and tetracaine. They are classified as mydriatic and cycloplegic agents. They dilate the pupil and paralyze the ciliary muscle, which prevents accommodation. Atropine is used for cycloplegic refraction and for iris and uveal tract inflammation. The usual dose (0.5% and 1%) for uveitis in children and adults is 1 to 2 drops or 0.3 to 0.5 cm of ointment 2 to 3 times daily. The adult dose for refraction is 1 drop (1% solution) 1 hour before the procedure.

TETRACAINE

Tetracaine (Pontocaine) is a local anesthetic of the ester type. It is used to numb the eye for cataract extraction, tonometry, gonioscopy, removal of foreign objects, corneal suture removal, and glaucoma surgery. Tetracaine begins to work in about 25 seconds and lasts for about 30 minutes. It is available in both an ophthalmic ointment and a solution. It comes as a 0.5% ointment and solution.

☣ PHARMACOKINETICS

HALF-LIFE	ONSET	PEAK	DURATION
Short	<30 sec	1-5 min	15-20 min

MISCELLANEOUS DRUGS
ARTIFICIAL TEARS

An array of over-the-counter (OTC) products is available to use as lubrication or moisture for the eyes. Artificial tears are isotonic and contain buffers for pH control. In addition they contain preservatives for microbial control and may contain viscosity agents for extended ocular activity. Selected OTC brand names include Cellafresh, Moisture Drops, Murine, Nutears, and Tears Plus.

⚓ ATROPINE SULFATE

Atropine sulfate solution 0.5%, 1.2%, and 3% and ophthalmic ointment 0.5% and 1% are used as mydriatic and cycloplegic agents. They dilate the pupil and paralyze the ciliary muscle, which prevents accommodation. Atropine is used for cycloplegic refraction and for iris and uveal tract inflammation. The usual dose (0.5% and 1%) for uveitis in children and adults is 1 to 2 drops or 0.3 to 0.5 cm of ointment 2 to 3 times a day. The adult dose for refraction is 1 drop (1% solution) one hour before the procedure.

⚓ CROMOLYN

Cromolyn sodium (Opticrom) is an antiallergic agent that inhibits the release of inflammation-producing mediators from sensitized inflammatory cells called mast cells. It is used in the treatment of vernol keratoconjunctivitis. The usual dose for children over 4 years of age and adults is one drop 4 to 6 times per day.

CHYMOTRYPSIN

Chymotrypsin (Alpha Chymar, Catarese) is a proteolytic enzyme used as an aid in intracapsular lens extraction. Cataract extraction or removal is facilitated by injecting 0.2 to 0.5 ml of a freshly prepared solution behind the iris into the posterior chamber. Enzymatic activity dissolves the zonules that hold the lens so that it can be removed. After the procedure a miotic drug is administered to contract the pupil.

CYCLOPENTOLATE

Cyclopentolate solution (Cyclogyl) 0.5, 1, and 2% is used as a diagnostic mydriatic and cycloplegic drug. The usual adult dose is 1 to 2 drops (0.5, 1, or 2%). This is repeated in 5 to 10 minutes if needed. The dose for children is the same as that for adults. Infants require one drop of the 0.5% solution.

⚓ FLUORESCEIN

Fluorescein sodium (AK-Fluor, Flu-Glo Strips) is an ophthalmic diagnostic dye used to identify corneal defects and to locate foreign objects in the eye. It is also used in fitting hard contact lenses. After instillation of fluorescein, various defects are highlighted. They are distinguished according to the following criteria:

- Corneal defects are colored bright green.
- Conjunctival lesions are colored yellow-orange.
- Foreign objects have a green halo around them.
- A contact lens that touches the cornea will appear black with UV light.

HYPEROSMOLAR SODIUM CHLORIDE

Hyperosmolar sodium chloride preparations (Adsorbonac, Muro 128 [2% and 5% solution], and Muro 128 ointment) are used to reduce corneal edema caused by osmotic pressure. They are available as ointments or solutions. One to two drops of 2% to 5% solution is applied every 3 to 4 hours. The 0.5% ophthalmic ointment is applied once daily.

NURSING PROCESS

ASSESSMENT

Before administering an ophthalmic agent per doctor's orders, the nurse should conduct a baseline assessment of the eye and its structures to help document specific data about possible causes of the eye disorder and to measure success of treatment. Any redness, swelling, pain, tearing, eye discharge, decrease in visual acuity, or any other unusual symptoms should be noted, documented, and reported to the patient's physician. Hypersensitivity to the specific medication, contraindications and cautions, and preexisting diseases should also be noted and documented.

Specific contraindications and cautions to the use of each specific ophthalmic agent are as follows:

Parasympathomimetic agents or miotics (often used for glaucoma) are usually contraindicated in patients with bradycardia, hyperthyroidism, coronary artery disease, GI or urinary obstructive problems or disease, peptic ulcers, epilepsy or convulsive disorders, parkinsonism, and asthma. Cautious use with careful monitoring is recommended in patients who are pregnant or have hypertension or bronchial asthma. Baseline vital signs and an assessment of the respiratory system should be documented and unusual (abnormal) findings reported to the physician.

The indirect-acting parasympathomimetics such as echothiophate iodide used for glaucoma are contraindicated in patients allergic to the drug or those with uveitis. Cautious use is recommended in patients with asthma, bradycardia, or peptic ulcer disease and in those who are pregnant. See Table 54-5 for drug interactions.

The principal use of sympathomimetic ophthalmic agents is dilation of the eye before ophthalmic examination and related procedures. Dipivefrin is used in the treatment of open-angle glaucoma because the agent is converted to epinephrine, which acts to decrease aqueous humor production and increase outflow. Contraindications include patients with allergic reaction to the drugs and those with narrow-angle glaucoma. Cautious use is recommended in patients who are pregnant or breastfeeding, and in patients with aphakia.

Beta-adrenergic blockers are contraindicated in patients who are allergic to these agents, and in those who have chronic obstructive pulmonary disease (COPD), asthma, heart block, right pump failure, and congenital glaucoma.

Carbonic anhydrase inhibitors should be administered cautiously in patients who have adrenocortical insufficiency because they are at higher risk for associated fluid and electrolyte disturbances. Cross allergies are possible in those individuals sensitive to sulfonamide drugs, such as thiazide diuretics and oral sulfonylureas and sulfonamide antibiotics, since they may be at risk for allergic reactions to the CAIs. CAIs are contraindicated in patients with hyponatremia or hypokalemia or who have renal or liver dysfunction. In addition, it is important to question the patient

NURSING ■ CARE ■ PLAN

Glaucoma

Ms. A.B. is at the physician's office today for instructions about self-administration of pilocarpine via ocusert dosage form. Although 82 years old, she is healthy and all senses are intact. Her motor and cognition skills are intact with no deficits noted. She is eager to learn and has many questions regarding her glaucoma and associated care. She lives alone, but her 21-year-old niece helps her out quite a bit and has come with her today so that she may also learn how to help with this medication.

Assessment with nursing diagnoses	Planning with goals and outcome criteria	Implementation and patient education	Evaluation

Subject
 	
Complaint of blurred vision, decreased vision acuity, and difficulty with "close up" vision
Frequent headaches and eye pain
States "I live all alone but I do pretty good."
 	
Objective
 	
82-year-old woman who is having annual eye exam
Increased IOP
Good health otherwise and without significant medical problems
 	
Nursing diagnoses
 	
Knowledge deficit related to new dosage technique for pilocarpine
	Goals
	
	Patient will remain compliant and have therapeutic response to Pilocarpine Ocusert technique within 1 mo of therapy
	
	Outcome criteria
	
	Patient will demonstrate proper instillation technique of Ocusert dosage form before leaving physician's office as evidenced by:
	  Proper technique and accurate skill of pulling down lid and inserting med
		To insert the ocusert form of pilocarpine you must first wash your hands and then follow these instructions:
		
		Pull down lower lid of eye
		
		Apply ocusert med pouch into conjunctival sac
		
		Change weekly, but it is good to check each evening before bedtime
		
		If the med comes out then rinse it and reinsert as directed
		
		Teach a significant other, friend, or relative how to insert medication too, just in case
			Patient will show therapeutic response to medication regimen as evidenced by:
			  Decreased IOP
			  Decreased headaches and eye pain

about current medications because of the possibility of interactions with amphetamines, quinidine, mecamyaline, and methenamine. Baseline vital signs and an assessment of the patient's vision, intraocular pressure, serum electrolytes, urinalysis, and platelet and complete blood cell count are also recommended before initiation of drug therapy.

Osmotic agents such as glycerin ophthalmic solution and glycerin oral solution are contraindicated in patients who have cardiac, renal, or hepatic disease because the sudden fluid volume shifts may precipitate circulatory overload and possible heart failure. The elderly patient may be subject to dehydration with these agents because of rapid fluid shifts and subsequent diuretic action. Blood sugars must be monitored more closely in patients who are diabetic and taking osmotic agents since glycerin has been found to cause transient hyperglycemia and glucosuria as a result of metabolism of glycerin to carbohydrates.

With the ophthalmic antibiotics, each drug carries its own contraindications or cautions. Chloramphenicol, erythromycin, tetracycline, neomycin, gentamicin, and tobramycin drops are contraindicated in patients who are allergic to the medication, and cautious use is recommended in patients who are pregnant or have antibiotic hypersensitivity.

Mydriatic agents, such as atropine, are contraindicated in patients with a history of severe reactions to atropine and should be used extremely cautiously in patients who have primary glaucoma. The dilation of the pupil results in narrowing of the canal of Schlemm and restriction of the drainage of intraocular fluids, which increases intraocular pressure that may result in precipitation of an acute glaucoma attack. It is also important to obtain and document baseline vital signs and vision status.

Sympathomimetic agents (epinephrine, phinylephrine, and tetrahydrozoline) cause mydriasis and help decrease the congestion of conjunctival vessels. These agents cause vasoconstriction, pupil dilation, relaxation of the ciliary muscle, an increase in the outflow of aqueous humor, and a decrease in aqueous humor formation. Most of these agents, as previously mentioned in this chapter, are used to treat wide-angle glaucoma secondary to uveitis or to produce mydriasis for ocular examination. It is important to remember contraindications and cautions to sympathomemetic use such as patients with coronary heart disease, angina, tachycardia, and hypertension. **As with other ophthalmic agents, there is always the risk of systemic absorption, which can cause systemic effects and many drug interactions.**

The antiviral agents are contraindicated in pregnancy. Antiseptics are rarely used because they do not completely sterilize the eye. There are limited cautions and contraindications with the use of antifungal agents because they are not systemically absorbed. Topical corticosteroid ophthalmic agents are contraindicated in patients with pyogenic infections or minor corneal abrasions. Ophthalmic steroids may also increase incidence of fungal infections of the eye and are to be used only as directed with the advice of a physician. Antiinflammatory agents may also mask allergic reactions or hypersensitivity to other agents. Artificial tears and lubricants are usually safe, so there are no major contraindications or cautions to their use. Baseline vital signs and a visual assessment should be performed before starting therapy with any of these agents.

NURSING DIAGNOSES

Nursing diagnoses associated with the use of ophthalmic agents include:
- Risk for infection related to eye disorder or noncompliance to therapy.
- Risk for self-injury related to side effects of therapy.
- Pain related to eye disorder.
- Sensory alteration (visual) related to eye disorder and effects of medication.
- Knowledge deficit related to lack of information about medication and disorder.

PLANNING

Goals related to administration of ophthalmic medications include:
- Patient remains free of signs and symptoms of infection of the eye with therapy.
- Patient remains compliant to therapy.
- Patient remains free from self-injury related to side effects of therapy.
- Patient will be without eye pain related to eye disorder.

- Patient regains normal visual patterns or preinfection or pre-disorder vision.

Outcome Criteria

Outcome criteria for the patient receiving ophthalmic agents include:
- Patient states signs and symptoms of infection of the eye such as eye pain, drainage, redness, and decreased activity and to report immediately to physician.
- Patient states ways to become more compliant to therapy by taking medications as prescribed.
- Patient minimizes self-injury related to side effects of therapy such as a safe environment and assistance at home while experiencing decreased vision.
- Patient minimizes eye pain related to eye disorder with use of compresses or use of nonaspirin analgesics as ordered.
- Patient shows improvement in visual patterns with increased activity and tolerance to reading, ADLS, etc.

IMPLEMENTATION

Since it is important to administer only clear solutions, the nurse should shake the medication vial before use. Any excess medication must be removed promptly and pressure applied to the inner canthus for 1 minute to avoid systemic symptoms or side effects. Ointments should be applied as a thin layer. All ophthalmic agents should be administered in the conjunctival sac. Be sure you administer all eye medications as ordered and in the proper order if more than one medication is ordered by the physician. See an appropriate drug resource or handbook for specific instructions.

The following medications are discussed because of their special characteristics (all other agents and associated nursing implications are presented in Table 54-12). Atropine is an antidote for myotics and should be available. Echothiophate iodide, an indirect-acting parasympathomimetic agent, should be administered only after you carefully check the vial's concentration amount and after proper reconstitution of the powder.

Dipivefrin, a sympathomimetic and mydriatic, should be instilled as the previous agents with pressure to the lacrimal sac, inner canthus area for 1 minute. Although they have different mechanisms of action, beta-adrenergic blockers such as timolol maleate should be instilled as other optic agents.

Topical anesthetics should be administered exactly as ordered for foreign body removal or treatment of eye injury. You should avoid repeated and continuous use because of the risk of delayed wound healing, possible corneal perforation, permanent corneal opacification, and visual loss. When used, the eye should be

-12 Ophthalmic Agents: Nursing Implications

DRUG GROUP	DRUG EXAMPLES	NURSING IMPLICATIONS
Beta-adrenergic blocking agents	Timolol	Use nasolacrimal pressure to prevent possible systemic absorption, as with all other topical ophthalmic solutions or ointments; monitor for bradycardia, heart block, and wheezing.
Carbonic anhydrase inhibitors (CAIs)	Acetazolamide Dichlorphenamide Methazolamide	Administer as ordered and with meals if necessary to decrease GI upset; fluid volume should be monitored carefully; monitor affected eye closely for therapeutic effects; check for drug interactions.
Osmotic agents	Mannitol Urea Glycerin	Mannitol use may result in digitalis toxicity when given concurrently; if crystallized, may dissolve in warm water; adequate hydration is important—up to 2000 ml/day; Urea, if given at a rate >4 ml/min may result in hemolysis and cerebral vasomotor symptoms; monitor fluid volume status closely; preparation and administration varies; read instructions closely. Glycerin should be used with extreme caution; flavor with lemon or lime juice over cracked ice; monitor for signs of cerebral dehydration.
Mydriatics and cyclopegics	⚓Atropine Cyclopentolate	Atropine: Monitor for side effects such as irregular pulse, confusion, dry mouth, and fever; causes blurred vision and photosensitivity, so sunglasses should be worn outside until effect is gone. Cyclopentolate: Use with caution and give as ordered; same nursing management as with atropine.
Sympathomimetics	Epinephrine Phenylephrine Hydroxyamphetamine Tetrahydrozoline	Monitor for serious side effects that may occur if systemically absorbed such as tachycardia and elevated blood pressure. With corticosteroid agents, report blurred vision or visual disturbances, eye pain, ptosis (lid drooping), or enlarged pupils.
Antiinfective/anti-inflammatory		Prophylactic use is potentially dangerous and is not recommended; may cause local reactions such as redness, itching, edema and dermatitis. Follow instructions for instillation.
Antibacterials	Chloramphenicol ⚓Erythromycin Neomycin Tetracycline ⚓Gentamicin Tobramycin Sulfonamides	With chloramphenicol monitor for drop in CBC, fever, sore throat, and unusual bleeding; With erythromycin make sure to administer as ordered and apply only a thin ointment strip; With neomycin combination agents and tetracycline, be sure to follow instructions; Gentamicin and similar agents should be given as ordered; Cleanse eye with use of sulfonamide agents such as sulfacetamide and sulfisoxazole because they will be inhibited by purulent drainage or exudate; discard any darkened solution; may cause mild pain on instillation.
Antifungals	Natamycin	May cause irritation of the eye.
Antivirals	Idoxuridine Trifluridine Vidarabine	Notify physician if the patient complains of blurred vision, visual disturbances or photosensitivity if not present before therapy; notify the physician about any blurred vision, eye irritations, or visual changes not previously experienced; apply as ordered and, if ointment, apply only a thin strip; always instill drops and ointments into conjunctival sac.
Antiseptics	Silver nitrate	Used for gonococcal infections and may inactivate bacitracin if used concurrently; should leave in contact with sac for at least 3 sec; irrigation afterward not recommended.
Topical anesthetic	Proparacaine Teracaine	These are not recommended for long-term use because they could lead to possible irreversible eye damage; eye should be patched until injury healed; CNS excitation and subsequent depression are potential systemic side effects if absorbed.
Artificial tears	Lacrisert; Lacri-Lube, Duratears and Hypo Tears are ointment forms;	Instill as directed; Ocusert forms given daily.

continued

Table 54-12 | Ophthalmic Agents: Nursing Implications—cont'd

DRUG GROUP	DRUG EXAMPLES	NURSING IMPLICATIONS
Antiallergics	↓Cromolyn sodium	Instill as ordered; therapeutic effects in 4 wk if given regularly.
Enzyme preparation	Chymotrypsin	May result in postoperative glaucoma for about 1 wk, which can be reversed with parasympathomimetics.
Hyperosmolar preparations	Sodium chloride ointment	Apply as ordered.
Nonsteroidal anti-inflammatory	Flurbiprofenn Suprofen Diclofenac ↓Ketorolac	Use only as prescribed; solutions preferred for eye infections because ointments often decrease healing.
Ophthalmic surgery aids	Sodium hyaluronate	Used to protect the eye from damage and is to be given exactly as ordered.

Patient Teaching TIPS

Ophthalmic Agents

✔ Patients taking parasympathomimetic ophthalmic agents should be informed (with demonstrations) about the adequate procedure for instilling eye drops and for applying pressure to the inner canthus. Solutions and the eye dropper should be kept sterile. Long-term therapy is usually necessary, and compliance is important to prevent eye damage.

✔ Indirect parasympathomimetics, such as echothiphate iodide, should be given to patients only after they demonstrate adequate knowledge of the medication and technique for administration and after explanation of side effects associated with most direct- and indirect-acting agents (e.g., blurred vision, bronchospasm, nausea, vomiting, bradycardia, hypotension, and sweating). Patients should be informed that they may experience decreased night visual acuity, stinging sensation, dull ache, or tearing upon instillation and that they should call the physician if these symptoms worsen.

✔ Patients taking sympathomimetics, such as dipivefrin HCL and epinephrine, should be instructed on instillation procedure and told to report any stinging, burning, itching, lacrimation, or puffiness of the eye.

✔ Beta-adrenergic blocking agents such as timolol should be administered as any other optic agent, and pressure should be applied to the inner canthus for 1 full minute after administration. Patients should be encouraged to report any of the following symptoms to their physician: blurred vision, difficulty breathing, wheezing, sweating, flushing, or loss of sight.

✔ Patients should be encouraged to eat a high-potassium, low-sodium diet while taking carbonic anhydrase inhibitors and to drink at least 2 liters of fluid per day to reduce the risk of renal stone formation. Daily weights should be recorded, and patients should be informed of signs and symptoms of fluid and electrolyte imbalances.

✔ Patients taking osmotic agents should drink at least 2000 ml of fluid per day. Patients on glycerin should be informed that lying flat during and after the oral administration will help diminish any headache caused by cerebral dehydration.

✔ Patients taking atropine should be informed that the next dose should be omitted if they are experiencing dry mouth and tachycardia. Photosensitivity is an expected side effect; sunglasses will help ease the discomfort.

✔ With topical anesthetics, patients should not rub or touch the eye while it is numb because of possible eye damage. They should also wear a patch to protect the eye because of loss of blink reflex.

✔ Patients should take antiinfectives, antiinflammatory, and antibacterial ophthalmic solutions as prescribed and individual instructions followed. Increase in eye pain, discharge, and fever should be reported to the physician.

✔ Patients should take ophthalmic corticosteroids cautiously and not overuse or abuse them. The medication should not be stopped without consulting the physician because of the possibility of adverse reactions. Contact lenses should not be worn while taking these medications. All suspensions should be well mixed before use. Stinging is usually experienced after instillation of drops.

✔ Patients taking cromolyn sodium drops should not wear contact lenses until the medication has been discontinued.

TAKE HOME POINTS

Antiglaucoma Drugs
- Glaucoma = disorder of the eye caused from inhibition of the normal flow and drainage of aqueous humor.
- Treatment = reduce IOP either by increasing aqueous humor drainage or decreasing its production.
- Drugs that increase acqueous humor drainage are direct parasympathomimetics, indirect parasympathomimetics, sympathomimetics, and beta blockers.
- Drugs that decrease aqueous humor production are sympathomimetics, beta blockers, carbonic anhydrase inhibitors, and osmotic diuretics.

Ocular Antiinfectives
- Treat bacterial, viral, and fungal infections of the eye.
- A large proportion of the inflammatory diseases seen in ophthalmology are caused by viruses.
- Common ocular infections include conjunctivitis, hordeolum (sty), keratitis, uveitis, and endophthalmitis.

Antiinflammatory Ophthalmic Agents
- Many of the same antiinflammatory drugs that are used systemically are used ophthalmically.
- NSAIDs and corticosteroids are used.

- Corticosteroids = used to inhibit inflammatory response to mechanical, chemical, or immunologic agents.
- NSAIDs = decrease inflammation, relieve pain, and reduce fever associated with tissue damage.

Topical Anesthetics
- Used to prevent pain to the eye.
- Beneficial during surgery, ophthalmic examinations, and removal of foreign bodies.
- Two currently available topical anesthetic drugs for ophthalmic use are proparacaine and tetracaine.

Nursing Considerations
- All ophthalmic preparations need to be administered *exactly* as ordered and using safe, accurate application or instillation technique.
- Report increase in symptoms, such as eye pain and drainage, to the physician immediately.

patched because of the loss of blink reflex. See the box on p. 875 for patient education guidelines.

EVALUATION

Therapeutic responses to miotics include decreased aqueous humor of the eye with resultant decreased IOP and decreased signs, symptoms, and long-term effects associated with glaucoma. Possible side effects are included in the discussion of patient education.

Beta-adrenergic blockers, such as timolol maleate optic solution, have been therapeutic if there is a resultant decrease in IOP. Possible side effects include weakness, depression, anxiety, nausea, confusion, eye irritation, rash, bradycardia, hypotension, and arrhythmias.

Therapeutic responses to antibiotic, antifungal, or antiviral ophthalmic agents include elimination of the infection and resolution of symptoms.

Therapeutic response to ophthalmic anesthetic topical agents include healing of the eye without permanent damage and a decrease in symptoms associated with the damage. Side effects include CNS excitation if systemically absorbed, causing blurred vision, dizziness, tremors, nervousness, and restlessness. Drowsiness, dyspnea, and cardiac arrhythmias may occur secondary to CNS depression.

Cromolyn sodium ophthalmic solution, if therapeutic, will lead to decreased allergic reactions such as decreased itching, tearing, redness, and eye discharge. Potential complications of this agent include hypersensitivity to it and swelling of the conjunctiva (chemosis).

All of the agents discussed have different effects and are associated with various nursing implications. Close monitoring is essential with these and all medications to prevent possible complications and injury to the patient.

Critical Thinking **A C T I V I T I E S**

1. A therapeutic response to cyanocobalamin includes which of the following:
   a. Deyspnea on exertion.
   b. Anorexia at midday.
   c. Decreased urinary output.
   d. Increased activities of daily living.

2. Glaucoma is caused by _____ of the normal flow and drainage of _____.
   1. Stimulation   2. Inhibition   3. Acqueous humor   4. Mucus

   a. 1 and 4   b. 2 and 4   c. 1 and 3   d. 2 and 3

3. A large proportion of the inflammatory diseases seen in ophthalmology are caused by:
   a. Bacteria
   b. Viruses
   c. Fungi

▲▲

BIBLIOGRAPHY

Albanese J, Nutz P: *Mosby's 1995 nursing drug cards,* St Louis, 1995, Mosby.

Johnson KB: *Harriet Lane handbook,* ed 13, St Louis, 1993, Mosby.

Keen JH: *Critical care and emergency drug reference,* St Louis, 1994, Mosby.

Knoben JE, Anderson PO: *Handbook of critical drug data,* ed 6, Hamilton, Ill, 1988, Drug Intelligence Publications.

McEvoy GK: *AHFS drug information,* Bethesda, Md, 1994, American Society of Hospital Pharmacists.

McKenry L, Salerno E: *Mosby's pharmacology in nursing,* ed 19, St Louis, 1995, Mosby.

Skidmore-Roth L: *Mosby's 1995 nursing drug reference,* St Louis, 1995, Mosby.

Hahn, K: Administering eye medications, *Nursing, 89* 19(9):80, 1989.

Schein OD et al: Eye drops and infection, *Arch Ophthalmol* 110:82, 1992.

Chapter 55

Otic Agents

Objectives

When you reach the end of this chapter, you will be able to:

1 Describe the anatomy of the ear.
2 Cite the various ear disorders in the two categories of such disorders and explain their causes.
3 Name the various types of otic preparations and explain the mechanism of action of each.
4 Discuss the nursing process as it relates to the administration of otic preparations.
5 Develop a nursing care plan as it relates to the administration of otic preparations.

CHAPTER OUTLINE

The Ear and Ear Disorders

Treatment of Ear Disorders
  Antibacterial and antifungal otic agents
    Chloramphenicol
  Antibiotic and steroid combination products
  Miscellaneous otic agents
  Antifungal agents
  Local anesthetic agents
    Pramoxine and Benzocaine
  Wax emulsifiers
    Carbamide peroxide

Nursing Process
Assessment
Nursing Diagnoses
Planning
  Outcome criteria
Implementation
Evaluation

Glossary

Cerumen (sə roo' mən) A yellowish or brownish waxy excretion produced by vestigial apocrine sweat glands in the external ear canal. Also called *earwax*. (p. 880)

Otic agents (o' tik) Drugs applied locally to treat inflammation of the external ear canal or to remove excess cerumen (earwax). Also called *otics*. (p. 879)

Otitis media (o ti' tis mēd ē ə) Inflammation or infection of the middle ear, a common affliction of childhood. It is often preceded by an upper respiratory tract infection. (p. 879)

Wax emulsifiers (ē' mul' si fyers) Products that loosen and help in the removal of cerumen. (p. 880)

The Ear and Ear Disorders

The ear consists of three portions: the outer, middle, and inner ear. The outer, or external, ear is made up of the pinna, or outer projecting part of the ear, and the external auditory meatus. The middle ear comprises the tympanic cavity, mastoid appendages (e.g., malleus, incus), and the auditory, or eustachian tube. The inner ear is made up of such structures as the cochlea and semicircular canals. The ear and its associated structures are illustrated in Fig. 55-1.

The disorders of the ear can be categorized according to the portion of the ear affected. Those of the outer and middle ear are the ones pertinent to the discussion here because these are the disorders that are usually treated with the agents discussed in this chapter. In general the most common disorders of these portions of the ear are bacterial and fungal infections, inflammatory disorders that cause pain, and earwax accumulation. Such disorders tend to be self-limiting, and if treatment is needed, it is generally easy to accomplish. However, if problems persist or are left untreated, more serious problems such as hearing loss may eventuate.

External ear disorders are generally the result of

▼ FIG. 55-1 Structure of the ear.

physical trauma to the ear and consist of disorders such as lacerations or scrapes to the skin and localized infection of the hair follicles that usually results in the development of a boil. These are examples of the self-limiting types of disorders just mentioned. They are often minor and heal with time. Other, more serious disorders may initially appear to be minor but, if left untreated, can become more serious. Such "minor" irritations are dermatitis of the ear, itching, local redness, weeping, or drainage, but they may be the result of inflammation caused by seborrhea, psoriasis, or contact dermatitis. They may also be the first signs of a more serious underlying disease process such as head trauma. Drainage, pain, and dizziness are sure indications of the need for prompt medical care.

By far the most common middle ear disorder is infection caused by various microorganisms, a condition commonly called **otitis media.** This disorder most commonly afflicts children and usually occurs after an upper respiratory tract infection. It may also occur in adults, but it is then generally associated with trauma to the middle ear stemming from trauma to the tympanic membrane. Foreign objects and water sports are the usual sources of such trauma. Common symptoms of middle ear disorders such as otitis media are pain, fever, malaise, pressure, a sensation of fullness in the ears, and hearing loss. If left untreated, tinnitus (ringing in the ears), nausea, vertigo, and mastoditis may occur. Hearing deficits and even hearing loss may eventuate if appropriate and prompt therapy is not started.

TREATMENT OF EAR DISORDERS

Some of the minor ailments that affect the outer ear can be treated with over-the-counter (OTC) medications, but persistent, painful conditions always require a physician's care. Middle ear disorders are rarely treated with OTC medications, unless they are prescribed by a physician after referral. The drugs commonly used to treat the relatively minor disorders of the external and middle ear are called **otic agents** and are topically applied. Following is a list of these agents:

- Antibiotics
- Antifungals
- Antiinflammatory agents
- Wax emulsifiers
- Steroids
- Local anesthetics
- Local analgesics

More serious problems than those just mentioned may require treatment with potent, systemically administered medications such as antimicrobial agents, analgesics, antiinflammatory drugs, and antihistamines. These medications have been discussed in earlier chapters.

Antibacterial and Antifungal Otic Agents

Many of the antibacterial and antifungal agents that are given systemically also come in topical formulations that are applied to the external ear, chloramphenicol and gentamicin being two commonly used ones. Several of these agents are also combined with steroids to take advantage of their additional antiinflammatory, antipruritic, and antiallergic drug effects. The antimicrobial drugs used as otic agents are effective in the treatment of mastoidectomy infections and infections of the external auditory canal. Middle ear infections such as otitis media, generally require treatment with systemically administered antibiotics, however.

CHLORAMPHENICOL

Chloramphenicol (Chloromycetin Otic and Pentamycetin) has the advantage of possessing a very broad spectrum of activity. It is effective against *Staphylococcus aureus, Escherichia coli, Pseudomonas aeruginosa, Enterobacter aerogenes, Haemophilus influenzae*, and many others. It can cause adverse effects very similar to those caused by many of the topically applied antibiotics. These include burning, redness, rash, swelling, and other signs of topical irritation. Chloramphenicol otic is available as a 0.5% solution that is usually instilled in the ear. Two to three drops three times daily is the recommended dosage for both adults and children.

Antibiotic and Steroid Combination Products

The steroid most commonly used in combination with antibiotics is hydrocortisone, and it is added to reduce the inflammation and itching associated with ear infections. The antibiotics contained in the most popular combination products and the various trade names of these products are given in Table 55-1. These products are most commonly used for the treatment of bacterial infections of the external auditory canal caused by susceptible bacteria such as *S. aureus, E. coli, Klebsiella* spp., and others.

Miscellaneous Otic Agents

There is a wide variety of single-agent and combination-agent products that are used to treat fungal and bacterial infections, inflammation, ear pain, and other minor or superficial problems of the external ear. An additional problem is the accumulation and eventual impaction of earwax, or **cerumen,** which can be the cause of many of these symptoms. Products that soften and help eliminate earwax are referred to as **wax emulsifiers** and are therefore also discussed with the miscellaneous agents.

Antifungal Agents

Although fungal infections of the ear are uncommon, there are some otic agents that are available for their treatment. The agents contained in two commonly used antifungal combination products and the trade names of each are listed in the box below. These combination products include drugs from several classes of agents—steroids, local anesthetics, and topical antiseptics—and hence the therapeutic effect is a combination of the respective effects of the individual agents. They are used as antibacterial, antifungal, local anesthetic, and antiinflammatory otic drugs.

Local Anesthetic Agents

There are numerous otic combination products that contain local anesthetic agents. Many common ear disorders are associated with some degree of pain and inflammation, and the numbing or anesthetic effect

---

Antifungal Combination Otic Products

INGREDIENTS	TRADE NAMES
1% Hydrocortisone 1% Pramoxine 0.1% Chloroxylenol Propylene glycol Acetic acid Benzalkonium	Ear-Eze, Otic-HC Ear Drops, Tega-Otic
1% Hydrocortisone 2% Acetic acid 3% Propylene glycol diacetate 0.02% Benzethonium chloride	VōSol HC Otic

---

Table 55-1 Steroid and Antibiotic Combinations for Otic Use

STEROID	ANTIBIOTIC (DOSE/ML)	TRADE NAME
1% Hydrocortisone (solution)	5 mg of neomycin and 10,000 units of polymyxin B 10,000 units of polymyxin B	Cortisporin Otic, Otocort Otobiotic Otic, Pyocidine Otic
1% Hydrocortisone (suspension)	5 mg of neomycin and 10,000 units of Polymyxin B 3.3 mg of neomycin and 3 mg of colistin	Cortisporin Otic, Otocort Coly-Mycin S Otic

provided by the local anesthetic makes it very beneficial in the relief of the pain. The same characteristics of the local anesthetics that were discussed in Chapter 9 apply to the topically applied local anesthetics used in these preparations.

PRAMOXINE AND BENZOCAINE

One combination product that contains local anesthetics has been mentioned in the box on the previous page, and the local anesthetic it contains is pramoxine. Pramoxine is structurally similar to dyclonin and does not contain the usual ester or amide linkage of the procaine-type drugs. Besides its otic use, it is also applied topically for the temporary relief of the pain and itching associated with dermatoses, minor burns, anogenital pruritus or irritation, anal fissures, and hemorrhoids.

Another local anesthetic otic agent that is used in combination with analgesics and emollients is benzocaine. This combination consists of:

- 1.4% Benzocaine
- 5.4% Antipyrine
- Glycerin
- Oxyquinoline sulfate

It may be used as an antiinflammatory, analgesic, or emollient. Common trade names for this combination product are: Allergen Ear Drops, Auralgan Otic, and Auromid.

Benzocaine differs from pramoxine in that it is a local anesthetic of the ester type. It is also used for the temporary relief of pain and itching, either alone or in combination with other drugs.

Wax Emulsifiers

Wax or cerumen is a natural product of the ear and is produced by modified sweat glands in the auditory canal. However, it can occasionally build up and become impacted, resulting in pain and temporary deafness. The wax emulsifiers can loosen and help remove such impacted cerumen.

CARBAMIDE PEROXIDE

One commonly used wax emulsifier is carbamide peroxide. It is customarily combined with other agents that work together to loosen and help remove cerumen. One such combination product contains:

- 6.5% Carbamide peroxide
- Glycerin
- Propylene glycol

Trade names for combination products that contain these ingredients are Debrox Drops, Murine Ear Drops, and Auro Ear Drops.

As a source of hydrogen peroxide, carbamide per-oxide slowly releases hydrogen peroxide and oxygen when exposed to moisture such as that on the skin or the mouth. This release of oxygen imparts a weak antibacterial action to the otic agent. In addition, the effervescence resulting from the release of oxygen has the mechanical effect of removing cerumen from inaccessible spaces such as the ear canal. Agents such as the glycerin soften the cerumen, making it easier to remove.

NURSING PROCESS

ASSESSMENT

Before administering any of the otic preparations, the nurse should make sure the patient's baseline hearing or auditory status is evaluated and the findings documented. There should also be a thorough evaluation of the patient's symptoms, and any other related medical information should be elicited. Any drug and food allergies should be noted and documented. In addition, it is important for the nurse to understand the specific indication for or the intended use of the medication so that it can be given exactly as ordered. An understanding of the anatomy of the ear is important as well, especially as it relates to patients in different age groups. This understanding should extend to the specific administration technique used as well. Contraindications to the use of chloramphenicol otic preparations include hypersensitivity and eardrum perforation.

Drug hypersensitivity to hydrocortisone, neomycin sulfate, or polymyxin B sulfate would be a contraindication to the use of any of the individual agents or to any of the combination products containing these agents. A perforated eardrum would be a contraindication to the use of these agents as well.

NURSING DIAGNOSES

Nursing diagnoses related to patients receiving otic agents include:

- Impaired communication as the result of hearing loss stemming from an ear disorder.
- Risk for injury related to symptoms of the ear disorder and possible vestibular dysfunction.
- Risk for infection related to inadequate treatment.
- Sensory loss (auditory) related to ear infection.

NURSING ■ CARE ■ PLAN

Otitis Media

Karen, an 11-year-old with otitis media, has been placed on cefaclor (Ceclor) 250 mg tid. She has tolerated Ceclor in the past, but her grandmother brought her into the physician's office and needs instructions for administration of the medicine, since Karen's mother is out of town. Use of AuroEar drops has been recommended as well.

Assessment with nursing diagnoses	Planning with goals and outcome criteria	Implementation with patient education	Evaluation
Subjective "I don't remember much about how to take this medicine" **Objective** Successful therapy before with cefaclor Mother out of town Grandmother caregiver for now **Nursing diagnoses** Knowledge deficit related to teaching needs on cefaclor	**Goals** Patient and grandmother verbalize instructions associated with taking cefaclor before leaving physician's office **Outcome criteria** Before leaving the physician's office, patient and grandmother: State dosing times and amounts State side effects of medication State side effects to report to the physician Demonstrate adequate technique for installing AuroEar drops as ordered	It is important to take medication exactly as prescribed and until all medication is gone Eating yogurt while on antibiotics will help to maintain normal bacteria in the intestines and decrease diarrhea Contact the physician should you experience sore throat, bleeding, easy bruising, joint pain Side effects to possibly expect include headache, dizziness, nausea, vomiting, diarrhea,* loss of appetite,* and rash AuroEar drops to be used daily	Patient will display the following therapeutic responses to cefaclor: Decreased ear pain Decreased fever Patient will experience minimal side effects, such as diarrhea Patient's pain of the ear area will decrease with adequate response to Ceclor and with daily use of AuroEar drops

*Most common side effects.

PLANNING

Goals pertaining to patients receiving otic agents include:
■ Patient regains normal patterns of hearing and communicating.
■ Patient will be free of discomfort and symptoms related to the ear disorder.
■ Patient remains free of or experiences minimal signs and symptoms of ear infection with course of treatment.
■ Patient will be free of adverse reactions or side effects.
■ Patient will be free of complications associated with medication therapy.

Outcome Criteria

Outcome criteria for patients receiving otic agents include:

■ Patient openly verbalizes feelings related to problems with communication (decreased hearing).
■ Patient reports increased hearing loss and increased symptoms of ear pain, redness and swelling of the ear canal, and fever to the physician immediately.
■ Patient states measures to take to increase the effectiveness of the medication regimen such as accurate application or instillation.
■ Patient demonstrates accurate medication administration techniques.

IMPLEMENTATION

Chloramphenicol drops should be instilled only after the ear has been thoroughly cleansed, all cerumen removed by irrigation, and the stopper cleaned with alcohol. Eardrops should generally be warmed to body temperature before instillation but not higher than the body temperature because this may affect the potency of the medication. Steroid and antibiotic combination otic preparations, wax emulsifiers, and ear-drying agents should all be administered according to these same guidelines. See the box above for patient teaching tips.

EVALUATION

The therapeutic effects of the otic preparations include less pain, redness, and swelling in the ear; a reduction in fever and the WBC counts; and negative culture findings if previous culture has yielded positive findings. The ear canal should be watched for the occurrence of rash or contact dermatitis with a rash. Life-threatening reactions such as bone marrow suppression may occur in association with chloramphenicol use, but these are rare.

Critical Thinking A C T I V I T I E S

1. Chloramphenicol drops should be:
   a. administered at a cool temperature.
   b. instilled in the ear regardless of the amount of cerumen present.
   c. instilled only if ordered with a steroid otic drop.
   d. administered at a warm, approximately body, temperature.

BIBLIOGRAPHY

Albanese J, Nutz P: *Mosby's 1995 nursing drug cards,* St Louis, 1995, Mosby.

Johnson KB: *Harriet Lane handbook,* ed 13, St Louis, 1993, Mosby.

Keen JH: *Critical care and emergency drug reference,* St Louis, 1994, Mosby.

Knoben JE, Anderson PO: *Handbook of critical drug data,* ed 6, Hamilton, Ill, 1988, Drug Intelligence Publications.

McEvoy GK: *AHFS drug information,* Bethesda, Md, 1994, American Society of Hospital Pharmacists.

Skidmore-Roth L: *Mosby's 1995 nursing drug reference,* St Louis, 1995, Mosby.

Appendix

Canadian Trade Names

Canadian Trade Name	Generic Equivalent	Canadian Trade Name	Generic Equivalent
Activase rt-PA	alteplase	M.O.S.-S.R.	morphine
Alloprin	allopurinol	Novaniacin	nicotinic acid
Apo-Allopurinol	allopurinol	Novochlorhydrate	chloral hydrate
Apo-Amitriptyline	amitriptyline	Novocimetine	cimetidine
Apo-Cimetidine	cimetidine	Novo-Diltiazem	diltiazem
Apo-Diltiaz	diltiazem	Novodipiradol	dipyridamole
Apo-Dipyridamole	dipyridamole	Novoflupam	flurazepam
Apo-Flurazepam	flurazepam	Novomethacin	indomethacin
Apo-Haloperidol	haloperidol	Novometoprolol	metoprolol tartrate
Apo-Ibuprofen	ibuprofen	Novo-Nifedin	nifedipine
Apo-Indomethacin	indomethacin	Novoperidol	haloperidol
Apo-Metoclop	metoclopramide	Novo-Pranol	propranolol
Apo-Metoprolol	metoprolol tartrate	Novoprofen	ibuprofen
Apo-Nifed	nifedipine	Novo-Purol	allopurinol
Apo-Propanolol	propranolol	Novoquinidin	quinidine sulfate
Apo-Verap	verapamil	Novoreserpine	reserpine
Astrin	aspirin	Novorythro	erythromycin estolate
Atropisol	atropine	Novo-Veramil	verapamil
Balminil Expectorant	guaifenesin	Nu-Diltiaz	diltiazem
Betaloc	metoprolol tartrate	Nu-Loraz	lorazepam
Calcilean	heparin calcium	Nu-Nifed	nifedipine
Clozaril	clozapine	Nu-Verap	verapamil
Detensol	propranolol	PMS-Amitriptyline	amitriptyline
Dixarit	clonidine	PMS Levazine	amitriptyline
Elavil Plus	amitriptyline	Pentacarinat	pentamidine isethionate
Eldisine	vindesine sulfate	Peptol	cimetidine
Eltroxin	levothyroxine	Peridol	haloperidol
Emex	metoclopramide	Pneumopent	pentamidine isethionate
Epimorph	morphine	Pressyn	vasopressin
Eprex	epoetin	Prochlorperacine	prochlorperazine
Erybid	erythromycin base	Procytox	cyclophospamide
Erythromid	erythromycin base	Prorazine	prochlorperazine
Euglucon	glyburide	Pulmophylline	theophylline
GBH	lindane	Purimol	allopurinol
Heparin Leo	heparin sodium	Quinate	quinidine gluconate
Hepalean	heparin sodium	Regulex	docusate sodium
Imferon	iron dextran	Reserfia	reserpine
Indocid	indomethacin	Resyl	guaifenesin
Isopto Atropine	atropine	Robidex	dextromethorphan
Isotamine	isoniazid	Serpasil	reserpine
Koffex	dextromethorphan	Sotacor	sotalol
Kwellada	lindane	Stemetil	prochlorperazine
Larodopa	levodopa	Sulcrate	sucralfate
Levate	amitriptyline	Syn-Diltiazem	diltiazem
Lorazepam	lorazepam	Tamofen	tamoxifen
Losec	omeprazole	Tamone	tamoxifen
Maxeran	metoclopramide	Tamoplex	tamoxifen
Minims Atropine	atropine	Transderm-V	scopolamine (hyoscine)
Morphine H.P.	morphine	Tri-B$_3$	nicotinic acid
Morphitec	morphine	Trikacide	metronidazole
M.O.S.	morphine	Xylocard	lidocaine

Disorders Index

A

Absence seizure, 141
Acne, 557
Acquired immunodeficiency syndrome, 672
Acromegaly, 459
Actinic keratosis, 837
Acute angle-closure glaucoma, 849
Acute lymphoblastic leukemia
    antimetabolites for, 689, 691
    asparaginase for, 701
    cytotoxic antibiotics for, 693, 695
    mitotic inhibitors for, 696, 698
Acute myeloid leukemia, 689, 691
Acute renal failure, 391
Addison's disease, 491, 494
Adrenocortical insufficiency
    adrenal agents for, 494
    pituitary drugs for, 459
Adult respiratory distress syndrome, 407
Affective disorders, 164, 169-193
    antidepressant agents for, 170-173
    antimanic agents for, 179-180
    antipsychotic agents for, 180-186
    monoamine oxidase inhibitors for, 173-176
    nursing process in, 186-193
    second-generation antidepressants for, 176-179
Akinetic seizure, 141
Alcoholism, 167
Allergic asthma, 521
Allergic rhinitis, 507
Amebiasis, 611, 616
Amebic dysentery, 559
Amenorrhea, 429
Anaphylaxis, 216
Anemia, 718, 819-820, 821
Angina, 231, 300-318
    beta-blockers for, 233, 305-308
    calcium channel blockers for, 308-311
    coronary artery disease and, 301-302
    nitrates and nitrites for, 302-305
    nursing process in, 312-317
Angle-closure glaucoma, 849
Ankylosing spondylitis, 641
Anxiety, 164, 184
Arrhythmia, 231
    beta-blockers for, 233
    cardiac glycosides for, 265-266
    digitalis toxicity and, 271
    vasoactive adrenergics for, 216
    ventricular, 282, 285, 286, 287
Arterial thrombosis, 358
Arthritis
    azathioprine for, 659
    sulfonamides for, 545
Ascariasis, 618
Ascites, 390
Asthma
    beta-agonists for, 524-528
    bronchodilators for, 522-524
    corticosteroids for, 528-531
    cromolyn and nedocromil for, 532
    immune globulins for, 672
    nursing process in, 533-537
Athlete's foot, 833
Atrial dysrhythmia, 285
Atrial fibrillation, 282, 285, 286
Atrial flutter, 286
Atropic vaginitis, 425, 426
Attention deficit disorder, 195, 198, 200-201, 213
Autoimmune disorders, 656
    immune globulins for, 672
    interferon for, 714

B

Bacterial infection
    aminoglycosides for, 559

Bacterial infection—cont'd
    cephalosporins for, 552
    macrolides for, 564
    penicillins for, 548
    quinolones for, 562
    sulfonamides for, 546
    tetracyclines for, 557
    vancomycin for, 568
Balantidiasis, 557
Bancroft's filariasis, 621
Benign prostatic hyperplasia, 446, 449
Beriberi, 787
Bile duct tumor, 689
Biliary obstruction, 371
Bladder cancer
    alkylating agents for, 685, 687
    antimetabolites for, 689
    interferon for, 714
Blastomycosis, 598
Body louse infestation, 836
Bradycardia, 250
Brain tumor
    alkylating agents for, 685, 687
    antimetabolites for, 689
Braxton Hicks contractions, 432
Breast cancer
    alkylating agents for, 685, 687
    androgens for, 449
    antimetabolites for, 689
    cytotoxic antibiotics for, 693, 695
    estrogenic agents for, 425, 426
    interleukin-2 for, 717
    mitotic inhibitors for, 696
    nursing care plan for, 708
    progestational agents for, 429
Bronchial asthma, 521
Bronchitis, 526
Brucellosis, 557
Burn, 407

C

Cancer, 676-709
    alkylating agents for, 683-688
    altretamine for, 699, 700
    antimetabolites for, 688-692
    asparaginase for, 699, 700-701
    biologic response modifiers for, 710-724
        colony-stimulating factors, 718, 719-722
        immune system and, 711-712
        interferons, 712-716
        interleukins, 717-719
        nursing process and, 722-723
    cell growth cycle and, 681-683
    cytotoxic antibiotics for, 692-695
    etiology of, 679-681
    hydroxyurea for, 701
    mitotic inhibitors for, 695-698
    nursing care plan for, 708
    nursing process in, 701-707
Candidiasis, 598, 603, 833, 834
Carcinoid tumor, 459
Cardioversion, 167
Cataract, 846
Cerebral edema, 391, 494
Cervical cancer, 693, 695
Cestode infection, 618
Chancroid, 557
Chemotherapy emesis, 770, 771
Chickenpox, 579, 580
Chlamydial infection
    macrolides for, 564
    ocular, 863
    sulfonamides for, 546
    tetracyclines for, 557
Cholera, 557
Chronic bronchitis, 521, 522
Chronic granulomatous disease, 716

Chronic lymphocytic leukemia, 669, 672
    alkylating agents for, 685, 687
    antimetabolites for, 689, 691
Chronic myelocytic leukemia
    alkylating agents for, 685, 687
    cytotoxic antibiotics for, 693, 695
    hydroxyurea for, 701
    interferon for, 714
Chronic obstructive pulmonary disease, 521, 538
Chronic stable angina, 301
Cirrhosis, 395
Clonorchiasis, 621
Coccidioidomycosis, 598
Cold, common, 509
Colorectal cancer
    antimetabolites for, 689
    interleukin-2 for, 717
Common cold, 509
Community-acquired infection, 627
Condyloma acuminatum (condylomata acuminata), 714, 716
Congestive heart failure
    cardiac glycosides for, 265-266
    digitalis for, 269
    diuretics for, 385, 388, 395
Conjunctivitis, 862
    allergic, 869
    bacterial, 863
Constipation, 752-762
    bulk-forming laxatives for, 755-756
    emollient laxatives for, 756-758
    hyperosmotic laxatives for, 758-759
    nursing process in, 760-762
    saline laxatives, 759
    stimulant laxatives for, 759-760
Convulsions, 141
Corneal inflammation, 869
Coronary artery disease, 301-302
Coronary artery thrombus, 358
Cough, 511
Crohn's disease, 545
Cryptococcosis, 598
Cryptorchidism, 438
Cushing's syndrome, 491, 494
Cystic fibrosis, 672
Cytomegalovirus, 578, 580

D

Deep vein thrombosis, 358, 407
Dehydration, 406
Depression, 172, 176, 178
Dermatitis herpetiformis, 546
Dermatophytosis, 598, 834
Diabetes insipidus
    desmopressin for, 355
    diuretics in, 395
    pituitary drugs for, 459
Diabetes mellitus, 475-488
    glucose-elevating drugs for, 484-485
    insulin-dependent, 477-478
    insulins for, 478-481
    investigational drugs for, 484
    non–insulin dependent, 478
    nursing process in, 485-487
    oral antidiabetic agents for, 481-484
Diabetic ketoacidosis, 477
Diabetic neuropathy, 641
Diarrhea, 745-752
    adsorbents for, 749
    antacids and, 732
    anticholinergics for, 749-750
    belladonna-alkaloid combinations for, 750-751
    intestinal flora modifiers for, 751-752
    nursing process in, 760-762
    opiates for, 751
Diphtheria, 669
Diphyllobothriasis, 618

...35, 738
...uterine bleeding
...ic agents for, 425
...gestational agents for, 429
...uterine stimulants for, 434
Dysmenorrhea, 641, 648
Dysrhythmia, 285-287, 413

E

Ear disorders, 878-884
    antibacterial and antifungal agents for, 879-880
    local anesthetic agents for, 880-881
    nursing process in, 881-883
Edema
    cerebral, 494
    diuretics in, 388, 391, 394, 396
    pulmonary, 390
Embolism, 358
Emphysema, 521, 522
Endometrial cancer, 429
Endometriosis, 429, 449
Endophthalmitis, 862
Enterobacter infection, 546
Enterobiasis, 618, 621
Enterococcus infection
    penicillins for, 548
    vancomycin for, 568
Enterocolitis, 568
Enuresis, 459
Epilepsy, 135-147
    antiepileptic agents for, 136-144
    diuretics in, 388
    immune globulins for, 672
    nursing process in, 144-145
Erythema multiforme, 424
Escherichia coli infection
    aminoglycosides for, 559
    sulfonamides for, 546
Esophageal candidiasis, 603
Esophagitis
    antacids for, 732, 734
    omeprazole for, 738
Essential fatty acid deficiency, 811
Essential tremor, 233
Ewing's sarcoma, 693, 695

F

Familial hypophosphatemia, 781
Fibrocystic breast disease, 449
Filariasis, 621
Flatworm infection, 618
Flatulence, 733
Folate deficiency, 823
Folic acid deficiency, 823
Follicular lymphoma, 687
Fungal infection, 834, 863

G

Gallbladder cancer, 689
Gastric hyperacidity, 732
Gastritis, 732
Gastroesophageal reflux disease, 734
Generalized anxiety disorder, 165
Genital herpes, 580
Genital warts, 716
Giardiasis, 612
Gilles de la Tourette syndrome, 184
Glaucoma, 387, 388, 847-848, 852
Glial tumor, 717
Glucose-6-phosphate dehydrogenase deficiency, 545
Gonorrhea
    macrolides for, 564
    tetracyclines for, 557

Gout, 641, 644, 647, 648
Gram-negative bacteria
    aminoglycosides for, 559
    cephalosporins for, 552
    quinolones for, 562
Gram-positive bacteria
    aminoglycosides for, 559
    cephalosporins for, 552
    penicillins for, 548
    quinolones for, 562
    vancomycin for, 568
Granuloma inguinale, 557
Graves' disease, 466
Growth failure, 459

H

Haemophilus influenzae infection, 564, 669
Hairy cell leukemia
    cytotoxic antibiotics for, 693, 695
    interferon for, 714, 716
Hantavirus infection, 578
Head and neck cancer
    alkylating agents for, 685
    antimetabolites for, 689
    cytotoxic antibiotics for, 693, 695
    interleukin-2 for, 717
Head louse infestation, 836
Headache
    alpha-adrenergic blocking agents for, 229
    nonsteroidal antiinflammatory drugs for, 641
Heartburn, 732
Helicobacter pylori infection, 557
Helminthic infection, 617-622
Hemophilia, 459
Hepatitis, 669, 672, 714, 716
Hereditary angioedema, 449
Herpes simplex virus infection, 578, 580
Hiatal hernia, 732
Hiccups, 184
High-altitude sickness, 388
Histiocytosis, 696
Histoplasmosis, 598
Hodgkin's disease
    alkylating agents for, 685, 687
    cytotoxic antibiotics for, 693, 695
    interleukin-2 for, 717
    mitotic inhibitors for, 696, 698
Hookworm infection, 621
Hordeolum, 862
Hospital-acquired infection, 627
Human immunodeficiency virus infection, 578
Hyperacidity, 734
Hyperaldosteronism, 392
Hyperbilirubinemia, 125
Hypercalcemia
    cytotoxic antibiotics for, 693, 695
    digitalis toxicity and, 271
    diuretics in, 389
Hypercalciuria
    cytotoxic antibiotics for, 693, 695
    diuretics in, 395
Hypercapnia, 198
Hypercholesterolemia, 369
Hyperkalemia, 412, 526
Hyperlipidemia, 370-371
Hypernatremia, 415
Hypersecretory conditions, 738
Hypertension, 319-340
    adrenergic agents for, 322-326
    alpha-adrenergic blocking agents for, 229
    angiotensin-converting enzyme inhibitors for, 326-329
    beta-blockers for, 233
    calcium channel blockers for, 330
    diuretics for, 330, 389
    ganglionic-blocking agents for, 257
    nonsteroidal antiinflammatory drugs for, 641

Hypertension—cont'd
    nursing process in, 332-340
    vasodilators for, 330-332
Hyperthyroidism, 466, 471
Hypertrophic subaortic stenosis, 233
Hypochromic anemia, 819
Hypoglycemia, 478, 815
Hypogonadism
    androgens for, 449
    estrogenic agents for, 425, 426
    fertility agents for, 438
Hypokalemia, 268, 271, 413
Hypomagnesia, 797
Hyponatremia, 415
Hypoparathyroidism, 781, 782
Hypoproteinuria, 407
Hypotension
    beta-agonists for, 526
    vasoactive adrenergics for, 216
Hypothyroidism, 271, 466, 468

I

Idiopathic thrombocytopenic purpura, 669, 672
Immunodeficiency diseases, 669, 672
Infertility, 436-439
Influenza, 509, 578, 580
Insecticide poisoning, 250
Intestinal candidiasis, 603
Iron deficiency, 823
Irritable bowel syndrome, 250
Ischemic heart disease, 301

J

Jock itch, 833

K

Kaposi's sarcoma
    interferon for, 714, 716
    mitotic inhibitors for, 696
Kawasaki syndrome, 672
Keratitis, 580, 856, 862, 863
Keratoconjunctivitis, 580
Klebsiella infection
    aminoglycosides for, 559
    sulfonamides for, 546
Kraurosis vulvae, 425, 426

L

Lassa virus infection, 578
Lennox-Gastaut seizure, 141
Leukemia, 678-679
    alkylating agents for, 685, 687
    antimetabolites for, 689, 691
    cytotoxic antibiotics for, 693, 695
    mitotic inhibitors for, 696, 698
Lice infestation, 836
Liver
    cancer of, 689
    disease of, 389, 390
    failure of, 407
    peliosis of, 447
Lung cancer
    alkylating agents for, 685, 687
    antimetabolites for, 689
    cytotoxic antibiotics for, 695
    interleukin-2 for, 717
    mitotic inhibitors for, 696, 698
Lyme disease
    macrolides for, 564
    tetracyclines for, 557

Lymphogranuloma venereum, 557
Lymphoma, 678-679
    alkylating agents for, 685, 687
    cytotoxic antibiotics for, 693, 695
    mitotic inhibitors for, 696
Lymphosarcoma
    alkylating agents for, 687
    cytotoxic antibiotics for, 693, 695
    mitotic inhibitors for, 698

M

Macrocytic anemia, 820
Malaria, 546, 608-612
Malnutrition, 804
Mania, 184
Measles, 669, 672
Melanoma
    alkylating agents for, 685
    cytotoxic antibiotics for, 693, 695
    interferon for, 714
    interleukin-2 for, 717
    mitotic inhibitors for, 696
Meningitis, 603
Menopause, 425, 426
Microcytic anemia, 819
Migraine, 233
Motion sickness, 250, 507, 770
Multiple myeloma
    alkylating agents for, 685, 687
    antimetabolites for, 689
    interferon for, 714
Multiple sclerosis
    interferon for, 714, 716
    pituitary drugs for, 459
Mumps, 669
Muscle spasm, 167
Myasthenia gravis
    cholinergic agents for, 241
    pituitary drugs for, 459
    potassium replacement therapy in, 413
Mycoplasma infection
    macrolides for, 564
    tetracyclines for, 557
Mycosis fungoides
    alkylating agents for, 687
    antimetabolites for, 691
    mitotic inhibitors for, 696
Myocardial infarction
    antidysrhythmic agents for, 286
    antiplatelet agents for, 352
    beta-blockers for, 233
    digitalis toxicity and, 271
    thrombolytics for, 358
Myoclonic seizure, 141
Myxedema, 468

N

Narcolepsy, 196, 198, 213
Nausea, 764-774
    antiemetic agents for, 765-771
    antipsychotic agents for, 184
    hydroxyzine for, 168
    nursing process in, 772-774
Nematode infection, 618
Neonatal pulmonary hypertension, 229
Neonatal sepsis, 672
Nephropathy, diabetic, 477
Nephrosis, 407
Nephrotic syndrome, 390
Neuroblastoma
    alkylating agents for, 687
    cytotoxic antibiotics for, 693, 695
    mitotic inhibitors for, 696, 698
Neuropathy, diabetic, 477
Neutropenia, 718
Nocardiosis, 546, 547
Nocturnal enuresis, 459

Non-Hodgkin's lymphoma
    alkylating agents for, 687
    antimetabolites for, 689
    interleukin-2 for, 717
    mitotic inhibitors for, 696
Normochromic anemia, 820
Nosocomial infection, 627

O

Obesity, 198, 213
Obsessive-compulsive disorder, 165
Ocular hypertension, 857
Open-angle glaucoma, 387, 388, 849, 855, 857
Ophthalmia neonatorum, 863
Opisthorchiasis, 621
Oral candidiasis, 598, 603
Oropharyngeal candidiasis, 603
Orthostatic hypertension, 229
Osteoarthritis, 640, 641, 647
Osteomalacia, 781
Osteoporosis, 425, 426
Otitis media, 879, 882
Ovarian cancer
    alkylating agents for, 685, 687
    altretamine for, 701
    antimetabolites for, 689
    interleukin-2 for, 717
    mitotic inhibitors for, 696, 698
Ovarian failure, 425, 426

P

Pancreatic cancer
    antimetabolites for, 689
    cytotoxic antibiotics for, 693, 695
Panic disorder, 165
Papillomavirus infection, 714
Paraneoplastic syndrome, 679
Parkinson's disease, 148-161
    anticholinergic therapy in, 156-158
    dopaminergic therapy in, 152-156
    neuroprotective therapy in, 150-152
    nursing process in, 158-161
Paroxysmal atrial flutter, 286
Paroxysmal supraventricular tachycardia, 216, 282, 286
Partial seizure, 141
Patent ductus arteriosus, 644
Pediculosis, 836
Peliosis of liver, 447
Penile cancer, 693, 695
Peptic esophagitis
    antacids for, 732
    histamine₂ antagonists for, 735
Peptic ulcer, 250
    antacids for, 732
    nursing care plan for, 742
    sucralfate for, 739
    tetracyclines for, 557
Pericardial effusion, 557
Peripheral arterial disease, 352
Pernicious anemia, 823
Pheochromocytoma, 227, 233
Phlebitis, 809
Phobia, 165
Platyhelminthes infection, 618
Pleural effusion, 557
Plummer's disease, 466
Pneumocystis carinii pneumonia, 616
Pneumocystosis, 612
Polio, 669
Polycythemia vera, 687
Polydipsia, 476
Polyphagia, 476
Polyuria, 476
Porphyria, 184
Postpartum uterine atony and hemorrhage, 434
Posttraumatic stress disorder, 165

Premature atrial contractions, 282
Premature ventricular beats, 233
Premature ventricular contractions, 282
Preterm labor, 436
Priapism, 447
Primary nocturnal enuresis, 459
Prinzmetal's angina, 301
Prostate cancer, 425, 426, 427
Proteus infection
    aminoglycosides for, 559
    sulfonamides for, 546
Protozoal infection, 612-617
Pseudomembranous colitis, 568
Pseudomonas infection, 559, 560
Psittacosis, 557
Psychomotor seizure, 141
Psychosis, 164
Pubic louse infestation, 836
Pulmonary edema, 390
Pulmonary embolism, 358
Pulmonary hypertension, 229

Q

Q fever, 557

R

Rectal cancer, 689
Recurrent epithelial keratitis, 580
Relapsing fever, 557
Renal cancer, 429
Renal cell carcinoma
    interferon for, 714
    interleukin-2 for, 717, 718
Renal disease, 389
Respiratory disease, 520-522
Respiratory syncytial virus, 578, 580, 672
Reticulum cell sarcoma
    alkylating agents for, 687
    cytotoxic antibiotics for, 693, 695
    mitotic inhibitors for, 698
Retinitis, 580
Retinoblastoma, 687
Retinopathy, 477, 782
Retrovirus infection, 714
Rhabdomyosarcoma
    cytotoxic antibiotics for, 693, 695
    mitotic inhibitors for, 696, 698
Rheumatoid arthritis
    azathioprine for, 659
    nonsteroidal antiinflammatory drugs for, 640, 644-645, 647
    sulfonamides for, 545
Rhinovirus infection, 509, 714
Rickets, 781, 796
Rickettsia rickettsii infection, 543-544
Rickettsial pox, 557
Ringworm infection, 833
Rocky Mountain spotted fever, 557
Roundworm infection, 621
Rubella, 669

S

Salt-losing adrenogenital syndrome, 494
Sarcoma, 678
    alkylating agents for, 685
    cytotoxic antibiotics for, 693, 695
    mitotic inhibitors for, 696
Scabies, 836
Schistosomiasis, 621
Schizophrenia, 184
Scrub typhus, 557
Scurvy, 793
Seizures, 135-147
    antiepileptic agents for, 136-144
    nursing process in, 144-145

Serratia infection, 559
Shigellosis, 557
Shingles, 579, 580
Shock
    beta-agonists for, 526
    crystalloid solutions for, 407
    vasoactive adrenergics for, 216
Simple phobia, 165
Social phobia, 165
Spirochetal infection, 557, 564
Staphylococcus infection
    penicillins for, 548
    quinolones for, 562
    sulfonamides for, 546
    vancomycin for, 568
Status asthmaticus, 521
Status epilepticus, 138-139, 167
Steroid psychosis, 493
Stomach cancer
    alkylating agents for, 685
    antimetabolites for, 689
    cytotoxic antibiotics for, 693, 695
Streptococcus infection, 543-544
    macrolides for, 564
    penicillins for, 548
Stress ulcer
    histamine$_2$ antagonists for, 735
    sucralfate for, 739
Stroke, 352
Sty, 862
Supraventricular tachyarrhythmia, 282, 286, 287
    beta-blockers for, 233
    digitalis for, 269
    vasoactive adrenergics for, 216
Syndrome of inappropriate antidiuretic hormone, 557
Syphilis
    macrolides for, 564
    tetracyclines for, 557

T

Tachyarrhythmia, 413
    supraventricular, 282, 286, 287
        beta-blockers for, 233
        digitalis for, 269
        vasoactive adrenergics for, 216
Tachycardia
    paroxysmal supraventricular, 216, 282, 286
    ventricular, 282, 286

Taeniasis, 618
Tapeworm infection, 618, 621
T-cell lymphoma, 714
Testicular cancer
    alkylating agents for, 685, 687
    cytotoxic antibiotics for, 693, 695
    mitotic inhibitors for, 696, 698
Tetanus, 167, 669, 670
Thallium poisoning, 413
Thrombosis
    coronary artery, 358
    deep vein, 358, 407
    nonsteroidal antiinflammatory drugs for, 644
Thrush, 598, 603, 833
Thyroid storm, 466
Tinea, 598, 833, 834
Tonic-clonic seizure, 141
Tourette syndrome, 184
Toxic nodular disease, 466
Toxoplasmosis, 546, 547, 611
Transient ischemic attack, 352
Trematode infection, 618
Trichomoniasis, 612
Trigeminal-glossopharyngeal neuralgia, 141
Tuberculosis, 587-596
    antitubercular agents for, 588-593
    bacille Calmette-Guéerin for, 669
    nursing process in, 593-595
Typhus, 557

U

Ulcerative colitis, 545
Unstable angina, 301
Upper respiratory tract infection, 509
Urinary tract infection
    aztreonam for, 567
    quinolones for, 562
    sulfonamides for, 545, 547
Uterine bleeding
    estrogenic agents for, 425
    progestational agents for, 429
    uterine stimulants for, 434
Uveitis, 862

V

Vaginal candidiasis, 603
Vaginitis, 425, 426

Varicella-zoster infection, 578, 672
Vasospastic angina, 301
Ventricular arrhythmia, 233, 282, 285, 286,
Ventricular fibrillation, 271, 282
Ventricular tachycardia, 282, 286
Vertigo, 770
VIPoma, 459
Viral infection
    cytomegalovirus, 578, 580
    Hantavirus, 578
    herpes simplex, 578, 580
    human immunodeficiency virus, 578
    immune globulins for, 672
    interferons for, 714
    Lassa virus, 578
    ocular, 863
    papillomavirus, 714
    respiratory syncytial virus, 578, 580, 672
    retrovirus, 714
    rhinovirus, 509, 714
Vomiting, 764-774
    antiemetic agents for, 765-771
    antipsychotic agents for, 184
    hydroxyzine for, 168
    nursing process in, 772-774
von Willebrand's disease, 459
Vulvar cancer, 693, 695

W

Wernicke's encephalopathy, 787
Wilms' tumor
    cytotoxic antibiotics for, 693, 695
    mitotic inhibitors for, 696, 698
Wolff-Parkinson-White syndrome, 282
Worm infection, 617-622

Y

Yeast infection, 833

Z

Zollinger-Ellison syndrome, 735

Index

A

A fiber, 90-91
Abbokinase; see **urokinase**
Absence seizure, 141
Absorption of drug, 13-16
  geriatric considerations, 29, 30
  neonatal and pediatric considerations, 27
Accommodation, 846
Accupril; see **quinapril**
ACE inhibitors; see Angiotensin-converting enzyme inhibitors
acebutolol, 232, 233, 283
acetaminophen, 347, 645, 650
acetazolamide, 388, 858-859
Acetic acids, 630
  antiinflammatory, 646
  for ear disorders, 880
acetophenetidin, 680
Acetyl coenzyme A reductase, 369
Acetylation, 592
Acetylcholine, 239, 851
  anticholinergics and, 156, 247, 528
  in glaucoma, 850
  nausea and vomiting and, 765, 766
  parasympathetic nervous system and, 848
  parietal cell and, 730
  Parkinson's disease and, 149
acetylsalicylic acid, 352, 353, 645-646
  angiotensin-converting enzyme inhibitors and, 328
  anticoagulants and, 347
  platelets and, 349-350
ACh; see Acetylcholine
achromycin, 865
Acid agents, 630
Acid-related disorders, 729-731
Acne agents, 557, 832-833, 840
Acquired immunodeficiency syndrome, 672
Acromegaly, 459
Acthar; see Corticotropin
Actidil; see **triprolidine**
Actimmune; see Interferon gamma-1b
Actinic keratosis, 837
Action potential, 277-278
Activase; see **alteplase**
Activated charcoal, 283, 733-735, 747
Activated partial thromboplastin time, 362
Active immunization, 664-665
Active immunizing agents, 666-671
Acular; see **ketorolac**
Acute angle-closure glaucoma, 849
Acute diarrhea, 746
Acute lymphoblastic leukemia
  antimetabolites for, 689, 691
  asparaginase for, 701
  cytotoxic antibiotics for, 693, 695
  mitotic inhibitors for, 696, 698
Acute myeloid leukemia, 689, 691
Acute pain, 90
Acute renal failure, 391
Acute therapy, 20-21
Acutrim; see **phenylpropanolamine**
acyclovir, 577, 578, 579-581, 835
Acylaminopenicillins, 552
Adalat; see **nifedipine**
Addison's disease, 491, 494
Adenocard; see **adenosine**
Adenohypophysis, 455
adenosine, 293
  dosage range, 287
  management of overdose, 283
Adenosine diphosphate
  phosphorus and, 798
  platelet adhesion and, 348-349
Adenosine monophosphate, 798
Adenosine triphosphate, 731, 798
Adenosylcobalamin, 791
Adenylate cyclase, 731

Adjuvant agents
  in anesthesia, 107, 108
  in relieving pain, 93
Adrenal agents, 489-499
  adrenal system and, 490-491
  antiadrenals, 495
  corticosteroids, 491-493
  nursing process and, 495-498
Adrenal cortex, 490
Adrenal gland, 490-491
Adrenal medulla, 490
Adrenalin; see Epinephrine
Adrenergic agents, 194-203, 206-223
  amphetamines, 200-201
  analeptics, 197-199
  anorexiants, 199-200, 213-215
  antiglaucoma, 853-855, 874
  bronchodilators, 215-217
  cardiac glycosides and, 268
  cyclic antidepressants and, 172
  decongestant, 510
  hydralazine and, 331
  for hypertension, 322-325
  monoamine oxidase inhibitors and, 174
  nasal decongestants, 217
  nursing process and, 201-203, 219-223
  ophthalmic decongestants, 218
  patient teaching, 336
  sympathetic nervous system and, 207-209
  vasoactive, 216, 218-219
Adrenergic receptors, 208-209, 225
Adrenergic-blocking agents, 224-237
  alpha-blockers, 225-230
  beta-blockers, 230-234
  nursing process and, 234-237
Adrenocortical insufficiency
  adrenal agents for, 494
  pituitary drugs for, 459
Adrenocorticotropic hormone, 456
Adriamycin; see **doxorubicin**
Adsorbents, 747, 748
Adsorbonac; see Hyperosmolar sodium chloride
Adult respiratory distress syndrome, 407
Adverse drug reaction, 22
Aerobic bacillus, 587
AeroBid; see **flunisolide**
Aerosol foam, 831
Aerosol spray, 831
Affective disorders, 164, 169-193
  antidepressant agents for, 170-179
  antimanic agents for, 179-180
  antipsychotic agents for, 180-186
  monoamine oxidase inhibitors for, 173-176
  nursing process in, 186-193
Afferent arteriole, 386
Affinity, drug-receptor interaction and, 19
Aflatoxin, 680
Afrin; see **pseudoephedrine**
Age
  cancer and, 679
  digitalis toxicity and, 271
  host factors and, 545
Agonist, 92
  drug-receptor interaction and, 20
  stimulation of sympathetic nervous system, 225
Agonist-antagonist, 92, 98
Agoral Plain; see Mineral oil
Agoraphobia, 164
Agranulocyte, 529
Air-lock technique, 61
AK-Chlor; see **chloramphenicol**
AK-Dex; see **dexamethasone**
AK-Fluor; see **fluorescein**
Akinesia, 152
Akinetic seizure, 141
Akineton; see **biperiden**
AK-Mycin; see **erythromycin**
AK-Sulf; see **sulfacetamide**
AK-Tracin; see **bacitracin**
AK-Zol; see **acetazolamide**

Alazine; see **hydralazine hydrochloride**
Albumin, 410
  colloids and, 408, 409
  drug distribution and, 16
  geriatric considerations, 30
Albuminar; see Albumin
Albutein; see Albumin
albuterol, 214, 217, 525, 526-527, 536
Alcohol
  anticholinergics and, 157
  antidiarrheals and, 749
  antiemetics and, 769
  antifungal drugs and, 602
  for antisepsis, 630
  barbiturates and, 124
  benzodiazepines and, 166, 167
  chloral hydrate with, 130
  clonidine and, 324
  narcotic analgesics and, 95
  nonsteroidal antiinflammatory drugs and, 644
  pituitary drugs and, 458
  reserpine and, 324
Alcohol cholesterol, 490
Alcoholism, 167
Aldactone; see **spironolactone**
Aldehyde agents, 631-632
aldesleukin, 719
Aldose reductase inhibitors, 484
Aldosterone, 490
  angiotensin-converting enzyme inhibitors and, 327
  loop of Henle and, 386
Aldosterone-inhibiting diuretics, 392-394
Alfenta; see **alfentanil**
alfentanil, 108
Alferon N; see Interferon alfa-n3
Alkaloids
  belladonna, 249-250, 750-751
  ergot, 432
  Rauwolfia, 326, 337
  vinca, 695-696
Alkets; see Magnesium-containing antacids
Alkylamines, 505
Alkylating agents, 683-688
  carmustine, 687, 688
  cisplatin, 687, 688
  cyclophosphamide, 687, 688
  mechlorethamine, 686-688
Alkylation, 684
Allergen, 521
Allergen Ear Drops; see **benzocaine**
Allergic asthma, 521
Allergic rhinitis, 507
allopurinol, 647-648
Aloe, 759
Alophen; see **phenolphthalein**
Alpha Chymar; see **chymotrypsin**
Alpha-adrenergic receptors, 208-209, 225
Alpha-blockers, 225-230
  for hypertension, 323, 326
  patient teaching, 336
5-Alpha-dihydrotestosterone, 446
5-Alpha-reductase, 446
alprazolam, 167, 168
Alredase; see **tolrestat**
Altace; see **ramipril**
alteplase, 357-358
Altered amino acid formulations, 806, 808
AlternaGel; see Aluminum-containing antacids
altretamine, 700
Alum, 671
Aluminum-containing antacids, 733
Alupent; see **metaproterenol**
Alurate; see **aprobarbital**
Alveolus, 520
amantadine, 153, 155
  anticholinergics and, 157
  antidiarrheals and, 749
  antiviral effects, 577, 578, 581
Amebiasis, 611, 613, 616

Amebic dysentery, 559
Amen; *see* **medroxyprogesterone**
Amenorrhea, 429
Americaine; *see* **benzocaine**
American Nurses' Association Code of Ethics, 40
Amicar; *see* **aminocaproic acid**
Amidate; *see* **etomidate**
amikacin, 560, 561
Amikin; *see* **amikacin**
amiloride, 393-394
Amin-Aid, 806, 808
Amino acids, 810
aminocaproic acid, 354-355
aminoglutethimide, 347, 495
Aminoglycosides, 559-562
  assessment of, 570
  interleukins and, 718
  loop diuretics and, 390
  ocular, 862-864
  penicillins and, 549
Aminopenicillins, 548, 551
4-Aminoquinoline derivatives, 608
Aminosalicylates, 591
Aminosyn, 810
amiodarone, 291-292
  cardiac glycosides and, 268
  dosage range, 287
  indications for, 282
  management of overdose, 283
amitriptyline, 173
amlodipine, 311
Ammoniated mercury ointment, 632
ammonium chloride, 514
amoxapine, 173
amphetamine, 200
  as anorexiant, 213
  monoamine oxidase inhibitors and, 174
Amphetamines, 200-201
  carbonic anhydrase inhibitors and, 858
  clonidine and, 324
  stimulant effects of, 195
Amphocin; *see* **amphotericin B**
Amphojel; *see* Aluminum-containing antacids
amphotericin B, 600, 602
  cardiac glycosides and, 268
  patient teaching, 605
  pituitary drugs and, 458
  topical, 834
ampicillin, 550, 551
Ampicillin sodium; *see* **sodium ampicillin**
Ampule, 55-58
Anabolic activity, 446
Anabolic steroids, 446, 450, 680
Anabolism, 810
Analeptics, 195, 197-199
Analgesics
  antiemetics and, 769
  geriatric complications, 31
  narcotic; *see* Narcotic analgesic agents
  nonsteroidal; *see* Nonsteroidal antiinflammatory
    drugs
Anaphylaxis
  immunizing agents and, 668
  vasoactive adrenergics for, 216
Anatomic site of infection, 545
Ancef; *see* **cefazolin sodium**
Androgen inhibitors, 446, 450
Androgenic activity, 446
Androgens, 446, 450
Android; *see* **methyltestosterone**
Anemia, 718, 819-820, 821
Anesthetics, 106-119
  adrenergics and, 212
  clonidine and, 324
  ganglionic blockers and, 257
  general, 107-111
  laxatives and, 756
  local, 111-114
  miotics and, 851
  mydriatic drugs and, 854
  nursing process and, 115-119

Anesthetics—cont'd
  ocular topical, 869-870, 874
  stages of anesthesia, 109, 115
  topical, 835-836
Angina, 231, 300-318
  beta-blockers for, 233, 305-308
  calcium channel blockers for, 308-311
  coronary artery disease and, 301-302
  nitrates and nitrites for, 302-305
  nursing process in, 312-317
Angiotensin II, 327
Angiotensin-converting enzyme inhibitors, 326-329
  patient teaching, 337
  potassium-sparing diuretics and, 393
Angle-closure glaucoma, 849
Anhydron; *see* **cyclothiazide**
anhydrous ampicillin, 551
Aniline dye, 680
anisindione, 347-348
anistreplase, 358-359
Anisylated plasminogen streptokinase activator
    complex, 356
Ankylosing spondylitis, 641
Anorexiants, 195, 199-200, 211, 213-215
Antacids, 728-744
  acid-related pathophysiology, 729-731
  aluminum-containing, 733
  angiotensin-converting enzyme inhibitors and,
    328
  anticholinergics and, 157
  antidiarrheals and, 749
  antifungal drugs and, 602
  antipsychotic agents and, 182
  antitubercular drugs and, 591
  beta-blockers and, 232
  calcium-containing, 733
  cardiac glycosides and, 268
  didanosine and, 579
  histamine₂ antagonists, 735-737
  iron preparations and, 822
  laxatives and, 756
  magnesium-containing, 733-735
  misoprostol, 740
  nursing process and, 740-743
  proton pump inhibitors, 737-738
  sucralfate, 738-739
Antagonist, 92
  competitive, 247
  drug-receptor interaction and, 20
  inhibition of sympathetic nervous system, 225
Anterior pituitary, 455
Anthracycline cytotoxic antibiotics, 694
Anthraquinones, 759
Antiadrenals, 495
Antiallergics, ocular, 875
Antianginal agents
  beta-blockers, 305-308
  calcium channel blockers, 308-311
  coronary artery disease and, 301-302
  nitrates and nitrites, 302-305
  nursing process and, 312-317
Antianxiety agents, 164-169
Antibacterials; *see* Antibiotics; Antiinfective
    therapy
Antibiotics, 542-574
  aminoglycosides, 559-562
  anticoagulants and, 347
  aztreonam, 567
  cephalosporins, 552-556
  cytotoxic, 692-695
  for ear disorders, 880
  general principles of therapy, 544-545
  imipenem-cilastatin, 568
  infection and, 543-544
  laxatives and, 756
  macrolides, 564-566
  nursing process and, 569-574
  penicillins, 547-552
  quinolones, 562-564
  sulfonamides, 545-547
  tetracyclines, 556-559

Antibiotics—cont'd
  topical, 627-630, 840
  vancomycin, 568-569
Antibody, 521, 659, 666, 712
Anticholinergics, 246-254
  amantadine and, 579
  as anesthetic adjuvants, 108
  antifungal drugs and, 602
  for asthma, 528
  atropine, 250-251
  beta-blockers and, 232, 307
  cardiac glycosides and, 268
  cholinergic agents and, 242
  cyclic antidepressants and, 172
  decongestant, 510
  for diarrhea, 747, 748, 749-750
  dicyclomine, 251
  geriatric complications, 31
  glycopyrrolate, 251
  for nausea and vomiting, 766, 769
  nursing process and, 251-253
  in Parkinson's disease, 156-158, 159
  scopolamine, 251
Anticholinesterase, 250
Anticoagulants, 343-348
  antidiarrheals and, 749
  antidysrhythmic drugs and, 284
  antifungal drugs and, 602
  antitubercular drugs and, 591
  aspirin and, 352
  barbiturates and, 124
  geriatric complications, 31
  laxatives and, 756
  nonsteroidal antiinflammatory drugs and,
    644
  nursing process and, 359-362
Anticonvulsants, 136-144
  benzodiazepines, 142
  carbamazepine, 142-143
  ethosuximide, 143
  mechanism of action, 137-138
  phenobarbital, 143
  phenytoin, 143-144
  therapeutic uses, 138-139
  valproic acid, 144
Antidepressants, 170-179
  adrenergics and, 212
  antiemetics and, 769
  patient teaching, 190
  second-generation, 176-179
  tricyclic, 170-173
    adrenergics and, 212, 324
    anticholinergics and, 157, 249
    antidiarrheals and, 749
    antiemetics and, 769
    central nervous system stimulants and, 197
    fertility agents and, 438
    monoamine oxidase inhibitors and, 174
    mydriatics and, 854
    physostigmine reversal of, 242
Antidiabetic agents, 475-488
  aspirin and, 352
  glucose-elevating drugs, 484-485
  insulin-dependent diabetes mellitus, 477-478
  insulins, 478-481
  investigational, 484
  non–insulin dependent diabetes mellitus, 478
  nursing process and, 485-487
  oral, 481-484
  pancreas and, 476
Antidiarrheals, 746-752
  adsorbent, 749
  anticholinergic, 749-750
  belladonna-alkaloid combinations, 750-751
  cardiac glycosides and, 268
  intestinal flora modifiers, 751-752
  nursing process and, 760-762
  opiate, 751
Antidiuretic hormone, 456
  collecting duct and, 386
  pituitary agents and, 455

Antidysrhythmic agents, 276-299
  cardiac electrophysiology and, 277-280
  class Ia drugs, 283-287
  class Ib drugs, 287-288
  class Ic drugs, 288-289
  class II drugs, 289-291
  class III drugs, 291-292
  class IV drugs, 282-293
  dosage ranges, 285-287
  indications for, 282
  nursing process and, 293-299
  Vaughan Williams classification of, 280-281
Antiemetic agents, 764-774
  anticholinergic, 769
  neuroleptic, 769-771
  nursing process and, 772-774
  prokinetic, 771
  serotonin blockers, 771
Antiepileptic drugs, 136-144
  benzodiazepines, 142
  carbamazepine, 142-143
  ethosuximide, 143
  mechanism of action, 137-138
  phenobarbital, 143
  phenytoin, 143-144
  therapeutic uses, 138-139
  valproic acid, 144
Antifibrinolytics, 353-355, 364
Antiflatulents, 728-744
  acid-related pathophysiology, 729-731
  aluminum-containing, 733
  calcium-containing, 733
  histamine₂ antagonists, 735-737
  magnesium-containing, 733-735
  misoprostol, 740
  nursing process and, 740-743
  proton pump inhibitors, 737-738
  sucralfate, 738-739
Antifungal agents, 597-606
  ocular, 874
  otic, 879-880
  for skin disorders, 833-834, 840
Antigen, 664, 712
  in asthma, 521
  tumor, 711
Antiglaucoma drugs, 847-861
  beta-blockers, 855-857
  carbonic anhydrase inhibitors, 857-859
  nursing implications, 874
  osmotic diuretics, 859-861
  parasympathomimetics, 848-853
  sympathomimetics, 853-855
Antigout agents, 647, 649
Antihelmintics, 622-623
Antihistamines, 503-509
  adrenergics and, 212
  anticholinergics and, 157, 249
  antidiarrheals and, 749
  antiemetics and, 769
  as anxiolytics, 165
  barbiturates and, 124
  cholinergic agents and, 242
  efficacy and side effects of, 504
  narcotic drug interaction, 95
  for nausea and vomiting, 766, 769
  nonsedating, 506-508
  nursing process and, 515-517
Antihypertensive agents, 319-340
  adrenergic, 212, 322-326
  angiotensin-converting enzyme inhibitors, 326-329
  antipsychotic agents and, 182
  beta-blockers and, 307
  calcium channel blockers, 330
  diuretics, 330
  fertility agents and, 438
  ganglionic blockers, 257
  general anesthetics and, 110
  geriatric complications, 31
  interleukins and, 718

Antihypertensive agents—cont'd
  nursing process and, 332-340
  vasodilators, 330
Antiinfective therapy
  antibiotics, 542-574
    aminoglycosides, 559-562
    anticoagulants and, 347
    aztreonam, 567
    cephalosporins, 552-556
    cytotoxic, 692-695
    for ear disorders, 880
    general principles of therapy, 544-545
    imipenem-cilastatin, 568
    laxatives and, 756
    macrolides, 564-566
    nursing process and, 569-574
    penicillins, 547-552
    quinolones, 562-564
    sulfonamides, 545-547
    tetracyclines, 556-559
    topical, 840
    vancomycin, 568-569
  antifungal agents, 597-606
    ocular, 874
    otic, 879-880
    for skin disorders, 833-834, 840
  antihelmintics, 622-623
  antimalarial, 608-612, 622-623
  antiprotozoal, 613-617, 622-623
  antiseptics and disinfectants, 626-636
    acid agents, 630
    alcohol agents, 630
    aldehyde agents, 631-632
    biguanide agents, 632
    chlorine compounds, 632
    dyes, 632
    iodine compounds, 632-633
    mercurial agents, 632
    nursing process and, 634-636
    ocular, 874
    oxidizing agents, 633
    phenolic compounds, 633
    surface-active agents, 634
    topical antimicrobials, 627-630
  antitubercular agents, 587-596
    ethambutol, 591-592
    isoniazid, 592
    Mycobacterium tuberculosis and, 587-588
    nursing process and, 593-595
    pyrazinamide, 592-593
    rifampin, 593
    streptomycin, 593
  antiviral agents, 575-586
    acyclovir, 579-581
    amantadine, 581
    ganciclovir, 581
    nursing process and, 582-584
    ocular, 866, 874
    ribavirin, 581-582
    topical, 835, 840
    trifluridine, 582
    zidovudine, 582
  ocular, 861-866, 874
  otic, 879-880
  for skin disorders, 832
  topical, 627-630, 831-835, 840
Antiinflammatory agents
  nonsteroidal, 637-653
    acetaminophen, 650
    acetic acids, 646
    angiotensin-converting enzyme inhibitors and, 328
    anticoagulants and, 347
    antigout agents, 647-649
    arachidonic acid pathway and, 638-639
    aspirin, 352, 645-646
    carboxylic acids, 643-645
    enolic acids, fenamic acids, and nonacidic compounds, 647
    geriatric complications, 31

Antiinflammatory agents—cont'd
  gold compounds, 649-650
  as narcotic analgesic adjuvants, 93
  nursing process and, 650-652
  opthalmic, 866-871, 895
  penicillins and, 549
  propionic acids, 646-647
  ocular, 866-869, 874
  topical, 835-836, 840
Antilipemic agents, 367-381
  bile acid sequestrants, 371-372
  fibric acid derivatives, 374-376
  HMG-CoA reductase inhibitors, 373-374
  lipids and lipid abnormalities, 368-371
  nicotinic acid, 376-378
  nursing process and, 379-380
  probucol, 378-379
Antilirium; *see* **physostigmine**
Antimalarial drugs, 608-612, 622-623
Antimanic agents, 179-180
Antimetabolites, 599, 688-692
  cytarabine, 692
  mercaptopurine, 691-692
  methotrexate, 690-691
Antimicrobials; *see* Antiinfective therapy
Antiminth; *see* **pyrantel**
Antimuscarinic agents, 246-254
  as anesthetic adjuvants, 108
  atropine, 250-251
  beta-blockers and, 232
  cholinergic agents and, 242
  cyclic antidepressants and, 172
  dicyclomine, 251
  geriatric complications, 31
  glycopyrrolate, 251
  for nausea and vomiting, 766, 769
  nursing process and, 251-253
  in Parkinson's disease, 156-158, 159
  scopolamine, 251
Antinausea agents, 764-774
  anticholinergic, 769
  neuroleptic, 769-771
  nursing process and, 772-774
  prokinetic, 771
  serotonin blockers, 771
Antineoplastic agents, 676-709
  alkylating agents, 683-688
    carmustine, 687, 688
    cisplatin, 687, 688
    cyclophosphamide, 687, 688
    mechlorethamine, 686-688
  altretamine, 700
  antimetabolites, 688-692
    cytarabine, 692
    mercaptopurine, 691-692
    methotrexate, 690-691
  asparaginase, 699, 700-701
  cancer etiology and, 679-681
  cell growth cycle and, 681-683
  cytotoxic antibiotics, 692-695
    bleomycin, 694-695
    doxorubicin, 694, 695
  hydroxyurea, 701
  mitotic inhibitors, 695-698
    etoposide, 697-698
    paclitaxel, 698
    vincristine, 698
  topical, 837
Antiparasitics, 840
Antiparkinsonian agents, 148-161
  amantadine, 155
  anticholinergics, 156-158
  benztropine mesylate, 158
  bromocriptine and pergolide, 155-156
  levodopa, 153-155
  levodopa-carbidopa, 155
  nursing process and, 158-161
  selegiline, 150-152
  trihexyphenidyl, 158
Antiplatelet agents, 348-353, 362-364

Antiprotozoal agents, 613-617, 622-623
Antipruritic agents, 835-836
Antipsychotic agents, 180-186
  adrenergics and, 212
  antidiarrheals and, 749
  barbiturates and, 124
  laxatives and, 756
Antiseptics, 626-636
  acid agents, 630
  alcohol agents, 630
  aldehyde agents, 631-632
  biguanide agents, 632
  chlorine compounds, 632
  in community-acquired and nosocomial
    infections, 627
  dyes, 632
  iodine compounds, 632-633
  mercurial agents, 632
  nursing process and, 634-636
  ocular, 874
  oxidizing agents, 633
  phenolic compounds, 633
  surface-active agents, 634
  topical antimicrobials, 627-630
Antithrombin III, 343
Antithyroid agents, 469-471, 472
Antitubercular agents, 587-596
  ethambutol, 591-592
  isoniazid, 592
  Mycobacterium tuberculosis and, 587-588
  nursing process and, 593-595
  pyrazinamide, 592-593
  rifampin, 593
  streptomycin, 593
Antitussives, 511-514
Antivenin, 667
Antivert; *see* **meclizine**
Antiviral agents, 575-586
  acyclovir, 579-581
  amantadine, 581
  ganciclovir, 581
  nursing process and, 582-584
  ocular, 866, 874
  ribavirin, 581-582
  topical, 835, 840
  trifluridine, 582
  zidovudine, 582
Anturane; *see* **sulfinpyrazone**
Anxiety, 164, 184
Anxiolytics, 120, 126, 190
A.P.L.; *see* Chorionic gonadotropin
Apocrine gland, 830
Apolipoproteins, 368
Apoproteins, 368
Apothecary system, 46
Appetite suppressants, 324
apraclonidine, 855
Apresoline; *see* **hydralazine hydrochloride**
aprobarbital, 125, 126, 131
aprotinin, 354
APSAC; *see* **anistreplase**
Aqua-MEPHYTON; *see* Vitamin K
Aquasol A; *see* Vitamin A
Aquasol E; *see* Vitamin E
Aquatensen; *see* **methyclothiazide**
Aqueous humor, 846
Ara-C; *see* **cytarabine**
Arachidonic acid pathway, 638-639
Aralen; *see* **chloroquine**
Arfonad; *see* **trimethaphan**
Arm-a-med; *see* **isoetharine**
Armour Thyroid, 468
Arrhythmia, 231, 277
  beta-blockers for, 233
  cardiac glycosides for, 265-266
  digitalis toxicity and, 271
  vasoactive adrenergics for, 216
Artane; *see* **trihexyphenidyl**
Arterial thrombosis, 358
Arthritis
  azathioprine for, 659

Arthritis—cont'd
  nonsteroidal antiinflammatory drugs for, 640,
    644-645, 647
  sulfonamides for, 545
Artificial tears, 870, 874
Artificially acquired passive immunity, 666
ASA; *see* **acetylsalicylic acid**
Asbestos, 680
Ascariasis, 618
Ascites, 390
Ascorbic acid, 793-794, 822
Asendin; *see* **amoxapine**
asparaginase, 699, 700-701, 718
aspirin, 352, 353, 645-646
  angiotensin-converting enzyme inhibitors and,
    328
  anticoagulants and, 347
  platelets and, 349-350
Assessment in nursing process, 9
astemizole, 504, 505, 507
  antifungal drugs and, 602
  macrolides and, 565
Asthma, 521, 527
  beta-agonists for, 524-528
  bronchodilators for, 522-524
  corticosteroids for, 528-531
  cromolyn and nedocromil for, 532
  immune globulins for, 672
  nursing process in, 533-537
Asthma attack, 521
Atarax; *see* **hydroxyzine**
atenolol, 232-234, 290
  for angina, 307
  dosage range, 286
  indications for, 282
Atherosclerosis, 370
Athlete's foot, 833
Ativan; *see* **lorazepam**
atovaquone, 613-616
Atrial action potential, 280
Atrial dysrhythmia, 285
Atrial fibrillation, 282, 285, 286
Atrial flutter, 286
Atrioventricular block, 271
Atrioventricular node, 278-280
  adrenergic receptor responses to stimulation, 207
  congestive heart failure and, 265
Atromid-S; *see* **clofibrate**
Atropa belladonna, 249
Atropic vaginitis, 425, 426
atropine, 250-251
  as anesthetic adjuvant, 108
  for antidysrhythmic drug reversal, 283
  for diarrhea, 749-750
  diphenoxylate with, 751
  ophthalmic, 870
A/T/S; *see* **erythromycin**
attapulgite, 749, 750
Attention deficit disorder, 195, 198, 200-201, 213
Attenuvax; *see* Measles vaccine
Auralgan Otic; *see* **benzocaine**
auranofin, 649
Auro Ear Drops; *see* **carbamide peroxide**
Auromid; *see* **benzocaine**
aurothioglucose, 649-650
Autoimmune disorders, 656
  immune globulins for, 672
  interferon for, 714
Autoinduction, 135
Automaticity, 265, 279
Autonomic nervous system, 225
  adrenergic agents, 194-203, 206-223
    amphetamines, 200-201
    analeptics, 197-199
    anorexiants, 199-200, 213-215
    antiglaucoma, 853-855, 874
    bronchodilators, 215-217
    cyclic antidepressants and, 172
    hydralazine and, 331
    for hypertension, 322-325
    monoamine oxidase inhibitors and, 174

Autonomic nervous system—cont'd
    nasal decongestants, 217
    nursing process and, 201-203, 219-223
    ophthalmic decongestants, 218
    patient teaching, 336
    sympathetic nervous system and, 207-209
    vasoactive, 216, 218-219
  adrenergic receptors and, 208-209, 225
  adrenergic-blocking agents, 224-237
    alpha-blockers, 225-230
    beta-blockers, 230-234
    nursing process and, 234-237
  cholinergic agents, 238-246
    nursing process and, 243-245
    parasympathetic nervous system and, 239-240
  cholinergic-blocking agents, 246-254
    as anesthetic adjuvants, 108
    atropine, 250-251
    beta-blockers and, 232, 307
    cholinergic agents and, 242
    cyclic antidepressants and, 172
    dicyclomine, 251
    geriatric complications, 31
    glycopyrrolate, 251
    for nausea and vomiting, 766, 769
    nursing process and, 251-253
    in Parkinson's disease, 156-158, 159
    scopolamine, 251
  ganglionic-blocking agents, 255-261
    mecamylamine, 258
    nicotinic receptor and, 256
    nursing process and, 259-261
    sodium nitroprusside and, 331
    trimethaphan, 258
Autonomy, 40
Aventyl; *see* **nortriptyline**
Avoirdupois system, 46
Axid; *see* **nizatidine**
Aygestin; *see* **norethindrone**
Azactam; *see* **aztreonam**
azatadine, 505, 508-509
azathioprine, 658
azithromycin, 566
Azmacort; *see* **triamcinolone**
Azo-Gantanol; *see* **sulfamethoxazole**
Azogantrisin; *see* **sulfisoxazole**
AZT; *see* **zidovudine**
aztreonam, 567

B

B cell, 712
Bachmann's bundle, 279
Baciguent; *see* **bacitracin**
Bacille Calmette-Guérin, 668, 669
bacitracin, 832, 864
Bactericidal antibiotics, 559
Bacteriostatic antibiotics, 545, 556
Bactrim; *see* **sulfamethoxazole**
Balanced anesthesia, 93, 107, 127
Balantidiasis, 557
Bancroft's filariasis, 621
Barbiturates
  anticoagulants and, 347
  antiemetics and, 769
  cardiac glycosides and, 268
  for epilepsy, 139, 140
  laxatives and, 756
  mitotane and, 700
  narcotic analgesics and, 95
  phenobarbital, 124-126
  reserpine and, 324
  as sedative-hypnotic agents, 121-124
Basaljel; *see* Aluminum-containing antacids
Basophil, 529
BCNU; *see* **carmustine**
beclomethasone dipropionate, 510, 530-531
Beclovent; *see* **beclomethasone dipropionate**
Beconase; *see* **beclomethasone dipropionate**
Beef tapeworm, 618

Beepen-VK; *see* **penicillin V potassium**
Beesix; *see* Pyridoxine
Belladonna alkaloids, 249-250, 750-751
Benadryl; *see* **diphenhydramine**
benazepril, 327
bendroflumethiazide, 396
Beneficence, 40
Benemid; *see* **probenecid**
Benign prostatic hyperplasia, 446, 449
Benign tumor, 678
Bentyl; *see* **scopolamine**
benzalkonium, 631, 634, 880
Benzedrex inhaler; *see* **propylhexedrine**
Benzene, 680
benzethonium chloride, 880
benzocaine, 112, 881
Benzodiazepines
    as anesthetic adjuvants, 108
    for anxiety, 168-169
    barbiturates and, 124
    for epilepsy, 142
    narcotic analgesics and, 95
    as sedative-hypnotic agents, 126-130
Benzoic acid, 630
benzonatate, 513
Benzothiazepines, 311
benzoyl peroxide, 832
benzphetamine, 199, 213
benzthiazide, 396
benztropine, 157, 158
Benzyl peroxides, 633
bepridil, 311
Beriberi, 787
Beta-2; *see* **isoetharine**
Beta-adrenergic receptors, 208-209, 225
Beta-agonists, 524-528
Beta-blockers, 230-234, 280-291
    adrenergics and, 212
    alpha-blockers and, 228
    for angina, 305-308
    antiglaucoma, 855-857, 874
    antimalarial agents and, 612
    calcium channel blockers and, 310
    central nervous system stimulants and, 197
    general anesthetics and, 110
    indications for, 282
    patient teaching, 316
    reserpine and, 324
    uterine relaxants and, 435
Beta-carotene, 779
Betadine; *see* **povidone-iodine**
Beta-lactam penicillins, 547-548
Beta-lactam ring, 548
Betalin S; *see* Thiamine
Betalin-12; *see* Cyanocobalamin
betamethasone, 492, 835
Betapace; *see* **sotalol**
Betaseron; *see* Interferon beta-1B
betaxolol, 234, 856-857
bethanechol, 242, 243
Betopic; *see* **betaxolol**
Biamine; *see* Thiamine
Biaxin; *see* **clarithromycin**
Bicarbonate, 732
    carbonic anhydrase inhibitors and, 387
    sucralfate and, 739
BiCNU; *see* **carmustine**
Biguanide agents, 632
Bile acid sequestrants, 371-373
Bile acid-binding resins, 371
Bile duct tumor, 689
Biliary excretion, 18
Biliary obstruction, 371
Biltricide; *see* **praziquantel**
Biogenic amine hypothesis, 170
Biologic response modifiers, 710-724
    colony-stimulating factors, 718, 719-722
    immune system and, 711-712
    interferons, 712-716
    interleukins, 717-719
    nursing process and, 722-723

Biologicals, 664
Biotransformation, 16-17
biperiden, 158
Biphasic oral contraceptives, 431
Bipolar affective disorder, 164
bisacodyl, 759
bisacodyl tannex, 759
bismuth subsalicylate, 747, 749, 750
Bisodol powder; *see* Magnesium-containing
    antacids
bisoprolol, 234
bitolterol, 214, 525
Bladder cancer
    alkylating agents for, 685, 687
    antimetabolites for, 689
    interferon for, 714
Blastomycosis, 598
Bleach, 632
Bleeding
    anticoagulation therapy and, 346
    blood products for, 412
    dehydration and fluid loss in, 406
    thrombolytics and, 357
Blenoxane; *see* **bleomycin**
bleomycin, 693, 694-695
Bleph; *see* **sulfacetamide**
Blind placebo-controlled study, 38
Blood
    androgens and, 447
    anticoagulants and, 346
    antidiarrheals and, 748
    antifungals and, 601
    antiplatelet drugs and, 351
    antiprotozoal agents and, 614
    antipsychotic agents and, 182
    antithyroid drugs and, 470
    barbiturates and, 123
    beta-blockers and, 231
    dopaminergic agents and, 154
    histamine₂ blockers and, 736
    immunosuppressants and, 658
    interferons and, 714
    loop diuretics and, 389
    nonsteroidal antiinflammatory drugs and, 641
    omeprazole and, 737
    penicillins and, 549
    sulfonamides and, 546
    thiazide diuretics and, 395
    tumor origin in, 678
    whole, 410, 411, 412
Blood cholesterol, 370
Blood pressure, 338
    cholinergic agents and, 241
    classification of, 321
    normal regulation of, 322
Blood products, 410-412
Blood vessels
    adrenergic receptor responses to stimulation, 207
    antihistamines and, 506
    cholinergic agents and, 241
    fluid in, 405
    nitrates and, 303
    tumor origin in, 678
Blood-brain barrier, 230-231
Blood-forming agents, 818-827
    in anemia, 819-820, 821
    folic acid, 823-824
    hematopoiesis and, 819
    iron, 820-822
Body louse, 836
Body surface area, 27
Bolus intravenous administration, 67-69
Bonamine; *see* **meclizine**
Bone marrow suppression, 682-683
    alkylating agents and, 685
    antimetabolites and, 690
    cytotoxic antibiotics and, 693
    hydroxyurea and, 699
    mitotic inhibitors and, 696
Bonine; *see* **meclizine**
Booster shot, 664

Boric acid, 630
Bowel movement, 752
Bowel obstruction, 406
BPH; *see* Benign prostatic hyperplasia
Brachial nerve block, 114
Bradycardia, 250
Bradykinesia, 150
Bradykinin, 327
Brain
    anticholinergics and, 248
    antiepileptic drugs and, 138
    pain and, 90-91
    Parkinson's disease and, 149
Brain tumor
    alkylating agents for, 685, 687
    antimetabolites for, 689
Braxton Hicks contractions, 432
Breast cancer
    alkylating agents for, 685, 687
    androgens for, 449
    antimetabolites for, 689
    cytotoxic antibiotics for, 693, 695
    estrogenic agents for, 425, 426
    interleukin-2 for, 717
    mitotic inhibitors for, 696
    nursing care plan for, 708
    progestational agents for, 429
Brethaire; *see* **terbutaline**
Brethine; *see* **terbutaline**
bretylium, 286, 291
bretyllium, 282, 283
Bretylol; *see* **bretylium**
Brevibloc; *see* **esmolol**
Brevicon, 431
Brevital; *see* **methohexital**
Bricanyl; *see* **terbutaline**
Brilliant green, 632
bromocriptine, 153, 155-156
brompheniramine, 504, 505, 509
Bronchial asthma, 521
Bronchial muscles, 207
Bronchitis, 526
Bronchodilators, 215-217, 522-539
    anticholinergic, 528
    for asthma, 521
    beta-agonist, 524-528
    for chronic bronchitis, 522
    corticosteroid, 528-531
    cromolyn, 532
    dosage ranges, 214
    for emphysema, 522
    indirect-acting antiasthmatic agents, 531-532
    nedocromil, 532
    nursing process and, 533-537
    respiratory system and, 520
    sympathomimetic, 524-528
    xanthine derivatives, 522-524
Bronitin; *see* **epinephrine**
Bronkaid; *see* Epinephrine
Bronkephrine; *see* **ethylnorepinephrine**
Bronkodyl; *see* **theophylline**
Bronkometer; *see* **isoetharine**
Brucellosis, 557
buclizine, 509
Bulk-forming laxatives, 753, 755-756
bumetanide, 347, 388, 390, 391
Bumex; *see* **bumetanide**
Buminate; *see* Albumin
Bundle of His, 280
bupivacaine, 113
buprenorphine, 98, 100
bupropion, 178-179
Burn, 407
Burn products, 840
busulfan, 685
butabarbital, 125, 126, 131
Butalan; *see* **butabarbital**
butamben, 112
Butazolidin; *see* **phenylbutazone**
Butesin; *see* **butamben**
Buticaps; *see* **butabarbital**

Butisol; *see* **butabarbital**
butoconazole, 834
butorphanol, 98, 100
Butyrophenones, 184-185, 438

C

C fiber, 90-91
caffeine, 197-199, 283, 522
CAIs; *see* Carbonic anhydrase inhibitors
Calan; *see* **verapamil**
Calcifediol, 783
Calcijex; *see* Calcitriol
Calcitriol, 783-784
Calcium, 778, 794-797
calcium carbonate, 732
Calcium channel blockers, 292-293
    alpha-blockers and, 228
    for angina, 308-311
    antimalarial agents and, 612
    for hypertension, 330
    indications for, 282
    patient teaching, 316, 337
Calcium salts, 796, 797
    in antacids, 732
    for constipation, 758
Calcium-containing antacids, 733
Calderol; *see* Calcifediol
Canadian Food and Drugs Act, 38-39
Canadian Narcotic Control Act, 39
Canadian Nurses Association Code of Ethics, 41
Canal of Schlemm, 846
Cancer, 676-709
    alkylating agents for, 683-688
    altretamine for, 699, 700
    antimetabolites for, 688-692
    asparaginase for, 699, 700-701
    biologic response modifiers for, 710-724
        colony-stimulating factors, 718, 719-722
        immune system and, 711-712
        interferons, 712-716
        interleukins, 717-719
        nursing process and, 722-723
    cell growth cycle and, 681-683
    cytotoxic antibiotics for, 692-695
    etiology of, 679-681
    hydroxyurea for, 701
    mitotic inhibitors for, 695-698
    nursing care plan for, 708
    nursing process in, 701-707
Candida albicans, 598
Candidiasis, 598, 603, 627, 833, 834
Capillary leak syndrome, 717
Capoten; *see* **captopril**
capreomycin
    as antitubercular agent, 589, 590
    loop diuretics and, 390
captopril, 327, 329
Carafate; *see* **sucralfate**
carbachol, 850
Carbamates, 165
carbamazepine
    anticoagulants and, 347
    for epilepsy, 139-143
    macrolides and, 565
    pituitary drugs and, 458
    second-generation antidepressants and, 178
carbamide peroxide, 881
carbenicillin, 552
carbidopa, 153, 155
Carbocaine; *see* **mepivacaine**
Carbohydrates
    in modular formulations, 806, 808
    in nutritional support, 810-811
carbolic acid, 631
Carbonic anhydrase inhibitors, 387-388
    miotics and, 851
    ophthalmic, 857-859, 874
carboplatin, 685

Carboxylic acids, 643-645
Carboxypenicillins, 552
Carcinogen, 23, 680
Carcinoid tumor, 459
Carcinoma, 678
Cardene; *see* **nicardipine**
Cardiac Arrhythmia Suppression Trial, 288-289
Cardiac gland, 729-731
Cardiac glycosides, 264-275
    in congestive heart failure and arrhythmias, 265-266
    digoxin, 269
    digoxin immune Fab, 269-270
    geriatric complications, 31
    mydriatics and, 854
    nursing process and, 270-275
Cardiac output, 321
Cardiac pacemaker, 271
Cardioprotective beta-blockers, 231
Cardioquin; *see* **quinidine**
Cardioselective beta-blockers, 230
Cardioselective sympathomimetics, 211
Cardiovascular system
    adrenergic receptor responses to stimulation, 207
    antianginal agents
        beta-blockers, 305-308
        calcium channel blockers, 308-311
        coronary artery disease and, 301-302
        nitrates and nitrites, 302-305
        nursing process and, 312-317
    antidysrhythmic agents, 276-299
        cardiac electrophysiology and, 277-280
        class Ia drugs, 283-287
        class Ib drugs, 287-288
        class Ic drugs, 288-289
        class II drugs, 289-291
        class III drugs, 291-292
        class IV drugs, 282-293
        dosage ranges, 285-287
        indications for, 282
        nursing process and, 293-299
        Vaughan Williams classification, 280-281
    antihypertensive agents, 319-340
        adrenergic, 212, 322-326
        angiotensin-converting enzyme inhibitors, 326-329
        antipsychotic agents and, 182
        beta-blockers and, 307
        calcium channel blockers, 330
        diuretics, 330
        fertility agents and, 438
        ganglionic blockers as, 257
        general anesthetics and, 110
        geriatric complications, 31
        hypertension and, 320-321
        interleukins and, 718
        nursing process and, 332-340
        vasodilators, 330
    antilipemic agents, 367-381
        bile acid sequestrants, 371-372
        fibric acid derivatives, 374-376
        HMG-CoA reductase inhibitors, 373-374
        lipids and lipid abnormalities, 368-371
        nicotinic acid, 376-378
        nursing process and, 379-380
        probucol, 378-379
    cardiac glycosides, 264-275
        in congestive heart failure and arrhythmias, 265-266
        digoxin, 269
        digoxin immune Fab, 269-270
        geriatric complications, 31
        mydriatics and, 854
        nursing process and, 270-275
    chronic salicylate intoxication and, 642
    coagulation modifier agents, 341-366
        anticoagulants, 343-348
        antifibrinolytics, 353-355
        antiplatelet agents, 348-353
        hemostasis and, 343, 344, 345

Cardiovascular system—cont'd
        nursing process and, 359-365
        thrombolytics, 356-359
    interactions and adverse effects
        alpha-blockers and, 227
        anticholinergics and, 248, 249
        antidiarrheals and, 748
        antiemetic agents and, 768
        antifibrinolytics and, 354
        antifungals and, 601
        antihistamines and, 506
        antiplatelet drugs and, 351
        antiprotozoal agents and, 614
        antipsychotic agents and, 182
        antiseptic and disinfectant agents and, 630
        barbiturates and, 123
        beta-blockers and, 231, 307
        calcium channel blockers and, 309
        calcium salts and, 796
        cardiac glycosides and, 267
        central nervous system stimulants and, 197
        cholinergic agents and, 241
        colony-stimulating factors and, 720
        corticosteroids and, 493
        cyanocobalamin and, 792
        cyclic antidepressants and, 171
        desmopressin, lypressin, and vasopressin and, 457
        dopaminergic agents and, 154
        estrogens and, 425
        fertility agents and, 437
        ganglionic blockers and, 257
        immunosuppressants and, 658
        insulin and, 479
        interferons and, 714
        macrolides and, 565
        miotics and, 850
        monoamine oxidase inhibitors and, 174
        narcotic analgesic agents and, 93
        niacin and, 789
        nonsteroidal antiinflammatory drugs and, 641
        oral contraceptives and, 430
        osmotic diuretics and, 860
        oxytocic agents and, 433
        selegilene and, 151
        thyroid drugs and, 467
        tocolytic agents and, 435
        vitamin D and, 783
Cardioversion, 167
Cardizem; *see* **diltiazem**
Cardura; *see* **doxazosin**
carmustine, 685, 687, 688, 705
Carotene, 779
Carpuject syringe, 53
casanthrol, 759
Cascara sagrada, 759
Casec, 806
Catabolism, 810
Catapres; *see* **clonidine**
Cataract, 846
Catarese; *see* **chymotrypsin**
Catecholamines, 207, 209-210, 256-257
Catechol-*O*-methyltransferase, 209
Cathartics, 760
Caudal obstetrical analgesia, 114
Caudal surgical anesthesia, 114
CD4 cell, 657
cefazolin sodium, 553
cefixime, 554, 555-556
cefoxitin, 554, 555
ceftazidime, 554, 556
Ceftin; *see* **cefuroxime**
ceftriaxone, 554, 556
cefuroxime, 554, 555
Cell, fluid in, 405
Cell cycle-nonspecific agent, 681
Cell cycle-specific agent, 681
Cell growth cycle, 681-683
Cell-mediated immune system, 666
Cellular immunity, 711

Central nervous system
  anesthetics, 106-119
    adrenergics and, 212
    clonidine and, 324
    general, 107-111
    local, 111-114
    miotics and, 851
    mydriatic drugs and, 854
    nursing process and, 115-119
    ocular topical, 869-870, 874
    stages of anesthesia, 109, 115
    topical, 835-836
  antiepileptic drugs, 136-144
    benzodiazepines, 142
    carbamazepine, 142-143
    ethosuximide, 143
    mechanism of action, 137-138
    phenobarbital, 143
    phenytoin, 143-144
    therapeutic uses, 138-139
    valproic acid, 144
  antiparkinsonian agents, 148-161
    amantadine, 155
    anticholinergics, 156-158
    benztropine mesylate, 158
    bromocriptine and pergolide, 155-156
    levodopa, 153-155
    levodopa-carbidopa, 155
    nursing process and, 158-161
    selegiline, 150-152
    trihexyphenidyl, 158
  chronic salicylate intoxication and, 642
  interactions and adverse effects
    alpha-blockers and, 227
    androgens and, 447
    anticholinergics and, 156, 248, 249
    antidiarrheals and, 748
    antiemetic agents and, 768
    antifibrinolytics and, 354
    antifungals and, 601
    antihistamines and, 506
    antimalarial drugs and, 610
    antiplatelet drugs and, 351
    antiprotozoal agents and, 614
    antipsychotic agents and, 182
    antiseptic and disinfectant agents and, 630
    antithyroid drugs and, 470
    barbiturates and, 123
    benzodiazepines and, 166
    beta-blockers and, 231, 307
    carbonic anhydrase inhibitors and, 858
    cardiac glycosides and, 267
    central nervous system stimulants and, 197
    cholinergic agents and, 241
    corticosteroids and, 493
    corticotropin and, 457
    cyanocobalamin and, 792
    cyclic antidepressants and, 171
    desmopressin, lypressin, and vasopressin and, 457
    dopaminergic agents and, 154
    fertility agents and, 437
    growth hormone and, 458
    histamine$_2$ blockers and, 736
    HMG-CoA reductase inhibitors and, 374
    immunizing agents and, 668
    immunosuppressants and, 658
    insulin and, 479
    interferons and, 714
    loop diuretics and, 389
    macrolides and, 565
    miotics and, 850
    monoamine oxidase inhibitors and, 174
    narcotic analgesic agents and, 93
    niacin and, 789
    omeprazole and, 737
    oral contraceptives and, 430
    osmotic diuretics and, 860
    oxytocic agents and, 433
    penicillins and, 549
    potassium-sparing diuretics and, 393

Central nervous system—cont'd
    pyridoxine and, 790
    quinolones and, 563
    second-generation antidepressants and, 177
    selegilene and, 151
    thiazide diuretics and, 395
    thyroid drugs and, 467
    tocolytic agents and, 435
    vitamin A and, 780
    vitamin D and, 783
    vitamin E and, 784
    vitamin K and, 786
  narcotic analgesic agents, 88-105
    agonist-antagonist, 98
    antiemetics and, 769
    barbiturates and, 124
    chemical structure of, 92
    clonidine and, 324
    codeine sulfate, 95
    dosages, 95, 96
    fentanyl, 97-98
    mechanism of action, 92
    meperidine hydrochloride, 98
    methadone hydrochloride, 98
    morphine sulfate, 95
    naloxone hydrochloride, 98
    naltrexone hydrochloride, 99
    nursing process and, 99-103
    physiology and psychology of pain, 89-92
    propoxyphene hydrochloride, 98
    side and adverse effects, 93-94
    therapeutic uses, 93
    toxicity and overdose, 94-95
  psychotherapeutic agents, 162-193
    antianxiety, 164-169
    antidepressant, 170-179
    antimanic, 179-180
    antipsychotic, 180-186
    nursing process and, 186-193
  sedatives and hypnotics, 120-134
    as anesthetic adjuvants, 108
    antiemetics and, 769
    aprobarbital, 126
    barbiturates, 121-124
    benzodiazepines, 126-130
    butabarbital, 126
    clonidine and, 324
    estazolam, 129
    flurazepam, 129
    geriatric complications, 31
    nursing process in, 130-133
    pentobarbital, 126
    phenobarbital, 124-126
    quazepam, 129-130
    secobarbital, 126
    sleep and, 121
    temazepam, 130
    triazolam, 130
Central nervous system depressants
    anticholinergics and, 157
    antidiarrheals and, 749
    antipsychotic agents and, 182
    benzodiazepines and, 128, 167
    cyclic antidepressants and, 172
    mitotane and, 700
Central nervous system stimulants, 194-203
    amantadine and, 579
    amphetamines, 200-201
    analeptics, 197-199
    anorexiants, 199-200
    nursing process and, 201-203
Central total parenteral nutrition, 812
Centrality, 808
Centrally acting adrenergic agents, 322-323, 325
cephalexin, 553
Cephalosporins, 552-556
    anticoagulants and, 347
    assessment of, 570
    first-generation, 553
    implementation of, 572
    nutritional supplements and, 807

Cephalosporins—cont'd
    second-generation, 553-555
    third-generation, 555-556
Ceptaz; see ceftazidime
Cerebral edema, 391, 494
Cerumen, 880
Cervical cancer, 693, 695
Cestode, 618
cetylpyridinium chloride, 633
Chancroid, 557
Chelation, 733
Chemoreceptor trigger zone, 765
Chemotherapy; see Antineoplastic agents
Chemotherapy emesis, 770, 771
Chest pain, 231, 301
Chickenpox, 579, 580
Chief cell, 729-731
Child
    anticonvulsant therapy for, 146
    antidiarrheals for, 760
    beta-adrenergic agonists for, 221
    cardiac glycosides for, 273
    cromolyn sodium for, 537
    drug effects on, 26-27
    general anesthesia and, 116
    human immunodeficiency virus and, 583
    narcotic analgesics and, 102
    nursing process and, 31-33
    psychotherapeutic agents for, 186
    recommended daily dietary allowances, 778
    thiazide diuretics and, 398
Chimney soot, 680
Chlamydial infection
    macrolides for, 564
    ocular, 863
    sulfonamides for, 546
    tetracyclines for, 557
chloral hydrate, 130
chlorambucil, 685
chloramphenicol
    for ear disorders, 880
    ocular, 866
chlordiazepoxide, 167, 168
chlorhexidine gluconate, 631, 632
Chlorine, 795
Chlorine compounds, 632
Chloromycetin; see chloramphenicol
chloroprocaine, 113
chloroquine, 390, 610, 611
Chloroseptic; see carbolic acid
chlorothiazide, 396
chlorotrianisene, 426
chloroxylenol, 880
chlorpheniramine, 504, 505, 509
chlorpromazine, 172, 183
chlorpropamide, 83, 458
chlorthalidone, 268, 396
Chlor-Trimeton; see chlorpheniramine
Cholera, 557
Cholesterol
    bile acid sequestrants and, 371
    coronary artery disease and, 370
    fibric acid derivatives and, 374-375
    HMG-CoA reductase inhibitors and, 373
    homeostasis of, 368-369
    niacin and, 788-789
cholestyramine, 268, 371-373
Cholinergic agents, 238-246
    nursing process and, 243-245
    parasympathetic nervous system and, 239-240
Cholinergic-blocking agents, 246-254
    as anesthetic adjuvants, 108
    atropine, 250-251
    beta-blockers and, 232, 307
    cholinergic agents and, 242
    cyclic antidepressants and, 172
    dicyclomine, 251
    geriatric complications, 31
    glycopyrrolate, 251
    for nausea and vomiting, 766, 769
    nursing process and, 251-253

Cholinergic-blocking agents—cont'd
  in Parkinson's disease, 156-158, 159
  scopolamine, 251
Cholinesterase, 240
Cholinesterase inhibitors, 851
Chorea, 150
Chorex-5; see Chorionic gonadotropin
Chorionic gonadotropin, 437, 439
Choroid, 846
Chromium, 795
Chronic bronchitis, 521, 522
Chronic diarrhea, 746
Chronic granulomatous disease, 716
Chronic lymphocytic leukemia, 669, 672
  alkylating agents for, 685, 687
  antimetabolites for, 689, 691
Chronic myelocytic leukemia
  alkylating agents for, 685, 687
  cytotoxic antibiotics for, 693, 695
  hydroxyurea for, 701
  interferon for, 714
Chronic obstructive pulmonary disease, 521, 538
Chronic pain, 90
Chronic salicylate intoxication, 642-643
Chronic stable angina, 301
Chronotropic agents, 265
Chronulac; see Lactulose
Chylomicron, 368-369
chymotrypsin, 870-871
ciclopirox olamine, 834
Cidex; see formaldehyde
Ciliary body, 846
cimetidine, 736-737
  altretamine and, 700
  benzodiazepines and, 128, 167
Cipro; see ciprofloxacin
ciprofloxacin, 562, 563-564, 865
Cirrhosis, 395
cisplatin, 685, 687, 688, 697, 702
Citrucel; see methylcellulose
clarithromycin, 566
Claritin; see loratadine
Clark's rule, 27
Class Ib antidysrhythmic drugs, 287-288
  indications for, 282
  nursing process and, 293-295
Class Ic antidysrhythmic drugs, 288-289
  indications for, 282
  nursing process and, 293-295
Class II dysrhythmic drugs, 289-291
  indications for, 282
  nursing process and, 295-296
Class III dysrhythmic drugs, 291-292
  indications for, 282
  nursing process and, 296-297
Class IV dysrhythmic drugs, 282-293
  indications for, 282
  nursing process and, 297-299
Classic angina, 301
clavulanic acid, 549
clemastine, 505, 509
Cleocin; see clindamycin
clindamycin, 567-568
  antidiarrheals and, 749
  assessment of, 570
  implementation of, 573
clioquinol, 834
clofibrate, 374-376, 458
Clomid; see clomiphene
clomiphene, 439
clonazepam, 141, 142
clonidine, 324, 325
Clonorchiasis, 621
clorazepate dipotassium, 141, 142
Clot specific, term, 356
clotrimazole, 605, 833, 834
Clotting factors, 345
clozapine, 185-186
Clozaril; see clozapine
Coagulation modifier agents, 341-366
  anticoagulants, 343-348

Coagulation modifier agents—cont'd
  antifibrinolytics, 353-355
  antiplatelet agents, 348-353
  hemostasis and, 343, 344, 345
  nursing process and, 359-365
  thrombolytics, 356-359
Coagulation system, 343, 344
Coal tar preparations, 680
Cobalt, 795
cocaine
  stimulant effects, 195
  as topical anesthetic, 112
Coccidioidomycosis, 598
Cocoa, 199
codeine sulfate, 95, 96, 100, 514
Coenzyme, 777
Coffee, 199
Cogentin; see benztropine
Cogwheel rigidity, 156
Colace; see Docusate salts
colchicine, 648
Cold medications, 509-517
  adrenergics and, 212
  antitussives, 511-514
  decongestants, 510-511
  expectorants, 514-515
  nursing process and, 515-517
Colestid; see colestipol
colestipol, 268, 371-373
colistin, 880
Collagen, platelet adhesion and, 348-349
Collecting duct, 386
Colloid oncotic pressure, 405-406
Colloids, 405, 408-410
Colon, 752
Colon cancer, 689, 717
Colony-stimulating factors, 718, 719-722
CoLyte; see polyethylene glycol
Coma, phenobarbital, 123
Common cold, 509
Community-acquired infection, 627
Compazine; see prochlorperazine
Competitive antagonist, 20, 247
Complete-B, 806
Complex seizure, 137
Comprehensive Drug Abuse Prevention and
      Control Act, 36, 37
Computer-controlled dispensing system, 50
COMT; see Catechol-O-methyltransferase
Condyloma acuminatum (condylomata acuminata),
      714, 716
Cone, 846
Confidentiality, 40
Congestive heart failure
  angiotensin-converting enzyme inhibitors for,
      327
  cardiac glycosides for, 265-266
  digitalis for, 269
  diuretics in, 385, 388, 395
  hypertension and, 320
Conjugated estrogens, 424, 425
Conjunctiva, 845
Conjunctivitis, 862
  allergic, 869
  bacterial, 863
Consciousness, stages of anesthesia and, 109
Constipation, 752-762
  bulk-forming laxatives for, 755-756
  emollient laxatives for, 756-758
  hyperosmotic laxatives for, 758-759
  narcotic analgesics and, 94
  nursing process in, 760-762
  saline laxatives for, 759
  stimulant laxatives for, 759-760
Controlled substances
  barbiturates, 124
  dispensing restrictions, 37
  schedule categories, 36
Controlled Substances Act, 36, 37
Controlyte, 806
Convulsion, 136, 141

Copper, 795
Cordarone; see amiodarone
Corgard; see nadolol
Cornea, 846
Corneal inflammation, 869
Coronary artery, 301
Coronary artery disease
  angina and, 301-302
  cholesterol and, 370
Coronary artery thrombus, 358
Cortan; see prednisone
Cortef; see hydrocortisone
Corticosteroid-binding globulin, 16
Corticosteroids, 491-493
  adrenal cortex and, 490
  for asthma, 528-531
  carbonic anhydrase inhibitors and, 858
  interleukins and, 718
  loop diuretics and, 390
  nasal decongestant, 510
  nonsteroidal antiinflammatory drugs and, 644
  ocular, 866-871
  thiazide diuretics and, 396
  topical, 835
Corticosterone, 455
Corticotropin, 455, 458, 461, 462
Cortisol, 456, 476
Cortisone, 492
cotrimoxazole, 546
Cough suppression
  antitussives for, 511
  narcotics for, 93
Coumadin; see warfarin
Cream, 831
Crescendo angina, 301
cresol, 631
Crohn's disease, 545
cromolyn sodium
  for asthma, 531-532
  for conjunctivitis, 870
  pediatric implications, 537
Cross-sensitivity, 552
Cryoprecipitate, 410, 411
Cryptococcosis, 598
Cryptorchidism, 438
Cryptosporidium, 612
Crystal violet, 631, 632
Crystalloids, 406-408
CSFs; see Colony-stimulating factors
CTZ; see Chemoreceptor trigger zone
Cultural aspects, 41, 42
  of hypertension, 322
  of pain, 89
  of premature birth, 439-440
Cushing's syndrome, 491, 494
Cyanocobalamin, 791-793, 824
Cyanoject; see Cyanocobalamin
Cyclic adenosine monophosphate, 731
  beta-agonists and, 525
  central nervous system stimulants and, 195
  theophylline and, 523
Cyclic antidepressants, 170-173
Cyclogyl; see cyclopentolate
cyclopentolate, 871
cyclophosphamide, 685, 687, 688, 702, 704
Cycloplegia, 247, 846
Cycloplegics, 846, 874
cycloserine, 589, 590
cyclosporin A, 658-659
  antifungal drugs and, 602
  macrolides and, 565
  nonsteroidal antiinflammatory drugs and, 644
cyclothiazide, 396
Cycrin; see medroxyprogesterone
cyproheptadine, 505, 509
Cystic fibrosis, 672
Cytadren; see aminoglutethimide
cytarabine, 692
Cytokines, 715
Cytomegalovirus, 578, 580
Cytomel; see liothyronine

Index

Cytoplasmic maturation, 819
Cytosar-U; see cytarabine
Cytotec; see misoprostol
Cytotoxic antibiotics, 692-695
    bleomycin, 694-695
    doxorubicin, 694, 695
Cytotoxic T-cell, 712
Cytovene; see ganciclovir
Cytoxan; see cyclophosphamide

D

dacarbazine, 685
dactinomycin, 693
Dakin's solution, 631, 632
Dalmane; see flurazepam
danazol, 448
Danocrine; see danazol
danthron, 759
dapsone, 579
Daraprim; see pyrimethamine
Datura stramonium, 249
daunorubicin, 693
DDAVP; see desmopressin
DDP; see cisplatin
Deadly nightshade, 249
Debrox Drops; see carbamide peroxide
Decadron; see dexamethasone
Declomycin; see demeclocycline
Decongestants, 510-511
    nasal, 217
    ophthalmic, 218
Deep sleep, 123
Deep vein thrombosis, 345, 358
    crystalloid solutions for, 407
    thrombolytic agents for, 358
Defecation, 752
Dehydration, 406
Delestrogen; see Estradiol valerate
Deltalin; see Ergocalciferol
Deltasone; see prednisone
Deltoid injection site, 61
demecarium, 850, 853
demeclocycline, 458, 558
Demodex; see torsemide
Demulen, 431
Deoxyribonucleic acid, 576-577
Dep Gynogen; see Estradiol cypionate
Depakene; see valproic acid
Depakote; see valproic acid
Dependence and tolerance, 22
Depolen; see Estradiol cypionate
Depo-Provera; see medroxyprogesterone
Depression, 164, 172, 176, 178
Dermatitis herpetiformis, 546
Dermatologic agents, 828-841
    anatomy of skin, 829, 830
    antiviral, 835
    nursing process and, 837-841
    topical anesthetic, antipruritic, and
        antiinflammatory, 835-836
    topical antiinfectives, 831-835
    topical antineoplastic, 837
    topical ectoparasiticidal, 836-837
Dermatophytes, 598
Dermatophytosis, 834
Dermis, 829, 830
Dermoplast; see benzocaine
desmopressin, 457, 460, 461
    in diabetes insipidus, 355
    patient teaching, 462
    pituitary drugs and, 458
desoxyephedrine, 510
Desoxyn; see methamphetamine
Desyrel; see trazodone
Dexaject-LA; see dexamethasone
dexamethasone, 492, 495
    for asthma, 530
    intranasal, 510
    ocular, 869

Dexatrim; see phenylpropanolamine
dexchlorpheniramine, 505, 509
Dexedrine; see dextroamphetamine
Dexone; see dexamethasone
Dextran, 409, 410
dextroamphetamine, 213, 215
dextromethorphan, 512-513
5% Dextrose, 407
dezocine, 98, 100
DiaBeta; see glyburide
Diabetes insipidus
    desmopressin for, 355
    diuretics in, 395
    pituitary drugs for, 459
Diabetes mellitus, 475-488
    aspirin and, 352
    glucose-elevating drugs for, 484-485
    insulin for, 478-481
    insulin-dependent, 477-478
    insulins for, 478-481
    investigational drugs for, 484
    non–insulin dependent, 478
    nursing process in, 485-487
    oral antidiabetic agents for, 481-484
    oral hypoglycemics for, 481-484
    pancreas and, 476
Diabetic ketoacidosis, 477
Diabetic neuropathy, 641
Diabinase; see chlorpropamide
Dialose; see Docusate salts
Dialysis
    for antidysrhythmic drug reversal, 283
    in chronic salicylate intoxication, 642
    crystalloid solutions for, 407
Diaminopyrimidines, 609, 612
Diamox; see acetazolamide
Diapid; see lypressin
Diarrhea, 745-752
    adsorbents for, 749
    antacids and, 732
    anticholinergics for, 749-750
    belladonna-alkaloid combinations for, 750-
        751
    dehydration and fluid loss in, 406
    intestinal flora modifiers for, 751-752
    milk of magnesia and, 732
    nursing process in, 760-762
    opiates for, 751
diazepam
    as anesthetic adjuvant, 108
    for antidysrhythmic drug reversal, 283
    for anxiety, 167, 169
    in status epilepticus, 138-139, 142
diazoxide, 331, 332, 396, 484-485
Dibenzodiazepines, 185-186
Dibenzoxazepines, 185
Dibenzyline; see phenoxybenzamine
        hydrochloride
dibrecaine, 112
dicyclomine, 251
didanosine, 577, 578
Didrex; see benzphetamine
dienestrol, 426
diethylcarbamazine, 619, 620
diethylpropion, 199-200
diethylstilbestrol, 426-427, 680
Diflucan; see fluconazole
Digibind; see digoxin immune Fab
digitalis, 266
    adrenergics and, 212
    amphotericin B and, 602
    carbonic anhydrase inhibitors and, 858
    loop diuretics and, 390
    patient teaching, 272
    thiazide diuretics and, 396
digitoxin, 266
digoxin, 266, 269
    antidiarrheals and, 749
    calcium channel blockers and, 310
    central nervous system stimulants and, 197
    geriatric complications, 31

digoxin—cont'd
    laxatives and, 756
    management of toxicity, 267-268
digoxin immune Fab, 269-270
Dihydroindolones, 185
Dihydropeptidase, 568
Dihydropyridines, 311
Dihydrotachysterol, 784
Dilacor; see diltiazem
Dilantin; see phenytoin
Dilator muscle, pupillary, 846
Dilatrate SR; see isosorbide dinitrate
diltiazem, 292
    for angina, 311
    dosage range, 287
    indications for, 282
dimenhydrinate, 505, 509
Dimensional analysis, 48
Dimetane; see brompheniramine
Dimetane-DC; see codeine sulfate
dinoprostone, 433
Diocto-K; see Docusate salts
diphenhydramine, 504, 505, 508
diphenidol hydrochloride, 774
diphenoxylate, 751
Diphtheria, 669
Diphtheria vaccine, 668-670
Diphyllobothriasis, 618
dipivefrin, 855
Diprivan; see propofol
dipyridamole, 350, 352-353
Di-Quinol; see iodoquinol
Direct-acting miotics, 851-852
Disinfectants, 626-636
    acid agents, 630
    alcohol agents, 630
    aldehyde agents, 631-632
    biguanide agents, 632
    chlorine compounds, 632
    in community-acquired and nosocomial
        infections, 627
    dyes, 632
    iodine compounds, 632-633
    mercurial agents, 632
    nursing process and, 634-636
    oxidizing agents, 633
    phenolic compounds, 633
    surface-active agents, 634
    topical antimicrobials, 627-630
disopyramide, 282, 283, 284-287
Distal tubule, 386
Distribution of drug, 16
    geriatric considerations, 30
    neonatal and pediatric considerations, 27
disulfiram, 167
Diucardin; see hydroflumethiazide
Diulo, metolazone
Diuretic ceiling effect, 397
Diuretics, 384-402
    adrenergic drugs and, 324
    alpha-blockers and, 228
    angiotensin-converting enzyme inhibitors and,
        328
    beta-blockers and, 232, 307
    carbonic anhydrase inhibitors, 387-388, 858
    ganglionic blockers and, 257
    for hypertension, 330
    kidney function and, 385-386
    loop, 388-390
    nonsteroidal antiinflammatory drugs and,
        644
    nursing care plan for, 401
    nursing process and, 398-399
    osmotic, 390-392
    patient teaching, 333
    pituitary drugs and, 458
    potassium-sparing, 392-394
    to reduce intraocular pressure, 859-861
    thiazide, 395-397
        amphotericin B and, 602
        cardiac glycosides and, 268

Diuretics—cont'd
    direct-acting vasodilators and, 331
    geriatric complications, 31
Diuril; *see* **chlorothiazide**
divalproex
    antimalarial agents and, 612
    for epilepsy, 139, 140
Dizmiss; *see* **meclizine**
DKA; *see* Diabetic ketoacidosis
dobutamine, 216, 218
    for antidysrhythmic drug reversal, 283
    dose-response relationship, 210
Dobutrex; *see* **dobutamine**
Documentation of medication order, 50-51
Docusate salts, 758
Domeboro; *see* Acetic acid
Done nomogram, 642
Donnatal; *see* Belladonna alkaloids
Dopamine, 218
    for antidysrhythmic drug reversal, 283
    antipsychotic agents and, 182
    dosage, 216
    dose-response relationship, 210
    nausea and vomiting and, 765
    Parkinson's disease and, 149-150
Dopaminergic receptor, 209
Dopaminergic therapy, 152-156, 160
Dopram; *see* **doxapram**
Doral; *see* **quazepam**
Dorsal horn of spinal cord, pain and, 90-91
Dorsogluteal injection site, 60
Doryx; *see* **doxycycline**
Dose calculations, 26-27, 47-48
Dose-limiting side effects, 682
Double-blind, placebo-controlled study, 38
doxapram, 199
doxazosin, 229
doxorubicin, 693, 694, 695, 718
Doxy-Caps; *see* **doxycycline**
doxycycline, 558-559
doxylamine, 509
Doxy-Tabs; *see* **doxycycline**
Dramamine; *see* **dimenhydrinate**
Drisdol; *see* Ergocalciferol
Dromotropic agents, 265
dronabinol, 771
Drug administration, 49-85
    absorption and, 13-14
    adding medications to IV fluid containers, 69-70
    eardrops, 81
    injections, 62-64
    intravenous bolus, 67-69
    intravenous medications by piggyback or
        volume administration sets, 65-66
    medication orders and documentation, 50-51
    nasal drops, 82
    nasogastric tube in, 83-85
    ophthalmic, 80
    oral, 14-16, 78-79
    patient-controlled analgesia, 71-77
    preparing injections from ampules and vials, 55-
        58
    sites for, 59-61
    syringes for, 52-54
    topical, 16
        anesthetics, 111, 112, 113, 835-836
        antiinfectives, 831-835
        antineoplastics, 837
        antiviral agents, 835
        ectoparasiticidal drugs, 836-837
        ocular anesthetics, 869-870, 874
Drug concentration, 21
Drug legislation
    Canadian, 38-39
    United States, 35-36
Drug weights and measures, 45-47
Drug-induced teratogenesis, 23
Drug-receptor interaction, 19-20
D.S.S. capsules; *see* Docusate salts
Duodenal ulcer, 735, 738
Duphalac; *see* Lactulose

Duragen; *see* Estradiol valerate
Duragesic; *see* **fentanyl**
Duralutin; *see* **hydroxyprogesterone caproate**
Dura-Tab; *see* **quinidine**
Duration of drug, 19
Durham-Humphrey Amendment, 36
DV; *see* **dienestrol**
Dwarf tapeworm, 618
Dyes, disinfectant, 632
DynaCirc; *see* **isradipine**
dyphylline, 523
Dyrenium; *see* **triamterene**
Dyskinesia, 150
Dysmenorrhea, 641, 648
Dysregulation hypothesis, 170
Dysrhythmia, 276-299
    cardiac electrophysiology and, 277-280
    class Ib drugs for, 287-288
    class Ic drugs for, 288-289
    class II drugs for, 289-291
    class III drugs for, 291-292
    class IV drugs for, 282-293
    nursing process and, 293-299
    potassium replacement therapy in, 413
Dystonia, 150

E

Ear
    antidiarrheals and, 748
    antiemetics and, 768
    antiprotozoal agents and, 614
    carbonic anhydrase inhibitors and, 858
    disorders of, 878-884
        antibacterial and antifungal agents for, 879-880
        local anesthetic agents for, 880-881
        nursing process in, 881-883
    miotics and, 850
    osmotic diuretics and, 860
    structure of, 878-879
Eardrops, 81
Earwax, 880
Eccrine gland, 830
echothiophate, 850, 852, 871
econazole nitrate, 834
Ecotrin; *see* Aspirin
Ectoparasiticidal drugs, 836-837
Edecrin; *see* **ethacrynic acid**
Edema, 405-406
    cerebral, 494
    diuretics in, 388, 391, 394, 396
Effective refractory period, 279
Efferent arteriole, 386
Effort angina, 301
Efudex; *see* **fluorouracil**
Ejection fraction, 265
Eldepryl; *see* **selegiline**
Elderly; *see* Geriatric patient
Electroencephalography, 136
Electrolytes, 403-420
    blood products and, 410-412
    colloids and, 408-410
    crystalloids and, 406-408
    nursing process and, 416-418
    osmotic diuretics and, 860
    physiology of fluid balance, 404-406
    plasma protein fractions and, 411-412
    potassium, 412-414
    sodium, 415-416
Elemental formulations, 806, 807
Elixophyllin; *see* **theophylline**
Elspar; *see* **asparaginase**
Embolism, 345, 358
Emesis, 764-774
    antiemetic agents for, 765-771
        anticholinergic, 769
        neuroleptic, 769-771
        prokinetic, 771
        serotonin blockers, 771

Emesis—cont'd
    antipsychotic agents for, 184
    dehydration and fluid loss in, 406
    hydroxyzine for, 168
    nursing process in, 772-774
Emetic potential, 682
Emetic laxatives, 753, 756-758
Emphysema, 521, 522
Empiric therapy, 21, 544
enalapril, 327, 329
encainide, 282, 286, 288-289
Encephalopathy, immunizing agents and, 668
Endep; *see* **amitriptyline**
Endocrine system, 454-455
    adrenal agents, 489-499
        adrenal system and, 490-491
        antiadrenals, 495
        corticosteroids, 491-493
        nursing process and, 495-498
    antidiabetic agents, 475-488
        aspirin and, 352
        glucose-elevating drugs, 484-485
        insulin-dependent diabetes mellitus, 477-478
        insulins, 478-481
        investigational, 484
        non-insulin dependent diabetes mellitus, 478
        nursing process and, 485-487
        oral, 481-484
        pancreas and, 476
    histamine₂ blockers and, 736
    interactions and adverse effects
        androgens and, 447
        antipsychotic agents and, 182
        central nervous system stimulants and, 197
        corticosteroids and, 493
        growth hormone and, 458
    ovary in, 422
    pituitary agents, 454-464
        endocrine system and, 454-455
        nursing process and, 460-463
    thyroid agents, 465-474
        adrenergics and, 212
        antithyroid agents and, 469-471
        iron preparations and, 822
        mydriatics and, 854
        nursing process and, 471-473
        thyroid function and, 466
Endometrial cancer, 429
Endometriosis, 429, 449
Endometrium, 422
Endophthalmitis, 862
Endorphins, 91
Enduron; *see* **methyclothiazide**
Energix-B; *see* Hepatitis B vaccine
enflurane, 110, 111
Enkaid; *see* **encainide**
Enkephalins, 91
Enolic acids, 647
enoxacin, 562
Ensure, 806, 807-808
Enteral nutrition, 804-808, 814
Enteral route, 14, 15
Enterobacter, 546
Enterobiasis, 618, 621
Enterococcus
    penicillins for, 548
    vancomycin for, 568
Enterocolitis, 568
Enterohepatic circulation, 18
Enulose; *see* Lactulose
Enuresis, 459
Environmental carcinogen, 680
Enzymes, 20, 777
    barbiturates and, 122
    ocular, 875
Eosinophil, 529
ephedrine, 510
    as bronchodilator, 525, 527-528
    guanadrel and, 324
Epidermal growth factor, 739
Epidermis, 829, 830

Epidermophyton, 598
Epilepsy, 135-147
  antiepileptic drugs for, 136-144
    benzodiazepines, 142
    carbamazepine, 142-143
    ethosuximide, 143
    phenobarbital, 143
    phenytoin, 143-144
    valproic acid, 144
  diuretics in, 388
  immune globulins for, 672
  nursing process in, 144-145
Epinephrine, 207, 217
  adrenal medulla and, 490
  beta-blockers and, 230
  as bronchodilator, 527-528
  dosage, 214, 216
  dose-response relationship, 210
  ganglionic blockers and, 256-257
  in glucose regulation, 476
  miotics and, 851
  vasoactive effects of, 218
EPO; *see* Erythropoietin
epoetin alfa, 721
Epogen; *see* **epoetin alfa; erythropoietin**
Epsom salts, 759
Equanil; *see* **meprobamate**
Ergocalciferol, 784
ergonovine, 433-434
Ergostat; *see* **ergotamine tartrate**
Ergosterol, 599
Ergot alkaloids, 432
ergotamine tartrate, 228, 229
Ergotrate; *see* **ergonovine**
EryDerm; *see* **erythromycin**
Erygel; *see* **erythromycin**
Erythema multiforme, 424
Erythrocyte
  formation of, 819
  pentoxifylline and, 350
erythromycin, 566, 567, 832
  formulations of, 564
  nutritional supplements and, 807
  ocular, 864
erythromycin estolate, 567
erythromycin ethylsuccinate, 567
erythromycin gluceptate, 567
erythromycin lactobionate, 567
erythromycin stearate, 567
Erythropoiesis, 819
Erythropoietic effect, 446
Erythropoietin, 719, 824
Escherichia coli
  aminoglycosides for, 559
  sulfonamides for, 546
Eserine sulfate; *see* **physostigmine**
Esidrix; *see* **hydrochlorothiazide**
esmolol, 233, 234, 290
  dosage range, 286
  indications for, 282
  management of overdose, 283
Esophageal candidiasis, 603
Esophagitis
  antacids for, 732, 734
  omeprazole for, 738
Essential amino acids, 810
Essential fatty acid deficiency, 811
Essential hypertension, 321
Essential tremor, 233
estazolam, 129, 131
Esterified estrogens, 425
Estinyl; *see* Ethinyl estradiol
Estrace; *see* Estradiol
Estraderm; *see* Estradiol
Estradiol, 423-424, 425
Estradiol cypionate, 426
Estradiol valerate, 426
Estratab; *see* Esterified estrogens
Estriol, 423-424
Estrogens, 423-427
  antifibrinolytics and, 355

Estrogens—cont'd
  carcinogenic effects of, 680
  patient teaching, 441
  replacement therapy, 425-427
Estrone, 423-424
estropipate, 426
Estrovis; *see* **quinestrol**
ethacrynic acid, 388, 390, 391
  anticoagulants and, 347
  cardiac glycosides and, 268
ethambutol, 589-592
Ethanol, 630
Ethanolamines, 505
Ethical practice, 39-42
Ethinyl estradiol, 424, 426
ethionamide, 589, 590
ethosuximide, 141, 143
ethoxzolamide, 268
Ethrane; *see* **enflurane**
Ethylenediamines, 505
ethylnorepinephrine, 525, 527-528
etidocaine, 113
etomidate, 108
etoposide, 697-698
Euthroid; *see* **liotrix**
Evac-U-Lax; *see* **phenolphthalein**
Evaluation in nursing process, 11
E-Vitamin Succinate; *see* Vitamin E
Ewing's sarcoma, 693, 695
Excretion of drug, 17-18, 30
Exelderm; *see* **sulconazole**
Ex-Lax; *see* **phenolphthalein**
ExNa; *see* **benzthiazide**
Exogenous lipids, 368
Expectorants, 514-515
Expedited drug approval, 38
Extended-spectrum penicillins, 548, 551-552
External ear disorders, 878-879
Extracellular volume, 405
Extravasation, 227
  alkylating agents, 686
  cytotoxic antibiotics, 694
  mitotic inhibitors, 697
Extravascular fluid, 405
Extravascular volume, 405
Eye
  anticholinergics and, 248, 249
  antidiarrheals and, 748
  antiemetics and, 768
  antiglaucoma agents, 847-861
    beta-adrenergic blockers, 855-857
    carbonic anhydrase inhibitors, 857-859
    osmotic diuretics, 859-861
    parasympathomimetics, 848-853
    sympathomimetics, 853-855
  antiinfective agents, 861-866
  antiinflammatory agents, 866-869
  antiprotozoal agents and, 614
  antiviral agents, 866
  cardiac glycosides and, 267
  cholinergic agents and, 241
  corticosteroids and, 493
  nursing process and, 871-876
  stages of anesthesia and, 109
  structure of, 844-847
  topical anesthetics, 869-870
Eyebrow, 844
Eyedrops, 80
Eyelash, 844
Eyelid, 844

F

Fallopian tube, 422
Familial hypophosphatemia, 781
famotidine, 736
fansidar, 612
Fast-channel cell, 278
Fast-response cell, 278

Fat
  in modular formulations, 806, 808
  in nutritional support, 811
  triglycerides and, 368
Fat emulsions, 811
Fat-soluble vitamins, 779-786
  recommended daily dietary allowances, 778
  vitamin A, 779-780
  vitamin D, 782-784
  vitamin E, 784-785
  vitamin K, 785-786
Fatty streak, 370
Feen-A-Mint; *see* **phenolphthalein**
felbamate, 139, 141-142
Feldene; *see* **piroxicam**
felodipine, 311
Female reproductive agents, 421-442
  female reproductive system and, 422-423
  fertility agents, 436-439
  labor and delivery drugs, 431-436
    uterine relaxants, 434-436
    uterine stimulants, 431-434
  nursing process and, 439-442
  oral contraceptives, 430-431
  sex hormones, 423-429
    estrogens, 423-427
    progestins, 427-429
Female reproductive system, 422-423
Femiron; *see* **ferrous fumarate**
Femstat; *see* **butoconazole**
Fenamic acids, 647
fenfluramine, 200, 213
fentanyl, 97-98, 100, 108
Feostat; *see* **ferrous fumarate**
ferrous fumarate, 822
Ferrous salts, 821
Fertility agents, 436-439, 442
Fetus
  benzphetamine and, 199
  teratogenic effects of drugs, 22-23
Fever
  dehydration and fluid loss in, 406
  nonsteroidal antiinflammatory drugs for, 640, 644-645
FFP; *see* Fresh frozen plasma
Fiberall; *see* Psyllium
Fibric acid derivatives, 374-376
Fibrin, 343
Fibrinogen, 408
Fibrinolysis, 343
Fibrinolytic system, 343, 345
Fibrocystic breast disease, 449
Filariasis, 621
filgrastim, 721
finasteride, 448
First-generation antidepressants, 172
First-generation cephalosporins, 553
First-pass effect, 14, 15
Fishworm, 618
Fixed-combination insulin, 481
Flagyl; *see* **metronidazole**
Flat worm, 618
Flatulence, 733
Flavin adenine dinucleotide, 788
Flavin mononucleotide, 788
flecainide, 286, 288-289
Fleet Babylax; *see* **glycerin**
Fleet Mineral Oil Enema; *see* Mineral oil
Flexical, 806
Flexical, 806
Florinef; *see* **fludrocortisone**
Floropryl; *see* **isoflurophate**
Floxin; *see* **ofloxacin**
fluconazole, 600, 602
flucytosine, 599
fludrocortisone, 495
Flu-Glo Strips; *see* **fluorescein**
Fluid balance, 404-406
Fluid overload, 815
Fluids and electrolytes, 403-420
  for antidysrhythmic drug reversal, 283
  blood products, 410-412

Fluids and electrolytes—cont'd
  colloids, 408-410
  crystalloids, 406-408
  nursing process and, 416-418
  osmotic diuretics and, 860
  physiology of fluid balance, 404-406
  plasma protein fractions, 411-412
  potassium, 412-414
  sodium, 415-416
Fluke, 618
flumazenil, 127-128, 167
flunisolide, 510, 530
fluorescein, 871
Fluorine, 795
Fluoroplex; *see* **fluorouracil**
Fluoroquinolones, 562-564
fluorouracil, 599, 701, 704, 837
Fluothane; *see* **halothane**
fluoxetine, 179
fluoxymesterone, 448
fluphenazine, 183
flurazepam, 129, 131
flurbiprofen, 868
fluvastatin, 373
Foam cell, 370
Folate antagonists, 690-691
Folate deficiency, 823
Folex PFS; *see* **methotrexate**
Folic acid, 823-824
  antagonism, 689
  recommended daily allowances, 778
Follicle-stimulating hormone, 423, 456
Follicular lymphoma, 687
Follutein; *see* Chorionic gonadotropin
Food
  monoamine oxidase inhibitors and, 175
  oral route of administration and, 14-15
Food, Drug, and Cosmetic Act of 1938, 35-36
Food and Drug Administration, 37
Food-drug interaction, 544
Forane; *see* isoflurane
formaldehyde, 631
Fortaz; *see* **ceftazidime**
foscarnet, 577, 578
fosinopril, 327
fosphenytoin, 142
Foxglove, 266
Fraction method, 48
Free-Amine III, 810
Fresh frozen plasma, 410, 411, 412
Fried's rule, 27
Fuchsin, 632
Fundic gland, 730
Fungal infection, 598
  antifungal agents for, 599-603
  nosocomial, 627
  nursing process in, 603-605
  ocular, 834, 863
Fungizone; *see* **amphotericin B**
Furacin; *see* **nitrofurazone**
Furane; *see* **isoforane**
furosemide, 390, 391
  anticoagulants and, 347
  aspirin and, 352
  cardiac glycosides and, 268

G

gabapentin, 142
Gallbladder cancer, 689
Gamma-aminobutyric acid
  barbiturates and, 121
  benzodiazepines and, 127, 165
  vitamin B_6 and, 790
Gammagard; *see* Immune globulin
Gammar; *see* Immune globulin
Gamulin Rh; *see* Rh_0 immune globulin
ganciclovir, 577, 578, 581

Ganglionic-blocking agents, 255-261
  mecamylamine, 258
  nicotinic receptor and, 256
  nursing process and, 259-261
  sodium nitroprusside and, 331
  trimethaphan, 258
Gantanol; *see* **sulfamethoxazole**
Gantrisin; *see* **sulfisoxazole**
Garamycin; *see* **gentamicin**
Gas, 729
Gastric gland, 729-731
Gastric hyperacidity, 729, 732
Gastrin, 730
Gastritis, 732
Gastrocrom; *see* **cromolyn**
Gastroesophageal reflux disease, 734
Gastrointestinal system
  adrenergic receptor responses to stimulation, 207
  antacids and antiflatulents, 728-744
    acid-related pathophysiology, 729-731
    aluminum-containing, 733
    angiotensin-converting enzyme inhibitors and, 328
    anticholinergics and, 157
    antidiarrheals and, 749
    antifungal drugs and, 602
    antipsychotic agents and, 182
    beta-blockers and, 232
    calcium-containing, 733
    cardiac glycosides and, 268
    didanosine and, 579
    histamine_2 antagonists, 735-737
    iron preparations and, 822
    laxatives and, 756
    magnesium-containing, 733-735
    misoprostol, 740
    nursing process and, 740-743
    proton pump inhibitors, 737-738
    sucralfate, 738-739
  antidiarrheals and laxatives, 746-752
    adsorbent, 749
    anticholinergic, 749-750
    belladonna-alkaloid combinations, 750-751
    intestinal flora modifiers, 751-752
    nursing process and, 760-762
    opiate, 751
  antiemetic agents, 764-774
    anticholinergic, 769
    neuroleptic, 769-771
    nursing process and, 772-774
    prokinetic, 771
    serotonin blockers, 771
  chronic salicylate intoxication and, 642
  interactions and adverse effects
    alpha-blockers and, 227
    anticholinergics and, 156, 248, 249
    anticoagulants and, 346
    antiemetic agents and, 768
    antifibrinolytics and, 354
    antifungals and, 601
    antihistamines and, 506
    antimalarial drugs and, 610
    antiplatelet drugs and, 351
    antiprotozoal agents and, 614
    antipsychotic agents and, 182
    antithyroid drugs and, 470
    barbiturates and, 123
    benzodiazepines and, 166
    beta-blockers and, 231
    bile acid sequestrants and, 372
    calcium channel blockers and, 309
    calcium salts and, 796
    carbonic anhydrase inhibitors and, 858
    cardiac glycosides and, 267
    central nervous system stimulants and, 197
    cholinergic agents and, 241
    colony-stimulating factors and, 720
    corticosteroids and, 493
    corticotropin and, 457
    cyanocobalamin and, 792

Gastrointestinal system—cont'd
  cyclic antidepressants and, 171
  desmopressin, lypressin, and vasopressin and, 457
  dopaminergic agents and, 154
  estrogens and, 425
  fertility agents and, 437
  fibric acid derivatives and, 375
  ganglionic blockers and, 257
  histamine_2 blockers and, 736
  HMG-CoA reductase inhibitors and, 374
  immunosuppressants and, 658
  interferons and, 714
  iron preparations and, 821
  loop diuretics and, 389
  macrolides and, 565
  miotics and, 850
  monoamine oxidase inhibitors and, 174
  narcotic analgesic agents and, 93
  niacin and, 789
  nicotinic acid and, 377
  nonsteroidal antiinflammatory drugs and, 641
  omeprazole and, 737
  oral contraceptives and, 430
  osmotic diuretics and, 860
  oxytocic agents and, 433
  penicillins and, 549
  potassium-sparing diuretics and, 393
  progestins and, 428
  quinolones and, 563
  second-generation antidepressants and, 177
  selegiline and, 151
  sulfonamides and, 546
  thiazide diuretics and, 395
  thyroid drugs and, 467
  tocolytic agents and, 435
  vitamin A and, 780
  vitamin D and, 783
  vitamin E and, 784
  vitamin K and, 786
  nutritional supplements, 803-815
    enteral nutrition, 804-808
    nursing process and, 813-815
    parenteral nutrition, 808-813
  vitamins and minerals, 777-798
    laxatives and, 756
    niacin, 788-790
    nursing process and, 799-802
    recommended daily dietary allowances, 778
    riboflavin, 787-788
    thiamine, 787
    vitamin A, 779-780
    vitamin B_6, 790-791
    vitamin B_12, 791-793
    vitamin C, 793-794
    vitamin D, 782-784
    vitamin E, 784-785
    vitamin K, 785-786
Gastrostomy, 805
Gate theory of pain transmission, 90-92
Gaviscon; *see* Antacids
G-CSF; *see* Granulocyte colony stimulating factor
Gel, 831
gemfibrozil, 374-376
General anesthetics, 107-111
Generalized anxiety disorder, 165
Generation time, 681
Genetic abnormality
  antibiotic effects and, 545
  cancer and, 679-680
Genital herpes, 580
Genital warts, 716
Genitourinary system
  adrenergic receptor responses to stimulation, 207
  female reproductive agents, 421-429
    estrogens, 423-427
    fertility agents, 436-439
    nursing process and, 439-442
    oral contraceptives, 430-431

Genitourinary system—cont'd
　　progestins, 427-429
　　uterine relaxants, 434-436
　　uterine stimulants, 431-434
　interactions and adverse effects
　　anticholinergics and, 156, 248, 249
　　antidiarrheals and, 748
　　antiemetic agents and, 768
　　antifungals and, 601
　　antiprotozoal agents and, 614
　　antipsychotic agents and, 182
　　calcium salts and, 796
　　carbonic anhydrase inhibitors and, 858
　　central nervous system stimulants and,
　　　197
　　cholinergic agents and, 241
　　corticotropin and, 457
　　desmopressin, lypressin, and vasopressin and,
　　　457
　　estrogens and, 425
　　fibric acid derivatives and, 375
　　growth hormone and, 458
　　histamine₂ blockers and, 736
　　narcotic analgesic agents and, 93
　　niacin and, 789
　　omeprazole and, 737
　　oral contraceptives and, 430
　　osmotic diuretics and, 860
　　oxytocic agents and, 433
　　progestins and, 428
　　vitamin D and, 783
　　vitamin E and, 784
　male reproductive agents, 445-451
Genoptic; see gentamicin
Genora, 431
gentamicin, 560, 561-562
　ocular, 862-864
Gentian violet, 631, 632
Gentran; see Dextran
Geriatric patient
　antiparkinsonian agents and, 159
　beta-adrenergic agonists and, 221
　digitalis toxicity and, 271
　diuretic therapy and, 398
　drug effects on, 27-31
　general anesthesia and, 116
　iron agents and, 826
　narcotic analgesics and, 103
　nursing process and, 31-33
　Parkinson's disease and, 149
　psychotherapeutic agents for, 186
　thyroid hormones and, 471
Gesterol; see hydroxyprogesterone caproate
GFR; see Glomerular filtration rate
Giardiasis, 612, 613
Gilles de la Tourette; see Tourette syndrome
Glandular secretions
　anticholinergics and, 248, 249
　cholinergic agents and, 241
Glaucoma, 847-848, 852
　diuretics in, 387, 388
Glial tumor, 717
glipizide, 483, 484
Globin, 819
Globulin, 408
Glomerular filtration rate, 385-386
Glomerulus, 385
Glucagon, 476, 484-485
Glucocorticoids, 490, 491
Glucose, 476
Glucose-6-phosphate dehydrogenase deficiency, 22,
　545
Glucose-elevating drugs, 484-485
Glucotrol; see glipizide
Glutaraldehyde, 631
glutethimide, 347
glyburide, 483, 484
glycerin, 759, 860
Glycogen, 476
Glycogenolysis, 230, 476
glycopyrrolate, 108, 251

Glynase Prestab; see glyburide
GM-CSF; see Granulocyte-macrophage colony
　stimulating factor
Goals in nursing process, 7, 9-10
Gold compounds, 649-650
gold sodium thiomalate, 649-650
GoLYTELLY; see polyethylene glycol
Gonadorelin, 437
Gonadotropins, 422
Gonadotropin-stimulating hormone, 423
Gonic; see Chorionic gonadotropin
Gonorrhea
　macrolides for, 564
　tetracyclines for, 557
Gout, 641, 644, 647, 648
Gram-negative bacteria
　aminoglycosides for, 559
　cephalosporins for, 552
　in nosocomial infection, 627
　quinolones for, 562
Gram-positive bacteria
　aminoglycosides for, 559
　cephalosporins for, 552
　penicillins for, 548
　quinolones for, 562
　vancomycin for, 568
granisetron, 771
Granulocyte, 529
Granulocyte colony stimulating factor, 719
Granulocyte-macrophage colony stimulating factor,
　719
Granuloma inguinale, 557
Graves' disease, 466
griseofulvin, 599, 600, 605
Group A beta-hemolytic streptococci, 356, 627
Growth failure, 459
Growth fraction, 681
Growth hormone, 456
　alpha-blockers and, 323
　pituitary agents and, 455
guaifenesin, 514, 515
guanadrel, 324, 326
guanethidine, 326, 331
Guiatuss; see guaifenesin
Gyne-Lotrimin; see clotrimazole

H

Haemophilus influenzae, 564, 669
Haemophilus influenzae type B conjugate vaccine,
　669, 670-671
Hairy cell cancer, 693, 695, 714, 716
halazone, 632
Halcion; see triazolam
Haldol; see haloperidol
Half-life of drug, 18-19
haloperidol
　dopaminergic agents and, 154
　patient teaching, 191
　for psychosis, 184-185
haloprogin, 834
Halotestin; see fluoxymesterone
Halotex; see haloprogin
halothane, 110, 111
Hantavirus, 578
H-BIG₂; see Hepatitis B immune globulin
Head and neck cancer
　alkylating agents for, 685
　antimetabolites for, 689
　cytotoxic antibiotics for, 693, 695
　interleukin-2 for, 717
Head louse, 836
Headache
　alpha-adrenergic blocking agents for, 229
　nonsteroidal antiinflammatory drugs for, 641
Heart; see Cardiovascular system
Heart rate
　beta-blockers and, 306
　cholinergic agents and, 241

Heartburn, 732
Height, child dosage calculation and, 27
Helicobacter pylori, 557
Helminthic infection, 617-622
Hematologic system; see Blood
Heme, 819
Hemocyte; see ferrous fumarate
Hemoglobin, 819
Hemolytic agents, 612
Hemophilia, 459
Hemorrhage
　anticoagulation therapy and, 346
　blood products for, 412
　dehydration and fluid loss in, 406
　thrombolytics and, 357
Hemorrheologic drugs, 343
Hemostasis, 343, 344, 345
Hemostatic agents, 343
Henbane, 249
heparin, 348
　geriatric complications, 31
　intravenous, 361
　pituitary drugs and, 458
　protamine reversal, 346
　subcutaneous, 360
Heparin flush, 68
Hepatic-Aid, 806, 808
Hepatitis, 714, 716
Hepatitis A, 672
Hepatitis B, 669
Hepatitis B immune globulin, 672
Hepatitis B vaccine, 669, 671
Hep-Lock; see heparin
Hep-N-Gammagee; see Hepatitis B immune
　globulin
Herd immunity, 667
Hereditary angioedema, 449
Herpes simplex virus, 578, 580
　antivirals for, 578, 580
　in nosocomial infection, 627
Hespan; see Hetastarch
Hetastarch, 409, 410
Hetrazan; see diethylcarbamazine
HexaBetalin; see Pyridoxine
Hexachlorophenes, 633
Hexadrol; see dexamethasone
Hexalen; see altretamine
Hiatal hernia, 732
Hib vaccine; see Haemophilus influenzae type B
　conjugate vaccine
Hibiclens; see chlorhexidine gluconate
Hiccups, 184
High-altitude sickness, 388
High-density lipoprotein, 368-369
　fibric acid derivatives and, 375
　nicotinic acid and, 377
　probucol and, 378
Hismanal; see astemizole
Histamine
　antihistamines and, 503-509
　narcotic analgesics and, 93
　nausea and vomiting and, 765
　parietal cell and, 730
Histamine receptors, 182, 503
Histamine₁ antagonists, 504
Histamine₁ receptor, 503
Histamine₂ blockers, 503-504, 735-737
　antifungal drugs and, 602
　calcium channel blockers and, 310
　laxatives and, 756
　patient teaching, 740
Histamine₂ receptor, 503
Histanil; see promethazine
Histiocytosis, 696
Histoplasmosis, 598
HMG-CoA reductase inhibitors, 373-374
Hodgkin's disease
　alkylating agents for, 685, 687
　cytotoxic antibiotics for, 693, 695
　interleukin-2 for, 717
　mitotic inhibitors for, 696, 698

Home health
albuterol, 536
after anesthesia, 117
antidysrhythmics, 295
antineoplastic agents, 706
digitalis, 273
narcotic analgesic agents, 101
phenothiazines, 187
Hookworm, 621
Hordeolum, 862
Hormones, 454-455
anterior and posterior pituitary, 456
in ovulation, 423
pancreatic, 476
Hospital-acquired infection, 627
Host factors, 544-545
Household bleach, 632
Household system, 46
H.P. Acthar Gel; *see* Corticotropin
5-HT₃ receptor blockers, 771
Human immunodeficiency virus infection, 578, 583
Humatin; *see* **paromomycin**
Humatrope; *see* **somatropin**
Humibid; *see* **guaifenesin**
Humoral immune system, 712
Humoral immunity, 711
Humorsol; *see* **demecarium**
Humulin, 479, 480
Hurricaine; *see* **benzocaine**
Hydantoins
dopaminergic agents and, 154
for epilepsy, 139, 140
hydralazine hydrochloride, 331, 332
Hydrea; *see* **hydroxyurea**
Hydrochloric acid, 729-730
hydrochlorothiazide, 396, 397
hydrocortisone, 492, 493, 880
Hydrocortone; *see* **hydrocortisone**
Hydro-Diuril; *see* **hydrochlorothiazide**
hydroflumethiazide, 396
hydrogen peroxide, 631, 633
hydromorphone, 100
Hydromox; *see* **quinethazone**
Hydrostatic pressure, 405
hydroxyprogesterone caproate, 429
hydroxyurea, 701
hydroxyzine
as anesthetic adjuvant, 108
for anxiety, 168, 169
effects of, 505
Hygroton; *see* **chlorthalidone**
Hylorel; *see* **guanadrel**
Hymenolepiasis, 618
hyoscine, 749-750
hyoscyamine, 749-750
Hyoscyamus niger, 249
Hyperacidity, 734
Hyperaldosteronism, 392
Hyperalimentation, 808-813
Hyperbilirubinemia, 125
Hypercalcemia
cytotoxic antibiotics for, 693, 695
digitalis toxicity and, 271
diuretics in, 389
Hypercalciuria
cytotoxic antibiotics for, 693, 695
diuretics in, 395
Hypercapnia, 198
Hypercholesterolemia, 369
Hyperglycemia, 476-478
HyperHep; *see* Hepatitis B immune globulin
Hyperkalemia, 412, 526
Hyperlipidemia, 370-371
Hypernatremia, 415
Hyperosmolar sodium chloride, 871, 875
Hyperosmotic laxatives, 753, 758-759
Hypersecretory conditions, 738
Hypersensitivity reaction, 22
Hyperstat; *see* **diazoxide**
Hypertension, 319-340
adrenergic agents for, 322-326

Hypertension—cont'd
alpha-adrenergic blocking agents for, 229
angiotensin-converting enzyme inhibitors for, 326-329
beta-blockers for, 233
calcium channel blockers for, 330
diuretics for, 330, 389
ganglionic-blocking agents for, 257
monoamine oxidase inhibitor-induced, 150
nonsteroidal antiinflammatory drugs for, 641
nursing process in, 332-340
vasodilators for, 330-332
Hyperthyroidism, 466, 471
Hypertonic dehydration, 406
Hypertonic saline, 407
Hypertrophic subaortic stenosis, 233
Hyphae, 598
Hypnotics; *see* Sedatives and hypnotics
Hypochlorous acid, 632
Hypochromic anemia, 819
Hypodermic needle, 52
Hypodermis, 829
Hypoglycemia, 478
insulin overdose and, 479
total parenteral nutrition and, 815
Hypoglycemic agents, 475-488
antidiarrheals and, 749
aspirin and, 352
glucose-elevating drugs, 484-485
insulin-dependent diabetes mellitus, 477-478
insulins, 478-481
investigational, 484
non–insulin dependent diabetes mellitus, 478
nursing process and, 485-487
oral, 481-484
pancreas and, 476
Hypogonadism
androgens for, 449
estrogenic agents for, 425, 426
fertility agents for, 438
Hypokalemia, 268, 271, 413
Hypomagnesia, 797
Hyponatremia, 415
Hypoparathyroidism, 781, 782
Hypoproteinemia, 407
Hypotension
angiotensin-converting enzyme inhibitors and, 328
beta-agonists for, 526
vasoactive adrenergics for, 216
Hypotensive agents
ganglionic blockers and, 257
nonsteroidal antiinflammatory drugs and, 644
Hypothalamic-pituitary dopamine system, 181
Hypothalamus, 454-455
Hypothalamus-pituitary-adrenal axis, 490-491
Hypothyroidism, 271, 466, 468
Hypotonic dehydration, 406
HypRho-D Mini-Dose; *see* Rh₀ immune globulin
Hytakerol; *see* Dihydrotachysterol
Hytrin; *see* **terazosin**

I

ibuprofen, 644, 646
idarubicin, 693
IDDM; *see* Insulin-dependent diabetes mellitus
Idiopathic asthma, 521
Idiopathic hypertension, 321
Idiopathic thrombocytopenic purpura, 669, 672
Idiosyncratic drug reaction, 22
idoxuridine, 577, 578, 866
ifosfamide, 685
Iletin, 479, 480
Ilotycin; *see* **erythromycin**
Imdur; *see* **isosorbide mononitrate**
Imidazoles, 599
imipenem-cilastatin, 568, 579

Immune globulin, 672
hepatitis B, 672
Rh₀, 669, 673
tetanus, 670, 673
Immune system, 656
antihistamines and, 506
biologic response modifiers, 710-724
colony-stimulating factors, 718, 719-722
interferons, 712-716
interleukins, 717-719
nursing process and, 722-723
cancer and, 681
cell-mediated, 666
immunizing agents, 663-675
active immunization and, 664-665
bacille Calmette-Guérin, 668, 669
diphtheria and tetanus, 668-670
Haemophilus influenzae, 669, 670-671
hepatitis B, 669, 671, 672
immune globulin, 672-673
measles, mumps, and rubella, 669, 671
nursing process and, 673-675
passive immunization, 665-666
polio, 669, 671, 672
immunosuppressant agents, 656-662
azathioprine, 658
cyclosporin A, 658-659
muromonab-CD3, 659
nursing process and, 660-661
Immunity, 664-666
Immunization, 664-666
Immunizing agents, 663-675
active immunization and, 664-665
bacille Calmette-Guérin, 668, 669
diphtheria and tetanus, 668-670
Haemophilus influenzae, 669, 670-671
hepatitis B, 669, 671, 672
immune globulin, 672-673
measles, mumps, and rubella, 669, 671
nursing process and, 673-675
passive immunization, 665-666
polio, 669, 671, 672
Immunizing biologicals, 664
Immunodeficiency diseases, 669, 672
Immunoglobulin, 666
Immunoglobulin E, 521
Immunosuppressant agents, 656-662
azathioprine, 658
cyclosporin A, 658-659
muromonab-CD3, 659
nursing process and, 660-661
Imodium; *see* **loperamide**
Implantation of ovum, 422
Implementation in nursing process, 10-11
Imuran; *see* **azathioprine**
Increased work load, 266
indapamide, 396
Inderal; *see* **propranolol**
Indirect-acting antiasthmatic agents, 531-532
Indirect-acting cholinergic drugs, 240
Indirect-acting miotics, 852-853
Indirect-acting sympathomimetics, 209
Indocin; *see* **indomethacin**
indomethacin, 644, 646
angiotensin-converting enzyme inhibitors and, 328
interleukins and, 718
loop diuretics and, 390
Infant
drug effects on, 26-27
enteral nutrition supplements for, 807
general anesthesia and, 116
recommended daily dietary allowances, 778
Infection, 543-544
INFeD; *see* **iron dextran**
Infertility, 436-439
Infiltrating IV, 64
Infiltration anesthesia, 113
Inflammation
leukocytes and, 529
nonsteroidal antiinflammatory drugs for, 640

Influenza, 509
Influenza A, 578, 580
Informed consent, 37-38
Inhalation of drug, 16
Inhaled corticosteroids, 529
Inhaled general anesthetics, 107
Injection
    preparing from ampules and vials, 55-58
    sites for, 59-61
Inner ear, 878
Inotropes, 211, 265, 283
Insecticide poisoning, 250
Insulin, 478-481
    fixed-combination, 481
    intermediate-acting, 479-480
    long-acting, 480-481
    pancreatic secretion of, 476
    rapid-acting, 479, 480
Insulin syringe, 52
insulin zinc, 480
Insulin-dependent diabetes mellitus, 477-478
Intal; *see* **cromolyn**
Integumentary system; *see* Skin
Intensol; *see* Dihydrotachysterol
Intercalation, 692
Intercostal nerve block, 114
Interferon alfa-2a, 715
Interferon alfa-2b, 715
Interferon alfa-n3, 715
Interferon beta-1B, 715
Interferon gamma-1b, 716
Interferons, 712-716
Interleukin-2, 657, 717-719
Interleukin-3, 719
Intermediate-acting insulin, 479-480
Intermediate-density lipoprotein, 368-369
International Classification of Seizures, 136, 137
International units, 47
Internodal pathway, 279
Interstitial fluid, 404, 405
Intestinal candidiasis, 603
Intestinal flora modifiers, 747-752
Intestine, drug excretion and, 18
Intracellular fluid, 404
Intradermal injection
    administration of, 62-64
    sites for, 59-61
Intralipid, 811
Intramuscular injection, 14
    administration of, 62-64
    sites for, 59-61
Intranasal steroids, 510
Intraocular pressure
    beta-blockers and, 855-856
    carbonic anhydrase inhibitors and, 857
    glaucoma and, 847
    indirect-acting miotics and, 849
    osmotic diuretics and, 859
    sympathomimetic agents and, 853
Intravascular fluid, 405
Intravenous administration
    adding medications to IV fluid containers, 69-70
    anesthetic agents, 107, 108
    bolus, 67-69
    heparin, 361
    by piggyback or volume administration sets, 65-66
Intrinsic asthma, 521
Intrinsic factor, 791, 792
Intrinsic sympathomimetic activity, 230
Intron A; *see* Interferon alfa-2b
Intropin; *see* Dopamine
Inversine; *see* **mecamylamine**
Investigational new drug, 37
Iodinated glycerol, 514
Iodine, 795
    compounds for antisepsis, 631, 632-633
    recommended daily dietary allowances, 778
Iodophors, 633
iodoquinol, 613-616, 617
Ion-exchange resins, 371

Ionizing radiation, 681
Iopidine; *see* **apraclonidine**
Ipecac syrup, 514
ipratropium bromide, 528
Iris, 845
Iron, 795, 820-822
    deficiency of, 823
    recommended daily dietary allowances, 778
iron dextran, 822
Irreversible cholinesterase inhibitors, 240
Irritable bowel syndrome, 250
Ischemia, 301
Ischemic heart disease, 301
Islets of Langerhans, 476
Ismelin; *see* **guanethidine**
ISMO; *see* **isosorbide mononitrate**
Isocal, 806
isoetharine, 214, 525
isoflurane, 110, 111
isoflurophate, 850, 852
isoniazid, 588-592
    antifungal drugs and, 602
    enflurane and, 110
isophane insulin, 480
isopropanol, 630
Isopropyl alcohol, 630
isoproterenol, 214, 216, 217, 218-219, 525
Isoptin; *see* **verapamil**
Isopto Carpine; *see* **pilocarpine**
Isopto Eserine; *see* **physostigmine**
Isopto P-ES; *see* **physostigmine**
Isordil; *see* **isosorbide dinitrate**
isosorbide dinitrate, 304-305
isosorbide mononitrate, 305
Isospora belli, 612
Isotonic dehydration, 406
isradipine, 311
Isuprel; *see* **isoproterenol**
Itching, 168
itraconazole, 579, 600
Iveegam; *see* Immune globulin

J

Jejunostomy, 805
Jelly, 831
Jimsonweed, 249
Jock itch, 833
Joint National Committee on Detection, Evaluation, and Treatment of High Blood Pressure, 321
Justice, 40

K

Kabikinase; *see* **streptokinase**
Kaliuretic diuretics, 392
kanamycin, 560, 589, 590
Kaopectate; *see* **attapulgite**
Kaposi's sarcoma
    interferon for, 714, 716
    mitotic inhibitors for, 696
Kappa opioid receptor, 92
Kasof; *see* Docusate salts
Kawasaki syndrome, 672
Kefauver-Harris Amendment, 36
Keflex; *see* **cephalexin**
Keftab; *see* **cephalexin**
Kefurox; *see* **cefuroxime**
Kefzol; *see* **cefazolin sodium**
Keratitis, 580, 856, 862, 863
Keratoconjunctivitis, 580, 870
Keratolytics, 832, 840
Ketalar; *see* **ketamine**
ketamine, 108
ketoconazole, 600
    didanosine and, 579
    mitotic inhibitors and, 697
    topical, 834
Ketones, 477

ketorolac, 645, 646-647, 868
Kidney
    cancer of, 429
    carbonic anhydrase system in, 387
    changes in geriatric patient, 29
    diuretics, 384-402
        carbonic anhydrase inhibitors, 387-388, 858
        for hypertension, 330
        loop, 388-390
        nursing care plan for, 401
        nursing process and, 398-399
        osmotic, 390-392, 859-861
        patient teaching, 333
        potassium-sparing, 328, 392-394
        renal function and, 385-386
        thiazide, 395-397
    drug excretion and, 17-18
    fluids and electrolytes, 403-420
        blood products, 410-412
        colloids, 408-410
        crystalloids, 406-408
        nursing process and, 416-418
        physiology of fluid balance, 404-406
        plasma protein fractions, 411-412
        potassium, 412-414
        sodium, 415-416
    function of, 385-386
    interactions and adverse effects
        antifungals and, 601
        antitubercular agents and, 593
        immunosuppressants and, 658
        interferons and, 714
        nonsteroidal antiinflammatory drugs and, 641
    neonatal and pediatric pharmacokinetic considerations, 27
    tumor origin in, 678
Kinesed; *see* Belladonna alkaloids
Klebsiella
    aminoglycosides for, 559
    sulfonamides for, 546
Klonopin; *see* **clonazepam**
Konakion; *see* Vitamin K
Kondremul; *see* Mineral oil
Kraurosis vulvae, 425, 426
Kwell; *see* **lindane**
Kytril; *see* **granisetron**

L

labetalol, 233, 234
Labor and delivery drugs, 431-436
    uterine relaxants, 434-436
    uterine stimulants, 431-434
Lacrimal caruncle, 845
Lacrimal glands, 845-846
Lactated Ringer's solution, 407, 408
Lactic acid, 630
Lactobacillus acidophilus, 750, 751-752
Lactulose, 758
LAK cell; *see* Lymphokine-activated killer cell
Lamisil; *see* **terbinafine**
Laniazid; *see* **isoniazid**
Lanocaine; *see* **benzocaine**
Lanosterol, 599
LanoxiCaps; *see* **digoxin**
Lanoxin; *see* **digoxin**
Lariam; *see* **mefloquine**
Lasix; *see* **furosemide**
Lassa virus, 578
Lateral canthus, 845
Latin terms and abbreviations, 45
Laughing gas, 110, 111
Laxatives, 752-762
    bulk-forming, 755-756
    cardiac glycosides and, 268
    emollient, 756-758
    hyperosmotic, 758-759
    narcotic analgesics and, 94
    nursing process and, 760-762

Laxatives—cont'd
  saline, 759
  stimulant, 759-760
Lax-Pills; *see* **phenolphthalein**
Ledercillin VK; *see* **penicillin V potassium**
Lee-White whole blood clotting time, 362
Left ventricular end-diastolic volume, 265
Legal issues, 39, 40, 64
Legend drugs, 36
Lennox-Gastaut seizure, 141
Lens, 846
Lente insulin, 479-480
Lescol; *see* **fluvastatin**
Leukemia, 678-679
  alkylating agents for, 685, 687
  antimetabolites for, 689, 691
  cytotoxic antibiotics for, 693, 695
  mitotic inhibitors for, 696, 698
Leukine; *see* **sargramstim**
Leukocyte, 528-530
Levlen, 431
levodopa, 153-155
  antiemetics and, 769
  selegiline with, 151
levodopa-carbidopa, 155
Levophed; *see* Norepinephrine
levorphanol, 100
Levothroid; *see* **levothyroxine**
levothyroxine, 469
Levoxine; *see* **levothyroxine**
Librium; *see* **chlordiazepoxide**
Lice, 836
Licensure, 40
lidocaine, 112, 113, 114, 287-288
  dosage range, 285
  indications for, 282
  management of overdose, 283
lincomycin, 573
lindane, 836
liothyronine, 469
liotrix, 469
Lipid emulsions, 811
Lipids, 368-371
Lipolysis, 230
Lipophylicity, 231
Lipoprotein lipase, 375
Lipoproteins, 368
Liposyn, 811
Liquaemin sodium; *see* **heparin**
Liquid systems of measurement, 46
lisinopril, 327
lithium, 191
  angiotensin-converting enzyme inhibitors and,
    328
  carbonic anhydrase inhibitors and, 858
  loop diuretics and, 390
  pituitary drugs and, 458
  potassium-sparing diuretics and, 393
Liver
  acetaminophen and, 650
  antiseptic and disinfectant agents and, 630
  antitubercular agents and, 593
  barbiturates and, 123-124
  biotransformation and, 17
  cancer of, 689
  changes in geriatric patient, 29
  crystalloid solutions for hepatic failure, 407
  diuretics for disease, 389, 390
  immunosuppressants and, 658
  insulin and, 476
  interferons and, 714
  lipid metabolism and, 368-369
  nonsteroidal antiinflammatory drugs and,
    641
  peliosis of, 447
LMD; *see* Dextran
Local anesthetics, 111-114, 880-881
Local treatment, 668
Lofen; *see* **diphenoxylate**
Logen; *see* **diphenoxylate**
lomefloxacin, 562

Lomenate; *see* **diphenoxylate**
Lomotil; *see* **diphenoxylate**
lomustine, 685, 705
Lonalac, 806
Long-acting insulin, 480-481
Loniten; *see* **minoxidil**
Loop diuretics, 388-390
Loop of Henle, 386
Lo/Orval, 431
loperamide, 750, 751
Lopid; *see* **gemfibrozil**
Lopressor; *see* **metoprolol**
Loprox; *see* **ciclopirox olamine**
loratadine, 505, 507-508
lorazepam
  for anxiety, 168, 169
  in status epilepticus, 139, 142
Lorelco; *see* **probucol**
Lotensin; *see* **benazepril**
Lotion, 831
Lotrimin; *see* **clotrimazole**
lovastatin, 374
Low-density lipoprotein, 368-369
  bile acid sequestrants and, 371
  fibric acid derivatives and, 374-375
  HMG-CoA reductase inhibitors and, 373
  nicotinic acid and, 377
  probucol and, 378
Lower respiratory tract, 520
loxapine, 185
Loxitane; *see* **loxapine**
Lozol; *see* **indapamide**
Lubricant laxatives, 753
Lumbar anesthesia, 114
Lung; *see also* Respiratory system
  antifungals and, 601
  cancer of, 678
    alkylating agents for, 685, 687
    antimetabolites for, 689
    cytotoxic antibiotics for, 695
    interleukin-2 for, 717
    mitotic inhibitors for, 696, 698
  cholinergic agents and, 241
Luteinizing hormone
  function of, 456
  ovulation and, 423
Lyme disease
  macrolides for, 564
  tetracyclines for, 557
Lymphocyte, 529
Lymphogranuloma venereum, 557
Lymphokine-activated killer cell, 717
Lymphokines, 717
Lymphoma, 678-679
  alkylating agents for, 685, 687
  cytotoxic antibiotics for, 693, 695
  mitotic inhibitors for, 696
Lymphosarcoma
  alkylating agents for, 687
  cytotoxic antibiotics for, 693, 695
  mitotic inhibitors for, 698
Lyphocin; *see* **vancomycin**
lypressin, 457, 460, 461, 462
Lysol, 633
Lysozyme, 846

M

Maalox; *see* Aluminum-containing antacids
Macrocytic anemia, 820
Macrolides, 564-566
  assessment of, 570-571
  ocular, 864
Macrominerals, 795
mafenide, 837
Magnacal, 806
Magnesium, 778, 795, 797-798
Magnesium citrate, 759
Magnesium hydroxide, 759

Magnesium laxatives, 759
Magnesium salts, 759
Magnesium-containing antacids, 733-735
Mag-Ox; *see* Magnesium-containing antacids
Maintenance therapy, 21
Malaria, 546, 608-612
Malassezia furfur, 598
Male reproductive agents, 445-451
Male reproductive system, 445-446
Malignancy, 678
Malignant hyperthermia, 117
Malignant neoplasm, 678
Malnutrition, 804
Malpractice, 40
Manganese, 795
Mania, 164, 184
mannitol, 390-392, 860-861
Marijuana, 767
Marinol; *see* **dronabinol**
Mast cell stabilizers, 531
Mathematical calculations, 44-48
Maxair; *see* **pirbuterol**
Maxaquin; *see* **lomefloxacin**
Maxolon; *see* **metoclopramide**
MCT Oil, 806, 808
Measles, 669, 672
Measles vaccine, 669, 671
mebendazole, 618, 619, 620
mecamylamine, 258
Mechanism of action, 19-20
mechlorethamine, 685, 686-688, 702, 704
meclizine, 509, 769
meclofenamic acid, 647, 648
Meclomen; *see* **meclofenamic acid**
Medial canthus, 845
Medication history, 9
Medication order, 50-51
Medication record, 51
Medihaler-Epi; *see* **epinephrine**
Medihaler-Iso; *see* **isoproterenol**
Medilax; *see* **phenolphthalein**
medroxyprogesterone, 428, 429
mefenamic acid, 647, 648
mefloquine, 609, 610-612
Mefoxin; *see* **cefoxitin**
Megace; *see* **megestrol**
megestrol, 428
Melanoma
  alkylating agents for, 685
  cytotoxic antibiotics for, 693, 695
  interferon for, 714
  interleukin-2 for, 717
  mitotic inhibitors for, 696
melphalan, 685
Memory cell, 712
Menadione, 785-786
Menaquinone, 785-786
Menarche, 422
Menest; *see* Esterified estrogens
Meningitis, 603
Menopause, 422, 425, 426
Menotropins, 439
Menses, 424
Menstrual cycle, 422-423
meperidine, 98
  administration guidelines, 100
  as anesthetic adjuvant, 108
  dosage, 96
  monoamine oxidase inhibitors and, 174
Mephyton; *see* Vitamin K
mepivacaine, 112
meprobamate, 168, 169
Mepron; *see* **atovaquone**
merbromin, 632
mercaptopurine, 691-692, 700
Mercurial agents, 632
Meritene, 806
Merthiolate; *see* **thimerosal**
Mesocortical dopamine system, 181
Mesolimbic dopamine system, 181
Mestinon; *see* **pyridostigmine**

Metabolic system
  antiprotozoal agents and, 614
  antipsychotic agents and, 182
  calcium salts and, 796
  carbonic anhydrase inhibitors and, 858
  chronic salicylate intoxication and, 642
  cyanocobalamin and, 792
  insulin and, 479
  penicillins and, 549
  thiazide diuretics and, 395
  tocolytic agents and, 435
  vitamin A and, 780
  vitamin E and, 784
Metabolism of drug, 16-17
  geriatric considerations, 30
  neonatal and pediatric considerations, 27
Metahydrin; *see* **trichlormethiazide**
Metamucil; *see* Psyllium
Metaprel; *see* **metaproterenol**
metaproterenol, 525, 527
Metastasis, 678
methadone hydrochloride, 96, 98, 100
methamphetamine, 213
methdilazine, 509
Methemoglobinemia, 303
Methergine; *see* **methylergonovine**
methicillin, 550, 551
methimazole, 470, 471
methohexital, 108
methotrexate, 690-691
  antidiarrheals and, 749
  asparaginase and, 700
  assessment of, 701-702
  interleukins and, 718
  mitotic inhibitors and, 697
  nursing implications, 704
methoxyflurane, 110, 111
methyclothiazide, 396
Methycobalamin, 791
Methyl violet, 632
1-Methyl-4-phenyl-1,2,3,6-tetrahydropyridine, 149, 151
1-Methyl-4-phenylpyridine, 149, 151
methylcellulose, 756
methyldopa, 438
methylergonovine, 433-434
methylphenidate hydrochloride, 200-201, 213, 215
methylprednisolone, 492
methyltestosterone, 448
Meticorten; *see* **prednisone**
metoclopramide, 771
metolazone, 396, 397
metoprolol, 233, 234, 282, 290
  for angina, 307-308
  dosage range, 286
Metric 21; *see* **metronidazole**
Metric system, 46
metronidazole, 613-616, 617
Mevacor; *see* **lovastatin**
mexiletine, 288
  dosage range, 285
  indications for, 282
  management of overdose, 283
Mexitil; *see* **mexiletine**
Mextard, 481
mezlocillin, 552
MicaTin; *see* **miconazole**
Mickey Finn, 130
miconazole, 600, 833-834
MICRhoGam; *see* Rh$_0$ immune globulin
Microcytic anemia, 819
Microlipid, 806, 808
Microminerals, 795
Micronase; *see* **glyburide**
Microorganisms, 543-544
  antimicrobial agents and, 628
  immune system and, 656
Microsporum, 598
Midamor; *see* **amiloride**
midazolam, 108

Middle ear disorders, 879
Migraine, 233
Mild hypertension, 321
Milk of magnesia, 735, 759
Milliequivalents, 47
Miltown; *see* **meprobamate**
Mineral oil, 347, 756-758
Mineralocorticoids, 490, 491
Minerals, 794-798
  nursing process and, 799-802
  recommended daily dietary allowances, 778
Minipress; *see* **prazosin**
minoxidil, 331, 332, 836-837
Miochol; *see* Acetylcholine
Miotics, 846, 850
Miradon; *see* **anisindione**
misoprostol, 641, 740
mitomycin, 693
Mitosis, 681
mitotane, 700
Mitotic index, 681
Mitotic inhibitors, 695-698
  etoposide, 697-698
  paclitaxel, 698
  vincristine, 698
mitoxantrone, 693
Mixed-acting sympathomimetic, 209
MMR II; *see* Measles vaccine
Moban; *see* **molindone**
Modane; *see* **phenolphthalein**
Modane Soft; *see* Docusate salts
Modular formulations, 806, 808
Mold, 598
molindone, 185
Molybdenum, 795
Monistat; *see* **miconazole**
Monitoring, 21-23
Monoamine oxidase, 209
Monoamine oxidase inhibitors
  adrenergic agents and, 212, 324
  anticholinergics and, 249
  antidepressants and, 173-176
  antidiarrheals and, 749
  barbiturates and, 124
  benzodiazepines and, 128, 167
  central nervous system stimulants and, 197
  dopaminergic agents and, 154
  hydralazine and, 331
  narcotic analgesics and, 95
  nasal decongestants and, 511
  in Parkinson's disease, 150-152
Monoclonal antibody, 712
Monocyte, 529
Monoket; *see* **isosorbide mononitrate**
Monophasic oral contraceptives, 431
Monopril; *see* **fosinopril**
moricizine, 282, 283
morphine, 95
  administration guidelines, 100
  as anesthetic adjuvant, 108
  dosage, 96
Mosquito bite, 608
Motilin, 564
Motion sickness, 250, 507, 770
Motrin; *see* **ibuprofen**
MPP; *see* 1-Methyl-4-phenylpyridine
MPTP; *see* 1-Methyl-4-phenyl-1,2,3,6-tetrahydropyridine
MRVAX II; *see* Measles vaccine
Mu opioid receptor, 92
Mucoid cell, 729-731
Mucus
  expectorants and, 514
  sucralfate and, 739
Multi-drug resistant tuberculosis, 588
Multipax; *see* **hydroxyzine**
Multiple myeloma
  alkylating agents for, 685, 687
  antimetabolites for, 689
  interferon for, 714

Multiple sclerosis
  interferon for, 714, 716
  pituitary drugs for, 459
Mumps vaccine, 669, 671
Murine; *see* **tetrahydrozoline**
Murine antibody, 659
Murine Ear Drops; *see* **carbamide peroxide**
Muro 128; *see* Hyperosmolar sodium chloride
muromonab-CD3, 659
Muscarinic receptors, 182, 239-240
Muscle
  adrenergic receptor responses to stimulation, 207
  aging and, 30
  cholinergic agents and, 241
Muscle spasm
  antianxiety agents for, 167
  diazepam for, 167
Musculoskeletal system
  antithyroid drugs and, 470
  corticosteroids and, 493
  vitamin A and, 780
  vitamin D and, 783
  vitamin E and, 784
Mustargen; *see* **mechlorethamine**
Mustine; *see* **mechlorethamine**
Mutagen, 23
Myambutol; *see* **ethambutol**
Myasthenia gravis
  cholinergic agents for, 241, 242
  pituitary drugs for, 459
  potassium replacement therapy in, 413
Mycelex; *see* **clotrimazole**
Mycelium, 598
Mycobacterium tuberculosis, 587-590
Mycoplasma
  macrolides for, 564
  tetracyclines for, 557
Mycosis, 598
Mycosis fungoides
  alkylating agents for, 687
  antimetabolites for, 691
  mitotic inhibitors for, 696
Mycostatin; *see* **nystatin**
Mydriasis
  anticholinergics and, 247
  ganglionic blockers and, 257
Mydriatics, 846, 854, 874
Mykrox; *see* **metolazone**
Mylanta; *see* Aluminum-containing antacids
Myocardial deficiency, 266
Myocardial infarction
  antidysrhythmic agents for, 286
  antiplatelet agents for, 352
  beta-blockers for, 233, 306
  digitalis toxicity and, 271
  streptokinase for, 356
  thrombolytic agents for, 358
  thrombolytics for, 358
Myochrysine; *see* **gold sodium thiomalate**
Myoclonic seizure, 141
Mysoline; *see* **primidone**
Myxedema, 468

N

nabumetone, 647, 648
nadolol, 308
naftifine, 834
Naftin; *see* **naftifine**
nalbuphine, 98, 100
naloxone hydrochloride, 94, 96, 98, 100
naltrexone hydrochloride, 94, 96, 99
naphazoline, 510, 511
Naphthalene dye, 680
Naqua; *see* **trichlormethiazide**
Narcan; *see* **naltrexone hydrochloride**
Narcolepsy, 196, 198, 213
Narcotic analgesic agents, 88-105
  agonist-antagonist, 98
  antidiarrheals and, 749

Narcotic analgesic agents—cont'd
  antiemetics and, 769
  barbiturates and, 124
  chemical structure of, 92
  clonidine and, 324
  codeine sulfate, 95
  dosages, 95, 96
  fentanyl, 97-98
  laxatives and, 756
  mechanism of action, 92
  meperidine hydrochloride, 98
  methadone hydrochloride, 98
  morphine sulfate, 95
  naloxone hydrochloride, 98
  naltrexone hydrochloride, 99
  nursing process and, 99-103
  physiology and psychology of pain, 89-92
  propoxyphene hydrochloride, 98
  side and adverse effects, 93-94
  therapeutic uses, 93
  toxicity and overdose, 94-95
Narcotic antagonists, 98-99
  naloxone hydrochloride, 98
  naltrexone hydrochloride, 99
Narcotic withdrawal, 94-95
Nardil; see phenelzine
Nasal decongestants, 217, 510-511
Nasal drops, 82
Nasalchrom; see cromolyn
Nasalide; see flunisolide
Nasoduodenal tube feeding, 805
Nasogastric tube
  drug administration via, 83-85
  feeding through, 805, 814
Nasojejunal tube feeding, 805
Natacyn; see natamycin
natamycin
  ocular, 864
  topical, 834
National Cholesterol Education Program, 370-371
National High Blood Pressure Coordinating
    Committee, 320-321
Natural killer cell, 713
Naturally acquired passive immunity, 666
Naturetin; see bendroflumethiazide
Nausea, 764-774
  antiemetic agents for, 765-769, 765-771
    anticholinergic, 769
    neuroleptic, 769-771
    prokinetic, 771
    serotonin blockers, 771
  antipsychotic agents for, 184
  hydroxyzine for, 168
  nursing process in, 772-774
Navane; see thiothixene
NCEP; see National Cholesterol Education Program
ND27; see tolnaftate
Nebupent; see pentamidine
nedocromil, 531-532
Negative chronotropic effect, 266
Negative dromotropic effect, 266
Negative feedback, hormone secretion and, 455
Negligence, 40
Nelova LO/11, 431
Nematode, 618
Nembutal; see pentobarbital
neomycin, 560, 880
Neonate
  diuretic therapy and, 398
  drug effects on, 26-27
  general anesthesia and, 116
  pulmonary hypertension in, 229
  sepsis in, 672
Neoplasm, 678
Neosar; see cyclophosphamide
neostigmine, 283
Neosynephrine; see phenylephrine
Nephron, 385
Nephropathy, diabetic, 477
Nephrosis, 407
Nephrotic syndrome, 390

Nerve block, 113
Nerve fiber
  pain and, 90-91
  stimulation of, 208
  tumor origin in, 678
netilmicin sulfate, 560
Neupogen; see filgrastim
Neuroblastoma
  alkylating agents for, 687
  cytotoxic antibiotics for, 693, 695
  mitotic inhibitors for, 696, 698
Neuroeffector junction, 209
Neuroendocrine system, 455
Neurohypophysis, 455
Neuroleptic agents, 766, 769-771
Neuromuscular blocking agents
  antidiarrheals and, 749
  beta-blockers and, 232
  ganglionic blockers and, 257
  laxatives and, 756
  reversal of, 250
Neuron
  antiepileptic drugs and, 138
  Parkinson's disease and, 149
Neuropathy, diabetic, 477
Neuroprotective therapy, 150-152
Neurotin; see gabapentin
Neurotransmitters
  antidepressants and, 170
  ganglionic blockers and, 256-257
  in nausea and vomiting, 765
  pain and, 91
  Parkinson's disease and, 149
Neutral protamine Hagedorn insulin, 479-480
Neutropenia, 718
Neutrophil, 529
New drug application, 38
New drug development, 36-38
Nia-Bid; see Niacin
Niac; see Niacin
Niacels; see Niacin
Niacin, 788-790
  as lipid-lowering agent, 376-378
  recommended daily dietary allowances, 778
Niacinamide, 789
Niacor; see Niacin
Niaplus; see Niacin
nicardipine, 311
Niclocide; see niclosamide
niclosamide, 619, 620
Nico-400; see Niacin
Nicobid; see Niacin
Nicolar; see Nicotinic acid
Nicor; see Nicotinic acid
Nicotinamide adenine dinucleotide, 788
Nicotinamide adenine dinucleotide phosphate, 788
Nicotinex; see Niacin
Nicotinic acid, 376-378
Nicotinic receptors, 239
NIDDM; see Non–insulin dependent diabetes
    mellitus
nifedipine, 311
Nightshade, 249
Nigrostriatal dopamine system, 181
Nilstat; see nystatin
nimodipine, 311
Nimotop; see nimodipine
Nipride; see Sodium nitroprusside
Nitrates
  for angina, 302-305
  clonidine and, 324
  patient teaching, 315
nitric oxide, 110, 111
Nitrites, 302-305
Nitro-bid; see nitroglycerin
nitrofurantoin, 756
nitrofurazone, 837
Nitrogen mustard; see mechlorethamine
nitroglycerin, 303-304
Nitrong; see nitroglycerin
Nitropress; see sodium nitroprusside

Nitrosoureas, 685, 705
Nitrostat; see nitroglycerin
nizatidine, 736
Nizoral; see ketoconazole
Nocardiosis, 546, 547
Noctec; see chloral hydrate
Nocturnal enuresis, 459
Nö-Döz; see caffeine
Noncompetitive antagonist, 20
Nonessential amino acids, 810
Non-Hodgkin's lymphoma
  alkylating agents for, 687
  antimetabolites for, 689
  interleukin-2 for, 717
  mitotic inhibitors for, 696
Non–insulin dependent diabetes mellitus, 478
Nonmalfeasance, 40
Nonprescription drugs, 36
Non–rapid eye movement sleep, 121, 122
Nonseasonal asthma, 521
Nonsedating antihistamines, 506-508
Nonspecific beta-blockers, 230
Nonspecific interactions, 20
Nonsteroidal antiinflammatory drugs, 637-653
  acetaminophen, 650
  acetic acids, 646
  angiotensin-converting enzyme inhibitors and,
      328
  anticoagulants and, 347
  antigout agents, 647-649
  arachidonic acid pathway and, 638-639
  aspirin, 352, 645-646
  carboxylic acids, 643-645
  enolic acids, fenamic acids, and nonacidic
      compounds, 647
  geriatric complications, 31
  gold compounds, 649-650
  as narcotic analgesic adjuvants, 93
  nursing process and, 650-652
  ophthalmic, 866-871, 895
  penicillins and, 549
  propionic acids, 646-647
Norepinephrine, 207, 219
  adrenal medulla and, 490
  alpha-blockers and, 225
  for antidysrhythmic drug reversal, 283
  beta-blockers and, 230
  dosage, 216
  ganglionic blockers and, 256-257
norethindrone, 429
norfloxacin, 562
Norinyl, 431
Norlutate; see norethindrone
Norlutin; see norethindrone
Normal saline, 407, 408
Normochromic anemia, 820
Normodyne; see labetalol
Noroxin; see norfloxacin
Norpace; see disopyramide
nortriptyline, 173
Norvasc; see amlodipine
Nose
  antidiarrheals and, 748
  antiemetics and, 768
  antiprotozoal agents and, 614
  carbonic anhydrase inhibitors and, 858
  miotics and, 850
  osmotic diuretics and, 860
Nosocomial infection, 627
Novahistine DH; see codeine
Novocain; see procaine
Novolin, 481
NPH insulin; see Neutral protamine Hagedorn
    insulin
Nucleic acid, 424
Nupercainal; see dibrecaine
Nurse practice acts, 40
Nursing care plan
  asthma, 5334
  breast cancer, 708
  chest pain, 313-314

Nursing care plan—cont'd
  congestive heart failure, 270
  hypertension, 334-335
  peptic ulcer disease, 742
Nursing diagnosis, 9
Nursing process, 7-11
Nutrients, 804
Nutritional supplements, 803-815
  enteral nutrition, 804-808
  nursing process and, 813-815
  parenteral nutrition, 808-813
Nutritional support, 804
Nutropin; see somatropin
Nydrazid; see isoniazid
Nystat; see nystatin
nystatin, 600, 602-603, 834
Nystex; see nystatin

O

Obesity
  amphetamines for, 213
  central nervous system stimulants for, 198
Objective data, 9
Obsessive-compulsive disorder, 165
Occupational carcinogen, 680
OCL; see polyethylene glycol
Octamide; see metoclopramide
octreotide, 457, 462
Ocu-Chlor; see chloramphenicol
Ocufen Liquifilm; see flurbiprofen
Ocular antiinfectives, 861-866
Ocular hypertension, 857
Ocu-Mycin; see erythromycin
Ocusert Pilo; see pilocarpine
ofloxacin, 562
Ogen; see estropipate
Oil, 831
Ointment, 80, 831
OKT3; see muromonab-CD3
omeprazole, 602, 738
Omnipen; see anhydrous ampicillin
Omnipen-N; see sodium ampicillin
Oncogenic virus, 680
Oncovin; see vincristine
ondansetron, 771
Onset of drug, 19
Open-angle glaucoma, 387, 388, 849, 855, 857
Operand; see povidone-iodine
Ophthalgan; see glycerin
Ophthalmia neonatorum, 863
Ophthalmic agents, 842-877
  administration of, 80
  adrenergic, 211
  antiglaucoma, 847-861
    beta-adrenergic blockers, 855-857
    carbonic anhydrase inhibitors, 857-859
    osmotic diuretics, 859-861
    parasympathomimetics, 848-853
    sympathomimetics, 853-855
  antiinfective, 861-866
  antiinflammatory, 866-869
  antiviral, 866
  eye structure, 844-847
  nursing process and, 871-876
  topical anesthetics, 869-870
Ophthalmic decongestants, 218
Ophthalmoscopic examination, 849-850
Opiates, 92, 747, 748, 751
Opioid abstinence syndrome, 94-95
Opioid tolerance, 94
Opioids, 92
  as anesthetic adjuvants, 108
  geriatric complications, 31
Opisthorchiasis, 621
Opticrom; see cromolyn; cromolyn sodium
Optimine; see azatadine
OPV; see Poliovirus vaccine
Oral candidiasis, 598, 603

Oral contraceptives, 430-431
  antifibrinolytics and, 355
  penicillins and, 549
Oral drug administration, 14-16, 78-79
Oral hypoglycemic agents, 481-484
  antifungal drugs and, 602
  beta-blockers and, 232
  thiazide diuretics and, 396
Orasone; see prednisone
Oreton-M; see methyltestosterone
Orimune; see Poliovirus vaccine
Oropharyngeal candidiasis, 603, 834
OROS; see Osmotically released oral system
Orthoclone OKT3; see muromonab-CD3
Ortho-Novum, 431
Orthostatic hypertension, 229, 324
Orval, 431
Osmitrol; see mannitol
Osmoglyn; see glycerin
Osmolite, 806
Osmotic diuretics, 390-392, 859-861, 874
Osmotic pressure, 405
Osmotically released oral system, 142
Osteoarthritis, 640, 641, 647
Osteomalacia, 781
Osteoporosis, 425, 426
Otic agents, 878-884
  antibacterial and antifungal, 879-880
  local anesthetic, 880-881
  nursing process and, 881-883
Otitis media, 879, 882
Outcome criteria in nursing process, 7, 9-10
Ova, 422
Ovarian cancer
  alkylating agents for, 685, 687
  altretamine for, 701
  antimetabolites for, 689
  interleukin-2 for, 717
  mitotic inhibitors for, 696, 698
Ovarian failure, 425, 426
Ovary, 422
Over-the-counter drugs
  antihistamines, 508
  artificial tears, 870
  caffeine-containing, 199
  Durham-Humphrey Amendment and, 36
  polypharmacy and, 28
Overton-Meyer theory, 107-108
oxamnoquine, 618, 619
oxazolidinediones, 139, 140
oxiconazole nitrate, 834
Oxidizing agents, 633
Oxistat; see oxiconazole nitrate
oxtriphylline, 523
oxycodone, 100
Oxygen therapy, 117
Oxygen-carrying resuscitation fluids, 410-412
oxymetazoline, 510
oxymorphone, 98, 100
oxyphenbutazone
  cardiac glycosides and, 268
  loop diuretics and, 390
Oxytocic agents, 226, 432
Oxytocin, 434, 456

P

Pacemaker, digitalis toxicity and, 271
Pacemaker activity, 279
Pacific yew tree derivative, 696
Packed red blood cells, 410, 411, 412
paclitaxel, 698
Pain
  anginal, 301
  nonsteroidal antiinflammatory drugs for, 640
  physiology and psychology of, 89-92
Pain threshold, 89-90
Pain tolerance, 90
Painkillers, 89; see also Analgesics

Palliative therapy, 21
Palpebral fissure, 844
Pamelor; see nortriptyline
Pancreas, 476
Pancreatic cancer
  antimetabolites for, 689
  cytotoxic antibiotics for, 693, 695
Panic disorder, 165
Papillomavirus, 714
para-aminosalicylic acid, 589, 590
Paracervical obstetrical analgesia, 114
Paraneoplastic syndrome, 679
Parasites, 608, 612
Parasympathetic nervous system, 239-240
  cholinergic-blocking agents and, 247
  nicotinic receptor and, 256
Parasympatholytics, 246-254
  as anesthetic adjuvants, 108
  atropine, 250-251
  beta-blockers and, 232, 307
  cholinergic agents and, 242
  cyclic antidepressants and, 172
  decongestant, 510
  dicyclomine, 251
  geriatric complications, 31
  glycopyrrolate, 251
  for nausea and vomiting, 766, 769
  nursing process and, 251-253
  in Parkinson's disease, 156-158, 159
  scopolamine, 251
Parasympathomimetic agents, 238-246
  antiglaucoma, 848-853
  nursing process and, 243-245
  parasympathetic nervous system and, 239-240
Paravertebral nerve block, 114
Parenteral anesthetics, 111, 112
Parenteral nutrition, 808-813
Parenteral route, 14
Parietal cell, 729-731
Parkinson's disease, 148-161
  antiparkinsonian agents for, 150-158
  nursing process in, 158-161
Parlodel; see bromocriptine
Parnate; see tranylcypromine
paromomycin, 613-616, 617
paromomycin sulfate, 560
paroxetine, 179
Paroxysmal atrial flutter, 286
Paroxysmal supraventricular tachycardia, 216, 282, 286
Partial agonist, 20, 92
Partial opiate agonists, 98
Partial seizure, 137, 141
Passive immunization, 664, 665-666
Passive immunizing agents, 667, 669, 671-673
Paste, 831
Patent ductus arteriosus, 644
Pathologic fungi, 598
Patient-controlled analgesia, 71-77
Paxil; see paroxetine
PBZ; see tripelennamine
PCA; see Patient-controlled analgesia
PD; see Parkinson's disease
Peak effect, 19
Pec-Dec, diethylcarbamazine
Pediazole; see sulfisoxazole
Pediculosis, 836
PEG; see polyethylene glycol
Peliosis of liver, 447
Pellagra, 788, 789-790
Penetrex; see enoxacin
penicillin G, 549-551
penicillin G benzathine, 549, 550
penicillin G potassium, 549, 550
penicillin G procaine, 549, 550
penicillin G sodium, 549, 550
penicillin V potassium, 550, 551
Penicillinase-resistant penicillins, 548, 550, 551
Penicillins, 547-552
  aminopenicillins, 548, 551
  assessment of, 570

Penicillins—cont'd
cephalosporins and, 552-553
extended-spectrum, 548, 551-552
implementation of, 571-572
natural, 549-551
nutritional supplements and, 807
penicillinase-resistant, 548, 550, 551
Penis
adrenergic receptor responses to stimulation, 207
cancer of, 693, 695
pentaerythritol tetranitrate, 305
Pentam; *see* **pentamidine**
pentamidine, 613-616, 617
Pentamycetin; *see* **chloramphenicol**
pentazocine, 98, 100
Penthrane; *see* **methoxyflurane**
pentobarbital, 108, 125, 126, 131
pentostatin, 693
Pentothal; *see* **thiopental**
pentoxifylline, 350, 353
Pen-Vee; *see* **penicillin V potassium**
Pepcid; *see* **famotidine**
Pepsin, 729-731
Peptic esophagitis
antacids for, 732
histamine₂ antagonists for, 735
Peptic ulcer, 729-730
antacids for, 732
anticholinergics for, 250
nursing care plan for, 742
sucralfate for, 739
tetracyclines for, 557
Pepto-Bismol; *see* **bismuth subsalicylate**
Percutaneous infiltration, 114
pergolide, 153, 155-156
Pergonal; *see* Menotropins
Periactin; *see* **cyproheptadine**
Pericardial effusion, 557
Peridem; *see* Psyllium
Peripheral arterial disease, 352
Peripheral total parenteral nutrition, 809-810
Peripherally acting adrenergic agents, 323, 325-326, 333
Peripherally acting antihistamines, 506-508
Peritrate; *see* **pentaerythritol tetranitrate**
Periwinkle plant, 695
Permax; *see* **pergolide**
Permissive hypothesis, 170
Pernicious anemia, 823
Persantine; *see* **dipyridamole**
Pharmaceutical abbreviations, 45
Pharmacodynamics, 19-20
Pharmacogenetics, 22
Pharmacognosy, 24
Pharmacokinetics, 13-19
absorption in, 13-16
distribution in, 16
excretion in, 17-18
geriatric considerations, 29-30
half-life in, 18-19
metabolism in, 16-17
neonatal and pediatric considerations, 26
onset, peak, and duration in, 19
Pharmacology, 2-85
cultural aspects, 41, 42
defined, 13
drug administration, 49-85
absorption and, 13-14
adding medications to IV fluid containers, 69-70
eardrops, 81
injections, 62-64
intravenous bolus, 67-69
intravenous medications by piggyback or volume administration sets, 65-66
medication orders and documentation, 50-51
nasal drops, 82
ophthalmic, 80

Pharmacology—cont'd
oral, 14-16, 78-79
patient-controlled analgesia, 71-77
preparing injections from ampules and vials, 55-58
sites for, 59-61
syringes for, 52-54
topical, 16
via nasogastric tube, 83-85
ethical practice, 39-42
legal issues, 39, 40
mathematical calculations, 44-48
medication administration, 7-11
neonatal, pediatric, and geriatric considerations, 25-33
pharmacodynamics, 19-20
pharmacognosy, 24
pharmacotherapeutics, 20-23
study skills for, 2-6
Pharmadine; *see* **povidone-iodine**
phenacetin, 680
phenelzine, 175-176
Phenergan; *see* **promethazine**
phenindamine, 505
phenobarbital, 124-126, 131
for epilepsy, 140, 143
in status epilepticus, 139
Phenobarbital coma, 123
Phenolic compounds, 633
phenolphthalein, 759-760
Phenothiazines, 183
anticholinergics and, 157, 249
beta-blockers and, 307
dopaminergic agents and, 154
effects of, 505
fertility agents and, 438
guanadrel and, 324
narcotic analgesics and, 95
patient teaching, 191
for psychosis, 183
Phenotyping, 370
phenoxybenzamine hydrochloride, 228, 229
phentolamine, 228, 229
Phenylalkylamines, 311
phenylbutazone, 268, 647, 648
Phenyl-E; *see* Vitamin E
phenylephrine, 216, 219, 510
phenylpropanolamine, 200, 324, 510
phenytoin
antidysrhythmic drugs and, 284
antifungal drugs and, 602
antitubercular drugs and, 591
for epilepsy, 141, 143-144
management of overdose, 283
mitotane and, 700
mitotic inhibitors and, 697
in status epilepticus, 139
Pheochromocytoma, 227, 233
Phlebitis, 809
Phobia, 165
Phosphajel; *see* Aluminum-containing antacids
Phosphate Respihaler; *see* **dexamethasone**
Phosphate Turbinase; *see* **dexamethasone**
Phospholine iodide; *see* **echothiophate**
Phospholipase, 867
Phosphorus, 778, 795, 798
Physical dependence, 22, 94-95
Physiologic changes in geriatric patient, 28-29
physostigmine, 242, 243, 850, 853
phytonadione, 346, 785-786
Pilocar; *see* **pilocarpine**
pilocarpine, 850, 851-852
Pilopine HS; *see* **pilocarpine**
Piperadines, 505
piperazine, 619
pipercillin, 552
pirbuterol, 525
piroxicam, 647, 648
Pitocin, 432
Pitressin; *see* Vasopressin

Pituitary agents, 454-464
endocrine system and, 454-455
nursing process and, 460-463
Pituitary gland, 454-455
Placebo, 38
Placebo-controlled study, 38
Planning in nursing process, 9
Plaque formation, atherosclerotic, 370
Plasbumin; *see* Albumin
Plasma, 405
Plasma cell, 712
Plasma expanders, 409
Plasma protein fractions, 410, 411-412
Plasma volume, 404
Plasmalyte, 407
Plasmin, 343, 356
Plasminogen, 343, 356
Plasmodium falciparum, 608, 609
Platelet, 348
Platinol; *see* **cisplatin**
Platyhelminthes infection, 618
Plendil; *see* **felodipine**
Pleural effusion, 557
plicamycin, 693
Plummer's disease, 466
Pneumocystis carinii pneumonia, 612, 616
Pneumocystosis, 612, 613
Podophyllotoxin derivatives, 696
Polaramine; *see* **dexchlorpheniramine**
Polio, 669
Poliovirus vaccine, 669, 671, 672
Polycillin; *see* **trihydrate ampicillin**
Polycose, 806, 808
Polycythemia vera, 687
Polydipsia, 476
Polyenes, 599
polyethylene glycol, 758
Polyfunctional alkylating agents, 684
Polygam; *see* Immune globulin
Polymeric formulations, 806, 807-808
polymyxin B
for ear disorders, 880
ocular, 864
Polypeptide antibiotics, ocular, 864
Polyphagia, 476
Polypharmacy, 28
polythiazide, 396
Polyuria, 476
Polyvinyl chloride, 680
Pondimin; *see* **fenfluramine**
Ponstel; *see* **mefenamic acid**
Pontocaine; *see* **tetracaine**
Pork tapeworm, 618
Porphyria, 184
Portagen, 806
Positive chronotropic effect, 210
Positive dromotropic effect, 210
Positive inotropic effect, 210, 266
Posterior horn of spinal cord, pain and, 90-91
Posterior pituitary, 455
Postpartum uterine atony and hemorrhage, 434
Posttraumatic stress disorder, 165
Postural instability in Parkinson's disease, 150
Potassium, 412-414, 795
Potassium iodide, 514
Potassium-sparing diuretics, 328, 392-394
povidone-iodine, 631, 633
Powder, 831
PPF; *see* Plasma protein fractions
pralidoxime, 850
pramoxine, 112, 880, 881
pravastatin, 373
praziquantel, 618, 619, 621
prazosin, 229-230, 324, 326
PRBCs; *see* Packed red blood cells
Precision LR, 806
prednisolone, 492
prednisone, 492, 493-495, 700
Pregnancy-related host factors, 545
Pregnyl; *see* Chorionic gonadotropin
Preinfarction angina, 301

Premarin, 424
Premature atrial contractions, 282
Premature birth, 439-440
Premature ventricular contractions, 233, 282
Prepodyne; *see* Iodophors
Prescription drugs, 36
Pressors, 211
Preterm labor, 436
Priapism, 447
Prilosec; *see* **omeprazole**
primaquine, 609, 610
Primary epilepsy, 136
Primary hypertension, 321
Primary nocturnal enuresis, 459
Primatene; *see* Epinephrine
Primaxin; *see* **imipenem-cilastatin**
primidone, 141
Principen; *see* **trihydrate ampicillin**
Prinivil; *see* **lisinopril**
Printer's ink, 680
Prinzmetal's angina, 301
Priscoline; *see* **tolazoline**
Privine; *see* **naphazoline**
probenecid, 648-649
    alkylating agents and, 687
    antidiarrheals and, 749
    antitubercular drugs and, 591
    penicillins and, 549
probucol, 378-379
procainamide, 284
    dosage range, 285
    indications for, 282
    management of overdose, 283
    reserpine and, 324
procaine, 112
Pro-Cal-Sof; *see* Docusate salts
Procan SR; *see* **procainamide**
procarbazine, 685
Procardia; *see* **nifedipine**
prochlorperazine, 769-771
Procrit; *see* **epoetin alfa**
Procytox; *see* **cyclophosphamide**
Pro-Depo; *see* **hydroxyprogesterone caproate**
Prodrug, 328
Profasi HP; *see* Chorionic gonadotropin
Progesterone, 427, 429
Progestins, 427-429, 441
Prokinetic agents, 767, 771
Prolactin, 456
Proleukin; *see* **aldesleukin**
Prolixin; *see* **fluphenazine**
Proloid; *see* **thyroglobulin**
promethazine, 108, 505, 509
Prompt insulin zinc, 480
Pronestyl; *see* **procainamide**
propafenone, 289
    dosage range, 286
    indications for, 282
    management of overdose, 283
Prophylactic therapy, 21, 544
Propine; *see* **dipivefrin**
Propionic acids, 646-647
propofol, 108
propoxyphene hydrochloride, 96, 98, 100
propoxyphene napsylate, 96, 98
propranolol, 232, 233, 290-291
    for angina, 308
    dosage range, 286
    indications for, 282
    management of overdose, 283
propylene glycol, 880
propylhexedrine, 510
propylthiouracil, 470, 471
Proscar; *see* **finasteride**
Prosom; *see* **estazolam**
Prostacyclin, 350
Prostaglandins
    biosynthesis of, 638-639
    nausea and vomiting and, 765
    oxytocic agents and, 432

Prostaglandins—cont'd
    platelet adhesion and, 348-349
    sucralfate and, 739
Prostate cancer, 425, 426, 427
Prostin E₂; *see* **dinoprostone**
protamine, 346
protamine-zinc insulin, 480
Protapam; *see* **pralidoxime**
Protein
    in modular formulations, 806, 808
    recommended daily dietary allowances, 778
Proteus
    aminoglycosides for, 559
    sulfonamides for, 546
Proton pump inhibitors, 737-738
Protostat; *see* **metronidazole**
Protozoal infection, 612-617
Protropin; *see* **somatrem**
Proventil; *see* **albuterol**
Provera; *see* **medroxyprogesterone**
Proximal tubule, 386
Prozac; *see* **fluoxetine**
Pruritus, 168
pseudoephedrine, 215, 217, 510
Pseudomembranous colitis, 568
Pseudomonas
    aminoglycosides for, 559, 560
    in nosocomial infection, 627
Psittacosis, 557
Psychologic dependence, 22
Psychomotor seizure, 141
Psychosis, 164
Psychotherapeutic agents, 162-193
    antianxiety, 164-169
    antidepressant, 170-179
    antimanic, 179-180
    antipsychotic, 180-186
    nursing process and, 186-193
Psyllium, 756
PTU; *see* **propylthiouracil**
Puberty, 424
Pubic louse, 836
Pulmonary edema, 390
Pulmonary embolism, 345, 358
Pulmonary hypertension, 229
Pupil, 247, 845, 846
Pure Food and Drug Act of 1906, 35
Purine analogue antivirals, 584
Purine antagonists, 689, 691-692
Purine nucleosides, 576, 577
Purinethol; *see* **mercaptopurine**
Purkinje cell, 278
Purkinje fiber action potential, 279
PURR mnemonic, 2-6
pyrantel, 619, 620-621
pyrazinamide, 589, 590, 592-593
Pyridine analogue antivirals, 584
Pyridine nucleosides, 577
pyridostigmine, 242, 243
Pyridoxal, 790
Pyridoxine, 154, 790-791
pyrilamine, 505
pyrimethamine, 611, 612
Pyrimidine antagonists, 689, 692

Q

Q fever, 557
quazepam, 129-130, 131
Questran; *see* **cholestyramine**
Quibron-T; *see* **theophylline**
Quinaglute; *see* **quinidine**
quinapril, 327
quinestrol, 426
quinethazone, 396
Quinidex; *see* **quinidine**
quinidine, 284
    antidiarrheals and, 749
    antiemetics and, 769

quinidine—cont'd
    cardiac glycosides and, 268
    dosage range, 285
    indications for, 282
    management of overdose, 283
    reserpine and, 324
quinine, 609, 610
Quinolones, 562-564
    assessment of, 570
    didanosine and, 579
    implementation of, 573
    iron preparations and, 822
    ocular, 865

R

Radiation as carcinogen, 681
ramipril, 327
ranitidine, 736
Rapid eye movement sleep, 121, 122, 123
Rapid-acting insulin, 479, 480
Rauwolfia alkaloids, 326, 337
Reassessment, pharmacotherapeutic, 23
Receptor interaction, 19-20
Recombinant tissue plasminogen activator, 356
Recombivax HB; *see* Hepatitis B vaccine
Recommended daily dietary allowances, 778
Rectal cancer, 689
Rectum, 752
Recurrent epithelial keratitis, 580
Red blood cell
    formation of, 819
    pentoxifylline and, 350
Redisol; *see* Cyanocobalamin
Reese's Pinworm Medicine; *see* **pyrantel**
Reflex, stages of anesthesia and, 109
Reflex stimulation, 514
Reflex tachycardia, 303
Refractory period, 265
Regional anesthetics, 111-114
Regitine; *see* **phentolamine**
Reglan; *see* **metoclopramide**
Regutol; *see* Docusate salts
Relafen; *see* **nabumetone**
Relative refractory period, 279
Renal cell carcinoma
    interferon for, 714
    interleukin-2 for, 717, 718
Renal system; *see* Kidney
Renese; *see* **polythiazide**
Renin angiotensin-aldosterone system, 306, 327
Reproductive agents
    female, 421-424
        estrogens, 423-427
        female reproductive system and, 422-423
        fertility agents, 436-439
        nursing process and, 439-442
        oral contraceptives, 430-431
        progestins, 427-429
        uterine relaxants, 434-436
        uterine stimulants, 431-434
    male, 445-451
        male reproductive system and, 445-446
        nursing process and, 448-451
Resectial; *see* **mannitol**
reserpine, 326
    beta-blockers and, 856
    carcinogenic effects of, 680
    cardiac glycosides and, 268
    drug interactions, 324
    fertility agents and, 438
resorcinol, 633
Respiratory agents, 519-539
    anticholinergics, 528
    for asthma, 521
    beta-agonists, 524-528
    bronchodilators, 522-524
    for chronic bronchitis, 522
    corticosteroids, 528-531
    cromolyn, 532

Respiratory agents—cont'd
  for emphysema, 522
  indirect-acting antiasthmatic agents, 531-532
  nedocromil, 532
  nursing process and, 533-537
Respiratory syncytial virus, 580
  antivirals for, 578
  immune globulins for, 672
Respiratory system, 520
  adrenergic receptor responses to stimulation, 207
  antihistamines, 503-509
    efficacy and side effects of, 504
    narcotic analgesics and, 95
    nonsedating, 506-508
    nursing process and, 515-517
  bronchodilators, 215-217, 522-539
    anticholinergic, 528
    for asthma, 521
    beta-agonist, 524-528
    for chronic bronchitis, 522
    corticosteroid, 528-531
    cromolyn, 532
    dosage ranges, 214
    for emphysema, 522
    indirect-acting antiasthmatic agents, 531-532
    nedocromil, 532
    nursing process and, 533-537
    sympathomimetic, 524-528
    xanthine derivatives, 522-524
  cold medications, 509-517
    adrenergics and, 212
    antitussives, 511-514
    decongestants, 510-511
    expectorants, 514-515
    nursing process and, 515-517
  decongestants, 510-511
  interactions and adverse effects
    anticholinergics and, 248, 249
    antidiarrheals and, 748
    antiprotozoal agents and, 614
    barbiturates and, 123
    cholinergic agents and, 241
    colony-stimulating factors and, 720
    immunizing agents and, 668
    miotics and, 850
    narcotic analgesic agents and, 93
    omeprazole and, 737
    selegilene and, 151
Resting membrane potential, 277, 278
Reticulocyte, 819
Reticulum cell sarcoma
  alkylating agents for, 687
  cytotoxic antibiotics for, 693, 695
  mitotic inhibitors for, 698
Retin-A; see tretinoin
Retinitis, 580
Retinoblastoma, 687
Retinoic acid, 832
Retinol, 779-780
Retinopathy, 477, 782
Retrovir; see zidovudine
Retrovirus, 714
Reversible cholinesterase inhibitors, 240
Rh₀ immune globulin, 669, 673
Rhabdomyosarcoma
  cytotoxic antibiotics for, 693, 695
  mitotic inhibitors for, 696, 698
Rheomacrodex; see Dextran
Rhesonativ; see Rh₀ immune globulin
Rheumatoid arthritis
  azathioprine for, 659
  nonsteroidal antiinflammatory drugs for, 640, 644-645, 647
  sulfonamides for, 545
Rheumatrex; see methotrexate
Rhinovirus, 509, 714
Rhodopsin, 779
Rhythmol; see propafenone
ribavirin, 577, 578, 581-582
Riboflavin, 778, 787-788

Ribonucleic acid, 576-577
Rickets, 781, 796
Rickettsia rickettsii, 543-544
Rickettsial pox, 557
Ridaura; see auranofin
rifabutin, 589, 590
Rifadin; see rifampin
rifamate, 592
rifampin, 593
  anticoagulants and, 347
  antifungal drugs and, 602
  as antitubercular agent, 589, 590
  penicillins and, 549
Rimactane; see rifampin
rimantadine, 577, 578, 581
Ringworm, 833
Ritalin; see methylphenidate hydrochloride
ritodrine, 436
Robinul; see glycopyrrolate
Robitussin; see guaifenesin
Robitussin A-C; see codeine
Robitussin-DM; see dextromethorphan
Rocaltrol; see Calcitriol
Rocephin; see ceftriaxone
Rocky Mountain spotted fever, 557
Rodex T.D.; see Pyridoxine
Rods, 846
Roferon-A; see Interferon alfa-2a
Rogaine; see minoxidil
Romazicon; see flumazenil
Rosaniline dyes, 632
Roundworm, 618, 621
Route of administration, absorption and, 13-14
Rubella vaccine, 669, 671
Rubex; see doxorubicin
Rubramin PC; see Cyanocobalamin
Ru-Vert-M; see meclizine

S

Salbutamol; see albuterol
Salicylates, 639
  antitubercular drugs and, 591
  carboxylic acids, 643-645
  laxatives and, 756
  toxicity of, 642-643
Salicylic acid, 638
Salicylism, 642-643
Saline flush, 68
Saline laxatives, 753, 759
salmeterol, 515
Salt, 408
Salt-losing adrenogenital syndrome, 494
Saluron; see hydroflumethiazide
Sandimmune; see cyclosporin A
Sandoglobulin; see Immune globulin
Sandostatin, se octreotide
Sani-Supp; see glycerin
Sarcoma, 678
  alkylating agents for, 685
  cytotoxic antibiotics for, 693, 695
  mitotic inhibitors for, 696
sargramstim, 721-722
Scabene; see lindane
Scabies, 836
Schistosomiasis, 621
Schizophrenia, 184
Sclera, 844-845
scopolamine, 251
  as anesthetic adjuvant, 108
  for nausea and vomiting, 769
Scrub typhus, 557
Scurvy, 793-794
Seasonal asthma, 521
Sebaceous gland, 830
secobarbital, 108, 125, 126, 131
Seconal; see secobarbital
Secondary epilepsy, 136

Secondary hypertension, 321
Second-generation antidepressants, 176-179
Second-generation cephalosporins, 553-555
Sectral; see acebutolol
Sedatives and hypnotics, 120-134
  as anesthetic adjuvants, 108
  antidiarrheals and, 749
  antiemetics and, 769
  aprobarbital, 126
  barbiturates, 121-124
  benzodiazepines, 126-130
  butabarbital, 126
  clonidine and, 324
  estazolam, 129
  flurazepam, 129
  geriatric complications, 31
  nursing process and, 130-133
  pentobarbital, 126
  phenobarbital, 124-126
  quazepam, 129-130
  secobarbital, 126
  sleep and, 121
  temazepam, 130
  triazolam, 130
Seizures, 135-147
  antiepileptic drugs for, 136-144
    benzodiazepines, 142
    carbamazepine, 142-143
    ethosuximide, 143
    phenobarbital, 143
    phenytoin, 143-144
    valproic acid, 144
  nursing process in, 144-145
Seldane; see terfenadine
Selective serotonin-reuptake inhibitors, 176-178
selegiline, 150-152
Selenium, 795
Semiessential amino acids, 810
Semilente, 480
Seminiferous tubule, 445
Semisynthetic opioids, 92
Senna, 759
Septisol; see triclosan
Sequential nephron blockade, 389
Serevent; see salmeterol
Serophene; see clomiphene
Serotonin, 765
Serotonin blockers, 767, 771
Serratia, 559
sertraline, 179
Serum sickness, 667
Sex hormones, female, 423-429
Shigellosis, 557
Shingles, 579, 580
Shock
  beta-agonists for, 526
  crystalloid solutions for, 407
  immunizing agents and, 668
  vasoactive adrenergics for, 216
Sigma opioid receptor, 92
Silvadene; see silver sulfadiazine
silver nitrate, 866
silver sulfadiazine, 837
simethicone, 733
Simple phobia, 165
Simple seizure, 137
simvastatin, 373
Sinemet; see levodopa-carbidopa
Sinex Long-Acting; see oxymetazoline
Sinoatrial node, 278-279, 280
  adrenergic receptor responses to stimulation, 207
  congestive heart failure and, 265
6-MP; see mercaptopurine
Skin
  anatomy of, 829, 830
  antidiarrheals and, 748
  antiemetic agents and, 768
  antifungals and, 601
  antiprotozoal agents and, 614
  antipsychotic agents and, 182

Skin—cont'd
  antiseptic and disinfectant agents and, 630
  antithyroid drugs and, 470
  carbonic anhydrase inhibitors and, 858
  colony-stimulating factors and, 720
  corticosteroids and, 493
  cyanocobalamin and, 792
  histamine$_2$ blockers and, 736
  immunizing agents and, 668
  iron preparations and, 821
  macrolides and, 565
  niacin and, 789
  nicotinic acid and, 377
  nursing process and, 837-841
  omeprazole and, 737
  pyridoxine and, 790
  quinolones and, 563
  sulfonamides and, 546
  thiazide diuretics and, 395
  tumor origin in, 678
  vitamin A and, 780
  vitamin K and, 786
Sleep, 121, 122
Sleep architecture, 121
Slo-bid; see **theophylline**
Slo-Niacin; see Niacin
Slow acetylators, 545, 592
SLUDGE acronym, 156, 240
Social phobia, 165
Sodium, 415, 795
sodium ampicillin, 551
Sodium channel, 278
Sodium chloride, 408
  hyperosmolar, 871, 875
  replacement of, 416
sodium hypochlorite, 631, 632
Sodium laxatives, 759
sodium nitroprusside, 283, 332
Sodium sulamyd; see **sulfacetamide**
sodium thiosulfate, 834
Sodium-potassium ATPase pump, 277
Soft drinks, 199
Solarcaine; see **benzocaine**
Solfoton; see **phenobarbital**
Solganal; see **aurothioglucose**
Solid systems of measurement, 46
Solu-Cortef; see **hydrocortisone**
Solurex; see **dexamethasone**
Somatic nervous system, 239
Somatic pain, 90
somatrem, 455, 457, 458, 461
somatropin, 455, 457, 458, 461, 462
sorbinil, 484
Sorbitol, 759
Sorbitrate; see **isosorbide dinitrate**
sotalol, 233, 234, 291
  dosage range, 286
  indications for, 282
  management of overdose, 283
Span-FF; see **ferrous fumarate**
Spectazole; see **econazole nitrate**
Spherocyte, 820
Spinal anesthesia, 113
Spirochetal infection, 557, 564
spironolactone, 394
S-P-T, 468
Standards of care, 40
Staphcillin; see **methicillin**
Staphylococcus
  in nosocomial infection, 627
  penicillins for, 548
  quinolones for, 562
  sulfonamides for, 546
  vancomycin for, 568
statil, 484
Status asthmaticus, 521
Status epilepticus, 138-139, 167
Stem cell, 720
Step-care approach to hypertension, 320
Sterapred; see **prednisone**
Steroid psychosis, 493

Steroids
  anabolic, 446, 450
  aspirin and, 352
  cardiac glycosides and, 268
  for ear disorders, 880
  estrogens, 423-427
  intranasal, 510
  nutritional supplements and, 807
Sterols, 599
Stevens-Johnson syndrome, 424
  estrogen and, 424
  loop diuretics and, 389
Stilphostrol; see **diethylstilbestrol**
Stimulant laxatives, 753, 759-760
Stomach, 729-731
Stomach cancer
  alkylating agents for, 685
  antimetabolites for, 689
  cytotoxic antibiotics for, 693, 695
Stool softeners, 753
Streptase; see **streptokinase**
Streptococcus, 543-544
  group A beta-hemolytic, 356
  macrolides for, 564
  penicillins for, 548
streptokinase, 356, 357, 358
streptomycin, 560, 589, 590
streptozocin, 685
Stress ulcer
  histamine$_2$ antagonists for, 735
  sucralfate for, 739
Stresstein, 806
Stroke, 345
  antiplatelet agents for, 352
  hypertension and, 320
Study skills, 2-6
Sty, 862
Subcutaneous injection, 14
  administration of, 62-64
  heparin, 360
  sites for, 59-61
Subjective data, 9
Sublimaze; see **fentanyl**
Sublingual route, 14
Subtherapeutic response, 544
Succinimides, 139, 140
succinylcholine, 117
sucralfate, 738-739
Sudafed; see **pseudoephedrine**
Sudden cardiac death, 289
sufentanil, 100, 108
sulconazole, 834
sulfacetamide, 865
sulfamethoxazole, 546-547, 697
Sulfamylon; see **mafenide**
Sulfate, 739
sulfinpyrazone, 649, 687
sulfisoxazole, 547
Sulfonamides, 545-547
  assessment of, 570
  implementation of, 572
  ocular, 865
Sulfonylureas, 284, 481-484
Sulfur, 795
Superficial pain, 90
Superinfection, 544
Supplemental therapy, 21
Supportive therapy, 21
Supraventricular tachyarrhythmia, 282, 286, 287
  beta-blockers for, 233
  digitalis for, 269
  vasoactive adrenergics for, 216
Suprax; see **cefixime**
Surface-active agents, 634
Surfak; see Docusate salts
Surital; see **thiamylal**
Sustacal, 806
Sweat gland, 830
Symmetrel; see **amantadine**
Sympathetic cervical nerve block, 114
Sympathetic lumbar nerve block, 114

Sympathetic nervous system, 207-209
  nicotinic receptor and, 256
  relationship to parasympathetic nervous system, 239
Sympatholytics, 224-237
  alpha-blockers, 225-230
  beta-blockers, 230-234
  nursing process and, 234-237
Sympathomimetic agents, 194-203, 206-223
  amphetamines, 200-201
  analeptics, 197-199
  anorexiants, 199-200, 213-215
  antiglaucoma, 853-855, 874
  bronchodilators, 215-217, 524-528
  cholinergic agents and, 242
  cyclic antidepressants and, 172
  decongestant, 217, 510
  monoamine oxidase inhibitors and, 174
  nursing process and, 201-203, 219-223
  ophthalmic decongestants, 218
  sympathetic nervous system and, 207-209
  uterine relaxants and, 435
  vasoactive, 216, 218-219
Synaptic cleft, 209
Syndrome of inappropriate antidiuretic hormone, 557
Synthetic opioids, 92
Synthroid; see **levothyroxine**
Syntocinon; see Oxytocin
Syphilis
  macrolides for, 564
  tetracyclines for, 557
Syringe, 52-54
Systemic vascular resistance, 321
Sytobex; see Cyanocobalamin

T

T cell, 712, 713
T cell lymphoma, 714
T helper cell, 657, 712
T suppressor cell, 712
T$_3$; see Triiodothyronine
T$_4$; see Thyroxine
Tacaryl; see **methdilazine**
TACE; see **chlorotrianisene**
Tachyarrhythmia, 413
Tachyphylaxis
  chloral hydrate and, 130
  local anesthetics and, 112
Taeniasis, 618
Tagamet; see **cimetidine**
Tambocor; see **flecainide**
Tapazole; see **methimazole**
Tape, 831
Tapeworm, 618, 621
Tavist; see **clemastine**
Taxol; see **paclitaxel**
Tazicef; see **ceftazidime**
Tazidime; see **ceftazidime**
TBW; see Total body water
Tea, 199
Tears, 846
  artificial, 870
Tegretol; see **carbamazepine**
Temaril; see **trimeprazine**
temazepam, 130, 131
Tenormin; see **atenolol**
Tenuate; see **diethylpropion**
Teratogen, 22-23, 545
terazosin, 229
terbinafine, 834
terbutaline, 214, 436, 515
terfenadine, 504, 508
  antifungal drugs and, 602
  macrolides and, 565
terpin hydrate, 514
Tessalon; see **benzonatate**
Testes, 445

Testicular cancer
  alkylating agents for, 685, 687
  cytotoxic antibiotics for, 693, 695
  mitotic inhibitors for, 696, 698
Testosterone, 446, 450
Tetanus, 167, 669, 670
Tetanus immune globulin, 670, 673
tetracaine, 112, 870
Tetracannabinoids, 771
Tetracyclines, 556-559
  assessment of, 570
  didanosine and, 579
  general anesthetics and, 110
  implementation of, 572
  iron preparations and, 822
  laxatives and, 756
  nutritional supplements and, 807
  ocular, 865
tetrahydrocannabinoid, 767
tetrahydrozoline, 215, 218, 510
Thallium poisoning, 413
THC; see **tetrahydrocannabinoid**
Theo-24; see **theophylline**
theobromine, 522
Theo-Dur; see **theophylline**
theophylline, 523-524
  for antidysrhythmic drug reversal, 283
  macrolides and, 565
Therapeutic index, 21
Therapeutic response, 544
Therapeutic window, 267
thiabendazole, 619
Thiamine, 778, 787
thiamylal, 108
Thiazide diuretics, 395-397
  amphotericin B and, 602
  cardiac glycosides and, 268
  direct-acting vasodilators and, 331
  geriatric complications, 31
thiethylperazine maleate, 774
thimerosal, 631, 632
Thioamide derivatives, 469
thiopental, 108, 283
thiotepa, 685
thiothixene, 183-184
Thioxanthenes, 183-184
Third-generation cephalosporins, 555-556
Thoracic nerve block, 114
Thorazine; see **chlorpromazine**
Thorn apple, 249
Threshold potential, 279
Throat
  antidiarrheals and, 748
  antiemetics and, 768
  antiprotozoal agents and, 614
  carbonic anhydrase inhibitors and, 858
  miotics and, 850
  osmotic diuretics and, 860
Thrombin, 348-349
Thromboembolic events, 345
Thrombolytics, 356-359, 364-365
Thromboplastin, 343
Thrombosis, 644
Thromboxane A_2, 348-349
Thrombus, 345
Thrush, 598, 603, 833
Thyrar, 468
thyroglobulin, 469
Thyroid agents, 465-474
  adrenergics and, 212
  antithyroid agents and, 469-471
  iron preparations and, 822
  mydriatics and, 854
  nursing process and, 471-473
  thyroid function and, 466
Thyroid gland, 466
Thyroid storm, 466
Thyroid Strong, 468
Thyroid-stimulating hormone, 456, 466
Thyrolar; see **liotrix**
Thyrotropin, 466

Thyroxine, 466
ticarcillin disodium, 550, 552
Ticlid; see **ticlopidine**
ticlopidine, 350, 353
Tilade; see **nedocromil**
timolol, 851, 857, 874
Timoptic; see **timolol**
Tinactin; see **tolnaftate**
Tincture of iodine, 633
Tinea, 598, 833, 834
Ting; see **tolnaftate**
Tissue, fluid in, 405
Tissue plasminogen activator, 343, 356
tobramycin sulfate, 560
tocainide, 282, 283, 285, 288
Tocopherols, 784
tolazoline, 228-229
tolbutamide, 697
Tolerance and dependence, 22
tolnaftate, 834
tolrestat, 484
Tonic-clonic seizure, 141
Tonocard; see **tocainide**
Topical administration, 16
  anesthetics, 111, 112, 113, 835-836
    ocular, 869-870, 874
  antifungal, 599
  antiinfectives, 831-835
  antimicrobials, 627-630
  antineoplastics, 837
  antiviral agents, 835
  ectoparasiticidal drugs, 836-837
  intranasal steroids, 510
Toprol XL; see **metoprolol**
Toradol; see **ketorolac**
Tornalate; see **bitolterol**
torsemide, 388, 390, 391
Tort, 40
Totacillin; see **trihydrate ampicillin**
Totacillin-N; see **sodium ampicillin**
Total body water, 404-405
Total parenteral nutrition, 808-813
Tourette syndrome, 184
Toxic nodular disease, 466
Toxic response to antibiotics, 544
Toxicology, 13, 22
Toxoid, 664, 667, 673
Toxoplasma gondii, 612
Toxoplasmosis, 546, 547, 611, 613
Trace elements, 794, 795
  nursing process and, 799-802
  in nutritional support, 811, 812
Trandate; see **labetalol**
Tranquilizers; see Antipsychotic agents
Transdermal delivery, 16
Transderm-Scop; see Scopolamine
Transient ischemic attack, 352
Transplantation, 659
Tranxene; see **clorazepate dipotassium**
tranylcypromine, 176
Traum-Aid HBC, 806
Travasorb Renal, 806
trazodone, 179
Trematode, 618
Tremor, 150
Trental; see **pentoxifylline**
tretinoin, 832-833
Trexan; see **naltrexone hydrochloride**
triamcinolone, 492, 530
triamterene, 394
triazolam, 130, 131
trichlormethiazide, 396
Trichomoniasis, 612, 613
Trichophyton, 598
triclosan, 632
Tricyclic antidepressants, 170-173
  adrenergic agents and, 212, 324
  anticholinergics and, 157, 249
  antidiarrheals and, 749
  antiemetics and, 769
  central nervous system stimulants and, 197

Tricyclic antidepressants—cont'd
  fertility agents and, 438
  monoamine oxidase inhibitors and, 174
  mydriatics and, 854
  physostigmine reversal of, 242
trifluridine, 577, 578, 582, 866
Trigeminal-glossopharyngeal neuralgia, 141
Triglycerides, 368
trihexyphenidyl, 157, 158
trihydrate ampicillin, 551
Triiodothyronine, 466
Tri-Levlen, 431
trimeprazine, 505, 509
trimethaphan, 258
Tri-Norinyl, 431
Triostat; see **liothyronine**
tripelennamine, 505, 509
Triphasic oral contraceptives, 431
Triphasil, 431
triprolidine, 509
Tronolane; see **pramoxine**
TSH; see Thyroid-stimulating hormone
T-Stat; see **erythromycin**
Tube feeding, 804-808, 814
Tubercle bacilli, 588
Tuberculin syringe, 52
Tuberculosis, 587-596
  antitubercular agents for, 588-593
  bacille Calmette-Guérin for, 669
  nursing process in, 593-595
Tumor, 678
Tumor antigen, 711
Tums; see **calcium carbonate**
Tussar SF; see **codeine**
Tylenol; see **acetaminophen**
Typhus, 557
Tyzine; see **tetrahydrozoline**

U

Ulcerative colitis, 545
Ultralente insulin, 480-481
Uniphyl; see **theophylline**
Unisom; see **doxylamine**
United States drug legislation, 35-36
Units, 47
Unstable angina, 301
Upper respiratory tract, 520
Upper respiratory tract infection, 509
Urecholine; see **bethanechol**
Uric acid, 649
Urinary alkalizers
  adrenergics and, 212
  ganglionic blockers and, 257
Urinary retention, 242
Urinary tract infection
  aztreonam for, 567
  quinolones for, 562
  sulfonamides for, 545, 547
urokinase, 358, 359
Uterine bleeding
  estrogenic agents for, 425, 426
  progestational agents for, 429
  uterine stimulants for, 434
Uterine relaxants, 434-436, 442
Uterine stimulants, 431-434, 441
Uterus, 207, 422
Uvea, 846
Uveitis, 862

V

Vaccine, 664-665
  Bacille Calmette-Guérin, 668, 669
  diphtheria, 668-670
  Haemophilus influenzae type B conjugate, 669, 670–671
  hepatitis B virus, 669, 671

Vaccine—cont'd
    measles, mumps, rubella, 669, 671
    poliovirus, 669, 671, 672
    tetanus, 668-670
Vagina, 422
Vaginal candidiasis, 603
Vaginitis, 425, 426
Valergen; *see* Estradiol valerate
Valium; *see* **diazepam**
valproic acid
    antimalarial agents and, 612
    for epilepsy, 139, 141, 144
Vancenase; *see* **beclomethasone dipropionate**
Vanceril; *see* **beclomethasone dipropionate**
Vancocin; *see* **vancomycin**
Vancoled; *see* **vancomycin**
vancomycin, 568-569
    assessment of, 571
    implementation of, 573
    loop diuretics and, 390
Variant angina, 301
Varicella-zoster, 578, 672
Vascor; *see* **bepridil**
Vascular headache, 229
Vaseretic; *see* **enalapril**
Vasoactive adrenergics, 218
Vasoactive intestinal polypeptide, 457
Vasoactive sympathomimetics, 211
Vasodilators, 330, 337
Vasopressin, 455, 457, 461
Vasopressors, 283
Vasospastic angina, 301
Vasotec; *see* **enalapril**
Vastus lateralis injection site, 59
Vaughan Williams classification of
        antidysrhythmic drugs, 231, 280-281
V-Cillin; *see* **penicillin V potassium**
VCR; *see* **vincristine**
Veetids; *see* **penicillin V potassium**
Velosulin, 479, 480
Venoglobulin; *see* Immune globulin
Ventolin; *see* **albuterol**
Ventricular action potential, 280
Ventricular arrhythmia, 233, 282, 285, 286, 287
Ventricular fibrillation, 271, 282
Ventricular fibrillation threshold, 287
Ventricular septum, 280
Ventricular tachycardia, 282, 286
Ventrogluteal injection site, 60
VePesid; *see* **etoposide**
Veracity, 40
verapamil, 292-293
    for angina, 311
    beta-blockers and, 856
    cardiac glycosides and, 268
    dosage range, 287
    indications for, 282
    management of overdose, 283
Verelan; *see* **verapamil**
Vermox; *see* **mebendazole**
Versed; *see* **midazolam**
Vertigo, 770
Very-low-density lipoprotein, 368-369
    gemfibrozil and, 376
    niacin and, 788-789
    nicotinic acid and, 377
Vial, 55-58
Vibramycin; *see* **doxycycline**
Vibra-Tabs; *see* **doxycycline**
Vicks Formula 44; *see* **dextromethorphan**
Vicks inhaler; *see* **desoxyephedrine**
Vicks Vatronol; *see* **ephedrine**
vidarabine, 577, 578, 866
Vinca alkaloids, 695-696
Vincasar PFS; *see* **vincristine**

vincristine, 698
Vinegar, 630
Vioform; *see* **clioquinol**
viomycin, 390
VIPoma, 459
Vira-A; *see* **vidarabine**
Virazole; *see* **ribavirin**
Viroptic; *see* **trifluridine**
Virus, replication of, 576
Visceral pain, 90
Visine; *see* **tetrahydrozoline**
Vistaril; *see* **hydroxyzine**
Vital, 806
Vitamin A, 779-780
    laxatives and, 756
    nutritional supplements and, 807
    recommended daily dietary allowances, 778
Vitamin A acid, 832-833
Vitamin B$_1$, 787
Vitamin B$_2$, 787-788
Vitamin B$_3$, 376-378, 788-790
Vitamin B$_4$, 778
Vitamin B$_6$, 154, 790-791
Vitamin B$_{12}$, 791-793
    recommended daily dietary allowances, 778
    red blood cells and, 820, 824
Vitamin C, 793-794
    iron preparations and, 822
    recommended daily dietary allowances, 778
Vitamin D, 782-783
    laxatives and, 756
    nutritional supplements and, 807
    recommended daily dietary allowances, 778
Vitamin E, 784-785
    anticoagulants and, 347
    laxatives and, 756
    recommended daily dietary allowances, 778
Vitamin K, 785-786
    clotting factors and, 345
    laxatives and, 756
    in warfarin reversal, 346
Vitamins, 777-794
    fat-soluble, 779-786
    laxatives and, 756
    nursing process and, 799-802
    water-soluble, 786-794
Vita-Plus E; *see* Vitamin E
Vitreous humor, 846
Vivonex, 806, 807
Volmax; *see* **albuterol**
Volume administration sets, 65-66
Volume of distribution, 16
Vomiting, 764-774
    antiemetic agents for, 765-771
        anticholinergic, 769
        neuroleptic, 769-771
        prokinetic, 771
        serotonin blockers, 771
    antipsychotic agents for, 184
    dehydration and fluid loss in, 406
    hydroxyzine for, 168
    nursing process in, 772-774
Vomiting center, 765
von Willebrand factor, 355
von Willebrand's disease, 459
Vosol Otic; *see* Acetic acids
VP-16; *see* **etoposide**
Vulvar cancer, 693, 695

warfarin, 347-348
    clotting factors and, 345
    cyclic antidepressants and, 172

warfarin—cont'd
    geriatric complications, 31
    macrolides and, 565
    mitotane and, 700
    mitotic inhibitors and, 697
    penicillins and, 549
    second-generation antidepressants and, 178
Water-soluble vitamins, 786-794
    niacin, 788-790
    recommended daily dietary allowances, 778
    riboflavin, 787-788
    thiamine, 787
    vitamin B$_6$, 790-791
    vitamin B$_{12}$, 791-793
    vitamin C, 793-794
Wax emulsifiers, 880, 881
Weight, child dosage calculation and, 27
Wellbutrin; *see* **bupropion**
Wernicke's encephalopathy, 787
Westhroid, 468
White blood cell, 529, 678
Whole blood, 410, 411, 412
Whole blood activated partial thromboplastin time,
        362
Wilms' tumor
    cytotoxic antibiotics for, 693, 695
    mitotic inhibitors for, 696, 698
Withdrawal syndrome, 94-95
Wolff-Parkinson-White syndrome, 282
Worm infection, 617-622

X

Xanax; *see* **alprazolam**
Xanthine derivatives, 522-523
Xylocaine; *see* **lidocaine**

Y

Yeast, 598, 627, 833
Yellow mercuric oxide, 632
Yew, 696
Yodoxin; *see* **iodoquinol**
Young's rule, 27
Yutopar; *see* **ritodrine**

Z

zalcitabine, 577, 578
Zantac; *see* **ranitidine**
Zarontin; *see* **ethosuximide**
Zaroxolyn; *see* **metolazone**
ZDV; *see* **zidovudine**
Zephiran; *see* **benzalkonium**
Zestril; *see* **lisinopril**
zidovudine, 577, 578, 582
Zinacef; *see* **cefuroxime**
Zinc, 778, 795
Zithromax; *see* **azithromycin**
Zofran; *see* **ondansetron**
Zollinger-Ellison syndrome, 735
Zoloft; *see* **sertraline**
Zona fasciculata, 490
Zona glomerulosa, 490
Zona reticularis, 490
Zovirax; *see* **acyclovir**
Z-track method of injection, 61
Zyloprin; *see* **allopurinol**
Zymenol; *see* Mineral oil

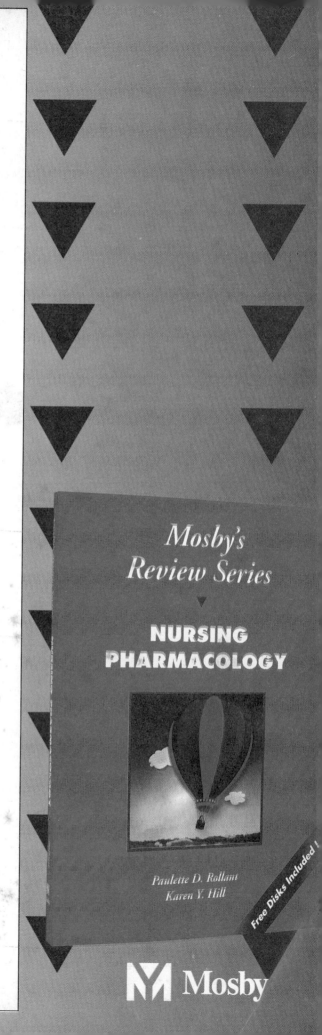